HANDBOOK OF MEDICAL HALLUCINOGENS

Handbook of
MEDICAL
HALLUCINOGENS

edited by

Charles S. Grob
Jim Grigsby

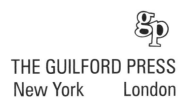

THE GUILFORD PRESS
New York   London

The authors have checked with sources believed to be reliable in their efforts to
provide information that is complete and generally in accord with the standards
of practice that are accepted at the time of publication. However, in view of the
possibility of human error or changes in behavioral, mental health, or medical
sciences, neither the authors, nor the editors and publisher, nor any other party
who has been involved in the preparation or publication of this work warrants that
the information contained herein is in every respect accurate or complete, and they
are not responsible for any errors or omissions or the results obtained from the use
of such information. Readers are encouraged to confirm the information contained
in this book with other sources.

Library of Congress Cataloging-in-Publication Data

Names: Grob, Charles S., 1950– editor. | Grigsby, Jim, editor.
Title: Handbook of medical hallucinogens / edited by Charles S. Grob,
    Jim Grigsby.
Description: New York, NY : The Guilford Press, [2021] | Includes
    bibliographical references and index.
Identifiers: LCCN 2020028890 | ISBN 9781462545445 (cloth ; alk. paper)
Subjects: LCSH: Hallucinogenic drugs—Therapeutic use. | Psychotherapy.
Classification: LCC RM324.8 .H355 2021 | DDC 615.7/883—dc23
LC record available at *https://lccn.loc.gov/2020028890*

About the Editors

Charles S. Grob, MD, is Professor of Psychiatry and Pediatrics at the David Geffen School of Medicine at the University of California, Los Angeles, and Director of the Division of Child and Adolescent Psychiatry at Harbor–UCLA Medical Center. He previously held faculty positions at the Johns Hopkins University and the University of California, Irvine. Dr. Grob has conducted approved clinical research with psychedelics since the early 1990s and has published numerous articles on psychedelics in the medical and psychiatric literatures, as well as several books. He is a founding board member of the Heffter Research Institute.

Jim Grigsby, PhD, is Professor in the Department of Psychology, and in the Division of Health Care Policy and Research of the Department of Medicine, at the University of Colorado Denver. His research and over 250 publications have focused on neuropsychology, cognitive neuroscience, telemedicine, and other areas of health services research. His work in neuroscience includes extensive research on executive functioning and on the clinical phenotypes of fragile X-associated tremor/ataxia syndrome (FXTAS), of which he was a co-discoverer. Dr. Grigsby's current research interests include the therapeutic use and mechanisms of psilocybin and MDMA.

Contributors

Gabrielle Agin-Liebes, PhD, Department of Psychiatry and Behavioral Sciences, Weill Institute for Neurosciences, University of California, San Francisco, San Francisco, California

Kenneth Alper, MD, Departments of Psychiatry and Neurology, New York University Grossman School of Medicine, New York, New York

Dráulio Barros de Araújo, PhD, Brain Institute, Federal University of Rio Grande do Norte, Natal, Brazil

Raquel Bennett, PsyD, KRIYA Institute, Berkeley, California

Michael P. Bogenschutz, PhD, Department of Psychiatry, New York University Grossman School of Medicine, New York, New York

Anthony P. Bossis, PhD, Department of Psychiatry, New York University Grossman School of Medicine, New York, New York

Gary Bravo, MD, KRIYA Institute, Berkeley, California

J. C. Callaway, PhD, Department of Medicinal Chemistry, University of Eastern Finland, Kuopio, Finland

Rob Colbert, PhD, The Nowak Society and Psychedelic Research and Training Institute, Fort Collins, Colorado

Mary Cosimano, LMSW, Center for Psychedelic and Consciousness Research, Johns Hopkins University School of Medicine, Baltimore, Maryland

Alan K. Davis, PhD, College of Social Work, The Ohio State University, Columbus, Ohio

Silvia Franco, MD, Department of Psychiatry, Columbia University and New York State Psychiatric Institute, New York, New York

Robert Grant, MD, MPH, Department of Pulmonary Medicine, School of Medicine, University of California, San Francisco, San Francisco, California; Healing Realms Psychotherapy, San Francisco, California

Jim Grigsby, PhD, Departments of Psychology and Medicine, University of Colorado Denver, Denver, Colorado

Shannon Hughes, PhD, School of Social Work, Colorado State University, Fort Collins, Colorado

Matthew W. Johnson, PhD, Department of Psychiatry and Behavioral Sciences, Johns Hopkins University School of Medicine, Baltimore, Maryland

Mendel Kaelen, PhD, Wavepaths, London, United Kingdom

David King, BSc, GKT School of Medical Education, King's College London, London, United Kingdom

Rafael Lancelotta, MS, Habituating to Wholeness, Lakewood, Colorado

Benjamin Malcolm, PharmD, MPH, College of Pharmacy, Western University of Health Sciences, Pomona, California

Maria Mangini, PhD, FNP, School of Nursing, Holy Names University, Oakland, California

Ana Elda Maqueda, PhD, Xka Pastora, Madrid, Spain

Jonny Martell, MD, Centre for Psychedelic Research, Imperial College London, London, United Kingdom

Dennis J. McKenna, PhD, Heffter Research Institute, Santa Fe, New Mexico

Sarah E. Mennenga, PhD, Department of Psychiatry, New York University Grossman School of Medicine, New York, New York

Annie Mithoefer, BSN, MAPS Public Benefit Corporation, Santa Cruz, California

Michael Mithoefer, MD, FAPA, MAPS Public Benefit Corporation, Santa Cruz California; Department of Psychiatry and Behavioral Sciences, Medical University of South Carolina, Charleston, South Carolina

Charles D. Nichols, PhD, Department of Pharmacology and Experimental Therapeutics, Louisiana State University Health Sciences Center, New Orleans, Louisiana

David E. Nichols, PhD, Eshelman School of Pharmacy, University of North Carolina at Chapel Hill, Chapel Hill, North Carolina

Kristine Panik, MD, Counseling and Psychological Services, University of California, Berkeley, California

Torsten Passie, MD, PhD, Department of Psychiatry and Psychotherapy, Hannover Medical School, Hannover, Germany; Institute for History and Ethics in Medicine, Goethe University, Frankfurt am Main, Germany

David Presti, PhD, Department of Molecular and Cell Biology, University of California, Berkeley, Berkeley, California

Stevens Rehen, PhD, D'Or Institute, Federal University of Rio de Janeiro, Rio de Janeiro, Brazil

Collin Reiff, PhD, Department of Psychiatry, New York University Grossman School of Medicine, New York, New York

Sidarta Ribeiro, PhD, Brain Institute, Federal University of Rio Grande do Norte, Natal, Brazil

William A. Richards, PhD, Center for Psychedelic and Consciousness Research, Johns Hopkins University School of Medicine, Baltimore, Maryland

Stephen Ross, MD, NYU Langone Health Program for Psychedelic Medicine, Department of Psychiatry, New York University Grossman School of Medicine, New York, New York

Emmanuelle A. D. Schindler, MD, PhD, Department of Neurology, Yale University School of Medicine, New Haven, Connecticut

Scott Shannon, MD, Psychiatric Research and Training Institute, Fort Collins, Colorado

Milan Scheidegger, MD, PhD, Department of Psychiatry, Psychotherapy and Psychosomatics, University Hospital of Psychiatry, Zurich, Switzerland

Candice L. Shelby, PhD, Department of Philosophy, University of Colorado Denver, Denver, Colorado

Enzo Tagliazucchi, PhD, Department of Physics, University of Buenos Aires, Buenos Aires, Argentina

Kelan Thomas, PharmD, MS, College of Pharmacy, Touro University California, Vallejo, California

Luís Fernando Tófoli, MD, PhD, School of Medical Sciences, University of Campinas, Campinas, Brazil

Will Van Derveer, MD, Integrative Psychiatry Institute, Boulder, Colorado

Michael Winkelman, MPH, PhD, School of Human Evolution and Social Change, Arizona State University, Tempe, Arizona

Preface

After decades of quiescence, the hallucinogen treatment model has returned. Once on the cutting edge of psychiatric research through the 1950s and early 1960s, the momentum of the growing field was derailed by the political and cultural turmoil of the late 1960s and early 1970s. Almost from the beginning, views toward the utility of this highly unusual treatment model were polarized. The enthusiastic belief possessed by some, that this had brought psychiatry and psychology to the threshold of an entirely new and novel paradigm, was dismissed by others as unrealistic and even messianic.

For nearly four decades, the field of hallucinogen studies went largely ignored in formal research and academic settings, as the prevailing psychiatric treatment model came to be increasingly reliant on antidepressants, antipsychotics, anxiolytics, and mood stabilizers. But early mainstream enthusiasm for successive generations of heavily marketed psychopharmaceuticals has waned in recent years, in step with a growing awareness of their limited efficacy, serious health considerations, and a dearth of new products in the pipeline. All of this has occurred in the face of growing public mental health crises, including, though not limited to, increased suicide rates and an extensive and refractory nationwide crisis of opioid addiction.

Given the limited effectiveness of conventional treatment options for many psychological disturbances, there is growing recognition of the need for innovation, and a willingness to examine even compounds once considered taboo, in the search for more efficacious treatments. With that in mind, our end goal with this volume is to create a comprehensive, transdisciplinary guide that describes the current status of research.

Before proceeding, the important matter of nomenclature should be addressed. Among the many controversies surrounding the field has been a disagreement regarding which word best categorizes these compounds. The three most common names currently in use are *psychedelic*, *entheogen*, and *hallucinogen*, but the history of the field is replete with a bewildering array of terms. Among others, these include *deliriants*, *delusionegens*, *eidetics*, *misperceptinogens*, *mysticomimetics*, *phanerothymes*, *phantasticants*, *psychodysleptics*, *psychogens*, *psychointegrators*, *psychosomimetics*, *psychotaraxics*, *psychoticants*, *psychotogens*, *psychotomimetics*, and *schizogens*. Each of these has its particular relevance, and at various times some achieved wider usage, yet all fall short of encompassing the range of actions these substances are known to induce.

Of the three conventional terms, the one most commonly recognized is *psychedelic*, translated from the ancient Greek and proposed in 1957 by the renowned British Canadian researcher Humphrey Osmond, in a famous exchange of letters with the writer Aldous Huxley, as *mind manifesting*. Subsequently, *psychedelic* became the term commonly identified with the widespread social use and abuse of lysergic acid diethylamide (LSD) during the 1960s, and its associations with the political activism then current.

The use of the word *entheogen* ("accessing the divine within") is of more recent derivation and was popularized by the religious scholar, Huston Smith, to draw attention to the innate capacity of some (though not all) of these compounds, under particular conditions, to induce profoundly altered psychospiritual states of consciousness.

Finally, while the name *hallucinogen* has often been dismissed as connoting psychopathology, and even as having right-wing and politically repressive overtones, the true meaning of the word *hallucinogen* is in point of fact derived from the ancient Latin *allucinari*, which translates into English as "mind wandering" or "mind journeying." If thus properly understood, the word *hallucinogen* should achieve greater acceptance and consequently provoke less controversy. In any event, the term *hallucinogen* has been and will continue to be the accepted term in formal medical parlance, and as such is used in this book's title. Contributing authors, nevertheless, were free to use their own preferred terminology.

In recent years the public and professional *zeitgeist* toward these novel compounds has begun to shift, with a growing appreciation that they represent a fascinating and valuable area of study. This book endeavors to provide an in-depth exploration of the current state of knowledge of hallucinogens, examining their ethnobotanical and anthropological origins, social and scientific history, neuropharmacological actions, range of indications and clinical effects, therapeutic potential, adverse reactions, and implications for the future.

This review of medical hallucinogens is necessarily selective, reflecting both the inclinations of the editors and the interests and expertise of the individual authors who have contributed to the volume. On the other hand, the research literature on hallucinogenic substances is large and growing rapidly. A February 2020 Medline search for the term *lysergic acid diethylamide* turned up 4,859 journal articles since 1943, the year that Albert Hofmann serendipitously discovered the psychoactive effects of the LSD molecule he had first synthesized in 1938. To review all of that literature would be impossible; moreover, it would produce what would likely be a tedious and interminable reading experience. Moreover, the study of hallucinogens is not limited to the medical–psychiatric–psychological fields, and this volume therefore draws on knowledge acquired across a range of scientific disciplines.

The book begins with a thorough discussion of the pharmacology of what are often called the "classic" or "serotonergic" hallucinogens, for which Nichols prefers the term *psychedelics*. These include LSD, psilocybin, mescaline, and dimethyltryptamine (DMT). The classic hallucinogens have much in common, including their affinity for certain serotonin receptors (most notably for 5-HT$_{2A}$) and the extraordinary phenomenology of the experiences they produce. All of these

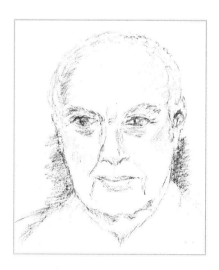

Albert Hofmann

have found niches as investigational psycho-therapeutic adjuncts.

Following this are several chapters exploring the social, cultural, and political contexts in which the hallucinogens have been used over time. Hallucinogens from a wide range of plant sources were used for perhaps as long as 9,000 years or more by pre-Neolithic shamans in what is now Algeria and, even today, indigenous peoples in many places around the world continue to use them. This volume provides an introduction to research conducted in the fields of anthropology and ethnobotany, which have made significant contributions to our understanding of how the discovery and use of naturally occurring hallucinogens evolved in a number of cultures, almost entirely outside mainstream Western societies. It is sobering to consider that many traditional healers must have sacrificed their livers or kidneys, not to mention their lives, in their empirical investigations of these drugs.

Over time, use and knowledge of these powerful mind-altering substances were relentlessly suppressed by emerging power structures, particularly state-sanctioned religions. With the advent of stratified and hierarchical societies, plant hallucinogens came to be viewed as threatening to the emerging commonweal, and restrictions were placed on such direct and revelatory access to the divine realms. In some societies (including the Aztec civilization), use of plant hallucinogens was restricted to the select castes of the religious priesthood. In others, including the progenitors of our own contemporary Euro-American culture, absolute proscriptions on the use of plant drugs for sacred purposes were enforced. Indeed, during the Middle Ages, indigenous healers, often practicing midwives with intimate knowledge of local plant pharmacopoeia, including those with hallucinogenic effects, were brutally persecuted by the Inquisition, which persisted well into the 17th century. During a span of 300 years, it has been estimated that several million women were accused of practicing witchcraft and condemned by tribunals of the Inquisition to die.

The history of hallucinogens in the 20th and 21st centuries is noteworthy for continuing controversy in the context of encouraging research results and sociopolitical turbulence, and chapters explore both the general sociopolitical environment and history of the time, and the evolution of these substances as tools for facilitating psychotherapeutic change. The two major approaches to LSD psychotherapy in the 1950s and 1960s—psycholytic therapy in Europe and the United Kingdom, and psychedelic therapy in North America—are reviewed in detail.

The mechanisms by which classic hallucinogens work in treating a surprisingly broad array of clinical disorders are largely unknown, although we do understand the importance of the 5-HT_{2A} receptor, and research is being done to elucidate the cascade of downstream effects on other serotonin receptors, as well as the dopaminergic system. Neuroimaging has become a widely used approach to understanding the psychological effects of LSD and psilocybin, and magnetic resonance imaging (MRI), electrophysiology (electroencephalograms and event-related potentials), positron emission tomography (PET), arterial spin labeling, and other techniques have been used for this purpose. One chapter addresses research on the nature of the psychedelic state from the perspectives of network connectivity, graph theory, information theory, and self-organization, and another focuses on the possible role of the reconsolidation of emotional memories in long-term, hallucinogen-assisted psychotherapy.

A considerable amount of research is dedicated to understanding the neurophysiological mechanisms underlying therapeutic efficacy. This is an important line of inquiry if we are to make sense of the kinds of change that are possible, and of the means for ensuring favorable and lasting change. However, it is remarkable that one of the most robust predictors of a positive outcome in many studies has been the occurrence—and the intensity—of what are referred to as *mystical-type experiences* or *psychedelic peak experiences*. How this is related to action at the molecular and neural levels is as yet unknown and remains a very interesting question for further investigation. Mystical experiences have long been associated with hallucinogen use not only among shamans of antiquity but also among contemporary researchers, and one chapter is dedicated to states of consciousness with potential religious or spiritual import, and their significance in the use of psychedelics.

Individual chapters are devoted to the classic hallucinogens (LSD, psilocybin, mescaline, and some of the tryptamines) and other drugs with apparently significant therapeutic potential. These include 3,4-methylenedioxymethamphetamine (MDMA), which has been found effective for treatment-resistant posttraumatic stress disorder (PTSD), and which is well into phase 3 clinical trials for U.S. Food and Drug Administration (FDA) approval. Others include *ketamine*, an N-methyl-D-aspartate (NMDA) receptor antagonist developed as a dissociative anesthetic and, more recently, utilized for treatment-resistant depression; *ibogaine*, derived from the African iboga tree and used experimentally for the treatment of addictions; *Salvia divinorum*, a plant originating in the Mexican state of Oaxaca that has long been used by Mazatec shamans; and *ayahuasca*, also known as yagé, an entheogen containing DMT and a number of alkaloids that function as monoamine oxidase inhibitors (MAOIs), used especially in Brazil, Peru, and Ecuador, and now widely used in North America.

The hallucinogens appear to have considerable potential as treatments for various emotional and behavioral disorders, but the drugs themselves are generally not sufficient to produce therapeutic effects. A good deal has been written on several determinants of outcome when hallucinogens are employed as adjuncts to psychotherapy. Most frequently discussed are the participant's psychological state (referred to as *set*) and the physical–aesthetic–emotional context of the experience, including preparation (referred to as *setting*). Dose and route of administration are similarly important factors, and music is almost universally employed as an emotionally evocative stimulus that helps to structure the experience.

The general consensus of clinicians and scientists in the field is that it is important to have one or two trained persons present during a psychedelic session in order to keep patients' attention focused inward, and to provide physical and emotional support during the session. Especially when things become psychologically intense, as they often do, these *guides, sitters,* or *facilitators* play an important role. In a way analogous to the players in the sport of curling, who use brooms to influence the route taken by the polished granite stones that slide across the ice, the guides play an important role in nondirectively reducing impediments to patients' involvement in the session.

Given the profound changes they regularly induce in one's experience of self and of the world, it is striking that the classic hallucinogens are quite safe, especially when used in a carefully controlled therapeutic situation. Acute adverse reactions during a session are ordinarily transient, and the associated anxiety is typically a part of the therapeutic process. Adverse effects are sometimes encountered, and these, and their management, are discussed.

As noted, a wide range of conditions have been suggested as appropriate for and amenable to treatment with the classic hallucinogens. These include addictions (alcohol, tobacco, and opioids), in which the drugs appear to reduce craving, and for which they have demonstrated preliminary evidence of being very effective both in the short term and over long-term follow-up. Some researchers have studied the use of psychedelics for treating headaches, including cluster headaches, and there is currently considerable interest, on the part of several research teams as well as the FDA, in studying the effectiveness of psilocybin for treating depression, and a large clinical trial is getting underway. Another use of the psychedelics—a focus of research since the 1960s, and apparently effective—is the administration of psilocybin and LSD in palliative care with late-stage cancer patients. In addition, although outcomes have not been rigorously studied, *psycholytic psychotherapy*—long-term therapy involving multiple drug sessions in conjunction with nondrug psychotherapy—shows promise for effecting significant change in personality beyond the amelioration of circumscribed behavioral disorders such as alcohol dependence.

Finally, research with hallucinogens raises a number of questions that are not strictly empirical in nature, but are of a more philosophical character. In this field, the disciplined thinking of philosophy can be helpful in conceptualizing hallucinogens, their mechanisms, and the psychological changes with which they are associated. The issue of molecular mechanisms in contrast to mystical experience, for example, raises questions best addressed by considering Bertrand Russell's theory of logical types.

After decades of repression, both during the modern era and throughout much of our history, hallucinogens have resurfaced once again, though now as respectable and potentially valuable objects of formal scientific research. No longer the objects of derision or repression, hallucinogens are being examined seriously in academic research settings around the world as potential tools for learning and healing. Indeed, we may have finally attained that point in time at which the optimal use of hallucinogens can be thoroughly explored and understood, under legally sanctioned and culturally supported conditions. It will be essential, nevertheless, to learn from the lessons of the past and optimize conditions under which these compounds are administered. The greatest attention must be consistently given to establishing and maintaining strong safety parameters, and to that end ensure that investigator-therapists employ the highest ethical standards in their work. The nascent field must also guard against pathological narcissism and hubris. Adhering to proper standards of conduct and respecting personal boundaries will ultimately support the safe passage of the normal volunteer research subject and the healing of the patient seeking relief from suffering. It will also serve to protect the field from further obstructions to achieving its long hoped for but as yet unrealized potential.

Moving forward, the greatest attention needs to be directed at minimizing adverse outcomes. The lessons learned, not only by a prior generation of modern researchers but also from the shamanic traditions dating back to the dawn of time, will be of great value to both current research efforts and future practitioners. For those who have fully understood the value of these highly unusual compounds, they are never taken for recreational or hedonic purpose. Intention is a key factor, and will likely frame the content of the experience. Serious purposes for embarking on the hallucinogen experience, including healing and spiritual awakening, provide a structure that ensures protection and the optimal conditions under which to heal, to learn, and to grow. Attention to set and setting, as was fully understood by our predecessors, from those in the recent past all the way back to the ancients, will optimize the likelihood of safe and efficacious outcomes.

There is growing recognition that the judicious use of the hallucinogen treatment model, when administered under optimal conditions, may achieve successful therapeutic outcomes even among patients who are refractory to conventional treatments. The implications for the future of psychiatry—and even other fields in medicine—are compelling. An integrative approach will be required, incorporating all that has been learned from those who have explored this inner terrain from other times and other cultures, as well as from our scientific and clinical predecessors a half-century ago. In today's world, we also have access to an extraordinary neuroscientific and medical technology that allows us to examine comprehensively the effects of hallucinogens, their mechanisms of action, and putative models for healing. Recent interest in microdosing regimens, in which a classic hallucinogen may only be administered sporadically at supposedly subthreshold dosages, raises new questions that await answers. Future research into mechanisms of action, as well as the potential medical and psychiatric uses of the hallucinogen treatment model, may over time achieve a significant impact on how we facilitate health and healing for both the individual and the collective.

Contents

PART IV. **Therapeutic Considerations**

PART V. **Indications and Purpose**

PART I

Overview of Hallucinogens

CHAPTER 1

The Pharmacology of Psychedelics

DAVID E. NICHOLS and CHARLES D. NICHOLS

◼ Introduction

We focus in this chapter on what have been called *serotonergic hallucinogens, classic hallucinogens,* or more simply *psychedelics.* Many written reviews have included detailed discussion of the pharmacology of psychedelics (Halberstadt, 2015; Nichols, 2016; Passie, Halpern, Stichtenoth, Emrich, & Hintzen, 2008; Passie, Seifert, Schneider, & Emrich, 2002). Most of these include much of the historical understanding of the pharmacology of these substances, but in the context of this chapter, we do not believe it is particularly important to review historical studies extensively; the interested reader can consult the previously cited reviews for comprehensive discussions. Rather, it seems more useful to provide up-to-date knowledge derived from recent studies and to distill the information down into its essential points. Nonetheless, some brief background is warranted to place the chapter in context.

The earliest rigorous scientific work on a psychedelic was Dr. Arthur Heffter's (1898) classic experiment with the peyote cactus, *Lophophora williamsii.* Through systematic chemical investigations, he was able to isolate the major alkaloids from the peyote cactus. He subsequently self-administered

each of the individually isolated alkaloids, thereby identifying mescaline (Figure 1.1), as the psychoactive component. Following the synthesis of mescaline in 1919 (Späth, 1919), this substance was the subject of self-experiments by numerous artists, scientists, philosophers, writers, and others for the next 50 years.

The next chapter of this story involves the accidental 1943 discovery of the psychoactive properties of lysergic acid diethylamide (LSD) by Dr. Albert Hofmann (1979), a natural products chemist working at the Sandoz Laboratories in Basel, Switzerland). He had first synthesized LSD in 1938 while developing ergot derivatives that might have therapeutic utility. In subsequent years, Hofmann carried out numerous scientific studies of South American intoxicating plants, culminating in the identification and synthesis of psilocybin, the active component in psilocybin mushrooms, which had been known by the Aztecs as *teonanacatl*, translated as "flesh of the gods" (Hofmann, Frey, Ott, Petrzilka, & Troxler, 1958; Hofmann, Heim, Brack, & Kobel, 1958). He was then able to demonstrate that the Aztec preparation known as *ololuiqui*, the seeds from a species of morning glory (*Rivea corymbosa*), contained lysergic acid amide (ergine;

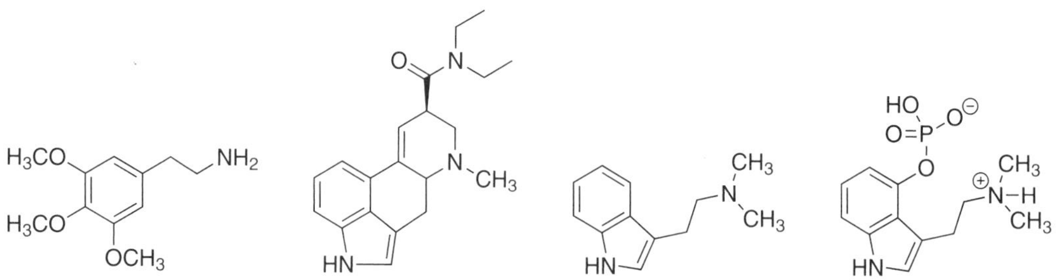

■ FIGURE 1.1. The chemical structures of mescaline, LSD, DMT, and psilocybin.

the ethyl groups of LSD have been replaced by hydrogen atoms) as its active psychoactive principle (Hofmann & Tscherter, 1960). Ergine has weak LSD-like properties, but *ololiuqui* was apparently used by the Aztecs when psilocybin mushrooms were in short supply.

A fourth hallucinogen, *N,N*-dimethyltryptamine (DMT), has gained recent popularity through the use of a plant decoction known as ayahuasca. This plant extract is prepared by boiling pounded *Banisteriopsis caapi* vines with leaves from *Psychotria viridis* (McKenna, Towers, & Abbott, 1984; Schultes & Hofmann, 1980). *Psychotria* leaves contain DMT, which is not orally active. However, *Banisteriopsis* contains beta-carboline alkaloids that inhibit liver monoamine oxidase (MAO), and ingestion of the mixture allows the DMT to enter the systemic circulation without being broken down in the liver. Ayahuasca has presumably been used for millennia by indigenous Amazonian peoples, but most recently it has been incorporated into syncretic religions that use it as a sacrament, in particular the União de Vegetal and the Santo Daime. Although DMT is a Schedule 1 controlled substance, the churches that use ayahuasca in their services have been given legal protection by a 2006 Supreme Court decision (*Gonzales v. O Centro Espírita Beneficente União do Vegetal*).

The psychological effects produced by psychedelics are highly subjective, usually including changes in thought and mood, depersonalization, and perceptual alterations that may include visual hallucinations, synesthesias, and tactile sensations. The subjective effects of serotonergic psychedelic hallucinogens are easily distinguished from those of other drug classes also called hallucinogens, such as N-methyl-D-aspartate (NMDA) receptor antagonists (e.g., phencyclidine, ketamine), κ-agonists (e.g., salvinorin A), and cannabinoids, which can also produce psychoactive effects. Because of these differences, we now distinguish serotonergic hallucinogens from other hallucinogens by categorizing them as psychedelics.

The profound psychoactive effects of these substances suggested that their biological target(s) must play an extremely important role in normal consciousness and perception, although elucidation of the nature of these targets took many years of research. Hints of their pharmacology were gleaned shortly after the discovery of the powerful psychoactive properties of LSD in 1943. In 1953, serotonin, which was first identified in 1949, was first detected in mammalian brain (Twarog & Page, 1953). Prior to that discovery, it was widely believed that serotonin was found only in the blood, and in the enteric nervous system, within chromaffin cells in the intestines where it was known to regulate vascular and intestinal tone. The realization that LSD was built upon a tryptamine molecular scaffold, as was serotonin (Figure 1.2), led to groundbreaking hypotheses that mental disorders like schizophrenia might be a result of disturbed serotonin function in the brain (Woolley & Shaw, 1954).

Soon after the discovery of LSD it was recognized that there are similarities between the effects of psychedelics and the symptomatology of schizophrenia, and LSD and mescaline were used experimentally to produce a model psychosis. Indeed, Sandoz laboratories distributed LSD as an experimental drug (Delysid) that mental health profes-

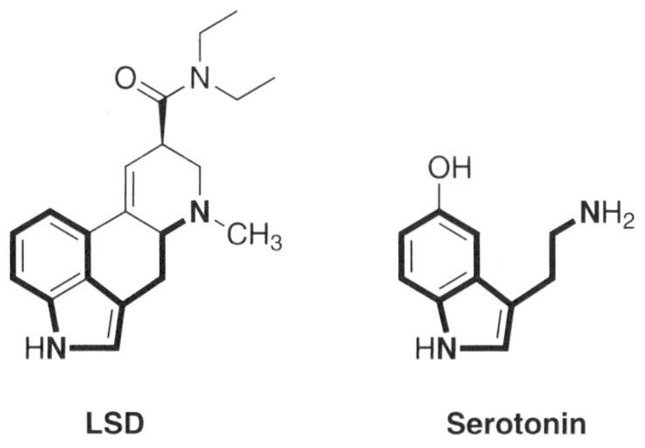

■ FIGURE 1.2. LSD and serotonin.

sionals could take to gain insight into the minds of their psychotic patients.

Research on the functions of serotonin in the brain rapidly increased in the subsequent years (see, e.g., Freedman, 1961; Rosecrans, Lovell, & Freedman, 1967). It also was discovered early on that LSD, mescaline, and psilocybin all produce a very rapid tolerance to their effects, known as tachyphylaxis, and generally produced cross-tolerance to each other (Appel & Freedman, 1968; Freedman, Aghajanian, Ornitz, & Rosner, 1958; Isbell, Wolbach, Wikler, & Miner, 1961). These findings led investigators to search for the common pharmacological target(s) of the various chemotypes.

Anden, Corrodi, Fuxe, and Hokfelt (1968) first proposed that LSD has a direct *agonist* action at brain serotonin receptors. It was soon discovered that LSD and other indoleamine psychedelics potently inhibit the firing of serotonergic neurons in the dorsal raphe nucleus (DRN) (Aghajanian, Foote, & Sheard, 1968, 1970). These cells send ascending serotonin projections to all parts of the forebrain and decreases in their rate of firing therefore attenuate serotonin biosynthesis and release throughout their projection areas. Indoleamine hallucinogens directly inhibit firing in many DRN target regions, but at low doses preferentially inhibit DRN cells while leaving downstream neurons virtually unaffected (DeMontigny & Aghajanian, 1977; Haigler & Aghajanian, 1974). The finding that hallucinogens are more potent at presynaptic than at postsynaptic sites led to the hypothesis that by depressing the activity of neurons in the DRN and thereby decreasing 5-hydroxy-

tryptamine (5-HT) outflow, psychedelic drugs removed the tonic inhibition of downstream neurons mediated by serotonin.

Further research, however, identified significant problems with this "presynaptic hypothesis" of hallucinogen action. One of the most serious problems was the finding that phenylalkylamine psychedelics such as mescaline did not consistently depress DRN firing (Haigler & Aghajanian, 1973; Penington & Reiffenstein, 1986). Although LSD and indoleamine psychedelics induced a dramatic reduction in nerve impulse flow of serotonergic neurons whether applied microiontophoretically or systemically, mescaline had a suppressant effect in the DRN only when given systemically (Haigler & Aghajanian, 1973). Penington and Reiffenstein (1986) concluded that because both LSD and mescaline can inhibit raphe cells when given systemically, but only LSD readily produced an inhibition in these cells when applied microiontophoretically, the two drugs differed in their mode of action on raphe cells. In addition, certain drugs that were not hallucinogenic also attenuated raphe call firing. For these reasons, the idea that psychedelics acted presynaptically to attenuate raphe cell firing was abandoned as a general mechanism of action.

The ability to inhibit DRN cell firing has proven to be a pharmacological effect unrelated to hallucinogenesis. Nonetheless, the 5-HT$_{1A}$ agonist activity of some indoleamines may contribute to their behavioral action. This effect will be explored in more detail later in this chapter.

■ The Key Role of the 5-HT$_{2A}$ Receptor

Early investigations sought to determine how interactions with specific neurotransmitter systems contribute to the effects of hallucinogens in humans. A few early studies addressed this issue by attempting to block the effects of LSD with serotonin, dopamine, and norepinephrine receptor antagonists (Isbell & Logan, 1957; Isbell, Logan, & Miner, 1959). Unfortunately, because of the lack of high-affinity receptor-selective antagonists, those studies failed to link the action of hallucinogens to any particular transmitter system.

Based on physiological preparations and crude pharmacological tools, two receptors for serotonin were initially identified and named D and M. As pharmacological tools became more sophisticated, it soon became apparent that there were several other forms of serotonin receptors. As these were identified, the D receptor was renamed the $5\text{-}HT_2$ receptor, and the M receptor became $5\text{-}HT_3$. Glennon, Young, and Rosecrans first proposed in 1983 that the behavioral effects of hallucinogens are mediated by activation of the $5\text{-}HT_2$ receptor. This proposal was based on the finding that the high-affinity, selective $5\text{-}HT_2$ antagonists pirenperone and ketanserin are highly effective in blocking the discriminative stimulus properties of 2,5-dimethoxy-4-methylamphetamine (DOM) and LSD (Colpaert & Janssen, 1983; Colpaert, Niemegeers, & Janssen, 1982), and of DOM-stimulus generalization to LSD, mescaline, and 5-methoxy-N,N-dimethyltryptamine (5-MeO-DMT; Glennon, Young, Jacyno, Slusher, & Rosecrans, 1983). It was subsequently demonstrated that a robust linear correlation ($r = .938$) exists between the $5\text{-}HT_2$ affinities of a series of phenylalkylamine hallucinogens and their effective dose 50 (ED_{50}) values for substitution in animals trained with DOM (Glennon, Titeler, & McKenney, 1984).

Molecular biology enabled the discovery that the $5\text{-}HT_2$ receptor was actually a family of three closely related receptors. Cloning of the $5\text{-}HT_{2C}$ (originally named the $5\text{-}HT_{1C}$) and $5\text{-}HT_{2A}$ receptors in 1988 and 1990, respectively, allowed for the development of antagonist ligands that were specific for one receptor or the other. An antagonist correlation analysis demonstrated a strong correlation between the $5\text{-}HT_{2A}$ affinity of a series of 5-HT antagonists and their potencies for blocking LSD stimulus generalization to R-(−)-2,5-dimethoxy-4-methylamphetamine (DOM) (Fiorella, Rabin, & Winter, 1995). Furthermore, stimulus control in animals trained with LSD (Winter, Eckler, & Rabin,

2004), 2,5-dimethoxy-4-iodoamphetamine (DOI) (Schreiber, Brocco, & Millan, 1994; Smith, Barrett, & Sanders-Bush, 1999), and DOM (Li, Rice, & France, 2008) was blocked by *M100907*, a highly selective $5\text{-}HT_{2A}$ antagonist. Figure 1.3 illustrates the structures of the R enantiomers of DOM, 2,5-dimethoxy-4-bromoamphetamine (DOB), and DOI. Taken together, these findings demonstrated that interactions with the $5\text{-}HT_{2A}$ receptor are required for psychedelics to induce discriminative stimulus effects. Clinical studies also have shown that the effects of psychedelics in humans are blocked by the antagonist ketanserin, which is selective for $5\text{-}HT_{2A}$ receptors in humans (Preller et al., 2017; Vollenweider, Vollenweider-Scherpenhuyzen, Babler, Vogel, & Hell, 1998).

Extensive research has clearly demonstrated that psychedelics are agonists or partial agonists at the brain serotonin $5\text{-}HT_{2A}$ receptor subtype (see recent review by Nichols, 2016). This receptor is a member of the Family A type G-protein-coupled receptors (GPCRs) and is widely expressed throughout the brain. The $5\text{-}HT_{2A}$ receptor is a $G_{q/11}$-coupled receptor that is linked to the phosphoinositide hydrolysis signaling cascade, with formation of diacylglycerol and mobilization of intracellular calcium (Barker, Burris, & Sanders-Bush, 1991; Nichols & Nichols, 2008). The $5\text{-}HT_{2A}$ receptor is excitatory and can cause neuronal cell depolarization when activated by a psychedelic. Members of both the indoleamine and phenylalkylamine classes of hallucinogens are high-affinity agonists or partial agonists at $5\text{-}HT_{2A}$ receptors. Phenylalkylamine hallucinogens such as DOM, DOI, and DOB are highly selective for $5\text{-}HT_2$ receptor subtypes (Pierce & Peroutka, 1989; Titeler, Lyon, & Glennon, 1988), and there is a consensus in the literature that the behavioral effects of

X = CH₃; (R)-DOM
X = Br; (R)-DOB
X = I; (R)-DOI

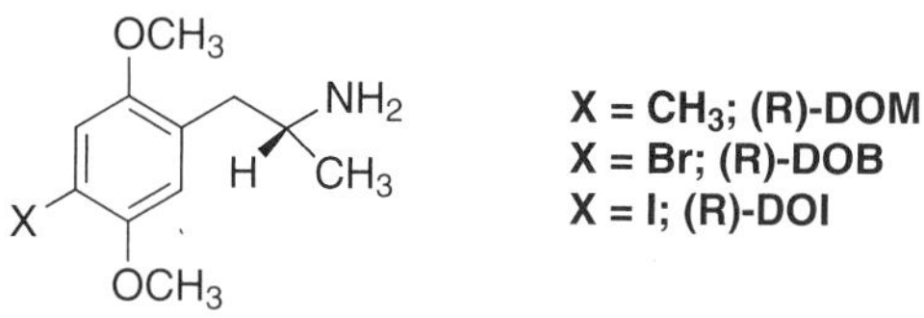

FIGURE 1.3. The structures of the (R)-(−)-enantiomers of DOM, DOB, and DOI.

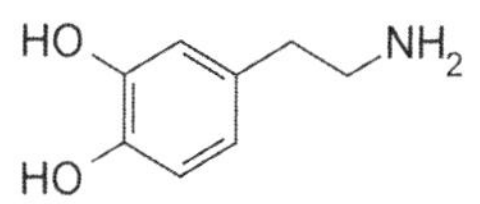

Dopamine (3,4-dihydroxyphenethylamine)

psychedelics are primarily mediated by the 5-HT$_{2A}$ receptor (Halberstadt, 2015; Nichols, 2016).

Expression of 5-HT$_{2A}$ receptors occurs throughout the brain, but their highest expression is found in an enigmatic structure known as the claustrum, a thin, irregular sheet of neurons that is attached to the underside of the neocortex in the center of the mammalian brain. There is also high expression of 5-HT$_{2A}$ receptors in apical dendrites of Layer 5 pyramidal cells in the medial prefrontal and anterior cingulate cortex, as well as in the reticular nucleus of the thalamus, ventral tegmental area, the locus coeruleus, amygdala, and several other important regions. Widespread changes in neuronal excitability resulting from activation of 5-HT$_{2A}$ receptors in these key brain areas would thus be expected to have marked effects on cognition and perception.

Activation of 5-HT$_{2A}$ receptors on glutamatergic pyramidal neurons within the brain by psychedelics, however, generally does not lead to depolarization and the generation of action potentials. Instead, the presence of psychedelics has been shown to increase glutamate release from depolarized neurons to generate what has been termed *recurrent activity* (Aghajanian & Marek, 2000). Interestingly, however, Beique, Imad, Mladenovic, Gingrich, and Andrade (2007) first reported on a subpopulation of large neurons in deep layers of the cortex that was highly sensitive to 5-HT and that responded with strong membrane depolarizations that were capable of initiating spiking activity. The nature of this cell population remained unknown until one of us (C. D. N.; see Martin & Nichols, 2016) was able to purify psychedelic-activated neurons from rat brain for the first time and demonstrate that psychedelics directly activated only a small subset of 5-HT$_{2A}$-expressing excitatory neurons (<5% of the total brain neuronal population) in key brain regions, including the prefrontal cortex (PFC) and the claustrum. Interestingly, the neurons activated by psychedelics express significantly higher levels of the gene for the 5-HT$_{2A}$ receptor and are therefore likely to be more sensitive to psychedelics than other neurons.

Martin and Nichols (2016) also found that the nature of how psychedelics activated these neurons differed depending on the specific brain region in which they were expressed. They hypothesize that this small population of directly responding neurons represents a "trigger population," and that activation of these neurons initiates cellular events that lead to recurrent activity, cortical network destabilization, and the host of perceptual and cognitive behaviors associated with psychedelics. For example, these activated neurons subsequently recruit other select cell types including small subpopulations (<10%) of inhibitory somatostatin- and parvalbumin-containing γ-aminobutyric acid (GABA)ergic interneurons. The differential activation of subsets of both excitatory and inhibitory neurons in ways that would not occur in a normal conscious brain likely alters the basic function of a given brain area and its ability to communicate with other regions. Because distinct regional cellular populations respond differently to psychedelics, different brain regions are more or less sensitive to their effects. These cellular effects of psychedelics, therefore, likely underlie the alterations in brain network communication observed by recent imaging studies.

Another interesting finding by Martin and Nichols (2016) is that psychedelics also activate astrocytes and glia. Astrocytes function as an interface between synaptic activity and the vasculature, helping to serve the metabolic needs of the neurons. One could speculate that the effects of psychedelics on astrocytes could be contributing to alterations in cortical blood flow and metabolism detected by blood oxygen level–dependent (BOLD) functional magnetic resonance imaging (fMRI) and positron emission tomography (PET), and that blood flow and metabolism may be decoupled through astrocyte activation.

The claustrum, with the highest density of 5-HT$_{2A}$ receptor expression in the entire brain, is an especially intriguing brain structure. Its exact functions remain unclear, but based on patterns of retrograde tracing in nonhuman primates, Reser and colleagues (2014) have suggested that the claustrum is ideally positioned as a modulator that could desynchronize or terminate correlated activation of default mode network (DMN)-related areas. Seeley and colleagues (2007) also propose that the connectivity and anatomy of the claustrum place it ideally to control temporal structure of network activity.

Most recently, the crucial role of the $5\text{-}HT_{2A}$ receptor in the clinical actions of psychedelics has been confirmed by clinical studies in which the psychoactive effects of psilocybin, and of LSD, have been blocked by preadministration of ketanserin, an antagonist that is selective for $5\text{-}HT_{2A}$ receptors in humans (Barrett, Preller, Herdener, Janata, & Vollenweider, 2018; Kometer, Schmidt, Jancke, & Vollenweider, 2013; Kraehenmann, Pokorny, Vollenweider, et al., 2017; Preller et al., 2017; Vollenweider et al., 1998).

■ Safety of Psychedelics

Surprisingly, despite the profound psychoactive effects that psychedelics produce, they are generally physiologically very safe. The classic serotonergic hallucinogens do not lead to dependence, and do not result in overdose deaths after reasonable dosages. Furthermore, single high-acute doses of psychedelics such as LSD do not lead to any molecular or genetic signs of toxicity in rodent models (Nichols & Sanders-Bush, 2002). The incidence of adverse effects is very low when these drugs are used in a controlled, supervised clinical environment (Strassman, 1984). LSD has led to only two reported overdose deaths, and those followed *massive* dosages (Nichols & Grob, 2018). Indeed, eight subjects who mistakenly insufflated LSD, believing it was cocaine, all fully recovered after a few days of medical treatment (Klock, Boerner, & Becker, 1975).

An exception to the safety of classic hallucinogens is the class of drugs referred to as "NBOMe" compounds (Figure 1.4). These compounds are N-benzyl derivatives of 2,5-dimethoxy-4-substituted phenethylamines, first discovered by Ralf Heim

(2003; Heim & Elz, 2000; Heim, Pertz, & Elz, 1999). They were found to have extraordinarily potent activity at the $5\text{-}HT_{2A}$ receptor (Braden & Nichols, 2007; Braden, Parrish, Naylor, & Nichols, 2006; Rickli et al., 2015). Extensive structure–activity studies on these molecules have been reported by Hansen and colleagues (2014).

Unfortunately, due to their extraordinary potency, as well as their relative ease of synthesis, these compounds are often misrepresented as LSD and have led to numerous emergency room admittances and deaths (Andreasen et al., 2015; Morini et al., 2017; Poklis et al., 2014; Suzuki, Poklis, & Poklis, 2014; Walterscheid et al., 2014). Although the exact cause of death following NBOMe ingestion is not known, 29 cases published in the literature of acute toxicity associated with the use of an NBOMe commonly reported symptoms that include tachycardia (96.6%), hypertension (62.0%), agitation/aggression (48.2%), seizures (37.9%), and hyperthermia (27.6%) (Wood, Sedefov, Cunningham, & Dargan, 2015). Acute kidney injury also has been reported. Because these are processes not normally controlled by $5\text{-}HT_{2A}$ receptor function, this toxicity is likely mediated by activity at other biological targets that remain unknown.

■ Animal Models to Study Psychedelics

A large amount of the knowledge we have about the mechanism of action of psychedelics has been derived from preclinical studies, either *in vitro* or *in vivo* animal models. The use of animal models to study these compounds has been recently reviewed (Hanks & Gonzalez-Maeso, 2013). Here we discuss only the most widely used and productive animal models: drug discrimination, the mouse head twitch response (HTR), and locomotor measures.

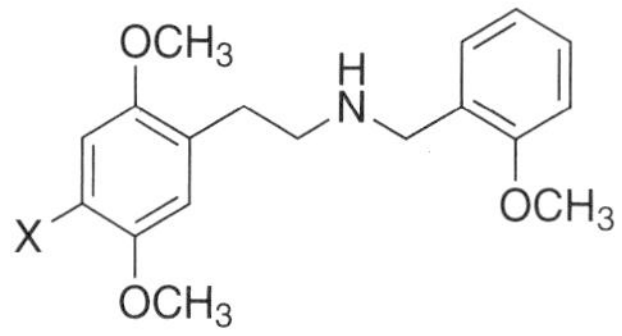

X = Cl; 25C-NBOMe
X = Br; 25B-NBOMe
X = I; 25i-NBOMe

■ FIGURE 1.4. Structures of the most common NBOMe compounds.

Drug Discrimination

Probably the most detailed information about the mechanism of action of psychedelic drugs has come from extensive drug discrimination studies. Rats can be trained to discriminate the subjective effects of drugs from saline using two-lever operant procedures (Glennon, Rosecrans, & Young, 1982, 1983; Hirschhorn & Winter, 1971). Drug discrimination is a sensitive and robust behavioral technique to assess the nature of the enteroceptive cue produced by central nervous system (CNS)-active drugs. Cross-generalization occurs between training drugs of different chemotypes (e.g., mescaline and LSD), indicating that they produce similar if not identical interoceptive stimulus effects. By contrast, other drug classes fail to evoke psychedelic-like stimulus effects reliably (Appel & Cunningham, 1986; Glennon et al., 1982; Glennon, Rosecrans, et al., 1983). The major limitation of drug discrimination is the need for several months of animal training prior to any testing experiments. Once animals have been trained to recognize a particular cue (e.g., LSD), other compounds can be tested to determine whether the LSD stimulus generalizes to the new test compound. If stimulus generalization occurs (i.e., the animals respond as if they had been given the training drug after administration of the test drug), it may be inferred that the test drug has pharmacological properties similar to the training drug (e.g., LSD). Animals can then be trained with the new drug and tests may be carried out to determine whether the new drug stimulus generalizes to the original training drug. In that event, symmetrical substitution is said to occur, and the inference that LSD and the new drug have similar or identical pharmacology is very strong. Various antagonists can be used to block the discriminative task, and depending on their degree of receptor selectivity, one can reach fairly strong conclusions about which receptor is the target of the training drug. For psychedelics, there is a reasonably good correlation between potency in rat drug discrimination and human potency (Nichols, 2004). False positives can occur, where stimulus generalization occurs with the test drug, when it actually differs in pharmacology from the training drug. When psychedelics are used as training drugs, however, false positives are rare.

HTR

Psychedelics evoke a HTR in mice, which is a paroxysmal rotational movement of the head (Corne & Pickering, 1967) and one of the best characterized of the psychedelic-induced stereotypies. Importantly, mice are inexpensive compared to other laboratory animals and, as contrasted with drug discrimination methods, the HTR does not require the animals to be trained. There is extensive evidence that the 5-HT_{2A} receptor mediates the psychedelic-induced HTR. The first evidence for a linkage between 5-HT_{2A} receptors and the HTR induced by psychedelics was the finding that the potencies of 19 5-HT antagonists to block the mescaline-induced mouse HTR is significantly correlated ($r = .88$) with their 5-HT_2 affinity (Leysen, Niemegeers, Van Nueten, & Laduron, 1982). Similar findings were later reported for the HTR induced by DOI (Schreiber et al., 1995). It also was demonstrated that ketanserin blocks the HTR to DOI (Darmani, Martin, Pandey, & Glennon, 1990). The HTR to DOI is completely blocked by *M100907*, a highly selective 5-HT_{2A} receptor antagonist, but not by the 5-HT_{2C} antagonist *SB 242,084*, confirming that the behavior is mediated by 5-HT_{2A} receptors (Vickers et al., 2001). Further evidence for a link between 5-HT_{2A} receptors and head twitch was provided by the finding that hallucinogens do not induce the HTR in $5\text{-HT}_{2A}^{-/-}$ knockout mice (Gonzalez-Maeso et al., 2007; Halberstadt, Koedood, Powell, & Geyer, 2011). Nevertheless, several drugs that can induce HTR do not activate the 5-HT_{2A} receptor, and some drugs that are reported to be nonhallucinogenic 5-HT_{2A} receptor agonists also can induce the HTR. Therefore, the HTR can only be used as a proxy for 5-HT_{2A} receptor activation and is not representative of interoceptive hallucinatory or psychedelic effects (Canal & Morgan, 2012).

Exploratory and Investigatory Behavior

In conventional open-field locomotor testing, hallucinogens produce inconsistent results that do not distinguish between the effects of hallucinogens and nonhallucinogenic agents (Brimblecombe, 1963; Cohen & Wakeley, 1968; Kabes, Fink, & Roth, 1972; Silva & Calil, 1975). The Behavioral Pattern Monitor (BPM), a combination of activity and holeboard chambers, was designed to overcome the shortcomings of open field measurements (Geyer, Russo, & Masten, 1986). The BPM provides both quantitative and qualitative measures of unconditioned locomotor and investigatory activity in rats and can be used to assess animals for changes in responsivity to environmental stimuli.

Psychedelics produce a characteristic profile of behavioral effects in the BPM. When phenylalkylamine (mescaline, DOM, DOI, and DOET) and indolealkylamine (psilocin, DMT, and 5-MeO-DMT) hallucinogens are tested in a novel environment, they decrease locomotor and investigatory behaviors (rearings and holepokes) and increase avoidance of the center of the chamber (Adams & Geyer, 1985a; Krebs-Thomson, Ruiz, Masten, Buell, & Geyer, 2006; Wing, Tapson, & Geyer, 1990). These effects have been attributed to exacerbation of the neophobia and agoraphobia normally exhibited by rats. When animals are tested in a familiar environment, these effects are not observed. LSD has similar effects on investigatory behavior and center entries (Adams & Geyer, 1985b), but it produces a biphasic locomotor pattern, with activity that initially is suppressed, then increases as time progresses (Mittman & Geyer, 1991).

M100907, but not the 5-HT$_{2C/2B}$ antagonist *SER-082*, can block most of the behavioral effects of DOI in the BPM paradigm, which are therefore likely mediated by activation of 5-HT$_{2A}$ receptors (Krebs-Thomson, Paulus, & Geyer, 1998). The pharmacology of the indoleamines is more complex. For example, both the mixed 5-HT$_1$/β-adrenergic antagonist propranolol (Mittman & Geyer, 1991), and the selective 5-HT$_{1A}$ antagonist *WAY-100635* (Krebs-Thomson & Geyer, 1998) block the initial LSD-induced suppression of locomotor activity, whereas the delayed LSD-induced hyperactivity is blocked by *M100907* (Ouagazzal, Grottick, Moreau, & Higgins, 2001) and the 5-HT$_2$ antagonist ritanserin (Mittman & Geyer, 1991). By contrast, the behavioral effects of 5-MeO-DMT are antagonized by

WAY-100635 but not by *M100907* (Krebs-Thomson et al., 2006), indicating a predominant role for 5-HT$_{1A}$ receptors.

■ The 5-HT$_{2C}$ Receptor

Phenylalkylamine and indoleamine hallucinogens also bind to 5-HT$_{2C}$ receptors with high-affinity and functionally are relatively nonselective for 5-HT$_{2A}$ versus 5-HT$_{2C}$ receptors (Nelson, Lucaites, Wainscott, & Glennon, 1999; Porter et al., 1999). The discovery that hallucinogens interact with 5-HT$_{2C}$ receptors confounded the hypothesis that activation of "5-HT$_2$ receptors" is the primary mechanism by which LSD-like drugs act (Glennon et al., 1984). This hypothesis was proposed prior to the discovery of 5-HT$_{2C}$ sites and was partially based on evidence demonstrating that ketanserin and other classical 5-HT$_2$ antagonists block the behavioral effects of hallucinogens in various animal paradigms. Unfortunately, many of the early serotonin antagonists are now known to bind at both 5-HT$_{2A}$ and 5-HT$_{2C}$ sites. For example, the antagonist ketanserin is selective for 5-HT$_{2A}$ receptors in humans but is nonselective between 5-HT$_{2A/C}$ in rodents, where many of the pharmacological studies of psychedelics have been and continue to be performed. The potent action of hallucinogens at both 5-HT$_{2A}$ and 5-HT$_{2C}$ receptors led some authors to speculate that hallucinogenesis may be mediated by interactions with both of these receptor populations (Glennon, 1990; Titeler et al., 1988). Indeed, Sanders-Bush and others had even suggested that 5-HT$_{2C}$ receptor occupation plays a primary mechanistic role in the action of hallucinogenic drugs (Burris, Breeding, & Sanders-Bush, 1991).

There is a significant correlation between the affinities of phenylalkylamine hallucinogens for 5-HT$_{2C}$ receptors and their potencies to evoke psychoactive effects in humans and to substitute in DOM-trained animals (Titeler et al., 1988). That can be explained by the fact that 5-HT$_{2A}$ and 5-HT$_{2C}$ receptors display parallel structure–activity relationships for ligand binding (Nelson et al., 1999), so it is possible that the observed correlation between 5-HT$_{2C}$ receptor affinity and hallucinogen potency merely reflects a correlation between affinities of 5-HT$_{2A}$

and 5-HT$_{2C}$ ligands. Importantly, for a series of structurally diverse 5-HT$_2$ antagonists, the rank order of potencies for blocking LSD-like stimulus effects (Fiorella et al., 1995) and DOI-induced HTR (Schreiber et al., 1995) does not parallel their 5-HT$_{2C}$ affinity. These findings strongly indicate that interactions with 5-HT$_{2C}$ receptors are not primarily responsible for mediating the behavioral effects of hallucinogens. Furthermore, 5-HT$_{2C/2B}$ antagonists (e.g., *SB 200,646A, SB 206,553,* and *SER-082*) and the selective 5-HT$_{2C}$ antagonist *SB 242,084,* consistently fail to block the effects of hallucinogens in a variety of behavioral paradigms (Halberstadt et al., 2016; Ouagazzal et al., 2001; Schreiber et al., 1994; Sipes & Geyer, 1995; Smith et al., 1999; Wettstein, Host, & Hitchcock, 1999; Winter, Rice, Amorosi, & Rabin, 2007). Although some findings suggesting that 5-HT$_{2C}$ receptor interactions may contribute to or modify the effects of some hallucinogens have occasionally been reported (Krebs-Thomson et al., 1998, 2006; Smith, Barrett, & Sanders-Bush, 2003), the vast majority of evidence demonstrates that the behavioral effects of these drugs are not dependent on the 5-HT$_{2C}$ receptor.

■ A Role for the 5-HT$_{1A}$ Receptor?

The 5-HT$_{1A}$ receptor was the first of the many serotonin receptors to be cloned and characterized (Kobilka et al., 1987). In the brainstem, 5-HT$_{1A}$ receptors are expressed presynaptically on cells in the dorsal and median raphe nuclei, where they act as somatodendritic autoreceptors to inhibit cell firing. The presynaptic 5-HT$_{1A}$ receptors expressed on raphe cells couple to G$\alpha_{i/o}$ proteins that activate inwardly rectifying potassium channels (GIRKs), causing neuronal membrane hyperpolarization (Aghajanian, 1995), which leads to a decreased rate of cell firing. Following the characterization of the 5-HT$_{1A}$ receptor, LSD and indoleamines were found to be potent agonists at this receptor type. Thus, the raphe cell suppression by LSD and indoleamines discussed earlier could be attributed to their agonist activity at presynaptic 5-HT$_{1A}$ receptors.

Furthermore, the effects of LSD and 5-MeO-DMT in the BPM are partially mediated by the 5-HT$_{1A}$ receptor. There is also considerable evidence that the 5-HT$_{1A}$ receptor plays a role in the discriminative stimulus effects of LSD and 5-MeO-DMT. For example, in mice trained to discriminate LSD from saline, the 5-HT$_{1A}$ receptor antagonist *WAY 100635* produced a 50% blockade of the LSD drug lever selection (Benneyworth, Smith, Barrett, & Sanders-Bush, 2005). In rats, LSD elicits intermediate levels of drug lever selection in animals trained with the 5-HT$_{1A}$ agonist *8-OH-DPAT,* and the 5-HT$_{1A}$ agonist ipsapirone elicits partial substitution in LSD-trained animals (Arnt, 1989). Likewise, the LSD stimulus completely generalizes to the mixed 5-HT$_{1A}$ agonist/α_2-adrenoceptor antagonist yohimbine (Colpaert, 1984; Marona-Lewicka & Nichols, 1995). Ipsapirone and *8-OH-DPAT* produce full substitution in animals trained with 5-MeO-DMT (Schreiber & de Vry, 1993; Spencer, Glaser, & Traber, 1987; Winter, Filipink, Timineri, Helsley, & Rabin, 2000). Indeed, it has been reported that *WAY-100635* and the mixed 5-HT$_{1A}$/β-adrenergic antagonist pindolol are more effective than pirenperone and ketanserin at blocking stimulus control by 5-MeO-DMT, indicating that the 5-MeO-DMT discriminative stimulus involves a substantial 5-HT$_{1A}$ receptor-mediated component (Spencer et al., 1987; Winter et al., 2000). These observations are consistent with evidence that the behavioral response to 5-MeO-DMT in rodents is mediated predominantly by the 5-HT$_{1A}$ receptor (Halberstadt et al., 2011; Krebs-Thomson et al., 2006; Tricklebank, Forler, Middlemiss, & Fozard, 1985). In addition, as noted earlier, psychedelics suppress raphe cell firing in the brain stem either directly (LSD and indoleamine compounds) or indirectly (by phenethylamines), an effect that also could lead to cortical cell excitation. As demonstrated by Puig, Artigas, and Celada (2005), electrical stimulation of the raphe increases serotonin release into cortical terminal fields, where it activates 5-HT$_{1A}$ receptors on the axon hillock of pyramidal cells, resulting in hyperpolarization. Thus, it seems possible that direct 5-HT$_{2A}$ receptor activation of cortical pyramidal cells could be synergistic with reduced release of serotonin in cortical terminal fields from hallucinogen-induced decreased raphe cell firing. That could be one pharmacological feature that differs between phenethylamine- and indoleamine-type psychedelics.

Pokorny and colleagues (2016) assessed the potential interaction between psilocybin and the 5-HT$_{1A}$ partial agonist buspirone. Subjects treated with 20 mg buspirone orally (p.o.) prior to a moderate dose of psilocybin (0.17 mg/kg p.o.) showed a significant diminution of effects on the visionary restructuralization (VR) dimension of the Five-Dimensional Altered States of Consciousness Questionnaire (5D-ASC), especially on the item clusters related to elementary and complex visual hallucinations. Although buspirone did not attenuate the effect of psilocybin on the OB dimension, buspirone did reduce the effect of psilocybin on several oceanic boundlessness (OB) dimension item clusters (positive depersonalization, positive derealization, altered sense of time, positive mood, and mania-like experiences). These results are consistent with evidence that the 5-HT$_{1A}$ receptor can modulate 5-HT$_{2A}$-induced responses.

By contrast, there is evidence that activation of 5-HT$_{1A}$ receptors can inhibit 5-HT$_{2A}$ receptor-induced behavioral effects. Pretreatment with the 5-HT$_{1A}$ agonist *8-OH-DPAT* dose-dependently attenuated the HTR to DOI in rats and mice (Arnt & Hyttel, 1989; Berendsen & Broekkamp, 1990; Darmani et al., 1990) and the reciprocal hindleg body scratch induced by DOI in the gerbil (Eison & Wright, 1992). The LSD analogue lysergic acid morpholide (LSM-775) does not induce head twitches in mice unless administered in combination with the 5-HT$_{1A}$ antagonist *WAY-100635*, indicating that 5-HT$_{1A}$ activation by LSM-775 masks its ability to induce the HTR (Brandt et al., 2018). Similarly, the mixed 5-HT$_{1A/1B}$/β-adrenergic antagonist pindolol was used to assess the involvement of 5-HT$_{1A}$ receptors in the response to DMT (Strassman, 1996). Pretreatment with pindolol intensified the subjective effects of DMT, suggesting that activation of 5-HT$_{1A}$ receptors by DMT acts to attenuate the psychedelic effects of the drug.

▪ MDMA

3,4-Methylenedioxymethamphetamine (MDMA; ecstasy) is a novel substituted amphetamine that has some similarity in its effects to phenethylamine psychedelics. It also has been claimed to have value as an adjunct to psychotherapy. MDMA produces mood elevation and an increased sense of empathy, with little sensory disruption. The effects of MDMA are distinct from those typically produced by psychedelics, however, and it has been proposed that MDMA is an entactogen, a distinct class of drugs (Nichols, 1986; Nichols, Hoffman, Oberlender, Jacob, & Shulgin, 1986). MDMA has been demonstrated to have promise in the treatment of patients with posttraumatic stress disorder (PTSD) (Sessa, 2017, 2018), and is now entering U.S. Food and Drug administration (FDA)–approved Phase 3 clinical studies. Its primary mechanism of action is indirect, by activation of serotonin receptors through release of 5-HT from presynaptic terminals. In addition, MDMA also induces release of dopamine and norepinephrine from presynaptic neuron terminals; it is unclear what contribution(s) the catecholamines make to the overall effect of MDMA. Nonetheless, the uniqueness of the psychopharmacology of MDMA compared to other structurally similar stimulants such as methamphetamine is apparently due to the addition of the robust serotonergic component.

▪ Clinical Pharmacology of Psychedelics

In the past three decades, there has been renewed interest in the possibility that psychedelics may be useful therapeutic drugs. In order to assess the acute clinical effects of psychedelics, one requires appropriate instruments to characterize and quantify changes in consciousness. Common psychedelic effects can be reliably measured using validated psychometric instruments consisting of self-report questionnaires and rating scales. The most widely used and validated instrument for that is the Altered States of Consciousness (APZ) Rating Scale (Dittrich, 1998). It measures three primary and one secondary dimension of altered states of consciousness (ASCs) that are believed to be invariant across types of ASC induction methods. This self-administered questionnaire was developed by Adolph Dittrich (1998) to assess alterations of consciousness in an etiology-independent manner. Numerous clinical trials have confirmed that the APZ Rating Scale is sensitive to the effects of psychedelics, including psilocybin, DMT, ayahuasca, mescaline, and LSD (Gouzoulis-Mayfrank et al., 1999, 2005; Hermle et al., 1992; Liechti, Dolder, & Schmid, 2017; Riba, Rodriguez-Fornells, & Barbanoj, 2002; Vollenweider et al., 1997, 1998).

Dittrich proposed that the subjective effects of hallucinogens could be divided into three major dimensions: (1) "oceanic boundlessness" (OB), (2) "anxious ego dissolution" (AED), and (3) "visionary restructuralization" (VR). The OB dimension is similar to classical mystical experiences and involves a pleasant state of depersonalization and derealization. The AED dimension incorporates dysphoric effects such as anxiety, thought disorder, delusions, fear of losing control, and ego disintegration. The VR dimension includes perceptual phenomena such as visual hallucinations and illusions, synesthesia, and changes in the meaning of percepts. The OB, AED, and VR dimensions contain multiple clusters of items from the APZ questionnaire. Studies that employed an updated version of the APZ, the 5D-ASC, have shown that psilocybin and LSD also increase scores in a dimension known as "reduction of vigilance" (RV), which includes measures of drowsiness, cognitive impairment, and decreased alertness (Carter et al., 2007; Hasler, Grimberg, Benz, Huber, & Vollenweider, 2004; Liechti et al., 2017; Vollenweider, Csomor, Knappe, Geyer, & Quednow, 2007). A fluorodeoxyglucose [^{18}F]FDG PET study demonstrated that psilocybin increases cerebral glucose metabolic activity in PFC, anterior cingulate, temporomedial cortex, and putamen, and the increased metabolic rate within those regions was found to be significantly correlated with subjective effects in the OB, VR, and AED dimensions (Vollenweider et al., 1997).

The Hallucinogen Rating Scale (HRS) is another instrument that has been used to assess the subjective effects of hallucinogens. The HRS contains 99 items in six clusters: (1) *Somaesthesia* (interoceptive effects), (2) *Affect* (changes in mood and emotion), (3) *Perception* (visual, auditory, tactile, and olfactory experiences), (4) *Cognition* (modification of thought and cognitive processes),

(5) *Volition* (the degree to which the subject is incapacitated by the drug), and (6) *Intensity* (overall strength of the drug effect). Although the HRS was designed specifically to measure the response to intravenous DMT (Strassman, Qualls, Uhlenhuth, & Kellner, 1994), it also has been employed in studies of ayahuasca (Riba, Rodriguez-Fornells, Strassman, & Barbanoj, 2001; Riba et al., 2003), psilocybin (Gouzoulis-Mayfrank et al., 1999; Griffiths et al., 2011; Griffiths, Richards, McCann, & Jesse, 2006), and 2,5-dimethoxy-4-bromophenethylamine (2C-B; Papaseit et al., 2018).

After a hiatus of more than 20 years, the first clinical studies of a psychedelic were reported by Strassman (Strassman & Qualls, 1994; Strassman, Qualls, & Berg, 1996; Strassman et al., 1994). These studies focused on basic physiological and hormonal changes following intravenous injection of different doses of DMT fumarate, and no attempt was made to assess its potential therapeutic actions. Interestingly, at the highest doses, subjects reported encounters with "alien" beings and landscapes, which led to a book and a movie by Strassman (2001) titled *DMT: The Spirit Molecule*.

The first modern attempt to identify a therapeutic use for a psychedelic was a study of the efficacy of psilocybin in the treatment of obsessive–compulsive disorder (OCD) (Moreno, Wiegand, Taitano, & Delgado, 2006). Nine subjects diagnosed with OCD were given a total of 29 doses of psilocybin, including a low, a medium, and a high dose in a double-blind procedure that lacked a placebo control. Marked but variable decreases in symptoms were observed in all subjects during one or more testing sessions. Most subjects experienced symptom reduction beyond 24 hours and beyond the pharmacological half-life of psilocybin, but only one subject reported symptom reduction at 6 months. These promising results indicate that the utility of psilocybin therapy should be investigated further, using a larger number of participants in a standard randomized controlled trial.

That same year, Griffiths and colleagues (2006), at Johns Hopkins University, reported on effects of psilocybin in normal volunteers. Thirty hallucinogen-naive adult volunteers reporting regular participation in religious or spiritual activities were enrolled in the study. Two or three sessions were conducted at 2-month intervals in which volunteers received orally administered psilocybin (30 mg/70 kg) and methylphenidate hydrochloride (40 mg/70 kg) in counterbalanced order. Psilocybin produced a range of acute perceptual changes, subjective experiences, and labile moods. Psilocybin also increased measures of mystical experience. At 2 months, 67% of the volunteers rated the experience with psilocybin to be either the single most meaningful experience of their lives or among the top five most meaningful experiences of their lives. Thirty-three percent of the volunteers rated the psilocybin experience as being the single most spiritually significant experience of their lives, with an additional 38% rating it to be among the top five most spiritually significant experiences.

At the 14-month follow-up, 58 and 67%, respectively, of volunteers rated the psilocybin-occasioned experience as being among the five most personally meaningful and among the five most spiritually significant experiences of their lives. Of the volunteers, 64% indicated that the experience increased their well-being or life satisfaction, and 58% met criteria for having had a "complete" mystical experience. Correlation and regression analyses indicated a central role of the mystical experience assessed on the session day in the high ratings of personal meaning and spiritual significance at follow-up (Griffiths, Richards, Johnson, McCann, & Jesse, 2008). It had been known since the 1960s that psychedelics can induce mystical and spiritual experiences (Pahnke, 1969; Pahnke & Richards, 1966), but this work documented significant positive, long-term benefits to the use of psychedelics in normal volunteers.

In a similar follow-up study (Griffiths et al., 2011), participants were 18 adults, 17 of whom were hallucinogen naïve. Five 8-hour sessions were conducted individually for each participant at 1-month intervals. Participants were randomized to receive the four active doses in either ascending or descending order (nine participants each). This double-blind study evaluated psilocybin at 0, 5, 10, 20, and 30 mg/70 kg (p.o.). Placebo was scheduled quasi-randomly. One month after sessions at the two highest doses, volunteers rated the psilocybin experience as having substantial personal and spiritual significance, and attributed to the experience sustained positive changes in attitudes, mood, and behavior, with the ascending dose sequence showing greater positive effects.

Results from these two Griffiths studies were then combined and analyzed by MacLean, Johnson, and Griffiths (2011). They reported potential changes in five generally recognized broad personality domains: neuroticism, extroversion, openness, agreeableness, and conscientiousness. Personality change was assessed 1–2 months after a high-dose psilocybin session and again more than 1 year later to determine the persistence of personality change. Although there were no significant changes in the personality domains of neuroticism, extroversion, agreeableness, or conscientiousness, the trait of openness increased significantly from screening to posttest. Taken together, their results indicate predominantly stable personality traits, but with specific increases in openness following the high-dose psilocybin session.

MacLean and colleagues (2011) further examined the relationship between mystical experience and increases in openness by comparing participants who met the criteria for having had a complete mystical experience during their high-dose session with participants who did not meet the criteria. ANOVA revealed a significant interaction between time (screening vs. posttest) and group (complete mystical experience vs. no complete mystical experience). Follow-up t-tests confirmed that the complete mystical experience group showed significant increases in openness from screening to posttest. They observed a significant linear correlation between the degree of mystical experience and change in openness. Interestingly, openness includes a relatively broad range of intercorrelated traits covering aesthetic appreciation and sensitivity, fantasy and imagination, awareness of feelings in self and others, and intellectual engagement. People with high levels of openness are "permeable to new ideas and experiences" and "motivated to enlarge their experience into novel territory" (see references in MacLean et al., 2011). Openness is also strongly associated with creativity, and some of its facets are correlated with general fluid intelligence and cognitive ability.

In another study by Griffiths and colleagues (2018) psilocybin was administered in a double-blind paradigm to 75 healthy participants who undertook a program of meditation/spiritual practices. Healthy participants were randomized to three groups of 25 each: (1) very low dose (1 mg/70 kg on Sessions 1 and 2) with moderate-level ("standard") support for spiritual practice (LD-SS); (2) high dose (20 and 30 mg/70 kg on Sessions 1 and 2, respectively) with standard support (HD-SS); and (3) high dose (20 and 30 mg/70 kg on Sessions 1 and 2, respectively) with high support for spiritual practice (HD-HS). Psilocybin was administered 1 and 2 months after spiritual practice initiation. Outcomes at 6 months included rates of spiritual practice and persisting effects of psilocybin. Compared with low-dose, high-dose psilocybin produced greater acute and persisting effects. At 6 months, compared with LD-SS, both high-dose groups showed large, significant positive changes on longitudinal measures of interpersonal closeness, gratitude, life meaning/purpose, forgiveness, death transcendence, daily spiritual experiences, religious faith and coping, and community observer ratings. The authors concluded that a mystical experience and/or its neurophysiological or other correlates are likely determinants of the enduring positive attitudinal, dispositional, and behavioral effects of psilocybin when administered under spiritually supported conditions. Recent studies by Liechti and colleagues (2017) and Schmid and Liechti (2018) indicated similar benefits resulting from LSD-induced mystical experiences.

Recently, antidepressant and anxiolytic effects in patients with terminal cancer have been demonstrated in clinical trials (Griffiths et al., 2016; Grob et al., 2011; Ross et al., 2016). In addition, in small pilot studies, psilocybin-assisted therapy has shown promise for disruption of addiction to alcohol (Bogenschutz et al., 2015) and nicotine (Johnson, Garcia-Romeu, Cosimano, & Griffiths, 2014; Johnson, Garcia-Romeu, & Griffiths, 2017). In the studies assessing the efficacy of psilocybin as a po-tential treatment for anxiety and depression in patients with cancer and tobacco addiction, the therapeutic response was correlated with the intensity of psilocybin-induced mystical experience.

■ Mechanism of Psychedelic Effects in Humans

As part of a series of studies of the effects of psilocybin in human volunteers, Vollenweider and colleagues (1998) assessed the effect of pretreatment with the 5-HT_{2A} antagonist ketanserin, the mixed $D_2/5\text{-HT}_{2A}$ antagonist risperidone, and the dopamine (D_2) antagonist haloperidol. The effects of psilocybin on the OB, AED, and VR dimensions of the APZ were reduced by pretreatment with 20 mg ketanserin (p.o.) and almost completely blocked by pretreatment with either 40 or 50 mg ketanserin (Carter et al., 2007; Vollenweider et al., 1998). Likewise, pretreatment with 0.5 and 1.0 mg risperidone (p.o.) produced partial and complete blockade, respectively, of the subjective effects of psilocybin (Vollenweider et al., 1998). Conversely, haloperidol was much less effective, producing only partial blockade of psilocybin effects in the OB dimension, while actually increasing scores in the AED dimension. Taken together, these findings confirm that the hallucinogenic effects of psilocybin in humans are primarily mediated by actions at the 5-HT_{2A} receptor, with D_2 receptor interactions playing only a minor role.

Vollenweider and colleagues also have examined whether the neurophysiological effects of psilocybin are affected by 5-HT_{2A} receptor blockade. Reductions in N170 visual-evoked potentials and α oscillatory activity in visual cortex are thought to play an important role in the visual hallucinations produced by psilocybin and other hallucinogens (Kometer & Vollenweider, 2018). Thus, it is notable that ketanserin completely blocks the effect of psilocybin on N170 potentials and α oscillations (Kometer et al., 2013), consistent with the absence of psilocybin-induced visual hallucinations in subjects pretreated with ketanserin (Carter et al., 2007; Vollenweider et al., 1998). Pretreatment with ketanserin also reportedly attenuates the reduction of prepulse inhibition

(PPI) produced by psilocybin (Quednow, Kometer, Geyer, & Vollenweider, 2012).

Several fairly recent studies have examined whether ketanserin also can block the effects of LSD in human subjects. As found previously with psilocybin, 40 mg ketanserin (p.o.) pretreatment completely blocked the subjective effects produced by 100 μg (p.o.) doses of LSD free base (Kraehenmann, Pokorny, Aicher, et al., 2017; Kraehenmann, Pokorny, Vollenweider, et al., 2017; Preller et al., 2017). Ketanserin fully inhibited the misattribution of personal relevance observed in subjects administered LSD, as well as the BOLD signal increase induced by LSD in frontal cortical areas involved in self-referential processing (Preller et al., 2017). Furthermore, ketanserin blocked the ability of LSD to increase *primary process thinking* (a dreamlike cognitive state characterized by seemingly unorganized sequences of thoughts and images) in subjects performing a guided mental imagery task (Kraehenmann, Pokorny, Aicher, et al., 2017).

In an fMRI study, Barrett, Preller, Herdener, Janata, and Vollenweider (2018) examined the effect of LSD on music processing in the brain. The relationships between the 24 major and minor keys of Western tonal music (e.g., how many notes they have in common, their relative perceptual "fit") can be represented on the surface of a torus (Krumhansl, 1990; Krumhansl & Kessler, 1982; Toiviainen & Krumhansl, 2003). As music progresses, the sequence of melodies and chord progressions creates specific patterns of activity on the toroidal surface. According to previous fMRI studies, these activity patterns in tonal space are tracked in the rostromedial PFC and other cortical regions (Janata, 2005; Janata et al., 2002), a phenomenon known as *tonality tracking*. Administration of LSD (100 μg p.o.) enhanced tonality tracking in medial PFC, superior temporal gyrus, inferior temporal gyrus, angular gyrus, and amygdala, brain regions involved in processing speech and music, as well as associated autobiographical and emotional responses (Barrett et al., 2018). Most of the effects of LSD on tonality tracking were blocked when subjects were pretreated with ketanserin (40 mg p.o.), consistent with the involvement of 5-HT$_{2A}$ receptors.

As noted earlier, ayahuasca is a brew prepared from a mixture of plants. *Banisteriopsis caapi* vines, which contain β-carboline alkaloids such as harmine and harmaline, are extensively boiled together with leaves of *Psychotria viridis,* which contain DMT (McKenna et al., 1984; Schultes & Hofmann, 1980). Although DMT is not orally active due to first-pass metabolism (Szara, 1957; Turner & Merlis, 1959), the β-carboline alkaloids act as reversible inhibitors of liver MAO, allowing DMT to possess oral activity. Similar to other psychedelics, administration of ayahuasca to human subjects reduces alpha oscillatory activity in occipital and parietal cortices (Riba, Anderer, Jane, Saletu, & Barbanoj, 2004; Schenberg et al., 2015; Valle et al., 2016). As with psilocybin and LSD, pretreatment with ketanserin (40 mg p.o.) blocks the effect of ayahuasca on alpha activity (Valle et al., 2016). Interestingly, however, ketanserin only partially attenuated the subjective experience produced by a dose of ayahuasca containing 0.75 mg/ kg DMT. Therefore, although 5-HT$_{2A}$ receptor agonist activity can fully account for the subjective effects of psilocybin and LSD (see earlier discussion), the same may not be true for ayahuasca. In addition to inhibiting MAO, the beta-carboline alkaloids in ayahuasca can interact with a variety of molecular targets and recognition sites, including voltage-dependent Na$^+$ channels (Deecher et al., 1992), imidazoline I$_2$ sites (Husbands et al., 2001), dual-specificity tyrosine phosphorylated and regulated kinase 1A (DYRK1A) (Bain et al., 2007), N-methyl-D-aspartate (NMDA) receptors (Du, Aloyo, & Harvey, 1997), and the σ$_1$ receptor (Bowen et al., 1995). Further studies are required to characterize fully the receptor mechanisms responsible for ayahuasca-induced phenomenology.

Although other chapters in this volume deal extensively with how psychedelics affect brain dynamics, it may be helpful here to comment briefly on this topic. We have noted that psychedelics depolarize cortical cells, and that action potentials are generated in claustral glutamate cells. Claustral projections are widespread throughout the brain, so the generation of action potentials that release glutamate onto already-sensitized cortical cells would be expected to produce changes in brain dynamics. We have recently proposed that claustral cell firing may be catalytic in engendering changes in resting state network communication (Nichols, Johnson, & Nichols, 2017). Recent studies using BOLD fMRI and magnetoencephalography (MEG) imaging methods after psychedelic administration in humans have given powerful insight into the networks that the brain employs for communication (Barrett et al., 2018; Carhart-Harris et al., 2012, 2016; Muthukumaraswamy et al., 2013; Preller et al., 2017, 2018; Tagliazucchi et al., 2016). In essence, the brain can be thought of as comprising anatomically distinct regions called nodes or hubs. Normally, communication occurs mostly within these nodes (i.e., integration), which are largely (but not completely) segregated from other nodes. After a psychedelic, however, the integration within, and segregation between different nodes is lost, and new communication networks are formed that allow widespread (global) communication between many other nodes or hubs. One of the key hubs that is disrupted is the DMN. This network is normally highly organized and active when a person is not carrying out a mental task. It has been proposed that collapse of integrity within the DMN leads to "ego loss" and the mystical experience after taking a psychedelic (Carhart-Harris et al., 2014; Tagliazucchi et al., 2016). Thus, 5-HT_{2A} receptor agonism leads to desynchronization of oscillatory activity, disintegration of intrinsic integrity in the DMN and related brain networks, and an overall brain dynamic characterized by increased between-network global functional connectivity, expanded signal diversity, and a larger repertoire of structured neurophysiological activation patterns. Crucially, these characteristic traits of psychedelic brain activity have been correlated with the phenomenological dynamics and intensity of subjective psychedelic effects (Swanson, 2018).

Psychedelics as Anti-Inflammatory Agents

The protein target of psychedelics, the 5-HT_{2A} receptor, is the most widely expressed serotonin receptor throughout the mammalian body. It is found in nearly all cell types of every organ. These include epithelial, endothelial, muscle, and immune-related cells. Despite that, nearly all research into the function of this receptor has focused on the CNS and its role in brain activity and behavior. Given the near ubiquitous expression of this receptor, it was somewhat unexpected that the genetic knockout mouse was found to be relatively normal. Furthermore, there are no known diseases associated with polymorphisms or mutations in the *HTR2A* gene locus. One potential role identified for this receptor in the periphery was as a participant in serotonin-mediated inflammation. Serotonin has long been recognized as a mediator of inflammation, and its levels have been found to be elevated at sites of inflammation (Shajib & Khan, 2015). Antagonists of the 5-HT_{2A} receptor have been shown to have anti-inflammatory effects in several animal models (Hayashi et al., 2003; Nishiyama, 2009). The anti-inflammatory effect of antagonists is presumably achieved by blocking the proinflammatory effects of serotonin itself on the target tissues, and prevention of activation of 5-HT_{2A} receptors. Interestingly, certain polymorphisms in the *HTR2A* gene locus have been associated with a protective effect against certain inflammatory disorders (Snir et al., 2013).

Therefore, it was a surprising discovery when one of us (C. D. N.) found that psychedelics are capable of producing an extremely potent anti-inflammatory effect: specifically, that psychedelics can prevent the inflammatory response induced by tumor necrosis factor-α (TNF-α) in cultures of cells isolated from vascular tissues (Yu et al., 2008). Several psychedelics were tested, including LSD, with a potency to block inflammation about that of corticosteroids for their targets. One drug, (R)-DOI, was especially potent and blocked TNF-α-mediated inflammation at much lower concentrations of the drug. The structural basis for the superpotency of (R)-DOI to inhibit inflammation compared to other psychedelics like LSD is not yet known, but it is the subject of active study.

Significantly, the ability of psychedelics to block inflammation in cell culture was translated to the whole animal. A single pretreatment with low subbehaviorally active doses of (R)-DOI was able to block completely the inflammation produced by systemic injection of TNF-α in mice (Nau, Yu, Martin, & Nichols, 2013). That included prevention of increased intercellular adhesion molecule 1 (ICAM1), vascular cell adhesion molecule 1 (VCAM1), interleukin 1b (IL1b), and monocyte chemoattractant protein-1 (MCP1) in tissues and interleukin 6 (IL6) in tissues and circulation (Nau et al., 2015). Moving to a rodent model of a human inflammatory disease, allergic asthma, a psychedelic once again proved to be a potent anti-inflammatory. In this model, (R)-DOI is able to prevent the hallmark symptoms of asthma, including airways hyperresponsiveness, eosinophilia, mucus overproduction, and recruitment of activated T helper 2 (Th2) cells to the lung at subbehavioral doses (Nau et al., 2015). Additionally, bronchial inflammation is suppressed, as are levels of inflammatory cytokines and chemokines in the lung of sensitized animals exposed to allergens (Nau et al., 2015). Further work has established that several other psychedelics in addition to (R)-DOI can potently suppress the development of asthma, whereas other psychedelics are less potent, in both mouse and rat models of allergic asthma (unpublished data C. D. N.). These compounds and assays are currently being utilized to examine functionally selective mechanisms downstream of receptor activation leading to behavioral and/or anti-inflammatory pathways.

The anti-inflammatory effects of additional psychedelics and 5-HT$_{2A}$ receptor agonists have been reported. The primary psychedelic component of ayahuasca, mentioned earlier, is DMT. Recently, there have been reports that this decoction has anti-inflammatory properties that are mediated through the σ-1 receptor (Szabo, Kovacs, Frecska, & Rajnavolgyi, 2014; Szabo et al., 2016). DMT was shown to reduce proinflammatory cytokine expression in human induced pluripotent stem cell (iPSC)–derived cortical neuron- and microglia-like cells in culture, and RNA interference (RNAi) knockdown of the σ-1 receptor gene eliminated these anti-inflammatory effects (Szabo et al., 2014, 2016). It remains to be seen, however, whether these interesting results can be translated to animal models of inflammation. In another relatively recent study, extracts of Australian cane toad skins were tested for anti-inflammatory effects in a human monocyte cell line, and were found to suppress lipopolysaccharide (LPS)–induced expression of several pro-inflammatory cytokines including TNF-α and IL6 (Zulfiker, Hashimi, Qi, Grice, & Wei, 2016). Although there are many bioactive compounds in the extracts, their positive control was bufotenine, a tryptamine drug related in structure to psilocin that is an agonist of the serotonin 5-HT$_{2A}$ receptor and a major component of the extracts. Bufotenine had roughly the same efficacy as the skin extracts, suggesting that this tryptamine was responsible for the observed anti-inflammatory effects (Zulfiker et al., 2016). Additional experiments will need to be performed to examine whether or not activity at the 5-HT$_{2A}$ receptor is the underlying anti-inflammatory mechanism of bufotenine and the Australian cane toad skin extracts.

Together, these *in vitro* and *in vivo* preclinical data support the idea that psychedelics may one day serve as potent steroid-sparing anti-inflammatory agents for a variety of disorders, including atherosclerosis, asthma, and inflammatory bowel disease. Importantly, levels of drug needed may be several orders of magnitude lower than necessary to influence behaviors.

■ Psychedelics and Gene Expression

In the late 1960s through the mid-1970s, a series of publications from a few different groups claimed that LSD produced chromosomal damage. Whereas the first of these examined the effects of LSD on leukocytes in culture, subsequent reports claimed chromosomal damage in human users of the drug (Egozcue, Irwin, & Maruffo, 1968; Long, 1972). It is now generally recognized that psychedelics, including LSD, do *not* produce chromosomal damage. They can, however, alter gene expression in their target tissues. Acute changes in expression may impact the immediate subjective experience, and long-lasting changes may underlie their therapeutic potential to treat depression and addiction. Two psychedelics have received significantly more study than others with respect to gene expression: LSD and DOI, the first likely due to its widespread use as a recreational drug, and the second because it is a selective receptor agonist of 5-HT$_2$ receptors that has been available as a valuable research tool to explore the pharmacology of this receptor family.

Initial studies using *in situ* hybridization and immunohistochemistry demonstrated that LSD and DOI are able to induce rapidly the expression of immediate early genes (IEGs) and their encoded proteins that include *c-fos* and *arc* in specific regions of rodent brain (Frankel & Cunningham, 2002; Gresch, Strickland, & Sanders-Bush, 2002; Pei et al., 2000; Scruggs, Patel, Bubser, & Deutch, 2000; Tilakaratne & Friedman, 1996). IEGs in general rapidly respond to various stimuli by increasing their messenger RNA (mRNA) expression. The majority, like *c-fos*, encode for a transcription factor that will subsequently activate several downstream target genes, depending on the nature of the stimuli. Interestingly, the cells that had increased IEG expression were not found to be the 5-HT$_{2A}$ receptor expressing neuronal population (Gresch et al., 2002; Pei, Tordera, Sprakes, & Sharp, 2004; Scruggs et al., 2000). Because IEG expression could be blocked by selective 5-HT$_{2A}$ receptor antagonists, it was believed that activation of the unidentified cells with increased IEG expression was indirect. Why the 5-HT$_{2A}$ positive neurons were not seemingly transcriptionally responding remained elusive for several more years.

The first unbiased screen of the effects of a psychedelic, LSD, in rodent brain was reported by Nichols and Sanders-Bush (2002). Using newly developed microarray technology, a single dose of LSD was found to increase only a small cohort of genes in rat PFC. A subsequent screen identified a few more up-regulated genes (Nichols & Sanders-Bush, 2004). Each of these genes had their expression either completely or partially mediated by 5-HT$_{2A}$ receptor activation. The majority were IEGs that had been implicated by others in the process of synaptic plasticity. One previously unknown transcript was identified and named *ilad1* (Nichols & Sanders-Bush, 2004). *Ilad1* and its predicted protein have significant homology to beta arrestin, with two arrestin-like domains for protein–protein interactions. *Ilad1* was subsequently renamed *arrdc2*

(arrestin domain containing protein 2) and represented the first member of a new class of proteins later termed α-arrestins (Alvarez, 2008). Of these genes, all were found to return to baseline expression levels within 3 hours with the exception of *nor1*, which remained at maximal levels for at least 5 hours after drug administration (Nichols & Sanders-Bush, 2004). Subsequent microarray screens by González-Maeso and co-workers (2003) identified a similar response in mouse cortical tissues. Interestingly, they noted that different agonists at the receptor could produce differing genetic responses.

The effects of psychedelics on long-term gene expression changes were examined in a new proposed potential rat model of psychosis. In this model, rats administered a low dose of LSD every other day over 6 months developed aberrant behaviors that are conserved with those of other models of psychosis, including increased locomotion, increased reactivity, anhedonia, and aggression (Marona-Lewicka, Nichols, & Nichols, 2011). Remarkably, these abnormal behaviors persisted for at least several weeks after discontinuation of the drug. An RNA-sequencing screen of the PFC of these rats 4 weeks after the final drug administration revealed about 700 genes significantly altered in expression (Martin, Marona-Lewicka, Nichols, & Nichols, 2014). Functional clustering highlighted groups of genes involved in synaptic plasticity, GPCR signaling, and metabolic function, among others (Martin et al., 2014). Furthermore, there was a significant enrichment of genes previously implicated by others in both schizophrenia and bipolar depression (Martin et al., 2014). Although this study examined gene expression after 3 months of drug administration, it highlighted the fact that LSD can influence gene expression for a long time after drug administration has stopped.

More recently, new tools have allowed for the examination of the molecular and genetic responses of individual cell types within the brain that respond to psychedelics (Martin, Xu, Porretta, & Nichols, 2017). With a focus on the medial PFC, a small subpopulation (~3–5%) of neurons was found that directly respond to LSD and DOI with increased IEG expression (Martin & Nichols, 2016). Transcripts that rapidly increased in expression include *c-fos*, ΔfosB, krox20/erg2, and *per1* (Martin & Nichols, 2016). Rapid and increased IEG expression in neurons highly correlates with depolarization, and these neurons may be similar to those identified earlier by electrophysiology that depolarize in response to 5-HT and 5-HT$_{2A}$ receptor agonists (Beique et al., 2007). All directly activated neurons expressed four times the level of *HTR2A* transcript than was measured for the nonactivated neuronal pool. Therefore, these neurons may be directly responding because they are more sensitive to 5-HT$_{2A}$ receptor agonists due to their increased receptor level compared to the nonresponding neurons. These directly responding neurons, named the trigger population, were discussed earlier. Interestingly, the transcriptional response of the trigger population of neurons differs between brain regions. For example, the immediate early gene *krox20/egr2* was induced in neurons purified from somatosensory cortex but not in neurons purified from the medial PFC. These regional transcriptional differences may underlie differential regional responses to psychedelics that manifest as differences in network connectivity between regions observed by imaging studies.

References

Adams, L. M., & Geyer, M. A. (1985a). Effects of DOM and DMT in a proposed animal model of hallucinogenic activity. *Prog Neuro-Psychopharmacol Biol Psychiatry, 9*(2), 121–132.

Adams, L. M., & Geyer, M. A. (1985b). A proposed animal model for hallucinogens based on LSD's effects on patterns of exploration in rats. *Behav Neurosci, 99*(5), 881–900.

Aghajanian, G. K. (1995). Electrophysiology of serotonin receptor subtypes and signal transduction pathways. In F. R. Bloom & D. J. Kupfer (Eds.), *Psychopharmacology: The fourth generation of progress* (pp. 1451–1459). New York: Raven Press.

Aghajanian, G. K., Foote, W. E., & Sheard, M. H. (1968). Lysergic acid diethylamide: Sensitive neuronal units in the midbrain raphe. *Science, 161*, 706–708.

Aghajanian, G. K., Foote, W. E., & Sheard, M. H. (1970). Action of psychotogenic drugs on single midbrain raphe neurons. *J Pharmacol Exp Therapeut, 171*(2), 178–187.

Aghajanian, G. K., & Marek, G. J. (2000). Serotonin model of schizophrenia: Emerging role of glutamate mechanisms. *Brain Res Rev, 31*(2–3), 302–312.

Alvarez, C. E. (2008). On the origins of arrestin and rhodopsin. *BMC Evolution Biol, 8*, 222.

Anden, N. E., Corrodi, H., Fuxe, K., & Hokfelt, T. (1968). Evidence for a central 5-hydroxytryptamine receptor stimulation by lysergic acid diethylamide. *Brit J Pharmacol, 34*(1), 1–7.

Andreasen, M. F., Telving, R., Rosendal, I., Eg, M. B., Hasselstrom, J. B., & Andersen, L. V. (2015). A fatal poisoning involving 25C-NBOMe. *Forensic Sci Int, 251*, e1–e8.

Appel, J. B., & Cunningham, K. A. (1986). The use of drug discrimination procedures to characterize hallucinogenic drug actions. *Psychopharmacol Bull, 22*(3), 959–967.

Appel, J. B., & Freedman, D. X. (1968). Tolerance and cross-tolerance among psychotomimetic drugs. *Psychopharmacologia, 13*(3), 267–274.

Arnt, J. (1989). Characterization of the discriminative stimulus properties induced by 5-HT1 and 5-HT2 agonists in rats. *Pharmacol Toxicol, 64*(2), 165–172.

Arnt, J., & Hyttel, J. (1989). Facilitation of 8-OHDPAT-induced forepaw treading of rats by the 5-HT2 agonist DOI. *Eur J Pharmacol, 161*(1), 45–51.

Bain, J., Plater, L., Elliott, M., Shpiro, N., Hastie, C. J., McLauchlan, H., et al. (2007). The selectivity of protein kinase inhibitors: A further update. *Biochem J, 408*(3), 297–315.

Barker, E. L., Burris, K. D., & Sanders-Bush, E. (1991). Phosphoinositide hydrolysis linked 5-HT2 receptors in fibroblasts from choroid plexus. *Brain Res, 552*(2), 330–332.

Barrett, F. S., Preller, K. H., Herdener, M., Janata, P., & Vollenweider, F. X. (2018). Serotonin 2A receptor signaling underlies LSD-induced alteration of the neural response to dynamic changes in music. *Cereb Cortex, 28*(11), 3939–3950.

Beique, J. C., Imad, M., Mladenovic, L., Gingrich, J. A., & Andrade, R. (2007). Mechanism of the 5-hydroxytryptamine 2A receptor-mediated facilitation of synaptic activity in prefrontal cortex. *Proc Natl Acad Sci USA, 104*(23), 9870–9875.

Benneyworth, M. A., Smith, R. L., Barrett, R. J., & Sanders-Bush, E. (2005). Complex discriminative stimulus properties of (+)lysergic acid diethylamide (LSD) in C57Bl/6J mice. *Psychopharmacology (Berl), 179*(4), 854–862.

Berendsen, H. H., & Broekkamp, C. L. (1990). Behavioural evidence for functional interactions between 5-HT-receptor subtypes in rats and mice. *Brit J Pharmacol, 101*(3), 667–673.

Bogenschutz, M. P., Forcehimes, A. A., Pommy, J. A., Wilcox, C. E., Barbosa, P. C., & Strassman, R. J. (2015). Psilocybin-assisted treatment for alcohol dependence: A proof-of-concept study. *J Psychopharmacol, 29*(3), 289–299.

Bowen, W. D., Vilner, B. J., Williams, W., Bertha, C. M., Kuehne, M. E., & Jacobson, A. E. (1995). Ibogaine and its congeners are sigma 2 receptor-selective ligands with moderate affinity. *European Journal of Pharmacology, 279*(1), R1–R3.

Braden, M. R., & Nichols, D. E. (2007). Assessment of the roles of serines 5.43(239) and 5.46(242) for binding and potency of agonist ligands at the human serotonin 5-HT2A receptor. *Mol Pharmacol, 72*(5), 1200–1209.

Braden, M. R., Parrish, J. C., Naylor, J. C., & Nichols, D. E. (2006). Molecular interaction of serotonin 5-HT2A receptor residues Phe339(6.51) and Phe340(6.52) with superpotent N-benzyl phenethylamine agonists. *Mol Pharmacol, 70*(6), 1956–1964.

Brandt, S. D., Kavanagh, P. V., Twamley, B., Westphal, F., Elliott, S. P., Wallach, J., et al. (2018). Return of the lysergamides: Part IV. Analytical and pharmacological characterization of lysergic acid morpholide (LSM-775). *Drug Test Anal, 10*(2), 310–322.

Brimblecombe, R. W. (1963). Effects of psychotropic drugs on open-field behaviour in rats. *Psychopharmacologia, 4*, 139–147.

Burris, K. D., Breeding, M., & Sanders-Bush, E. (1991). (+)Lysergic acid diethylamide, but not its nonhallucinogenic congeners, is a potent serotonin 5HT1C receptor agonist. *J Pharmacol Exp Ther, 258*(3), 891–896.

Canal, C. E., & Morgan, D. (2012). Head-twitch response in rodents induced by the hallucinogen 2,5-dimethoxy-4-iodoamphetamine: A comprehensive history, a re-evaluation of mechanisms, and its utility as a model. *Drug Test Anal, 4*(7–8), 556–576.

Carhart-Harris, R. L., Erritzoe, D., Williams, T., Stone, J. M., Reed, L. J., Colasanti, A., et al. (2012). Neural correlates of the psychedelic state as determined by fMRI studies with psilocybin. *Proc Natl Acad Sci USA, 109*(6), 2138–2143.

Carhart-Harris, R. L., Leech, R., Hellyer, P. J., Shanahan, M., Feilding, A., Tagliazucchi, E., et al. (2014). The entropic brain: A theory of conscious states informed by neuroimaging research with psychedelic drugs. *Front Hum Neurosci, 8*, 20.

Carhart-Harris, R. L., Muthukumaraswamy, S., Roseman, L., Kaelen, M., Droog, W., Murphy, K., et al. (2016). Neural correlates of the LSD experience revealed by multimodal neuroimaging. *Proc Natl Acad Sci USA, 113*(17), 4853–4858.

Carter, O. L., Hasler, F., Pettigrew, J. D., Wallis, G. M., Liu, G. B., & Vollenweider, F. X. (2007). Psilocybin links binocular rivalry switch rate to attention and subjective arousal levels in humans. *Psychopharmacology (Berl), 195*(3), 415–424.

Cohen, M., & Wakeley, H. (1968). A comparative behavioral study of ditran and LSD in mice, rats, and dogs. *Arch Int Pharmacodyn Ther, 173*(2), 316–326.

Colpaert, F. C. (1984). Cross generalization with LSD and yohimbine in the rat. *Eur J Pharmacol, 102*(3–4), 541–544.

Colpaert, F. C., & Janssen, P. A. (1983). A characterization of LSD-antagonist effects of pirenperone in the rat. *Neuropharmacology, 22*(8), 1001–1005.

Colpaert, F. C., Niemegeers, C. J., & Janssen, P. A. (1982). A drug discrimination analysis of lysergic acid diethylamide (LSD): *In vivo* agonist and antagonist effects of purported 5-hydroxytryptamine antagonists and of pirenperone, a LSD-antagonist. *J Pharmacol Exp Ther, 221*(1), 206–214.

Corne, S. J., & Pickering, R. W. (1967). A possible correlation between drug-induced hallucinations in man and a behavioural response in mice. *Psychopharmacologia, 11*(1), 65–78.

Darmani, N. A., Martin, B. R., Pandey, U., & Glennon, R. A. (1990). Do functional relationships exist between 5-HT1A and 5-HT2 receptors? *Pharmacol Biochem Behav, 36*(4), 901–906.

Deecher, D. C., Teitler, M., Soderlund, D. M., Bornmann, W. G., Kuehne, M. E., & Glick, S. D. (1992). Mechanisms of action of ibogaine and harmaline congeners based on radioligand binding studies. *Brain Res, 571*(2), 242–247.

DeMontigny, C., & Aghajanian, G. K. (1977). Preferential action of 5-methoxytryptamine and 5-methoxydimethyltryptamine on presynaptic serotonin receptors: A comparative iontophoretic study with LSD and serotonin. *Neuropharmacology, 16*, 811–818.

Dittrich, A. (1998). The standardized psychometric assessment of altered states of consciousness (ASCs) in humans. *Pharmacopsychiatry, 31*(Suppl. 2), 80–84.

Du, W., Aloyo, V. J., & Harvey, J. A. (1997). Harmaline competitively inhibits [3H]MK-801 binding to the NMDA receptor in rabbit brain. *Brain Res, 770*(1–2), 26–29.

Egozcue, J., Irwin, S., & Maruffo, C. A. (1968). Chromosomal damage in LDsers. *JAMA, 204*(3), 214–218.

Eison, A. S., & Wright, R. N. (1992). 5-HT1A and 5-HT2 receptors mediate discrete behaviors in the Mongolian gerbil. *Pharmacol Biochem Behav, 43*(1), 131–137.

Fiorella, D., Rabin, R. A., & Winter, J. C. (1995). The role of the 5-HT2A and 5-HT2C receptors in the stimulus effects of hallucinogenic drugs: I. Antagonist correlation analysis. *Psychopharmacology (Berl), 121*(3), 347–356.

Frankel, P. S., & Cunningham, K. A. (2002). The hallucinogen d-lysergic acid diethylamide (d-LSD) induces the immediate-early gene c-Fos in rat forebrain. *Brain Res, 958*(2), 251–260.

Freedman, D. X. (1961). Effects of LSD-25 on brain serotonin. *J Pharmacol Exp Ther, 134,* 160–166.

Freedman, D. X., Aghajanian, G. K., Ornitz, E. M., & Rosner, B. S. (1958). Patterns of tolerance to lysergic acid diethylamide and mescaline in rats. *Science, 127,* 1173–1174.

Geyer, M. A., Russo, P. V., & Masten, V. L. (1986). Multivariate assessment of locomotor behavior: Pharmacological and behavioral analyses. *Pharmacol Biochem Behav, 25*(1), 277–288.

Glennon, R. A. (1990). Do classical hallucinogens act as 5-HT2 agonists or antagonists? *Neuropsychopharmacology, 3*(5–6), 509–517.

Glennon, R. A., Rosecrans, J. A., & Young, R. (1982). The use of the drug discrimination paradigm for studying hallucinogenic agents: A review. In F. C. Colpaert & J. L. Slangen (Eds.), *Drug discrimination: Applications in CNS pharmacology* (pp. 69–96). Amsterdam: Elsevier Biomedical Press.

Glennon, R. A., Rosecrans, J. A., & Young, R. (1983). Drug-induced discrimination: A description of the paradigm and a review of its specific application to the study of hallucinogenic agents. *Med Res Rev, 3*(3), 289–340.

Glennon, R. A., Titeler, M., & McKenney, J. D. (1984). Evidence for 5-HT2 involvement in the mechanism of action of hallucinogenic agents. *Life Sci, 35*(25), 2505–2511.

Glennon, R. A., Young, R., Jacyno, J. M., Slusher, M., & Rosecrans, J. A. (1983). DOM-stimulus generalization to LSD and other hallucinogenic indolealkylamines. *Eur J Pharmacol, 86*(3–4), 453–459.

Glennon, R. A., Young, R., & Rosecrans, J. A. (1983). Antagonism of the effects of the hallucinogen DOM and the purported 5-HT agonist quipazine by 5-HT2 antagonists. *Eur J Pharmacol, 91*(2–3), 189–196.

Gonzalez-Maeso, J., Weisstaub, N. V., Zhou, M., Chan, P., Ivic, L., Ang, R., et al. (2007). Hallucinogens recruit specific cortical 5-HT(2A) receptor-mediated signaling pathways to affect behavior. *Neuron, 53*(3), 439–452.

Gonzalez-Maeso, J., Yuen, T., Ebersole, B. J., Wurmbach, E., Lira, A., Zhou, M., et al.

(2003). Transcriptome fingerprints distinguish hallucinogenic and nonhallucinogenic 5-hydroxytryptamine 2A receptor agonist effects in mouse somatosensory cortex. *J Neurosci, 23*(26), 8836–8843.

Gouzoulis-Mayfrank, E., Heekeren, K., Neukirch, A., Stoll, M., Stock, C., Obradovic, M., et al. (2005). Psychological effects of (S)-ketamine and *N,N*-dimethyltryptamine (DMT): A double-blind, cross-over study in healthy volunteers. *Pharmacopsychiatry, 38*(6), 301–311.

Gouzoulis-Mayfrank, E., Thelen, B., Habermeyer, E., Kunert, H. J., Kovar, K. A., Lindenblatt, H., et al. (1999). Psychopathological, neuroendocrine and autonomic effects of 3,4-methylenedioxyethylamphetamine (MDE), psilocybin and d-methamphetamine in healthy volunteers: Results of an experimental double-blind placebo-controlled study. *Psychopharmacology (Berl), 142*(1), 41–50.

Gresch, P. J., Strickland, L. V., & Sanders-Bush, E. (2002). Lysergic acid diethylamide-induced Fos expression in rat brain: Role of serotonin-2A receptors. *Neuroscience, 114*(3), 707–713.

Griffiths, R. R., Johnson, M. W., Carducci, M. A., Umbricht, A., Richards, W. A., Richards, B. D., et al. (2016). Psilocybin produces substantial and sustained decreases in depression and anxiety in patients with life-threatening cancer: A randomized double-blind trial. *J Psychopharmacol, 30*(12), 1181–1197.

Griffiths, R. R., Johnson, M. W., Richards, W. A., Richards, B. D., Jesse, R., MacLean, K. A., et al. (2018). Psilocybin-occasioned mystical-type experience in combination with meditation and other spiritual practices produces enduring positive changes in psychological functioning and in trait measures of prosocial attitudes and behaviors. *J Psychopharmacol, 32*(1), 49–69.

Griffiths, R. R., Johnson, M. W., Richards, W. A., Richards, B. D., McCann, U., & Jesse, R. (2011). Psilocybin occasioned mystical-type experiences: Immediate and persisting dose-related effects. *Psychopharmacology (Berl), 218*(4), 649–665.

Griffiths, R., Richards, W., Johnson, M., McCann, U., & Jesse, R. (2008). Mystical-type experiences occasioned by psilocybin mediate the attribution of personal meaning and spiritual significance 14 months later. *J Psychopharmacol, 22*(6), 621–632.

Griffiths, R. R., Richards, W. A., McCann, U., & Jesse, R. (2006). Psilocybin can occasion mystical-type experiences having substantial and sustained personal meaning and spiritual significance. *Psychopharmacology (Berl), 187*(3), 268–283; discussion 284–292.

Grob, C. S., Danforth, A. L., Chopra, G. S., Hagerty, M., McKay, C. R., Halberstadt, A. L., et al. (2011). Pilot study of psilocybin treatment for anxiety in patients with advanced-stage cancer. *Arch Gen Psychiatry, 68*(1), 71–78.

Haigler, H. J., & Aghajanian, G. K. (1973). Mescaline and LSD: Direct and indirect effects on serotonin-containing neurons in brain. *Eur J Pharmacol, 21*(1), 53–60.

Haigler, H. J., & Aghajanian, G. K. (1974). Lysergic acid diethylamide and serotonin: A comparison of effects on serotonergic neurons and neurons receiving a serotonergic input. *J Pharmacol Exp Ther, 188*(3), 688–699.

Halberstadt, A. L. (2015). Recent advances in the neuropsychopharmacology of serotonergic hallucinogens. *Behav Brain Res, 277*, 99–120.

Halberstadt, A. L., Koedood, L., Powell, S. B., & Geyer, M. A. (2011). Differential contributions of serotonin receptors to the behavioral effects of indoleamine hallucinogens in mice. *J Psychopharmacol, 25*(11), 1548–1561.

Halberstadt, A. L., Sindhunata, I. S., Scheffers, K., Flynn, A. D., Sharp, R. F., Geyer, M. A., et al. (2016). Effect of 5-HT$_{2A}$ and 5-HT$_{2C}$ receptors on temporal discrimination by mice. *Neuropharmacology, 107*, 364–375.

Hanks, J. B., & Gonzalez-Maeso, J. (2013). Animal models of serotonergic psychedelics. *ACS Chem Neurosci, 4*(1), 33–42.

Hansen, M., Phonekeo, K., Paine, J. S., Leth-Petersen, S., Begtrup, M., Brauner-Osborne, H., et al. (2014). Synthesis and structure-activity relationships of *N*-benzyl phenethylamines as 5-HT2A/2C agonists. *ACS Chem Neurosci, 5*(3), 243–249.

Hasler, F., Grimberg, U., Benz, M. A., Huber, T., & Vollenweider, F. X. (2004). Acute psychological and physiological effects of psilocybin in healthy humans: A double-blind, placebo-controlled dose–effect study. *Psychopharmacology (Berl), 172*(2), 145–156.

Hayashi, T., Sumi, D., Matsui-Hirai, H., Fukatsu, A., Arockia Rani, P. J., Kano, H., et al. (2003). Sarpogrelate HCl, a selective 5-HT2A antagonist, retards the progression of atherosclerosis through a novel mechanism. *Atherosclerosis, 168*(1), 23–31.

Heffter, A. (1898). Ueber pellote: Beitrag zur chemischen und pharmakologischen kenntnis der cacteen [About peyote: Contribution to the chemical and pharmacological knowledge of the cacti]. *Naunyn Schmiedeberg's Arch Exp Path Pharmacol, 40*, 385–429.

Heim, R. (2003). *Synthese und Pharmakologie potenter 5-HT2A-Rezeptoragonisten mit N-2-Methoxybenzyl-Partialstruktur: Entwicklung eines neuen Struktur-Wirkungskonzepts* [Synthesis and pharmacology of potent 5-HT2A receptor agonists with N-2-methoxybenzyl partial structure: Development of a new structure-effect concept]. Unpublished doctoral thesis, Freien Universität, Berlin, Germany.

Heim, R., & Elz, S. (2000). Novel extremely potent partial 5-HT2A receptor agonists: Successful application of a new structure–activity concept. *Arch Pharm Pharm Med Chem, 333*, 39.

Heim, R., Pertz, H. H., & Elz, S. (1999). Preparation and in vitro pharmacology of novel secondary amine-type 5-HT2A receptor agonists: From submillimolar to subnanomolar activity. *Arch Pharm Pharm Med Chem, 332*, 34.

Hermle, L., Funfgeld, M., Oepen, G., Botsch, H., Borchardt, D., Gouzoulis, E., et al. (1992). Mescaline-induced psychopathological, neuropsychological, and neurometabolic effects in normal subjects: Experimental psychosis as a tool for psychiatric research. *Biol Psychiatry, 32*(11), 976–991.

Hirschhorn, I. D., & Winter, J. C. (1971). Mescaline and lysergic acid diethylamide (LSD) as discriminative stimuli. *Psychopharmacologia, 22*(1), 64–71.

Hofmann, A. (1979). How LSD originated. *J Psychedelic Drugs, 11*(1–2), 53–60.

Hofmann, A., Frey, A., Ott, H., Petrzilka, T., & Troxler, F. (1958). [Elucidation of the structure and the synthesis of psilocybin]. *Experientia, 14*(11), 397–399.

Hofmann, A., Heim, R., Brack, A., & Kobel, H. (1958). [Psilocybin, a psychotropic substance from the Mexican mushroom Psilicybe mexicana Heim]. *Experientia, 14*(3), 107–109.

Hofmann, A., & Tscherter, H. (1960). [Isolation of lysergic acid alkaloids from the Mexican drug ololiuqui (Rivea corymbosa [L.] Hall.f.)]. *Experientia, 16*, 414.

Husbands, S. M., Glennon, R. A., Gorgerat, S., Gough, R., Tyacke, R., Crosby, J., et al. (2001). Beta-carboline binding to imidazoline receptors. *Drug Alcohol Depend, 64*(2), 203–208.

Isbell, H., & Logan, C. R. (1957). Studies on the diethylamide of lysergic acid (LSD-25): II. Effects of chlorpromazine, azacyclonol, and reserpine on the intensity of the LSD-reaction. *AMA Arch Neurol Psychiatry, 77*(4), 350–358.

Isbell, H., Logan, C. R., & Miner, E. J. (1959). Studies on lysergic acid diethylamide (LSD-25): III. Attempts to attenuate the LSD-reaction in man by pretreatment with neurohumoral blocking agents. *AMA Arch Neurol Psychiatry, 81*(1), 20–27.

Isbell, H., Wolbach, A. E., Wikler, A., & Miner, E. J. (1961). Cross tolerance between LSD and psilocybin. *Psychopharmacologia (Berl), 2,* 147–159.

Janata, P. (2005). Brain networks that track musical structure. *Ann NY Acad Sci, 1060,* 111–124.

Janata, P., Birk, J. L., Van Horn, J. D., Leman, M., Tillmann, B., & Bharucha, J. J. (2002). The cortical topography of tonal structures underlying Western music. *Science, 298,* 2167–2170.

Johnson, M. W., Garcia-Romeu, A., Cosimano, M. P., & Griffiths, R. R. (2014). Pilot study of the 5-HT2AR agonist psilocybin in the treatment of tobacco addiction. *J Psychopharmacol, 28*(11), 983–992.

Johnson, M. W., Garcia-Romeu, A., & Griffiths, R. R. (2017). Long-term follow-up of psilocybin-facilitated smoking cessation. *Am J Drug Alcohol Abuse, 43*(1), 55–60.

Kabes, J., Fink, Z., & Roth, Z. (1972). A new device for measuring spontaneous motor activity—effects of lysergic acid diethylamide in rats. *Psychopharmacologia, 23*(1), 75–85.

Klock, J. C., Boerner, U., & Becker, C. E. (1975). Coma, hyperthermia, and bleeding associated with massive LSD overdose: A report of eight cases. *Clin Toxicol, 8*(2), 191–203.

Kobilka, B. K., Frielle, T., Collins, S., Yang-Feng, T., Kobilka, T. S., Francke, U., et al. (1987). An intronless gene encoding a potential member of the family of receptors coupled to guanine nucleotide regulatory proteins. *Nature, 329,* 75–79.

Kometer, M., Schmidt, A., Jancke, L., & Vollenweider, F. X. (2013). Activation of serotonin 2A receptors underlies the psilocybin-induced effects on alpha oscillations, N170 visual-evoked potentials, and visual hallucinations. *J Neurosci, 33*(25), 10544–10551.

Kometer, M., & Vollenweider, F. X. (2018). Serotonergic hallucinogen-induced visual perceptual alterations. *Curr Top Behav Neurosci, 36,* 257–282.

Kraehenmann, R., Pokorny, D., Aicher, H., Preller, K. H., Pokorny, T., Bosch, O. G., et al. (2017). LSD increases primary process thinking via serotonin 2A receptor activation. *Front Pharmacol, 8,* 814.

Kraehenmann, R., Pokorny, D., Vollenweider, L., Preller, K. H., Pokorny, T., Seifritz, E., et al. (2017). Dreamlike effects of LSD on waking imagery in humans depend on serotonin 2A receptor activation. *Psychopharmacology (Berl), 234,* 2031–2046.

Krebs-Thomson, K., Paulus, M. P., & Geyer, M. A. (1998). Effects of hallucinogens on locomotor and investigatory activity and patterns: Influence of 5-HT2A and 5-HT2C receptors. *Neuropsychopharmacology, 18*(5), 339–351.

Krebs-Thomson, K., Ruiz, E. M., Masten, V., Buell, M., & Geyer, M. A. (2006). The roles of 5-HT1A and 5-HT2 receptors in the effects of 5-MeO-DMT on locomotor activity and prepulse inhibition in rats. *Psychopharmacology (Berl), 189*(3), 319–329.

Krumhansl, C. L. (1990). *Cognitive foundations of musical pitch.* New York: Oxford University Press.

Krumhansl, C. L., & Kessler, E. J. (1982). Tracing the dynamic changes in perceived tonal organization in a spatial representation of musical keys. *Psychol Rev, 89*(4), 334–368.

Leysen, J. E., Niemegeers, C. J., Van Nueten, J. M., & Laduron, P. M. (1982). [3H]Ketanserin (R 41 468), a selective 3H-ligand for serotonin2 receptor binding sites: Binding properties, brain distribution, and functional role. *Mol Pharmacol, 21*(2), 301–314.

Li, J. X., Rice, K. C., & France, C. P. (2008). Discriminative stimulus effects of 1-(2,5-dimethoxy-4-methylphenyl)-2-aminopropane in rhesus monkeys. *J Pharmacol Exp Ther, 324*(2), 827–833.

Liechti, M. E., Dolder, P. C., & Schmid, Y. (2017). Alterations of consciousness and mystical-type experiences after acute LSD in humans. *Psychopharmacology (Berl), 234*(9–10), 1499–1510.

Long, S. Y. (1972). Does LSD induce chromosomal damage and malformations?: A review of the literature. *Teratology, 6*(1), 75–90.

MacLean, K. A., Johnson, M. W., & Griffiths, R. R. (2011). Mystical experiences occasioned by the hallucinogen psilocybin lead to increases in the personality domain of openness. *J Psychopharmacol, 25*(11), 1453–1461.

Marona-Lewicka, D., & Nichols, D. E. (1995). Complex stimulus properties of LSD: A drug discrimination study with alpha 2-adrenoceptor agonists and antagonists. *Psychopharmacology (Berl), 120*(4), 384–391.

Marona-Lewicka, D., Nichols, C. D., & Nichols, D. E. (2011). An animal model of schizophrenia based on chronic LSD administration: Old idea, new results. *Neuropharmacology, 61*(3), 503–512.

Martin, D. A., Marona-Lewicka, D., Nichols, D. E., & Nichols, C. D. (2014). Chronic LSD alters gene expression profiles in the mPFC relevant to schizophrenia. *Neuropharmacology, 83,* 1–8.

Martin, D. A., & Nichols, C. D. (2016). Psychedelics recruit multiple cellular types and produce complex transcriptional responses within the brain. *EBioMedicine, 11,* 262–277.

Martin, D., Xu, J., Porretta, C., & Nichols, C. D. (2017). Neurocytometry: Flow cytometric sorting of specific neuronal populations from human and rodent brain. *ACS Chem Neurosci, 8*(2), 356–367.

McKenna, D. J., Towers, G. H., & Abbott, F. (1984). Monoamine oxidase inhibitors in South American hallucinogenic plants: Tryptamine and beta-carboline constituents of ayahuasca. *J Ethnopharmacol, 10*(2), 195–223.

Mittman, S. M., & Geyer, M. A. (1991). Dissociation of multiple effects of acute LSD on exploratory behavior in rats by ritanserin and propranolol. *Psychopharmacology (Berl), 105*(1), 69–76.

Moreno, F. A., Wiegand, C. B., Taitano, E. K., & Delgado, P. L. (2006). Safety, tolerability, and efficacy of psilocybin in 9 patients with obsessive–compulsive disorder. *J Clin Psychiatry, 67*(11), 1735–1740.

Morini, L., Bernini, M., Vezzoli, S., Restori, M., Moretti, M., Crenna, S., et al. (2017). Death after 25C-NBOMe and 25H-NBOMe consumption. *Forensic Sci Int, 279*, e1–e6.

Muthukumaraswamy, S. D., Carhart-Harris, R. L., Moran, R. J., Brookes, M. J., Williams, T. M., Errtizoe, D., et al. (2013). Broadband cortical desynchronization underlies the human psychedelic state. *J Neurosci, 33*(38), 15171–15183.

Nau, F., Jr., Miller, J., Saravia, J., Ahlert, T., Yu, B., Happel, K. I., et al. (2015). Serotonin 5-HT(2) receptor activation prevents allergic asthma in a mouse model. *Am J Physiol Lung Cell Mol Physiol, 308*(2), L191–L198.

Nau, F., Jr., Yu, B., Martin, D., & Nichols, C. D. (2013). Serotonin 5-HT2A receptor activation blocks TNF-alpha mediated inflammation *in vivo. PLOS ONE, 8*(10), e75426.

Nelson, D. L., Lucaites, V. L., Wainscott, D. B., & Glennon, R. A. (1999). Comparisons of hallucinogenic phenylisopropylamine binding affinities at cloned human 5-HT2A, -HT(2B) and 5-HT2C receptors. *Naunyn Schmiedeberg's Arch Pharmacol, 359*(1), 1–6.

Nichols, C. D., & Sanders-Bush, E. (2002). A single dose of lysergic acid diethylamide influences gene expression patterns within the mammalian brain. *Neuropsychopharmacology, 26*(5), 634–642.

Nichols, C. D., & Sanders-Bush, E. (2004). Molecular genetic responses to lysergic acid diethylamide include transcriptional activation of MAP kinase phosphatase-1, C/EBP-beta and ILAD-1, a novel gene with homology to arrestins. *J Neurochem, 90*(3), 576–584.

Nichols, D. E. (1986). Differences between the mechanism of action of MDMA, MBDB, and the classic hallucinogens Identification of a new therapeutic class: Entactogens. *J Psychoactive Drugs, 18*(4), 305–313.

Nichols, D. E. (2004). Hallucinogens. *Pharmacol Ther, 101*(2), 131–181.

Nichols, D. E. (2016). Psychedelics. *Pharmacol Rev, 68*(2), 264–355.

Nichols, D. E., & Grob, C. S. (2018). Is LSD toxic? *Forensic Sci Int, 284*, 141–145.

Nichols, D. E., Hoffman, A. J., Oberlender, R. A., Jacob, P., III, & Shulgin, A. T. (1986). Derivatives of 1-(1,3-benzodioxol-5-yl)-2-butanamine: Representatives of a novel therapeutic class. *J Med Chem, 29*(10), 2009–2015.

Nichols, D. E., Johnson, M. W., & Nichols, C. D. (2017). Psychedelics as medicines: An emerging new paradigm. *Clin Pharmacol Ther, 101*(2), 209–219.

Nichols, D. E., & Nichols, C. D. (2008). Serotonin receptors. *Chem Rev, 108*(5), 1614–1641.

Nishiyama, T. (2009). Acute effects of sarpogrelate, a 5-HT2A receptor antagonist on cytokine production in endotoxin shock model of rats. *Eur J Pharmacol, 614*(1–3), 122–127.

Ouagazzal, A., Grottick, A. J., Moreau, J., & Higgins, G. A. (2001). Effect of LSD on prepulse inhibition and spontaneous behavior in the rat: A pharmacological analysis and comparison between two rat strains. *Neuropsychopharmacology, 25*(4), 565–575.

Pahnke, W. N. (1969). Psychedelic drugs and mystical experience. *Int Psychiatry Clin, 5*(4), 149–162.

Pahnke, W. N., & Richards, W. A. (1966). Implications of LSD and experimental mysticism. *J Relig Health, 5*(3), 175–208.

Papaseit, E., Farre, M., Perez-Mana, C., Torrens, M., Ventura, M., Pujadas, M., et al. (2018). Acute pharmacological effects of 2C-B in humans: An observational study. *Front Pharmacol, 9*, 206.

Passie, T., Halpern, J. H., Stichtenoth, D. O., Emrich, H. M., & Hintzen, A. (2008). The pharmacology of lysergic acid diethylamide: A review. *CNS Neurosci Ther, 14*, 295–314.

Passie, T., Seifert, J., Schneider, U., & Emrich, H. M. (2002). The pharmacology of psilocybin. *Addict Biol, 7*(4), 357–364.

Pei, Q., Lewis, L., Sprakes, M. E., Jones, E. J., Grahame-Smith, D. G., & Zetterstrom, T. S. (2000). Serotonergic regulation of mRNA expression of Arc, an immediate early gene selectively localized at neuronal dendrites. *Neuropharmacology, 39*(3), 463–470.

Pei, Q., Tordera, R., Sprakes, M., & Sharp, T. (2004). Glutamate receptor activation is involved in 5-HT2 agonist-induced Arc gene expression in the rat cortex. *Neuropharmacology, 46*(3), 331–339.

Penington, N. J., & Reiffenstein, R. J. (1986). Direct comparison of hallucinogenic phenethylamines and D-amphetamine on dorsal raphe neurons. *Eur J Pharmacol, 122*(3), 373–377.

Pierce, P. A., & Peroutka, S. J. (1989). Hallucinogenic drug interactions with neurotransmitter receptor binding sites in human cortex. *Psychopharmacology (Berl), 97*(1), 118–122.

Poklis, J. L., Devers, K. G., Arbefeville, E. F., Pearson, J. M., Houston, E., & Poklis, A. (2014). Postmortem detection of 25I-NBOMe [2-(4-iodo-2,5-dimethoxyphenyl)-*N*-[(2-methoxyphenyl)methylethanamine] in fluids and tissues determined by high performance liquid chromatography with tandem mass spectrometry from a traumatic death. *Forensic Sci Int, 234*, e14–e20.

Pokorny, T., Preller, K. H., Kraehenmann, R., & Vollenweider, F. X. (2016). Modulatory effect of the 5-HT1A agonist buspirone and the mixed non-hallucinogenic 5-HT1A/2A agonist ergotamine on psilocybin-induced psychedelic experience. *Eur Neuropsychopharmacol, 26*(4), 756–766.

Porter, R. H., Benwell, K. R., Lamb, H., Malcolm, C. S., Allen, N. H., Revell, D. F., et al. (1999). Functional characterization of agonists at recombinant human 5-HT2A, 5-HT2B and 5-HT2C receptors in CHO-K1 cells. *Brit J Pharmacol, 128*(1), 13–20.

Preller, K. H., Herdener, M., Pokorny, T., Planzer, A., Kraehenmann, R., Stampfli, P., et al. (2017). The fabric of meaning and subjective effects in LSD-induced states depend on serotonin 2A receptor activation. *Curr Biol, 27*(3), 451–457.

Preller, K. H., Schilbach, L., Pokorny, T., Flemming, J., Seifritz, E., & Vollenweider, F. X. (2018). Role of the 5-HT2A receptor in self- and other-initiated social interaction in lysergic acid diethylamide-induced states: A pharmacological fMRI study. *J Neurosci, 38*(14), 3603–3611.

Puig, M. V., Artigas, F., & Celada, P. (2005). Modulation of the activity of pyramidal neurons in rat prefrontal cortex by raphe stimulation *in vivo*: Involvement of serotonin and GABA. *Cereb Cortex, 15*(1), 1–14.

Quednow, B. B., Kometer, M., Geyer, M. A., & Vollenweider, F. X. (2012). Psilocybin-induced deficits in automatic and controlled inhibition are attenuated by ketanserin in healthy human volunteers. *Neuropsychopharmacology, 37*(3), 630–640.

Reser, D. H., Richardson, K. E., Montibeller, M. D. O., Zhao, S., Chan, J. M. H., Soares, J. G. M., et al. (2014). Claustrum projections to prefrontal cortex in the capuchin monkey, Cebus apella. *Front Syst Neurosci, 8*, 123.

Riba, J., Anderer, P., Jane, F., Saletu, B., & Barbanoj, M. J. (2004). Effects of the South American psychoactive beverage ayahuasca on regional brain electrical activity in humans: A functional neuroimaging study using low-resolution electromagnetic tomography. *Neuropsychobiology, 50*(1), 89–101.

Riba, J., Rodriguez-Fornells, A., & Barbanoj, M. J. (2002). Effects of ayahuasca on sensory and sensorimotor gating in humans as measured by P50 suppression and prepulse inhibition of the startle reflex, respectively. *Psychopharmacology (Berl), 165*(1), 18–28.

Riba, J., Rodriguez-Fornells, A., Strassman, R. J., & Barbanoj, M. J. (2001). Psychometric assessment of the Hallucinogen Rating Scale. *Drug Alcohol Depend, 62*(3), 215–223.

Riba, J., Valle, M., Urbano, G., Yritia, M., Morte, A., & Barbanoj, M. J. (2003). Human pharmacology of ayahuasca: Subjective and cardiovascular effects, monoamine metabolite excretion, and pharmacokinetics. *J Pharmacol Exp Ther, 306*(1), 73–83.

Rickli, A., Luethi, D., Reinisch, J., Buchy, D., Hoener, M. C., & Liechti, M. E. (2015). Receptor interaction profiles of novel *N*-2-methoxybenzyl (NBOMe) derivatives of 2,5-dimethoxy-substituted phenethylamines (2C drugs). *Neuropharmacology, 99*, 546–553.

Rosecrans, J. A., Lovell, R. A., & Freedman, D. X. (1967). Effects of lysergic acid diethylamide on the metabolism of brain 5-hydroxytryptamine. *Biochem Pharmacol, 16*(10), 2011–2021.

Ross, S., Bossis, A., Guss, J., Agin-Liebes, G., Malone, T., Cohen, B., et al. (2016). Rapid and sustained symptom reduction following psilocybin treatment for anxiety and depression in patients with life-threatening cancer: A randomized controlled trial. *J Psychopharmacol, 30*(12), 1165–1180.

Schenberg, E. E., Alexandre, J. F., Filev, R., Cravo, A. M., Sato, J. R., Muthukumaraswamy, S. D., et al. (2015). Acute biphasic effects of ayahuasca. *PLOS ONE, 10*(9), e0137202.

Schmid, Y., & Liechti, M. E. (2018). Long-lasting subjective effects of LSD in normal subjects. *Psychopharmacology (Berl), 235*(2), 535–545.

Schreiber, R., Brocco, M., Audinot, V., Gobert, A., Veiga, S., & Millan, M. J. (1995). (1-(2,5-dimethoxy-4 iodophenyl)-2-aminopropane)-induced head-twitches in the rat are mediated by 5-hydroxytryptamine (5-HT) 2A receptors: Modulation by novel 5-HT2A/2C antagonists, D1 antagonists and 5-HT1A agonists. *J Pharmacol Exp Ther, 273*(1), 101–112.

Schreiber, R., Brocco, M., & Millan, M. J. (1994). Blockade of the discriminative stimulus effects of DOI by MDL 100,907 and the "atypical" antipsychotics, clozapine and risperidone. *Eur J Pharmacol, 264*(1), 99–102.

Schreiber, R., & de Vry, J. (1993). Studies on the neuronal circuits involved in the discriminative stimulus effects of 5-hydroxytrypta-mine1A receptor agonists in the rat. *J Pharmacol Exp Ther, 265*(2), 572–579.

Schultes, R. E., & Hofmann, A. (1980). *The botany and chemistry of hallucinogens.* Springfield, IL: Charles C Thomas.

Scruggs, J. L., Patel, S., Bubser, M., & Deutch, A. Y. (2000). DOI-induced activation of the cortex: Dependence on 5-HT2A heteroceptors on thalamocortical glutamatergic neurons. *J Neurosci, 20*(23), 8846–8852.

Seeley, W. W., Menon, V., Schatzberg, A. F., Keller, J., Glover, G. H., Kenna, H., et al. (2007). Dissociable intrinsic connectivity networks for salience processing and executive control. *J Neurosci, 27*(9), 2349–2356.

Sessa, B. (2017). MDMA and PTSD treatment: "PTSD: From novel pathophysiology to innovative therapeutics." *Neurosci Lett, 649,* 176–180.

Sessa, B. (2018). Why MDMA therapy for alcohol use disorder?: And why now? *Neuropharmacology, 142,* 83–88.

Shajib, M. S., & Khan, W. I. (2015). The role of serotonin and its receptors in activation of immune responses and inflammation. *Acta Physiol (Oxf), 213*(3), 561–574.

Silva, M. T., & Calil, H. M. (1975). Screening hallucinogenic drugs: Systematic study of three behavioral tests. *Psychopharmacologia, 42*(2), 163–171.

Sipes, T. E., & Geyer, M. A. (1995). DOI disruption of prepulse inhibition of startle in the rat is mediated by 5-HT(2A) and not by 5-HT(2C) receptors. *Behav Pharmacol, 6*(8), 839–842.

Smith, R. L., Barrett, R. J., & Sanders-Bush, E. (1999). Mechanism of tolerance development to 2,5-dimethoxy-4-iodoamphetamine in rats: Down-regulation of the 5-HT2A, but not 5-HT2C, receptor. *Psychopharmacology (Berl), 144*(3), 248–254.

Smith, R. L., Barrett, R. J., & Sanders-Bush, E. (2003). Discriminative stimulus properties of 1-(2,5-dimethoxy-4-iodophenyl)-2-aminopropane [(±)DOI] in C57BL/6J mice. *Psychopharmacology (Berl), 166*(1), 61–68.

Snir, O., Hesselberg, E., Amoudruz, P., Klareskog, L., Zarea-Ganji, I., Catrina, A. I., et al. (2013). Genetic variation in the serotonin receptor gene affects immune responses in rheumatoid arthritis. *Genes Immun, 14*(2), 83–89.

Späth, E. (1919). Uber die Anhalonium-Alkaloide [About the anhalonium-alkaloids]. *Monatsh Chem, 40,* 129–154.

Spencer, D. G., Jr., Glaser, T., & Traber, J. (1987). Serotonin receptor subtype mediation of the interoceptive discriminative stimuli induced by 5-methoxy-N,N-dimethyltryptamine. *Psychopharmacology (Berl), 93*(2), 158–166.

Strassman, R. J. (1984). Adverse reactions to psychedelic drugs: A review of the literature. *J Nerv Ment Dis, 172*(10), 577–595.

Strassman, R. J. (1996). Human psychopharmacology of N,N-dimethyltryptamine. *Behav Brain Res, 73*(1–2), 121–124.

Strassman, R. (2001). *DMT: The spirit molecule.* Rochester, VT: Park Street Press.

Strassman, R. J., & Qualls, C. R. (1994). Dose–response study of N,N-dimethyltryptamine in humans: I. Neuroendocrine, autonomic, and cardiovascular effects. *Arch Gen Psychiatry, 51*(2), 85–97.

Strassman, R. J., Qualls, C. R., & Berg, L. M. (1996). Differential tolerance to biological and subjective effects of four closely spaced doses of N,N-dimethyltryptamine in humans. *Biol Psychiatry, 39*(9), 784–795.

Strassman, R. J., Qualls, C. R., Uhlenhuth, E. H., & Kellner, R. (1994). Dose–response study of N,N-dimethyltryptamine in humans: II. Subjective effects and preliminary results of a new rating scale. *Arch Gen Psychiatry, 51*(2), 98–108.

Suzuki, J., Poklis, J. L., & Poklis, A. (2014). "My friend said it was good LSD": A suicide attempt following analytically confirmed 25I-NBOMe ingestion. *J Psychoactive Drugs, 46*(5), 379–382.

Swanson, L. R. (2018). Unifying theories of psychedelic drug effects. *Front Pharmacol, 9,* 172.

Szabo, A., Kovacs, A., Frecska, E., & Rajnavolgyi, E. (2014). Psychedelic N,N-dimethyltryptamine and 5-methoxy-N,N-dimethyltryptamine modulate innate and adaptive inflammatory responses through the sigma-1 receptor of human monocyte-derived dendritic cells. *PLOS ONE, 9*(8), e106533.

Szabo, A., Kovacs, A., Riba, J., Djurovic, S., Rajnavolgyi, E., & Frecska, E. (2016). The endogenous hallucinogen and trace amine N,N-dimethyltryptamine (DMT) displays potent protective effects against hypoxia via sigma-1 receptor activation in human primary iPSC-derived cortical neurons and microglia-like immune cells. *Front Neurosci, 10,* 423.

Szara, S. (1957). The comparison of the psychotic effect of tryptamine derivatives with the effects of mescaline and LSD-25 in self-experiments. In S. Garattini & V. Ghetti (Eds.), *Psychotropic drugs* (pp. 460–467). Amsterdam: Elsevier.

Tagliazucchi, E., Roseman, L., Kaelen, M., Orban, C., Muthukumaraswamy, S. D., Murphy, K., et al. (2016). Increased global functional connectivity correlates with LSD-induced ego dissolution. *Curr Biol, 26*(8), 1043–1050.

Tilakaratne, N., & Friedman, E. (1996). Genomic responses to 5-HT1A or 5-HT2A/2C receptor activation is differentially regulated in four regions of rat brain. *Eur J Pharmacol, 307*(2), 211–217.

Titeler, M., Lyon, R. A., & Glennon, R. A. (1988). Radioligand binding evidence implicates the brain 5-HT2 receptor as a site of action for LSD and phenylisopropylamine hallucinogens. *Psychopharmacology (Berl), 94*(2), 213–216.

Toiviainen, P., & Krumhansl, C. L. (2003). Measuring and modeling real-time responses to music: The dynamics of tonality induction. *Perception, 32*(6), 741–766.

Tricklebank, M. D., Forler, C., Middlemiss, D. N., & Fozard, J. R. (1985). Subtypes of the 5-HT receptor mediating the behavioural responses to 5-methoxy-N,N-dimethyltryptamine in the rat. *Eur J Pharmacol, 117*(1), 15–24.

Turner, W. J., & Merlis, S. (1959). Effect of some indolealkylamines on man. *AMA Arch Neurol Psychiatry, 81*(1), 121–129.

Twarog, B. M., & Page, I. H. (1953). Serotonin content of some mammalian tissues and urine and a method for its determination. *Am J Physiol—Legacy, 175*(1), 157–161.

Valle, M., Maqueda, A. E., Rabella, M., Rodriguez-Pujadas, A., Antonijoan, R. M., Romero, S., et al. (2016). Inhibition of alpha oscillations through serotonin-2A receptor activation underlies the visual effects of ayahuasca in humans. *Eur Neuropsychopharmacol, 26*(7), 1161–1175.

Vickers, S. P., Easton, N., Malcolm, C. S., Allen, N. H., Porter, R. H., Bickerdike, M. J., et al. (2001). Modulation of 5-HT(2A) receptor-mediated head-twitch behaviour in the rat by 5-HT(2C) receptor agonists. *Pharmacol Biochem Behav, 69*(3–4), 643–652.

Vollenweider, F. X., Csomor, P. A., Knappe, B., Geyer, M. A., & Quednow, B. B. (2007). The effects of the preferential 5-HT2A agonist psilocybin on prepulse inhibition of startle in healthy human volunteers depend on interstimulus interval. *Neuropsychopharmacology, 32*(9), 1876–1887.

Vollenweider, F. X., Leenders, K. L., Scharfetter, C., Maguire, P., Stadelmann, O., & Angst, J. (1997). Positron emission tomography and fluorodeoxyglucose studies of metabolic hyperfrontality and psychopathology in the psilocybin model of psychosis. *Neuropsychopharmacology, 16*(5), 357–372.

Vollenweider, F. X., Vollenweider-Scherpenhuyzen, M. F., Babler, A., Vogel, H., & Hell, D. (1998). Psilocybin induces schizophrenia-like psychosis in humans via a serotonin-2 agonist action. *NeuroReport, 9*(17), 3897–3902.

Walterscheid, J. P., Phillips, G. T., Lopez, A. E., Gonsoulin, M. L., Chen, H. H., & Sanchez, L. A. (2014). Pathological findings in 2 cases of fatal 25I-NBOMe toxicity. *Am J Forensic Med Pathol, 35*(1), 20–25.

Wettstein, J. G., Host, M., & Hitchcock, J. M. (1999). Selectivity of action of typical and atypical anti-psychotic drugs as antagonists of the behavioral effects of 1-[2,5-dimethoxy-4-iodophenyl]-2-aminopropane (DOI). *Prog Neuropsychopharmacol Biol Psychiatry, 23*(3), 533–544.

Wing, L. L., Tapson, G. S., & Geyer, M. A. (1990). 5HT-2 mediation of acute behavioral effects of hallucinogens in rats. *Psychopharmacology (Berl), 100*(3), 417–425.

Winter, J. C., Eckler, J. R., & Rabin, R. A. (2004). Serotonergic/glutamatergic interactions: The effects of mGlu2/3 receptor ligands in rats trained with LSD and PCP as discriminative stimuli. *Psychopharmacology (Berl), 172*(2), 233–240.

Winter, J. C., Filipink, R. A., Timineri, D., Helsley, S. E., & Rabin, R. A. (2000). The paradox of 5-methoxy-N,N-dimethyltryptamine: An indoleamine hallucinogen that induces stimulus control via 5-HT1A receptors. *Pharmacol Biochem Behav, 65*(1), 75–82.

Winter, J. C., Rice, K. C., Amorosi, D. J., & Rabin, R. A. (2007). Psilocybin-induced stimulus control in the rat. *Pharmacol Biochem Behav, 87*(4), 472–480.

Wood, D. M., Sedefov, R., Cunningham, A., & Dargan, P. I. (2015). Prevalence of use and acute toxicity associated with the use of NBOMe drugs. *Clin Toxicol (Phila), 53*(2), 85–92.

Woolley, D. W., & Shaw, E. (1954). A biochemical and pharmacological suggestion about certain mental disorders. *Proc Natl Acad Sci USA, 40*(4), 228–231.

Yu, B., Becnel, J., Zerfaoui, M., Rohatgi, R., Boulares, A. H., & Nichols, C. D. (2008). Serotonin 5-hydroxytryptamine(2A) receptor activation suppresses tumor necrosis factor-alpha-induced inflammation with extraordinary potency. *J Pharmacol Exp Ther, 327*(2), 316–323.

Zulfiker, A. H., Hashimi, S. M., Qi, J., Grice, I. D., & Wei, M. Q. (2016). Aqueous and ethanol extracts of Australian cane toad skins suppress pro-inflammatory cytokine secretion in U937 cells via NF-kappaB signaling pathway. *J Cell Biochem, 117*(12), 2769–2780.

CHAPTER 2

Plants for the People
The Future of Psychedelic Therapies in the Age of Biomedicine

DENNIS J. McKENNA

■ Introduction

Psilocybin and 3,4 methylenedioxymeth-amphetamine (MDMA) are on the cusp of being approved for clinical use, having nearly completed the three-phase process to gain approval from the U.S. Food and Drug Administration (FDA) for use as prescription drugs. In this chapter I discuss some of the historical and cultural precedents and events that led to the current situation, and examine some of the moral and ethical challenges that must be overcome to ensure that therapy with naturally occurring psychedelics remains accessible to large numbers of people.

■ Historical and Cultural Context

Psychedelic plants and fungi are among the most ancient medicines known to humanity. They have occupied a central position in the religious and cultural lives of indigenous peoples for thousands of years. They are essential components of traditional ethnomedical pharmacopoeias, where they are utilized for the alleviation of both spiritual (mental) illnesses and physical illnesses. In nearly all cultures that use these substances, their use is conducted under the purview of specialists who oversee their applications according to a set of culturally sanctioned beliefs, rituals, and practices. In this chapter I use the term *shaman* or *shamanic practitioners* because it has become accepted nomenclature, but with the caveat that it is not an accurate term except in the context of Siberian shamanism.[1] The cultural role of shamanic practitioners combines the functions of a medical doctor, a psychotherapist, a priest, and (sometimes) a sorcerer or witch. With careful control and induced by psychedelics or other means, such traditional practitioners consult apparently nonhuman intelligences (spirits) that inhabit a plane of existence separate from ordinary, everyday reality, in order to obtain information that may be relevant to the diagnosis of disease, the use of particular plants for the treatment of diseases, or other practices related to the physical and spiritual well-being of their patients and, by extension, to the spiritual health of the community.

Over millennia, indigenous peoples have been the stewards of such traditions, as well as the plants and fungi that form the basis of shamanic practices. There has been considerable overlap and cross-fertilization of strictly indigenous traditions, which has accelerated as a result of globalization, and migrations of populations from jungle or rural areas to urban centers, where the "pure" indigenous traditions have become diluted by fusion with those of other indigenous groups. This has resulted in the emergence of syncretic shamanic traditions that combine ritual elements and beliefs (and often medicines) derived from various indigenous sources. This syncretic shamanic tradition is the kind most commonly encountered by Westerners from outside the culture. Another significant change affecting traditional practices has also been brought about by its accommodation to Western influence, as shamanic practices have attracted interest far beyond their original cultural context. As shamanism has "gone global," along with many of the plants and fungi used in shamanic practice, the already highly syncretic practices have changed in response to economic pressures. Significantly, one of the most important changes has arisen due to the expectations of outside participants in shamanic ceremonies. People travel to places such as South America to attend ceremonies and consume the medicines (often at considerable expense and inconvenience) under the guidance of shamanic practitioners. Formerly, in most ethnomedical traditions, the shamans took the psychedelic medicines as an aid in diagnosis and healing; only rarely were they given to the patients. That has now changed. Outsiders seek out these ceremonies, expecting to take the medicines. Moreover, many seek out shamanic practitioners in the hopes of apprenticing themselves to learn the craft and become shamans themselves. The resulting economic impact on the traditional practices has transformed it into a service industry serving a global clientele, and sometimes practitioners serving this clientele achieve "superstar status." Many who follow this path achieve economic remuneration well beyond that afforded to most other members of their community, and this can understandably elicit envy and resentment from other community members who are excluded from the economic windfalls (although some may benefit in other ways simply as a result of having more foreigners, with fat wallets and consumerist orienta-

tions, pass through their communities). An unfortunate consequence of these inevitable changes triggered by global economic influences is that the community can no longer benefit from the important role of shamanic practitioners, who formerly plied their trade for little or no compensation, usually supporting themselves by other means, such as farming or fishing. *Curanderos* catering to a Western clientele have priced themselves out of affordability for most members of their communities. It could also be argued that there is a growing need, on a global scale, for the type of spiritual healing that shamanism offers, and the commercialization of the shamans' trade is bringing benefits to a wider community that desperately needs it.

In the West, psychedelic plants and fungi have also been used in the context of religion, magic, and sorcery, but there is no historically ancient "shamanic tradition" that has survived in the face of the rise of the culturally dominant patriarchal Abrahamic religions, with their emphasis on salvation in a postulated afterlife, and human dominance over nature, and the consequent devaluation of ecstatic, direct spiritual experience and of nature itself. Practitioners of such shamanic arts were stigmatized in the West as being in league with demonic forces and driven underground. This can be seen in the historical suppression of the pagan, matriarchal traditions exemplified by the Gnostic mystery schools by the politically dominant "official" religion, Christianity (Lash, 2006). Under the aegis of political Christianity during the Inquisition, the same attitudes of cultural and environmental genocide were applied to the earliest encounters between European explorers and the indigenous peoples of the New World. Indigenous peoples were, by definition, not Christian and hence not human, and this attitude justified the brutal suppression of indigenous shamanic traditions and their practitioners, as well as anyone else who refused to acknowledge, and accede to, the superiority of Christianity over any indigenous, native spirituality. In both Europe, and the New World, this systematic campaign of cultural, spiritual, environmental, and demographic genocide resulted in the slaughter of tens, if not hundreds, of millions of indigenous people (Stannard, 1992). It also resulted in the near eradication of New World shamanic practices involving the use of psychedelic plants and fungi, which were seen as instruments of the Devil. For example, the use of psilocybin mushrooms among the Aztecs, who named it *teonanacatl,* "God's flesh," was seen by the Inquisitionists as an especially heinous blasphemy due to its similarity to the Christian Eucharist, in which God's flesh (i.e., the body of Christ) was consumed due to the "miracle" of Transubstantiation.

Of course, no dominator culture ever succeeds in completely eradicating indigenous religious or spiritual practices, and this was true of *teonanacatl.* Its use was marginalized and driven underground for nearly 400 years, until it was "rediscovered"[2] by the American banker and amateur mycologist R. Gordon Wasson and his wife Valentina, in the early 1950s. The Wassons, however, published their findings in *Life* magazine, a much more visible if not exactly peer-reviewed journal, in May 1957 (Wasson, 1957). Wasson's article reported on their trip to Oaxaca, and their participation in a mushroom *velada* with the *curandera* Maria Sabina. They brought back specimens for identification and eventually got spores into the hands of Sandoz chemist and discoverer of lysergic acid diethylamide (LSD), Albert Hofmann. Hofmann and his colleagues managed to cultivate the mushrooms under laboratory conditions and were able to isolate and synthesize the two primary active ingredients, psilocybin and psilocin.

The publication of the Wasson article in *Life* magazine marked, in some sense, the first eruption of psychedelics into mainstream culture in the West. Of course, peyote had been known since the late 19th century; Arthur Heffter and others had isolated mescaline and other alkaloids from it, and the compound was synthesized in 1919 (Heffter, 1898; Späth, 1919). Hofmann synthesized LSD in 1938 but did not discover its psychedelic properties until he accidentally (?)[3] ingested a small amount while resynthesizing it in 1943. During the same period, Schultes spent years in the Amazon and documented the use of ayahuasca and tryptamine-based snuffs among various tribes. Ayahuasca first came to the attention of Western science as a result of a report by the English botanist Richard Spruce on his discovery of its use by an indigenous tribe in 1858; his report, however, was not published until 50 years later, 8 years after his death, in a book edited by A. R. Wallace, *Notes of a Botanist on the Amazon and Andes* (Spruce, 1908).

The compounds that were discovered during the first part of the 20th century, mescaline and peyote extracts, and various fractions and isolates obtained from *Banisteriopsis caapi,* one of the components of ayahuasca, were objects of curiosity to a small number of physicians, psychologists, and philosophers for decades but did not attract attention beyond these circles. That began to change, however, after Hofmann synthesized LSD and it was made available to psychologists and medical practitioners under the auspices of Sandoz Pharmaceuticals. LSD became a curiosity of the laboratory and the clinic, and from the early 1950s to the mid-1960s, it was investigated by numerous researchers in biomedicine not only for its potential therapeutic applications but also as a tool of basic research. In fact, it is not an exaggeration to assert that the discovery of LSD, and its subsequent availability to medical researchers, marked a major milestone in the emergence of modern neuroscience and molecular neuropharmacology (Nichols, 2016).

While the 1957 *Life* magazine article on magic mushrooms might have brought psy-

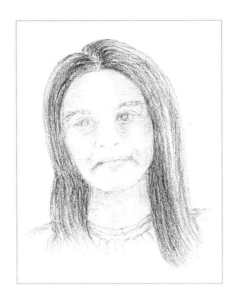

Maria Sabina

chedelics to the attention of the masses (*Life*, after all, was a common fixture on the coffee or kitchen tables of many American households during this period), it was really Timothy Leary's promotion of LSD as a catalyst for social change that put psychedelics at the center of the cultural conversation of the time. Leary's message to the youth of America to "turn on, tune in, and drop out" was not viewed as anything but threatening to the social order by the hegemons of cultural correctness. To an extent, Leary was right. LSD, once escaped from the laboratory, dropped like a bomb into Western society, which was already a seething broth of rapidly accelerating social, cultural, and political ferment. It was a time when many in society, especially the young, were questioning the conventional norms of their elders and the "establishment." The growing unpopularity of the war in Vietnam, and the decision by many young people to oppose it and in many cases to actively resist induction into military service, had much to do with the disruption of the social fabric and the widening divisions between young people and their parents, and others, in that generation. LSD, with its ability to completely reframe one's relationship to reality (at least temporarily) contributed to the emergence of a counterculture in which one was not only permitted, but expected, to question every aspect of societal norms, from politics to religion to morality. Entrenched authoritarian hegemonies, such as those that dominated society in the 1960s (and still do dominate it to a great extent), understandably did not take kindly to this disruption of accepted dogma and were particularly hostile to young people's insistence on thinking for themselves, which LSD encouraged. The backlash was predictably brutal. LSD, despite more than two decades of scientific investigation pointing to an array of likely therapeutic benefits, was stigmatized as the most dangerous drug in the world, even as Leary was branded the most dangerous man in America.[4] By the end the 1960s, in a depressing demonstration of political cowardice and thoughtlessness, all psychedelics had been prohibited as dangerous, addictive substances without any legitimate medical uses. The United States, which led the charge, persuaded the rest of the world to go along with this by applying political and economic pressure to other United Nations (UN; 1971) members, so that the global ban was fully in effect by 1971. An unintended (or perhaps intended) side effect of this legislative response was the immediate shutdown of all medical research on LSD and other psychedelics, much of it ongoing, much of it promising.

Another consequence of LSD's eruption into society and the subsequent backlash was that the connection of LSD and other psychedelics to millennia-old traditions of shamanic use were largely overlooked by both sides of the debate. If more attention had been paid to the historical and cultural antecedents of psychedelics, and their revered position in many indigenous societies, it might have mollified some of those concerned about their dangers, both as drugs and as agents of social change. Psychedelics, after all, are nothing new. They have been used safely and beneficially for thousands of years, in many societies, long before the FDA or other regulatory agencies existed to control, regulate, and in most cases prohibit their use. Indigenous societies that use psychedelics have managed to integrate them into their cultural fabric, as well as the insights that people derive from psychedelics, yet amazingly, to some, are neither morally or socially degenerate.[5]

■ The Psychedelic "Renaissance"

Society's efforts to ban and even to eradicate psychedelic plants, fungi, and compounds at the end of the 1960s were doomed to failure, as could have been predicted by a cursory look at similar attempts in the historical record. People are inherently resistant to the suppression of individual freedoms by authoritarian fiat, especially when directed at spiritual practices, and/or biological functions. Like the efforts to stamp out the Gnostic mystery schools of the fourth century C.E., or of the Inquisition to eradicate the "idolatrous" mushroom cults in Mexico in the 1500s, the legislative prohibition of psychedelics imposed in the 1960s succeeded only in driving the practices underground. The ritual and recreational use of psychedelics continued among already-marginalized subcultural segments of society, as did their therapeutic use by small numbers of renegade therapists willing to risk their professional careers and even possible incarceration in order to continue practicing therapies that many believed were far more effective than any other therapeutic modality available to them (Stolaroff, 1997). From the end of the 1960s to the early 1990s, psychedelics were in a kind of limbo; there was plenty of unsupervised ritual and recreational use going on, as well as underground therapeutic use. Some research with the substances in animals and in basic neuroscience research continued, but almost no clinical research was conducted under FDA-approved protocols. During this hiatus, between 1970 to the early 1990s, underground use continued but was not much discussed in public.[6] During this period, parts of society involved in psychedelics began to develop practices and rituals, often by integrating practices borrowed from indigenous traditions but appropriately adapted to the 20th century. Lacking a legitimate claim to ancient indigenous traditions, psychedelic practitioners nonetheless learned from them, and thereby learned how to utilize psychedelics in safe settings that minimized potential harms and maximized potential benefits.

Another factor that contributed to the survival of psychedelic practices during this prohibitionist era was the introduction about 1975 of simple techniques for cultivating *Psilocybe cubensis,* a potent species of magic mushrooms. Although various amateur mycologists were working on cultivation techniques at the time, Terence and Dennis McKenna were among the first to publish cultivation methods in the form of a small book, *Psilocybin: Magic Mushroom Grower's Guide,* which they published under pseudonyms, O. N. Oeric and O. T. Oss, under the imprint of And/Or Press, a small Berkeley publishing house (Oss & Oeric, 1976). This little book proved to be a societal game changer. Using the methods described in the book, any intelligent and reasonably persistent 10th grader could successfully grow small (and sometimes not so small) quantities of psilocybin mushrooms using readily available materials that could be purchased in any grocery or hardware store. Prior to this, psychedelics were difficult to access, and their production (usually of LSD) necessitated access to prohibited precursors, laboratory facilities, and at least a modicum of competency in synthetic organic chemistry, and the products originating from these underground operations depended on distribution networks that exposed producers and distributors to serious legal liabilities. Home cultivation of psilocybin mushrooms was much less risky. It attracted about as much attention as making sourdough starter and could be pursued by anyone as an enjoyable and often lucrative hobby. Although large-scale mushroom-growing operations did exist and were occasionally taken down by authorities, by and large, most mushroom cultivation was on small scales that attracted little attention. As a result, mushrooms penetrated society rather rapidly and very quietly, and no one took much notice. For the first time a potent, nontoxic, and safe psychedelic became readily available to anyone who wanted to make the effort. And, because mushrooms reliably elicited pleasant experiences that were nonthreatening, adverse reactions and "bad trips" were rare. As a result, most people's encounters with psychedelics during this prohibitionist era were through the consumption of cultivated psilocybin mushrooms. Gradually, widespread reports of positive experiences with mushrooms changed the tone of the cultural conversation. Mushrooms never rose to the level of the "most dangerous drug in America," as had LSD just a few years earlier. Cultural attitudes toward them were more tolerant, and people were more open to the idea of having extraordinary psychedelic experiences with the aid of mushrooms. There was a deeper level of acceptance, and most people, if they thought about magic mushrooms at all, were likely to regard them with bemusement. In this way, the self-fulfilling prophesy articulated by Terence McKenna in one of his public lectures, "We are involved in a symbiotic relationship with something that has disguised itself as an alien invasion, so as not to alarm us," came to be. The invasion was complete, not a shot was fired, and most people were just fine with it. Mushrooms quietly consolidated their occupation of many a nerd's basement and found a welcoming home in dormitory closets throughout the land, an occupation that continues to this day.[7]

Over time, this catalytic change in societal attitudes toward psychedelics engineered by fungal symbionts reframed the cultural conversation and enabled reconsideration of the heretical notion that psychedelics might be good for something after all. It forced the door open, ever so slightly, to the resumption of psychedelic research in human subjects; it triggered the recognition that the spasms of political hysteria that led to their blanket prohibition at the end of the 1960s might have been a bit hasty. The fog of collective amnesia that had obscured the considerable body of therapeutic research that preceded their prohibition began slowly to dissipate, as researchers began to rediscover this information. True, the earlier studies may not have had the most rigorous experimental designs, and there was often evidence of investigator bias, but this did not invalidate the entire corpus of research, and there was strong, indeed overwhelming, evidence that for certain conditions, such as alcoholism, psychedelics were at least as promising as any existing therapeutic modalities. This, combined with a renewed appreciation that psychedelics, used in the context of traditional ethnomedicine, also could result in therapeutic outcomes. The methods and assumptions underlying traditional use of psychedelics did not resemble in any way the protocols of biomedical psychiatry; nevertheless, the results were often as efficacious, if not more so, than conventional psychotherapy. Reports of individuals who were compelled to step out of the boundaries of conventional psychotherapy to seek healing for intractable conditions and had found relief either in visits to traditional shamanic healers or in neoshamanic ceremonies practiced by "underground" therapists began to emerge. It gradually became clear that it was time to set biases aside and take a second look at the therapeutic possibilities offered by psychedelics.

■ Psychedelics and Biomedicine

One of the pioneers of this reemerging psychedelic renaissance in the early 1990s was Dr. Rick J. Strassman, a psychiatrist in the School of Medicine at the University of New Mexico. Strassman's research had focused on the pineal gland and the functions of the pineal hormone, melatonin. This research interest led him to unconfirmed reports that the endogenous hallucinogen N,N-dimethyltryptamine (DMT), might be synthesized in the pineal gland and have some function as a neuromodulator or neurohormone. Scientific curiosity about this possibility led him to apply to the FDA for permission to conduct a clinical study in humans utilizing synthetic DMT administered intravenously. His application to the National Institute on Drug Abuse (NIDA) was approved, and in 1994 Strassman became the first investigator to legally administer a psychedelic to human subjects since prohibition had effectively shut down research at the end of the 60s (Strassman & Qualls, 1994; Strassman, Qualls, Uhlenhuth, & Kellner, 1994). Strassman's DMT research was a pivotal milestone in the revival of psychedelic research in human subjects. Unlike most of the research that followed, Strassman's clinical study was not oriented toward any therapeutic target. It was basically a descriptive study to document the physiological and psychological effects of DMT in humans. This absence of a therapeutic rationale may have accounted for its relatively easy approval by the FDA. No therapeutic claim was made, but it was a chance to investigate the properties of a putative endogenous hallucinogen.

Strassman's work started out as a fairly pedestrian clinical study, conducted according to standard clinical practice. But the outcomes of his research, and the bizarre reports of many of his subjects, particularly at higher doses, dramatically highlighted the inadequacies of conventional clinical protocols. Subjects commonly reported profound mystical experiences, often resembling published accounts of near-death experiences, and encounters with nonhuman entities that had striking parallels with accounts of alien abductions. These reports were difficult for Strassman, whose orientation was basically biomedical and reductionist, to interpret within the framework of a conventional clinical study. In his book *DMT: The Spirit Molecule*, published in 2001, Strassman wrote that these experiences "left me feeling confused and concerned about where the spirit molecule was leading us. It was at this point that I began to wonder if I was getting in over my head with this research. Eventually this cognitive dissonance, combined with the disapproval of his research by the Zen Buddhist group with which he had been affiliated for many years, led Strassman to abandon his clinical work. He has described the trials and challenges of his work in his well-known book and the short documentary of the same name, produced by filmmaker Mitch Schultz in 2010.

Although Strassman formally abandoned clinical research—a decision almost as courageous, or at least as honest, as his decision to navigate the regulatory maze presented by the FDA to become the first investigator in 20 years to conduct clinical research with psychedelics in the United States—he has remained active in the field and continues to write and speak about the Spirit Molecule.[8]

▣ Clinical Protocols

Strassman may not have succeeded in opening a portal to another dimension (which he never intended), but he certainly opened one to further and more rigorous clinical studies, most of which did have a therapeutic rationale. Strassman's research was very influential in making clinical psychedelic research respectable again, even though its outcomes were so outré as to challenge the very notion of reductionist clinical research with psychedelics.

The next clinical study with psychedelics under FDA-approved protocols did not take place until 2006, when Roland Griffiths and his group at Johns Hopkins University published a clinical study on psilocybin as a reliable inducer of so-called "mystical" experiences (Griffiths, Richards, McCann, & Jesse, 2006). This study was also remarkable. In common with Strassman's DMT studies, Griffith's clinical study of psilocybin did not have a therapeutic target. Rather it focused on psilocybin's ability to "occasion mystical-type experiences having substantial and sustained personal meaning and spiritual significance." Their paper attracted a great deal of notice in the biomedical and psychiatric worlds, and was generally praised for the rigor of its experimental design, as well as the novelty of applying a clinical research protocol to an aspect of human experience usually considered the provenance of religion and religious professionals. This paper, the first of many addressing this type of investigation, was significant for a number of reasons. For one thing, a *lack* of "sustained personal meaning and spiritual significance" in an individual's life has never been recognized in biomedical psychiatry as a "disorder" necessitating treatment. Yet the FDA approved the study, as it had earlier with Strassman's study. This speaks well of the FDA, as it implies that this regulatory body (or possibly some mavericks within it) recognized that psychedelics could be used to investigate, explore, understand, and possibly elicit "personally meaningful, spiritually significant experiences." In other words, psilocybin and other psychedelics, and the unique states of mind they can elicit, had applications beyond the merely therapeutic; they could be used to investigate the nature of consciousness itself and the outer limits of human experience. The study also represented a challenge to religious institutions; by boldly asserting that mystical experiences, which religious practitioners often seek through years of meditation and asceticism, could be reliably achieved by almost anyone with the judicious consumption of 25 milligrams or so of an indole alkaloid under the right circumstances. If it is possible to go to a clinic, ingest a chemical, and have a religious experience, who needs religion? But the study also presents a challenge to reductionist biomedicine because it means that not only is spirituality—spirit—"real," but it is a legitimate subject for scientific investigation. This represents a profound reframing of the reductionist conventions of biomedicine, which has sought to exorcise "spirit" from biomedicine for nearly 200 years. Now, suddenly, along comes a chemical that not only demonstrates the reality of spirit—or spiritual experiences—but it drags it out of the church or temple and places it firmly into the context of the clinical laboratory. The recognition of this fact must be as discomfiting for biomedicine as the co-optation of spiritual experience by biomedicine is for religion. Both require a fundamental reunderstanding of what it is to be human and conscious, and spiritual.

Roland Griffiths's initial clinical studies of psilocybin's ability to *occasion* (his term) "profoundly meaningful personal experiences" were not targeted to any specific therapeutic outcome; this property quickly became associated with a therapeutic application in the next round of clinical investigations: the relief of existential anxiety in the dying. Ironically, the first clinical study of psilocybin that specifically identified existential anxiety in the terminally ill as a treatment target did not originate in Griffiths's laboratory. Charles S. Grob, a psychiatrist in the Harbor UCLA Medical Center in California, conducted the first study of this sort (Grob et al., 2011). Grob, and one of the coauthors of the study, George Greer, also a psychiatrist, are both founding board members of the Heffter Research Institute, which was established as a nonprofit educational and scientific organization in 1992, with the mission to sponsor scientifically rigorous investigations of psychedelics "to contribute to a greater understanding of the mind, leading to the improvement of the human condition, and to alleviate suffering" (*www.heffter.org*). There was nothing in the original charter stating that Heffter would focus almost exclusively on psilocybin, in the same way that its sister organization, the Multidisciplinary Association for Psychedelic Studies (MAPS; *www.maps.org*) has focused almost exclusively on MDMA for the treatment of posttraumatic stress disorder (PTSD), among other disorders. Although neither organization had planned on this singular focus, the considerable drain placed on both financial and operational resources by the conduct of rigorous clinical trials, especially trials aimed at eventual regulatory approval of a new medicine to be made available to clinicians, necessitated that limited resources had to be deployed in the most cost-effective manner. As a result, though there was never any formal agreement, Heffter focused on psilocybin, while MAPS directed most of its resources toward MDMA. Both medicines address multiple therapeutic targets that have proven intractable for conventional psychiatric medicine, and for which the conventional psychopharmaceutical pharmacopoeia is largely ineffective.

Both Heffter and MAPS deserve recognition and credit for bringing these two psychedelic medicines, reviled and banned for decades, into the clinic and demonstrating through multiple rigorous clinical trials[9] that they can be used safely and effectively in the treatment of a range of mental disorders for which no other treatment or medicine is comparably efficacious.

The combination of multiple clinical studies on psilocybin and MDMA, conducted over the last two decades using rigorous study designs, with most yielding robust and in some cases spectacular (Johnson, Garcia-Romeu, Cosimano, & Griffiths, 2014) therapeutic responses for a variety of conditions, has brought these two medicines to a critical juncture in the development process. They have now reached a point at which both are about to be approved for at least one therapeutic application (PTSD in the case of MDMA, and intractable depression in the case of psilocybin). In other words, these two psychedelic medicines, once considered menaces to public health and given the most restricted status in the Drug Enforcement Administration's (DEA; 2019) classification of controlled substances (Schedule 1, substances that have no currently accepted medical use in the United States, a lack of accepted safety for use under medical supervision, and a high potential for abuse) are now on the cusp of being approved for clinical use. This is a remarkable turnaround for substances that were once so thoroughly marginalized, and it is even more remarkable that private benefactors to nonprofit organizations funded all of the clinical studies that produced the body of evidence that led to this transformation through donations; none of it was achieved with funding from either government research organizations such as the National Institutes of Health (NIH) or the pharmaceutical industry.

▨ Co-Optation and Corporatization

As a result of diligent and rigorous research by a growing number of investigators, it now appears assured that both psilocybin and MDMA will achieve regulatory approval for clinical use within the next 3–5 years. This represents a major paradigm shift in biomedical psychiatry. But the significance and impact of this approval go far beyond biomedical psychiatry. Acceptance of psychedelics into mainstream medicine has the potential to revolutionize biomedicine, in that it forces a change of the conceptual reference frame in which "spirit" and spirituality are recognized as essential elements of healing for both psychological and some physical disorders. This is a radical departure from the current reductionist approach in which physicians, due to the economic limitations imposed on the delivery of health care, are not able to spend sufficient time with patients to get to the root of mental disorders, and the expectations (of both the patient and the physician) are that the patient will leave the clinical interview with a prescription in hand that may or may not (and too often does not) have the efficacy to resolve the patient's problems. The unintended consequences of this are that neither party to the transaction, neither the therapist nor the patient, feels satisfied. Patients often leave with a feeling that they have not been heard, and that recommendations for treatment (almost invariably involving the prescription of one or more psychopharmaceuticals) are cursory, routine, and inadequate. Physicians, for their part, are frustrated that "the system" does not afford them the flexibility to provide real healing to an individual; there simply is not time to devote to conditions that require more than a 15-minute office visit. Introduction of psychedelics into biomedicine will inevitably (we hope) change that pattern because one thing that all psychedelic therapies have in common is that they are only effective within the context of intense psychotherapeutic support. To be effective, psychedelic therapy requires extensive and lengthy interactions between therapist and patient. This represents a challenge to the current economic models of health care, which, with rare exceptions, are predicated on the notion that insurance companies will cover only the bare minimum of treatments that may be indicated. Even after psychedelic medicines have achieved approval for clinical use, psychedelic therapies will likely be available only to those able to pay for them out of pocket because the modalities necessary for effective treatment are too costly to offer to patients without insurance, or with only minimal insurance. Thus, the therapies are at risk of being viewed as a self-indulgent option available only to "elites," those with

the money and time to pay for them, while excluding those unable to pay for them, even though they may need the treatments as much, if not more, than wealthier patients.

Another disturbing aspect of the coming acceptance of psychedelics into mainstream biomedicine is that now that the "heavy lifting" needed to bring these medicines into wider usage has been done by nonprofit organizations such as the Heffter Research Institute and MAPS, without the benefit of support from the government or the pharmaceutical industry, those with a capitalist orientation have woken to the fact that there are in fact significant profits to be made in the commercialization of psychedelic medicines. This has created a dilemma. On the one hand, if psychedelics are to achieve widespread clinical usage, it will be necessary to develop a production and distribution infrastructure. The medicines intended for clinical use must be manufactured under stringent quality control standards, as is necessary for any prescription medicine. This fact alone tilts the playing field. Only organizations with sufficient resources, that is, corporations, will be able to afford the millions in investment that will be required, even beyond the costs of Phase III clinical trials if they are to be brought to the market.

Organizations such as MAPS are already struggling with these challenges as MDMA nears approval as a breakthrough therapy. Also, there is already competition emerging between two for-profit companies working toward a similar regulatory approval of psilocybin. Compass (*https://compasspathways.com*), was founded by pharmaceutical entrepreneur George Goldsmith and is based in the United Kingdom, and Usona Institute (*www.usonainstitute.org*), founded by biotech entrepreneur Bill Linton, is based in Wisconsin. Linton is also on the board of the Heffter Research Institute. Each of these institutions is addressing the challenges posed by commercialization in different ways. Rick Doblin, founder of MAPS, is acutely aware of the potential for co-optation of decades of MAPS research by predatory corporations. MAPS has formed the MAPS public benefit corporation (PBC) in what appears to this writer to be a thoughtful and ethical response to the dilemma; PBCs combine the best aspects of nonprofit and for-profit corporate structures. They can be profitable, but they must also produce a public benefit, and this can provide a balance to the conventional for-profit corporate mandate, which is to provide maximum returns to stakeholders over all other considerations. Compass, though started as a nonprofit, has recently changed to a for-profit corporation and has raised alarms in some sectors by taking steps to protect its proprietary access to good manufacturing grade (GMP) psilocybin. Usona, on the other hand, which remains a nonprofit, has recently come into conflict with Compass because that company has forged an exclusive manufacturing agreement with a company for the manufacture of GMP-grade psilocybin, and has refused to share the product with Usona except under licensing agreements that Usona has so far deemed unacceptable. This is a rather complicated situation, and there is a temptation to view Compass as having a predatory corporate motive, namely, to control the supply of clinical grade psilocybin. To do so would be simplistic because neither Compass nor Usona is operating out of purely capitalist, profit-driven motives. The founders of both Compass and Usona are known to this writer as ethical, compassionate men whose primary motive is not profit. Both sincerely want to make these psychedelic medicines available to clinical practitioners. It is also true that both men are shrewd businessmen and good capitalists, not unaware of the opportunities for profit that may exist from commercialization. How all this will play out in the coming months and years as Usona and Compass jockey for position in the for-profit–nonprofit environment of psychedelic clinical medicine remains to be seen. It is my hope that there will be enough good will on both sides, and enough demand for psychedelic therapies, that all of these organizations can achieve a harmonious relationship in which all can benefit: the researchers who have struggled to conduct rigorous clinical investigations, often with inadequate funding and complete lack of funding from the government; the investors who have recognized the economic potential of clinical psychedelics and have stepped up to provide resources to support this next critical phase; the psychedelic community, which has dreamed for decades that this

day may come; and most importantly, the patients suffering from intractable illnesses who may be cured via psychedelic therapy.[10]

Return to the Roots

Most members of the psychedelic community will view the acceptance of psilocybin and MDMA into the pharmacopoeia of clinical medicine as a positive development; yet there remain troubling ethical issues that are perhaps more germane when the medicines under consideration are natural products. The concerns I discuss below are less of an issue for MDMA, which is a synthetic compound, not derived from any natural source.

In the case of psilocybin, however, or other naturally occurring psychedelics such as ayahuasca or mescaline, there are still unaddressed ethical and legal issues that beg for a clear articulation of policy. I discuss some of the main questions I identify as worthy of further discussion below.

What Is Not Patented Is Prohibited . . .

Psilocybin mushrooms, ayahuasca, peyote and San Pedro cactus, iboga, and DMT-containing snuffs are all natural psychedelics with long traditions of use in the shamanic practices of many indigenous groups. Only psilocybin has so far been positioned as a candidate for clinical use, necessitating a change in scheduling before it can be adopted into biomedicine. None of the others named here are currently candidates for development as clinically approved medicines under conventional FDA three-phase development protocols. This situation may change in the near future, as both ayahuasca and iboga/ibogaine have accrued a body of evidence indicating their efficacy for treatment of various disorders, though none has been advanced to formal three-phase clinical trials in the United States. Peyote and San Pedro cacti have in common that mescaline is the major active ingredient. Neither has been evaluated under formal clinical trials; mescaline was evaluated in several clinical trials in the late 1960s, but these were not intended to develop the drug as a medicine. Abundant ethnographic evidence supports the efficacy of peyote both as a treatment for alcoholism and as a prophylactic protection against alcoholism among Native American groups through the Native American Church, but it has not been approved by the FDA for this use (Halpern, Sherwood, Hudson, Yurgelun-Todd, & Pope, 2005). Further complicating matters is that the regulatory status of the natural forms of these shamanic or traditional medicines is murky at best. The confusion arises in part because the law is not clear on the legal status of the organisms that contain the active compounds; in most but not all instances, the law lists the active principles of the plants or fungi as Schedule 1 controlled substances, but not the organisms themselves. For example, psilocybin and psilocin, the active psychedelic occurring in over 200 species of mushrooms, are listed as controlled substances. The law makes no distinction between mushrooms containing psilocybin/psilocin, and both the compounds, and mushrooms containing them, are regarded as prohibited.[11,12] In the case of ayahuasca, the psychedelic compound that gives ayahuasca its visionary properties is DMT, which is derived not from the *Banisteriopsis* vine, which contains the monoamine oxidase (MAO)–inhibiting ß-carbolines, but from the admixture plants, *Psychotria viridis* or *Diplopterys caberana*. In most countries the ß-carbolines are not regulated, though Canada is an exception.[13] Under the UN Convention on Psychotropic Substances, the legal framework for the regulation of all psychotropics considered to have high abuse potential and no medical applications, ayahuasca is specifically exempt because it is a traditional medicine utilized in the spiritual and religious practices of indigenous peoples. Presumably, similar considerations would apply to other plants containing controlled substances that are also used in indigenous religious practices, but this is not explicitly stated. For example, DMT, the controlled substance in ayahuasca, under the UN convention can only be consumed by indigenous people in the context of religious practice. The law has yet to address the status of other DMT-containing plants, which number in the thousands; many of them contain sufficient levels of DMT to enable them to be utilized in the preparation of "ayahuasca analogues," which have phar-

macological properties similar to ayahuasca but incorporate none of its botanical ingredients (Ott, 1994). So far, the law is mute on the legal status of so-called "ayahuasca analogues." In the United States, only members of the União do Vegetal (UDV) or the Santo Daime may use ayahuasca; both Brazilian churches are permitted to use the preparation for religious purposes, as a result of Supreme Court decisions under the Religious Freedom Restoration Act.[14] In their decision, the Court did not address the question of whether ayahuasca may be consumed by indigenous people, but presumably it would be allowed, based on the rights of indigenous people to use it under the laws defined in the UN Convention on Psychotropic Substances. The Convention does not specify just which indigenous people this exemption covers, whether they have to be indigenous to a culture in which ayahuasca is traditionally used, or whether persons belonging to any indigenous group will qualify. This situation has created a legal conundrum that will probably be addressed in future court cases; as it stands now, apparently, ayahuasca is legal for members of ayahuasca churches of which the UDV and the Santo Daime are the largest and most visible; it may be legal for indigenous people (what specific ethnicities are allowed is not specified); but, apparently, it is definitely illegal for anyone who does not belong to one of the churches and is not indigenous. While I am not a lawyer, it seems clear to me that this law is unconstitutional because it violates equal protection under the law. It is not constitutional to require that a person be either a member of a particular church, and/or an indigenous person, to be permitted to consume ayahuasca.

Similar obfuscating and confusing rules also apply to the other natural psychedelics. Ibogaine is classified as a Schedule 1 controlled substance. The iboga plant is similarly explicitly prohibited, as is peyote, while San Pedro cactus,[15] which also contains mescaline, is not specifically prohibited, and, in fact, several *Echinopsis* species are popular ornamental cacti and often freely sold in nurseries throughout the United States. As the law is written, there is little distinction made between the plants that contain controlled substances and the substances themselves. The designation of specific plants as controlled substances is rare, but does include peyote (*Lophophora williamsii*), iboga (*Tabernanthe iboga*), the opium poppy (*Papaver somniferum*), coca (*Erythroxylum coca*), and *Cannabis* species (DEA, 2019).

The current less than clear legal guidelines governing scheduled substances and plants are in part a reflection of the policy decisions made at the end of the 1960s that culminated in the passage of the Controlled Substances Act. The law was drafted by politicians, not chemists or botanists, and in an atmosphere of haste and hysteria, in which basically every plant or substance that might possibly have been classified as a "dangerous" drug was swept up into legislation whether or not that designation was supported by evidence. Had the laws been drafted more thoughtfully, and perhaps with the benefit of advice from aforementioned scientific experts, the current legal murkiness might have been avoided.

■ Coevolution and Symbiosis

These distinctions between prohibited *substances* and prohibited *plants* may seem to be of little consequence, but they are actually important issues that should be clarified if the legal frameworks governing their regulation are to be appropriately and fairly revised. Such a reframing is needed and may even point to a way out of the current dilemma.

Consider the following points:

• Under current laws (in the United States) all psychedelic compounds are classified as Schedule 1 controlled substances; some, but not all, psychedelic plants or fungi or animals are similarly classified.[16]

• Clinical research on psilocybin has produced abundant scientific evidence of its efficacy for certain mental disorders.

• As a result, psilocybin is about to be approved for clinical use, and as a necessary preliminary step, must be moved from Schedule 1 to a less restrictive schedule. By definition, Schedule 1 controlled substances must have no evidence of medical applications; since psilocybin clearly does have medical utility, its Schedule 1 designation is invalid and should be revised.

• Once psilocybin becomes available for clinical use, the treatments are still likely to be unaffordable for most people. Insurance companies will probably not cover psychedelic therapies, at least for the foreseeable future. Accessibility will also become an issue; there is not enough clinical psilocybin to meet the need, and there is a shortage of qualified therapists.

• As a result, many if not most, people who wish to consume psychedelics for personal spiritual purposes or for therapeutic purposes will continue to turn to natural preparations; psilocybin in the form of mushrooms or DMT in the form of ayahuasca or iboga, peyote or San Pedro cacti consumed as natural preparations.

• Unless these legal issues are addressed, wealthy people will be able to avoid legal liability because they can pay for clinical psychedelic therapies. Those who cannot afford such therapies, or who prefer to use natural psychedelics, may continue to be branded as felons, while the natural medicines continue to be classified as dangerous Schedule 1 substances. Clearly, there is an inherent unfairness built into this situation that needs to be addressed through thoughtful revision of the regulatory schemas governing psychedelics.

A possible solution to this dilemma may require a fundamental reunderstanding of humanity's age-old relationship to plants in general and to psychoactive plants in particular. Over millennia of coevolution, humanity has utilized plants and fungi for a variety of purposes. Plants provide us with food, clothing, construction materials, aesthetic pleasure, and medicines. We value biologically active plants as medicines largely because of the chemicals they contain. Actually, the same is true of nutritive plants; the compounds they contain are nutrients. Some of those chemicals are psychoactive and may be used as stimulants, sedatives, analgesics, and anxiolytics, to name a few examples. The special kinds of plants known as psychedelics often are intrinsic elements of spiritual and religious practices.

Symbiosis in biology is defined as the living together of dissimilar organisms, as in mutualism, commensalism, amensalism, or parasitism.[17] The two subdefinitions of symbiosis that are most relevant to this discussion are mutualism and parasitism. It could be argued that humans' relationships with plants are a form of parasitism. Plants, through photosynthesis, produce nutrients and biologically active compounds, and virtually every organism in the biosphere that is not photosynthetic can be viewed as parasitic on the plants. Fungi are not photosynthetic; they subsist on dead or decaying matter, and in that sense fungi are also parasitic on plants (and sometimes this relationship is also pathogenic; e.g., when a plant is infected with a fungus that damages the plant in some way). Mutualism is the type of symbiosis most relevant to our discussion here; it is a close relationship between different species in which both partners benefit. This definition fits most human–plant (or fungal) symbioses. Plants provide humans with medicinal chemicals, nutrients, pigments, fibers, flavorings, and fragrances, all of which are beneficial to the human partner. Humans, in turn, provide benefits to plants by cultivating them, thereby ensuring that the species will survive and be protected to some extent from the vicissitudes of natural selection.[18]

This symbiotic, coevolutionary relationship between plants and humans is a fundamental, essential element of human biology and culture, found in all human societies, that has existed as long as humans (including the hominid ancestors of modern humans) have existed on this planet. Indeed, if it had not existed, and did not now exist, humans would not have survived.

From this perspective, symbiosis, and the "right to symbiose" should be recognized: "Any human has the right to form a symbiotic relationship with any plant, fungus or other non-human organism for purposes of mutual benefit." Codification of this simple statement into the regulatory frameworks governing access to psychoactive substances, starting with the UN Commission on Human Rights and incorporated into the laws of all member nations, would go a long way toward resolving this dilemma.

Humans and plants have engaged in this mutualistic partnership for hundreds of thousands of years. Within that time span,

humans have learned how to use psychoactive plants in beneficial ways (in most instances) and in the case of psychedelic plants, have developed spiritual traditions and technologies (shamanism) that provide a context for "set and setting," that is intended to optimize the benefits and minimize the risks associated with the use of such plants. The same variables that contemporary psychotherapists confront in developing their therapeutic protocols are the same ones that traditional healers have had to face for as long as these plants have been utilized in traditional medicine. And it should not come as a surprise that traditional healers have managed to accomplish this without benefit of oversight from the FDA or proscriptive regulation by political institutions. It is simply not true that psychedelics can only be safely administered by white-coated psychotherapists in highly structured clinical environments. To assert otherwise amounts to arrogance and medical hubris.

▪ Plants for the People: A New Paradigm

On the legal front, the solution to the problem of regulation of psychedelic and other psychoactive plants becomes straightforward and obvious once the primacy and the coevolutionary nature of plant–human symbiosis is recognized and widely accepted. The solution is simple: Codify into law the principle that plants (and fungi and other biologically active organisms) are not "drugs" in their natural form, and thus should not be regulated. When psychoactive substances are extracted from their natural sources, purified, and concentrated, they are then "drugs" and should be appropriately regulated as such. This simple change in jurisprudence, if adopted by the UN Commission on Controlled Substances, and accepted by all member nations, would go a long way toward solving the "Drug Problem" by empowering law enforcement and regulatory authorities to concentrate on regulating actual drugs rather than plants or crude plant extracts. No longer faced with the need to regulate organisms, the resources of regulatory and enforcement agencies could be used more effectively to concentrate on real drugs, chemicals (whether natural or synthetic) that may be problematic for human use and potentially harmful.

Fusion of Biomedical Psychotherapy and Traditional Medicine

In an ideal world in which this simple, obvious, and sorely needed change in regulatory practices has been accepted and implemented, psychedelic psychotherapists and their patients who wanted to receive therapy using pharmaceutical grade psilocybin or other medicines in highly structured clinical settings should be free to do so. The only limitations preventing such therapy would be its cost, but those who wish to have the extra reassurance and perceived greater safety of staging the experience in a clinical setting would have the choice to do so provided they accepted the cost. Those who, either because they lack the resources to pay for clinical therapies or because they prefer to use natural medicines, should also have that choice. Both approaches to psychedelic psychotherapy need not be in conflict. Let market forces decide which approach will become the most popular and accessible.

Under this new envisioned regulatory paradigm, one can imagine an eventual fusion of biomedical psychedelic psychotherapy and traditional shamanic practices, which themselves represent a kind of psychotherapy. If biomedical clinicians and traditional healers can work together, each borrowing and building on the best practices of the other (this is already happening in the community of "underground" psychedelic therapists), then the synthesis will result in the emergence of a new paradigm in psychedelic psychotherapy that will transform and enhance both practices in positive ways; it will be a true symbiosis, a mutualistic relationship that will realize the full potential of psychedelics to heal not only individuals but the entire human species.

Notes

1. These practitioners have various names that are usually culture-specific. Generically they are sometimes referred to as shamans and the practice as shamanism, but this is inaccurate. Strictly speaking, *shamanism*—a term that can be traced to various Siberian languages, is a practice that originated in Siberia in the late Paleolithic, while other cultures have their own terms for these practitioners, such as *curanderos, maestros, vegetalistas, ayahuasqueros,* and so forth. All of these "shamanic" traditions have in common that their practitioners deliberately induce altered states of consciousness, most often, but not always, with psychedelic or psychoactive plants or fungi, and in the trance state, are able to diagnose and treat illnesses, divine the future, retrieve "lost souls," and otherwise carry out various functions to support the religious and spiritual life of their communities (see *https:// en.wikipedia.org/wiki/shamanism*).

2. Actually, credit for the rediscovery of psychedelic mushrooms in use in the highlands of Mexico belongs to the ethnobotanist Richard Evans Schultes, who collected several specimens of *Paneolus* spp. in the mid-1930s, acting on information from a local informant, Blas Pablo Reko. Schultes (1939) published his findings in the Harvard Botanical Museum Leaflets (where he was the director of the Botanical Museum) and it was quickly forgotten.

3. Although whether this was really an accidental ingestion has been questioned (see *www. erowid.org/general/conferences/conference_ mindstates4_nichols.shtml*): Nichols's hypothesis is that it was not an accidental ingestion at all but a spontaneous mystical experience (which Hofmann writes that he was prone to have) that caused him to focus on LSD-25, the 25th in the series of ergoline derivatives, for whatever reason, and did not actually ingest it. So the "peculiar presentiment" that he refers to in *LSD: My Problem Child* (Hofmann, 2013) may have been a mystical intuition, which Hofmann then confirmed by deliberately ingesting 250 µg the next day.

4. Compare *www.commonwealthclub.org/ events/2018-02-08/timothy-leary-most-dangerous-man-america*.

5. Quite the contrary. Many indigenous societies have demonstrated positive benefits stemming from their use of psychedelics in the context of spiritual practices. It is widely acknowledged among anthropologists that the ritual use of peyote by members of the Native American Church is a bulwark against the diseases and societal dysfunctions attributed to alcoholism (McClusky, 1997). Similarly, members of the UDV, a Brazilian sect that uses ayahuasca sacramentally, insist that their use of the "tea" in religious rituals and in the context of the supportive community environment of the UDV, has enabled them to recover from dysfunctional lives, often marked by alcoholism, drug abuse, and domestic violence (Grob et al., 1996).

6. The notable exception to this was Terence McKenna, who maintained cultural visibility as the chief public advocate of psychedelics, especially psilocybin mushrooms and DMT. Some have cited McKenna as inheriting the mantle of Timothy Leary, but McKenna was less demagogic and far more intellectual than Leary in his approach, which may have insulated him from persecution by the authorities (cf. *http://articles. latimes.com/1996-05-03/news/ls-98_1_timothy-leary03/news/ls-98_1_timothy-leary*).

7. Although Terence, in his introduction to *Psilocybin: Magic Mushrooms Grower's Guide* (Oss, 1976) evoked the meme that the mushrooms had an extraterrestrial origin, they were in fact decidedly "terrestrial" invaders, even though the experiences they evoke often seem like science fiction, tinged with hints of cosmic dimensions and alien beings. I unpack this in my chapter in the book *DMT Dialogues: Encounters with the Spirit Molecule* (McKenna, 2018).

8. Compare, for example, Dr. Rick Strassman on whether psychedelic drugs prove we are more than our brain (*https://skeptiko.com/rick-strassman-psychedelic-drugs-prove-we-are-more-than-our-brain*).

9. Between 2006, the year in which Griffiths's initial study on psilocybin was published, there have been 32 clinical trials listed in the ClinicalTrials.gov database for disorders ranging from substance abuse to PTSD, to intractable depression. Similarly, MDMA has been evaluated in over 183 clinical trials since 1994. It is important to note that not all of the clinical trials listed in ClinicalTrials.gov were conducted under FDA-approved protocols. The database lists clinical trials conducted everywhere in the world. Investigators in the United Kingdom and the European Union have also conducted a comparable number of clinical studies. In particular, Franz Vollenweider's group at the Heffter Zurich Research Center, publishes frequently; it is based at the Psychiatric Hospital in Zurich. There are also very active research groups in the United Kingdom, primarily located at Imperial College London and King's College London.

10. For the backstory on this topic of the corporate co-optation of psychedelics, the reader is advised to consult the recent thoughtful interview with MAPS founder Rick Doblin on the Psychedelic Times website (Thoricatha, 2018). For a distinctly more negative view of Compass and potential improprieties that may have occurred, this article in Quartz is instructive (Goldhill, 2018).

11. This statement from Herbert Schaep, Secretary of the UN Narcotics Control Board, to the Dutch Ministry of Health in regard to a prosecution case in the Netherlands, is instructive: "As you are aware, mushrooms containing the above substances are collected and used for their hallucinogenic effects. As a matter of international law, no plants (natural material) containing psilocine and psilocybin are at present controlled under the Convention on Psychotropic Substances of 1971. Consequently, *preparations made of these plants are not under international control and, therefore, not subject of the articles of the 1971 Convention* [emphasis added]. Criminal cases are decided with reference to domestic law, which may otherwise provide for controls over mushrooms containing psilocine and psilocybin. As the Board can only speak as to the contours of the international drug conventions, I am unable to provide an opinion on the litigation in question" (Schaepe, 2001).

12. The question of whether psilocybin mushrooms themselves, as opposed to the alkaloids they contain, *should* be classed as controlled substances has been the subject of some court cases in the United Kingdom and The Netherlands, with no very satisfactory answer. The current legal status of psilocybin mushrooms in various forms varies widely in different countries. In most countries, mushrooms containing psilocybin are illegal, whether fresh or dried, cultivated or wild. In other countries, distinctions are made. In a few countries, mushrooms are not illegal or illegal, but not enforced. Wikipedia provides a useful chart of the legal status of psilocybin mushrooms in about 30 countries: *https://en.wikipedia.org/wiki/legal_status_of_psilocybin_mushrooms#_netherlands*.

13. In the Canadian Controlled Drugs and Substances Act (Government of Canada, 1996), harmaline and harmalol are both listed under Schedule III. Harmaline and harmol are trace constituents of ayahuasca; harmalol has been reported in one sample in the paper by McKenna, Towers, and Abbott (1984).

14. Compare *http://udvusa.org/supreme-court-case* and *https://scholar.google.com/scholar_case?case=4950416976993015546&q=church+of+the+holy+light+of+the+queen+v.+mukasey&hl=en&as_sdt=6,24&as_vis=1*.

15. San Pedro cactus is the common name for *Echinopsis* (formerly *Trichocereus*) *pachanoi*, one of about 10 species of *Echinopsis* that are utilized in Andean shamanic medicine (*www. erowid.org/plants/cacti/cacti.shtml*).

16. Although psychedelic mushrooms are not plants, they belong to a distinct taxonomic kingdom, but for purposes of this discussion, similar considerations apply when it comes to their regulation. Similar considerations apply to psychedelic animals such as *Bufo alvarius*, the Sonoran

desert toad, whose venom contains high levels of 5-methoxy-DMT.

17. Symbiosis has several technical subdefinitions: *Mutualism* is the close association of organisms of different species for mutual benefit; *commensalism* is a symbiotic relationship in which one species lives with, on, or within another without causing damage to either species; *amensalism* is a relationship between two different species, in which one species is adversely affected by the relationship while the other partner is unaffected; *parasitism* is a type of symbiosis in which one organism lives on or in another and obtains nutrients from it (the host).

18. One could make the case that this kind of mutualistic association between plants and humans, while beneficial to both partners, arises from a cynical self-interest on both sides. We cultivate plants, thus helping them to grow and spread, which seems to be a goal of most plants. We protect them from competition in the wild and ensure their survival as a species, but as part of this devil's bargain, they allow us to manipulate them through artificial selection, such as selective breeding or even direct modification of their genomes. And we may think that we are cultivating plants, which we are, but the plants might say that they are cultivating us! By providing humans with nutrients and other essentials of survival, plants ensure that we stick around to take care of them. Michael Pollan (2007) has written eloquently about this co-exploitation.

▨ References

Drug Enforcement Administration. (2019). Diversion Control Division. Retrieved January 3, 2019, from *www.deadiversion.usdoj.gov/schedules*.

Goldhill, O. (2018). QZ.com: A millionaire couple is threatening to create a magic mushroom monopoly. Retrieved January 3, 2019, from *https://qz.com/1454785/a-millionaire-couple-is-threatening-to-create-a-magic-mushroom-monopoly*.

Government of Canada. (1996). Controlled Drugs and Substances Act. Retrieved January 4, 2019, from *https://laws-lois.justice.gc.ca/eng/acts/C-38.8/page-1.html*.

Griffiths, R. R., Richards, W. A., McCann, U., & Jesse, R. (2006). Psilocybin can occasion mystical-type experiences having substantial and sustained personal meaning and spiritual significance. *Psychopharmacology (Berlin), 187*(3), 268–283; discussion 284–292.

Grob, C. S., Danforth, A. L., Chopra, G. S., Hagerty, M., McKay, C. R., Halberstadt, A. L., et al. (2011). Pilot study of psilocybin treatment for anxiety in patients with advanced-stage cancer. *Archives of General Psychiatry, 68*(1), 71–78.

Grob, C. S., McKenna, D. J., Callaway, J. C., Brito, G. S., Neves, E. S., Oberlaender, G., et al. (1996). Human psychopharmacology of hoasca, a plant hallucinogen used in ritual context in Brazil. *Journal of Nervous and Mental Disease, 184*(2), 86–94.

Halpern, J. H., Sherwood, A. R., Hudson, J. I., Yurgelun-Todd, D., & Pope, H. G., Jr. (2005). Psychological and cognitive effects of long-term peyote use among Native Americans. *Biological Psychiatry, 58*(8), 624–631.

Heffter, A. (1898). Ueber Pellote: Beitrag zue chemischen un pharmakologischen Kenntnis der Cacteen (Zweite MIttheilung) [About peyote: Contribution to the chemical and pharmacological knowledge of the cacti (second part)]. *Archives of Experimental Pathology and Pharmacology, 40,* 423.

Hofmann, A. (1980). *LSD: My problem child.* New York: McGraw-Hill.

Johnson, M. W., Garcia-Romeu, A., Cosimano, M. P., & Griffiths, R. R. (2014). Pilot study of the 5-HT2AR agonist psilocybin in the treatment of tobacco addiction. *Journal of Psychopharmacology, 28*(11), 983–992.

Lash, J. L. (2006). *Not in His image: Gnostic vision, sacred ecology and the future of belief.* White River Junction, VT: Chelsea Green.

McClusky, J. (1997). Native American Church peyotism and the treatment of alcoholism. *MAPS Bulletin, 7*(4), 3–5.

McKenna, D. J. (2018). Is DMT a chemical messenger from an extraterrestrial civilization? In D. Luke, R. Spowers, & A. Bilton (Eds.), *DMT dialogues: Encounters with the spirit molecule* (pp. 38–68). Rochester, VT: Park Street Press.

McKenna, D. J., Towers, G. H. N., & Abbott, F. (1984). Monoamine oxidase inhibitors in South American hallucinogenic plants: Tryptamine and beta-carboline constituents of ayahuasca. *Journal of Ethnopharmacology, 10*(2), 195–223.

Nichols, D. E. (2016). Psychedelics. *Pharmacological Reviews, 68*(2), 264–355.

Oss, O. T., & Oeric, O. N. (1976). *Psilocybin: Magic mushroom grower's guide.* Berkeley, CA: And/Or Press.

Ott, J. (1994). *Ayahuasca analogs: Pangaen entheogens.* Author.

Pollan, M. (2007). *The omnivore's dilemma: A natural history of four meals.* New York: Penguin Press.

Schaepe, H. (2001). UN's INCB Psilocybin Mushroom Policy. Retrieved January 7, 2012, from *erowid.org*.

Schultes, R. E. (1939). The identification of teonanacatl, a narcotic basidiomycete of the Aztecs. *Botanical Museum Leaflets, Harvard University, 7*(3), 37–56.

Schultz, M. (2010). DMT: The spirit molecule. Retrieved January 3, 2091, from *www.imdb.com/title/tt1340425/?ref_=fn_al_tt_1*.

Späth, E. (1919). Über die Anhalonium-Alkaloide: I. Anhalin und Mezcalin [About the anhalonium alkaloids: I. Anhaline and mescaline]. *Monatshefte für Chemie und verwandte Teile anderer Wissenschaften* [*Monthly Notebooks for Chemistry and Related Parts of Other Sciences*], *40*(3), s129–s154.

Spruce, R. (1908). Volume I. In A. R. Wallace (Ed.), *Notes of a botanist on the Amazon and Andes*. London: Macmillan.

Stannard, D. E. (1992). *American Holocaust: Columbus and the conquest of the New World*. Oxford, UK: Oxford University Press.

Stolaroff, M. J. (1997). *The secret chief: Conversations with a pioneer of the underground psychedelic therapy movement*. Sarasota, FL: MAPS.

Strassman, R. J. (2001). *DMT: The spirit molecule: A doctor's revolutionary research into the biology of near death and mystical experiences*. Rochester, VT: Park Street Press.

Strassman, R. J., & Qualls, C. R. (1994). Dose–response study of *N,N*-dimethyltryptamine in humans: I. Neuroendocrine, autonomic, and cardiovascular effects. *Archives of General Psychiatry, 51*(2), 85–97.

Strassman, R. J., Qualls, C. R., Uhlenhuth, E. H., & Kellner, R. (1994). Dose–response study of *N,N*-imethyltryptamine in humans: II. Subjective effects and preliminary results of a new rating scale. *Archives of General Psychiatry, 51*(2), 98–108.

Thoricatha, W. (2018). Let's talk about compass and psychedelic capitalism: An interview with Rick Doblin. Retrieved January 3, 2019, from *https://psychedelictimes.com/interviews/lets-talk-about-compass-and-psychedelic-capitalism-interview-with-rick-doblin*.

United Nations. (1971). International Narcotics Control Board. Retrieved December, 28, 2018, from *www.incb.org/incb/en/psychotropics/1971_convention.html*.

Wasson, R. G. (1957, May 13). Secret of "divine mushrooms." *Life*, pp. 100–120.

CHAPTER 3

Anthropology, Shamanism, and Hallucinogens

MICHAEL J. WINKELMAN

▓ Introduction

The modern encounter with hallucinogens was embedded in the distorted views of witchcraft when knowledge about these substances returned to the Western imagination. The European rediscovery of hallucinogens was distorted by Christian frameworks that labeled as devil worship the indigenous spiritual, healing, and ritual practices encountered during the European colonization of the world. Later, through the lens of anthropologists, the Western World began a rediscovery of the spiritual and therapeutic potentials embodied in the uses of hallucinogenic mushrooms, snuffs, brews, and enemas (see Rätsch, 2005; Schultes, Hofmann, & Rätsch, 1992; Schultes & Winkelman, 1996).

Anthropology has provided perspectives for understanding hallucinogens through ethnographic, cross-cultural, and biological approaches that have identified the diverse roles these substances have played across cultures and over time. As anthropologists, ethnobotanists, and historians documented the use hallucinogenic substances and shared their knowledge, they contributed to a revitalization of Western practices of healing using the alterations of consciousness produced by these substances. Their ancient applications for healing involved the shamanic ritual, which was the institutionalized context for most hallucinogen use found worldwide. To shamans, these plants are *entheogens,* agents for producing an experience of engagement with the spirit world. Given that modern medicine has discovered a wide range of conditions that can be effectively treated by these substances (see Winkelman & Roberts, 2007; Winkelman & Sessa, 2019), shamans undoubtedly also were able to exploit their effectiveness for many conditions.

Anthropology's cross-cultural and biological approaches provide an understanding of the biological basis of the cross-cultural similarities in shamanic healing practices and how they relate to psychedelics and their effects on our evolved social psychology (Winkelman, 2010b, 2013, 2017). Shamanic healing practices and beliefs exhibit cross-cultural similarities, common patterns manifested in communal ritual practices of foraging societies worldwide. Universal features of shamanism, such as alteration of consciousness, healing, and engagement with an animistic world reflect biological effects of psychedelics (Winkelman, 2010b, 2013).

Shamanic practices and beliefs are directly related to the principal neurological effects of psychedelics, a neurophenomenological relationship in which the phenomenological aspects of experience are directly related to the effects of psychedelics on brain operations and functions (see Winkelman, 2013, 2018). These neurophenomenological dynamics produced by shamanic use of hallucinogens involve activation of innate cognitive modules or intelligences (for discussion, see Winkelman, 2018). These neurological effects of psychedelics elicit underlying biological systems that provide a basis for the central elements of shamanism, such as an animistic worldview embracing the idea that spirits are a fundamental aspect of reality, an engagement with one's identity in relationship to an animal; a spiritual transformation manifested in a death-and-rebirth experiences; and an awareness of one's own soul or spirit, exemplified in out-of-body experiences.

Anthropology's biocultural approach has provided a platform for integration of biological and evolutionary perspectives in understanding the interaction of hallucinogens and shamanism in human evolution and the development of culture, healing, and spirituality (Winkelman, 2009, 2010b, 2014). This chapter addresses how hallucinogens have contributed to the evolution of an institution involving innate healing processes—shamanism—and how shamanic perspectives can provide guidelines for their therapeutic application. Shamanic engagement with hallucinogens involved their roles as entheogens or spiritual agents, and for facilitating integrative processes. The various shamanic practices for using these substances can provide guidelines for modern therapeutic applications (Winkelman, 2007).

Psychedelics and Humans' Evolved Ecopsychology

There is a long-term evolutionary relationship between humans and psychotropic plant substances that reflects their selective effects on our evolution (Sullivan, Hagen, & Hammerstein, 2008; Winkelman, 2014). Evolutionary paradigms propose that our ancestors acquired fitness benefits as a consequence of ingestion of psychoactive substances that enhanced neurotransmitter functions. Ancient environmental exposures to plant substances had effects on human evolution. Psychedelics have deep evolutionary roots with human's evolved ecopsychology through their relationship to our nervous system and their effects on personal awareness, social and environmental relations, and consciousness.

Ancient humans' engagement with psychedelics was an inevitable consequence of the presence of psilocybin-containing mushrooms in environments around the world. Species containing psilocybin are found across most ecozones around the world (Guzman, Allen, & Gartz, 1998), exposing hominins to their effects for millions of years. Adaptation to the fungi in their environment—especially distinctions among toxic, comestible, and psychedelic ones—was a significant feature affecting survival. We have a many million-year history of acquiring biological and cultural adaptations to distinguish those mushroom species, with fatal toxic effects from those that can serve as food sources or produce mystical experiences. The presence of psilocybin-containing genera and diverse species across many ecozones ensured that human ancestors encountered and ingested psilocybin-containing mushrooms, allowing these to act as environmental factors in the selection for the characteristics of the human brain and our innate ecopsychology. Selective effects of an environmental factor—psychedelic mushrooms—shaped the evolution of human psychology, sociality, and cognition.

A Shamanic Ecopsychology

Humanity's evolved psychology involves capacities that resulted from interaction with these exogenous sources of neurotransmitter analogues because their effects on neural transmission enhanced the operation of our neuromodulatory systems, especially serotonin and dopamine. The consequences of the augmentation of these neurotransmitter systems is a worldview of interconnectedness; social orientation to altruism, cooperation, and enhanced bonding; reductions in defensiveness, fear, and anxiety; an enhanced visual representation system that promoted cognitive integration; as well as connection and identity with nature in a sense of spirituality.

Psychedelics' Emotional Effects in Human Adaptation

Psychedelics' effects on cognition, emotions, and behavior provided mechanisms by which these substances played roles as environmental factors in affecting the dynamic of relationships with "others"—humans, as well as spirits. Psilocybin produces biases towards positive emotions in social relations (Kometer et al., 2012) and reduces threat responses by shifting emotional biases to positive evaluations by decreasing visual threat processing. Psilocybin reduces reactions of the amygdala in tuning of visual regions to threats, shifting emotional processing toward positive valence (Kraehenmann et al., 2014), decreasing top-down connectivity involved in visual threat processing, and shifting emotional biases away from negative interpretations. Lysergic acid diethylamide (LSD) has a similar dynamic in its acute effects on emotional processing, impairing recognition of sad and fearful faces, while increasing feelings of happiness and trust, closeness to others, emotional empathy and desire to be with others, and prosocial behavior (paraphrasing Dolder, Schmid, Muller, Borgwardt, & Liechti, 2016, p. 2638). Acute doses involving as little as one administration of a serotonergic psychedelic produces significant therapeutic changes in personality at least for the short term through producing changes in openness. A study by Erritzoe and colleagues (2018) reinforces these findings with results from a psilocybin therapy study that found significant reductions in scores on neuroticism scales and increases in extraversion and openness scores. These effects of enhancing positive interpersonal relations could have played a role in selecting for traits that increased social cohesion.

Shamanism: The Institutionalization of Hallucinogen Use

Shamanism is at the origins of the human engagement with hallucinogens use, provid-ing the ritual context within which humans' innate psychology was selected for qualities elicited by the psychedelics' neurological effects and exploited by ritual processes. This interaction of shamanism and psychedelics contributed to selection for a variety of features of human cognition and sociality, particularly relations with nature and in the qualities of our self and others. Entheogens shaped our evolved psychology through their intrinsic animistic and spiritual effects. These influences also contributed to the origins of ritual healing practices, the formation of our evolved sociality and psychology, and the evolution of society (Winkelman, 2013, 2015).

Psychedelics exercised their selective influences in the context of participation in ritual and healing activities, which were enhanced by the effects of psychedelics (enhanced serotonergic activation and secondary dopamine release) and the ability to benefit from the resultant psychological, emotional, and behavioral experiences. A shamanic ecopsychology reflects the selective influences exercised by psychedelic-induced visionary experiences for enhanced ritual participation through hypnotic and placebo susceptibility and enhanced fluidity of cognition. This interaction of psychedelic effects and shamanic ritual together contributed to the selection for ritual healing responses and the associated psychological, social, and cognitive tendencies that enhanced the elicitation of processes.

■ Shamanism as a Cross-Cultural Complex

The existence of a worldwide shamanic complex involving similar spiritual healing practices has been long noted in anthropology and comparative religion, and even in 18th-century Europe the concept informed the thinking about the foreign "other" (Flaherty, 1992). Long before the mid-20th-century publication of Eliade's (1954) now classic book entitled *Shamanism: Archaic Techniques of Ecstasy,* the notion of the shaman had become popularized in Western society, especially among intellectuals, and the term *saman,* borrowed from the Tungusic language of Siberia, acquired the status of a general concept. The shaman reflected widespread similarities in premodern spiritual healing practices that were inferred to be core aspects of prehistorical religion.

Eliade's intuitions about the fundamental similarity in ritual healers around the world were confirmed by empirical cross-cultural research (Winkelman, 1986, 1990, 1992). Using a formal cross-cultural sample and quantitative methods, Winkelman established the presence of virtually identical practices in the foraging cultures of the premodern world that survived even as societies evolved agriculture but soon disappeared with agricultural intensification, warfare, and political incorporation (integration). These common patterns of behavior and belief, which we call *shamanism*, were virtually universal in foraging societies but declined, transformed, and disappeared under the effects of agricultural transformation and political developments that eliminated the cultures with egalitarian foraging lifestyles that supported shamanic activities.

Cross-Cultural Features of Shamanism

Winkelman's formal cross-cultural research confirmed many of the features that Eliade alleged to be associated with shamanism in societies worldwide, revealing a biogenetic shamanic paradigm (Winkelman, 2010a, 2010b, 2015). These features included the following:

- The shaman's presence as the preeminent social leader with a central role in the group's political life, as well as spiritual and healing activities.
- The shaman's role as the leader of a communitywide nighttime ritual performance involving the shaman's charismatic enactment of an encounter with the spirit world.
- The ritual production of a dramatic alterations of consciousness interpreted as an engagement with and entry into the spirit world.
- The alteration of consciousness though physical austerities such as fasting water deprivation, avoidances of specific foods and sexual abstinence, and ritual drivers based in activities such as extensive drum-

ming, prolonged dancing, individual and collective chanting and singing, and frequently through the use of psychedelics and other vision-producing plants.

- A specific alteration of consciousness conceptualized as flight, similar to modern astral projection, out-of-body and near-death experiences, in which the shaman, while in a period of physical collapse and appearing unconscious, experienced an entry into the spirit world.
- An engagement with ritual activities of healing focused on divining the cause of illness and treating conditions attributed to soul loss, the extraction of internal objects sent by sorcerers to cause illness and death, and the removal of the negative spirit influences.
- A selection for the position through special encounters with spirits in the forest, hallucinations, illness, and special dreams.
- A period of training involving austerities and prolonged periods of solitude in the wilderness, often characterized as a vision quest that involved a visual encounter with spiritual entities that empowered the shaman.
- Typically, the use of special plants, particularly entheogens, emetics, and various power plants thought to provide teachings from their inherent spirit beings.
- An initiatory experience involving the experience of personal death, often involving being attacked, killed, and devoured by animals.
- A rebirth experience in which the initiate was reconstructed by animals that incorporated their powers into a new person who could use their abilities.
- The source of shamanic power deriving from special relations with animals.
- The shamanic ability to use relations with animal spirits to divine, heal, and kill.
- The ability of the shaman to experience a personal transformation into an animal.
- The belief and practices concerning the shamans' ability to cause harm to others and kill them magically through intrusive darts or soul theft.
- Other special abilities, including immunity to fire and power to control the weather and animals.

Entheogens in Shamanism

Central to many shamanic traditions were beliefs regarding the origins of shamanic power in the indwelling qualities of special plants some call hallucinogens. However, from a shamanic perspective, these plants are understood as sources of visionary inspiration and novel information, and as entheogens, substances that stimulate inherent spiritual properties. The concept of hallucinogen, implying false perceptions and distortions of reality, contradicts the bases of the shamanic engagement with these visionary experiences as accessing a superordinate reality. The shamanic engagement with vision-producing substances of the plant world was conceptualized as an engagement with a spirit world revealed in the visionary experiences. Spirit world visions and engagement with spiritual beings are central to shamanism, and the entheogens are powerful tools for inducing these experiences. The ritual performance during the darkness of night and with an eyes-closed, internal focus of attention facilitate this engagement with visionary experiences.

This notion of a spiritual contact through special plant deities is widely attested to in traditions of shamanism, among classical civilizations, and in many modern and postmodern contexts in which these substances are viewed as having intrinsic spiritual properties and a sentient intelligence. In the shamanic context, they are used as entheogens and are known for an ability to engage a personal experience of transformation into an animal. In mystical and meditative contexts, their ability to evoke visionary powers and transcendent realizations made them powerful tools for the expansion of consciousness.

The premodern uses of hallucinogens are almost coterminous with the practices of shamanism, where they were typically used to produce a direct engagement with the supernatural and the mythical world. Typically, these entheogenic engagements produced an experience of the separation of one's soul or spirit from the body, enabling one to travel to and interact with the beings of the supernatural world. For the shaman, these plants were teachers that enabled one to activate latent abilities and harness powers found within oneself and in the supernatural universe. Of particular significance were the relationships established with animals that permitted the experience of a personal transformation into an animal and the acquisition of its powers. These powers and the visionary experiences engaged through the entheogens permitted the shaman to divine the causes of illness and to heal them. In addition to shamanic training, entheogens were used for healing and in initiations and community ceremonies (Andritzky, 1989).

The parallels of shamanism with the effects of psilocybin reinforce the need to understand their roles in the creation of shamanism. Psychedelics, particularly psilocybin-containing mushrooms, but also a wide range of other substances, produce a specific spectrum of experiences summarized by Winkelman (2010b, 2013):

- A direct experience of a supernatural world of spirits and mythical entities.
- An experience of the separation of one's soul or spirit from the body and its travel to the supernatural world.
- A death of the ego and its rebirth, providing a process of self-transformation.
- Information manifested in visions.
- Powers activated within and outside of the person, including the incorporation of spirits into one's body.
- Relationships with animals, particularly carnivores, that provide a source of power.
- Experiences of transformation into an animal.

▨ Entheogenic Nature: Animism and the Origins of Shamanic Ecopsychology

Entheogenic experiences of spiritual qualities of nature reflect the concept of animism, a foundational principle of shamanism. The central effects of entheogens enhance the experience of animism, in which animals, plants and even rocks, water, and the wind are experienced as living, sentient beings. This experience of a living and personified essence to nature involves the projection of the fundamental structures of human consciousness and our intentional, cognitive, and self qualities to nature (Winkelman, 2004, 2013, 2019; Winkelman & Baker, 2016).

Shamanism elaborated this animistic perspective in the development of extended awareness of the sentience of nature, attributing the qualities of human consciousness, meaning, and intentionality to the natural world. The natural tendency of humans to attribute mind states, internal dispositions, and rational purpose to others is unavoidably attributed to nature as well. The universality of spiritual beliefs reflects this adaptive tendency, which was expanded into the attribution to nature of spirit beings operating with human-like features.

Animism expressed a foundational feature of shamanism that is manifested in sentient animal entities with human-like properties. This animistic perception of nature as a living entity is anthropomorphized, seen in human terms, exemplified in the entheogenic perspective of special relations with teaching spirits that are inherent to these plants and express themselves through humans when ingested. Shamanism is based in these personified influences of these plants, with the plant spirits fundamental to shamanic concepts of self powers and environmental relations, a shamanic ecopsychology that conceptualized psychedelic plants as embodying sentient beings with intelligence and purpose.

The animistic tendency expands on our basic propensity for detection of animate entities, with a special capacity for engaging animals, reflecting what evolutionary psychologists have identified as an innate natural intelligence of humans for recognizing species essences and categorizing species of animals (for discussion, see Winkelman, 2010b, 2019). Given the importance of animals to human survival, their species qualities are part of our unconsciousness mental capacity, an innate intelligence for recognizing species characteristics and responding to them. Shamans derived power from special relations with animals and the ability to control their spirits and used our innate capacities for recognizing animal features as a framework to enhance our conceptualization of our personal and social qualities.

This innate capacity for species recognition is a part of our evolved psychology that provides a basis for a natural symbol system that expresses metaphorical meanings embodied in the various qualities of animal species (Winkelman, 2010b). This specialized innate capacity for organizing knowledge about animal species provided a universal analogical system for creation of meaning. Capacities for recognizing animal species and their variant qualities were the natural framework for creating symbols for elaborating psychological and social identity.

These engagements exploit humans' innate social intelligence, our capacities for inferring the mental states of others and predicting their expectations (i.e., in social roles), as well as their future behavior. Psychedelics enhance this intuitive "theory of mind," engaging in attributions of mental states exemplified in the perception of the entheogenic others with messages and teachings.

Animism and Self-Development

Shamanism was the context within our innate animal intelligence that was elaborated as a symbol system for process of self-differentiation, manifested in animals and their qualities. This ability to use intrinsic features of species is exemplified in the shamanic animal guardian spirit powers, which involve representations of self qualities as involving an animal. Shamanic animal allies and guardian spirits engage self-development and self-representation through the capacity to incorporate others' perceptions into the self, extending this innate process of social internalization to internalizing the qualities of animal species into our self-identity. Consequently, the variant qualities of animal species were the natural intelligence context within which human psychological development was elaborated, incorporating the properties of animals in self-concept and social representations.

The shamanic self-identifications with a personified and sentient nature has entheogenic roots within shamanism, in which these plants were conceptualized as containing teachers, spirits, and even gods; they were often manifested as animals, exemplified in the association of ayahuasca with the jaguar and anaconda, of the peyote with the deer among the Huichol, and the association of *Amanita muscaria* with reindeer. Entheogens are known for stimulating this sense of an animal being incorporated within the body and expressed through the self or provoking an experience of one's transformation into an animal. This sense of animal presence and identity is frequently stimulated by psychedelics, which served as tools to enhance the incorporation of these animal qualities as personal capacities.

Engagement of these animal spirit constructs in shamanic practice provided representations of the personal unconscious, as well as the intrapsychic and social dynamics involved in the management of emotions (Winkelman, 2010b). This animistic dynamic is manifested in shamanic concepts such as guardian spirits, which serve as sources of power for the shaman, and represent personal and social identity, and other psychodynamic processes (i.e., self, id, ego, superego). The concept of animal spirits also reflects the dynamics of humans' lower brain processes, particularly those involving the paleomammalian and reptilian brains (see Winkelman, 2010b, for sources and discussion). Our tendency for self-representation as animals is deeply rooted in the human psyche, a neurophenomenological manifestation of the dynamics of these brain structures humans share with other animals (i.e., the reptilian complex and paleomammalian brain) and that produce the bodily forms of awareness we share with other animals. The ancient structures of the brain are experienced as spirits, externalized entities that reflect the dynamic processes of the subconscious.

These features of the emotional brain are the focus of the effects of shamanic ritual engagement, which manipulates and restructures their relations through alterations of consciousness. The ritual enactments of shamanism were designed to manipulate emotions and self-concept in order to heal through inducing vagal, personal, psychological and social integration. Animal spirits are a part of this natural psychology, providing powers and enhancing self-esteem and personal identity.

Animal spirits were the basis of shamanic power and were extended as a template in which the animal species of nature functioned as a natural model for understanding groups and society. The shamanic power animals that constitute basic aspects of the self were extended in the practices of totemism, which used these animal species concepts and their natural qualities as an innate template for conceptualizations of social groups, being symbols of lineages, clans, tribes and nations—and even sports team.

▪ Shamanic Uses of Entheogens

The ethnographic record illustrates that shamanic use of entheogenic substances engaged botanical diversity, a wide range of fungi and plant families that were used in shamanic contexts (see Rätsch, 2005; Schultes et al., 1992; Schultes & Winkelman, 1996). While evidence remains of the existence of ancient psychedelic use for their spiritual, entheogenic, and therapeutic properties in cultures around the world (Winkelman, 2019), the most complete descriptions available to modern anthropology were in the Americas: the Myristicaceae and Leguminosae families used for snuffs (i.e., *Anadenanthera* and *Virola*); the Cactaceae family, especially peyote (*Lophophora williamsii*) and San Pedro cactus (*Trichocereus* species); the enigmatic ayahuasca brews that combine the vines of *Banisteriopsis* with the leaves of *Psychotria* species or other *N,N*-dimethyltryptamine (DMT)-containing sources; and psilocybin-containing mushrooms of the Strophariaceae family, especially *Psilocybe* (Schultes & Winkelman, 1996).

In addition to the use of entheogens as therapeutic agents and for diagnostic procedures to determine the cause of illness, shamanistic practices incorporated them in the training of initiate shamans and in communal ceremonies for a ritual integration of the group for the enhancement of social cohesion. In many cultures, the training of shamans involved prolonged use of psychedelic plants by neophytes, generally under the supervision of their teachers. Luna (1986) describes this entheogenic use of ayahuasca during training among the *vegetalista* traditions of Amazonia, where, during long periods of isolation in the forest and under the influence of large doses of ayahuasca, the shaman-initiate learns directly from the spirits during visionary experiences. This supervision by an experienced practitioner was seen as protecting the novice from not just physical dangers but also particularly the dangers posed by evil spirits and sorcerers.

Training often involved repeated ingestion of large amounts of psychedelic plants while maintaining a strict diet. Initiates may ingest entheogens repeatedly over a period of months or even years as part of training and developing their personal power (Luna, 1986). This prolonged ingestion was seen as a necessary tool for entering into the spirit world. Key aspects of the effects of entheogens involve the manifestations of the "plant teachers" who represented the spirits of the plants and provided specific forms of knowledge and power. Shamanic traditions viewed these initiatory experiences with the plants as leading one to a higher level of reality, providing access to a knowledge of metaphysical and transcendent realms that gave the shaman a superhuman status. A widely noted cross-cultural use of psychedelics involves contexts in which elders guide ritual focused on the adult transition or resocialization for adult roles, often involving collective puberty or initiation rites.

■ Therapeutic Uses of Hallucinogens

The therapeutic use of hallucinogenic substances was central to shamanistic ritual healing practices in societies worldwide that constitute repositories for millennia of knowledge and clinical experience regarding their therapeutic applications. Shamanic ethnomedical traditions constitute a valuable set of guidelines regarding areas of clinical application, as well as best practices for the employment of these substances.

Shamanic entheogenic therapy generally involves the ingestion of the medicine by the therapist, in addition to the patient. The ingestion of the plant was seen as enhancing the shaman's diagnostic skills to identify the cause of illnesses and the procedures for resolving them, as well as activation of their healing powers. Entheogens were viewed as means to gain access to the spiritual and visionary dimensions, and the knowledge and power necessary to heal.

There are hundreds of entheogenic/hallucinogenic plants that have been used by humanity, only a few of which are well documented. Most of our knowledge of this ethnobotanical and ethnopharmacological diversity disappeared under the onslaught of Western colonial expansionism. Yet we do have a few well-documented traditions, among them the use of psilocybin in Mesoamerica and the trans-Amazonian ayahuasca practices.

Mescaline-Containing Cactus

Of the many cacti with hallucinogenic properties, the most widely known are *Lophophora williamsii* (peyote) and the *Trichocereus* species, known as San Pedro cactus. Peyote is considered to have general healing properties in cleansing the stomach, kidneys, liver, and blood (see Schultes & Winkelman, 1996). Peyote is also used for curing, protection against witches and ghosts, maintaining good health and mind, incentives to work, release from guilt, temperance from alcohol, transcendence, overcoming misfortunes, guidance and future good fortune, access to knowledge, foretelling future occurrences, and motivation. In the Native American Church, it serves to give purpose in life, internal peace and harmony, a reference group, meet needs for approval and esteem, validation of identity, and fostering an adaptation to the dominant society. *Trichocereus* species are used to solve many different kinds of problems—witchcraft and hexes, illness caused by resentment and envy, and imbalances in the spiritual and natural forces in the patient's life. The rituals serve as a means for integrating the ancient ancestral traditions into current adaptations through manipulation of aspects of the subconscious mind. Ritual processes transform individual personality and social relations through symbolic mediation that integrates psychological, social, and cosmological levels of meaning.

Snuffs

The snuffs used widely in the Andean highlands across the length of South America had a variety of medical, religious, and social purposes. The active principles in the snuffs made from species of *Virola* are tryptamines (various forms of DMT); similar bioactive constituents are found in the *Anadenanthera* (Schultes et al., 1992). *Virola* snuffs were employed for a variety of physical problems, especially stomach and bladder problems, malaria, intestinal worms, hemorrhoid,; mouth sores, cuts and wounds, rheumatism and swollen joints, and childbirth problems. In addition to traditional shamanic uses in the diagnosis and treatment of diseases and witchcraft, the snuffs had broader social functions when employed in intervillage feasts focused on building and solidifying alliances. The snuffs have been noted to provoke a release of the emotions and strains of everyday life, and also to stimulate antisocial behavior, including personal violence and homicide. The *Anadenanthera* snuffs had a central function in shamanistic practices, first in diagnosis for healing, and as a medicine. The snuffs were also used to induce courage, strength, and heighten vision, and alertness and stamina during hunting and battle. They had sorcery functions in rituals to cause illness and misfortune to enemies and for foretelling the future. *Anadenanthera* was also employed in social rituals such as fertility rites, annual harvest festivals, cremation ceremonies and ancestor worship, and other festive gatherings, such as mock intervillage battles.

Ayahuasca

Ayahuasca is a particularly complex hallucinogen that combines the MAO-inhibiting effects of the harmines of *Banisteriopsis* in order to protect from enzymatic degradation the DMT sources derived from leaves of *Psychotria* species or other DMT-containing plants. Ayahuasca has been used for many functions, including in divinatory and healing ceremonies (Dobkin de Rios, 1984). Shamanic uses include acquisition of protective spirits, prophesizing the future, sending messages to others or contacting distant relatives, and discovering enemies' plans. Ayahuasca was also used in preparation for war or hunting expeditions. A notable context of premodern ayahuasca involved cleansing ceremonies preceding and following the victory feast held to commemorate a successful head-hunting expedition. Collective ayahuasca ceremonies also marked male reunions of the extended nonresidential kinship groups, bringing together distant clans of a kin group. Ayahuasca was used

to reduce the potentially conflictive relations among the distant relatives. Ayahuasca was also used at funerals to facilitate the release of grief and anger, and transformation of these emotions into joy. Ayahuasca also had ritual functions in establishing intervillage relations; providing assistance in learning myths, art, chants, and dances; and for obtaining guidance in life. It is also used to treat a range of culture-bound syndromes— *susto* (fear), causing the loss of the person's soul; *daño* (harm), caused by sorcery, envy, or desire for vengeance; and *mal de ojo* (evil eye). In communal ritual it is consumed by adult group members in psycho- and sociotherapeutic treatments to deal with the problems of acculturation and to mediate between cultural worlds in creating a synthesis to manage culture change through symbolic confrontation. It is also used to treat social and sexual dysfunctions, emotional problems, and psychological, somatic, and physical problems, and as a preventative against all sorts of diseases. Contemporary uses of ayahuasca among modern peoples tend to focus more on psychological and spiritual issues (Winkelman, 2005).

Psilocybin-Containing Mushrooms

One of the widely recognized shamanistic therapeutic practices involves the use of mushroom species containing psilocybin, which are found in ancient cultures across most of the world (Winkelman, 2019). The best known of such practices involve numerous cultural groups in Mexico, ranging from prehistorical Mayan groups of the Yucatan peninsula, the historical Aztecs and the contemporary Mazatec, exemplified in the famous Maria Sabina. The Aztecs referred to this psychedelic fungus as *teonanacatl*, meaning "food of the gods." The shamanistic use of these mushrooms is documented across Mexico and Guatemala, with evidence of prehistoric use found in frescoes from central Mexico and the "mushroom stones" in highland Mayan areas of Guatemala dating back thousands of years.

The sensationalistic early European reports of Aztec cult uses of mushrooms generally offered little more than gross descriptions, failing to understand the cultural reasons for use. The European perspective viewed these substances as tools of the devil, and the practitioners were brutally tortured, and the practices repressed. The ritual use of the psychedelic mushrooms nonetheless survived and is still found across many areas of Mexico, with dozens of species of *Panaeolus, Psilocybe,* and *Stropharia* employed in shamanistic ritual activities.

Maria Sabina: The Mazatec "Wise Woman"

They indigenous use of psilocybin mushrooms returned to the attention of Western scholars in the early 20th century, when they were identified by anthropologists and ethnobotanists who encountered their magicoreligious use in Oaxaca, Mexico (for review, see Schultes & Winkelman, 1996; material in this section sourced there). The investigations of ritual mushrooms use among the Mazatec of Mexico by Schultes and others were the basis for the subsequent popularizations in the publications of Gordon Wasson (1980; Wasson, Cowan, & Rhodes, 1974). Prominent publications in *Life* magazine brought international attention to the Mazatec *sabia,* or wise woman, Maria Sabina, a shamanistic practitioner who used various psychedelic plant species for healing based in ancient traditions.

Maria Sabina's practices have obvious Christian influences, but her life and healing activities nonetheless illustrate some of the traits associated with the ancient pre-Columbian Mesoamerican use of mushrooms in healing rites. Among the features of her life that exhibit strong shamanistic elements are the processes of selection and training, the therapeutic practices, and the cosmologies regarding the causes of illness.

The life of Maria Sabina has many elements that reflect shamanic roots found worldwide in entheogenic traditions (see Estrada, 1981; Munn, 1973; Wasson, 1980; Wasson et al., 1974). Maria Sabina came from a lineage of "wise ones," with both paternal and maternal grandparents having worked as healers.

Maria Sabina began her learning at about age 6, when she began to ingest mushrooms out of hunger. Maria Sabina received a call to use to mushrooms, with these "saintly children" calling to her in her periods of hunger in the forest and telling her to eat

them for sustenance and inspiration. She experienced the mushrooms speaking to her, encouraging her, and giving her hope and sustenance in the visions and voices that offered her advice about how to address her life problems and eventually giving her the wisdom to cured illness. It was during one of these episodes that she received information about her sister's illness and how to heal her.

This direct interaction with the spirit power of the mushrooms was central to her personal development and healing practices. The ingestion of the mushrooms provides the spiritual contact that engages training for use of the sacred mushrooms, which are believed to be agents responsible for giving wisdom and enabling healing. The personification of the mushrooms is reflected in the terms used to refer to them, such as *saint children, little women, little nuns,* and *children who sprout.* These personifications also include Christian influences, with an equivalence reported between mushrooms and the Virgin Mary and Jesus Christ (Estrada, 1981; Wasson et al., 1974). In addition to the mushrooms, Maria Sabina and other Mazatec healers use other psychoactive plants, including *Salvia divinorum* and local tobacco (*Nicotiana rustica*).

Like shamans worldwide, Maria Sabina saw herself as having been selected from birth to be a healer, a potential that unfolded as consumption of the mushrooms gave her the wisdom necessary to perform the rituals of healing with the mushrooms. The idea that these plants contain sentient beings that communicate directly with the practitioner is evidenced in her extensive engagement with the "language of the mushrooms." These communications from the mushrooms are involved in both the training and professional practice of the wise ones, providing the information used to diagnose and heal. The wisdom of the mushroom healers is not learned from humans but is acquired directly from the mushrooms when their force enters into the healer's body and speaks directly to the person, telling the source of the problem and what to do to resolve it. In this sense, the formation of a mushroom healer involves a process of self-initiation in which the neophyte is taught directly by the spirits of the mushrooms. The visionary experiences induced by the mushrooms reveal the higher sources of spiritual authority and the knowledge embodied in a book of Wisdom or book of language. These spiritual texts are used to heal, a power derived from the "language of the mushrooms" that emerges in the songs of the healer when the mushrooms are consumed. The powers of the mushrooms are thought to act through the body of the shaman during the ritual, speaking and engaging in healing processes.

In the context of the ritual healing, an all-night vigil is held in the darkness in a remote house. There are generally a number of restrictions for those who wish to participate in the ceremonies that require a fast from breakfast on, a prohibition on sexual behavior and alcohol consumption for four days prior to and following the ceremony. The ill person, along with the family and other members of the community, gather together within the room, where they generally remain overnight. The healing *veladas* are normally held to seek a remedy to a persistent health problem, but they may be used for acquiring solutions to other family problems. The *velada* is typically focused on curing illness or to determine the possibility of recovery from some disease. It may also be employed in divinatory practices to locate lost animals or to discover the situation of family members who have traveled away.

While the healer always ingests the mushrooms, the healer decides whether the patients and others will ingest the mushrooms as well; this is often accompanied by a cup of *cacao* (chocolate). The mushrooms are normally eaten raw, but they may be pressed to release the juice, which is then drunk. When ingested, the mushrooms provide a vision of the cause of illness and the songs that the healer needs to sing to produce a cure. Among other ritual activities is the use of the local the San Pedro tobacco, which is mixed with lime and garlic, then rubbed on the sick person or ingested in order to increase the healing force of the mushrooms.

The healing *velada* involves singing and chanting, along with other vocalizations such as whistling, humming, and ventriloquistic effects, as well as dancing and percussive artistry by the healer. The healer chants monophonically during much of the night, starting with low moans that grow louder and emerge into sustained humming.

The humming is followed single-syllable chants that eventually coalesce into words, chanting, and oracular utterances that continue throughout the night. The healing force comes from the healer's and patient's visions that reveal the origin of the problem.

The *Psilocybe* species has a variety of shamanic, spiritual, and therapeutic applications, such as removing hexes and witchcraft, addressing soul/spirit loss and resolving spirit afflictions, and providing exorcism; it also is used for physical maladies, including fever and chills, toothache, pimples, and pain, and to address social problems in resolving quarrels and disputes (Schultes & Winkelman, 1996). The healer may address the actions of evil spirits, hexes performed by sorcerers and witches, or the consequence of the soul or spirit of the person being robbed or enchanted by evil spirits or sorcerers. These agents or influences are driven from the body by the healer, who clears away bad spirits or "airs," purifies the patient from sins, and undoes the effects of witchcraft. Ritual responses include evocation of the saints, application of herbal remedies, commanding evil influences to leave, and the direction of healing energies to the patient. Other healing effects come from the patient's visionary experiences, often of a terrifying nature that provokes vomiting, crying, and other emotional and cathartic reactions.

The mushrooms *veladas* incorporate a variety of therapeutic modalities to enhance the chanting and singing that occurs throughout the *velada*. The healers' use of sacred language is a "poetic art" (Munn, 1973) that uses the words and sounds as tools for the elicitation and catharsis of emotions. Maria Sabina's use of language in not only singing and chanting but also other kinds of utterances manifests a rhythmic quality that suggests that they function as procedures for altering consciousness and enhancing the healer's self-presentation as they unfold a dialogue in which she associates herself with both indigenous and Christian supernatural figures. These associations, along with the explicit content of the chants, reveal their therapeutic role in enhancing the patient's belief in the healer's power, encouraging positive expectations producing cathartic experiences.

▓ Shamanic Ritual Procedures for Managing Consciousness

Shamanic use of entheogens involves a variety of preparatory procedures and ritual practices designed to enhance and control alterations of consciousness. A part of the broader principles of entheogen use is a variety of ritualized contexts for collection, preparation, and consumption of the sacrament. Shamanic emphasis on ritual processes provides a context to engage our biogenetic mammalian adaptations for structured interactions that engage emotional and social coordination.

Shamanic traditions utilize a variety of mechanisms for inducing alterations of consciousness that help produce the entheogenic encounter, beginning with preparation involving fasting, periods alone in the wilderness, and vigorous drumming, singing, and dancing. These mimetic and enactive techniques of drumming, singing, and dancing evoke ancient structures of human consciousness involving communicative systems that are widespread in primates, and especially the great apes, in their nocturnal collective singing (Winkelman, 2015). This utilization of ancient expressive structures of the primate brain engages with our own animal nature in the powers of our unconscious (Winkelman, 2010b).

Food Restrictions

Diet is considered central to shamanic formation and practice, with dieting in general and restrictions on specific foods generally required for days to week or even months preceding and following the use of entheogens. These traditions of dieting and specific food restrictions are typified in the contemporary ayahuasca traditions that emphasize periods of restricted diet before and after the sessions, as well as specific restrictions on diet following the experiences (i.e., prohibitions on salt, sugar, alcohol, pork, beef, with permitted foods involving manioc, rice, plantains (bananas), and vegetables, along with a small amount of fish). General dietary restrictions prior to ingestion of entheogens help reduce the frequent experience of nausea and a sense of "blockage" in the abdominal area caused by food in the intestines, as well as permit enhanced absorption in the mostly empty intestines. These shamanic traditions indicate that that fasting or major food restrictions should be employed as basic preparatory procedures for entheogen use. Restriction of food and extreme fasting can provoke profound alterations of consciousness alone; as preparation for entheogenic sessions, they potentiate and augment the effects of the entheogens in significant ways.

Sexual Abstinence

A widespread aspect of spiritual and ascetic life is sexual abstinence; restrictions on sex were also central to foraging shamanic traditions, as well as many contemporary shamanistic traditions using ayahuasca. As was the case in shamanistic development around the world, sexual segregation during isolation in the forest is required during the training of *vegetalistas* and other *ayahuasqueros*. Shamanic training may require celibacy as well, before and after ceremonies. The lengthy and frequent periods of celibacy for shamans are often tied to concepts of purity and the belief that spirits are attracted to the sexually abstinent person.

Celibacy has physiological effects related to common physiological responses involved in sexual orgasm, as well as induction of altered states of consciousness (Maliszewski, Vaughan, Krippner, Holler, & Fracasso, 2011). Sexual response involves simultaneous activation of both the sympathetic and parasympathetic nervous systems leading to a peak of sexual excitation. Then a sympathetic collapse from exertion and exhaustion leads to a state of relaxation and parasympathetic dominance. The shamanic alteration of consciousness uses dancing and drumming to engage a similar pattern of excitation to the point of collapse, when the shaman enters the soul flight phase. Psychedelics also exhibit a pattern of initial sympathetic activation, leading to an eventual internal focus and parasympathetic dominant phase. Understanding this sympathetic to parasympathetic shift helps explain sexual restriction as preventing this shift and collapse via sex, saving a reserve of psychic energy for ceremonial release. Shamanic induction mechanisms are protected by preventing similar collapse occurring through sexual activity, which would produce a physiological response that could thwart a more profound parasympathetic collapse during the ritual.

Drumming, Singing, and Chanting

A universal aspect of shamanic ritual involves the use of drumming and other percussion, such as rattles. Similarly, singing and chanting is another shamanic universal, with vocalizations that reflect a widespread mammalian expressive communication mechanism (Winkelman, 2009, 2015). These songs and chants are considered to be a special language of the shaman, generally acquired from spirits or animals. These sounds are considered to have special powers that elicit both the spirits and the potential of the entheogens. Shamanic songs are often acquired in entheogenic experiences as gifts from the spirits. The songs are considered to have special moderating influences, enhancing the entheogens, guiding the shaman's divinatory perceptions, and activating the healing processes during the ritual. Songs are seen as evoking the therapeutic processes, constituting key aspects of the healing techniques through their ability to affect the participant's visions and emotions.

Overnight Rituals and "Dream Time"

A key aspect of shamanic practice is the integration of natural dream cycles within ritual period. The typically overnight performance of shamanic rituals and the late-night period of repose by the shaman during soul flight ensures the incorporation of the dream cycle into the ritual processes. Dream incubation during preparatory periods also enables shamans to integrate prior intentions into the ritual dream period visionary experiences. Dream experiences are fundamental to shamanism, explicitly recognized in many cultures as entering into "Dream Time."

The mammalian capacity for dreaming provides a preadaptation for uniquely human forms of consciousness. Dreaming constitutes an adaptation for learning during sleep through information consolidation, an engagement of ego awareness with the operational structures of the unconsciousness that shamanism manages through ritual (Winkelman, 2010b). Psychedelics are powerful agents for enhancing integration of these unconscious information consolidation processes. This shamanic incorporation of dream periods into shamanic experiences engages an innate mammalian capacity for information integration within a system of visual symbolism that reflects a fundamental process of the mind (Winkelman, 2010b). By linking the entheogenic experience with the functional capacities of dreaming and its visually based presentational symbolism, shamanism is able to extend and integrate the functional effects of psychedelics with innate emotional and cognitive processes and enhance the power of altered states of consciousness (ASC).

◼ Types of Shamanic ASC

Eliade emphasized the central role of alterations of consciousness as a defining feature of shamanism. The principal form of these experience involved the shaman's ability to "leave his body and ascend to the sky or descend to the underworld" (1964, p. 5). The shaman's soul flight allows travel both to distant places and to spirit worlds and levels of the universe. During these experiences. the shaman appears unconscious but experiences a persistence of consciousness and an active engagement with various spiritual levels of reality and their entities.

The initiatory activities of the shaman also involved an alteration of consciousness (Winkelman, 2011b), generally conceptualized as a period of involuntary psychological distress followed by a deliberate vision quest to engage a direct encounter with the spiritual powers. A typical feature was a death and rebirth experience that involved being killed by animals, which dismembered and ate the initiate, and subsequently reconstructed the shaman's body, incorporating themselves and new powers into the shaman. Another form of shamanic consciousness involved the personal experience of being transformed into an animal, experiencing the world through this animal from which they acquired power.

Shamanic Flight and Visionary Experiences

Entheogens are known for inducing experiences that are central to the shamanic spirit world encounter, a visionary engagement characterized as a "journey" or "flight," in which one experiences one's body traveling to spirit worlds. This shamanic soul journey is similar to out-of-body experience, astral projection, and near death or clinical death manifested cross-culturally, reflecting innate structures of the brain and self (Winkelman, 2010b, 2019). These shamanic experiences are based in our innate capacity for presentational symbolism, an imagistic symbolic modality that reflects the capacities of the nonverbal mind; Winkelman (2010b) has analyzed these experiences as a prelanguage system of representation based in mimesis, and in terms of the disassembling of modular structures of the protomind.

A central effect of hallucinogens is producing a strong internal orientation and engagement with a visual world, a mode of consciousness that enhances the processes of shamanic journeying. While shamans experience this as an engagement with spirits and various levels of reality, these shamanic journeys can also be seen as an engagement with various aspects of one's unconscious brain structures and processes. The journeying encounter with spirit beings can involve a variety of personal and social processes and unconscious structures that provide transactional entities for therapeutic relief, bonding experiences, and personal development. These visual experiences characteristic of many ASC involve the emergence of primary process thinking in visual symbols that manifest the emotional and social dynamics of pre-egoic levels. This emergence of unconscious content provides opportunity for transforming personal attachments and emotional traumas, enhancing awareness and overall well-being from the transfer of information from the unconscious into consciousness.

The content of visionary experiences provides both: content for diagnostic practices, reflecting repressed energies, unresolved conflicts, and development dynamics; and therapeutic processes, manifested in the connection with archetypal images. The entheogens are particularly powerful tools for eliciting what are considered to be natural symbols, the archetypes that connect the individual unconscious and biology with developmental goals and the social world. The psychedelics are powerful tools for eliciting these elements of the collective unconscious, often rendered as entities from the spirit world that express and release the archetypal energies. These entheogenic visionary experiences connect with this archetypal ground and engage therapeutic processes through connecting psyche with its ancient natural roots.

The visionary symbols convey the unconscious material that emerges and allows for a psychologically more integrated psychodynamics and consciousness through integrative processes occurring outside of conscious awareness. The psychedelics enhance this process, accelerating personal development and resolution of conflicts through the symbolic elevation of this embedded material into personal consciousness, where it can be transformed into a new self dynamic. Shamanic journeying can heal these developmental traumas and reestablish contact with one's true self.

The Shaman's Initiatory Crisis: Death and Rebirth

The seeking of the shamanic role is typically driven by a psychological crisis thought to be provoked by the spirits. This is their way to force the individual to become a shaman, with refusal thought to incur the risk of actual death. A central part of the shamanic development also involves an engagement with psychological death involving the transformation into a new self that emerges spontaneously, especially under influences of psychedelics. This shamanic experience involves a bodily death and dismemberment by animal forms. Shamanic approaches engage deaths without fear rather than fleeing and resisting, accepting the death-and-rebirth experience.

Walsh (1990) characterizes these encounters with images of one's own death within shamanic initiations and development as involving the stimulation of autonomous processes of the psyche. Walsh characterized the dismemberment experiences as involving "autosymbolic images" that manifest the breakdown of one's own psychological structures and psyche. The death-and-rebirth cycle reflects processes of psychological transformation involving an ego disintegration that allows for new developments, manifested as a rebirth or reformulation at higher levels of psychological integration.

Animal Transformation

The entheogenic encounter may also provoke an experience of personal transformation into an animal and the acquisition of specific animal powers. Animals provide representations of aspects of the person, functioning as a subconscious personality dynamic, and often representing lost souls or other aspects of identity or essence that become dissociated from central aspects of self. The ritual and entheogenic incorporation of power animals can provide a reintegration of the self and self development by instilling qualities and characteristics that help address a person's needs. Power animals constitute surrogate forms of the self that can nurture the traumatized self. Shamanic journeying through power animals can induce processes of transformation of one's personal and social nature, altering attitudes, behaviors, and social traits through incorporation of animal qualities. Representations of animal powers activate latent innate cognitive models, with ritual processes integrating them into emerging aspects of the self.

▓ A Psychedelic Neurophenomenology

Shamanic experiences, practices, and beliefs have substantial similarities across cultures, a reflection of underlying biological systems. Neurophenomenological perspectives (Laughlin, McManus and d'Aquili, 1992; Winkelman, 2010b) explain these similarities in shamanic practices and cosmologies through the effects of ritual practices on brain function. This model is extended (Winkelman 2013, 2018) to examine how basic effects of psychedelics on the human mind and psychology produce cognitive elements, such as embodied in the shamanic animistic, ecological, and spiritual worldview, and the inclusion of animal spirits in personal identity and powers.

Serotonergic Regulation and Psychedelic Deregulation

In spite of the diversity of entheogenic species and the broad range of psychoactive substances, the principal ones share similarities as tryptamines and indole alkaloids, which are sources of DMT and similar neurochemicals that function as agonists stimulating the serotonergic system. Serotonin has been considered the primary neurotransmitter system affected by psychedelics, especially through their effects at 5-HT_{2A} receptors (Nichols, 2016); action on other serotonin (5-HT) receptors is also established, as well as a wide range of other neurotransmitter systems.

The phasic effects of psychedelics (1) stimulate and enhance serotonin, (2) saturate and overload the serotonin system, and (3) release the habitual serotonin repression of the dopaminergic system. Psychedelics' resistance to normal reuptake mechanisms locks out serotonergic transmitter sites, habituating the receptors and reducing the regulatory processes of the serotonergic system. This results in a release of the dopamine system normally repressed by serotonin, causing a variety of visionary experiences (hallucinations, dreams, psychosis) and modifying control and coordination among the major brain subsystems. Psychedelics compromise the serotonergic inhibition of the ascending flow of information and emotional responses, resulting in the release of information from ancient levels of the brain that is normally inhibited by serotonin regulation. These effects are typified by psychedelics' interruption of cortico-striato-thalamo-cortical loops that inhibit the lower brain structures' sensory gating systems, providing an enhanced availability of information managed by these brain areas (Vollenweider, 1998; Vollenweider & Geyer, 2001).

These psychedelic effects in altering consciousness are illustrated by Vollenweider's (1998) research on the mechanisms of action of psychedelics on the major cortical loops. The frontal-subcortical circuits provide one of the principal organizational networks of the brain involving neuronal linkages and feedback loops of the cortical areas of the frontal brain with the thalamus of the brainstem region. Vollenweider attributes the consciousness-altering properties of psychedelics to their selective effects on the brain's cortico-striato-thalamo-cortical feedback loops that link the information gating systems of lower levels of the brain with the frontal cortex. The typical action of psychedelics interrupts the cortico-striato-thalamo-cortical loops that inhibit the lower brain structures' sensory gating systems that reduce the flow of information to the frontal areas of the brain (Vollenweider & Geyer, 2001). Psychedelic interruption of serotonergic inhibition of thalamic screening results in a flood of information from these ancient levels of the brain. This overwhelms the frontal processing capacities, alterations of experience of self and other, and creates internal focus on representations of psychological structures.

The inhibition of dopamine release by serotonin is central to neurochemical balance in the brain, with the serotonergic and noradrenergic systems of the right hemisphere inhibiting the dopamine system and the left hemisphere (Previc, 2009). This blockage of serotonin's inhibitory functions results in the disinhibition of the dopaminergic system, releasing a flood of information that is normally inhibited by serotonin. The reduction of serotonergic and noradrenergic modulation (control) results in the ascendance of the dopaminergic and acetylcholine systems that produce a variety of notable visual syndromes, especially hallucinations and dreaming (Hobson, 2001).

Psychointegration and the Integrative Mode of Consciousness

A common neurobiological basis for diverse "transcendent states" and their experiential properties derived from effects on the biogenic amine–temporal lobe limbic neurology and the mesolimbic serotonergic pathways that result in hypersynchronous discharges across the hippocampal-septal-reticular-raphe circuit (Mandell, 1980). Winkelman (2010b) has characterized this overall dynamic as "psychointegration," an integration of lower brain systems into the frontal cor-

tex. Hallucinogens and many other agents and conditions produce hypersynchronous slow-wave brain discharges in the serotonergic circuits that link the hypothalamus and limbic brain with the lower brain systems (for discussion, see Winkelman, 2011a, 2011b). This results in ascending discharges in the brain, manifested in slow-wave hypersynchronous discharges in the hippocampal-septal-reticular-raphe circuit that impose impulses from the ancient lower stratum of the brain on the frontal areas. These processes provided the framework for a general model of the alteration of consciousness involving an integrative mode of consciousness (see Winkelman, 2010b, 2011a). This integrative mode of consciousness is elicited by numerous physiological conditions, pharmacological agents and behaviors (i.e., long-distance running, drumming) that result in a loss of serotonin inhibition to the hippocampal cells, resulting in increase in hippocampal-septal slow-wave electroencephalographic (EEG) activity. Shamanic practices typify this dynamic by employing techniques such as fasting, exhausting exercise (dancing, drumming chanting), and various plants to induce this condition.

Psychointegration as Liberation of the "Animal Brains"

Psychedelics' interference with the principal regulatory functions of the serotonergic system are related to the triune model of the evolution of the brain. The effects of psychedelics on serotonin modify the control and coordination among the three major brain subsystems: the R-complex (reptilian brain), a behavioral brain that channels physiological information; the paleomammalian (limbic) emotional brain that manages self and affect; and the neomammalian brain (neocortex). These three brain systems provide the basis for behavioral, emotional, and informational functions called *protomentation, emotiomentation,* and *ratiomentation,* respectively. The activation of these ancient "animal" brains—the reptilian and paleomammalian complexes—has a direct correspondence with a central feature of shamanic experience—animal powers within the self (see Winkelman, 2010b, for sources and discussion; also see Winkelman, 2018).

Psychedelics reduce the inhibitory control of the serotonergic system on reptilian and paleomammalian brain activities. Serotonergic networks in the paleomammalian brain control both R-complex responses and inhibiting emotional functions of the limbic brain. Global effects of the 5-HT2 psychedelics on the serotonergic system include eventual compromise of serotonergic activity and control, resulting in enhanced reptilian and paleomammalian brain activity. The psychedelics' secondary effect produces systemic brain integration through liberating the reptilian brain's behavioral systems of communication and the paleomammalian brain's analogical and social bonding processes and material of an emotional, social, and personal nature. Deregulation of these brain areas by psychedelics and other alterations of consciousness results in the release of normally unconscious personal and emotional dynamics, which are transmitted by the ascending networks into the frontal brain and conscious awareness (see Winkelman, 2011a, 2017).

These dynamics of the reptilian and paleomammalian brains are directly related to the central features of shamanism involving animal powers and identities. An intuitive understanding of animal species qualities is part of our innate psychology, an innate intelligence embodied in an ancient structuring of cognitive categories (Winkelman, 2018, 2019). These animal concepts are core to the shamanic entheogenic encounter and are exploited in shamanic practices to produce cognitive and social evolution through the symbolic creation produced with the application of these categories of nature to the organization of society in practices of totemism (Winkelman, 2010b, 2015).

Psychedelics and other alterations of consciousness induce primary process thinking, an experience of a primordial reality involving an intimate connection of humans with animals and plants, and an innate internal communication with them. Psychedelics elicit experiences of a personified nature, manifested in an engagement with animals and other entities that could assist humans. These relations and experiences led to conceptions of these plant substances as "teachers," as well as the shamans' animal allies and powers.

Primary Process Thinking

Psychedelics contributed to formation of a shamanic worldview through effects on the experience of self. Views of the interconnectedness of humans and nature reflected biological effects of psychedelics in simultaneously disrupting the brain processes underlying the maintenance of the self, while also producing enhanced connectivity across brain regions (see Winkelman, 2017, for review).

Psychedelic disruption of the default mode network (DMN) results in an overall reduction of top-down brain control, a disruption of the functional control habitually exercised by the frontal cortex. In contrast, psychedelics increase functional connectivity among normally segregated networks, producing increases in cross-modular connectivity that provides more flexible communication across the brain. This increased functional connectivity among normally disconnected brain networks reflects the integration of the somatic and emotional networks that manage primary forms of consciousness. These and other networks are linked into dynamic patterns of coordinated oscillations and synchronization, producing coordination across the brain that enhance primary process thinking.

In their study, Kraehenmann and colleagues (2017) found that LSD lead to significant increases in primary process thinking (in comparison to placebo controls). Psychedelics produce intense visual imagery, positive emotions, and alterations in the sense of self and body through activation of 5-HT_{2A} receptors, stimulating primary process thinking exhibited in dreamlike imagery. These primary processing effects of LSD evoke a distinctive mode of psychological functioning that contrasts with secondary process, a reflective, rule-bound principle of thinking that inhibits lower-level motivation and emotion-driven primary process. Neuronal activation of primary process thinking involves subcortical and limbic brain regions, which manage instinctual drives, subcortical memory and primary emotions.

Novel Meaning and Symbolic Interpretation

The divinatory aspects of shamanism, involving the acquisition of novel information, are enhanced by several effects of psychedelic alterations of consciousness on the brain's information processing system. The loss of top-down brain coherence resulting from the interruption of serotonergic modulation control and feedback loops, combined with the increased neuronal excitability, disrupts normal perceptual processes and produces novel combinations of elements and information. The disruption of ordinary sensory binding creates a disordered and fluid state that results in novel cognitive combinations. The increase in entropy produces conceptual overlaps, novel blending, and new associations. These new and anomalous constructs are subjected to symbolic interpretations, providing new information.

Froese (2015) has shown that altering the brain's ordinary routines results in a greater randomization of brain activity, allowing for spontaneous synaptic plasticity that can reshape network connectivity and enhance overall neural coordination. This is exemplified in the effects of psychedelics that result in increased total brain connectivity. Froese proposes that disruptions in ordinary coping provokes a subject–object dualism, with potential for development into an observing attitude with detached reflection on one's circumstances. Such detached observation is found in mystical and near-death experiences, as well as shamanic and other alterations of consciousness.

Various factors stimulated the emergence of a reflective and symbolic mind across the course of hominin evolution, including both psychedelic ingestion and ritualized alterations of consciousness that induced this detached cognitive stance. The ability of ritual alteration of consciousness to enhance reflective cognitive processing was one of the adaptive advantages of mind alteration that promoted the emergence of the symbolic mind and an acceleration of cultural evolution (Winkelman, 2014).

Psychedelics provoke increases in cause-and-effect repertoires, entropy and integration, producing a conceptual overlap among concepts and novel conceptual blending. These effects help to explain increases in imagination, novel thinking, and creativity experienced during psychedelic states. The conceptual overlaps produced by psychedelics expand the bases for novel human cognition and facilitate creativity. Psychedelic experiences take randomized information from the perceptual system and subject it to abstract thinking mediated through visual symbols, enabling meaningful connections and producing new associations. Combined with the activation of emotional areas in the brain, these cognitions are imprinted with high significance. Psychedelic information is often perceived as having species-level importance because it elicits archetypal structures as a consequence of the deconstruction of ordinary consciousness, allowing for the emergence of earlier forms of cognitive processes ordinarily suppressed by the normal operation of the human brain.

Shamanic visionary practices contributed to human cognitive evolution through expanding ritual practices that enhanced engagement with these forms of knowing (see Rossano, 2009). The deliberate use of psychedelics to produce visual experiences expanded engagement with a special epistemological approach to knowledge and learning. Rock and Krippner (2011) characterize shamanic experiences as involving processes of deciphering images to infer meaning. Alterations of consciousness create heightened states of awareness, conceptualized as perceptions of a spiritual world; these experiences provide a visual symbol manifestation that is interpreted by the shaman to produce new knowledge. Across the course of human evolution, shamans engaged in the ritual exploration of innate image schemas to engage in survival-relevant decisions, providing a new area for adaptation, involving an enhanced ability to predict future conditions through enhanced integration of unconscious knowledge processes.

This human cognitive evolution involved the use of information acquired via normally unconscious processes for adaptations involving the prediction of future conditions and responding to those challenges. The forms of knowing accessed through psychedelic alterations of consciousness provided access to information embodied in prelanguage processes and consequently enabled the integration of information that is normally unconscious by making it available through the visual symbolic processes. Psychedelics provide experiences that engage analogical modeling processes, using image schemas to offer meaning. Psychedelic and shamanic perceptions are reflective of cognitive science perspectives on the interconnectedness of perception, cognition, and the universe (Winkelman, 2010b).

The visionary aspects of shamanism reflect the obvious: psychedelics stimulate the visual regions of the brain and their functional connectivity with other brain regions. The visionary restructuralization typical of shamanic psychedelic experiences reflects various mechanisms of action on the brain. In addition to direct stimulation of the visual system by psychedelics, there is the psychedelic effect of reduction of serotonergic and noradrenergic inhibitory effects on the mesolimbic temporal lobe structures. This inhibition permits the ascendance of the dopaminergic and acetylcholine systems, with the loss of serotonin's inhibitory effects and the ascendance of the dopaminergic system, resulting in a variety of visual syndromes, especially hallucinations and dreaming (Hobson, 2001; Previc, 2009). These typical visual and hallucinatory experiences produced by psychedelics are also a consequence of the enhanced connectivity between the visual cortex and memory centers, an increase of information input to the visual systems from internal information.

Presentational Symbolism: A Visual Epistemology

The visual experiences of shamanism are manifestations of a capacity for presentational symbolism, an ancient modality of cognition that engages forms of meaning making that preceded our now-dominant rational and language-based consciousness (Winkelman, 2010b). Presentational symbolism exhibits characteristics of complex synesthesia based in the integration of various perceptual modalities and presented primarily through the visual system that manifests an internal flow of complex images.

This visual cognition, manifesting a capacity for presentational symbolism, emerges spontaneously from unconscious brain processes, exemplified in dreams. These visionary experiences manifest involuntarily, especially as a consequence of the disinhibition of the habitual repressive regulation of the visual cortex, which results in

hyperactivity of the visual regions. These visual images may be induced by hyperactivation of dopamine receptors, stimulation of serotonin receptors, and the blockage of glutamate receptors (Rolland et al., 2014). A general mechanism underlying visionary experiences is provided by the effects of disruptions within the cortico-striato-thalamo-cortical loops that repress spontaneous visual images in order to modulate awareness and attention.

This ancient mode of imaginal consciousness also appears in dream processes, which provide integration of learning and engagement with problem-solving processes through the exploration of alternative scenarios in mental space. This ancient modality of cognition manifests in shamanic visions, mystical experiences, near-death experiences, out-of-body experiences, and a variety of other visual experiences. This nonverbal symbolism represents self, emotions, attachments, and their connection, with social life manifested in mechanisms operating at a pre-egoic level.

This mode of knowing has been well recognized for centuries but seldom studied because visions do not allow us to share information in any way that compares with the capacity of words to share our thoughts. These visual thinking capabilities nonetheless constitute an innate modular cognitive capacity that emerged over human evolution. This spatial–temporal reasoning capacity involves the ability to think though visualizing patterns, using visual images to think through a series of images and engaging in a mental manipulation of them.

Shamanic Imagery as Fantasy Consciousness

The visionary experiences of shamanism engage a representational system that also provides the substrate for fantasy, daydreaming, reverie, and mystical visions (Horváth, Szummer, & Szabo, 2017), forms of visual mentation based in the processes of perceiving, anticipating, planning, memories, and imagination. This is an affective representational system that functions at the basis of our daily experiences, an autonomic cognitive process that emerges spontaneously in consciousness. Visionary experiences are intimately related to personal affectivity and representations, a capacity for self-communication related to personal affective consciousness that is the foundation of all experience. This latent cognitive capacity is stimulated by psychedelics and takes dominance over our consciousness when activated by psychedelics. This expressive system is basically personal, an internal engagement with a deep narrative level of the mind that presents significant affective dynamics of our life. It also has a symbolic capacity for more complex thought, presenting material necessary for more advanced cognitive processes.

This system of multimodal thinking provides metacognitive elements for nonlinguistic thinking that enable assessment of a complex web of relations, combining multiple sources of information to represent complex relations by integrating memory with thinking with respect to the future (Lohmar, 2010). Psychedelic visions typify fantasy experiences in a polysemic manifestation combining visual information with affective responses and imagination, which provide intellectual realizations and personal awareness in a cognitive–affective system that is an ancient dimension of the human brain–mind.

Conclusions

The institutionalized roles of psychedelics in the religions of cultures around the world indicate that these substances were central to the evolution of spiritual experiences and religious institutions (see Ellens, 2014; Rush, 2013; Winkelman, 2014, 2019). Shamanism was central to that development. Psychedelics elevated this ancient mode of thought, one that has been long recognized in the philosophical and contemplative traditions, an intuitive mode of cognition rich in significance and meaning that is conveyed through visions and imagistic symbols. These features of knowing are liberated by psychedelics through interference with our normal top-down cognitive dynamics, compromising the dominance of higher cognitive functions and consequently releasing processes and information from ancient brain structures.

The shamanic use of psychedelics included a wide range of psychoactive agents with variable chemistry and divergent applications, a recognition of the selective effects of these diverse substances, and their potential applications in the treatment of a wide range of conditions. These treatment strategies and "best uses" included recognition of the importance of set and setting, embodied in the ritual structures developed for their use; the principles for preparation of healers and patients for their ingestion to produce optimal effects; preparations involving restrictions on diet and sexual abstinence; a group ritual context involving chanting and singing; incorporation of the ritual into overnight activities that integrate them with dream processes; and the cosmological perspectives on these substances and their nature that provide conceptual frameworks for managing the experiences.

References

Andritzky, W. (1989). Sociopsychotherapeutic functions of ayahuasca healing in Amazonia. *Journal of Psychoactive Drugs, 21*(1), 77–89.

Dobkin de Rios, M. (1984). *Hallucinogens: Cross-cultural perspectives.* Albuquerque: University of New Mexico Press.

Dolder, P. C., Schmid, Y., Müller, F., Borgwardt, S., & Liechti, M. E. (2016). LSD acutely impairs fear recognition and enhances emotional empathy and sociality. *Neuropsychopharmacology, 41*, 2638–2646.

Eliade, M. (1964). *Shamanism: Archaic techniques of ecstasy.* New York: Pantheon Books.

Ellens, H. (2014). *Seeking the sacred with psychoactive substances: Chemical paths to spirituality and God.* Santa Barbara, CA: Praeger/ABC-CLIO.

Erritzoe, D., Roseman, L., Nour, M., MacLean, K., Kaelen, M., Nutt, D., et al. (2018). Effects of psilocybin therapy on personality structure. *Acta Psychiatrica Scandinavica, 138*, 368–378.

Estrada, A. (1981). *Maria Sabina: Her life and chants* (H. Munn, Trans.). Santa Barbara, CA: Ross-Erickson.

Flaherty, G. (1992). *Shamanism and the eighteenth century.* Princeton, NJ: Princeton University Press.

Froese, T. (2015). The ritualised mind alteration hypothesis of the origins and evolution of the symbolic human mind. *Rock Art Research, 32*(1), 90–97.

Guzman, G., Allen, J., & Gartz, J. (1998). A worldwide geographical distribution of the neurotropic fungi, an analysis and discussion. *Annual Museo Civico Rovereto, 14,* 189–280.

Hobson, J. (2001). *The dream drugstore.* Cambridge, MA: MIT Press.

Horváth, L., Szummer, C., & Szabo, A. (2017). Weak phantasy and visionary phantasy: The phenomenological significance of altered states of consciousness. *Phenomenology and the Cognitive Sciences, 17,* 117–129.

Kometer, M., Schmidt, A., Bachmann, R., Studerus, E., Seifritz, E., & Vollenweider, F. X. (2012). Psilocybin biases facial recognition, goal-directed behavior, and mood state toward positive relative to negative emotions through different serotonergic subreceptors. *Biological Psychiatry, 72,* 898–906.

Kraehenmann, R., Pokorny, D., Aicher, H., Preller, K. H., Pokorny, T., & Bosch, O. G., et al. (2017). LSD increases primary process thinking via serotonin2A receptor activation. *Frontiers in Pharmacology, 8,* Article 814.

Kraehenmann, R., Preller, K., Scheidegger, M., Pokorny, T., Bosch, O., Seifritz, E., et al. (2014). Psilocybin-induced decrease in amygdala reactivity correlates with enhanced positive mood in healthy volunteers. *Biological Psychiatry, 78*(8), 516–518.

Laughlin, C., McManus, J., & d'Aquili, E. (1992). *Brain, symbol, and experience: Toward a neurophenomenology of consciousness.* New York: Columbia University Press.

Lohmar, D. (2010). The function of weak phantasy in perception and thinking. In S. Gallagher & D. Schmicking (Eds.), *Handbook of phenomenology and cognitive science* (pp. 159–177). London: Springer.

Luna, L. E. (1986). *Vegetalismo: Shamanism among the Mestizo population of the Peruvian Amazon.* Stockholm, Sweden: Almqvist & Wiksell International.

Maliszewski, M., Vaughan, B., Krippner, S., Holler, G., & Fracasso, C. (2011). Altering consciousness nultidisciplinary perspectives. In E. Cardeña & M. Winkelman (Eds.), *History, culture and the humanities* (Vol. 1, pp. 189–210). Santa Barbara, CA: Praeger/ABC-CLIO.

Mandell, A. (1980). Toward a psychobiology of transcendence: God in the brain." In D. Davidson & R. Davidson (Eds.), *The psychobiology of consciousness* (pp. 379–464). New York: Plenum Press.

Munn, H. (1973). The mushrooms of language. In M. Harner (Ed.), *Hallucinogens and shamanism* (pp. 86–122). London: Oxford University Press.

Nichols, D. E. (2016). Psychedelics. *Pharmacological Reviews, 68*(2), 264–355.

Previc, F. (2009). *The dopaminergic mind in human evolution and history.* Cambridge, UK: Cambridge University Press.

Rätsch, C. (2005). *The encyclopedia of psychoactive plants: Ethnopharmacology and its applications* (J. R. Baker, Trans.). Rochester, VT: Park Street Press. (Original work published 1998)

Rock, A., & Krippner, S. (2011). *Demystifying shamans and their world: A multidisciplinary study.* Charlottesville, VA: Imprint Academic.

Rolland, B., Renaud, J., Amad, A., Thomas, P., Cottencin, O., & Bordet, R. (2014). Pharmacology of hallucinations: Several mechanisms for one single symptom? *BioMed Research International, 2014,* Article ID 307106.

Rossano, M. (2009). Ritual behavior and the origins of modern cognition. *Cambridge Archaeological Journal, 19*(2), 243–256.

Rush, J. (Ed.). (2013). *Entheogens and the development of culture.* Berkeley, CA: North Atlantic Books.

Schultes, R., Hofmann, A., & Rätsch, C. (1992). *Plants of the gods: Their sacred, healing and hallucinogenic powers.* Rochester, VT: Healing Arts Press.

Schultes, R., & Winkelman, M. (1996). The principal American hallucinogenic plants and their bioactive and therapeutic properties. In M. Winkelman & W. Andritzky (Eds.), *Yearbook of cross-cultural medicine and psychotherapy: Vol. 6. Sacred plants, consciousness and healing* (pp. 205–240). Berlin: VWB Verlag.

Sullivan, R., Hagen, E., & Hammerstein, P. (2008). Revealing the paradox of drug reward in human evolution. *Proceedings of the Royal Society of London B: Biological Sciences, 275,* 1231–1241.

Vollenweider, F. (1998). Recent advances and concepts in the search for biological correlates of hallucinogen-induced altered states of consciousness. *Heffter Review of Psychedelic Research, 1,* 21–32.

Vollenweider, F., & Geyer, M. (2001). A systems model of altered consciousness: Integrating natural and drug psychoses. *Brain Research Bulletin, 56*(5), 495–507.

Walsh, R. (1990). *The spirit of shamanism.* Los Angeles: Tarcher.

Wasson, R. G. (1980). *The wondrous mushroom: Mycolatry in Mesoamerica.* New York: McGraw-Hill.

Wasson, R. G., Cowan, F., & Rhodes, W. (1974). *Maria Sabina and her Mazatec mushroom velada.* New York: Harcourt Brace Jovanovich.

Winkelman, M. (1986). Magico-religious practitioner types and socioeconomic analysis. *Behavior Science Research, 20*(1–4), 17–46.

Winkelman, M. (1990). Shaman and other "magico-religious healers": A cross-cultural study of their origins, nature, and social transformation. *Ethos, 18*(3), 308–352.

Winkelman, M. (1992). *Shamans, priests, and witches: A cross-cultural study of magicoreligious practitioners* (Anthropological Research Papers No. 44). Tempe: Arizona State University.

Winkelman, M. (2004). Shamanism as the original neurotheology. *Zygon Journal of Religion and Science, 39*(1), 193–217.

Winkelman, M. (2005). Drug tourism or spiritual healing?: Ayahuasca seekers in Amazonia. *Journal of Psychoactive Drugs, 37*(2), 209–218.

Winkelman, M. (2007). Shamanic guidelines for psychedelic medicines. In M. Winkelman & T. Roberts (Eds.), *Psychedelic medicine: New evidence for hallucinogenic substances as treatments* (Vol. 2, pp. 143–167). Westport, CT: Praeger/Greenwood.

Winkelman, M. (2009). Shamanism and the origins of spirituality and ritual healing. *Journal for the Study of Religion, Nature and Culture, 34*(4), 458–489.

Winkelman, M. (2010a). The shamanic paradigm: Evidence from ethnology, neuropsychology and ethology. *Time and Mind, 3*(2), 159–182.

Winkelman, M. (2010b). *Shamanism: A biopsychosocial paradigm of consciousness and healing.* Santa Barbara, CA: Praeger/ABC-CLIO.

Winkelman, M. (2011a). A paradigm for understanding altered consciousness: The integrative mode of consciousness. In E. Cardeña & M. Winkelman (Eds.), *Altering consciousness multidisciplinary perspectives: Vol. 1. History, culture and the humanities* (pp. 23–44). Santa Barbara, CA: Praeger/ABC-CLIO.

Winkelman, M. (2011b). Shamanism and the alteration of consciousness. In E. Cardeña & M. Winkelman (Eds.), *Altering consciousness multidisciplinary perspectives: Vol. 1. History, culture and the humanities* (pp. 159–180). Santa Barbara, CA: Praeger/ABC-CLIO.

Winkelman, M. (2013). Shamanism and psychedelics: A biogenetic structuralist paradigm of ecopsychology. *European Journal of Ecopsychology, 4*, 90–115.

Winkelman, M. (2014). Evolutionary views of entheogenic consciousness. In J. Harold Ellens (Ed.), *Seeking the sacred with psychoactive substances: Chemical paths to spirituality and to God* (Vol. 1, pp. 341–364). Santa Barbara, CA: Praeger/ABC-CLIO.

Winkelman, M. (2015). Shamanism as a biogenetic structural paradigm for humans' evolved social psychology. *Psychology of Religion and Spirituality, 7*(4), 267–277.

Winkelman, M. (2017). Mechanisms of psychedelic visionary experiences: Hypotheses from evolutionary psychology. *Frontiers in Neuroscience, 11*, 539.

Winkelman, M. (2018). An ontology of psychedelic entity experiences in evolutionary psychology and neurophenomenology. *Journal of Psychedelic Studies, 2*(1), 5–23.

Winkelman, M. (Ed.). (2019). Psychedelics in history and world religions [Special issue]. *Journal of Psychedelic Studies, 3*, 41–42.

Winkelman, M., & Baker, J. (2016). *Supernatural as natural.* New York: Routledge.

Winkelman, M., & Roberts, T. (Eds.). (2007). *Psychedelic medicine: New evidence for hallucinogenic substances as treatments.* Westport, CT: Praeger/Greenwood.

Winkelman, M., & Sessa, B. (2019). *Advances in psychedelic medicine: State of the art therapeutic applications.* Santa Barbara, CA: Praeger/ABC-CLIO.

CHAPTER 4

A Short, Strange Trip
LSD Politics, Publicity, and Mythology— from Discovery to Criminalization

MARIA MANGINI

During the decades during which they have been known in contemporary Western culture, the psychedelic drugs have been construed as agents that might assist in psychotherapy, produce spiritual transformation, enhance creativity, foster social chaos and moral breakdown, provide access to unexamined realms of a multifaceted reality, or provoke derangement, delusion, and toxic psychosis. Which of these possibilities is most likely to be expressed in a particular occasion of use is not entirely a private matter. The character of an individual experience is influenced and perhaps determined by the circumstances and surroundings of the user; his or her personal preferences, issues, and conflicts; scientific, journalistic, and cultural reports, and the expectations they may engender; and how the specific identity, quantity, and quality of the material ingested combine as drug, set, setting, and matrix. Once the pharmacological effects have dissipated, it remains for the user to find a way to assimilate his or her psychedelic experience, which may be radically dissimilar to any previous experience, into an integrated understanding of self, society, and reality. After a prolonged period of ne-

glect, psychedelics are once again a topic of mainstream societal interest, and psychedelic therapy is reemerging, but decades of misinformation and dysinformation about these substances present a formidable body of psychedelic mythology and propaganda that needs to be considered.

The use of psychoactive plants was once a common practice in Europe. The Eleusinian Mysteries, for example, were transformative rituals that took place in ancient Greece, extending out of Mycenaean traditions (approximately 1500 B.C.E.) and the Greek Dark Ages. For over two millennia this experience, which many claim may have been a psychedelic session, was not only tolerated by ancient civilization but also celebrated by it. Men, women, slaves, and emperors all went to Eleusis to drink the magical potion called *kykeon* and to experience healing and spiritual insights. The only requirements to participate in the rituals and drink the *kykeon* were to speak fluent Greek and never to have committed a murder. The effects of taking part in this intensely life-affirming and healing experience were felt by vast numbers of people over the 2,000 years that these rites took place. The 20th-century historian Will Durant (1989) states of the mysteries, "In this ecstasy of revelation . . . they felt the unity of God, and the oneness of God and the soul; they were lifted up out of the delusion of individuality and knew the peace of absorption into deity."

Many of the identified heretics of the Inquisition were practitioners of plant-based shamanism. During the European witch craze, the full force of the Inquisition was brought to bear on the users of psychoactive plants, preparers of potions and philtres, herbalists, "cunning men" and "witch women" of Western Europe, with a ferocity unmatched even in attempts to eradicate the practices of indigenous people of the Western Hemisphere (Walker, 1983) Although the genocidal pressures exerted on practitioners of indigenous religions of the Americas decimated the population and disrupted the orderly process of transmission of traditional skills, Native American populations are presently in a period of ethnic resurgence. Enough representatives of the traditional cultures of the past have survived to enable reemergence of previously suppressed traditions, values, rituals, and everyday practices.

The Inquisition was far more successful. By systematically eliminating the European "witches" and all who associated with them, supported them, defended them, or resembled them, most traces of indigenous European religions, and of the identities and uses of associated psychoactive plants, were successfully eradicated in Western Europe. By casting the healer as a witch and the hallucinogenic plants as tools of Satan, the Church succeeded in virtually eradicating knowledge of these elements of pagan and shamanic consciousness. The parts that remained were relabeled with negative markers that indicated their forbidden status, such as "deadly nightshade," "wolfbane," "toadstool," and "henbane" (Rudgley, 1995).

Fifty years before Albert Hofmann's discovery of the psychoactive properties of lysergic acid diethylamide (LSD), there was already European interest in the pharmacological properties of psychoactive plants, and the isolation and characterization of their chemical constituents. Louis Lewin, a German pharmacologist, published the first methodical analysis of the peyote cactus and established the presence of plant alkaloids in peyote samples in 1888. In his book *Phantastica*, Lewin (1924/1998) took on the task of classifying drugs and plants in accordance with their psychological effects. The classifications were Inebriantia (inebriants), Exitantia (stimulants), Euphorica (euphoriants), Hypnotica (tranquilizers), and Phantastica (hallucinogens).

In 1897, Arthur Heffter used a combination of animal studies and self-experimentation to demonstrate the psychoactive properties of one of these alkaloids, mescaline. He isolated mescaline from the peyote cactus, the first such isolation of a naturally occurring psychedelic substance in pure form. In addition, he conducted experiments on its effects by comparing the effects of peyote and mescaline on himself (Heffter Research Institute, 2018).

S. Weir Mitchell (1896) experimented with peyote in the United States and is usually considered the first to describe many of the characteristic visual phenomena associated with peyote: heightened sensitivity to light and color, and abstract visual pattern formation on closed eyelids. In early 1897 British psychologist Havelock Ellis obtained a supply of peyote from the firm of Potter & Clarke in London and also entered "unique, vast and enchanted realm[s]" of the mind and wrote enthusiastically about his experiences (Ellis, 1897, 1898; Zieger, 2008).

Ellis gave some peyote buttons to William Butler Yeats in April 1897, but the poet found the peyote's effect on his breathing unpleasant, and expressed a preference for hashish, which had been known and used by literary and artist groups for decades. The *Club des Hashischins* in Paris, for example, met monthly and included members such as Dr. Jacques-Joseph Moreau, Théophile Gautier, Charles Baudelaire, Gérard de Nerval, Honoré de Balzac, Eugène Delacroix, Aurthur Rimbaud, Victor Hugo, and Alexandre Dumas.

Ellis (1898) wrote that peyote is "the most democratic of the plants which lead men to an artificial paradise" because of the "the halo of beauty which it casts around the simplest and commonest things." Research on peyote was not pursued at this time, possibly because of the mixed results obtained (both Ellis and Mitchell gave it to people who experienced fear of dying) and perhaps because of criticism from people like the editors of the *British Medical Journal,* whose editorial suggested that peyote was in fact a "New Inferno" and not another "Artificial Paradise," such as that described by Baudelaire in his writings about hashish and opium in 1860.

Ellis was castigated by the *British Medical Journal* for a familiar concern: that a portion of the public that was fascinated by the prospect of new experiences might seek an encounter with what he called the "mescal button" ("which must not be confounded with the intoxicating drink of the same name made from an agave"; "Paradise or Inferno," 1898, p. 390) and experience injurious legal or medical consequences. Ellis was reprimanded for irresponsibility in "putting the temptation before the section of the public which is always in search of new sensation" (p. 390).

Although many of the early experimenters with peyote were aware of Native American peyote use, with its strong religious dimension, they did not share this experience. For them, peyote was experienced as something profane and fascinating, but with aesthetic and scientific implications. The peyote ceremony only reached the United States about 1870, but it was old in Mexico when the Spaniards arrived in the 1500s. It was brought to the United States by the Apaches in Texas, who gave it to the Kiowa and the Comanche, from whom it spread to become a pan-Indian practice, with varying ceremonial forms developed by the social environment and the specific leaders who influenced particular areas.

Quanah Parker, a war leader of a Comanche band, who advocated for the legal use of peyote, famously said, "The white man goes to his church house and talks *about* Jesus, the Indian goes into his tipi and talks *to* Jesus" (Hagen, 1993). Parker had been cured by a Mexican *curandera* using peyote and became one of two principal peyote leaders in North America, the other being John Wilson. Parker used the half-moon style and Wilson the more Christian-syncretic "cross-fire." The "peyote church" attracted a significant number of Native American members and is estimated to have about a quarter-million adherents today. Many of the ritual components are comparable to traditional Native American religious practices, such as the offering of tobacco to the peyote spirit, the use of peyote as a medicinal plant, vision experiences, and singing as an act of prayer. Several Christian elements have been added through vision experiences, including the use of Bibles, baptism of new members in peyote water, and Christian symbolism at the "altar." Native American Church theology centers on the belief that peyote can bring peace of mind, teach one to think good thoughts and know the difference between right and wrong, and heal illnesses if one sincerely believes and concentrates.

In the late 20th century, Al Smith, a drug-abuse counselor who advocated recovery for Native people through indigenous spirituality and culturally relevant practices, became the lead plaintiff in the Supreme Court case *Employment Division v. Smith,* which was decided in 1990. The issue was whether the First Amendment's Free Exercise Clause protected participants in peyote religious ceremonies from the disapproving arm of the state. The Court held that it does not. The *Smith* opinion evoked widespread disgust and led Congress to enact not one but two statutes to repudiate it. The Religious Freedom Restoration Act of 1993 (RFRA) was written very broadly: As we learned in in *Burwell v. Hobby Lobby,* it can be interpreted to protect powerful corporate employers from observing the statutory rights of their employees. Ironically, the drafters of RFRA excluded one key religious group— the Native American Church. Peyote, the sponsors thought, was "controversial." Native Americans and the mainstream religious community worked together to get another statute passed: the 1994 Amendments to the American Indian Religious Freedom Act. It provides that "the use, possession, or transportation of peyote by an Indian who uses peyote in a traditional manner for bona fide ceremonial purposes in connection with the practice of a traditional Indian religion is lawful, and shall not be prohibited by the United States or by any State."

In February 2016, official representatives of the National Council of Native American Churches met in Laredo, Texas, to discuss, among other business matters, the proliferation of organizations appropriating the "Native American Church" name, despite the fact that these appropriators had absolutely no ties to the indigenous worship of the holy sacrament Peyote.

The National Council comprised recognized, indigenous member organizations that included the Native American Church of North America, the Azzeé Bee Nahagá of Diné Nation, the Native American Church of the State of Oklahoma, the Native American Church of the State of South Dakota, and invited leaders of the Consejo Regional Wixárika of Mexico.

On February 13, 2016, the member organizations of the National Council signed a statement to make it publicly known that they do not condone the activities of what they deem illegitimate organizations, some comprised of non-Native people, who claim that cannabis, ayahuasca, and other substances are part of Native American Church theology and practice. They reiterated that the only plant that serves as a Native American Church sacrament is peyote, and rejected and condemned any claim that any other plant serves or has ever served as a sacrament in indigenous Native American Church ceremonies (Native American Rights Fund, 2016).

In 1914, on the eve of World War I, Mabel Dodge Luhan, an American heiress, literary patron, and member of the Greenwich Village *avant garde,* became interested in peyote. With her friends, she had a tiny bit of knowledge, an adventurous spirit, and a bag of peyote buttons. She wrote one of the first accounts of a peyote trip in white America, and the incident became legendary in counterculture circles.

Her trip, among nine friends, was chaotic and disorienting, even terrifying when one of the participants left the house, but Mabel later married a Native American man who gave her peyote medicine when she was very ill, and she had a classic transformative experience:

> Beginning: I in the room and the room I was in, the old building containing the room, the cool wet night space where the building stood and all the mountains standing out like sentries in their everlasting attitudes. So on and on into wider spaces farther than I could divine, where all the heavenly bodies were contented with the order of the plan, and system within system interlocked in grace. I was not

separate and isolated any more. The magical drink had revealed the irresistible delight of spiritual composition: the regulated relationship of one to all and all to one . . . all things are really related to each other. (Luhan, 2002, p. 163)

Mabel used the term "expansion of consciousness" long before it was to become idiomatic some 40 years later (Palmer & Horowitz, 1982).

After Albert Hofmann's recognition of the psychoactive properties of LSD in 1943, the therapeutic potential of psychedelic drugs once again became the subject of speculation, study, and controversy. LSD's exceptionally high activity, corresponding to that of endogenous trace substances that effect mental states, suggested the possibility of psychotherapeutic use to its earliest researchers.

Hoffman's reports of his self-experiments and Stoll's original systematic description of LSD-induced mental states in healthy volunteers and patients with schizophrenia were followed by more than 1,000 reports of therapeutic experimentation with LSD and related substances (Stoll, 1947).

After 25 years of study, a combination of flawed methodology, uneven results, and social reprehension led to the abandonment of this program of research, leaving many avenues of inquiry unexplored and many questions unanswered. Today, after a 50-year hiatus, research on the therapeutic potential of the psychedelic drugs is gradually being resumed, and there is renewed interest in the history of previous studies (Pollan, 2018).

The use of the word *psychedelic* to describe the class of drugs to be discussed here is sometimes construed to indicate a positive attitude toward their use, as opposed to the term *hallucinogen,* which was the more widely employed designation in law and medicine until the 1990's (Nichols, 1999). While the term *psychedelic* is used by, for example, *Goodman & Gilman's: The Pharmacological Basis of Therapeutics* (Brunton, Knollman, & Hilal-Dandan, 2018), the "gold standard" of authority and accuracy in describing the actions and uses of therapeutic agents, this class of drugs has been variously labeled hallucinogens, psychotomimetics, illusogens, entheogens (generating religious experience), phantasticants, psychezymics (mind fermenting) oneirogens (producing dreams), psychotogens, psychehormics (mind rousing), deliriants, psychodysleptics (disturbing the mind), psycholytics (breaking up mental structures), revelatiomimetics (seeming to reveal something), phanerothymes (making the soul visible), mysticomimetics (imitating an initiation), and apocalyptogens (uncovering a revelatory and/or apocalyptic eschatological experience) (Grinspoon & Bakalar, 1983; Osmond, 1957; Strassman, 1995; Werner, 1993). The variety of terms available is an indication of the diversity of viewpoints on these substances. Psychedelics have been variously described as causing a temporary and artificial psychosis, an analogue of transformative mystical experience, or an interruption of habitual psychological functioning that allows self-generated modification of patterns of behavior and reorganization of feelings and thoughts (Calabrese, 1994; Clark, 1985; Cohen, 1960a, 1964; Kurland, Savage, Panhke, Grof, & Olsson, 1971; Kurland, Unger, Shaffer, & Savage, 1967; Louria, 1966; Silverman, 1976; Strassman, 1995; Walsh, 1982; Zaehner, 1972; Zinberg, 1976).

The word *psychedelic,* derived from Greek roots meaning "manifesting the mind," was first used by Humphry Osmond in a letter to Aldous Huxley in 1956 (Huxley, 1956/1969). Osmond (1957) later offered this term as one that was "clear, euphonious and uncontaminated by other associations." That clarity was short-lived, and within the first 10 years after being coined by Huxley and Osmond, "the word 'psychedelic' [was] ruined; it might as well be scrapped by those who still wish to speak earnestly about their experience" (Bieberman, 1967).

Even so, what is understood to manifest in the psychedelic experience is the content of the user's unconscious, which may be exteriorized by psychedelics depending on the circumstances and condition of the user, often summed up as the essential elements of *set, setting,* and *matrix* (Aaronson & Osmond, 1970; Eisner, 1997).

As understood by psychedelic researchers, *set* is an individual-level phenomenon that has to do with the respondent's personality, personal history, life situation at the time of the drug exposure, psychological makeup, physical health, previous experience with unusual states of consciousness, and expectations and/or motivation for taking the psychedelic drug. *Setting,* the second essential element, encompasses the local social factors and includes the circumstances and environment in which the drug experience occurs; the people present and how they treat the user; the contributions of music, flowers, mirrors, photographs, and other objects at hand during the psychedelic session; and what the administrator of the drug expects the user's reaction to it to be (Hoffer & Osmond, 1967; Pahnke, 1969). The third essential element, *matrix,* has sometimes been subsumed under *setting* by psychedelic researchers. It includes the broad social setting and historic cultural and political circumstances in which the use occurs, the situation in which the user is living at the time of the experience, and the environment to which the user returns after the experience (Eisner, 1997; Grof, 1975). The element of matrix, the least understood and analyzed of these elements in most discussions of psychedelics, is the one that is currently most in a state of flux (Pollan, 2018). This chapter examines some of the specific interests and controversies that characterized the matrix of the last period of extensive psychedelic exploration and experimentation 50 or more years ago.

In 1953, researchers in Western Canada were engaged in a series of studies on schizophrenia involving the use of mescaline and LSD. Their aim was "start with the signs and symptoms and natural history of schizophrenia, and ask how these could be produced" (Osmond & Smythies, 1952). Compounds that were thought to produce mental disturbances similar to schizophrenia were administered to volunteers in order to construct biochemical and psychological models of psychoses. In an early report of this research, Humphry Osmond stated that it had "been known for fifty years that mescaline . . . produces symptoms almost identical with schizophrenia" (Osmond & Smythies, 1952). Actually, at that time, there were three theories of the effects of mescaline and LSD. They were variously described as "deliriants" that provoked a toxic delirium, "psychotomimetics," which caused an artificial psychosis similar to the experience of a psychotic break (Hoffer, 1967); or "psycholytics" which produced psychic states in which the subject recalled repressed memories and other unconscious material in a setting of clear consciousness (Sandison & Spencer, 1954). Mayer-Gross (1951), another early researcher in this area, had noted the differences between schizophrenia and the effects of mescaline:

> The symptoms of mescaline intoxication have been compared to those of schizophrenia, but it is much more the strangeness experienced by the patient suffering from schizophrenia and the difficulties of describing what is happening in the two conditions which is similar. Many typical schizophrenic symptoms are never seen in mescaline intoxication.

In a search for a naturally occurring trace substance that could induce a schizophrenia-like reaction, Osmond and Hoffer had studied the "schizogenic" properties of a group of materials, and had coined for them the name *hallucinogens*: mescaline, LSD or lysergide, harmine, ibogaine, and hashish (Hoffer, Osmond, & Smythies, 1954). Based on the speculation that the LSD experience could be akin to that of *delirium tremens,* a disorder involving visual and auditory hallucinations found in habitual and excessive users of alcoholic beverages, they began a series of studies of lysergide in the treatment of alcoholism at Saskatchewan Hospital in Weyburn, Saskatchewan, where the first two alcoholic patients were treated in 1953 (Hoffer, 1967; Thomas, 1977).

Because alcoholics who had experienced *delirium tremens* sometimes were noted to "hit bottom," an experience of surrender that is often considered to be the key to beginning recovery from alcoholism, Hoffer and Osmond wondered if a similar experience, therapeutically induced, would help alcoholics stay sober (Hoffer, 1967). They understood the LSD reaction to be similar in character to *delirium tremens*, but one that could be produced at a time and place when it could be directed and controlled. Hoffer and Osmond speculated that they could inspire an alcoholic patient to "mend his ways" by inducing such an experience (Osmond, 1969).

Hoffer and Osmond were familiar with the testimonies of "rapid abolition of an-

cient impulses and propensities" collected by William James (1902, p. 269) from the reformed drunkards of the Jerry McAuley Water Street Temperance Mission, and with James's observation that the only radical remedy known to medicine "for dipsomania is religiomania." They were aware that "a very remarkable experience" (Osmond, 1969, p. 217) of some kind had caused Bill W to begin to build AA (Delbanco & Delbanco, 1995; Osmond, 1969). They knew that some kind of "hitting bottom" experience was at the heart of the Weslyan Methodist sect's success in converting alcoholics and helping them to stop drinking through a process of catching them in the remorseful time after a drinking bout, scaring them thoroughly with the potential consequences of continued drinking, then offering hope for improvement in a program of abstinence (Osmond, 1969).

Hoffer and Osmond speculated that the experience of *delirium tremens* could be used to encourage alcohol abstinence. It is unpredictable, overwhelming, and frightening. In the early 1950s, it was fatal in about 10–15% of patients (Osmond, 1969). It is the last in a continuum of alcohol withdrawal symptoms that may begin soon after the cessation of drinking as the blood level of alcohol begins to drop. First described in 1813, it is sometimes referred to as "the horrors" and may be accompanied by "rum fits" or seizures (Sutton, 1813). It progresses erratically from agitation and autonomic hyperactivity to mental confusion, disorientation, delusions, and vivid hallucinations of colored shapes, snakes, dragons, and other fantastic objects. The patient may be amnestic for the experience (Adriani, 1976). Delirium tremens occurs in about 4–5% of patients withdrawing from alcohol. Advances in treatment have reduced mortality to less than 5% (Yost, 1996).

Hoffer and Osmond (Osmond, 1969) soon noted, however, that substances such as LSD and mescaline, which they had understood to be productive of hallucinations, could also produce "a particularly vivid and intense awareness of personality problems" that seemed to make the alcoholic more amenable to psychotherapy (Smith, 1958) For many patients, this was also an "admonitory" experience, in which they were profoundly shocked and frightened by their vision of themselves and how alcohol was affecting them. Hoffer and Osmond abandoned the idea of provoking a simulacrum of the *delirium tremens* in favor of encouraging patients' self-examination of personality problems and the development of insight into their "dismal present and appalling future" (Osmond, 1969). They made no deliberate attempt to produce fear in their patients, as they had noted early in their investigations that making alcoholics afraid "often produces a desperate resolution to go on drinking" (Osmond, 1969) and seemed to lead to severe anxiety and poor communication (Smith, 1958).

In 1956, Humphry Osmond presented a paper at the New York Academy of Sciences conference titled "The Pharmacology of Psychotomimetic and Psychotherapeutic Drugs." In this paper, "A Review of the Clinical Effects of Psychotomimetic Agents," Osmond described the major uses of this class of drugs. Some of these uses were the subject of ongoing research: the study of psychopathology through the production of "model psychoses," the experiential training and education of psychiatrists and psychologists, and use as an adjunct to conventional psychotherapy. Two of the potential uses that he proposed were less well known: exploration of the normal mind under unusual conditions and discoveries with social, philosophical, and religious implications made by means of LSD and other drugs of this class (Osmond, 1957). Osmond pointed out that continuing to consider these agents to be primarily "psychotomimetic" begged the question of their other potential uses. To prevent this, he proposed a name for the class of drugs that would include their capacity to enrich the mind and enlarge the vision: *psychedelic,* a term coined from Greek roots that mean "manifesting the mind." For the next 12 years, research on the potential therapeutic benefit of psychedelic drugs in the treatment of alcoholism continued, producing innumerable areas of controversy.

As well as being used in the treatment of alcoholism, U.S. researchers in the 1950s had begun to explore the possibility that LSD might be used to enhance creativity, or to facilitate psychotherapy (Eisner & Cohen, 1958). In their enthusiasm, some researchers began to share LSD with friends in their homes, and as publicity about the effects of LSD increased, so did the demand for LSD experiences (Abramson, 1967). Many prominent persons, including the founder of Alcoholics Anonymous, Bill Wilson, and Chuck Dederich, the founder of Synanon, were having LSD sessions. Television and newspaper coverage depicted LSD as a new wonder drug (Novak, 1997). A 1958 report in the *Journal of Nervous and Mental Disease* included "LSD-25 social parties" in a list of ways that LSD might be used (Feld, Goodman, & Guido, 1958).

The first systematic attempt to assess the potential side effects and complications of psychedelic therapy was Sidney Cohen's (1960a, 1960b) survey of 62 investigators using psilocybin or LSD in therapy. The 44 researchers who replied to his questionnaire had administered psychedelics to almost 5,000 individuals on more than 25,000 occasions. Based on the data they supplied, Cohen estimated that psychiatric reactions lasting over 48 hours occurred in 0.8 per 1,000 normal volunteers, and 1.8 per 1,000 patients undergoing therapy. Suicide was a less frequent complication, occurring in less than 0.4 per 1,000 patients. No suicides or suicide attempts were reported in volunteers.

Cohen concluded that untoward events were infrequent, and that the psychedelics were "safe when given to a selected healthy group" (1960a, p. 39) if used with proper precautions. Recommended precautions included constant supervision, hospitalization if doses greater than 1μg/kg were used, provision of trained and experienced support personnel during the experience, and the availability of consultation in the event of posttreatment symptom development (Cohen, 1960a).

Despite the relatively benign picture painted by Cohen's survey, by the end of 1961 a "climate of criticism" was developing around psychedelic research (Stevens, 1987). Psychopharmacologist Jonathan O. Cole (1961) expressed "very mixed feelings" about research with psychedelics, particularly the possibility that they might be used to "establish long-term control over minds" by "altering loyalties or changing moral attitudes or political beliefs." Sensational accounts of the LSD experiences of celebrities, the influence of LSD on creativity, and the superiority of LSD treatment to conventional psychotherapy spurred popular demand, and college students began experimenting with psychedelics (Novak, 1997).

In October 1961, the Harvard Psilocybin Research Project, run by Timothy Leary and Richard Alpert, was criticized by its sponsor, the Center for Research in Personality, for failure to adhere to guidelines similar to those described by S. Cohen. At a special faculty meeting, David MacClelland (1961), director of the Center, enumerated four "symptoms" he had noticed in the Project's participants, both researchers and experimental subjects. Disassociation and detachment, interpersonal insensitivity, religious and philosophical naiveté, and impulsivity were said to distinguish those who had those who had taken psychedelic drugs. MacClelland saw these as evidence that the chief effects of psilocybin and similar substances were to encourage withdrawal from social reality and concentration on one's inner life (Caldwell, 1968; Gordon, 1963). The Project was required to surrender its official supply of psilocybin to Dr. Dana Farnsworth, head of the University Health Service, to be released only for experiments approved by an ad hoc faculty committee. Reports of the disciplinary action were carried by the *Harvard Crimson,* then picked up by national news wire (Weil, 1963).

In the spring of 1962, when the faculty committee refused to provide Walter Pahnke, a doctoral student of Leary and Alpert, psilocybin for the carefully designed Marsh Chapel experiment on the ability of psilocybin to provoke mystical experience, supplies that had been withheld by the researchers from the University were used instead (Gordon, 1963; Pahnke, 1963; Stevens, 1987). University authorities protested that this was not the only occasion on which Leary and Alpert had failed to follow the newly agreed-upon procedure. Other psychedelic researchers defended the decision, pointing out that Pahnke's faculty-appointed doctoral committee had approved the experimental protocol, and that Farnsworth, like many of the other most critical voices, was "in no way equipped as an expert" on the use of psychedelic drugs (Clark, 1969). Soon afterward, Timothy Leary left Harvard without notice, and in May 1963, Richard Alpert became the only Harvard faculty member to be fired in the 20th century (Hiatt, 2016).

Lisa Bieberman, an honors graduate from Radcliffe with degrees in mathematics and philosophy, helped organize a public protest against the firing of Alpert. Bieberman (1967), one of the most eloquent writers on the psychedelic experience, became, what one *Harvard Crimson* article described as a "disciple" of Timothy Leary.

"I began to hang around Leary's office after classes," Bieberman (1967) said, "licking envelopes, tying letters, and running errands. I faithfully read all the papers [Leary and Alpert] put out." The next year she became the circulation manager for Leary's *Psychedelic Review.*

In an interview with the *Harvard Crimson,* Bieberman described her experience with psychedelic drugs in spiritual terms: "It's hard to explain to people who have not taken these drugs just what their good effects are. But they can give you a new perspective on the way you are living, and an increased sensitivity. You look at life in a completely different way and the important thing is to be able to apply this new perspective to your life when you come back" (Conrad, 1966).

This highly controversial episode was discussed in a special issue of the *Harvard Alumni Bulletin* on the university's professors and their work. Henry K. Beecher (1963), the Dorr Professor of Research in Anesthesia, refuted the accusation that University opposition was driving research underground, and maintained that, to the contrary, there was "an abundance of support in this field for the able, responsible investigator, at present more than ever before."

By July of 1962, Sidney Cohen and Keith Ditman had encountered the rapidly growing illicit use of LSD and had published an article describing "an increasing number of untoward events in connection with LSD-25 administration." Although they continued to support the investigational use of LSD for its potential to aid in the study of the mind, they pointed out that the unsupervised use of the drug enhanced its capacity to produce serious consequences (Cohen & Ditman, 1962). The complications mentioned included antisocial acting out behaviors, misuse of LSD as part of a larger pattern of multidrug use and "abuse of [the] euphoriant property" of LSD by marketing it as an item of underworld traffic (p. 161).

This was followed by a second report on adverse reactions to LSD, in which Cohen and Ditman (1963) foresaw that the problems that could occur after inexpert or casual experimentation could serve to further complicate the research environment. They reported on nine cases illustrating several types of untoward effects: prolonged psychotic decompensation, depressive reactions, release of preexisting psychopathic antisocial trends, abandonment of social responsibilities, and paranoid reactions in which the transcendental aspects of the LSD experience confirmed latent ideas of grandiosity. They still held that such reactions were infrequent, however; as long as the drug was employed with "carefully screened, maximally supervised patients, given the drug by responsible, experienced investigators." With considerable prescience, they noted that "when undesirable reactions and sensational publicity become associated with a drug, competent investigators are inclined to avoid participating in the careful, thoughtful studies that are necessary to evaluate it properly." By December 1962, when their article was submitted, new legislation had already been passed by the U.S. Congress that would restrict availability of LSD only to researchers engaged in federally approved studies.

This legislation, the Kefauver–Harris Amendments to the Cosmetic, Food, and Drug Act of 1938, created a class of "investigational new drugs." These were drugs that had not yet been marketed but were undergoing testing to demonstrate their safety and efficacy. These "new drugs" could not be distributed commercially without approval from the U.S. Food and Drug Administration (FDA). Despite the fact that they had been studied for almost two decades and had been the subject of more than 1,000 English-language articles (Cohen, 1968), several of the psychedelics fell under this classification, as the FDA was not satisfied that their safety and efficacy had been established.

The discovery of the teratogenic properties of thalidomide in the early 1960s had focused attention on the need for better regulation of the use of experimental drugs.

The special investigational new drug (IND) application for permission to use drugs classified as investigational was instituted in 1963, but until then, anyone could order LSD, psilocybin, or mescaline by submitting to Sandoz a signed statement that the person ordering had the training and facilities to conduct drug investigations, and that the supplies of the experimental drug obtained would be used only for research purposes.

Researchers and other interested users obtained LSD and psilocybin from Sandoz's branch office in New Jersey. LSD was supplied under the trade name Delysid, in the form of small, blue 25-µg tablets or 100-µg/cc ampules for parenteral use (Hollister, 1968). Mescaline could be ordered from several chemical supply firms for between $4 and $15/dose (Weil, 1963). These sources had provided the material with which therapists in Los Angeles, Vancouver, and the San Francisco Bay Area were providing LSD sessions to paying clients eager for the experience (Chandler & Hartman, 1960; Sherwood, Stolaroff, & Harman, 1962; Stevens, 1987).

Under the new IND regulations, Sandoz technically became the "sponsor" for all investigations of LSD and psilocybin. James Goddard of the FDA testified in 1966 that Sandoz had in 1963 filed a basic investigational plan for testing LSD, which indicated that a reasonably safe and rationally conducted program of experimentation would be required of researchers. There was as yet no direct relationship between investigators and the FDA (Lowinger, 1966). Jerome Levine, a University of Maryland psychiatric researcher who studied LSD for the National Institute of Mental Health, described Sandoz's role in relation to psychedelic researchers as more that of distributor of LSD than as the sponsor of research, and stated that researchers were using LSD from Sandoz in studies that were neither designed by Sandoz nor directed at exploration of particular properties of LSD (J. Levine, personal communication, September 1998). Sandoz's patent on LSD-25 expired in 1963, and manufacturers in Czechoslovakia and Italy began commercial production of the drug at about this time. Sandoz was becoming uneasy about the ability to continue to control the distribution of LSD (Christen, 1966).

A flurry of articles about LSD appeared in popular periodicals during 1963, until, as Abram Hoffer suggested, it was "hardly likely that any literate citizen has not heard something about it" (Hoffer, 1967). The *Ladies' Home Journal* quoted Jonathan Cole of the National Institute of Mental Health on LSD in an article called "Instant Happiness": "[LSD] can produce an unstable state varying—within five minutes—from horror to ecstasy" (Goldman, 1963). *Time* described spiritual experiences reported by users of psilocybin, LSD, and peyote as "instant mysticism" ("Instant Mysticism," 1963) *Cosmopolitan* reported:

> Suddenly LSD has become the sophisticated "fun thing" to try around the smart set, the fast set and the beat set, and if you haven't got a buddy who can run down to his friendly neighborhood LSD bootlegger and buy an ampoule of those little blue pills, you are simply not *in* my friend. (Gaines, 1963)

As the drug's official sponsor, Sandoz began in 1963 to restrict the U.S. distribution of LSD to National Institute of Mental Health-funded programs, Veteran's Administration (VA)-sanctioned programs in VA hospitals, government agencies, and programs in state universities with approval from state mental health commissioners (Caldwell, 1968). In Canada, transportation and sale of LSD were forbidden, and possession was permitted only by researchers with University appointments who were listed with the Ministry of Health (Hoffer, 1967). Private therapists without institutional affiliations were not included in the list of approved researchers for whom Sandoz would act as the IND application sponsor. Unlike the "neighborhood bootlegger," most therapists and clinics were unable to obtain the psychedelics, as they could not afford the time and expense the new regulations required them to invest (O. Janinger, personal communication, May 1996). Some therapists continued to do psychedelic work with their patients, but the patients had to obtain their own drugs on the black market (Abramson, 1967). Other therapists were forced to discontinue their work because of problems with funding. The International Foundation for Advanced Study in Menlo Park, California, operated by Robert Mogar, Willis Harmon, Charles and Ethyl Savage, James Fadiman, Al Hubbard, Myron Stolaroff, and others, closed in 1964 because the fee of $650 per person per session was not enough to cover costs, and hoped-for federal financial support was not forthcoming (Editorial, 1964).

As it was quite difficult to synthesize pure LSD-25, controls on importation and use were originally thought to be adequate for restricting the illicit supply. In the early 1960s, however, a new process for culturing the ergot fungus made the precursor chemicals much more available (Osmond, 1973). The 1962 White House Conference on Narcotics and Drug Abuse considered the psychedelics to be of only minor importance as drugs of abuse, largely because of their limited availability and high cost. Others foresaw that the publicity they had received and the possibility of profit would be likely to increase their distribution (Cohen & Ditman, 1962).

Theoretical and philosophical speculation about LSD was beginning to appear in the journal literature. Joel Elkes, who had been among the first to call attention to the potential for untoward reactions to LSD (Elkes, Elkes, & Mayer-Gross, 1954) reiterated the side effects, complications, and dangers of abuse of the psychedelics that had been noted earlier by Cohen's survey research (Elkes, 1963). In short editorial, Roy Grinker (1963), the editor of *Archives of General Psychiatry,* claimed that "latent psychotics are disintegrating under the influence of even single doses; long-continued LSD experiences are subtly creating a psychopathology. Psychic addiction is being developed . . ." (p. 425), necessitating greater controls on the use of LSD.

This editorial by Grinker, who never published any work on LSD and was, according to Abram Hoffer, "uncontaminated by firsthand experience with it" (Hoffer, 1967) appeared in the same issue of the *Archives of General Psychiatry* as Cohen and Ditman's study of prolonged adverse reactions to LSD, and was subsequently cited as a reference on the severity of the LSD problem by a September 1963 editorial in the *Journal of the American Medical Association,* among others. That editorial by Dana Farnsworth, of the Harvard University Health Service, admitted that research on the psychedelics was vital and should continue. While he decried the "hysterical attitude that could result in the adoption of unwarranted restrictive legislation," he also suggested that "regular use of the hallucinogens will prepare individuals to 'move up' to other and more powerful drugs such as morphine or heroin" and described psychedelics as substances that "have the power to damage the individual psyche, indeed to cripple it for life."

By March 1964, in the *Journal of the American Medical Association,* Jonathan Cole and Martin Katz, two senior NIMH psychopharmacologists, described the use and misuse of the psychedelics as "among the touchiest topics of recent months" and provided "a sober look at the present situation" (p. 758). They likened the "psychotomimetics" to the broom of the sorcerer's apprentice (in that they had walked out of the laboratory and turned on their researchers) and maintained that "rather than being the subject of careful scientific inquiry, these agents have become invested with an aura of magic" (p. 758). Nevertheless, Cole and Katz asserted the need for careful study of this class of drugs because of the potential importance of the therapeutic claims made for them in treatment of otherwise treatment-resistant psychiatric conditions.

Cole and Katz's (1964) article was accompanied by Roy Grinker's (1964) second editorial warning of the dangers of the drugs he described as "psychomimetic [*sic*]" (p. 768). Grinker complained that the use by therapists of LSD made it "impossible to find an investigator willing to work with LSD-25 who was not himself an 'addict.'" This usage is a classic example of a basic misconception described by Fort (1968): "Generally any socially disapproved drug comes to be referred to as narcotics or dope and the user as an addict." Nevertheless, Grinker's editorial was widely quoted in the popular press and used as evidence of the dangers of LSD research by the editors of the *New England Journal of Medicine* (Further Consideration of the Dangers of LSD, 1966).

Battle lines were being drawn. At the May 1964 convention of the American Psychiatric Association, the controversies about LSD became "a central point of interest, fear,

and warnings" (Godfrey, 1969). Advertisements announcing the publication of a new scholarly journal, *Psychedelic Review,* were refused by *The Progressive,* and by *American Psychologist* (Bunce, 1979). Despite the passion with which the psychedelics were discussed by both proponents and opponents, there still seemed to be consensus that what was needed was more and better designed research (Beecher, 1963; Cohen & Ditman, 1962, 1963; Cole & Katz, 1964; Farnsworth, 1963; Grinker, 1963). The complex machinery of experimental design and research funding was slowly moving to produce "detailed and carefully controlled studies designed to be free from possible distortions due to either bias or enthusiasm" (Cole & Katz, 1964, p. 759).

In their 1995 review of the status of psychedelic drug research, which predated the current "psychedelic renaissance," Grob and Harman noted that "it is very rare in the history of science that a government has explicitly and vigorously prohibited scientific research in any particular area." Research about psychedelic drugs has been one of these rare exceptions. The effect of the proscription of research was to keep psychedelics out of the hands of scientists, therapists, and spiritual teachers, while failing to prevent the development of a black market from which they have always been available for unsupervised self-experimentation. The use of psychedelic drugs was conflated in the public mind with the use of other kinds of illegal drugs with vastly differing effects. The many American adults who have themselves had direct experience with psychedelic drugs until recently have been largely silent. For some, these experiences have been a source of embarrassment and, potentially, of scandal.

All of the psychedelic drugs are still legally classified by the U.S. Drug Enforcement Administration (DEA) as controlled substances in Schedule 1: "No known medical or therapeutic use, high potential for abuse." Their use is completely prohibited other than in highly restricted research settings, and penalties for possession and transfer are severe. Despite this classification, the DEA has estimated that millions of Americans have tried what are probably the best known psychedelics, LSD and psilocybin. In 2017, approximately 17% of respondents, age 18 or older, to the National Survey of Drug Use and Health (NSDUH) had used "hallucinogens" (of which the National Institute on Drug Abuse [NIDA; 2017] surveys only the use of LSD and psilocybin) at some time in their lives. An analysis prepared from the 2010 NSDUH Substance Abuse and Mental Health Data Archive files estimated 32 million lifetime U.S. psychedelic users (95% confidence interval [CI]: 30–33 million). U.S. residents in 2010 surveys reported lifetime use of LSD (23 million, 95% CI: 22–25 million), psilocybin (21 million, 95% CI: 20–22 million), mescaline (11 million, 95% CI: 10–12 million), or peyote (6 million, 95% CI: 5–7 million). Lifetime rate of psychedelic use among people ages 50–64 years (the "baby boomer" generation) was similar to the rate among people ages 21–49 years (Krebs & Johansen, 2013)

The long-range effects of psychedelic drug use on the lives and futures of adolescent and young adult users was debated with great passion during the 1960s and 1970s in scores of articles in the popular press; in journals of social commentary; in the scholarly literature of education, medicine, sociology, and psychiatry; and in families throughout the country. James L. Goddard, commissioner of the FDA, wrote an impassioned official letter on the topic to more than 2,000 college deans of students, science department heads, and other faculty, in which he claimed that both "students and members of the faculty [were] being secretly approached to engage in hallucinogenic 'experiences'" (LSD: The Search for Definite Conclusions, 1966). While some found this approach to be overly dramatic, others praised Goddard for recognizing the gravity of the situation and working to combat an insidious and dangerous activity (Young & Hixson, 1966). A specially convened 1966 national conference on psychedelic dangers (Bunce, 1979) was attended by 1,450 college deans, and John U. Munro, Dean of Harvard College, declared that anyone who did not have better sense than to dabble in the use of psychedelic drugs should leave college to make room for more serious and motivated students (Chayet, 1969).

Several congressional select committees held hearings on various aspects of the emerging "LSD problem." Gubernatorial candidate Ronald Reagan and then-first-term governor Jerry Brown vied in California for the toughest anti-LSD position, and the state legislature was castigated by the popular press when it acted on expert testimony recommending against criminalizing LSD possession (McGlothlin, 1966). President Lyndon Johnson attacked LSD in his 1968 State of the Union message. In an era of racial tension, urban riots, and growing divisiveness about the war in Southeast Asia, the chair of the New Jersey Drug Study Commission sued to prevent popular magazines from publishing articles about LSD use, claiming that psychedelic drugs were the greatest problem then afflicting America (Bunce, 1979; McGlothlin, 1966).

Twenty-one expert witnesses in the United States Senate, including every medical doctor and every LSD researcher who testified, discouraged making simple possession of LSD a crime, as it was expected to have a damaging and counterproductive effect on the otherwise unremarkable lives of the numerous young adults who were drawn to experiment with psychedelics. Representative George Bush of Texas was the first member of Congress to go on record with the Subcommittee in favor of making possession illegal and penalties stiffer, and his position prevailed, supported by the testimony of sheriffs, chiefs of police, and persons identified as "concerned with promoting juvenile decency" (U.S. House of Representatives, 1968). Popular federal and state laws were enacted against possession for personal use, as well as for manufacture or sale.

Forbidden fruit, however, tends to be picked without oversight. Although research into the therapeutic and heuristic possibilities of these substances in the systematic study of brain and mind function was effectively dismantled by the effect of the new laws and regulations, large numbers of adolescents and young adults perpetuated the exploration of the nature and outcomes of the psychedelic experience in unsupervised self-experimentation (McGlothlin, 1974; National Clearinghouse for Drug Abuse Information, 1970). Adverse psychedelic reactions resulted in "psychiatric emergencies" among the early self-experimenters at rates far in excess of those observed in supervised research subjects or therapeutic populations (Robbins, Robbins, Frosch, & Stern, 1967; Ungerleider, Fisher, & Fuller, 1966). Reports of suicides and homicides "under the influence of psychedelic drugs" also multiplied during this time period (Stafford, 1992).

During what the *New York Times* called an "LSD spree," Stephen Kessler was accused of stabbing the mother of his estranged wife on April 11, 1967 ("A Slaying Suspect Tells of LSD Spree," 1967). At the time of his arrest, Kessler was reported to have dazedly inquired about what he might have done and claimed amnesia after "flying for three days on LSD" ("Murder by LSD?," 1967). His arrest prompted an emergency meeting of New York law enforcement officials, prosecutors, and representatives of the FDA, who recommended new legislation to make sale or distribution of LSD a felony in New York ("LSD Parley Called Here to Stem Increase in Use," 1967). Sensational news of the "first known LSD murderer" finally convinced Sandoz Pharmaceuticals, already reluctant to continue to sponsor investigations of its psychedelic chemicals in the face of increasing legal regulation, to stop distribution of LSD and psilocybin and to recall all supplies that the company had provided to researchers ("Murder by LSD?," 1967). It also provided a horrifying story about the potential of psychedelic drugs to cause harm, which was widely cited for years afterward.

At Kessler's trial in October 1967, he claimed to have taken doses of 10–50 µg of LSD on a total of five occasions between the summer of 1964 and March 1966, the month preceding the murder ("Murder Suspect Tells of LSD Use," 1967). On the 2 days before the murder, Kessler had taken 1½ grains of pentobarbital and had "drunk three quarts of laboratory alcohol, cut with water" (Bromberg, 1970; Stafford, 1992). Kessler made no mention of having taken LSD in the month before the murder, but a psychiatrist who had examined him after his arrest claimed that Kessler could have taken doses of LSD that he was unable to recall ("Jury Told Kessler Took an LSD Cube 0before the Slaying," 1967).

Defense claims of insanity due to LSD ingestion were mooted on the basis of Kessler's history of chronic paranoid schizophrenia,

for which he had previously been hospitalized twice at Bellevue. The jury did not consider his use of LSD when he was found not guilty by reason of insanity (Barter & Reite, 1969; "Jury Acquits Kessler in LSD Murder," 1967). Because of its notoriety, the Kessler case has been analyzed by legal and medical scholars in subsequent discussions of the status of the "LSD defense" (Barter & Reite, 1969; "Jury Acquits Kessler in LSD Murder," 1967). Forensic psychiatrists have suggested that the capacity to plan and execute complex crimes is significantly impaired under the influence of psychedelics, and have refuted claims of LSD-induced amnesia for events of a violent and dramatic nature (Bromberg, 1970), suggesting instead that defendants and trial attorneys might make such claims solely as a courtroom tactic (Ungerleider, 1970).

On October 4, 1969, Diane Linkletter, youngest daughter of radio and television personality Art Linkletter, died after jumping from her sixth-floor apartment. Her father held a press conference the day after her death in which he claimed that, rather than being a suicide, Diane "was murdered by the people who manufacture and sell LSD" ("Art Linkletter: 'It Wasn't Suicide,'" 1969). Linkletter blamed Diane's LSD experiments 6 months previously for leaving her in a despondent and depressed state. Not mentioned was her annulled teenage marriage, which the family had wanted kept quiet, or the suicide 3 months prior to Diane's death of her brother-in-law, husband of her eldest sister, Dawn ("Art Linkletter: 'It Wasn't Suicide,'" 1969). A personal friend of then-president Richard Nixon, Linkletter was invited 2 weeks after his daughter's death to give a presentation to congressional leaders, including the Speaker of the House, the Senate Majority leader, and Robert Finch, the Secretary of Health Education and Welfare (Johnson, 2010). At this meeting, Finch officially relinquished his department's role in "scheduling" drugs according to their potential for abuse and usefulness as medicines. This function became part of the responsibility of the Bureau of Narcotics and Dangerous Drugs under the Justice Department. The death of the well-educated, intelligent daughter of a well-known Christian family was not a ghetto or a campus problem. It was an ideal vehicle for gathering support for the drug bill that Nixon was planning on sending to Congress—the "War on Drugs" (Baum, 1996). Linkletter became a lifelong antidrug activist and later was named by Nixon to the National Advisory Council for Drug Abuse Prevention. No drugs were found in Diane Linkletter's system by toxicology studies (Johnson, 2010).

The potential of psychedelics to cause direct physical harm was exaggerated and, in some instances, was fabricated in the hope that fear of unpredictable physical consequences would limit their attractiveness. The *Los Angeles Times* published the first report of "permanent impairment of vision as a result of staring at the sun while under the influence of LSD," which was described as a permanent defect "burned" into the retinal area of central vision, and producing a disability similar to macular degeneration ("Four LSD Users Suffer Serious Eye Damage," 1967). The Associated Press circulated this story nationally and it appeared in *Time* magazine and the *New York Times* ("Four Students Under LSD Hurt Eyes by Sun-Gazing," 1967; "More Bad Trips on LSD," 1967). In the interval, although neither the affected students nor the spokesperson for the Santa Barbara Ophthalmological Society, who described the nature of the damage in the original story, were ever named, and no follow-up articles had explored, for example, how the affected students were coping with their new disability, the story resurfaced 8 months later (Mikkelson, 2007). This time the source was Norman M. Yoder, commissioner of the Office of the Blind for the State of Pennsylvania, who invented the story that six college students had burned their retinas so badly by staring at the sun for hours during an LSD trip that all six became totally blind. Dr. Yoder had heard the original story when he attended a lecture on the dangers of LSD several months earlier, and later falsified six case studies of blinded students, whom he reported were receiving state aid, to an official of the federal Department of Health, Education, and Welfare. Although the case studies contained significant factual inconsistencies, they prompted the FDA to seek to identify and prosecute the supplier of the LSD that the students had taken. Commissioner Yoder then admitted

that he had made up the story because of "concern over illegal LSD use by children" (Mikkelson, 2007). Yoder resigned his post in disgrace when an official review of the students' records revealed that, although the students were blind, LSD had nothing to do with their disability ("Another LSD Hallucination," 1968; "Darkness at Noon," 1969; Fuller, 1976; "LSD Blindness Case Faces F.D.A. Inquiry," 1968; "More Bad Trips on LSD," 1967; Schatz & Mendelblatt, 1973; "Six College Men Take LSD, Blinded by Sun," 1968). Two documented reports of severe and irreversible ocular damage that has resulted from prolonged staring at the sun by individuals under the influence of LSD have been reported (Fuller, 1976; Nichols, 2004; Schatz & Mendelblatt, 1973), but specious stories of eye injury probably outnumber verifiable incidents by a significant factor (Erowid, 1994)

Not just humans were thought to be at risk from adverse psychedelic effects. In a famous experiment, the details of which are still being debated, Tusko, a 7,000-pound male Indian elephant belonging to the Lincoln Park Zoo in Oklahoma, "died from an overdose of LSD," providing another sensational news feature with more than one possible interpretation. During an attempt to study *musth*, a form of cyclic elephant madness, a group of researchers headed by Louis Jolyon (Jolly) West, MD, former director of the UCLA Neuropsychiatric Institute, shot Tusko with a hypodermic dart containing a very large dose of LSD (West, Pierce, & Thomas, 1962).

The experimenters speculated in their report that the dose given may have been orders of magnitude too high (100.0 µg/kg vs. the 1.0–2.0 µg/kg that is considered to be an effective dose for humans). Using this model, the calculated dose for a 3,000-kg elephant would have been about 6–9 mg. If metabolic rate were used to calculate the dose, it would have been about 3.9 mg, and if brain size were used, about 0.64 mg, rather than the 297 mg that was actually administered. In any event, according to the report of the experiment by West and colleagues (1962), Tusko initially displayed trumpeting and restlessness within 3 minutes of the LSD injection, similar behavior to that he had exhibited the previous day when he was shot with a dart of penicillin to assess his baseline reaction to this method of medication administration. Although his mate tried to support him, he "began to sway, his hindquarters buckled, and it became increasingly difficult for him to maintain himself upright. Five minutes after the injection he trumpeted, collapsed, fell heavily onto his right side, defecated, and went into status epilepticus" (p. 1101) with labored breathing and cyanosis of the tongue. After 20 minutes, West injected him with a similarly calculated dose (2,800 mg) of promazine hydrochloride, a Thorazine-like major tranquilizer that only partially relieved the respiratory distress and seizure. An additional injection of pentobarbital sodium was given intravenously, but 1 hour and 40 minutes after the initial injection of LSD, the elephant died of laryngeal spasm after a prolonged tonic seizure. West and colleagues speculated that elephants might be uniquely sensitive to LSD and suggested the possibility of its use for animal control work in Africa. Debate about whether LSD was the cause of Tusko's death continues almost 40 years later, despite the replication of the experiment on two elephants who survived similar doses by Ronald Siegel (1984), a researcher studying animal states of awareness. The legend of Jolly the Elephant Killer is apparently too well established as a piece of psychedelic folklore to be completely supplanted by further research, but extrapolation from this experiment to an estimate of a possible lethal dose of LSD is impossible due to the mistakes made in scaling of the LSD dose, as well as the large amounts of promazine and the unknown amount of barbiturate that were subsequently administered (Erowid, 2012).

A "psychedelic syndrome" (D. Smith, 1969) of "dyssocial" (Cohen, 1966), unproductive (Carlin & Post, 1974), and alienated behavior (U.S. House of Representatives, 1968) was believed to afflict those who had become involved with the psychedelic drugs. Behaviors cited as evidence of this problem included rejection of Judeo-Christian roots for Eastern spirituality (Cole & Katz, 1964), political "passivism" (Schachter, 1968), adoption of patterns of magical and cosmic thinking (Smith, 1969), sexual license (Farnsworth & Weiss, 1969), and a preference for bizarre dress and inadequate personal hygiene (Bingham, 1967). The fearful question on the minds of spokespeople for the parental generation was whether these disaffiliated and deranged youngsters would ever be able to take up the responsibilities of adulthood and the reins of government, business and community responsibility in the future (Farnsworth, 1968; Robitscher, 1969; Watts, 1977; Wittenborn, 1969).

Unusual beliefs and unpopular attitudes have frequently been "scientifically" diagnosed as psychiatric illness, spiritual malaise, and community affliction based on personal and cultural value judgments. Persons whose beliefs did not conform to governmental norms have been incarcerated for cultural reeducation and alignment with the ideals of the Revolution during the Stalinist era in the USSR, and from the Cultural Revolution to the present-day treatment of the Uighur Muslims in China (Sudworth, 2018). Heretics and witches have been sought using the science of identifying the bedeviled detailed in the *Malleus Malleficarum (The Hammer of Witches)* (Kramer & Sprenger, 1486/1928), the medieval handbook for Inquisitors. Nazi social theories targeted not only Roma, Jews, and those of other "inferior races," but also physically disabled persons, homosexuals, and adherents of "eccentric" systems of belief and practice, such as Freemasons. An entire medico-moral movement developed in the 18th century around masturbation. *The Heinous Sin of Self Abuse* and other medical texts provided information on the signs, symptoms, and social ills resulting from this practice, and various forms of physical restraint that could be used to prevent it were widely available as medical appliances in the United States until the 1930s (Goodman, 2000; Greydanus & Geller, 1980; Hare, 1962).

Fears that psychedelics might corrupt youth, induce psychosis, harm elephants, or lead to unpredictable social consequences were eclipsed in March 1967 by reports of damage to human chromosomes caused by LSD. Maimon Cohen, a geneticist from State University of New York (SUNY), Buffalo, is reported to have become interested in the possible deleterious effects of LSD during a short visit to the Haight Ashbury district of San Francisco while attending a medical meeting in 1966 (Fort, 1970). In March 1967, Cohen and his associates published their first report of the frequencies of chromosome breaks in cultures of human peripheral leukocytes after exposure to various concentrations of LSD for 4, 24, and 48 hours. At least a twofold increase in chromosomal abnormalities was detected in all but the lowest concentration at the shortest exposure. In addition, the researchers noted a more than threefold excess in the number of damaged chromosomes over normal in a patient with schizophrenia who had received 15 treatments with LSD (Cohen, Marinello, & Back, 1967).

At the time that their work was first published, M. Cohen gave several interviews describing his team's work, in which he claimed that "our rationale was to show that LSD isn't as innocuous as people believe" (interviews in *Medical World News* and the *New York Times*, cited in Prince, 1967). Despite this display of bias, few questioned the objectivity of his observations.

Daniel X. Freedman, chair of the University of Chicago Department of Psychiatry, was one of those who advocated caution in the discussion. At a National Institutes of Mental Health (NIMH) conference on adverse reactions to psychedelics, he described his own "skepticism about the basic science and laboratory indications that there are somatic dangers to LSD" (Freedman, 1967). He admitted, however, "a deep wish that there would be a dire somatic consequence of the drug, because then we wouldn't have to spend all our time meeting about it, talking to parents, teachers, clubs, and churches. My social life has changed a good deal due to the accident that I happened to study LSD ten years ago." The published conference summary interpreted these remarks of Freedman's as a wish that the chromosome damage reports were true, as it might "stem the increase in illicit hallucinogenic drug use" (Meyer, 1967).

M. Cohen's findings of *in vitro* chromosome damage were quickly extrapolated to a potential for teratogenic effects *in vivo*. The teratogenic potential of drugs used during pregnancy had been fully appreciated for the first time with the occurrence in early 1960s of 12,000 cases of phocomelia, a rare congenital defect involving reduction of the proximal portion of the extremities, after pregnant women had ingested the sedative thalidomide. The possibility that LSD could have teratogenic effects was quickly and widely reported in the popular press. *McCall's* advertised an article on chromosome damage with a picture of a dismembered baby. The report, "LSD: Danger to Unborn Babies" actually cast doubt on the validity of M. Cohen's findings but advised against the casual use of any medications during pregnancy (Brecher, 1967). A *Saturday Evening Post* feature story (Davidson, 1967), "The Hidden Evils of LSD," claimed that new research indicated that LSD was "causing genetic damage that poses a threat of havoc now and appalling abnormalities for generations yet unborn" and that "if you take LSD even once your children may be born malformed or retarded" (p. 19). It is possible that the social utility of M. Cohen's chromosome studies contributed to their rapid dissemination. Jonathan Cole told the *Saturday Evening Post* that NIMH was so concerned about these findings that it was encouraging new research on chromosome damage. More than 60 studies in this area were completed in the next five years.

The lead article in the November 17, 1967 issue of the *New England Journal of Medicine* was a collaboration by Maimon Cohen, Kurt Hirschorn, and William Frosch, author of the account of adverse LSD effects seen as psychiatric emergencies at Bellevue. They presented the results of a comparison of the number of chromosome breaks found in a sample of 18 LSD users who had been admitted to the Bellevue psychiatric emergency service with 16 control subjects. Two controls with a very high percentage of breaks were dropped from the study before data analysis because of the onset of the symptoms of a viral infection soon after blood samples were obtained. With the exception of these two, the LSD patients had chromosome breakage rates two to four times higher than the controls. There was no mention of the occurrence of viral illness in the LSD patients. In addition, four children who had been exposed to LSD *in utero* were evaluated and found to have morphological rearrangements of their chromosomes.

The researchers recommended that a large epidemiological study be undertaken to evaluate the potential dangers they identified: a possible increase in leukemia and other neoplasms in LSD users; a potential for teratogenic effects on the fetus exposed *in utero*; and the risk of genetic translocations producing damage in future generations (Cohen, Hirschorn, & Frosch, 1967). An accompanying editorial described LSD as "radiomimetic"—causing somatic mutations and cell depletion similar to chronic whole-body radiation. The editorial emphasized that these findings would require users to reconsider their attitudes toward drug use. For the sake of the biological fitness of the next generation, it said, "the time [had] come to stress the negative attributes of psychotomimetic drugs" (Fitzgerald, 1968).

Others were not as quick to accept Cohen's conclusions. Daniel Freedman (1968) was one of the first to point out that "reports of chromosomal changes in preparations of lymphocytes raised in tissue culture are not identical with 'genetic damage.'" The Maryland Psychiatric Research Center, one of the few sites of ongoing LSD research on human subjects, took the opportunity to set up a double-blind, controlled study of before-and-after rates of chromosomal aberrations in patients exposed to pure LSD but found no definitive evidence of damage after LSD exposure (Tjio, Pahnke, & Kurland, 1969). In a Danish study, researchers administered massive LSD doses to mice (1mg/kg) and found definite evidence of bone marrow damage (Skakkebaek, Philip, & Rafaelson, 1968), but these results were not reproducible in subsequent studies (Waranky & Takacs, 1968). Other researchers questioned the teratogenicity of LSD (Jarvik & Kato, 1968), or pointed out the multitude of chemicals known to produce chromosome breakage in cultured cells, including salicylates, caffeine, theophylline, theobromine, hydrogen peroxide, calcium deficiency, penicillin, sulfas, tetracycline, and water, unless twice distilled in glass (Judd, Brandycamp, & McGlothlin, 1969).

Two extensive reviews of the literature published in the early 1970s attempted to synthesize the numerous conflicting findings of various studies. Dishotsky, Loughman, Mogar, and Lipscomb (1971) reviewed 68 studies and case reports published from 1967 to 1970, and concluded that "pure LSD ingested in moderate doses does not damage chromosomes *in vivo*, does not cause detectable genetic damage, and is not a teratogen or a carcinogen in man." They found no contraindication to the continued controlled experimental use of LSD other than pregnancy. In a review in *Teratology,* Sally Long (1972) examined the possibility of direct or indirect genetic or teratogenic effects on children, and concluded that the risk of such effects from research or treatment using LSD was small enough that it might be outweighed by potential therapeutic benefits, a decision that should be left to the researcher. Because of the curtailment of research on LSD with human subjects, few subsequent studies provide data on possible chromosome damage effects in humans. Research in animal models has continued to support the consensus that LSD is neither teratogenic nor oncogenic, and that it is, at most, a weak mutagen (Abraham & Aldridge, 1993; Richards, 2015). According to Katherine Bonson (2018) of the FDA's Controlled Substance Staff, Center for Drug Evaluation and Research, "to date, there are no credible data supporting the allegation that LSD alters genetic material."

Although LSD specifically is known to be medically safe and nontoxic when taken in the usual dosages of 50–200 µg (Nichols & Grob, 2018) it has the potential to cause disturbing psychological experiences of frightening hallucinations and confrontations with fear of death. These unpleasant episodes, which have been colloquially called "bad trips" or "bummers," have sometimes been blamed on presumed adulterants that were thought to taint some batches of LSD. Adulteration with strychnine is one of the most widely believed and persistent myths related to LSD, with even prominent professional publications mentioning it as an additive intended to increase its potency as a hallucinogen. Users have related unpleasant experiences to the presence of adulterants, with methamphetamine causing a "speedy" trip and strychnine being the basis for a bummer (Presti & Beck, 2001). Historic analyses of samples of street LSD, however, consistently showed that adulterants were not present (Grinspoon & Bakalar, 1979). The use of blotter paper to produce uniform doses from microgram quantities of high-potency LSD has historically made the inclusion of adulterants difficult (Presti & Beck, 2001). The emergence in this century of NBOMe (synthetic hallucinogen) derivatives, which are also potent in microgram quantities, has introduced the possibility of substitution of a substance with a significant range of adverse physical effects, including fatal overdose, for LSD in the blotter format (Suzuki, Poklis, & Poklis, 2014). Despite the possibility of prolonged psychotic reactions in vulnerable individuals, there are no known cases of fatal LSD overdose (Passie, Halpern, Stichtenoth, Emrich, & Hintzen, 2008).

The issue of chromosome damage presented the first rational reason not to engage in controlled scientific study of psychedelic drugs. Potential subjects of LSD research raised questions about genetic risks, and scientists raised ethical questions about the safety of research subjects (Dahlberg, Mechaneck, & Feldstein, 1968). Officials of the government agencies charged with programming and funding research experienced conflicts between the scientific approach and their personal opinions and morals (Freedman, 1969).

The kinds of studies considered to be useful and important by funding agencies were tied to social policy by dependence on congressional appropriations (Fort, 1970) The use of LSD was seen by some as symbolic of a social movement of rebellious opposition to government policies, predominant values, and conventional behaviors (Levine, 1968; Neill, 1987). Dramatic and exciting publicity, even when negative, acted as a lure for those disposed to use psychedelic drugs, and created hostility and anger in those who opposed their use. Drug policies depending primarily on prohibition and law enforcement for control increased the profit for those illegal entrepreneurs willing to take the increased risks and added the danger of adverse legal consequences to the list of possible harms resulting from psychedelic drug use. What did not deter the drug entrepreneur, however, demoralized many clinical investigators (Curran, 1967).

The social turbulence, psychiatric commotion, and medical controversy that surrounded the psychedelics in the 1960s and 1970s did not encourage much reservation of judgment on their long-range effects. Societies that had long histories of systematic alteration of consciousness for socially acceptable purposes were dismissed as primitive and pathetic (Grof, 1987; McClelland, 1961). The potential for genetic mutation of the future progeny of psychedelic experimenters was seized upon as a vital topic for further research (Meyer, 1967), despite serious limitations of sensational early studies (Prince, 1967). Decades of research that suggested possible therapeutic benefit from the psychedelics were dismissed as methodologically inadequate, and support for further studies that could have addressed these inadequacies was not forthcoming (Mangini, 1998). Even commentators who did not entirely condemn both supervised and unsupervised experimentation cautiously reserved judgment regarding any claims of potential benefit until the long-range effects of the psychedelics on the mind, the body, and the social fabric were better known (McGlothlin, 1985).

Much of the perplexed speculation on the possible long-range social outcomes of widespread experimentation with psychedelics focused on their potential effects on the cognitive structures of users. Fears expressed by social commentators of the 1960s and 1970s concerned the potential permanent changes in the epistemologies of drug users, which, it was speculated, might irreconcilably alienate them from traditional community standards of behavior, discourse, and reality (Allen, 1985; Kaiser & Gold, 1973; Louria, 1968). Psychedelic substances seem to facilitate the development of alternative perspectives on reality and soften conceptual boundaries (Cleckner, 1977). Rather than supporting participation in the accustomed cosmological and social order, observers feared that users' exposure to psychedelics would condition them to "variant models of time, space, and cause–effect which [would] result in epistemic [*sic*] organizations highly maladaptive to the demands of everyday 'normal' life" (Marsella & Price-Williams, 1974).

Whether or not the repeat user experienced any immediate adverse psychedelic effects, the combination of multiple psychedelic experiences and membership, in some kind of "psychedelic community" or social

world in which alternative beliefs, perceptions, and knowledge systems not based on
sense data were attended to and validated,
was thought to facilitate the development of
the "psychedelic syndrome" (Smith, 1969).
The clinical picture of those affected was
one of discernible changes in beliefs and values despite intact cognitive abilities. Chronic
users with multiple episodes of LSD ingestion were observed in one study to have an altered sense of time and a changed awareness
of themselves as separate entities from the
world around them (Blacker, Jones, Stone,
& Pfefferbaum, 1968). The immediate concern of some researchers was that, having rejected conventional epistemology, developed
eccentric belief systems and adapted to alternative social worlds, these individuals would
be unable or unwilling to reenter "straight"
society (Smith, 1967). The psychedelic experience might, it was feared, lead users to see
their accustomed culture and reality not as
self-evident and unquestioned, but "as arbi-
trary or one possible order among others"
(Thompson, 1987).

Sidney Cohen (1960b), who came to be
regarded as one of the principal spokesper-
sons on psychedelic experience in the United
States, wrote of the effects of LSD:

> Any attempt to communicate the total LSD
> experience will surely fail. Much of it occurs
> on a non-verbal level and is so highly variable
> that an over-all statement will not encompass
> the entire spectrum of possible reaction. Fur-
> thermore, it is so foreign to our everyday exis-
> tence that our vocabulary is lacking in words
> to describe precisely even that which could be
> described.

Early attempts at description of the effects
of psychedelics emphasized accounts of the
sensations experienced after taking psychedelic drugs, "to the detriment of the emphasis that should be placed on [their] role as
an integral part of an ongoing life, most of
which must be lived in a non-drugged condition" (Bieberman, 1968). Personal transformation following psychedelic experiences
was widely reported anecdotally but was not
confirmed by the measures used in previous
long-term studies. Many early attempts to
review the use of psychedelic drugs and report their impact on users were by persons
seeking adverse effects specifically. Failure

to recognize and investigate occasions of
positive transformation may have been an
artifact of the generally negative perception
of the psychedelic experience that predomi-
nated after use and possession of psychedelic
drugs were criminalized in our society. In
those studies that did seek to identify positive effects, it is possible that the measures
employed did not fully access the types of
changes that may have occurred.

As the use of illegal psychedelic drugs
was officially and publicly reprehended in
the modern American context (Jaffe, 1990),
harm reduction strategies aimed at those
who chose to use these drugs became a politically charged topic (Grove, 1996), and
acknowledgment of potential benefits of illegal drug use was rarely attempted (Walsh,
1982). Medically and legally, any use of a
psychedelic drug was far more likely to be
construed as drug abuse and labeled as de-
viant behavior than gross intoxication with,
or regular ingestion of, other abusable substances (Fort, 1968; Jacobs & Fehr, 1987;
Jaffe, 1971; Zinberg, 1984).

The orthodox public political stance in
relation to psychedelic drug use became so
unremittingly disapproving as to make it
difficult to maintain a balanced approach.
The prevailing social climate shifted very
much toward the negative after the peak
years of psychedelic drug use. Grove (1996)
described the response to drug use and drug
users as driven by a model of condemnation
that "relied almost exclusively for its authority on extreme manifestations of drug-related harm . . . [and did] not let us identify the
presence of drug use except where [it] has
already caused considerable harm or damage." Gotz suggested as early as 1972 that
"it would seem that the judgment has already been rendered: [psychedelic] drugs can
only be 'abused.'" He objected to the way in
which this foreclosed on the possibility that
the psychedelics might be used in a way that
was "moderate, guided, purposeful, and
conducive to [changes] of character that we
say we value." William McGlothlin, one of
the most prolific and most moderate of the
early LSD researchers, was also one of the
earliest to call for and conduct long-range
studies of psychedelic drug effects. In 1966,
he suggested that youthful "disaffiliates,"
who formed the majority of the "psychedelic

movement," were passing through an understandable developmental stage, one in which they were readily influenced to accept new attitudes, values, and beliefs. He noted that although there was "considerable individual variation, the most consistent personal pattern [was] a lessening of concern over status, competition, material possessions, and other pursuits of the achievement oriented society" (p. 5). He found it difficult to imagine how these young people would look in their 40s, but he suggested that the "capacity of hallucinogenic drugs for shaping personality and values (both adjustive and disruptive) [was] likely to have considerably more social impact" than more feared and scrutinized effects, such as acute psychotic reactions.

Jonathan O. Cole, former chief of the Psychopharmacology Service Center at NIMH, suggested at the 1969 Rutger's Symposium on Drug Abuse that a survey like the Kinsey report might provide new information about psychoactive drug use that would allow for more rational decision making on the subject. He maintained that while repressive legislation was justified by the immediate social crisis, attitudes and laws about drug use might soften if "socially competent and effective individuals" were later to be identified as nonproblematic drug users, and speculated that drug use "in stable middle-class society is far greater than one would imagine" (Cole, 1969).

Cole's speculation was never extensively explored, and very few efforts to study stable nonproblematic drug users or workable contexts for the use of illegal drugs were subsequently attempted. Rather than a softening and moderation of laws and attitudes about drug use, the next 50 years have produced increasingly rigid and draconian attempts to suppress all illicit drug use. Not only have these attempts been unsuccessful in eliminating drug use, but they also have disrupted the process of social learning whereby peer groups transmit rules and norms, and develop informal social controls, thereby increasing the associated risks (Becker, 1974; Bunce, 1979; Zinberg & Harding, 1979).

Early antipsychedelic crusaders maintained that harsh antidrug laws would later be modified if they proved unjustified. Jonas Robitscher (1969) provided a fairly typical medico-legal perspective for the time at the Rutgers Symposium, at which he suggested that strong and prompt action should be taken to restrict the "delusional and hallucinatory experiences" produced by LSD and other illegal drugs on the basis that the harm that they might do was not known. If the experiences proved not to be harmful, or to be of benefit, Robitscher argued, these measures could later be rescinded:

> If time proves that these substances are beneficial, we can adopt them when we know more about them. If time proves that users of these substances cannot participate in society as we know it, cannot use their abilities for the common welfare, become dependent on other segments of society for support and maintenance, and cannot provide a stable family unit in which children can grow up to take their place in society, it is important that we minimize the use of these [drugs] here and now. (p. 305)

Historically, the potential negative outcomes of psychedelic alterations in attitudes, beliefs, and values have been assigned much more public credibility than the positive ones. Despite statistical evidence that there are a large number of highly educated middle-aged and older persons who have used psychedelics, no distinctive ill-effects in this population have been traced to their history of drug use. On the contrary, "significant numbers of people feel that the psychedelics have made positive contributions to their personal psychological growth" (Walsh, 1982, p. 22). For these persons, there has been a disparity between the generally negative view of psychedelic drugs that was popularly presented and their personal experience.

According to psychedelic researchers Sidney Cohen and Stanley Krippner (1985), "At many times, in many places, groups have gathered to approach the Mysterium Tremendum. When drugs were used for this purpose, those gatherings could be called 'psychedelic clusters' of a small number of individuals who were entranced with their ineffable experiences." In the United States, in the second half of the 20th century, many psychedelic clusters have formed and dissolved, and some have endured.

The Native American Church is one highly visible cluster. Incorporated in 1918, it continues to be a significant spiritual movement with both Native and non-Native adherents. Other psychedelic clusters have formed around the work of some of the psychologists and psychiatrists who have administered psychedelics in therapy. Dr. Oscar Janiger, for example, administered psychedelics to roughly 900 patients and research subjects from 1954 until 1962, and 45 of these individuals participated in a 40-year follow-up study of their psychedelic experiences (Doblin, Beck, Obata, & Alioto, 1999). The work of another therapist, Leo Zeff, a "pioneer of the underground psychedelic therapy movement" who conducted psychedelic therapy with a psychedelic cluster numbering in the thousands during the 1960s and 1970s, has been described by Stolaroff (2004).

Timothy Leary and Richard Alpert established several centers for exploration of the psychedelic experience in Massachusetts, New York, and Mexico, and clusters of seekers sought them out, along with police and news reporters. The loosely organized cluster known as the Merry Pranksters traveled widely throughout the United States in the 1960s and spun off other ill-defined psychedelic clusters including Grateful Dead and the Hog Farm. Steven Gaskin so inspired the cluster of which he was the spiritual leader that they moved *en masse* from San Francisco to Tennessee in 1971 to found The Farm, a community that has been described as a psychedelic church. While the specific aims and methods of these groups differ extravagantly, members of each of these clusters have had in common a desire for personal transformation and an awareness that LSD and other psychedelics could be powerful facilitators for this purpose.

An intriguing perspective on the ability of psychedelics to produce profound personal transformation was that of Lisa Bieberman, publisher of the *Psychedelic Information Center Bulletin*, and one of the most thoughtful and articulate writers on early experimentation with consciousness-expanding drugs. Bieberman (1968) believed that profound psychedelic transformations are possible because the experience available from psychedelic drugs is potentially productive of a religious or mystical insight, "a conviction of a divine Reality based on personal encounter, plus interpretation and im-

plementation based on the individual's . . . background, personality and situation." She suggested that this might be more common than was generally thought, but that it tended to be obscured by the fashions, music, political postures and other countercultural baggage that had attached itself to the psychedelic drugs.

Bieberman (1967) rejected the word *psychedelic* as having been degraded as a referent to this extraordinary experience by its associations with "gaudy illegible posters, gaudy unreadable tabloids, loud parties, anything paisley, noisy crowded discotheques, trinket shops and the slum districts that patronize them." She preferred *phanerothyme*, a word coined by Aldous Huxley, which she defined as "(1) a state of mental and spiritual clarity, achieved through the responsible and reverent use of certain plants or drugs, such as peyote, mescaline, psilocybin and LSD; (2) certain drugs, when used for the sake of phanerothyme" (Bieberman, 1968, p. 4). She counseled that rather than trying to describe the effects of psychedelics, it would be preferable to describe what the psychedelic experience teaches. "The test," Bieberman wrote, "is not how magnificent the visions, but rather how clear is the understanding obtained, and the test of clarity is its applicability to daily life" (p. 4).

In Bieberman's view, it would only become possible to assess the quality of the original transformative experience over the long term. Those who had been fortunate enough to have experienced the full extent of the psychedelics' transformative potential would know themselves and be known to others by the fruits of that experience in their everyday existence. Thus, Bieberman seemed to suggest that those who were not transformed by the experience had not been exposed to its full manifestation, an explanation that was advanced by some psychedelic therapists as well (Chwelos, Blewett, Smith, & Hoffer, 1959; Savage, 1962; Terrill, 1964). She wrote, "Phanerothyme cannot be completely defined because there remains much that is recognized by the experiencer, who will know phanerothyme from any mere hallucination, intoxicant or stimulant. . . . [A] drug becomes phanerothyme only by the intent of the receiver" (Bieberman, 1968, p. 6).

Roberts (1999) has suggested that this usage is analogous to the sacramental use of altar wine; its sacramental status is derived not from its chemical structure, or its possible use as a medicine, food, or intoxicant, but the understanding with which it is used by the celebrant. This perspective suggests a multifactorial combination of experience, intention, social circumstance, and practice that interact in producing manifestations of the transformative potential of psychedelic drugs.

▓ References

A slaying suspect tells of LSD spree. (1967, April 12). *New York Times*, pp. 1, 32.

Aaronson, B. S., & Osmond, H. (1970). Introduction: Psychedelics, technology, psychedelics. In B. S. Aaronson & H. Osmond (Eds.), *Psychedelics* (pp. 3–18). Garden City, NY: Anchor.

Abraham, H. D., & Aldridge, A. M. (1993). Adverse consequences of lysergic acid diethylamide. *Addiction, 88*(10), 1327–1334.

Abramson, H. A. (Ed.). (1967). *The use of LSD in psychotherapy and alcoholism.* Indianapolis, IN: Bobbs-Merrill.

Adriani, J. (1976). Drug dependence in hospitalized patients. In P. Bourne (Ed.), *Acute drug abuse emergencies* (pp. 231–250). New York: Academic Press.

Allen, D. G. (1985). Nursing research and social control: Alternative models of science that emphasize understanding and emancipation. *Image: The Journal of Nursing Scholarship, 17*(2), 58–64.

Another LSD hallucination. (1968, January 26). *Time*, p. 66.

Art Linkletter: "It wasn't suicide, it was murder." (1969, October 6). *The Dispatch*, p. 4.

Barter, J., & Reite, M. (1969). Crime and LSD: The insanity plea. *American Journal of Psychiatry, 126*(4), 113–119.

Baum, D. (1996). *Smoke and mirrors.* Boston: Little, Brown.

Becker, H. S. (1974). Consciousness, power, and drug effects. *Journal of Psychoactive Drugs, 6*(1), 67–76.

Beecher, H. K. (1963). Science, drugs students. *Harvard Alumni Bulletin, 65*(8), 338.

Bieberman, L. (1967). The psychedelic experience. *New Republic, 157*, 17–19.

Bieberman, L. (1968). *Phanerothyme: A Western approach to the religious use of psychochemicals* [Pamphlet]. Psychedelic Information Center.

Bingham, J. (1967, September 24). The intelligent square's guide to hippieland. *New York Times Magazine*, pp. 68–76.

Blacker, K. H., Jones, R. T., Stone, G. C., & Pfefferbaum, D. (1968). Chronic users of LSD: The "Acidheads." *American Journal of Psychiatry, 125*(3), 341–351.

Bonson, K. R. (2018). Regulation of human research with LSD in the United States (1949–1987). *Psychopharmacology, 235*(2), 591–604.

Brecher, E. M. (1967, September). LSD: Danger to unborn babies. *McCall's*, pp. 70–71, 124.

Bromberg, W. (1970). LSD-induced amnesia. *American Journal of Psychiatry, 126*(8), 166.

Brunton, L., Knollman, B., & Hilal-Dandan, R. (2018). *Goodman and Gillman's the pharmacological basis of therapeutics* (13th ed.). New York: McGraw-Hill.

Bunce, R. (1979). Social and political sources of drug effects: The case of bad trips on psychedelics. *Journal of Drug Issues, 9*(2), 213–233.

Calabrese, J. D. (1994). Reflexivity and transformation symbolism in the Navajo Peyote meeting. *Ethos, 22*(4), 494–527.

Caldwell, W. V. (1968). *LSD psychotherapy.* New York: Grove Press.

Carlin, A., & Post, R. D. (1974). Drug use and achievement. *International Journal of the Addictions, 9*(3), 401–410.

Chandler, A., & Hartman, M. (1960). Lysergic acid diethylamide (LSD-25) as a facilitating agent in psychotherapy. *Archives of General Psychiatry, 2*, 286–299.

Chayet, N. L. (1969). Legal aspects of drug abuse. In J. R. Wittenborn, H. Brill, J. P. Smith, & S. Wittenborn (Eds.), *Drugs and youth: Proceedings of the Rutgers Symposium on Drug Abuse* (pp. 236–249). Springfield, IL: Charles C Thomas.

Christen, J. P. (1966, June 18). Lysergic acid diethylamide. *British Medical Journal*, p. 1540.

Chwelos, N., Blewett, D. B., Smith, C. M., & Hoffer, A. (1959). Use of d-lysergic acid diethylamide in the treatment of alcoholism. *Quarterly Journal of Studies on Alcohol, 20*(3), 577–590.

Clark, W. H. (1969). *Chemical ecstasy.* New York: Sheed & Ward.

Clark, W. H. (1985). Ethics and LSD. *Journal of Psychoactive Drugs, 17*(4), 229–234.

Cleckner, P. J. (1977). Hallucinogens in the United States: A diagnostic evaluation. *Journal of Psychedelic Drugs, 9*, 133–141.

Cohen, M. M., Hirschorn, K., & Frosch, W. A. (1967). *In vivo* and *in vitro* chromosomal damage induced by LSD-25. *New England Journal of Medicine, 277*(20), 1043–1049.

Cohen, M. M., Marinello, M. J., & Back, N. (1967). Chromosomal damage in human leukocytes induced by lysergic acid diethylamide. *Science, 155,* 1417–1419.

Cohen, S. (1960a). LSD: Side effects and complications. *Journal of Nervous and Mental Disease, 130,* 30–40.

Cohen, S. (1960b). Notes on the hallucinogenic state. *International Record of Medicine, 173*(6), 380–387.

Cohen, S. (1966). A classification of LSD complications. *Psychosomatics, 7,* 182–186.

Cohen, S. (1968). A quarter century of research with LSD. In J. T. Ungerleider (Ed.), *The problems and prospects of LSD.* Springfield, IL: Charles C Thomas.

Cohen, S., & Ditman, K. (1962). Complications associated with LSD-25. *Journal of the American Medical Association, 181*(2), 161–162.

Cohen, S., & Ditman, K. (1963). Prolonged adverse reactions to lysergic acid diethylamide. *Archives of General Psychiatry, 8,* 475–480.

Cohen, S., & Krippner, S. (1985). Editor's introduction. *Journal of Psychoactive Drugs, 17*(4), 213–217.

Cole, J. O. (1961). Drugs and control of the mind. In S. Farber & R. H. L. Wilson (Eds.), *Man and civilization: Control of the mind.* New York: McGraw-Hill.

Cole, J. O. (1969). LSD and marijuana: Research needs. In J. R. Wittenborn, H. Brill, J. P. Smith, & S. Wittenborn (Eds.), *Drugs and youth: Proceedings of the Rutgers Symposium on Drug Abuse* (pp. 212–216). Springfield, IL: Charles C Thomas.

Cole, J. O., & Katz, M. M. (1964). The psychotomimetic drugs. *Journal of the American Medical Association, 187*(10), 758–759.

Conrad, A. (1966, April 29). Local LSD PR-girl tells how to make (and take) those little sugar cubes. *The Harvard Crimson.*

Curran, W. J. (1967). *Current legal issues in clinical investigation with particular attention to the balance between the rights of the individual and the needs of society.* Paper presented at the sixth annual meeting of the American College of Neuropsychopharmacology, San Juan, Puerto Rico.

Dahlberg, C. C., Mechaneck, R., & Feldstein, S. (1968). LSD research: The impact of lay publicity. *American Journal of Psychiatry, 125*(5), 137–141.

Darkness at noon. (1969, January 22). *Newsweek.*

Davidson, B. (1967, August 12). The hidden evils of LSD. *Saturday Evening Post,* pp. 19–23.

Delbanco, A., & Delbanco, T. (1995, March 20). A.A. at the crossroads. *The New Yorker,* 50–63.

Dishotsky, N. I., Loughman, W. D., Mogar, R. E., & Lipscomb, W. R. (1971). LSD and genetic damage. *Science, 172,* 431–439.

Doblin, R., Beck, J. E., Obata, K., & Alioto, M. (1999). Dr. Oscar Janiger's pioneering LSD research: A forty year follow-up. *MAPS: Bulletin of the Multidisciplinary Association for Psychedelic Studies, 9*(1), 7–21.

Durant, W. (1989). *The story of civilization: Vol. II. The life of Greece.* New York: Simon & Schuster.

Editorial. (1964). *The Psychedelic Review, 1*(4), 372–377.

Eisner, B. G. (1997). Set, setting and matrix. *Journal of Psychoactive Drugs, 29*(2), 213–216.

Eisner, B. G., & Cohen, S. (1958). Psychotherapy with lysergic acid diethylamide. *Journal of Nervous and Mental Disease, 127,* 528–539.

Elkes, C., Elkes, J., & Mayer-Gross, W. (1954). Hallucinogenic drugs. *Lancet, 268,* 719.

Elkes, J. (1963). The dysleptics: Note on no man's land. *Comprehensive Psychiatry, 4*(3), 195–198.

Ellis, H. H. (1897, June 5). A note on the phenomena of mescal intoxication. *Lancet,* pp. 1540–1542.

Ellis, H. H. (1898). Mescal: A new artificial paradise. *Contemporary Review, 74,* 130–141.

Erowid. (1994). Urban folklore: LSD users stare at the sun until blind. Retrieved from *https://erowid.org/chemicals/lsd/lsd_myth6.shtml.*

Erowid. (2012). LSD related death of an elephant. Retrieved from *https://erowid.org/chemicals/lsd/lsd_history4.shtml.*

Farnsworth, D. L. (1963). Hallucinogenic agents. *Journal of the American Medical Association, 185*(11), 878–879.

Farnsworth, D. L. (1968, March 2). *Drug abuse: Legal and ethical implications of the nonmedical use of the hallucinogenic and narcotic drugs.* Paper presented at the 88th Mary Scott Newbold Symposium, Philadelphia, PA.

Farnsworth, D. L., & Weiss, S. T. (1969). Marijuana: The conditions and consequences of use and the treatment of users. In J. R. Wittenborn, H. Brill, J. P. Smith, & S. Wittenborn (Eds.), *Drugs and youth: Proceedings of the Rutgers Symposium on Drug Abuse* (pp. 168–177). Springfield, IL: Charles C Thomas.

Feld, M., Goodman, J., & Guido, J. A. (1958). Clinical and laboratory observations on LSD-25. *Journal of Nervous and Mental Disease, 126,* 176–183.

Fitzgerald, P. H. (1968). Radiomimetic properties of LSD. *New England Journal of Medicine, 278,* 1404.

Fort, J. (1968). LSD and the mind altering drug (M.A.D.) world. In J. T. Ungerleider (Ed.), *Problems and prospects of LSD* (pp. 5–21). Springfield, IL: Charles C Thomas.

Fort, J. (1970). Social aspects of research with psychedelic drugs. In J. A. Gamage & E. L.

Zerkin (Eds.), *Hallucinogenic drug research: Impact on science and society* (pp. 115–126). Beloit, WI: Stash Press.

Four LSD users suffer serious eye damage. (1967, May 18). *Los Angeles Times*, p. 1.

Four students under LSD hurt eyes by sun-gazing. (1967, May 19). *New York Times*.

Freedman, D. X. (1967, September 29). *Remarks*. Paper presented at the annual conference on Adverse Reactions to Psychedelic Drugs, Chevy Chase, MD.

Freedman, D. X. (1968). On the use and abuse of LSD. *Archives of General Psychiatry, 18*, 330–347.

Freedman, D. X. (1969). Panel discussion. In R. E. Meyer (Ed.), *Adverse reactions to psychedelic drugs*. Chevy Chase, MD: National Clearinghouse for Mental Health Information.

Fuller, D. G. (1976). Severe solar maculopathy associated with the use of lysergic acid diethylamide (LSD). *American Journal of Ophthalmology, 81*(4), 413–416.

Further consideration of the dangers of LSD. (1966). *New England Journal of Medicine, 274*, 836.

Gaines, B. (1963). LSD: Hollywood's status-symbol drug. *Cosmopolitan, 155*, 78–81.

Godfrey, K. E. (1969). Psychedelic drugs as therapeutic agents. In R. E. Hicks & P. J. Fink (Eds.), *Psychedelic drugs* (pp. 226–233). New York: Grune & Stratton.

Goldman, R. (1963). Instant happiness. *Ladies' Home Journal, 80*, 67–71.

Goodman, M. (2000). The sin of Onan. *Journal of the Royal Society of Medicine, 193*(3), 159.

Gordon, N. (1963). The hallucinogenic drug cult. *The Reporter, 29*(3), 35–43.

Gotz, I. (1972). *The psychedelic teacher: Drugs, mysticism, and schools*. Philadelphia: Westminster.

Greydanus, D. E., & Geller, B. (1980). Masturbation: Historic perspective. *New York State Journal of Medicine, 12*, 1892–1896.

Grinker, R. R. (1963). Lysergic acid diethylamide. *Annals of General Psychiatry, 8*(5), 425.

Grinker, R. R. (1964). Bootlegged ecstasy. *Journal of the American Medical Association, 187*(10), 768–769.

Grinspoon, L., & Bakalar, J. L. (1979). *Psychedelic drugs reconsidered*. New York: Basic Books.

Grinspoon, L., & Bakalar, J. L. (1983). *Psychedelic reflections*. New York: Human Sciences Press.

Grob, C., & Harman, W. (1995). Making sense of the psychedelic issue. *Noetic Sciences Review, 35*, 4–41.

Grof, S. (1975). *Realms of the human unconscious*. New York: Viking Press.

Grof, S. (1987). Spirituality, addiction, and Western science. *ReVision, 10*(2), 5–18.

Grove, D. (1996). Real harm reduction: Underground survival strategies. *Harm Reduction Communication, 1*(2), 1–8.

Hagen, W. T. (1993) *Quanah Parker, Comanche chief*. Norman: University of Oklahoma Press.

Hare, E. H. (1962). Masturbational insanity: The history of an idea. *Journal of Medical Science, 108*, 1–25.

Heffter Research Institute. (2018). About Dr. Arthur Heffter. Retrieved from *https://heffter. org/about-dr-heffter*.

Hiatt, N. (2016, May 23). A trip down memory lane: LSD at Harvard. Retrieved from *www. thecrimson.com/article/2016/5/23/trip-down-memory-lane*.

Hoffer, A. (1967). A program for the treatment of alcoholism: LSD, malvaria and nicotinic acid. In H. A. Abramson (Ed.), *The use of LSD in psychotherapy and alcoholism* (pp. 407–433). Indianapolis, IN: Bobbs-Merrill.

Hoffer, A., & Osmond, H. (1967). *The hallucinogens*. New York: Academic Press.

Hoffer, A., Osmond, H., & Smythies, J. (1954). Schizophrenia: A new approach: II. Result of a year's research. *Journal of Mental Science, 100*, 29–45.

Hollister, L. E. (1968). *Chemical psychosis*. Springfield, IL: Charles C Thomas.

Huxley, A. (1969). #744: To Dr. Humphry Osmond. In G. Smith (Ed.), *Letters of Aldous Huxley* (pp. 795–796). London: Chatto & Windus. (Original work published 1956)

Instant mysticism. (1963). *Time, 82*, 86–87.

Jacobs, M. R., & Fehr, K. O. B. (1987). *Drugs and drug abuse* (2nd ed.). Toronto: Addiction Research Foundation.

Jaffe, J. H. (1971). Pharmacological effects of drugs. In Joint Committee on Continuing Legal Education (Ed.), *ALI-ABA course of study on defense of drug cases* (pp. 62–89). Philadelphia: American Law Institute and American Bar Association.

Jaffe, J. H. (1990). Drug addiction and drug abuse. In A. G. Gilman, L. S. Goodman, & A. Gilman (Eds.), *The pharmacologic basis of therapeutics* (8th ed., pp. 522–569). New York: Pergamon/Macmillan.

James, W. (1902). *The varieties of religious experience: A study in human nature*. Longmans, Green & Co.

Jarvik, L. F., & Kato, T. (1968, February 3). Is LSD a teratogen? *Lancet, 1*, 250.

Johnson, T. (2010, May 27). Art Linkletter's war on drugs. *Variety*.

Judd, L. L., Brandycamp, W. W., & McGlothlin, W. H. (1969). Comparison of the chromosomal patterns obtained from groups of continued users, former users, and nonusers of LSD-25. *American Journal of Psychiatry*, 126(5), 72–81.

Jury acquits Kessler in LSD murder. (1967, October 26). *New York Times*, p. 63.

Jury told Kessler took an LSD cube before the slaying. (1967, October 12). *New York Times*, p. 46.

Kaiser, C., & Gold, R. (1973). Perception, psychedelics and social change. *Journal of Drug Issues*, 3(2), 141–151.

Kramer, H., & Sprenger, J. (1928). *Malleus maleficarum (the hammer of witches)*. New York: Citadel. (Original work published 1486)

Krebs, T., & Johansen, P.-O. (2013). Over 30 million psychedelic users in the United States. *F1000 Research, 2*, 98.

Kurland, A. A., Savage, C., Panhke, W. N., Grof, S., & Olsson, J. E. (1971). LSD in the treatment of alcoholics. *Pharmakopsychiatrie und Neuro-Psychopharmakologie, 4*, 83–94.

Kurland, A., Unger, S., Shaffer, J. W., & Savage, C. (1967). Psychedelic therapy utilizing LSD in the treatment of the alcoholic patient: A preliminary report. *American Journal of Psychiatry, 123*(10), 1202–1209.

Levine, J. (1968, December 12–15). *Some LSD controversies revisited*. Paper presented at the sixth annual meeting of the American College of Neuropsychopharmacology, San Juan, Puerto Rico.

Lewin, L. (1998). *Phantastica: A classic survey on the use and abuse of mind-altering plants.* Rochester, VT: Park Street Press. (Original work published 1924)

Long, S. (1972). Does LSD induce chromosomal damage and malformations?: A review of the literature. *Teratology, 6*, 72–90.

Louria, D. B. (1966). *Nightmare drugs.* New York: Pocket Books.

Louria, D. B. (1968). Lysergic acid diethylamide. *New England Journal of Medicine, 278*(8), 435–438.

Lowinger, P. (1966). Drug tests, integrity and courage. *Science, 153*, 121.

LSD blindness case faces F.D.A. inquiry. (1968, January 14). *New York Times*.

LSD parley called here to stem increase in use. (1967). *New York Times*, pp. 1, 30.

LSD: The search for definite conclusions. (1966). *Journal of the American Medical Association, 196*(4), 32–33.

Luhan, M. D. (2002) Edge of the Taos desert. In L. Anderson & T. S. Edwards (Eds.), *At home on this earth: Two centuries of U.S. women's nature writing* (pp. 156–168). Hanover, NH: University Press of New England.

Mangini, M. (1998). Treatment of alcoholism using psychedelic drugs: A review of the program of research. *Journal of Psychoactive Drugs, 30*(4), 381–418.

Marsella, A., & Price-Williams, D. (1974). A note on epistemic organization and hallucinogens. *Bulletin of the Menninger Clinic, 38*(1), 70–72.

Mayer-Gross, W. (1951, August 11). Experimental psychoses and other mental abnormalities produced by drugs. *British Medical Journal*, pp. 317–320.

McClelland, D. C. (1961). *Some social reactions to the psilocybin research project.* Cambridge, MA: Harvard Center for Research in Personality.

McGlothlin, W. H. (1966). Toward a rational view of hallucinogenic drugs (MR-83). Retrieved from *https://files.eric.ed.gov/fulltext/ED030131.pdf.*

McGlothlin, W. H. (1974). Amphetamines, barbiturates and hallucinogens (J-70-33). Washington, DC: U.S. Department of Justice, Bureau of Narcotics and Dangerous Drugs.

McGlothlin, W. H. (1985). A chemistry for world peace. *Journal of Drug Issues, 14*(2), 225–245.

Meyer, R. E. (1967, September 29). *Summary of the conference.* Paper presented at the Conference on Adverse Reactions to Hallucinogenic Drugs, Chevy Chase, MD.

Mikkelson, D. (2007). LSD users stare at sun. Retrieved from *www.snopes.com/fact-check/blinded-by-the-light.*

Mitchell, S. W. (1896, December 5). Remarks on the effects of Anhelonium Lewinii (the mescal button). *British Medical Journal*, pp. 1625–1628.

More bad trips on LSD. (1967, May 26). *Time.* Retrieved from *http://content.time.com/time/magazine/article/0,9171,843820,00.html.*

Murder by LSD? (1967, April 25). *Newsweek*, pp. 29–30.

Murder suspect tells of LSD use. (1967, October 10). *New York Times*, p. 37.

National Clearinghouse for Drug Abuse Information. (1970). Answers to the most frequently asked questions about drug abuse. Retrieved from *https://babel.hathitrust.org/cgi/pt?id=uc1.$b170496&view=1up&seq=3.*

National Institute on Drug Abuse. (2017). Trends in prevalence of various drugs. Retrieved from *www.drugabuse.gov/national-survey-drug-use-health.*

Native American Rights Fund. (2016). National Council of Native American Churches speak out against illegitimate organizations.. Retrieved from *www.narf.org/national-council-of-native-american-churches-speak-out-against-illegitimate-organizations.*

Neill, J. R. (1987). "More than medical significance": LSD and American psychiatry. *Journal of Psychoactive Drugs, 19*(1), 39–45.

Nichols, D. (1999). From Eleusis to PET scans:

The mysteries of psychedelics. *MAPS Bulletin,* 9(4), 50–55.

Nichols, D. (2004). Hallucinogens. *Pharmacology and Therapeutics, 101,* 131–181.

Nichols, D., & Grob, C. S. (2018). Is LSD toxic? *Forensic Science International, 284,* 141–145.

Novak, S. J. (1997). LSD before Leary. *Isis, 88,* 87–110.

Osmond, H. (1957). A review of the clinical effects of psychotomimetic agents. *Annals of the New York Academy of Science, 66*(3), 418–434.

Osmond, H. (1969). Alcoholism: A personal view of psychedelic treatment. In R. E. Hicks & P. J. Fink (Eds.), *Psychedelic drugs* (pp. 217–225). New York: Grune & Stratton.

Osmond, H. (1973). Medical and scientific importance of the hallucinogens. *The Practitioner, 210*(235), 112–119.

Osmond, H., & Smythies, J. (1952). Schizophrenia: A new approach. *Journal of Mental Science, 98,* 309–315.

Pahnke, W. N. (1963). *Drugs and mysticism: An analysis of the relationship between psychedelic drugs and mystical consciousness.* Unpublished doctoral dissertation, Harvard University, Cambridge, MA.

Pahnke, W. N. (1969). The psychedelic mystical experience in the human encounter with death. *Harvard Theological Review, 62*(1), 1–21.

Palmer, C., & Horowitz, M. (1982). *Sisters of the extreme: Women writing on the drug experience: Charlotte Brontë, Louisa May Alcott, Anaïs Nin, Maya Angelou, Billie Holiday, Nina Hagen, Diane di Prima, Carrie Fisher, and many others.* Rochester, VT: Park Street Press.

Paradise or inferno. (1898, February 5). *British Medical Journal, 1,* 390. Retrieved September 24, 2020, from *www.jstor.org/stable/20253365.*

Passie, T., Halpern, J. H., Stichtenoth, D. O., Emrich, H. M., & Hintzen, A. (2008). The pharmacology of lysergic acid diethylamide: A review. *CNS Neuroscience and Therapeutics, 14*(4), 295–314.

Pollan, M. (2018). *How to change your mind.* New York: Penguin/Random House.

Presti, D., & Beck, J. (2001). Strychnine and other enduring myths: Expert and user folklore surrounding LSD. In T. Roberts (Ed.), *Pstychoactive sacramentals: Essays on entheogens and religion* (pp. 125–137). San Francisco: Council on Spiritual Practices.

Prince, A. M. (1967). LSD and chromosomes. *Psychedelic Review, 9,* 38–40.

Richards, W. (2015). *Sacred knowledge: psychedelics and religious experiences.* New York: Columbia University Press.

Robbins, E., Robbins, L., Frosch, W. A., &

Stern, M. (1967). Implications of untoward reactions to hallucinogens. *Bulletin of the New York Academy of Medicine, 43*(11), 985–999.

Roberts, T. (1999). Psychedelics, peak experiences and wellness: Do entheogen-induced mystical experiences boost the immune system? *MAPS: Bulletin of the Multidisciplinary Association for Psychedelic Studies, 9*(3), 23–29.

Robitscher, J. (1969). The right of society to protect its members. In J. R. Wittenborn, H. Brill, J. P. Smith, & S. Wittenborn (Eds.), *Drugs and youth: Proceedings of the Rutgers Symposium on Drug Abuse* (pp. 299–305). Springfield, IL: Charles C Thomas.

Rudgley, R. (1995) The archaic use of the hallucinogens in Europe. *Addiction, 90,* 163–164.

Sandison, R. A., & Spencer, A. M. (1954). The therapeutic value of lysergic acid diethylamide in mental illness. *Journal of Mental Science, 100,* 491–507.

Savage, C. (1962). Summary: LSD, transcendence and a new beginning. *Journal of Nervous and Mental Disease, 135*(5), 425–439.

Schachter, B. (1968). Psychedelic drug use by adolescents. *Social Work, 13*(3), 33–39.

Schatz, H., & Mendelblatt, F. (1973). Solar retinopathy from sun-gazing under the influence of LSD. *British Journal of Ophthalmology, 57*(4), 270–273.

Sherwood, J. N., Stolaroff, M. J., & Harman, W. W. (1962). The psychedelic experience—a new concept in psychotherapy. *Journal of Neuropsychiatry, 4*(2), 69–80.

Siegel, R. K. (1984). LSD-induced effects in elephants: Comparisons with musth behavior. *Bulletin of the Psychonomic Society, 22*(1), 53–56.

Silverman, J. (1976). On the effects and uses of psychedelic drugs. *Journal of Altered States of Consciousness, 2*(2), 133–146.

Six college men take LSD, blinded by sun. (1968, January 13). *Los Angeles Times,* p. 1.

Skakkebaek, N. E., Philip, J., & Rafaelson, O. J. (1968). LSD in mice: Abnormalities in meiotic chromosomes. *Science, 160,* 1246–1248.

Smith, C. M. (1958). A new adjunct to the treatment of alcoholism: The hallucinogenic drugs. *Quarterly Journal of Studies on Alcohol, 19*(3), 406–417.

Smith, D. E. (1969). LSD and the psychedelic syndrome. *Clinical Toxicology, 2*(1), 69–73.

Smith, J. P. (1967). LSD: The false illusion. *FDA Papers, 1*(6), 10–18.

Stafford, P. (1992). *Psychedelics encyclopedia* (3rd ed.). Berkeley, CA: Ronin.

Stevens, J. (1987). *Storming heaven.* New York: Harper & Row.

Stolaroff, M. (2004). *The Secret Chief revealed:*

Conversations with a pioneer of the underground psychedelic therapy movement. Sarasota FL: Multidisciplinary Association for Psychedelic Studies.

Stoll, W. A. (1947). Lysergic acid diethylamide, a phantasticum from the ergot group. *Schweitzer Archiv für Neurologie und Psychiatrie, 60*, 1–45.

Strassman, R. J. (1995). Hallucinogenic drugs in psychiatric research and treatment: Perspectives and prospects. *Journal of Nervous and Mental Disease, 183*(3), 127–138.

Sudworth, J. (2018). China Uighurs: Xinjiang legalises "reeducation" camps. Retrieved from *www.fbcnews.com.fj/world/china-uighurs-xinjiang-legalises-reeducation-camps*.

Sutton, T. (1813). *Tracts on delirium tremens and some other internal inflammatory affections*. London: Thomas Underwood.

Suzuki, J., Poklis, J., & Poklis, A. (2014). "My friend said it was good LSD": A suicide attempt following analytically confirmed 25I-NBOMe ingestion. *Journal of Psychoactive Drugs, 46*(5), 379–382.

Terrill, J. (1964). The nature of the LSD experience. In D. Solomon (Ed.), *LSD: The consciousness-expanding drug* (pp. 175–182). New York: Putnam.

Thomas, C. L. (1977). *Taber's cyclopedic medical dictionary* (13th ed.). Philadelphia: F. A. Davis.

Thompson, J. L. (1987). Critical scholarship: The critique of domination in nursing. *Advances in Nursing Science, 10*(1), 27–38.

Tjio, J.-H., Pahnke, W., & Kurland, A. A. (1969). LSD and chromosomes. *Journal of the American Medical Association, 210*(5), 849–856.

Ungerleider, J. T. (1970). LSD and the courts. *American Journal of Psychiatry, 126*(8), 1179.

Ungerleider, J. T., Fisher, D. D., & Fuller, M. (1966). The dangers of LSD. *Journal of the American Medical Association, 197*(6), 109–112.

U.S. House of Representatives, Committee on Interstate and Foreign Commerce, Subcommittee on Public Health and Welfare. (1968). *Increased controls over hallucinogens and other dangerous drugs: Hearings before the Subcommittee on Public Health and Welfare of the Committee on Interstate and Foreign Commerce, House of Representatives, 90th Congress, Second Session*. Washington, DC: U.S. Goverment Printing Office.

Walker, B. G. (1983). *The woman's encyclopedia of myths and secrets*. San Francisco: Harper & Row.

Walsh, R. (1982). Psychedelics and psychological well-being. *Journal of Humanistic Psychology, 22*(3), 22–32.

Waranky, J., & Takacs, E. (1968). LSD: No teratogenicity in rats. *Science, 159*, 731–732.

Watts, D. (1977, September 4). *Social definitions of the psychedelic drug experience*. Paper presented at the annual meeting of the Society for the Study of Social Problems, Chicago, IL.

Weil, A. (1963, November 5). The strange case of the Harvard drug scandal. *Look Magazine*, p. 27.

Werner, M. J. (1993). Hallucinogens. *Pediatrics in Review, 14*(12), 466–472.

West, L. J., Pierce, C. M., & Thomas, W. D. (1962). Lysergic acid diethylamide: Its effects on a male Asiatic elephant. *Science, 138*, 1100–1102.

Wittenborn, J. R. (1969). The problem of drug abuse in middle class youth. In J. R. Wittenborn, H. Brill, J. P. Smith, & S. Wittenborn (Eds.), *Drugs and youth: Proceedings of the Rutgers Symposium on Drug Abuse* (pp. 5–7). Springfield, IL: Charles C Thomas.

Yost, D. (1996). Alcohol withdrawal syndrome. *American Family Physician, 54*(2), 657–664.

Young, W. R., & Hixson, J. R. (1966). *LSD on campus*. New York: Dell Books.

Zaehner, R. C. (1972). *Zen, drugs, and mysticism*. New York: Vintage.

Zieger, S. (2008). Victorian hallucinogens. Retrieved from *https://id.erudit.org/iderudit/017857ar*.

Zinberg, N. (1976). Observations on the phenomenology of consciousness change. *Journal of Psychedelic Drugs, 8*(1), 59–76.

Zinberg, N. (1984). *Drug, set, and setting: The basis for controlled intoxicant use*. New Haven, CT: Yale University Press.

Zinberg, N., & Harding, W. (1979). Control and intoxicant use: A theoretical and practical overview. *Journal of Drug Issues, 9*(2), 21–43.

CHAPTER 5

History of the Use of Hallucinogens in Psychiatric Treatment

TORSTEN PASSIE

▦ Introduction

This chapter covers the history of psychotherapeutic treatment methods that use some hallucinogens (and entactogens) to facilitate psychotherapy. Because of their ability to intensify and restructure inner experience, the psychoactive substances typically used today as adjuncts to psychotherapy include lysergic acid diethylamide (LSD), psilocybin, and 3,4-methylenedioxymethamphetamine (MDMA). Investigation and development of these procedures in psychiatry began about 100 years ago. However, if one looks further back into the past, it is obvious that psychedelic agents have been used for religious and healing purposes by shamans and other healers for more than 10,000 years (Furst, 1972; Schultes & Hofmann, 1979).

After a period of broad and fruitful research (cf. Passie, 1997; Grof, 1980a, 1980b; Leuner, 1962), the use of hallucinogens as aids to psychotherapy was neglected and all but forgotten from about 1970 to 2000, due to unfortunate historical circumstances. Nevertheless, prior to that hiatus, the more than 700 scientific papers published on the topic clearly demonstrate how actively physicians and psychologists were involved in investigating the therapeutic potential of psychedelics during the 1950s and 1960s (Passie, 1997).

Associated with the social restlessness of the 1960s was an increasing prevalence of uncontrolled use at the end of the decade—a phenomenon that developed independently from medical use. A statutory prohibition of these substances was first enacted in 1966 in the United States. and Europe. Although the laws allowed for exceptional exemptions, the de facto result was a nearly complete cessation of the previously prolific study of their effectiveness (Grinspoon & Bakalar, 1979; U.S. Food and Drug Administration, 1975).

Central to the widespread use of hallucinogens in the 1960s was the group that formed around Harvard psychologists Timothy Leary, Richard Alpert, and Ralph Metzner, who initially discussed the evocation and implications of the psychedelic experience in a scientific manner. Starting in 1964, however, they began promoting these substances as agents for the "illumination of the human mind," and as a means to become free of the constraints of the Western worldview and its attitude toward self-awareness (Dass, Metzner, & Bravo, 2010).

This promotion of hallucinogens for "consciousness expansion" coincided with, and contributed to, the mass protest movement among young people in Western industrialized countries against existing cultural norms and values, which, according to them, were outdated, and against racial and other injustices. In the context of this this international movement, the use of psychedelics became a mass phenomenon (Lee & Shain, 1985; Stevens, 1987), intensifying social turbulence, especially in the United States (Keniston, 1968/1969). Complications that can arise from taking psychedelics under poorly controlled conditions were reported, and played a major role in how the media portrayed hallucinogens. These included traumatic internal experiences or "bad trips," often resembling severe panic attacks, "flashback" phenomena, triggering of latent psychosis in vulnerable individuals, and more.

Press coverage became even more negative with a single-case report of possible chromosome damage, published in 1967 by Cohen, Marinello, and Back—a report that did not stand up to meticulous scientific examination (see review by Grof, 1980a). Nevertheless, the resulting bad publicity instigated a sudden retreat of scientists and therapists active in the field, who feared being caught in the undertow of negative headlines. As psychiatrist Oscar Janiger, who was involved in LSD psychotherapy in Los Angeles described it, "The whole goddamn climate changed. Suddenly you were conspirators out to destroy people."

Two basic approaches to the use of psychedelics have been developed over time, and these have been described as *psycholytic* (soul-loosening) and *psychedelic* (mind-manifesting). I focus in this chapter on these methods and also discusses the historical context of their development. I also deal with two modified approaches: *psychedelytic* therapy, and *MDMA-assisted psychotherapy*. Some rather unconventional approaches are also addressed.

■ The Psychotomimetic Paradigm

The first phase of clinical research with psychedelics was marked by the *psychotomi-metic* paradigm. Encouraged by the Swiss pharmaceutical firm Sandoz, most researchers until the 1950s thought that the primary effect of LSD was to induce states that resemble an acute psychosis. It was presumed that LSD could be used to give psychiatrists firsthand experiences of their psychotic patients. In the mid-1950s, psychiatrists began to suspect metabolic aberrations as the cause of psychosis, especially after the discovery of the neurotransmitter serotonin, with which LSD primarily interacts (Green, 2008). In the following two decades, a large number of biochemical, physiological, and psychological experiments were carried out on animals and humans involving LSD. The number of scientific publications on LSD in the years from 1943 to 1970 approached 10,000, causing LSD to be described as "the most researched pharmacological substance ever" (Hintzen & Passie, 2010).

In the mid-1950s it became apparent that the argument that LSD produces a reasonable model psychosis had some major shortcomings. The consensus was stated well by the prominent Swiss psychiatrist Manfred Bleuler (1958), who observed the following:

1. Schizophrenia cannot be characterized by the presence of any particular isolated symptom. Only a combination of symptoms, including thought disorder, ego disturbance, depersonalization, and hallucinations, progressing gradually to render the individual incapable of controlling his or her life, is characteristic of schizophrenia.
2. The symptoms induced by LSD differ from the usual syndrome characterizing schizophrenia. For example, visual phenomena are predominant with LSD, whereas auditory hallucinations are predominant in schizophrenia.
3. The alienating and unharmonious, the *Uneinfühlbare,* typical for schizophrenia, is absent with LSD.
4. Schizophrenics can easily discriminate between chemically induced (toxic) phenomena and naturally occurring psychotic phenomena.

These insights marked the end of the era of LSD as a psychotomimetic. However, some more recent studies have tried to elucidate neurophysiological pathways of psychotic states (e.g., Gouzoulis-Mayfrank et al., 1999; Riba et al., 2006; Vollenweider & Geyer, 2001).

▓ A Prehistory of the Use of Drugs in Psychotherapy

The first pharmacological attempts to influence an individual's state of consciousness in Western psychotherapy date back to the 19th century, when ether, chloroform, and hashish were used to deepen hypnotic states (Schrenck-Notzing, 1891). Beginning in the 1920s, physicians used subnarcotic doses of barbiturates to decrease cortical control in an attempt to make suppressed psychological material accessible. This was referred to as *narcoanalysis* (Horsley, 1943).

Since the 1920s, a variety of human experiments with hallucinogens, especially mescaline, have been conducted. Interestingly, most researchers concluded that the experiences do not reflect the psychodynamics of their experimental subjects (Passie, 1993/1994). However, they remained interesting for other reasons, and the Italian psychoanalyst Baroni (1931) was the first to use mescaline in a psychotherapeutic setting.

▓ A Short History of Psycholytic Therapy

In the first clinical study of LSD, Stoll (1947) noted that most subjects experienced strong personal emotions and memories during their sessions. Busch and Johnson (1950) were the first to report on the use of LSD in psychotherapy. They were followed by Chandler and Hartmann (1950) and British psychiatrist Ronald Sandison, who found intensification of affect and abreactive memory activation leading to significant improvements in neurotic patients after a single dose of LSD (Sandison, Spencer, & Whitlaw, 1954).

Around 1950, Sandoz issued a prospectus, stating that small doses of their new product Delysid (the brand name for what they also called LSD-25) caused transitory disturbances of affect, hallucinations, depersonalization, reliving of repressed memories, and mild neurovegetative symptoms. The indications mentioned for its use were "analytical psychotherapy, to elicit release of repressed material and provide mental relaxation, particularly in anxiety states and obsessional neuroses." Hence, the clinicians who first explored the therapeutic use of LSD had a psychoanalytic orientation and attempted to integrate Delysid into their practice of psychoanalytic psychotherapy.

Also in the early 1950s, German psychiatrist Hanscarl Leuner (1984) developed guided affective imagery, a daydream technique used in psychotherapy. Concluding that small doses of hallucinogens may intensify imagery and induce regression and catharsis, Leuner (1959) began to use low-dose LSD with his psychotherapy patients. German psychoanalyst Walter Frederking (1953/1954, 1955) was another early proponent of LSD as an adjunct to psychotherapy.

Psychoanalysis as a theoretical orientation was prominent in psychiatry in the 1950s, and the psycholytic method was grounded in what at the time were widely accepted analytic concepts. With psycholytic therapy, serial individual treatment sessions (5–20) with low doses of LSD or psilocybin were conducted at weekly intervals to produce a dream-like experience. These sessions were embedded in a conventional psychotherapeutic process.

The general approach was designated "psycholytic therapy," or "psycholysis," by Sandison at the First European Symposium for Psychotherapy under LSD-25 in 1960 (Barolin, 1960). Although the original use and development of psycholytic therapy occurred among psychoanalytic therapists mainly in Europe, some work along these lines was also conducted in the United States and in South America (e.g., Fontana, 1965). At one point, the psycholytic method was used at 18 academic centers in Europe, and by more than a hundred outpatient therapists (cf. Caldwell, 1968; Malleson, 1971). During the 1960s, due to a continuous process of refinement, psycholytic therapists arrived at what might be considered today as a fully developed method (cf. Abramson, 1967; Grof, 1980b; Leuner, 1981). Between 1953 and 1968, more than 7,000 patients were treated with psycholytic therapy, and at that time there were approximately 400 scientific publications on the approach (Passie, 1997).

At the end of the 1960s, research and therapeutic work with hallucinogens came to a halt in both Europe and the United States. This was a consequence of legislation banning these substances, initiated in the United States but adopted in most of Europe as well. Among the few exceptions were therapists in what was then Czechoslovakia. Several clinics there were active through the 1970s, and about 40 LSD therapists worked with outpatients. In 1968, the United Kingdom saw 40 LSD therapists protesting against the prohibition of their method (Sandison et al., 1954), arguing that hallucinogens were safe and effective when used in a therapeutic context. One survey in the United Kingdom showed that the risks are no greater with LSD than with conventional psychotherapy (Malleson, 1971). This confirmed the findings of an earlier similar survey of Cohen (1960) in the United States.

Hanscarl Leuner in Germany and Jan Bastiaans (1917–1997) in the Netherlands were the only two university chairs in psychiatry who still held licenses for the use of LSD in psychotherapy. Both focused on treatment-resistant patients. Leuner treated neurotic inpatients. Bastiaans, who had worked with narcoanalysis since 1946, reported in 1961 that LSD was significantly more effective than standard therapy among the treatment-resistant survivors of concentration camps and prisoners of World War II with whom he worked (cf. Snelders, 1998). In LSD sessions, while patients lay on a couch in his office, Bastiaans (1974, 1983) took the position of a father figure who gave his patients the warmth and understanding they required. However, this made more traditional psychoanalytic colleagues, who worked with more emotional detachment, somewhat wary. After Leuner and Bastiaans retired in the late 1980s, no university researchers were left.

In 1986, the Swiss Physicians Society for Psycholytic Therapy (SÄPT) was started by physicians interested in the therapeutic use of LSD (Baumann, 1986). Five members were able to get a special permit to use LSD and MDMA in their offices, which lasted until 1993, when an accident unrelated to their work with LSD and MDMA led to the revocation of their permits. Nevertheless, members of this group were able to gain considerable experience, and created a new kind of group work with psychedelics (Gasser, 1996; Styk, 1994; Widmer, 1997).

Principles of Psycholytic Therapy

The first psycholytic psychotherapists were all psychoanalytically trained and used conventional treatment settings. Preparation for the administration of LSD was done in the course of long-term psychotherapy, so that a good relationship and some understanding of patients' problems could be achieved prior to use of hallucinogens. Patients were informed that LSD is just an aid to therapy, that the LSD experience is not the curative process itself, as much of the integration still has to be done in subsequent psychotherapy sessions and everyday life.

While under the influence of LSD, the patient lies on a couch in a darkened room. The therapist stays with the patient for the session. The dosage is individually adjusted so that the patient remains aware of the therapeutic character of the situation. The patient is asked to surrender without reservation to the impressions, emotions, and visions that appear. Under the influence of LSD, all conventional psychotherapeutc mechanisms are amplified—the successive reliving of traumatic experiences from childhood, associated with emotional abreaction, rational integration, and resulting insights. The therapeutic relationship is usually greatly intensified, and analysis of transference is an essential part of psycholytic treatment. The occasional remarks of patients are recorded with a tape recorder or in writing, and are given to them afterwards to prepare a summary report of their experience. The LSD experiences are subsequently interpreted and worked through in drug-free sessions, usually within a psychodynamic framework. The typical number of sessions is 5–50 (usually 10–20), incorporated in the course of 100–200 conventional psychotherapy sessions. However, some researchers have treated patients with less time and fewer sessions. Others found that a few LSD sessions conducted at the right time can be very effective.

It became obvious early on that the conventional treatment setting was not appropriate for this type of therapeutic work. Psycholytic therapy requires a "more humane approach, genuine support, and personal involvement" (Grof, 1980b, p. 31). Obviously, a more direct approach was necessary, along with occasional physical support (albeit with caveats—e.g., Leuner warned against touching a patient below the shoulders), no immediate interpretations, some psychodramatic involvement in the patient's experience, and a higher tolerance for acting-out behavior. This shift from a detached attitude to more direct participation on the part of the therapist has led to criticism by many psychiatric professionals.

The use of LSD places greater demands on the therapist than does conventional psychotherapy. The patient's increased regression and anxiety, as well as potentially stronger transference and countertransference reactions, can be challenging for the therapist.

Modifications of Psycholytic Therapy

Psycholytic therapy underwent a number of modifications during its active years. Some European therapists experimented with shorter-acting psilocybin derivatives such as CZ-74 (4-hydroxy-N,N-diethyltryptamine, also known as 4-HO-DET; Baer, 1967; Shulgin & Shulgin, 2014), which has a duration of 4–6 hours and is phenomenologically similar to LSD; CEY-19 (phosphoryloxy-N,N-diethyltryptamine, also known as 4-PO-DET or *ethocybin*), which has a duration of 2–4 hours and is also similar to LSD, and the mescaline derivative 2-CD (2,5-dimethoxy-4-methylphenethylamine; Schlichting, 1989). Therapists in the United States experimented with the short-acting dipropyltrytamine (DPT) in psycholytic therapy (Soskin, 1975; Soskin, Grof, & Richards, 1973), as well as in psychedelic therapy (Richards, Rhead, DiLeo, Yensen, & Kurland, 1977).

In the 1960s, Ling and Buckman (1963), Leuner (1967), and others promoted the additional administration of methylphenidate to increase emotional responses and abreaction. Methylamphetamine was also tried, but its use was found to be detrimental. For the most part, stimulants were found not to add much of value to psycholytic therapy, and their supplemental use was later abandoned.

Other modifications of psycholytic therapy included group sessions, attempted by Leuner (1971) and Sandison and colleagues (1954), who worked with multiple inpatients in individual treatment rooms, with an attending nurse and a visiting physician as sitters, to minimize costs. With this technique, up to five patients could be treated at the same time (Figure 5.1). After the acute effects of LSD diminish, the patients met in a group room to discuss their experiences and insights with the physician and nurse. Leuner also developed what he called the "interval inpatient treatment," in which patients were treated as outpatients, but with brief overnight stays in the clinic, limited to 2 days, for psycholytic sessions.

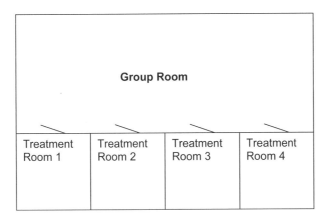

FIGURE 5.1. Typical clinical facility for individual sessions as used by Leuner et al. (1983) and Sandison et al. (1954).

Especially noteworthy was the work of Czech psychiatrist Milan Hausner (1929–2000), who began his work with LSD in 1954 and continued until 1980. Hausner's approach was developed in Sadska hospital near Prague, where many inpatients and outpatients were administered LSD for as many as 60 sessions (Hausner & Dolezal, 1963; Hausner & Segal, 2009). The therapy protocol was variable. Typically, patients were treated during a hospital stay for 5–7 weeks in conjunction with group therapy, sociotherapy, occupational therapy, sports, psychodrama, and autogenic training, plus follow-up care after discharge from hospital. In many cases, patients spent 3–6 months on the ward, during which time they had weekly LSD sessions, followed by art therapy and group discussions of the patients' experiences (Hausner & Segal, 2009). The clinic also worked with patients who stayed for weekend LSD sessions every 3–4 weeks.

On the weekends, groups of five to six patients underwent LSD therapy in individual rooms, in the presence of a specially trained nurse. Patients were divided into two groups, one of which underwent LSD therapy while the other served as "co-guides." This was reversed the following day. The "weekend clinic" approach had several advantages. Patients could live in their homes and keep their jobs, and they could immediately integrate experiences in everyday life, which is important for therapeutic success. According to Hausner, no adverse effects were encountered with this approach.

Assessing the Effectiveness of Psycholytic Therapy

During the years when psycholytic therapy was developed and researched (1950s and 1960s), the methods of scientific research on psychotherapy were rudimentary. Most psycholytic therapists reported improvement in about two-thirds of their usually difficult-to-treat neurotic patients (Mascher, 1967). Assessed from a current perspective, their studies and findings may have been compromised by methodological biases (cf. Pletscher & Ladewig, 1994). However, some psychedelic therapists were more rigorous in their methodology (e.g., Kurland, Savage,

Pahnke, Grof, & Olsson, 1971; Ludwig, Levine, & Stark, 1970). The assessment of the effectiveness of psycholytic therapy is further complicated by the fact that in Europe, psycholytic treatment was primarily used for patients resistant to conventional psychotherapy, which may have biased treatment samples toward persons with more severe psychopathology. Moreover, several researchers used these patients as their own controls (e.g., Geert-Jorgensen, 1968; Leuner, 1994).

In only a few studies was psycholytic therapy performed with at least a few controlled variables (Denson & Sydiaha, 1970; Robinson, Davis, Sack, & Morrissey, 1963; Soskin 1973; Soskin et al., 1973; Vourlekis, Faillace, & Szara, 1967). Their results yielded little evidence for the superiority of psycholytic therapy over conventional psychotherapy. Nevertheless, double-blind studies performed by Vourlekis and colleagues (1967) and Soskin and colleagues (1973) indicate, congruent with many uncontrolled studies, that specific actions of psychedelics may enhance and deepen the psychotherapeutic process.

A Short History of Psychedelic Therapy

Another major approach to the therapeutic use of hallucinogens, one that differs significantly from the psycholytic method, was developed in North America and termed the "psychedelic method." The development of this procedure can be attributed to the rather disparate work of several researchers.

Beginning around 1950, prompted by the observation that many alcoholics remain abstinent after the traumatic experience of an hallucinatory and anxiety-provoking delirium tremens episode, Hoffer and Osmond set out to produce delirium tremens using high doses of LSD, with the objective of effecting abstinence. Their results suggested that, in contrast to their initial hypothesis, the apparent lasting therapeutic effects of LSD were associated with expanded self-awareness and religious experiences (Hoffer, 1967).

In 1955, anesthesiologist Eric Kast conducted a comparative study of analgesics among terminal cancer patients, in which

LSD was used as an active placebo. To his surprise, he found that patients who received LSD reported a decrease in pain and a more relaxed attitude toward death, along with deepened self- and situational insight (Kast, 1963, 1966).

In addition to these reports of the therapeutic use of hallucinogens by clinicians, ethnographic reports suggested that ingestion of certain hallucinogenic plants in the context of an indigenous religious ritual (e.g., peyote, Brazilian ayahuasca religion) led to dramatic, positive personality changes in sociopathic and alcohol-dependent individuals (cf. Andritzky, 1989; La Barre, 1989; MacRae, 1992).

Informed by their early experiments, Hoffer and Osmond (1966) developed and started using the *psychedelic* treatment technique, which made induction of mystical–religious experiences the focus of therapeutic action (Blewett & Chwelos, 1959). This approach uses a quasi-religious preparation of the patient, affecting both set and setting: high doses, specific surroundings, and music to evoke insights and mystical experiences. These investigators emphasized the apparent transformative power of mystical states of consciousness. The LSD experience "forced [patients] to reconsider their patterns of behavior by an enhanced self-understanding" (Smith, 1958).

Duncan Blewett, the supervising psychologist of Osmond's treatment team in Canada, concluded that patients experienced themselves and the world

> through immediate intuition or insight in a way differing from ordinary sense perception or the use of logical reasoning. . . . In such an experience there appears always to be a feeling of some direct contact with the infinite and the eternal, a feeling of being at one with the world's Author and all His Works, a complete abandonment of the self and all its motives. Also frequently noted are tremendous infusions of love, feelings of remarkably enhanced understanding, and an awareness of very great beauty all about one. There is a feeling of being outside the bounds of time, space, and the self. (Blewett, 1958/2016, p. 240)

Because the idea that a "constructive" experience beyond the boundaries of the "ego" could help to overcome illness and personal-

ity problems marked a significant and seemingly unscientific paradigm change, Blewett was harshly criticized by some colleagues at the time.

One individual who contributed significantly to interest in the hallucinogens in the 1950s and 1960s, although he was neither a physician nor a psychologist, was Alfred M. Hubbard, who was influential among the early investigators of LSD. He played a significant role in the evolution of the psychedelic method. He developed and promulgated a technique to induce a transcendental or "psychedelic experience" in a large percentage of participants. Osmond and his associates began to learn from Hubbard, and implemented his insights and techniques into their own approach to psychedelic therapy (Blewett & Chwelos, 1959).

By the early 1960s, LSD treatment programs were operational in four medical facilities in Canada (Dyck, 2008). The researchers from Saskatchewan began treating their patients mainly in small group settings, with three or four patients at a time. With their approach, Hoffer and Osmond reckoned their program was "faster, cheaper, and twice as effective as any other program" (Hoffer & Osmond, 1966, p. 36). Based on, and guiding, their extensive experience in Saskatchewan, their colleagues, psychologist Duncan Blewett and psychiatrist Nick Chwelos, wrote the *Handbook for the Therapeutic Use of Lysergic Acid Diethylamide-25*. This was the first psychedelic treatment manual. The group also published the results of several studies (cf. synoptic review in Krebs & Johansen, 2012).

Early findings suggested that LSD might be one of the most innovative and successful approaches to the treatment of alcoholism, and the methods of these Canadian researchers were adopted especially by researchers in the United States. Eventually, the psychedelic treatment model came to be used, and refined, at about 10 facilities in the United States. This line of research continued through the 1960s, culminating in controlled studies at the Maryland Psychiatric Research Center in Catonsville, Maryland (e.g., Grof, 1975; Pahnke, Kurland, Unger, Savage, & Grof, 1970; Kurland, 1985; Yensen & Dryer, 1993/1994). Although the results of those studies were favorable and encouraging, with very few exceptions, the use of the psychedelic method remained limited to North America, while the psycholytic approach remained dominant in Europe.

Beginning around the year 2000, clinical studies of hallucinogens resumed in the United States. Psychedelic therapy underwent a resurgence, encouraged by the findings of projects conducted at a handful of academic centers, especially work involving research with psilocybin in normal volunteers at Johns Hopkins University. In a number of carefully designed and conducted clinical studies, researchers at Johns Hopkins have shown that mystical-type experiences can be reliably induced, with lasting psychological improvement, and without serious adverse effects (Griffiths et al., 2016; Griffiths, Richards, McCann, & Jesse, 2008). More recently, a pilot study to treat alcoholism with psilocybin-assisted psychedelic therapy was successfully completed at New York University (Bogenschutz et al., 2015), and psychedelic therapy has also been shown to be an effective means to facilitate smoking cessation (Johnson, Garcia-Romeu, Cosimano, & Griffiths, 2014).

One indication for psychedelic therapy that has been discussed since the 1950s is the use of hallucinogens to improve quality of life among people who are terminally ill. This theme appeared in the writings of author Aldous Huxley, who was introduced to mescaline by Humphrey Osmond, and

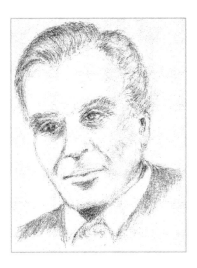

Aldous Huxley

found the experience very useful. In his later novel *Island,* the inhabitants use the *Moksha medicine* to induce a mystical vision that had the effects of freeing them from the fear of death and enabling them to live more fully. Through his own experiments with psychedelics, Huxley concluded that the LSD experience could make dying easier, and in 1958 Huxley wrote a letter to Osmond arguing for the administration of LSD to dying patients. He took the idea seriously enough that in 1963, before he died, Huxley asked his wife Laura to inject him with LSD during his last hours.

In the same year, anesthesiologist Eric Kast set out to examine the potential analgesic propertifes of LSD in people with severe pain. In a study comparing morphine and meperidine, with LSD used as an active placebo, Kast (1963) found that patients coped better with pain and existential issues after they had received LSD. When he asked his patients about the effects of LSD, they often reported profound experiences, which had changed their perspectives on life and death (Kast, 1966). Inspired by Huxley and Kast, Sidney Cohen (1965) conducted further trials along these lines.

In 1965, a member of the treatment team of the psychedelic research group at the Maryland Psychiatric Research Center (MPRC) developed cancer that was associated with marked psychological distress. It was suggested that her distress might be effectively treated with a psychedelic session. The outcome was sufficiently encouraging that the team decided to further explore this treatment, administering LSD and DPT to more than 100 MPRC patients (Grof & Halifax, 1978; Kurland, 1985; Kurland, Grof, Pahnke, & Goodman, 1973; Pahnke, 1969; Pahnke, Kurland, Goodman, & Richards, 1969; Richards et al., 1977). The shorter-acting DPT was found to be especially useful, as LSD could be exhausting, especially with this population of patients (Grof, Goodman, Richards, & Kurland, 1973). Following a lengthy hiatus in clinical studies of hallucinogens, Grob and colleagues (2011) published a pilot study in which they successfully treated terminal cancer patients with psychotherapy and psilocybin. Gasser and colleagues (2014; Gasser, Kirchner, & Passie, 2016), Griffiths and colleagues

(2016), and Ross and colleagues (2016) subsequently replicated these favorable results in larger trials.

In addition, the results of a small pilot study suggested that psilocybin might be an effective treatment for depression (Carhart-Harris et al., 2016). Beginning in 2018, the psychedelic treatment of depression became the focus of Phase 2 clinical trials in Europe and North America.

■ Principles of Psychedelic Therapy

Psychedelic therapy is a highly specialized form of brief, intensive psychotherapy, facilitated by the administration of hallucinogens. It has three different phases: preparation, the psychedelic session, and working through.

Preparation involves conversations in which patient and therapist discuss the patient's difficulties in living (past and present) and his or her goals, aspirations, frustrations, and relationship to religion. The patient is seen from three to five times a week for 2–4 weeks. It can be helpful to incorporate family members into the preparatory phase.

During the *psychedelic session,* the patient is given a high dose of LSD (250–450 micrograms [µg]) or a similar substance. The hallucinogen causes a loosening of defenses and leads to reliving, abreaction, and insight. An integral part of a successful session is the dissolution of the ego and a mystical experience of oneness, accompanied by feelings of sacredness and joy.

Following the psychedelic session is the phase of *working through,* in which new insights and discoveries are sorted out. Old maladaptive defenses are shed or discarded, and new ways of experiencing, looking at, and reacting to events are explored. Without this posthallucinogen reinforcement, the LSD experience may gradually fade away, becoming just a memory.

In psychedelic therapy, ideally, the patient has been supported by the therapist's en-

TABLE 5.1. Traditional Approaches to the Psychotherapeutic Use of Hallucinogens (Passie, 1997)

Psycholytic therapy	Psychedelic therapy
• Low doses of LSD (50–150 µg), psilocybin (7–15 mg), CZ 74 (10–20 mg), MDMA, etc., producing symbolic dream images, regressions, and transference phenomena.	• High doses LSD (250–1,500 µg) leading to so-called cosmic–mystical experiences often marked by oneness and ecstatic joy.
• Activation and deepening of the psychoanalytic process.	• Modern transpersonal approaches used to explain structure and effects of experiences.
• Numerous sessions required (5–30).	• The goal is one to three "overwhelming" experiences with a mystical connotation.
• Analytic discussion of experienced material in individual and group sessions (focus on ego psychology, transference, and defense mechanisms).	• Suggestive quasi-religious preparation and use of specific surroundings and music. Usually not a very detailed discussion of the experience.
• Reality comparison and attempt to adapt experience to everyday life.	• Adaption to reality not the main purpose. Enhancing the meaning of the "psychedelic" experience.
• Goal: Cure through restructure of personality via a maturational process and loosening of infantile parental attachments.	• Goal: Symptomatic cure involving behavior change.
• Classical indications for psychotherapy: neuroses, psychosomatic disorders, psychopaths, sexual neuroses, borderline cases. Neither alcoholism nor psychoses.	• Alcoholism, psychoneuroses, terminal cancer patients.

couragement, permissiveness, and warmth, while learning to communicate his or her innermost feelings with another fellow human. A positive, trusting therapeutic relationship is required to lead the patient though the often-difficult experiences that may emerge. Patients are given headphones and eye shades, and are instructed to surrender to the flow of the experience. Music helps to structure the experience, furthering catharsis, and enabling the patient to "let go." A specific music playlist for psychedelic therapy was developed by Bonny and Pahnke (1972).

During the psychedelic session, the patient is encouraged to express negative feelings if they occur. Resistance is identified as such but not interpreted. If the patient is avoiding a particular problem, he or she is told that he or she is avoiding it. Though feelings are identified and accepted, no transference interpretations are attempted. Therapists are chosen for their capacity to be warm and giving without endangering their own egos. In a well-prepared patient with good ego resources, a session may almost run itself, while others might need varying degrees of support and help. In the late afternoon, it can be helpful for the patient to be taken outdoors to experience nature's beauty.

An example of a psychedelic mystical experience may be helpful here. According to one study participant,

> Sound ceased and I seemed to be floating in a great, very, very still void or hemisphere. Peace and contentment seemed to flow through my entire body. It is impossible to describe the overpowering peace, contentment, and being part of goodness itself that I felt. My body felt as if it were dissolving and actually becoming a part of the goodness and peace that was all around me. Words can't describe this. A tremendous feeling of exaltation came over me. I felt rapture and ecstasy. . . . It was overwhelming! There are no words to describe my feelings then. I seemed to be transported to the top of the highest mountains. All was still and quiet. A sense of cleanliness and purity swept over me. I felt humble and insignificant. I was completely awed! . . . I felt as though I had been reborn. (in Unger, 1974, p. 213)

It is important that patients remain in psychotherapy and have appropriate social support for the postsession integration of the psychedelic experience. As results have shown, when patients are "left alone" after such experiences, the effects of treatment may disappear rapidly.

It would be a misconception to view psychedelic therapy as making psychotherapy "easier." The procedures not only require special training and competence for the therapist, but also conducting this type of therapy can be fatiguing and place the therapist under a considerable strain. It can be an arduous and stressful procedure for patient and therapist alike (Unger, 1974, p. 214).

The systematic and rigorous evaluation of psychedelic therapy has been difficult. Results differ widely as a function of how the drug is administered, and how the therapist interacts with the volunteer. Smart and Storm (1964), for example, were concerned about the different protocols for a psychedelic session, and questioned the favorable results of psychedelic therapy reported among alcoholics. They conducted what they described as a "strictly controlled" evaluation to address this issue, attempting to eliminate positive, supportive behavior on the part of therapists. In their study, alcoholics received no predrug (preparatory) treatment and were not informed ahead of time about the drug's effects. Participants were injected with 800 μg of LSD (a large dose) or 20 mg of ephedrine as placebo, and were then "attached to the bed by a light but strong belt for security" (Smart, Storm, Baker, & Solursh, 1967). They were then "interviewed" by a doctor and nurse for 3 hours. The results of this study were (predictably) unfavorable, and the critical comments made by MacLean and Wilby (1967) explain why this was so.

The problem, as Smart and associates (1967) viewed it, is that the results of psychedelic therapy are so dependent on set and setting that an objective observer might wonder whether the outcome is not primarily a function of suggestion, of the therapist's encouragement of a positive attitude toward the session. There have been significant improvements in research methodology since the 1960s, and more methodologically sound studies in recent years have yielded consistently good results, which have been replicated recently with careful attention to both clinical and experimental protocols (e.g., Bogenschutz et al., 2015; Griffiths, Richards, McCann, & Jesse, 2006; Griffiths et al., 2016; Grob et al., 2011; Ross et al., 2016).

Psychedelytic Therapy

It was not an easy task for therapists to merge such very different approaches as psychedelic and psycholytic therapy. The Atlantic Ocean also came between the therapists using these different approaches, with distinctly European and North American allegiances to one or the other. As leading LSD psychotherapist Grof has pointed out, the difference is not in the nature of the experience but in the qualitative incidence of certain elements in the sessions characteristic of each approach. Many patients in psychedelic therapy, for example, experience childhood memories and other material of biographical significance—such phenomena are not unique to psycholytic treatment. On the other hand, many psycholytic therapists have observed experiences of a mystical nature among their patients but have tended to view them as resistance against painful psychodynamic issues.

Nevertheless, it appeared to many researchers that both methods could make significant contributions to individual outcomes, and that a merger of the two might be beneficial. A combination of the psycholytic and psychedelic approaches was first suggested by Alnaes (1965) and by Grof (1967). This "psychedelytic" approach integrates both the processing of psychodynamic material in low-dose, serial psycholytic session, and the intense and profoundly transformational experiences of high-dose psychedelic sessions (Yensen, 1994). An amalgam of psychedelic and psycholytic processes has been applied in several studies, with beneficial effects (Benz, 1989; Fontana, 1965; Gasser et al., 2014).

Contrary to popular belief, high-dose psychedelic sessions may be safer than low-dose sessions. With a high dose, a decreased ability to resist the effects of the drug is associated with a more complete surrender, along with more complete resolution and integration. On the other hand, psychedelic sessions may involve more potential problems during the acute effects of the drug, as psychic defenses collapse, reality testing and self-control are compromised, and an individual experiences large-scale emergence of unconscious emotions and feelings. In psycholytic therapy, a more gradual, successive uncovering of unconscious material is feasible. However, unwilling subjects might easily generate maladaptive psychic defenses and intense anxiety reactions, and emotional lability between sessions can result from closely spaced serial LSD sessions. An additional limitation of low-dose psycholytic therapy is that sometimes doses are insufficient to facilitate access to intense emotional material.

The SÄPT, founded in 1985 in Switzerland, received a special permit allowing its physician members to conduct psychotherapy with LSD and MDMA between 1988 and 1993. SÄPT therapists treated patients primarily in group settings and developed some specific therapeutic group techniques (Benz, 1989; Styk, 1994). Congruent with the psychedelytic approach, higher doses were used than in psycholytic therapy (e.g., 100–200 µg LSD), along with full dose MDMA. The setting allowed for individual experiences, as well as permissive group interaction, especially in later stages of the drug sessions. The use of music was alternated with periods of quiet. A similar treatment model has been developed by European underground therapists in the last 25 years (cf. Passie, 2012). It is possible that psychedelytic therapy, applied in group settings, might become the predominant approach in the future, as it both supports the therapeutic process through the interpersonal field and reduces professional time and thereby the cost of treatment.

Anaclitic Therapy

Anaclitic therapy was apparently developed and conducted by only two London psychiatrists, Joyce Martin and Pauline McCririck. They took advantage of the deep regression that can occur under the influence of a medium dose of LSD (100–200 µg), and gave their patients an element of direct satisfaction of infantile needs for physical affection by providing close physical contact during the sessions. They sometimes held their patients, fed them warm milk, and caressed and held their clients' heads in their laps. The patients' subjective reports revealed authentic feelings of a symbiotic union with the mother image, with an experience of a "good breast" (Martin, 1957).

According to Grof (1980b), who has observed anaclitic sessions, these can be "extremely healing experiences." He theorizes that this kind of intensive care under the influence of LSD can "fill the vacuum caused by deprivation and frustration," providing what is sometimes referred to as a "corrective emotional experience" (Alexander & French, 1946). The anaclitic approach fueled a great controversy, both because of concern about a therapist touching a patient in such an intimate way, and because it is contradictory to tenets of conventional therapy, which focus instead on acceptance of and appropriate coping with early frustrations. Anaclitic therapy was never widely practiced, but elements have been used by Azima (1963), and by therapists of the SÄPT in group therapy sessions (Gasser, 1996; Widmer, 1997).

Hypnodelic Therapy

Ludwig and associates experimented with the use of hypnosis in conjunction with LSD (125–200 μg), in order to channel the unstructured aspects of the psychedelic state in a somewhat more structured therapeutic direction (Ludwig & Levine, 1965). They tested this in a controlled study designed to treat a group of opioid addicts, comparing hypnodelic therapy and treatment involving only LSD. Subjects were hypnotized within the first half-hour after LSD administration, before the drug began to take effect. In the hypnotic state, subjects were encouraged to examine and understand their current difficulties. They were helped to work through problems, to overcome resistances, and to relive relevant childhood memories, and therapists attempted to facilitate catharsis and abreaction. After 3 hours, they were brought out of the hypnotic state, having been given a posthypnotic suggestion to remember what occurred during the session, and to continue working on their problems.

Persons in the LSD group (without hypnosis) were reported to have had good outcomes, but less positive than was the case for the group with the additional hypnotic induction (Levine & Ludwig, 1967). Hypnodelic therapy was never widely used.

The Psychosynthesis of Salvador Roquet

Salvador Roquet (1920–1995) was a Mexican physician who studied a number of psychotropic drugs used by indigenous peoples, including psychedelics, in therapy. He worked at the Albert Schweitzer Institute in Mexico City, an institution conducting psychotherapy outcome research. During the early 1970s, Roquet and his associates developed a system of psychotherapy which he called *psychosynthesis* (Roquet, Favreau, Ocana, & Velasco, 1975; Roquet & Favreu, 1981; Villoldo, 1977). In addition to conventional psychoanalytically oriented therapy, this system included group therapy sessions using psychedelics. These sessions lasted for about 20 hours, and were held in a large room, equipped with large posters and music, as well as slide and film projectors. The visual material, which was intended to induce sensory overload, encompassed a wide variety of situations in life, ranging from some that were funny or beautiful to scenes that were often cruel or disturbing (e.g., concentration camps). Slides were presented to stimulate a broad spectrum of emotions and cathartic reactions.

In groups with 15–30 participants and a few professional psychotherapists, 12 sessions were held per year, per patient. An integral part of psychosynthesis was the administration of different psychoactive drugs, including LSD, ketamine, 3,4-methylene-dioxy-amphetamine (MDA), mescaline, *Rivea corymbosa, Datura* species, *Salvia divinorum,* and ayahuasca, in a specific order. This was another way to confront patients with a broad spectrum of experiences and emotions. Among the people treated by Roquet were patients with diagnoses of neurosis and personality disorders, but some people with addictions were also treated, as well as some asymptomatic, healthy individuals. In 1974, Mexican authorities raided the Institute. Roquet was arrested, charged with drug trafficking and endangering his patients, and imprisoned. He was eventually acquitted, but his work with psychedelic therapy was prohibited, and Roquet settled in California.

According to Roquet, between 1968 and 1974, he worked with 388 patients using his method. Roquet and Favreau (1981) attempted to evaluate the therapeutic results of psychosynthesis; Roquet maintained that 85% of his patients improved.

MDMA-Assisted Psychotherapy

Mescaline and some of its derivatives have been studied for their hallucinogenic activity since the beginning of the 20th century (Passie, 1993/1994). It was Californian pharmacologist Gordon A. Alles (1959) who first described the specific psychopharmacological effects of MDA, which was found to induce a state of intensified emotion with less hallucinatory activity and cognitive alteration than mescaline. For this reason, in the early 1960s MDA was tested by Chilean psychiatrist Claudio Naranjo as an agent that might facilitate psychotherapy (Naranjo, 1973; Naranjo, Shulgin, & Sargent, 1967).

In a continuing search for a "psychotherapeutic drug," Naranjo and his associate, American chemist Alexander T. Shulgin, studied derivatives of the essential oils of nutmeg. In 1962, Shulgin synthesized 3-methoxy-4,5-methylenedioxyamphetamine (MMDA), which appeared promising in part because it had fewer hallucinogenic effects (Shulgin, Sargent, & Naranjo, 1973). Nevertheless, MDA—but not MMDA—became the drug of choice for many underground psychotherapists from the mid-1960s onward (e.g., Stolaroff, 2004). MDA was also used in studies of drug-assisted psychotherapy (Turek, Soskin, & Kurland, 1974; Yensen et al., 1976).

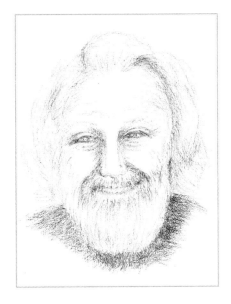

Alexander Shulgin

In 1977, Shulgin introduced psychologist and Jungian psychotherapist Leo Zeff to MDMA, which looked like a better and less toxic alternative to MDA (Benzenhöfer & Passie, 2010). Zeff introduced MDMA to a number of other therapists, and it became the new drug of choice for those seeking a legal approach to psychedelic-assisted psychotherapy. While MDMA was still legal,

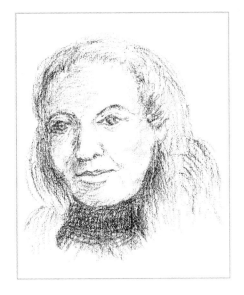

MDA (3,4-methylenedioxyamphetamine)

Ann Shulgin

MDMA (3,4-methylenedioxymethamphetamine)

Zeff and a number of other therapists working with it developed recommendations for specific settings, precautions, guidelines, and indications (Passie, 2018).

Despite the apparent utility of MDMA and the protests of physicians and psychologists who believed it was beneficial to their patients, in 1985, MDMA was classified as a Schedule 1 drug. An expert committee of the World Health Organization (WHO; 1985) recommended international prohibition of MDMA as an adjunct to psychotherapy. The committee was not, however, opposed to the study of MDMA, and its report noted that

> the expert Committee held extensive discussions concerning the reported therapeutic usefulness of MDMA. [It was] felt that the studies lacked the appropriate methodological design. There was, however, sufficient interest expressed to recommend that investigations be encouraged to follow up these preliminary findings. The Expert Committee urged countries to use the provisions of article 7 of the Convention on Psychotropic Substances to facilitate research on this interesting substance. (WHO, 1985)

In the United States, in 1986, Rick Doblin, who had an interest in hallucinogens and a doctorate in public policy, and was eager to promote further research with MDMA, founded the Multidisciplinary Association for Psychedelic Studies (MAPS). Doblin and MAPS promoted research into MDMA for more than 30 years, and their efforts led to the first clinical studies in 1992 (Grob, Poland, Chang, & Ernst, 1996; Liester, Grob, Bravo, & Walsh, 1992). Several laboratories have laid groundwork for the use of MDMA with clinical and pharmacological research.

It became apparent in early exploratory studies of MDMA in psychotherapy that the drug might be especially useful for people with PTSD (Passie, 2018a), and this is the diagnosis on which MAPS has since focused

attention. Since 2000, several Phase II studies, funded by MAPS, have been completed as part of the organization's long-term plan for approval and marketing of MDMA for therapy with people who have treatment-resistant PTSD (Mithoefer et al., 2011, 2018, 2019; Ot'alora G et al., 2018). MDMA as an adjunct to psychotherapy was also given breakthrough drug designation from the FDA, and FDA-approved Phase III clinical trials got underway in 2018 and 2019.

Principles of MDMA-Assisted Therapy for Posttraumatic Stress Disorder

MAPS developed a treatment manual and training curriculum to educate therapists in performing MDMA-assisted therapy. The procedures have been standardized, and the treatment is conducted by a female–male team in individual settings. Patients are given eyeshades, low-volume music is played, and patients are instructed to focus attention inward. The nondirective attitude of the therapists is somewhat similar to psychedelic therapy, as their role is to further, but not interfere with, patients' inner process. Therapists are, however, expected to gently focus patients' attention on their traumatic experiences, if necessary.

Slightly different mechanisms may be involved in the healing with MDMA than appears to be the case with the classic hallucinogens (Passie, 2012). The alteration of psychological functioning is not as extreme as with the hallucinogens, and it has been shown that MDMA significantly reduces the activity of the brain's fear networks (Gamma et al., 2000; Gouzoulis-Mayfrank et al., 1999). This may enable patients to confront and work through painful and dissociated memories or other aspects of traumatic experience, and to find new insights and adaptations. Because of its effects on the brain's fear network, MDMA might be conceptualized as a "trust booster." This is important insofar as the basic feeling of safety and trust tends to be adversely affected in patients with posttraumatic stress disorder (PTSD; Williamson, Porges, Lamb, & Porges, 2014). An important aspect of the mechanism of MDMA could be a disruption of the reconsolidation of fear memory. In a rodent model of fear learning, Hake and colleagues (2019, p. 343) obtained results suggesting that MDMA "could augment psychotherapy by modifying fear memories during reconsolidation without necessarily enhancing their extinction." If this underlies therapeutic change in humans, it could account for the persistent changes observed in patients with PTSD in clinical trials (e.g., Mithoefer et al., 2013).

While MDMA was used at first mainly in individual sessions (as was LSD), it quickly became obvious that it can easily be used in group settings. MDMA has advantages for group settings because of its capacity to reduce interpersonal distrust, without interfering with sensory perception or cognition. Two approaches to group therapy were established. One involved instructing the participants to focus on themselves and to engage in inward-directed reflection as the major purpose of the session. The other approach (Adamson & Metzner, 1988; Naranjo, 1989) views interpersonal contact during the session as a major part of the therapeutic process. A similar approach has been used by the SÄPT therapists (Gasser, 1996; Passie, 2007). Because MDMA also seems to facilitate communication, especially in close relationships, MDMA has also been used in couple therapy (Greer & Tolbert, 1990).

▨ Group Treatment with Psychedelics

Treatment sessions with classic hallucinogens have the disadvantage of being very time-intensive for the therapist(s). Hence, since the early days of research with hallucinogen-assisted psychotherapy, there has been interest in the possibility of conducting sessions with several patients simultaneously. At first, some therapists simply tried to treat patients under the influence of LSD in conventional group settings, in which patients were expected to interact with one another verbally. These attempts were abandoned when it became obvious that the nature of the psychedelic experience was incompatible with conventional group process (e.g., Tenenbaum, 1961). Such proponents of psycholytic therapy as Leuner, Hausner, and Sandison eventually concluded that it would be feasible to have group sessions

during the preparation and integration phases, but when a patient was under the drug's effects, an individual session with an attending nurse and a physician who drops by the medication session from time to time was preferable. Nevertheless, some investigators have reported successful group work with low doses of LSD (e.g., Derbolowski, 1967/1968; Rojo Sierra, 1960), in a more regressive setting.

The psychedelic therapists who worked with Osmond and Blewett in treating alcoholics in Saskatchewan developed an approach in which patients took LSD in groups of three or four, with one therapist present. Drawing in part on the manual by Blewett and Chewlos (1959), patients were asked to recline in a darkened room, focus their attention inward, and stay by themselves listening to music for most of the session, with occasional contact by the therapist. A European proponent of a somewhat similar approach was Alnaes (1965).

A new phase of group treatments began in the early 1960s, using a more permissive setting that encourages regression. Patients were allowed to act out emotions and experience transference reactions during the session (e.g., Fontana, 1965; Spencer, 1963, 1964). Arendsen-Hein (1963), Derbolowski (1967/1968), Hausner and Dolezal (1963), and Tenenbaum (1961) also used a similar group approach successfully. Spencer (1963) experimented with a special kind of permissive group therapy for treatment-resistant "neurotic" patients. On Sandison's LSD ward at Powick Hospital (United Kingdom), patients were encouraged to be noisy, tip over tables and bedsteads, and smash dummies and toys that had been provided. Clay and a sand trays were available for modeling, and patients were also allowed to wander around the hospital grounds. In a variation on this theme, Eisner (1964, 1967) allowed patients to "abreact" by destroying cartons or other "inexpensive or useless objects" (1967, p. 546).

If one looks back into the history of psychedelics, group approaches were rather unusual. It seems that a main factor for the comeback of the group setting was the appearance of entactogens such as MDMA. Some initial group work was done when MDMA was still legal (Passie, 2018a). A more systematic use of groups was associated with the work of the SÄPT (Styk, 1994). These therapists learned that group settings can be very productive for facilitating psychotherapy, especially with MDMA (Benz, 1989; Gasser, 1996). They came to believe that it was advantageous if participants under MDMA and others under LSD were mixed because in contrast to LSD, MDMA seemed to "stabilize the groups." In addition to the economic advantages, other benefits of using these substances in group settings include (1) greater feelings of safety and trust; (2) making public one's own inconsistencies and traumas; (3) revealing transferences and defense mechanisms; (4) space for experiencing oneself and others in a new way; and (5) a feeling of belonging to a larger framework. It was also found that fewer transference problems emerged in a group when more than one therapist was present (Passie, 2012). It should be mentioned that a number of underground therapists have developed similar approaches to group therapy (Marsden, 2001; Passie, 2007).

The SÄPT and some other therapists have developed a useful group approach over the last two decades. After patients have been treated with 10–20 conventional (drug-free) individual psychotherapy sessions, they are invited to take part in psycholytic group sessions. These take place in a separate facility on weekends. Patients meet on Friday evening and become accustomed to the rooms and the other patients through some simple rituals. These are framed to focus on patients' actual problems. The dose is typically in the range of 100–150 mg MDMA or 75–200 μg LSD. Patients are asked to lie down on mattresses and to wear headphones and eyeshades. A music playlist is available for the session, and periods of music alternate with periods of quiet. Two to three therapists of both sexes are usually available to look after eight to 15 patients (more details in Benz, 1989; Passie, 2012).

During the first 3–4 hours of the session, people are expected to focus on themselves and not engage in communication with other group members. Therapists may be recruited to talk with a patient whenever it is necessary. Therapeutic interventions include talking and other supportive behaviors. After 6 or 7 hours, the therapists may do a

"round," talking to each patient separately to check on his or her state, focusing on his or her problems, and perhaps giving further advice. At that time, a small meal is offered to patients, and after this "closing ritual," the group is left with an opportunity for communication with each other. This is thought to be therapeutically effective because by then, people were open and free of anxiety, and that emotional state might lead to new experiences in communication. After breakfast the next morning, a so-called "integration circle" is held. At this time, every participant shares a summary of personal experiences and insights from the session. Therapists and other participants provide support, joining in discussing and interpreting the experience. The therapists focus on possible lessons that can be transferred to everyday life.

For the reasons described earlier, and for economic reasons, group approaches may become common options for the future. This treatment approach has been described as safe and effective (Gasser, 1996). The groups offer much interpersonal stimulation, and facilitate trust and new interpersonal experiences, in addition to the individual psycholytic process, which does not appear to be disturbed by the group setting.

Recent experience with these methods suggests that the group approach is beneficial. The new options produced by the specific effects of the *entactogens* (MDMA, MDE, etc.) seem to the effectiveness may allow for cost-effective treatment of neurotic disorders, specific addictions, personality disorders, eating disorders, obsessive–compulsive disorders, and PTSD.

▓ Education of Therapists

There has never been a standardized program to train therapists. Every group has its own way, usually just educating a few research therapists. It is unknown how the psychotherapists who were using LSD therapy with outpatients have been trained. Leuner at Göttingen University in Germany has worked on a curriculum to educate psycholytic thrapists, which includes sitting in the sessions facilitated by an experienced therapist, and after several sessions as an observer, the roles are changed, so that the experienced therapist observes the new therapist. There are self-experiences with LSD or the like for the therapist, in addition to theoretical seminars, and participation in the clinical work on the ward, where the patients are taken care of between the drug sessions and non-drug psychotherapy sessions (Leuner, 1992). In an effort to establish MDMA-assisted psychotherapy as a treatment for PTSD, MAPS (2019) has established a training curriculum for their therapists, including online courses, one self-experience with MDMA, discussion of videotaped therapeutic MDMA sessions, and discussion of videotapes of MDMA sessions they facilitated themselves. More recently, SÄPT (2018) has outlined a comprehensive curriculum for the education of psycholytic therapists. A main requirement is to be licensed as a psychotherapist, psychiatrist, or psychologist. The curriculum includes 10 theoretical seminars, some self-experience with MDMA and LSD, and peer supervision groups, in which patients under treatment are discussed with other psycholytic therapists. More recently it has become necessary to educate therapists for conducting Phase II trials for psilocybin as a treatment for depression. The managers of these trials designed a short-term educational course for their research therapists, including online courses, a weekend workshop, and a self-experience with psilocybin (COMPASS Pathways, 2019). Phelps (2016) has provided a comprehensive description of the attributes and features of a therapist for psychedelic therapy.

In 2019, the International Society for Substance-Assisted Psychotherapy (ISSP) was incorporated, with the intention to systematize knowledge of these new treatments, discuss standards for patient selection, establish procedures for patient safety, and support development of treatment manuals and educational curricula, as well as procedures for certification and quality assurance (cf., *www.is-sp.org*).

It is obvious to every clinician experienced with the use of psychedelics that their use in psychotherapy involves some risks that should not be overlooked. Therefore, it is necessary to educate therapists very carefully, and in a systematic fashion, on theoretical as well as practical levels. More than

three self-experiences of the effects of the psychedelics used are recommended.

A main danger from my perspective is that the educational processes might not be taken seriously and that given adequate time, complications (e.g., unusual or aggressive/self-destructive behaviors, traumatic bad trips) cannot be handled appropriately by insufficiently trained therapists, especially when it comes to LSD and psilocybin. Their effects cannot be empathically understood by a therapist without sufficient self-experience and education, and that could lead to serious complications that once again might halt the development of psychedelics as medicines.

▣ Synopsis and Outlook

The distinction between the psycholytic and psychedelic approaches is likely not to persist. A number of therapists (e.g., Grof, 1967, 1975) have tried carefully and successfully to combine advantages of both approaches in some form of the psychedelytic approach. Furthermore, it seems probable that in large part because of the constraints of medical economics, the group treatment approach will become more prevalent, if circumstances allow for it. However, group treatments may not be suitable for severely traumatized patients, and perhaps for those with more serious mental health problems.

Another relevant development has been the introduction of entactogenic substances that seem to be especially suitable for psychedelytic treatments, and may offer new options for treating a broader spectrum of conditions (Holland, 2001; Passie, Hartmann, Schneider, & Emrich, 2005). These new potential therapeutic directions stem in part from illegal psycholytic work carried out by a number of therapists worldwide, some of which have been incorporated to a certain extent into legal (research) contexts.

In addition to providing significant benefit to people with psychiatric/emotional disorders, it seems likely that many basically healthy people, albeit perhaps with some personal problems, will greatly benefit from psychedelic-assisted treatments that may provide them with new opportunities to learn about themselves. As Sidney Cohen (1967, p. 1), one of the prominent early LSD researchers, puts it, LSD "does not construct character, educate the emotions, or improve intelligence. It is not a spiritual labor-saving device, salvation, instant wisdom, or a shortcut to maturity. However, it can be an opportunity to experience oneself and the world in a new way—and to learn from it."

From the perspective of nearly seven decades of clinical research, it appears that psychotherapeutic treatments assisted by hallucinogens and entactogens work in a general sense by activating endogenous self-healing mechanisms. Among the factors involved are the evocation and intensification of feelings, visual imagery, activation of repressed memories, and a broadening of perception, combined with new patterns of association and the generation of new perspectives. Another therapeutically important element in the higher-dose psychedelic therapy approach is the experience of ego dissolution of a mystical kind, which seems to be correlated with treatment success (Roseman, Nutt, & Carhart-Harris, 2018). Although hallucinogens and entactogens may be beneficial for a wide range of clinical disorders, people with an essentially healthy inner structure may be able to profit more because they can activate more self-healing resources. Psychiatric contraindications for psycholytic treatments include patients with weak ego structures, borderline personality disorders, and possibly some severe addictions. Contraindications for somatic diseases have to be considered individually and carefully.

If these methods were used on a broader scale, many patients might benefit, and what the founder of psychoanalysis, Sigmund Freud (1939/2001), stated might come true: "The future may teach us to exercise a direct influence, by means of particular chemical substances, on the amounts of energy and their distribution in the mental apparatus. It may be that there are other still undreamt-of possibilities of therapy."

▓ References

Abramson, H. A. (Ed.). (1967). *Use of LSD in psychotherapy and alcoholism.* Indianapolis, IN: Bobbs-Merrill.

Adamson, S., & Metzner, R. (1988). The nature of the MDMA experience and its role in healing, psychotherapy, and spiritual practice. *Re-Vision, 10,* 59–72.

Alexander, F. A., & French, T. M. (1946). *Psychoanalytic therapy: Principles and application.* New York: Ronald Press.

Alles, G. A. (1959). Some relations between chemical structure and physiological action of mescaline and related compounds. In H. A. Abramson (Ed.), *Neuropharmacology* (pp. 181–268). New York: Josiah Macy Foundation.

Alnaes, R. (1965). Therapeutic application of the change in consciousness produced by psycholytica (LSD, psilocybin, etc.). *Acta Psychiatrica Scandinavica, 40*(Suppl. 180), 397–409.

Andritzky, W. (1989). Sociotherapeutic functions of ayahuasca healing in Amazonia. *Journal of Psychoactive Drugs, 21,* 77–89.

Arendsen-Hein, G. W. (1963). LSD in the treatment of criminal psychopaths In R. Crocket, R. A. Sandison, & A. A. Walk (Eds.), *Hallucinogenic drugs and their psychotherapeutic use* (pp. 101–106). Springfield, IL: Charles C Thomas.

Azima, H. (1963). Anaclitic therapy: Outline of therapeutic techniques based upon the concept of regression. In Canadian Psychiatric Association (Ed.), *Proceedings of the Third World Congress of Psychiatry* (Vol. 2, pp. 1070–1074). Toronto, ON: University of Toronto Press.

Baer, G. (1967). Statistical results on reactions of normal subjects to the psilocybin derivatives CEY 10 and CZ 74. *Neuropsychopharmacology, 129,* 400–404.

Barolin, G. S. (1960). Erstes Europäisches symposion für psychotherapie unter LSD-25, Göttingen, November. *Wiener Medizinische Wochenschrift, 111,* 266–268.

Baroni, D. (1931). Geständnisse im Meskalimrausch. *Psychoanalytische Praxis, 1,* 145–149.

Bastiaans, J. (1974). The KZ-syndrome: A thirty-year study of the effects on victims of Nazi concentration camps. *Revista Medico-chirurgicata a Societatii de Medici si Naturalis li diu Jasi, 78,* 573–578.

Bastiaans, J. (1983). Mental liberation facilitated by the use of hallucinogenic drugs. In L. Grinspoon & J. B. Bakalar (Eds.), *Psychedelic reflections* (pp. 143–152). New York: Human Sciences Press.

Baumann, P. (1986). "Halluzinogen"—unterstützte Psychotherapie heute. *Ärztezeitung, 67*(47), 2202–2205.

Benz, E. (1989). *Halluzinogen—unterstützte Psychotherapie.* Doctoral dissertation, Zürich University, Zürich, Switzerland.

Benzenhöfer, U., & Passie, T. (2010). Rediscovering MDMA (ecstasy): The role of the American chemist Alexander T. Shulgin. *Addiction, 105,* 1355–1361.

Bleuler, M. (1958). Comparison of drug-induced and endogenous psychoses in man. In P. B. Brvetly, R. Deniker, & D. Raduco-Thomas (Eds.), *Proceedings of the First International Congress of Neuropsychopharmacology.* Amsterdam, the Netherlands: Elsevier.

Blewett, D. (2016). The psychedelic experience in the Native American Church. In F. Kahan (Ed.), *A culture's catalyst: Historical encounters with peyote and the Native American Church in Canada.* Manitoba: University of Manitoba Press. (Original work published 1958)

Blewett, D., & Chwelos, N. (1959). *Handbook for the therapeutic use of lysergic acid diethylamide-25: Individual and group procedures.* Unpublished manuscript, Regina, Saskatchewan, Canada.

Bogenschutz, M., Forcehimes, A. A., Pommy, J. A., Wilcox, C. E., Barbosa, P. C. R., & Strassman, R. J. (2015). Psilocybin-assisted treatment for alcohol dependence: A proof-of-concept study. *Journal of Psychopharmacology, 29,* 289–299.

Bonny, H., & Pahnke, W. N. (1972). The use of music in psychedelic (LSD) psychotherapy. *Journal of Music Therapy, 9,* 64–87.

Busch, A. K., & Johnson, W. C. (1950). LSD as an aid in psychotherapy. *Diseases of the Nervous System, 11,* 241–243.

Caldwell, W. V. (1968). *LSD psychotherapy: An exploration of psychedelic and psycholytic therapy.* New York: Grove Press.

Carhart-Harris, R. L., Bolstridge, M., Rucker, J., Day, C. M. J., Erritzoe, D., Kaelen, M., et al. (2016). Psilocybin with psychological support for treatment-resistant depression: An open-label feasibility study. *Lancet Psychiatry, 3,* 619–627.

Chandler, A. L., & Hartmann, M. A. (1950). Lysergic acid diethylamide (LSD-25) as a facilitating agent in psychotherapy. *Archives of General Psychiatry, 2,* 286–299.

Cohen, M. M., Marinello, M. J., & & Back, N. (1967). Chromosomal damage in human leukocytes induced by lysergic acid diethylamide. *Science, 155,* 1417–1419.

Cohen, S. (1960). Lysergic acid diethylamide: Side effects and complications. *Journal of Nervous and Mental Disease, 130,* 30–40.

Cohen, S. (1965). LSD and the anguish of dying. *Harper's Magazine, 231,* 69–72, 77–78.

Cohen, S. (1967). *The beyond within.* New York: Atheneum.

COMPASS Pathways. (2019). Psilocybin therapy. Retrieved September 9, 2019, from *https:// compasspathways.com/research-clinical-trials.*

Dass, R., Metzner, R., & Bravo, G. (2010). *Birth of a psychedelic culture: Conversations about Leary, the Harvard experiments, Millbrook and the sixties.* Santa Fe, NM: Synergetic Press.

Denson, R., & Sydiaha, D. (1970). A controlled study of LSD treatment in alcoholism and neurosis. *British Journal of Psychiatry, 116,* 443–445.

Derbolowski, G. (1967/1968). Dealing and working with materials in group-analysis and with "LSD 25." *British Journal of Social Psychiatry, 2,* 67–72.

Dyck, E. (2008). *Psychedelic psychiatry: LSD from clinic to campus.* Baltimore: Johns Hopkins University Press.

Eisner, B. G. (1964). Notes on the use of drugs to facilitate group psychotherapy. *Psychiatric Quarterly, 38,* 310–328.

Eisner, B. G. (1967). The importance of the non-verbal. In H. A. Abramson (Ed.), *The use of LSD in psychotherapy and alcoholism* (pp. 542–560). Indianapolis, IN: Bobbs-Merrill.

Fontana, A. E. (1965). Clinical use of hallucinogenic drugs. In Canadian Psychiatric Association (Ed.), *Proceedings of the Third World Congress of Psychiatry, Vol. II* (pp. 942–944). Toronto, ON: University of Toronto Press.

Frederking, W. (1953/1954). Über die Verwendung von Rauschdrogen (Meskalin und Lysergsäurediaethylamid) in der Psychotherapie. *Psyche, 7,* 342–364.

Frederking, W. (1955). Intoxicant drugs (mescaline and lysergic acid diethylamide) in psychotherapy. *Journal of Nervous and Mental Disease, 131,* 262–266.

Freud, S. (2001). An outline of psycho-analysis. In *Standard edition of the complete psychological works of Sigmund Freud* (Vol. 23, pp. 144–208). London: Vintage. (Original work published 1939)

Furst, P. T. (1972). *Flesh of the gods: The ritual use of hallucinogens.* Westport, CT: Praeger.

Gamma, A., Buck, A., Berthold, T., Liechti, M. W., & Vollenweider, F. X. (2000). 3,4-methylenedioxymethamphetamine (MDMA) modulates cortical and limbic brain activity as measured by [H(2)(15)O]PET in healthy humans. *Neuropsychopharmacology, 23,* 388–395.

Gasser, P. (1996). Die psycholytische Psyhotherapie in der Schweiz von 1988–1993. *Schweizer Archiv für Neurologie und Psychiatrie, 147,* 59–65.

Gasser, P., Holstein, D., Michel, Y., Doblin, R., Yazar-Klosinski, B., Passie, T., et al. (2014). Safety and efficacy of LSD-assisted psychotherapy for anxiety associated with life-threatening diseases. *Journal of Nervous and Mental Disease, 202,* 513–520.

Gasser, P., Kirchner, K., & Passie, T. (2016). LSD-assisted psychotherapy for anxiety associated with a life-threatening disease: A qualitative study of acute and sustained subjective effects. *Journal of Psychopharmacology, 29,* 1–12.

Geert-Jorgensen, E. (1968). Further observations regarding hallucinogenic treatment. *Acta Psychiatrica Scandinavica, 203*(Suppl.), 195–200.

Gouzoulis-Mayfrank, E., Schreckenberger, M., Sabri, O., Arning, C., Thelen, B., Spitzer, M., et al. (1999). Neurometabolic effects of psilocybin, 3,4-methylenedioxyethylamphetamine (MDE) and d-methamphetamine in healthy volunteers: A double-blind, placebo-controlled PET study with [^{18}F]FDG. *Neuropsychopharmacology, 20,* 565–581.

Green, A. R. (2008). Gaddum and LSD: The birth and growth of experimental and clinical neuropharmacology research on 5-HT in the UK. *British Journal of Pharmacology, 154,* 1583–1599.

Greer, G. R., & Tolbert, R. (1990). The therapeutic use of MDMA. In S. J. Peroutka (Ed.), *Ecstasy: The clinical, pharmacological and neurotoxicological effects of the drug MDMA* (pp. 21–36). Boston: Kluwer.

Griffiths, R. R., Johnson, M. W., Carducci, M. A., Umbricht, A., Richards, W. A., Cosimano, M. P., et al. (2016). Psilocybin produces substantial and sustained decreases in depression and anxiety in patients with life-threatening cancer: A randomized double-blind trial. *Journal of Psychopharmacology, 30,* 1181–1197.

Griffiths, R. R., Richards, W. A., Johnson, M. W., McCann, U. D., & Jesse, R. (2008). Mystical-type experiences occasioned by psilocybin mediate the attribution of personal meaning and spiritual significance 14 months later. *Journal of Psychopharmacology, 22,* 621–632.

Griffiths, R. R., Richards, W. A., McCann, U., & Jesse, R. (2006). Psilocybin can occasion mystical-type experiences having substantial and sustained personal meaning and spiritual significance. *Psychopharmacology (Berlin), 187,* 268–283; discussion 284–292.

Grinspoon, L., & Bakalar, J. B. (1979). *Psychedelic drugs reconsidered.* New York: Basic Books.

Grob, C. S., Danforth, A. L., Chopra, G. S., Hagerty, M., McKay, C. R., Halberstadt, A. L., et al. (2011). Pilot study of psilocybin treatment for anxiety in patients with advanced-stage cancer. *Archives of General Psychiatry, 68,* 71–78.

Grob, C. S., Poland, R. E., Chang, L., & Ernst, T. (1996). Psychobiologic effects of 3,4-methylenedioxymethamphetamine in humans: Methodologic considerations and preliminary observations. *Behavioural Brain Research, 73,* 103–107.

Grof, S. (1967). *Psycholytic and psychedelic therapy with LSD: Toward an integration of approaches.* Paper presented at the Fifth Congress of the European Medical Society of Psycholytic Therapy (EPT), Frankfurt, Germany.

Grof, S. (1975). *Realms of the human unconscious: Observations from LSD research.* New York: Viking Press.

Grof, S. (1980a). The effects of LSD on chromosomes, genetic mutation, fetal development and malignancy. In S. Grof (Ed.), *LSD psychotherapy* (pp. 320–347). Pomona, CA: Hunter House.

Grof, S. (1980b). *LSD psychotherapy.* Pomona, CA: Hunter House.

Grof, S., Goodman, L. E., Richards, W. A., & Kurland, A. A. (1973). LSD-assisted psychotherapy in patients with terminal cancer. *International Pharmacopsychiatry, 8,* 129–144.

Grof, S., & Halifax, J. (1978). *The human encounter with death.* New York: Dutton.

Hake, H. S., Sanchez, A., Loetz, E. C., Ostrovskyy, M., Wood, R. R., Oleson, E. B., et al. (2019). 3,4-methylenedioxymethamphetamine (MDMA) impairs the extinction and reconsolidation of fear memory in rats. *Physiology and Behavior, 199,* 343–350.

Hausner, M., & Dolezal, V. (1963). Group and individual psychotherapy under LSD. *Acta Psychotherapeutica et Psychosomatica, 11,* 39–59.

Hausner, M., & Segal, E. (2009). *LSD: The highway to mental health.* Malibu, CA: ASC Books.

Hintzen, A., & Passie, T. (2010). *The pharmacology of LSD.* Oxford, UK: Oxford University Press.

Hoffer, A. (1967). A program for the treatment of alcoholism: LSD, malvaria and nicotinic acid. In H. A. Abramson (Ed.), *The use of LSD in psychotherapy and alcoholism* (pp. 343–406). New York: Bobbs-Merrill.

Hoffer, A., & Osmond, H. (1966). *New hope for alcoholics.* New York: University Books.

Holland, J. (Ed.). (2001). *Ecstasy: The complete guide.* Rochester, VT: Park Street Press.

Horsley, J. S. (1943). *Narco-analysis: A new technique in short-cut psychotherapy: A comparison with other methods and notes on the barbiturates.* Oxford, UK: Oxford University Press.

International Society for Substance-Assisted Psychotherapy. (2019). *Statement of purpose*. Retrieved from *www.is-sp.org*.

Johnson, M. W., Garcia-Romeu, A., Cosimano, M. P., & Griffiths, R. R. (2014). Pilot study of the 5-HT$_{2A}$R agonist psilocybin in the treatment of tobacco addiction. *Journal of Psychopharmacology, 28*, 983–992.

Kast, E. C. (1963). The analgesic action of lysergic acid diethylamide compared with dihydromorphinone and meperidine. *Bulletin on Drug Addiction and Narcotics, 27*, 3517–3529.

Kast, E. C. (1966). LSD and the dying patient. *Chicago Medical School Quarterly, 26*, 80–87.

Keniston, K. (1968/1969). Heads and seekers: Drugs on campus, counterculture and American society. *American Scholar, 38*, 97–112.

Krebs, T. S., & Johansen, P. Ø. (2012). Lysergic acid diethylamide (LSD) for alcoholism: Meta-analysis of randomized controlled trials. *Journal of Psychopharmacology, 26*, 994–1002.

Kurland, A. A. (1985). LSD in the supportive care of the terminally ill cancer patient. *Journal of Psychoactive Drugs, 17*, 279–290.

Kurland, A. A., Grof, S., Pahnke, W. N., & Goodman, L. E. (1973). Psychedelic drug-assisted psychotherapy in patients with terminal cancer: Part One. In I. K. Goldberg, S. Malitz, & A. H. Kutscher (Eds.), *Psychopharmacological agents for the terminally ill and bereaved* (pp. 86–90). New York: Columbia University Press.

Kurland, A. A., Savage, C., Pahnke, W. N., Grof, S., & Olsson, J. E. (1971). LSD in the treatment of alcoholics. *Pharmacopsychiatry, 2*, 83–94.

La Barre, W. (1989). *The peyote cult* (5th ed.). London: Norman.

Lee, M. A., & Shlain, B. (1985). *Acid dreams: The complete social history of LSD*. New York: Grove Press.

Leuner, H. (1959). Psychotherapie in Modellpsychosen. In E. Speer (Ed.), *Kritische Psychotherapie* (pp. 94–102). Stuttgart, Germany: Enke.

Leuner, H. (1962). *Die experimentelle Psychose*. Berlin: Springer.

Leuner, H. (1967). Basic functions involved in the psychotherapeutic effect of psychotomimetics. In H. Brill (Ed.), *Neuro-psycho-pharmacology* (pp. 445–448). Amsterdam, the Netherlands: Excerpta Medica.

Leuner, H. (1971). Halluzinogene in der Psychotherapie. *Pharmakopsychiatrie und Neuropsychopharmakologie, 4*, 333–351.

Leuner, H. (1981). *Halluzinogene*. Bern, Germany: Huber.

Leuner, H. (1984). *Guided affective imagery*. New York: Grune & Stratton.

Leuner, H. (1992). *Entwurf einer Ausbildungsordnung für die psycholytische Therapie*. Unpublished manuscript, Göttingen University, Göttingen, Germany.

Leuner, H. (1994). Hallucinogens as an aid in psychotherapy: Basic principles and results. In A. Pletscher & D. Ladewig (Eds.), *50 years of LSD: Current status and perspectives of hallucinogens* (pp. 175–190). New York: Parthenon.

Levine, J., & Ludwig, A. M. (1967). The hypnodelic treatment technique. In A. H. Abramson (Ed.), *The use of LSD in psychotherapy and alcoholism.* (pp. 533–541). Indianapolis, IN: Bobbs-Merrill.

Liester, M. B., Grob, C. S., Bravo, G. L., & Walsh, R. N. (1992). Phenomenology and sequelae of 3,4-methylenedioxymethamphetamine use. *Journal of Nervous and Mental Disease, 180*, 345–352.

Ling, T. M., & Buckman, J. (1963). *Lysergic acid (LSD 25) and Ritalin in the treatment of neurosis*. London: Lambarde Press.

Ludwig, A. M., & Levine, J. (1965). A controlled comparison of five brief treatment techniques employing LSD, hypnosis, and psychotherapy. *American Journal of Psychotherapy, 19*, 417–435.

Ludwig, A. M., & Levine, J. (1967). Hypnodelic therapy. *Current Psychiatric Therapies, 7*, 130–141.

Ludwig, A. M., Levine, J., & Stark, L. H. (1970). *LSD and alcoholism: A clinical study of treatment efficacy*. Springfield, IL: Charles C Thomas.

MacLean, R., & Wilby, W. E. (1967). Treatment of alcoholism with Lysergide: Comment on the article by Smart et al., with special reference to issues of responsibility in research reporting. *Quarterly Journal of Studies on Alcohol, 28*, 140–147.

MacRae, E. (1992). *Guiado pela luna: Xamanismo e uso ritual da Ayahuasca no culto de Santo Daime*. Sao Paulo, Brazil: Editora Brasiliense.

Malleson, N. (1971). Acute adverse reactions to LSD in clinical and experimental use in the United Kingdom. *British Journal of Psychiatry, 118*, 229–230.

Marsden, R. D. (2001). *Structured group use of psychedelic or entheogenic substances: Experiences of guide and participants*. Doctoral dissertation, California Institute for Integral Studies, San Francisco, CA.

Martin, J. A. (1957). L.S.D. (lysergic acid diethylamide) treatment of chronic psychoneurotic patients under day-hospital conditions. *International Journal of Social Psychiatry, 3*, 188–195.

Mascher, E. (1967). Psycholytic therapy: Statistics and indications. In H. Brill (Ed.), *Neuropsycho-pharmacology* (pp. 441–444). Amsterdam, the Netherlands: Excerpta Medica.

Mithoefer, M. C., Feduccia, A. A., Jerome, L., Mithoefer, A., Wagner, M., Walsh, Z., et al. (2019). MDMA-assisted psychotherapy for treatment of PTSD: Study design and rationale for phase 3 trials based on pooled analysis of six phase 2 randomized controlled trials. *Psychopharmacology, 236,* 2735–2745.

Mithoefer, M. C., Mithoefer, A. T., Feduccia, A. A., Jerome, L., Wagner, M., Wymer, J., et al. (2018). 3,4-methylenedioxymethamphetamine (MDMA)-assisted psychotherapy for post-traumatic stress disorder in military veterans, firefighters, and police officers: A randomised, double-blind, dose-response, phase 2 clinical trial. *Lancet Psychiatry, 5,* 486–497.

Mithoefer, M. C., Wagner, M. T., Mithoefer, A. T., Jerome, L., & Doblin, R. (2011). The safety and efficacy of [±]3,4-,methylenedioxymethamphetamine-assisted psychotherapy in subjects with chronic, treatment-resistant posttraumatic stress disorder: The first randomized controlled pilot study. *Journal of Psychopharmacology, 25,* 439–452.

Mithoefer, M. C., Wagner, M. T., Mithoefer, A. T., Jerome, L., Martin, S. F., Yazar-Klosinski, B., et al. (2013). Durability of improvement in post-traumatic stress disorder symptoms and absence of harmful effects or drug dependency after 3,4-methylenedioxymethamphetamine-assisted psychotherapy: A prospective long-term follow-up study. *Journal of Psychopharmacology, 27,* 28–39.

Multidisciplinary Association for Psychedelic Studies. (2019). MDMA therapy training program. Retrieved September 9, 2019, from *https://maps.org/training.*

Naranjo, C. (1973). *The healing journey: New approaches to consciousness.* New York: Pantheon.

Naranjo, C. (1989). Psychedelic experiences in the light of meditation. In C. Rätsch (Ed.), *Gateway to inner space* (pp. 75–90). Bridport, UK: Prism Unity.

Naranjo, C., Shulgin, A., & Sargent, T. (1967). Evaluation of 3,4-methylenedioxyamphetamine (MDA) as an adjunct to psychotherapy. *Pharmacology, 17,* 359–364.

Pahnke, W. N. (1969). The psychedelic mystical experience in the human encounter with death. *Harvard Theological Review, 62,* 1–21.

Pahnke, W. N., Kurland, A. A., Goodman, L. E., & Richards, W. A. (1969). LSD-assisted psychotherapy with cancer patients. *Current Psychiatric Therapies, 9,* 144–152.

Pahnke, W. N., Kurland, A. A., Unger, S., Savage, C. C., & Grof, S. (1970). The experimental use of psychedelic (LSD) psychotherapy. *Journal of the American Medical Association, 212,* 1856–1863.

Passie, T. (1993/1994). Ausrichtungen, Methoden und Ergebnisse früher Meskalinforschungen im deutschsprachigen Raum. *Yearbook of the European College for the Study of Consciousness 1993/1994,* 103–112.

Passie, T. (1997). *Psycholytic and psychedelic therapy research 1931–1995: A complete international bibliography.* Hanover, Germany: Laurentius.

Passie, T. (2007). Contemporary psychedelic therapy: An overview. In M. J. Winkelman & T. B. Roberts (Eds.), *Psychedelic medicine* (Vol. 1, pp. 45–68). London: Praeger.

Passie, T. (2012). *Healing with entactogens.* Sarasota FL: MAPS.

Passie, T. (2018). The early use of MDMA in psychotherapy. *Drug Science, Policy, and Law, 4,* 1–19.

Passie, T. (2019). *The science of microdosing psychedelics.* London: PsyPress.

Passie, T., Hartmann U., Schneider, U., & Emrich, H. M. (2005). Was sind Entaktogene? *Suchtmedizin, 7,* 235–245.

Phelps, J. (2016). Developing guidelines and competencies for the training of psychedelic therapists. *Journal of Humanistic Psychology, 57,* 450–487.

Pletscher, A., & Ladewig, D. (Eds.). (1994). *50 years of LSD—Current status and perspectives of hallucinogens.* New York: Parthenon.

Riba, J., Romero, S., Grasa, E., Mena, E., Carrio, I., & Barbanoj, M. J. (2006). Increased frontal and paralimbic activation following ayahuasca, the pan-Amazonian inebriant. *Psychopharmacology (Berlin), 186,* 93–98.

Richards, W. A., Rhead, J. C., DiLeo, F. B., Yensen, R., & Kurland, A. A. (1977). The peak experience variable in DPT-assisted psychotherapy with cancer patients. *Journal of Psychedelic Drugs, 9,* 1–10.

Robinson, J. T., Davis, L. S., Sack, E. L., & Morrissey, J. D. (1963). A controlled trial of abreaction with lysergic acid diethylamide. *British Journal of Psychiatry, 109,* 46–53.

Rojo Sierra, M. (1960). Fármacos psic-activos y ontoterapia jasperiana. *Libro de Actas del VI Congreso Nacional de Neuro-Psiquiatría,* 437–447.

Roquet, S., & Favreau, P. (1981). *Los Alucinógenos: De la concepción indígena a una nueva psicoterapia.* México City: Ediciones Prisma S.A.

Roquet, S., Favreau, P. L., Ocana, R., & Velasco, M. R. (1975). *Lo existencial a traves de psicodyslepticos: una nueva psicoterapia.* Mexico City: Instituto de Psicosintesis.

Roseman, L., Nutt, D., & Carhart-Harris, R. (2018). Quality of acute psychedelic experience predicts therapeutic efficacy of psilocybin for treatment-resistant depression. *Frontiers in Pharmacology, 17,* 974.

Ross, S., Bossis, A., Guss, J., Agin-Liebes, G., Malone, T., Cohen, B., et al. (2016). Rapid and sustained symptom reduction following psilocybin treatment for anxiety and depression in patients with life-threatening cancer: A randomized controlled trial. *Journal of Psychopharmacology, 30,* 1165–1180.

Sandison, R. A., Spencer, A. M., & Whitlaw, J. D. A. (1954). The therapeutic value of lysergic acid diethylamide in mental illness. *Journal of Mental Science, 100,* 491–507.

Schlichting, M. (1989). *Psychotrope Eigenschaften des Phenäthylamins DMM-PEA (2,5-dimethoxy-4-methyl-phenathylamin).* Unpublished doctoral thesis, Göttingen University, Göttingen, Germany.

Schrenck-Notzing, F. V. (1891). *Die Bedeutung narcotischer Mittel für den Hypnotismus.* Leipzig, Germany: Abel.

Schultes, R. E., & Hofmann, A. (1979). *Plants of the gods: Origins of hallucinogenic use.* New York: McGraw-Hill.

Shulgin, A. T., Sargent, T., & Naranjo, C. (1973). Animal pharmacology and human psychopharmacology of 3-methoxy-4,5-methylenedioxyphenylisopropylamine (MMDA). *Pharmacology, 10,* 12–18.

Shulgin, A., & Shulgin, A. (2014). *PiHKAL: A chemical love story.* Berkeley, CA: Transform Press.

Smart, R., & Storm, T. (1964). The efficacy of LSD in the treatment of alcoholism. *Quarterly Journal of Studies of Alcohol, 25,* 333–338.

Smart, R. G., Storm, T., Baker, E. F. W., & Solursh, L. (1967). *Lysergic acid diethylamide in the treatment of alcoholism.* Toronto, ON: University of Toronto Press.

Smith, C. M. (1958). A new adjunct to the treatment of alcoholism: The hallucinogenic drugs. *Quarterly Journal of Studies on Alcohol, 19,* 406–417.

Snelders, S. (1998). The LSD therapy career of Jan Bastiaans, M.D. *Bulletin of the Multidisciplinary Association for Psychedelic Studies, 8,* 18–20.

Soskin, R. A. (1973). The use of LSD in time-limited psychotherapy. *Journal of Nervous and Mental Disease, 157,* 410–419.

Soskin, R. A. (1975). Dipropyltryptamine in psychotherapy. *Current Psychiatrics Therapies, 15,* 147–156.

Soskin, R. A., Grof, S., & Richards, W. A. (1973). Low doses of dipropyltryptamine in psychotherapy. *Archives of General Psychiatry, 28,* 817–821.

Spencer, A. M. (1963). Permissive group therapy with lysergic acid diethylamide. *British Journal of Psychiatry, 109,* 37–45.

Spencer, A. M. (1964). Modifications in the technique of LSD therapy. *Comprehensive Psychiatry, 5,* 232–252.

Stevens, J. (1987). *Storming heaven: LSD and the American dream.* New York: Grove Press.

Stolaroff, M. (2004). *The secret chief revealed.* Sarasota, FL: MAPS.

Stoll, A. W. (1947). Lysergsäure-diäthylamid, ein Phantastikum aus der Mutterkorngruppe. *Schweizer Archiv für Neurologie und Psychiatrie, 60,* 279–323.

Styk, J. (1994). Rückblick auf die letzten sieben Jahre der Schweizerischen Ärztegesellschaft für Psycholytische Therapie (SÄPT). In A. Dittrich, A. Hofmann, & H. Leuner (Eds.), *Welten des Bewusstseins* (Vol. 4, pp. 149–154). Berlin: Verlag für Wissenschaft und Bildung.

Swiss Physicians Society for Psycholytic Therapy. (2018). *Weiterbildung zur Begleitung von Menschen in substanz-induzierten veränderten Bewusstseinszuständen.* Solothurn, Switzerland: Author.

Tenenbaum, B. (1961). Group therapy with LSD-25. *Diseases of the Nervous System, 22,* 459–492.

Turek, I. S., Soskin, R. A., & Kurland, A. A. (1974). Methylenedioxyamphetamine (MDA): Subjective effects. *Journal of Psychedelic Drugs, 6,* 7–14.

Unger, S. (1974). Brief comments on the clinical use of psychodysleptic drugs. In S. Radouco-Thomas, A. Villeneuve, & C. Radouco-Thomas (Eds.), *Pharmacology, toxicology and abuse of psychotomimetics (hallucinogens).* Quebec: Les Presses de l'Université Laval.

U.S. Food and Drug Administration. (1975, September). FDA lists approved LSD research projects. *FDA Consumer,* pp. 24–25.

Villoldo, A. (1977). An introduction to the psychedelic psychotherapy of Salvador Roquet. *Journal of Humanistic Psychology, 17,* 45–58.

Vollenweider, F. X., & Geyer, M. A. (2001). A systems model of altered consciousness: Integrating natural and drug-induced psychoses. *Brain Research Bulletin, 56,* 495–507.

Vourlekis, A., Faillace, L. A., & Szara, S. (1967). Psychotherapy combined with psychodysleptic tryptamine derivatives and an active placebo.

In H. Brill (Ed.), *Neuro-psycho-pharmacology* (pp. 1116–1118). Amsterdam, the Netherlands: Excerpta Medica.

Widmer, S. (1997). *Listening into the heart of things: The awakening of love on MDMA and LSD: The undesired psychotherapy.* Gerolfingen, Switzerland: Basic Editions.

Williamson, J. B., Porges, E. C., Lamb, D. G., & Porges, S. W. (2014). Maladaptive autonomic regulation in PTSD accelerates physiological aging. *Frontiers in Psychology, 5,* 1571.

World Health Organization. (1985). *Expert Committee on Drug Dependence: Twenty-second report* (Technical Report Series #729). Geneva, Switzerland: Author.

Yensen, R. (1994). Perspectives on LSD and psychotherapy: The search for a new paradigm. In A. Pletscher & D. Ladewig (Eds.), *50 years of LSD: Current status and perspectives of hallucinogens* (pp. 191–202). New York: Parthenon.

Yensen, R., DiLeo, F., Rhead, J. C., Richards, W. A., Soskin, S. A., Turek, B., et al. (1976). MDA-assisted psychotherapy with neurotic outpatients: A pilot study. *Journal of Nervous and Mental Disease, 163,* 233–245.

Yensen, R., & Dryer, D. (1993/1994). Thirty years of psychedelic research: The Spring Grove experiment and its sequels. In *Yearbook of the European College for the Study of Consciousness* (pp. 73–102). Berlin: Verlag für Wissenschaft und Bildung.

PART II

Neuroscience of Hallucinogens

CHAPTER 6

Human Neuroimaging Studies of Serotonergic Psychedelics

ENZO TAGLIAZUCCHI

■ Introduction and Scope

Serotonergic psychedelics are known to elicit changes in conscious awareness, including perception of the environment and the self, as well as in mood, emotion, and different aspects of cognition (Nichols, 2016). The effect of these compounds is complex and resists a straightforward classification that is useful for other drugs, such as "stimulants" or "sedatives." While the effects of certain psychedelics do have a stimulant dimension, their defining characteristic is the capacity to temporarily induce a state of altered consciousness. Because of this, the study of psychedelics cannot be based only on animal models, since humans are alone in their capacity to explicitly report the contents of their conscious awareness. Psychedelic research with healthy human subjects necessitates techniques for the noninvasive recording of brain activity or its physiological and metabolic correlates. These techniques are referred to as "neuroimaging" and in this chapter I review their application in the study of the neural correlates of altered consciousness induced by serotonergic psychedelics.

Psychedelics share agonism at the serotonin 5-HT$_{2A}$ receptor as a common mechanism of action and are found in two different families of chemical compounds. Substituted tryptamines include psilocybin, psilocin, and dimethyltryptamine (DMT), and substituted phenethylamines include mescaline and its analogues. The chemical structure of lysergic acid diethylamide (LSD) includes both the tryptamine and phenethylamine moieties and belongs to the ergotamines (Nichols, 2016). These particular compounds (psilocybin, DMT, mescaline and LSD) are frequently called "classic psychedelics," since they were encountered by the Western scientific mainstream before the proliferation of hundreds of synthetic psychedelics with similar effects and mechanisms of action (Shulgin et al., 2011). The classic psychedelics are extremely safe drugs and are therefore most frequently investigated in human neuroimaging experiments. The scope of this chapter is limited to experiments using these compounds, with the understanding that virtually no studies of interest have been left out due to the popularity of classic psychedelics in human neuroimaging experiments.

In terms of experimental techniques, this chapter adopts a broad definition of what constitutes neuroimaging, including not only functional magnetic resonance imaging (fMRI), positron emission tomography (PET) and single-photon emission computed tomography (SPECT), but also electroencephalography (EEG) and magnetoencephalography (MEG). While these last two methods are frequently not considered neuroimaging techniques, advances in source imaging algorithms allow them to perform relatively accurate localization of source activity, justifying their inclusion in this chapter (Michel et al., 2004).

This chapter beings with a brief overview of early studies of serotonergic psychedelics, mainly performed in the 1950s and 1960s and using EEG to record brain activity. While advances in neuroimaging methods and data analyses algorithms have rendered these studies for the most part obsolete, some of them anticipated well-established results and thus deserve a place in this review. Afterwards, studies using metabolic imaging (PET and SPECT), fMRI and EEG/MEG are reviewed, including the most common variations in experimental protocols (e.g., resting-state and task-based studies). In recent years, the number of neuroimaging studies using psychedelics has grown considerably. Thus, I did not attempt an exhaustive systematic review of all articles; instead, my aim in this chapter is to review the majority of studies, with a focus on those that are considered most influential or representative. See dos Santos and colleagues (2016) for a systematic review of studies (excluding articles using EEG and MEG) up to the year 2016.

▓ Early EEG Studies and Their Limitations

Scientific research with psychedelics during the 1950s and 1960s was aligned with the cultural *zeitgeist* of those decades, revolving mainly around LSD and mescaline. The advantages and idiosyncrasies of psilocybin and DMT (including ayahuasca, the Amazonian DMT-containing concoction) were not recognized and explored until decades later. The vast majority of early studies addressed the EEG correlates of the acute effects of LSD, anticipating an interesting

knowledge gap, which I discuss later in this chapter: Even though some of most heavily used and abused psychedelics are substituted phenethylamines, virtually no studies addressed the neurophysiological effects of psychedelic phenethylamines, since neuroimaging research has almost systematically excluded mescaline up to the present day.

It is difficult—and most likely unnecessary—to pinpoint the first EEG study of the acute effects of LSD in humans. Early studies converged on two findings that have been replicated by contemporary research: LSD decreases the power of α (8–12 Hz) scalp oscillations, and increases the average peak of the alpha rhythm (Bradley et al., 1953; Bradley & Elkes, 1957; Gastaut et al., 1953; Goldstein et al., 1963). EEG captures electric displacement currents reaching the scalp; these currents are caused by the transport of ions across the cell membrane that is required to generate an action potential (neural spike) (Da Silva, 2009). Even though currents generated by a single cell are impossible to measure, those generated by large synchronized cell assemblies can lead to scalp potentials in the range of 1 μV (i.e., one-millionth of a volt), which can be recorded using EEG. Thus, LSD was shown to affect cell assemblies synchronously activated at a frequency between 8 and 12 Hz; this is known as the α rhythm and it is the landmark feature of eyes-closed resting-state human EEG.

Since artefacts of muscular origin are known to increase high-frequency power in EEG recordings, it remains difficult to the present day to determine whether LSD or other psychedelics cause fast oscillations. However, an early study using implanted electrodes in cats was likely to overcome these limitations, finding low-voltage fast cortical EEG, and disorientation, howling, periodic pacing and starring associated with slow-wave high-voltage EEG recordings (Horovitz et al., 1965). Other studies directly addressed the effects of LSD and mescaline in intracranial human EEG recordings, corroborating the decreases in the α rhythm, but also finding increased activity in the β range (12–30 Hz) in cortical and subcortical regions, predominantly in the caudate nucleus, the amygdala, and the hippocampal and septal areas (Monroe, 1974; Monroe et al., 1957; Monroe & Heath, 1961). These studies display two characteristic features of early research with human subjects: a tendency to consider psychedelics chiefly as psychotomimetic agents (i.e., drugs leading to a transient state of psychosis, as seen in psychiatric diseases such as schizophrenia), and ethical standards that would be inadmissible according to present guidelines.

Early human research with psychedelics and EEG was not limited to the frequency content of resting-state EEG, but also addressed the modulation of responses elicited by sensory stimulation. For instance, Rodin and Luby (1966) investigated how LSD affected visual evoked potentials arising due to photic stimulation at different frequencies. They reported the disappearance of the "rhythmic after discharge" and a decrease in amplitude of the major positive component of the evoked potential; however, they did not report changes in the latency of the components. Chapman and Walter (1965) found that responses to flashes of light were reduced in amplitude under the acute effects of LSD, with late rhythmic components reduced or abolished. Inconsistencies were found concerning EEG potentials evoked by ulnar (or cubital) nerve stimulation, with reports of preserved response (Shagass et al., 1962) and increased second negative component (Shagass & Schwartz, 1964). Shagass (1967) also reported increased frequency of visually evoked "after rhythms", without correlation between changes in background EEG and those in evoked potentials. This work also reported reduced amplitudes of both somatosensory and visual responses, and earlier onset of the former.

Two studies of high contemporary interest addressed how infusion of LSD altered sleep and, in particular, the EEG patterns indicating the presence of different sleep stages (Muzio et al., 1964, 1966). These studies can be summarized by the observation that LSD can shift EEG patterns from those indicative of deep sleep/reduced awareness to those representative of dreaming (rapid eye movement [REM] sleep). These studies are a good example of pioneering human research with psychedelic drugs that should be replicated using contemporary experimental and data analysis techniques. The relevance of this work is manifest in the recent proposal of exploring psychedelics to restore conscious awareness in patients with brain injuries (Scott & Carhart-Harris, 2019).

The contribution of early EEG studies to our knowledge of the neurophysiological bases of the psychedelic state is difficult to evaluate. On the one hand, many studies anticipated contemporary findings obtained using more advanced experimental methods, such as those concerning the changes in amplitude and peak frequency of the α rhythm under LSD (Carhart-Harris et al., 2016). Many studies addressed relevant and timely problems that should be revisited and replicated using modern technologies. Other studies produced interesting results that remain to be validated by current research, such as the lateralization of EEG amplitudes under LSD (Goldstein & Stoltzfus, 1973). On the other hand, it is difficult to estimate the number of false positives resulting from inadequate data analysis and experimental design. While we now take computerized data analysis for granted, this was far from the standard during the 1950s and 1960s, as expressed by Rodin and Luby when discussing the status of the field in 1966: "Most studies were carried out by simple visual inspection of the recordings except for that by Grey Walter who used toposcopic analysis and that by Goldstein and colleagues who used Drohocki's integrator." It should be obvious that simple visual inspection cannot meet the strict methodological and statistical requirements of contemporary scientific research. Perhaps more problematic is experimental design, with several open-label and unblinded studies. Expectation effects are strongly suggested, for instance, by a study reporting hypomania and dysphoria induced by 7 µg of LSD (Greiner et al., 1958), while modern research failed to detect self-reported changes in perception, mentation, or concentration at this dose (Yanakieva et al., 2019). Finally, some of the early studies using LSD in humans should serve as a warning against relaxing ethical standards in current research with serotonergic psychedelics and psychoactive drugs in general.

■ Metabolism and Binding Affinity

Before the development of fMRI in the early 1990s, the most common neuroimaging techniques were based on the direct quantification of metabolism by means of cerebral blood flow and glucose consumption. Imaging methods such as PET and SPECT offer relatively good anatomical localization but very poor temporal resolution. The static view of brain metabolism provided by these tools is insufficient to investigate dynamic interareal synchronization (functional connectivity). However, they provide insights that are often complementary to other imaging techniques and have been used to establish some long-standing results concerning the neural correlates of the psychedelic state in humans.

Studies using psilocybin, PET, and SPECT provided new insights on the neuroanatomical bases of the psychedelic state. Administration of psilocybin led to lobal increases in the cerebral metabolic rate of glucose (CMRglu), especially in regions belonging to the frontomedial and frontolateral cortex, anterior cingulate, and temporomedial cortex (Vollenweider et al., 1997). Some of these changes in CMRglu (assessed with PET) correlated with the dose and the reported subjective effects of the participants. Another study investigating glucose metabolism under psilocybin reported increases regional CMRglu in the right anterior cingulate and right frontal operculum and decreased regional CMRglu in the thalamus and precentral cortex (Gouzoulis-Mayfrank et al., 1999). The latter correlated with reports of anxiety and depression, while the former correlated positively with stereotyped thoughts.

Cerebral blood flow under the acute effects of oral DMT (ayahuasca) was investigated by Riba and colleagues (2006), and more recently by Sanches and colleagues (2016). The first of these two articles reported that ayahuasca increased activation in the anterior cingulate and the frontal gyrus (right hemisphere), the amygdala and parahippocampal gyrus (left hemisphere), and the anterior insula and inferior frontal gyrus (bilateral) (Riba et al., 2006). The second study, investigating a population of patients suffering from major depression, reported increased blood perfusion in the subgenual anterior cingulate that correlated with reductions in depressive and anxiety scores (Sanches et al., 2016). SPECT was also used to demonstrate increased blood flow in frontal regions under mescaline, which correlated with the intensity of the subjective effects (Hermle et al., 1992).

In many applications, PET has been superseded by fMRI blood oxygen level-dependent (BOLD) imaging; however, the use of different radioligands in PET imaging can provide information not available from fMRI experiments alone. The use of a radiolabeled glucose analogue (fludeoxyglucose [FDG]) allows the quantification of changes in CMRglu, but other tracers can be used to investigate the binding affinity of selected compounds and how it is modified by the administration of psychedelics. Vollenweider and colleagues (1999) studied how psilocybin modulated the *in vivo* binding of radioactive [^{11}C]raclopride to dopamine D_2 receptors, finding decreases in binding affinity located in the caudate nucleus and the putamen. These decreases were attributed to competition with increased levels of endogenous dopamine, suggesting that stimulation of serotonin receptors 5-HT$_{2A}$ and 5-HT$_{1A}$ by psilocybin leads to striatal dopamine release. Finally, PET imaging can be used to map the density of 5-HT$_{2A}$ receptors (e.g., using [^{11}C]Cimbi-36 as a radioligand; Ettrup et al., 2014, 2016), the active site of serotonergic psychedelics, yielding a fronto-temporo-parietal distribution that presents some overlap with networks associated with conscious information access and self-referential thought (Davey et al., 2016; Koch et al., 2016; Rees et al., 2002). The reviewed articles using PET and SPECT to investigate changes in brain metabolism under the effects of psychedelics reported results consistent with the distribution of 5-HT$_{2A}$ receptors, agreeing in the observation of increased frontal and parietal metabolism.

Changes in Spontaneous Activity and Functional Connectivity

fMRI provides excellent spatial resolution (≈1 mm) combined with a temporal resolution that is acceptable for many applications (≈1 second). Currently, fMRI is the predominant imaging method for functional brain mapping and for the study of spontaneous brain activity and statistical associations between activity time series measured at different brain regions (i.e., functional connectivity). The sequence of physiological changes leading to the BOLD signal is complex and beyond the scope of this chapter; however, it is important to note that fMRI provides indirect measurements of brain activity. Increased flow of oxygenated blood is required to meet the metabolic demands required by ion pumps located in the cell membrane. These pumps must operate to restore the membrane potential to its resting value after depolarization and require the hydrolysis of adenosine triphosphate, a chemical reaction that consumes oxygen. fMRI provides a signal related to the presence of oxygenated hemoglobin in the blood; thus, it is sensitive to a combination of blood flow and its level of oxygenation (BOLD signal). This signal is delayed for some seconds with respect to neuroelectric activity, and its response to a single electrical event is deformed by the hemodynamic response function (Logothetis & Wandell, 2004).

fMRI can be used to investigate changes in blood flow related to sensory stimulation or task execution, or to quantify changes in spontaneous or resting-state activity. In this section I review resting-state fMRI studies, while in the next I address how psychedelics affect human cognition in task-based fMRI experiments.

The Imperial College group pioneered the use of resting-state fMRI under the effects of psychedelics, beginning with psilocybin (Carhart-Harris et al., 2016). This study produced an interesting but counterintuitive result: Psilocybin decreased cerebral blood flow in several regions, including the thalamus, putamen, hypothalamus, posterior cingulate cortex, precuneus, bilateral angular gyrus, supramarginal gyrus. anterior cingulate cortex, frontoinsular cortex, and orbitofrontal cortex, among others. These regions present partial overlap with the default mode network (DMN), a fronto-parieto-temporal network associated with spontaneous (i.e., as opposed to elicited) thought and introspection (Raichle, 2015). These changes in cerebral blood flow correlated with the intensity of the reported subjective effects of psilocybin, leading the authors to hypothesize an effect akin to the disengagement of a "reducing valve" associated with the key hubs of the DMN. The concept of a scrambling or dysregulating effect of psychedelics can be traced to this publication and was subsequently developed by the Imperial College group in following articles.

Further analysis of the psilocybin fMRI data provided evidence supporting the aforementioned hypothesis. Psilocybin increased the variability of BOLD oscillations within the limbic system, leading to an enhanced repertoire of functional connectivity motifs and increased disorder (i.e., entropy) of the time series representing the temporal alternation of these motifs (Tagliazucchi et al., 2014). Petri and colleagues (2014) applied more sophisticated methods to show consistent results, with psilocybin reducing the stability of transient functional connectivity patterns, creating an ampler repertoire of less stable functional connectivity motifs. These articles, together with others that I mention below, led Carhart-Harris and colleagues to propose that the subjective effects of psychedelics can be understood in terms of increased entropy of brain activity fluctuations (Carhart-Harris, 2018; Carhart-Harris et al., 2014a). Other reanalyses of the 2012 psilocybin fMRI experiment showed increased functional connectivity between DMN and task-positive regions (Carhart-Harris et al., 2012a), and generally increased coupling between groups of regions that synchronize during rest, termed *resting-state networks* (RSNs; Roseman et al., 2014).

Experiments with other psychedelic drugs yielded results partially consistent with those of Carhart-Harris and colleagues (2012a). Ayahuasca also decreased the fMRI signal at key DMN hubs and disrupted the functional connectivity of the posterior cingulate cortex (Palhano-Fontes et al., 2015). A multimodal investigation of the effects of LSD by the Imperial College group found increased blood flow and functional connectivity of the visual cortex, correlating with reported changes in visual imagery (Carhart-Harris et al., 2016). Functional connectivity decreased between the parahippocampal gyrus and the retrosplenial cortex, with the prefrontal cortex and the posterior cingulate cortex, and within regions belonging to the DMN. The global functional connectivity of fronto-parietal regions increased under LSD; these increases were also found for psilocybin, presented a significant overlap with maps of 5-HT$_{2A}$ receptor density, and correlated with the self-reported intensity of ego dissolution (Tagliazucchi et al., 2016)—complementing the functional connectivity correlates under psilocybin previously reported in Lebedev and colleagues (2015).

It is important to note that a recent article reported findings seemingly in contradiction with those reported in Tagliazucchi and colleagues (2016), namely, reduced global functional connectivity of fronto-parietal regions under LSD (Preller et al., 2018). However, direct comparison of both results is difficult given the application of global signal regression by Preller and colleagues. Removal of the global signal is known to shift the distribution of BOLD signal correlations toward balanced positive–negative correlations (Murphy et al., 2009); thus, this preprocessing step could have displaced positive correlations of fronto-parietal regions toward negative values. Also, in line with Tagliazucchi and colleagues (2016), Müller and colleagues (2018) demonstrated increased functional connectivity between connectivity hubs (i.e., thalamus, striatum, precuneus, anterior cingulate cortex) under the acute effects of LSD. Another study by the same group also showed that functional connectivity increases under LSD correlate with drug-induced hallucinations (Müller et al., 2017).

While data collection is relatively straightforward in resting-state fMRI experiments, analyses are frequently highly exploratory, incorporating novel and more sophisticated methods to extract meaningful information from high-dimensionality spatiotemporal data. Some examples are mentioned in the previous paragraphs (e.g., Petri et al., 2014; Tagliazucchi et al., 2014). Atasoy and colleagues (2017) applied connectome-harmonic decomposition to investigate dynamic changes in brain states under LSD and found an expansion in the repertoire of active brain states. Lord and colleagues (2019) investigated how the dynamical exploration of the repertoire of brain networks at rest is modulated by psilocybin, finding a destabilization of frontoparietal subsystems under psilocybin, consistent with Petri and colleagues (2014). All studies mentioned in this and previous paragraphs investigated functional connectivity between BOLD signals and were therefore incapable of estimating causal relationships between them. Preller and colleagues (2018) applied dynamic causal modeling to resting-state fMRI data

acquired during the acute effects of LSD, and found that LSD increased effective connectivity from the thalamus to posterior cingulate cortex in a way directly modulated by serotonin 5-HT$_{2A}$ receptor activation, and decreased effective connectivity from the ventral striatum to the thalamus, independent of serotonin 5-HT$_{2A}$ receptor activation. This study adds support to the thalamic filter model, suggesting that the core effects of psychedelics result from gating deficits within cortico-striato-thalamo-cortical feedback loops. Finally, computational modeling has been applied to link functional connectivity changes under LSD with 5-HT$_{2A}$ receptor density (Deco et al., 2018). By combining anatomical data from diffusion MRI and fMRI with 5-HT$_{2A}$ receptor density maps obtained using PET imaging, the authors constructed a semiempirical dynamical mean-field quantitative description of populations of excitatory and inhibitory neurons that allowed them to identify the mechanisms for the nonlinear interactions between fMRI data and serotonin receptor activation.

Changes in Cognition Informed by Task-Based Experiments

Psychedelics induce idiosyncratic changes in the way the world is perceived and acted upon. The most salient features of the altered state of consciousness relate to perception (Kometer & Vollenweider, 2016); accordingly, the first EEG studies performed with subjects under the effects of LSD investigated extensively the modulation of visual and somatosensory evoked potentials. However, the effects of psychedelics extend far beyond the sensory domain and affect other aspects of human cognition. Understanding the cognitive modifications induced by psychedelics, together with their neurophysiological underpinnings, remains one of the most fascinating challenges in the field.

Protocols such as event-related and block designs are, in combination with BOLD fMRI, very powerful tools to map the functional changes associated with task execution and sensory stimulation. In the study of psychedelics, the design of tasks is frequently influenced by the psychotomimetic hypothesis. Deficits in attentional functions observed in patients with schizophrenia led Daumann and colleagues (2010) to investigate the cerebral correlates of alertness under the effects of DMT and ketamine, a glutamatergic dissociative presenting some overlaps with psychedelics in terms of subjective effects. DMT led to decreased BOLD response during the performance of an alertness task (especially in regions related to visual processing) (Daumann et al., 2010). In a different study, Daumann and colleagues (2008) investigated the effects of DMT in the neural correlates that underlie orienting of attention, finding significant behavioral effects without changes in brain activation. In a related experiment, Schmidt and colleagues (2018) investigated the effect of LSD on response inhibition networks using a go/no-go task, finding that LSD impaired inhibitory performance and reduced brain activation in the right middle temporal gyrus, superior/middle/inferior frontal gyrus and anterior cingulate cortex, and in the left superior frontal and postcentral gyrus and cerebellum.

The Basel and Zurich groups investigated how psychedelics affect emotion, social cognition, and the processing of fearful stimuli. This research is relevant both for the psychotomimetic model (since schizophrenics suffer from social and emotional deficits) and the potential therapeutic use of psychedelics in certain psychiatric conditions, such as depression and anxiety. In this domain, current evidence suggests that psychedelics act by modulating the activation and functional connectivity of the amygdala, a deep brain structure related to the processing of emotional stimuli. LSD reduced reactivity of the left amygdala and the right medial prefrontal cortex during the presentation of fearful faces, with a negative correlation between the activation of the amygdala and the subjective effects of the drug (Mueller et al., 2017). The application of dynamic causal modeling to fMRI data acquired under the effects of psilocybin revealed that the drug decreased the threat-induced modulation of top-down connectivity from the amygdala to primary visual cortex, suggesting a mechanism underlying emotional regulation during the psychedelic state (Kraehenmann et al., 2016). In another study, Kraehenmann

and colleagues (2015) found that amygdala reactivity to negative and neutral stimuli was lower after psilocybin administration, with changes in reactivity correlated with psilocybin-induced increases in positive mood state. Grimm and colleagues (2018) investigated the effects of psilocybin on emotion processing networks by assessing the effects on the functional connectivity of the amygdala during a face discrimination task. They found that psilocybin decreased the connectivity between the amygdala and the striatum during angry face discrimination and increased the connectivity between the amygdala and the frontal pole during happy face discrimination. Importantly, Roseman and colleagues (2018) investigated the response of the amygdala to neutral, fearful, and happy faces in a group of depressive patients who received a single dose of psilocybin with psychological support. Increased responses to fearful and happy faces were observed in the right amygdala posttreatment, and these differences predicted clinical improvement at 1 week. Taken together, these studies suggest that psilocybin—as opposed to other drugs used to treat mood disorders—do not blunt the emotional response but allow patients to successfully confront their emotions.

Further evidence supporting the therapeutic mechanism of action of psilocybin emerges from a study addressing how the drug modulates the processing of negative social interactions (e.g., social rejection). Psilocybin led to reduced feelings of social exclusion, presenting correlations with decreased anterior cingulate cortex and middle frontal gyrus activation, both regions involved in the processing of social pain (Preller et al., 2016). The authors proposed that these results are relevant in the context of the social stigma suffered by psychiatric patients.

Also relevant in the context of the therapeutic effects of psychedelics are studies investigating the processing of autobiographical information. Preller and colleagues (2017) found that LSD increases the attribution of personal meaning to previously meaningless music, an effect mediated by cortical midline structures. Carhart-Harris and colleagues (2016) found that psilocybin induced activations in the amygdala, hippocampus, putamen, cingulate cortex, precuneus and temporal and frontal poles, among others, when subjects were cued with personal memories. Furthermore, significant positive correlation was observed between vividness and subjective well-being in a 2-week follow-up. These studies suggest that psilocybin modulates the processing of autobiographical information by increasing the response in a distributed network of brain regions, including the amygdala and midline structures.

fMRI has been used to investigate the neural correlates of altered sensory perception elicited by psychedelic drugs, using both simple and complex visual and auditory stimuli. In a pioneering study using ayahuasca, de Araujo and colleagues (2012) showed that during an imagery task, the drug-induced activations in visual regions were comparable to those elicited by natural images with the eyes opened, with additional activations in the cuneus, lingual gyrus, parahippocampal gyrus, retrosplenial and frontopolar cortices. Roseman and colleagues (2016) combined a retinotopic localizer with functional connectivity analyses to identify the patches of V1 and V3 representing vertical and horizontal meridians of the visual field, and showed that LSD increased connectivity between patches with incongruent specificity. This result supports that LSD leads to a functional organization of the visual cortex less dependent on its retinotopic organization. Taken together, these two studies show that psychedelics induced vivid visual imagery related to the activation of visual regions with eyes closed, and that they reorganize the low-level processing of visual information.

The processing of musical stimuli has received attention from two independent experiments. LSD increased the functional connectivity between the parahippocampus and the visual cortex, with positive correlation with subjective ratings of eyes-closed visual imagery (including autobiographical imagery) (Kaelen et al., 2016). These results support previous links between the parahippocampal cortex, music evoked emotion, and psychedelic-induced mental imagery. In a different study, tonality-tracking analysis of BOLD data revealed that LSD alters neural responses in regions associated with low- and high-level musical and auditory processing, as well as in other areas related to

memory, emotion, and self-referential processing (Barrett et al., 2018). Both studies converge in the finding that the interaction between music and the psychedelic states transcends networks involved with auditory processing and involves other cognitive systems as well.

▪ Contemporary Electrophysiological Studies

Many results from early studies have been revisited and replicated using modern imaging technologies such as MEG and EEG with source estimation. Also, these methods can yield novel insights not available to early researchers. MEG recordings during the acute effects of psilocybin revealed a broadband decrease in oscillatory power, localized in posterior association cortices for 1–50 Hz, and in frontal association cortices for 8–100 Hz (Muthukumaraswamy et al., 2013). Consistent with fMRI studies, large decreases in spectral power appeared within the DMN. Computational modeling showed that desynchronization in the posterior hub of the DMN could be explained by increased excitability of deep-layer pyramidal neurons, rich in 5-HT_{2A} receptors. An independent article hypothesized that decreases in activity and spectral power due to excitation of these neurons may be related to secondary excitation of inhibitory interneurons (Carhart-Harris et al., 2014b). MEG recordings showed consistent results for LSD data: Broadband decreases in spectral power were observed, with changes in different bands and anatomical locations correlating with the subjective effects (Carhart-Harris et al., 2016). Decreases in occipital α correlated with the intensity of visual imagery, decreases in parietal (midline) and temporal α and δ correlated with reports of ego-dissolution. This study also showed that LSD increases the peak frequency of the α rhythm, consistently with early EEG studies (Bradley et al., 1953; Bradley & Elkes, 1957; Gastaut et al., 1953; Goldstein et al., 1963).

An attractive hypothesis is that diminished α power under serotonergic psychedelics reflects loss of cortical inhibition; α oscillations have been repeatedly linked to the inhibition of neural processes irrelevant for the current cognitive demands (Klimesch et al., 2007). Loss of inhibition may imply facilitated access to consciousness, for instance, of spontaneous activity fluctuations in visual areas that are otherwise filtered out from awareness. This hypothesis is consistent with reports of correlations between α decreases under LSD and increased visual imagery (Carhart-Harris et al., 2016), and has received direct support by a study with ayahuasca and EEG (Valle et al., 2016). Ayahuasca decreased EEG power in the δ, θ, and α bands; source imaging showed that occipital α decreases correlated with the intensity of visual imagery, and pretreatment with a 5-HT$_{2A}$ receptor antagonist (ketanserin) inhibited both changes in EEG and the correlation with visual imagery. Further studies with ayahuasca using EEG produced novel insights on psychedelic action on the human brain. Riba and colleagues (2006) mapped the time series of EEG spectral power changes, finding that ayahuasca decreased absolute power in all frequency bands (most prominently in the θ band), that these changes began as early as 15–30 minutes, peaked between 45 and 120 minutes, and returned to baseline levels at 4–6 hours. Schenberg and colleagues (2015) investigated the time series of spectral power changes, as well as the blood level of DMT, β-carbolines and their metabolites, reporting a biphasic effect. After 50 minutes from ingestion, they reported reduced power in the α band (located at the parieto-occipital cortex), together with increased γ power between 75 and 125 minutes (located at frontal, parietal and central regions). These effects correlated with circulating levels of the active compounds in ayahuasca (i.e., DMT, harmine, harmaline, and tetrahydroharmine).

An EEG study with psilocybin reproduced the α power decreases, and also found that lagged phase synchronization between a network of brain regions correlated with subjective reports of drug-induced spritual experiences (Kometer et al., 2015). Other studies with psilocybin addressed various aspects of cognition. Bernasconi and colleagues (2013) investigated the EEG visual evoked potentials elicited by emotional faces and found that psilocybin modulated the 168- to 189-microsecond poststimulus potential, with a second period of modulation between 211 and 242 microseconds poststimulus. Source imaging localized these changes to limbic areas, including the amygdala and the parahippocampal gyrus. Convergent evidence from EEG experiments suggests that psilocybin, compared to ketamine, fails to disrupt the potentials evoked by mismatch negativity (Heekeren et al., 2008; Umbricht et al., 2003). An MEG study using LSD, however, found results conflicting with those of the aforementioned articles: LSD decreased the neural response to novel stimuli and increased that for familiar stimuli, and dynamic causal modeling showed that top-down connectivity was modulated under the effects of LSD (Timmermann et al., 2018).

Future Directions of Research

The results reviewed in this chapter present important consistencies in terms of findings across drugs and imaging modalities. However, variability in the results remains, and this variability may indicate promising future lines of research.

All the compounds mentioned in this chapter (psilocybin, mescaline, DMT, and LSD) share agonism at 5-HT$_{2A}$ receptors as a common mechanism of action. However, these molecules bind and act at other serotonin receptor subtypes, as well as at receptors of other neurotransmitters and neuromodulators. Preliminary research shows that action at these other sites can influence the subjective effects of psychedelics (Zamberlan et al., 2018). Differences can be found between substituted tryptamines and phenethylamines: The former present higher binding affinities for 1A/1B receptors, while the latter are more selective for 2A receptors (Nichols, 2016). Many of the currently most widespread psychedelics for recreational use belong to the family of substituted phenethylamines, such as 2,5-dimethoxy-4-methylamphetamine (DOM), 2,5-dimethoxy-4-bromophenethylamine (2C-B), and 25I-NBOMe (Shulgin et al., 2011). However, very few neuroimaging studies have addressed the acute effects of mescaline, the prototypical psychedelic phenethylamine. More generally, placebo-controlled neuroimaging studies can fail to reveal changes specific to certain compounds. Future studies could formally compare the neural correlates elicited by psychedelics with different chemical structures and binding affinity profiles. First steps have been performed using multivariate machine learning classifiers trained and tested using different serotonergic psychedelics and ketamine, revealing that changes in α power and connectivity are specific to 5-HT$_{2A}$ receptor agonists (Pallavicini et al., 2019). Also, the predictions of the entropic brain hypothesis (Carhart-Harris et al., 2014a, 2018) are corroborated not only for LSD and psilocybin but also for ketamine (Schartner et al., 2017).

While experiments using independent imaging modalities can provide important information on psychedelic action on the human brain, future studies must combine imaging modalities to overcome certain limitations. Techniques that measure variables related to cerebral blood flow can be affected by vasoconstriction, an established effect of serotonergic psychedelics (Nichols, 2016). Combined EEG–fMRI recordings could facilitate the localization of the prominent decreases in the α rhythm caused by these compounds. Simultaneous acquisition of fMRI and PET is a promising tool to investigate changes in brain activity related to *in vivo* measurements of 5-HT$_{2A}$ receptor occupancy (Madsen et al., 2019).

For all the variety in imaging modalities, experimental protocols, and investigated compounds, the studies cited in this chapter are homogeneous in a dimension highly relevant in the context of psychedelic action: the context surrounding the experience. Since psychedelic experiences are highly sensitive to contextual factors ("setting"), we do not know to which extent knowledge gathered in imaging facilities located in hospitals and research centers generalize to natural or "ecological" settings (Carhart-Harris et al., 2018). This is an important topic, since recreational use (and, potentially, future therapeutic use) takes place in extremely different surroundings, such as private houses, ceremonies and retreats, with external influencing factors such as scents, chants, and music. Many psychedelic experiences are, in fact, social experiences undertaken by a group and supervised by a guide. While some studies have attempted recordings in natural settings, these have been limited by underde-

veloped mobile EEG technology (Hoffmann et al., 2001; Stuckey et al., 2005). However, this technology has advanced considerably in recent years and appears ripe for field recordings of psychedelic use.

Finally, neuroimaging studies should be employed to investigate the mechanism underlying the therapeutic effects of psychedelics. The promise of this approach is highlighted by a study investigating the changes in fMRI before and after a single dose of psilocybin in patients suffering from depression (Carhart-Harris et al., 2017). Functional imaging could also be used to predict the likelihood of successful treatment, an application of high relevance considering the financial costs and regulatory hurdles involved in clinical research with psychedelic compounds.

▓ References

Atasoy, S., et al. (2017). Connectome-harmonic decomposition of human brain activity reveals dynamical repertoire re-organization under LSD. *Scientific Reports, 7*(1), Article 17661.

Barrett, F. S., et al. (2018). Serotonin 2A receptor signaling underlies LSD-induced alteration of the neural response to dynamic changes in music. *Cerebral Cortex, 28*(11), 3939–3950.

Bernasconi, F., et al. (2013). Spatiotemporal brain dynamics of emotional face processing modulations induced by the serotonin 1A/2A receptor agonist psilocybin. *Cerebral Cortex, 24*(12), 3221–3231.

Bradley, P. B., et al. (1953). On some effects of lysergic acid diethylamide (LSD 25) in normal volunteers. *Journal of Physiology, 121*(2), 50P–51P.

Bradley, P. B., & Elkes, J. (1957). The effects of some drugs on the electrical activity of the brain. *Brain, 80*(1), 77–117.

Carhart-Harris, R. L., et al. (2012a). Functional connectivity measures after psilocybin inform a novel hypothesis of early psychosis. *Schizophrenia Bulletin, 39*(6), 1343–1351.

Carhart-Harris, R. L., et al. (2012b). Implications for psychedelic-assisted psychotherapy: Functional magnetic resonance imaging study with psilocybin. *British Journal of Psychiatry, 200*(3), 238–244.

Carhart-Harris, R. L., et al. (2014a). The entropic brain: A theory of conscious states informed by neuroimaging research with psychedelic drugs. *Frontiers in Human Neuroscience, 8*, 20.

Carhart-Harris, R. L., et al. (2014b). How do

hallucinogens work on the brain? *Journal of Psychophysiology, 71*(1), 2–8.

Carhart-Harris, R. L., et al. (2016). Neural correlates of the LSD experience revealed by multimodal neuroimaging. *Proceedings of the National Academy of Sciences of the USA, 113*(17), 4853–4858.

Carhart-Harris, R. L., et al. (2017). Psilocybin for treatment-resistant depression: fMRI-measured brain mechanisms. *Scientific Reports, 7*(1), Article 13187.

Carhart-Harris, R. L., et al. (2018). Psychedelics and the essential importance of context. *Journal of Psychopharmacology, 32*(7), 725–731.

Chapman, L. F., & Walter, R. D. (1965). Actions of lysergic acid diethylamide on averaged human cortical evoked responses to light flash. *Recent Advances in Biological Psychiatry, 7*, 23–36.

Da Silva, F. L. (2009). EEG: Origin and measurement. In C. Mulert & L. Lemieux (Eds.), *EEG–fMRI* (pp. 19–38). Berlin: Springer.

Daumann, J., et al. (2008). Pharmacological modulation of the neural basis underlying inhibition of return (IOR) in the human 5-HT 2A agonist and NMDA antagonist model of psychosis. *Psychopharmacology, 200*(4), 573–583.

Daumann, J., et al. (2010). Neuronal correlates of visual and auditory alertness in the DMT and ketamine model of psychosis. *Journal of Psychopharmacology, 24*(10), 1515–1524.

Davey, C. G., et al. (2016). Mapping the self in the brain's default mode network. *NeuroImage, 132*, 390–397.

de Araujo, D. B., et al. (2012). Seeing with the eyes shut: Neural basis of enhanced imagery following ayahuasca ingestion. *Human Brain Mapping, 33*(11), 2550–2560.

Deco, G., et al. (2018). Whole-brain multimodal neuroimaging model using serotonin receptor maps explains non-linear functional effects of LSD. *Current Biology, 28*(19), 3065–3074.

dos Santos, R. G., et al. (2016). Classical hallucinogens and neuroimaging: A systematic review of human studies: Hallucinogens and neuroimaging. *Neuroscience and Biobehavioral Reviews, 71*, 715–728.

Ettrup, A., et al. (2014). Serotonin 2A receptor agonist binding in the human brain with [11C] Cimbi-36. *Journal of Cerebral Blood Flow and Metabolism, 34*(7), 1188–1196.

Ettrup, A., et al. (2016). Serotonin 2A receptor agonist binding in the human brain with [11C] Cimbi-36: Test–retest reproducibility and head-to-head comparison with the antagonist [18F] altanserin. *NeuroImage, 130*, 167–174.

Gastaut, H., et al. (1953). Action de la diéthylamide de l'acide d-lysergique (LSD 25) sur les fonctions psychiques et l'électroencéphalogramme.

Stereotactic and Functional Neurosurgery, 13(2), 102–120.

Goldstein, L., et al. (1963). Quantitative electroencephalographic analysis of naturally occurring (schizophrenic) and drug-induced psychotic states in human males. *Clinical Pharmacology and Therapeutics, 4*(1), 10–21.

Goldstein, L., & Stoltzfus, N. W. (1973). Psychoactive drug-induced changes of interhemispheric EEG amplitude relationships. *Agents and Actions, 3*(2), 124–132.

Gouzoulis-Mayfrank, E., et al. (1999). Neurometabolic effects of psilocybin, 3, 4-methylenedioxyethylamphetamine (MDE) and d-methamphetamine in healthy volunteers: A double-blind, placebo-controlled PET study with [18F] FDG. *Neuropsychopharmacology, 20*(6), 565–581.

Greiner, T., et al. (1958). Psychopathology and psychophysiology of minimal LSD-25 dosage: A preliminary dosage–response spectrum. *AMA Archives of Neurology and Psychiatry, 79*(2), 208–210.

Grimm, O., et al. (2018). Psilocybin modulates functional connectivity of the amygdala during emotional face discrimination. *European Neuropsychopharmacology, 28*(6), 691–700.

Heekeren, K., et al. (2008). Mismatch negativity generation in the human 5HT 2A agonist and NMDA antagonist model of psychosis. *Psychopharmacology, 199*(1), 77–88.

Hermle, L., et al. (1992). Mescaline-induced psychopathological, neuropsychological, and neurometabolic effects in normal subjects: Experimental psychosis as a tool for psychiatric research. *Biological Psychiatry, 32*(11), 976–991.

Hoffmann, E., et al. (2001). Effects of a psychedelic, tropical tea, ayahuasca, on the electroencephalographic (EEG) activity of the human brain during a shamanistic ritual. *MAPS Bulletin, 11*(1), 25–30.

Horovitz, Z. P., et al. (1965). Behavioral and electroencephalographic effects of LSD. *Journal of Pharmaceutical Sciences, 54*(1), 108–110.

Kaelen, M., et al. (2016). LSD modulates music-induced imagery via changes in parahippocampal connectivity. *European Neuropsychopharmacology, 26*(7), 1099–1109.

Klimesch, W., et al. (2007). EEG alpha oscillations: The inhibition–timing hypothesis. *Brain Research Reviews, 53*(1), 63–88.

Koch, C., et al. (2016). Neural correlates of consciousness: Progress and problems. *Nature Reviews Neuroscience, 17*(5), 307.

Kometer, M., et al. (2015). Psilocybin-induced spiritual experiences and insightfulness are associated with synchronization of neuronal oscillations. *Psychopharmacology, 232*(19), 3663–3676.

Kometer, M., & Vollenweider, F. X. (2016). Serotonergic hallucinogen-induced visual perceptual alterations. In A. Halberstadt, F. X. Vollenweider, & D. E. Nichols (Eds.), *Behavioral neurobiology of psychedelic drugs* (pp. 257–282). Berlin: Springer.

Kraehenmann, R., et al. (2015). Psilocybin-induced decrease in amygdala reactivity correlates with enhanced positive mood in healthy volunteers. *Biological Psychiatry, 78*(8), 572–581.

Kraehenmann, R., et al. (2016). The mixed serotonin receptor agonist psilocybin reduces threat-induced modulation of amygdala connectivity. *NeuroImage: Clinical, 11*, 53–60.

Lebedev, A. V., et al. (2015). Finding the self by losing the self: Neural correlates of ego-dissolution under psilocybin. *Human Brain Mapping, 36*(8), 3137–3153.

Logothetis, N. K., & Wandell, B. A. (2004). Interpreting the BOLD signal. *Annual Review of Physiology, 66*, 735–769.

Lord, L.-D., et al. (2019). Dynamical exploration of the repertoire of brain networks at rest is modulated by psilocybin. *NeuroImage, 199*, 127–142.

Madsen, M., et al. (2019). Psychedelic effects of psilocybin correlate with serotonin 2 A receptor occupancy and plasma psilocin levels. *Neuropsychopharmacology, 44*, 1328–1334.

Michel, C. M., et al. (2004). EEG source imaging. *Clinical Neurophysiology, 115*(10), 2195–2222.

Monroe, R. R. (1974). Drug effects on subcortical electrograms in humans. In T. M. Itil (Ed.), *Psychotropic drugs and the human EEG* (Vol. 8, pp. 228–237). Basel, Switzerland: Karger.

Monroe, R. R., et al. (1957). Correlation of rhinencephalic electrograms with behavior: A study of humans under the influence of LSD and mescaline. *Electroencephalography and Clinical Neurophysiology, 9*(4), 623–642.

Monroe, R. R., & Heath, R. G. (1961). Effects of lysergic acid and various derivatives on depth and cortical electrograms. *Journal of Neuropsychiatry, 3*, 75–82.

Mueller, F., et al. (2017). Acute effects of LSD on amygdala activity during processing of fearful stimuli in healthy subjects. *Translational Psychiatry, 7*(4), e1084.

Müller, F., et al. (2017). Increased thalamic resting-state connectivity as a core driver of LSD-induced hallucinations. *Acta Psychiatrica Scandinavica, 136*(6), 648–657.

Müller, F., et al. (2018). Altered network hub connectivity after acute LSD administration. *NeuroImage: Clinical, 18*, 694–701.

Murphy, K., et al. (2009). The impact of global signal regression on resting state correlations: Are anti-correlated networks introduced? *NeuroImage, 44*(3), 893–905.

Muthukumaraswamy, S. D., et al. (2013). Broadband cortical desynchronization underlies the human psychedelic state. *Journal of Neuroscience, 33*(38), 15171–15183.

Muzio, J., et al. (1964). *Alteration in the young adult human sleep EEG configuration resulting from d-LSD-25*. Report to the Association for the Psychophysiological Study of Sleep, Palo Alto, CA.

Muzio, J., et al. (1966). Alterations in the nocturnal sleep cycle resulting from LSD. *Electroencephalography and Clinical Neurophysiology, 21*(4), 313–324.

Nichols, D. E. (2016). Psychedelics. *Pharmacological Reviews, 68*(2), 264–355.

Palhano-Fontes, F., et al. (2015). The psychedelic state induced by ayahuasca modulates the activity and connectivity of the default mode network. *PLOS ONE, 10*(2), e0118143.

Pallavicini, C., et al. (2019). Spectral signatures of serotonergic psychedelics and glutamatergic dissociatives. *NeuroImage, 200*, 281–291.

Petri, G., et al. (2014). Homological scaffolds of brain functional networks. *Journal of the Royal Society Interface, 11*(101), Article 20140873.

Preller, K. H., et al. (2016). Effects of serotonin 2A/1A receptor stimulation on social exclusion processing. *Proceedings of the National Academy of Sciences of the USA, 113*(18), 5119–5124.

Preller, K. H., et al. (2017). The fabric of meaning and subjective effects in LSD-induced states depend on serotonin 2A receptor activation. *Current Biology, 27*(3), 451–457.

Preller, K. H., et al. (2018). Changes in global and thalamic brain connectivity in LSD-induced altered states of consciousness are attributable to the 5-HT2A receptor. *eLife, 7*, e35082.

Raichle, M. E. (2015). The brain's default mode network. *Annual Review of Neuroscience, 38*, 433–447.

Rees, G., et al. (2002). Neural correlates of consciousness in humans. *Nature Reviews Neuroscience, 3*(4), 261–270.

Riba, J., et al. (2002). Topographic pharmaco-EEG mapping of the effects of the South American psychoactive beverage ayahuasca in healthy volunteers. *British Journal of Clinical Pharmacology, 53*(6), 613–628.

Riba, J., et al. (2006). Increased frontal and paralimbic activation following ayahuasca, the pan-Amazonian inebriant. *Psychopharmacology, 186*(1), 93–98.

Rodin, E., & Luby, E. (1966). Effects of LSD-25 on the EEG and photic evoked responses. *Archives of General Psychiatry, 14*(4), 435–441.

Roseman, L., et al. (2014). The effects of psilocybin and MDMA on between-network resting state functional connectivity in healthy volunteers. *Frontiers in Human Neuroscience, 8,* 204.

Roseman, L., et al. (2016). LSD alters eyes-closed functional connectivity within the early visual cortex in a retinotopic fashion. *Human Brain Mapping, 37*(8), 3031–3040.

Roseman, L., et al. (2018). Increased amygdala responses to emotional faces after psilocybin for treatment-resistant depression. *Neuropharmacology, 142,* 263–269.

Sanches, R. F., et al. (2016). Antidepressant effects of a single dose of ayahuasca in patients with recurrent depression: A SPECT study. *Journal of Clinical Psychopharmacology, 36*(1), 77–81.

Schartner, M. M., et al. (2017). Increased spontaneous MEG signal diversity for psychoactive doses of ketamine, LSD and psilocybin. *Scientific Reports, 7,* Article 46421.

Schenberg, E. E., et al. (2015). Acute biphasic effects of ayahuasca. *PLOS ONE, 10*(9), e0137202.

Schmidt, A., et al. (2018). Acute LSD effects on response inhibition neural networks. *Psychological Medicine, 48*(9), 1464–1473.

Scott, G., & Carhart-Harris, R. L. (2019). Psychedelics as a treatment for disorders of consciousness. *Neuroscience of Consciousness, 2019*(1), niz003.

Shagass, C. (1967). Effects of LSD on somatosensory and visual evoked responses and on the EEG in man. In J. Wortis (Ed.), *Recent advances in biological psychiatry* (pp. 209–227). Boston: Springer.

Shagass, C., et al. (1962). Some drug effects on evoked cerebral potentials in man. *Journal of Neuropsychiatry, 3,* S-49.

Shagass, C., & Schwartz, M. (1964). Evoked potential studies in psychiatric patients. *Annals of the New York Academy of Sciences, 112,* 526–542.

Shulgin, A. T., et al. (2011). *The Shulgin index: Psychedelic phenethylamines and related compounds.* Berkeley, CA: Transform Press.

Stuckey, D. E., et al. (2005). EEG gamma coherence and other correlates of subjective reports during ayahuasca experiences. *Journal of Psychoactive Drugs, 37*(2), 163–178.

Tagliazucchi, E., et al. (2014). Enhanced repertoire of brain dynamical states during the psychedelic experience. *Human Brain Mapping, 35*(11), 5442–5456.

Tagliazucchi, E., et al. (2016). Increased global functional connectivity correlates with LSD-induced ego dissolution. *Current Biology, 26*(8), 1043–1050.

Timmermann, C., et al. (2018). LSD modulates effective connectivity and neural adaptation mechanisms in an auditory oddball paradigm. *Neuropharmacology, 142,* 251–262.

Umbricht, D., et al. (2003). Effects of the 5-HT 2A agonist psilocybin on mismatch negativity generation and AX-continuous performance task: Implications for the neuropharmacology of cognitive deficits in schizophrenia. *Neuropsychopharmacology, 28*(1), 170–181.

Valle, M., et al. (2016). Inhibition of alpha oscillations through serotonin-2A receptor activation underlies the visual effects of ayahuasca in humans. *European Neuropsychopharmacology, 26*(7), 1161–1175.

Vollenweider, F. X., et al. (1997). Positron emission tomography and fluorodeoxyglucose studies of metabolic hyperfrontality and psychopathology in the psilocybin model of psychosis. *Neuropsychopharmacology, 16*(5), 357–372.

Vollenweider, F. X., et al. (1999). 5-HT modulation of dopamine release in basal ganglia in psilocybin-induced psychosis in man—a PET study with [^{11}C] raclopride. *Neuropsychopharmacology, 20*(5), 424–433.

Yanakieva, S., et al. (2019). The effects of microdose LSD on time perception: A randomised, double-blind, placebo-controlled trial. *Psychopharmacology, 236*(4), 1159–1170.

Zamberlan, F., et al. (2018). The varieties of the psychedelic experience: A preliminary study of the association between the reported subjective effects and the binding affinity profiles of substituted phenethylamines and tryptamines. *Frontiers in Integrative Neuroscience, 12,* 54.

CHAPTER 7

Memory Reconsolidation in Psycholytic Psychotherapy

JIM GRIGSBY

Introduction

This chapter is concerned with possible mechanisms for the therapeutic effects of the classic hallucinogens, which include lysergic acid diethylamide (LSD), psilocybin, and mescaline, along with the shorter-acting dimethyltryptamine (DMT). In particular, the focus is on LSD and psilocybin when they are used as adjuncts to intermediate and long-term psychotherapy (Grof, 1980). This application of hallucinogens is a derivative of the *psycholytic* approach that was used primarily in Europe during the 1950s and 1960s (Leuner, 1963; Sandison, 1954), and further developed by Stanislav Grof (1980) during his early work in Czechoslovakia. It differs in important ways from clinical applications of hallucinogens that have been studied since the early years of the 21st century and has not yet been rigorously researched.

The classic (serotonergic) hallucinogens, for which Nichols reserves the term *psychedelics,* are 5-HT$_{2A}$ receptor agonists (Nichols & Nichols, Chapter 1, this volume). 5-HT$_{2A}$ receptors are widely distributed in the brain but are especially concentrated throughout the neocortex, claustrum, mammillary bodies, and the lateral nucleus of the amygdala, with a somewhat lower density in the hippocampus, caudate, putamen, and nucleus accumbens (Zhang & Stackman, 2015). According to Nichols, LSD is a "relatively nonselective serotonin and dopamine receptor ligand" (2016, p. 289), and variation among these hallucinogens with respect to their strength and precise effects is presumably a function of not only their differential affinity for the 5-HT$_{2A}$ receptor but also the extent to which they bind to other serotonin receptor subtypes (e.g., 5-HT$_{2C}$, 5-HT$_{1A}$), and to the receptors of other neurotransmitters (e.g., especially dopamine).

The effects of the classic hallucinogens are determined by not only the specific receptors to which they bind but also the location of those receptors in the brain, as well as the differential effects each has on gene expression (e.g., *c-fos, egr1, egr2*), guanine nucleotide-binding protein (G-protein) coupling in multiple signaling pathways, glutamate signaling, and other biochemical processes (Nichols, 2016; Nichols & Nichols, Chapter 1, this volume). Finally, the set and setting, as well as the personality of the individual

LSD user, and of the guide/facilitator, are crucial determinants of the psychological reaction to LSD and related drugs.

Nichols (2016) noted that much of the gene expression induced by LSD affects synaptic strength and regulation, and hence memory consolidation, through metabotropic glutamate receptor (mGluR)-mediated plasticity, for example, or the effects of cytosine–cytosine–adenosine–adenosine–thymidine (CCAAT)/enhancer-binding protein β (C/EBP-β). Downstream pathways remain "poorly understood," although it appears possible that LSD may have two phases of action. The first, an early, serotonergic psychedelic phase, appears to peak between 3 and 5 hours after oral administration. This is followed by a delayed-onset phase—probably dopaminergic—typically appearing about 4–6 hours after administration (Freedman, 1984; Nichols, 2016).

What is known about the action and effects of the classic hallucinogens, and of their therapeutic effectiveness for different indications, suggests that they operate via multiple, complex therapeutic mechanisms. This is in part a function of the diversity of the biochemical pathways activated by these molecules, as well as the extraordinary psychological states associated with the psychedelic experience, which are themselves determined to a large extent by the vagaries of set and setting within and between individuals (Cohen, 1960; Leary, Litwin, & Metzner, 1963). The hallucinogens are not inherently therapeutic by themselves; rather, the benefits accrued by users are dependent on a session conducted in a safe, structured, and supportive social and physical environment. Hence, the nonpharmacological effects of hallucinogens (e.g., set, setting, therapeutic goals, personalities of subject and sitter/facilitator, therapeutic approach) are widely recognized as key determinants of the course and outcome of a psychedelic session.

It is unclear whether the therapeutic mechanisms of psychedelics are best understood physiologically, psychologically, or even spiritually. Although the psychedelic experience is initiated at 5-HT_{2A} and related serotonin receptor sites (Preller et al., 2018), it has been found that specific brain structures are somehow involved, and neuroimaging research has identified what appear to

be profound alterations of the brain's state overall. At the same time, data from a number of clinical studies provide evidence that the occurrence of a "mystical-type experience" (Griffiths, Richards, Johnson, McCann, & Jesse, 2008; Griffiths, Richards, McCann, & Jesse, 2006; Pahnke, Kurland, Goodman, & Richards, 1969; Pahnke & Richards, 1969; Ross et al., 2016), or a psychedelic "peak experience" (Maslow, 1964), is strongly correlated with positive therapeutic outcomes.

Therapeutic Use of Hallucinogens: Psycholytic and Psychedelic Approaches

Of the classic hallucinogens, LSD and psilocybin are those most commonly used to treat a heterogeneous range of conditions, with considerable success. Most early research, beginning in the 1950s, used LSD. In recent years, it has been supplanted by psilocybin, which is less psychologically intense, has a somewhat shorter duration of action, and does not have the checkered social, political, and legal reputation of LSD.

The first clinical article on the use of a classic hallucinogen as a therapeutic agent appears to have been published by Busch and Johnson (1950), who used LSD as an adjunct to psychodynamic psychotherapy. That article was soon followed by others (e.g., Abramson, 1955, 1956; Frederking, 1955; Katzenelbogen & Fang, 1953; Sandison, 1954). None of these authors reported research with a rigorous scientific design, but their publications nevertheless described the early development of the practice of LSD-assisted psychotherapy. Despite the absence of outcome studies, by the mid- to late 1960s, there was considerable enthusiasm for the therapeutic use of hallucinogens, LSD in particular.

With some exceptions, much of the initial wave of research was conducted in Europe, and the basic premise was that LSD might serve to facilitate or expedite the process of long-term psychotherapy or psychoanalysis (e.g., Leuner, 1963, 1967). This line of research became known as *psycholytic psychotherapy*, and it typically involved the incorporation of low doses of LSD at 1- to

2-week intervals into ongoing, relatively long-term psychodynamic psychotherapy or psychoanalysis. The objective was to facilitate personality change rather than to focus narrowly on treating specific behavioral symptoms such as alcohol dependence. A course of psycholytic therapy might involve somewhere between 10 and over 100 drug sessions (Leuner, 1963, 1967; Sandison & Whitelaw, 1957), with doses typically in the range of 50–200 μg of LSD (Eisner & Cohen, 1958; Leuner, 1967; Sandison, 1963).

Patients in psycholytic therapy were asked "to stay in the reclining position with their eyes closed. However, LSD subjects may on occasion remain silent for long periods of time or, conversely, scream and produce inarticulate sounds; they might toss and turn, sit up, kneel, put their head in one's lap, pace around the room, or even roll on the floor" (Grof, 1980, pp. 31–32). For some patients, such apparently cathartic motor discharges, sometimes extreme and possibly autonomic in origin, could occur in different forms for extended periods in a number of psychedelic sessions. These might include unusual "postures, movements, grimaces, sounds, shaking, crying, coughing, or gagging" (p. 156), as well as "extreme tension tremors, cramps, jerks and complex twisting movements" (p. 164).

A second approach to the therapeutic use of hallucinogens came to be known as *psychedelic psychotherapy*. Originating in North America in the 1950s and 1960s, psychedelic therapy was developed by Hoffer, Osmond, Blewett, and Hubbard in Saskatchewan, and later adapted by investigators in the United States (e.g., Leary et al., 1963; Pahnke et al., 1969; Pahnke & Richards, 1969). Early use of the psychedelic approach focused especially on the treatment of alcoholism (Hoffer, 1967). The psychedelic method employs high doses of LSD (500–1,500 μg) administered on one or possibly two or three occasions. Rather than incorporating LSD into a long-term course of therapy as an adjunct, in psychedelic therapy patients were prepared for the administration of LSD in one or a few brief, nondrug therapy sessions focused on a specific, circumscribed behavioral condition or disorder. After the psychedelic experience, additional nondrug therapy sessions might be conducted with the goal of integrating the drug experience into the individual's sense of self and daily life. To this day, a manual outlining the psychedelic method, written in collaboration with Abram Hoffer and Humphrey Osmond by Duncan Blewett and Nick Chwelos in 1959, with a good deal of input from Al Hubbard, remains the foundation for most current treatment protocols.

Over time, both the psycholytic and psychedelic approaches have undergone refinements and modifications, in some cases spawning significantly different methods (Grof, 1980; Passie, Chapter 5, this volume). One rather controversial modification that had an enduring effect on LSD therapy was the anaclitic method, introduced by British psychoanalysts Joyce Martin (1957) and Pauline McCririck (n.d.). Using a conceptual framework that was psychoanalytic in its understanding of development and psychopathology, these clinicians "assumed an active mothering role and entered into close physical contact with their patients to help them to satisfy primitive infantile needs reactivated by the drug" (Grof, 1980, p. 38). This violated basic psychoanalytic tenets regarding touch, transference, and countertransference, but physical contact as a therapeutic technique in LSD sessions appeared beneficial when used sparingly in certain situations. Having observed anaclitic work, and from his own experience, Grof concluded that "the importance of physical contact in LSD psychotherapy is unquestionable" (p. 39).

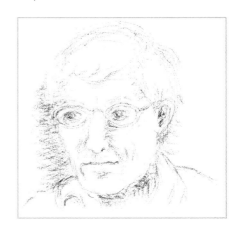

Duncan Blewett

Although early psychedelic psychotherapy outcome studies had small samples and methodological limitations, the results were generally positive. Some conditions have been found amenable to a brief intervention with a classic hallucinogen administered on only one or a few occasions—depression, posttraumatic stress disorder (PTSD), and existential distress associated with terminal illness, for example. Lasting change in personality, however, appears to require repeated dosing with hallucinogens, frequently in the context of intermediate- or long-term psychotherapy.

In addition to older studies, more recent research with psilocybin provides encouraging evidence of the efficacy of hallucinogens in treating addiction to alcohol, tobacco, and opioids, and the same can be said for the effectiveness of psilocybin in treating other conditions (Bogenschutz et al., 2015; Bogenschutz & Johnson, 2016; Griffiths et al., 2016; Grob et al., 2011; Krebs & Johansen, 2011; Ross et al., 2016; Savage & McCabe, 1973). Other researchers found that a psychedelic approach using LSD or psilocybin could be effective for improving quality of life among terminally ill cancer patients (Griffiths et al., 2016; Grob et al., 2011; Grof, Goodman, Richards, & Kurland, 1973; Kast, 1966, 1967; Pahnke et al., 1969; Ross et al., 2016). This is a striking finding: that one session involving administration of a psychopharmacological agent may be adequate to cause a reduction or cessation of alcohol consumption or other addictive substance use, or decrease depression and existential distress in palliative care. How this might happen is not clear, although potential mechanisms have been suggested, and improvement is correlated with the occurrence of mystical-type experiences. The research, however, is insufficient for definitive conclusions.

In contrast to psychedelic therapy, the data supporting psycholytic therapy are not especially compelling, although some anecdotal reports are intriguing. Most of the early papers on this method were clinical reports or case presentations, and even when research was attempted, it was generally neither well designed nor carefully conducted. This is not surprising, as work with the psycholytic approach largely took place in the 1950s and 1960s, a time when psychotherapy outcome research methods were not especially rigorous. Even today, for a number of reasons, it is difficult to conduct outcome research in the context of long-term therapy, especially when the objective is change in sense of self or personality rather than a discrete, observable behavior such as drinking alcohol. This was especially true 60 or 70 years ago.

The relative effectiveness of psychedelic and psycholytic therapies has never been evaluated, and such a comparison may not be feasible, as the goals of psycholytic and psychedelic treatment typically differ considerably. However, a durable, long-lasting change in personality (the usual objective of the psycholytic method) is not a likely outcome of two or three high-dose sessions with LSD or psilocybin. Moreover, even a high-dose psychedelic session does not ensure the occurrence of a mystical or peak experience, the incidence of which Grof estimated at between 25 and 78%, as a function of the population undergoing treatment. The low doses used in psycholytic therapy are "less conducive to" the peak experiences commonly observed in the "single overwhelming dose" approach (Grof, 1980), so there is a good chance that few psycholytic drug sessions would be associated with a mystical-type experience.

Comparing these two major approaches, Grof (1980, p. 37) concluded that "in general, psychedelic therapy seems to be most effective in the treatment of alcoholics, narcotic-drug addicts, depressed patients, and individuals dying of cancer. In patients with psychoneuroses, psychosomatic disorders and character neuroses, major therapeutic changes usually cannot be achieved without systematically working through various levels of problems in serial LSD sessions."

Even within one or the other approach, different mechanisms may be important depending on a given patient's condition and goals. In psychedelic psychotherapy, both addiction and depression in late-stage cancer patients, for example, seem to improve as a function of the occurrence and intensity of a "mystical-type" or "peak" experience (Bogenschutz & Johnson, 2016; Bogenschutz et al., 2015; Griffiths et al., 2008, 2011). Why either condition would improve following a single psychedelic experience is not known, and why people with two rather different disorders—addiction and a mood disturbance—might obtain similar benefits is also unknown. Moreover, it is not apparent whether it is the peak experience *per se* that is the mechanism that effects change; perhaps that experience itself is an emergent property of a biochemical process that is responsible for the change.

Grof's Amalgam of Psycholytic and Psychedelic Psychotherapies

The psycholytic, psychedelic, and to some extent the anaclitic therapies find a kind of integration in the approach to LSD psychotherapy developed by Stan Grof, who began his research on LSD in Czechoslovakia in the 1950s and 1960s. Grof treated individuals with a wide range of psychiatric diagnoses, from schizophrenia, major depression, and obsessive–compulsive disorder, to people with less severe disorders, as well as persons with no psychiatric diagnosis. Many of these patients were on an inpatient psychiatric unit, and they often underwent several dozen, or in some cases over 100, psychedelic sessions (Grof, 1980). The outcomes of this method have not been studied systematically, but it is this approach to which we now turn our attention in an attempt to elucidate, at least in part, its effectiveness.

Grof concluded that "it is possible to reduce the phenomena involved in both approaches to certain common denominators and to formulate a comprehensive general theory of LSD psychotherapy" (1980, pp. 122–123). Psycholytic therapy typically took place in the context of ongoing nondrug psychotherapy sessions that were done one or more times a week. When done with psychoanalytic patients, there might be three or even four such sessions in a week. The dosage of LSD, which was administered at 1- or 2-week intervals, was usually small, and the number of LSD sessions varied as a function of the clinical problem and therapy goals from as few as 15 to over 100, with an average of "somewhere around forty" (p. 31). The therapist was present much of the time, but patients also spent time alone, with a therapist or nurse available as needed. In psycholytic therapy, the content of LSD

sessions was "approached and interpreted using the basic principles and techniques of dynamic psychotherapy." The basic stance of the therapist was relatively nondirective, and while the therapeutic techniques were similar to those of standard psychodynamic psychotherapy, somewhat more activity, in the form of being more supportive and at times more direct, was required of the therapist. For most psycholytic practitioners, the hallucinogen was considered an adjunct to the traditional psychotherapy process, intended to accelerate therapeutic progress (Leuner, 1967; Sandison & Whitelaw, 1957).

In Grof's adaptation of psycholytic therapy, LSD was administered in conjunction with nondrug preparatory and integrative therapy sessions, both before and after administration of the hallucinogen, but it was not necessarily in the context of ongoing psychodynamic psychotherapy, and the emphasis was on the LSD experience. Hence, while the psycholytic method might be considered as hallucinogen-assisted psychotherapy, the method developed by Grof may be thought of as the psychotherapy-assisted use of hallucinogens. Grof's patients generally underwent a relatively large number of drug sessions at intervals of one to several weeks, using moderately large doses (200–500 µg) of LSD. As with most other methods, the hallucinogen sessions took place in a dimly lit room, with the patient wearing eyeshades

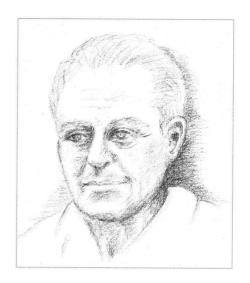

Stan Grof

to encourage an inward focus of attention, and with music providing an important evocative structure to the experience.

The therapist's role in this approach is largely nondirective, becoming more active primarily when the patient requires support, is having difficulty with the emerging experience, or during later stages of the session. "The task of the sitters is to give support and protection to the subjects, take care of their various psychological and physiological needs, facilitate the full unfolding of the experience, and deal with various forms of resistance as they occur during the session" (Grof, 1980, p. 150). Transference phenomena are common, and the therapist sometimes must deal with transferential situations as they arise. The aim, however, is not to use the patient's perceptions and emotional reactions as a therapeutic tool so much as to prevent the transference from interfering with the patient's awareness of and involvement in his or her internal process. Interpretations and cognitive processing are best minimized or avoided altogether, as they tend to be counterproductive, and conversation is kept to a minimum until after the peak of the hallucinogenic experience, about 4–5 hours into a session.

This approach is relatively open-ended, and any individual patient's course of treatment may encompass dozens of drug sessions. Although peak experiences may occur with this method, they are not the primary objective. Instead, Grof (1980, p. 123) maintained that the open-ended character of psycholytic therapy "gives a better opportunity for the patient to work through and resolve important problems of his or her life than the hit-or-miss approach of psychedelic therapy, which is limited to just one or a few high-dose LSD sessions."

Certain specific aspects of the therapeutic approach are essential for a favorable outcome in an LSD or psilocybin session. According to Grof (1980, p. 145), "a basic rule that is of critical importance in LSD psychotherapy is to keep the sessions internalized," as this enables "maximum awareness of the inner process and its full emotional, perceptual and physical expression" (p. 146). As he noted, "the most common problem in psychedelic sessions is resistance to the emerging unconscious material and an unwilling-

ness to 'go with the experience.'" For this reason, conversation between guide(s) and patient is best kept to a minimum, especially during the early, most intense hours of a session, whereas it may be beneficial in the waning hours. Instead, the sitters "ask the subject to pay attention to his or her body and surrender fully to the experience that starts unfolding" (1980, p. 156).

Chaos, Entropy, Criticality, and the Psychedelic State

The brain is a self-organizing system, a complex network of networks that has no homunculus, no administrator, no architect, no driver, in which order emerges from local interactions within and among different parts of the system. This concept is similar to what Prigogine (1980) referred to as a *dissipative structure*, a type of system that functions "far from equilibrium, whose departure from conditions of equilibrium leads both to instability and the development of new, complex behaviors" (Grigsby & Stevens, 2000, p. 121). Such complex systems are postulated to function "in two broad regimes separated by a third-phase transition regime . . . *chaotic* and *ordered*" (Kauffman, 1992, p. 305; original emphasis). The transitional regime is also referred to variously as *complex*, "poised on the boundary of chaos" (Kauffman, 1992), or as being in a self-organized *critical state* (Bak, 1996).

Neurodynamic processes have been studied using functional magnetic resonance imaging (fMRI) in the context of connectionist models of brain functioning based on graph theory, network analysis (Sporns, 2011), and information theory. Shannon, one of the developers of information theory (1948), adopted the concept of *entropy* from the second law of thermodynamics as a measure of the uncertainty or disorder of a system. Dissipative structures—such as the brain—are self-organizing, and they "consume energy from the environment and use it in such a way that they maintain a high degree of organization in the face of entropy" (Grigsby & Stevens, 2000, p. 121; Prigogine, 1980). They "operate 'on the edge of chaos,' in 'far-from-equilibrium conditions,' or in states of 'self-organized criticality'" (p. 106). This state–space, the activity of which changes during the transition between ordered and chaotic network activity, "reflects a delicate balance between repetitive, stereotyped activity and a tendency to engage in rather different, orderly, and yet sometimes apparently random and basically unpredictable activity" (p. 106).

Skarda and Freeman (1987, p. 171) noted the adaptive value of complex brain states that are poised between the routines of habit and relatively hardwired processing, and a more loosely structured, unpredictable state: "We postulate that the process of state change leading to the unstructured chaotic domain is essential for preventing convergence to previously learned patterns, and hence for the emergence of new patterned activity." Our ordinary waking consciousness is typically relatively ordered, consistent, and predictable. In contrast, the general state induced by the classic hallucinogens can lead one in entirely unanticipated directions, profoundly altering the likelihood of experiencing otherwise obscure or inaccessible thoughts, perceptions, memories, and behaviors. Such a far-from-equilibrium neuropharmacologically induced state may be associated with a slip into cognitive and affective disorganization or "ego loss" on one side, or into a more ordered psychological attractor state that may be familiar or novel, frightening or pleasurable, or sometimes perseverative, hellish, and seemingly inescapable (Schmid et al., 2015).

The basic physiological–psychological state induced by the classic hallucinogens is a prerequisite for the therapeutic effectiveness of these drugs. Whether, and for what indications, a hallucinogen session will result in beneficial effects, an interesting aesthetic experience, a mystical experience, or a panic attack characterized by paranoia and delusional thinking, is a function of this state, and of a number of other aspects of set and setting. The specific drug, along with the dose and route of administration, are the most fundamental determinants of the direction in which an experience might go. For example, as noted earlier, the high doses used in psychedelic psychotherapy appear to have a relatively high probability of inducing a central state that is conducive to

mystical or other types of peak experience. In contrast, the state induced by the low doses associated with psycholytic therapy is more likely to lead to experiences having a psychodynamic character, often activating intense emotional memories. But beyond these basic considerations, variations of set and setting play a major role in determining both the process and outcome of a session.

After facilitating a very large number of LSD sessions, Grof (1980, p. 52) stated that he had observed no "distinct pharmacological effects that are constant and invariant and can therefore be considered drug-specific." He therefore concluded that LSD is "a powerful unspecific amplifier or catalyst of the biochemical and neurophysiological processes in the brain. It seems to create a situation of general undifferentiated activation that facilitates the emergence of unconscious material from various levels of the personality," their precise nature being associated with "extrapharmacological factors."

■ The Ego, the Self, and the Default Mode Network

The terms *ego* and *self* tend to be used more or less interchangeably in discussions of hallucinogens. The ego, although it came to be reified and assigned a leading role in what is often called his "structural theory," was initially conceptualized by Freud in *The Ego and the Id* (1923) not as an entity or a structure, but as *a set of processes* that represented an adaptive evolutionary advantage. The ego per se has no locus in the brain but is instead a complex dynamical process, a continually changing state of the brain that is associated with the spontaneous, self-organized activity of a network comprising a number of widely distributed, interconnected neuroanatomic modules, or nodes. For Freud, "the ego represents what may be called reason and common sense" (p. 25), and although it encompasses the self, he did not consider the two identical. The concept of the ego was rather broad, such that its functions included attention, judgment, reasoning, memory, and reality testing. Current use of the term *ego* outside the psychoanalytic community tends to equate it with Freud's German word for the ego, *das Ich* ("the I"), which conveys a meaning more closely aligned with the *self*.

The *self* is a "complex, hierarchically organized functional system composed of many representations, each of which is a complex hierarchical system with many sub-components of its own" (Grigsby & Stevens, 2000, p. 329). There is no unitary self, nor could there be such a thing in a strict sense given the architecture of the brain. Instead, the self comprises a large number of internal representations of whom one takes oneself to be. Because of constraints on the capacity of consciousness, people are ordinarily able to experience fully only one self-representation at a time, so that we tend to have a "phenomenological sense of unitary self-hood" (Grigsby & Stevens, 2000).

As is the case with the ego, the term *self* is likewise somewhat loosely defined, but cognitive neuroscience tends to favor an idea of the self such as that proposed by Gallagher (2000, p. 14), who made a distinction between two different but related selves: These are "the 'minimal self,' a self devoid of temporal extension, and the 'narrative self,' which involves personal identity and continuity across time." Jeannerod (2006, pp. 64–65) emphasized the *minimal self* as an "embodied self," functioning on a "moment-to-moment basis," with an "implicit mode of consciousness, where consciousness becomes manifest only when required by the situation," and associated with the body's immediate experience (e.g., the extent of one's body in space). Gallagher (2005, p. 83) also refers to this as "a proprioceptive self—a sense of self that involves a sense of one's motor possibilities, body postures, and body powers, rather than one's visual features."

While the minimal self is needed to navigate and negotiate the physical environment, the *narrative self* has a sense of continuity across time. It is aware of its history and has the capacity to experience its actions and the events that happen to it self-consciously, making attributions about its behavior and experience. Self-concepts (e.g., the implicit feeling that "I am a kind person" or "I'm always self-sufficient and look after my own needs") are associated with the narrative self, which is active in social interactions with other people.

Carhart-Harris and colleagues (2014) roughly equate the concepts of self and ego, and maintain, as do other investigators (e.g., Brewer, Garrison, & Whitfield-Gabrieli, 2013; Northoff et al., 2006) that many of the brain regions or structures that are nodes in the networks that mediate the ego are found in what is frequently referred to as the *default mode network* (DMN; Raichle et al., 2001). In 2010, Carhart-Harris "nominated the DMN as the primary biologic substrate of the Freudian ego," and "with some qualifications . . . we still largely maintain these views" (2019, p. 322; Carhart-Harris & Friston, 2010). The major anatomical regions of the DMN, the exact nature and emergent properties of which remain somewhat unclear, include (1) the ventral medial prefrontal cortex (VMPFC), (2) the dorsomedial prefrontal cortex (DMPFC), and (3) the posterior cingulate cortex, precuneus, and angular gyrus. According to Carhart-Harris and colleagues (2014, p. 9), "it is through the development of self-organized activity in the DMN (and concomitant entropy/uncertainty/disorder minimization) that a coherent sense of self or 'ego' emerges."

The dynamic contribution of each of these nodes to the expression of the DMN is variable over time, but in ordinary waking consciousness, the probability is high that the network will be characterized by order. The self-organizing subcomponents of the DMN, following no plan and having no goal, and poised in the vicinity of a critical state, ordinarily interact as a functional system that has relatively consistent plans and goals, with a narrative self that can act in association with a sense of agency. Each node of the DMN makes a unique contribution to what might be identified as the ego, but the precise nature and degree of these contributions varies over time, in a probabilistic manner, in large part as a function of the individual's central physiological state (Grigsby & Stevens, 2000). Nevertheless, specific perturbations or disturbances of the network's dynamic state, such as those induced by sleep, anesthesia, certain neurological diseases, or the classic hallucinogens, are often associated with significant changes in the experience and expression of one's self or ego (Raichle, 2015; Seitzman, Snyder, Leuthardt, & Shimony, 2019).

Functional neuroimaging studies have shown an interesting and relatively reproducible dynamical pattern of functional connectivity in association with the administration of LSD and psilocybin (e.g., Atasoy et al., 2017; Carhart-Harris, 2018; Carhart-Harris et al., 2016; Lebedev et al., 2015; Tagliazucchi, 2014, and Chapter 5, this volume; Tagliazucchi et al., 2014, 2016; Vollenweider & Kometer, 2010). In particular, there appears to be a change in both global and local interactions in the brain, and a disruption of different *resting-state networks (RSNs)*. These widely distributed neural networks, characterized by intrinsic synchronous activity, are observed during normal awake resting states during the acquisition of blood oxygen level-dependent (BOLD) magnetic resonance images from individuals who are "at rest" in the magnet, performing no particular cognitive or perceptual task.

Among several higher-order cognitive RSNs are the salience network (SN), right and left executive control networks, the ventral attention network (VAN), the medial temporal lobe network (MTL), and the default mode network (DMN). Among these, according to Raichle (2015, p. 440), the DMN apparently "instantiates processes that support emotional processing, self-referential mental activity, and the recollection of prior experiences." In this way, it plays a "commanding role" in the large-scale functional organization of the brain. To a certain extent, the cognition associated with the DMN tends to involve "thoughts about one's personal past and future" (p. 440). Hence, the DMN may be associated with Gallagher's narrative self, a conclusion tentatively reached by Lebedev and colleagues (2015).

The DMN is thought to mediate a number of higher-order functional systems, including social cognition, prospective memory, and episodic memory (Seitzman et al., 2019). Raichle (2015, p. 443) suggests that the DMN is a major player "in the organization and expression of preplanned, reflexive behaviors that are critical to our existence in a complex world when unconstrained by the social and physical constraints of the envi-

ronment become impulsive and destructive." Comparative imaging studies have yielded data suggesting that many species, from rodents through infrahuman primates and humans, have a DMN.

The region of the posterior cingulate cortex (PCC) and precuneus is considered a major hub of the DMN. Research indicates that increased activity in this area is associated with "self-referential processing," mind wandering, craving, lapses of attention, and evaluation or judgment of experience. Decreased PCC activity is correlated with present-centered awareness or attention, meditation, and focused attention in general (Brewer et al., 2013). Northoff and colleagues (2006) concluded that self-referential processing, and the PCC and medial prefrontal cortex, are key components of both the minimal self and the narrative self.

▨ The DMN, Entropy, and Ego Dissolution

The state induced by LSD differs profoundly from ordinary waking consciousness, in a way that facilitates a very different way of thinking, feeling, and perceiving. Preller and colleagues (2019) have proposed the "thalamic filter" model, which asserts that "core effects of psychedelics may result from gating deficits, based on a disintegration of information processing within cortico-striato-thalamo-cortical (CSTC) feedback loops" (p. 2743). This model differs somewhat from that of Carhart-Harris and associates (2014), but the thinking of the two groups is in several respects similar, and even complementary. The precise model is immaterial to this chapter, as my emphasis is primarily on emotional memory reconsolidation as a potential key mechanism, so I emphasize neuroimaging research on the psychedelic state conducted by Carhart-Harris and his associates.

One phenomenon commonly experienced under the influence of hallucinogens is referred to as *ego dissolution*, which is essentially the loss of a coherent, consistent, individual sense of self that is experienced as separate from other people. This may occur to varying degrees under the influence of the classic hallucinogens, and may be associated with an affective valence ranging from a pleasant loosening of the boundaries of the ego, through transcendental states of oceanic boundlessness, or occasional panic associated with psychotic or severely disorganized states (Preller & Vollenweider, 2016). Mystical or psychedelic peak experiences represent variations on this theme. The range of manifestations of ego dissolution is broad, variable, and unpredictable.

During states of apparent ego dissolution, there is greater global connectivity, which means that there is an increase in communication among regions of the brain that ordinarily show little or no functional connectivity. At the same time, among those nodes in what are, in ordinary waking consciousness, consistently active modules of the DMN or certain other RSNs, connectivity is decreased (e.g., Tagliazucchi et al., 2016). Hence, for example, there are reports of alterations in the DMN marked by decreased coupling of the PCC and the MTL or VMPFC (Carhart-Harris et al., 2014; Lebedev et al., 2015). Carhart-Harris and colleagues (2012) therefore suggested that such changes in connectivity represent a diminution, or even an absence, of the narrative self, a finding consistent with the results of Tagliazucchi and colleagues (2016), but in contrast with an earlier report by Lebedev and colleagues (2015), who found that ego dissolution is associated with decreased connectivity within the salience network, but not within the DMN.

In the fully developed psychedelic state, LSD and psilocybin "can intensify all forms of affective responses and may activate vivid memory traces with pronounced emotional undertones" (Preller & Vollenweider, 2016, p. 236). According to Grof (1980, p. 62), it is especially likely that the classic hallucinogens will "selectively activate unconscious material that has the strongest emotional charge" at any given time.

In a general sense, this occurs because "heightened brain criticality enables the brain to be more sensitive to intrinsic and extrinsic perturbations which may translate as a heightened susceptibility to 'set' and 'setting'" (Carhart-Harris, 2018, p. 167). While it occupies the chaotic regime, the brain is in a "primary" or "high-entropy state of consciousness" (Carhart-Harris et al., 2014). In other words, the psychedelic state is charac-

terized by entropy (as intended in information theory); disorder is maximized; routine patterns of thinking and perception are disrupted; and thoughts, feelings, memories, and perceptions that typically have little or no access to consciousness may enter awareness. The probability that one will experience aspects of oneself that previously were inaccessible, which approaches zero in ordinary states of consciousness, increases significantly.

This high-entropy psychedelic state may be associated with ego dissolution, although the precise nature and degree to which the ego/self disappears is variable and uncertain. There is currently no neuroimaging biomarker that will identify the nature and measure the intensity of ego dissolution. Entropic changes in connectivity represent a rather general indicator, as increased entropy may occur in association with a number of different states and conditions, probably most of which remain to be identified. Furthermore, it is not known whether there are consistent and measurable differences in the connectivity of the DMN and/or the salience network when one experiences the selfless state of oceanic oneness characteristic of many volunteers in psilocybin studies (e.g., Griffiths et al., 2006), as compared with a more nonspecific "loosening" of the boundaries of the ego/self that is experienced by many individuals. It is difficult to put it much more concisely than did Tagliazucchi and colleagues (2016, p. 1045), who noted that "a decrease in brain modularity under the drug [indicates] a reduction in the separation of intrinsic brain networks." Nevertheless, connectionist modeling of the BOLD signal strongly suggests that under the influence of psilocybin or LSD, local network connectivity (e.g., including within the DMN) is weakened, while global connectivity is increased.

Carhart-Harris and colleagues (2014, p. 14) proposed that "psychedelics work by dismantling reinforced patterns of negative thought and behavior by breaking down the stable spatiotemporal patterns of brain activity upon which they rest." They argued that this "basic mechanism" of psychedelics is initiated by 5-HT$_{2A}$ agonism, leading to disintegration of ordinarily stable brain networks, increased network metastability,[1] and increased randomness of limbic/paralimbic connectivity. This is then thought to reduce the "precision weighting" placed on prior beliefs, with the result that they are "relaxed in an enduring way" after successful psychedelic treatment (Carhart-Harris, 2019, p. 320). Their contention thus seems to be that what is therapeutic about psychedelics is the shift in brain state from one characterized by more ordered, "pathologically subcritical styles of thought," toward a critical/chaotic state. Hence, these authors suggested that this alteration in brain state itself is what produces an enduring change in psychological functioning. Carhart-Harris (2019) recently updated this relatively complex model, though the details are too involved and not directly relevant to this discussion to consider in depth here. Moreover, the primary focus of this chapter is on the effect of classic hallucinogens on emotional memory, and not the brain's overall state itself.

Nevertheless, something about the psychedelic state is clearly essential to the therapeutic effectiveness of hallucinogens. But how does it account for differences in the effectiveness of psychedelic (as opposed to psycholytic) psychotherapy for certain applications? The dose alone certainly affects the intensity of the state, and probably the duration of the experience. However, especially for psycholytic therapy, this entropic state itself is an insufficient explanation. One or more additional mechanisms must be involved. Based on previous work (e.g., Grof, 1976, 1980; Preller & Vollenweider, 2016), there is evidence that the effect of these drugs on the neural substrate of emotional memory is crucial.

▓ Emotional Memory: Systems of Condensed Experience

According to Grof (1980, p. 63), in the course of psycholytic therapy, "sequential LSD sessions can be understood as a process of progressive activation and unfolding of the content of dynamic matrices in the unconscious." The dynamic matrices to which he refers are emotional memories, for which he proposed the term *systems of condensed experience,* or COEX systems. Though they

are similar in important respects, through the remainder of this chapter, I use the term *COEX system* when discussing Grof's model, and the term *emotional memory* to refer to recent research in cognitive neuroscience.

Grof defines a COEX system (1980, p. 66) as "a specific constellation of memories (and associated fantasies) from different life periods of the individual. The memories belonging to a particular COEX system have a similar basic theme or contain similar elements, and are accompanied by a strong emotional charge of the same quality." These COEX systems are relatively independent of one another. Each is dominated by a specific affective state—fear, anxiety, anger, hopelessness, sadness, shame, disgust, grief, joy, sexual excitement, and so on. They are not necessarily associated with any single event, and it may be that a detailed episodic memory of the event is not what is important. Instead, a COEX system is a set of neural networks, an aggregation of the affect associated with many events that involved similar emotions, or as Grof wrote, "the excessive emotional charge which is attached to COEX systems (as indicated by the powerful abreaction often accompanying the unfolding of these systems in LSD sessions) seems to represent a summation of the emotions belonging to all the constituent memories of a particular kind" (p. 66).

As Grof (1980) describes it, the therapeutic effectiveness of hallucinogens is a result of their effects on emotional, rather than episodic, memories. Memory for the details of an event is of secondary importance to memory of the affect associated with that event. Recall of the events themselves (autobiographical memory) is a type of declarative memory that is consolidated relatively independently of the emotions associated with them. Moreover, we remember little of our early years, as the declarative memory system is as yet immature, but even at a very young age we seem to have the capacity to recall the emotions evoked by experience (Rudy & Morledge, 1994).

From Grof's (1976, p. 72) perspective, those early life experiences that are characterized by intense emotion become "the core experience . . . the first experience of a particular kind that was registered in the brain and laid the foundations for a specific COEX system." Later experiences with a similar emotional valence are subsequently associated with those prior memories, strengthening both the synaptic strength of those neural networks, and the intensity of the emotion. These COEX systems are typically intense, most often (but not always) aversive, and the emotions that constitute them are especially strong during infancy and early childhood. COEX systems are typically inaccessible to ordinary awareness and are unavailable to consciousness most of the time. In their raw and unadulterated manifestations, they may be painful and even psychologically disabling, and as children we acquire a number of habitual cognitive, perceptual, emotional, and behavioral processes (e.g., defense mechanisms) via procedural learning and classical conditioning to avoid awareness of them—they are dissociated. In psycholytic therapy, it is on these COEX systems that hallucinogens do their work.

The classic hallucinogens allow (and sometimes demand) one to encounter different COEX systems repeatedly. The reexperiencing of intensely painful or traumatic emotions "is often followed by far-reaching changes in the clinical symptomatology, behavior patterns, values, and attitudes" of a person (Grof, 1976, p. 71). There may be a systematic pattern of returning to an emotional memory over a series of psychedelic sessions, representing repeated, deeper exposure to the COEX system on each occasion, in what Grof (1980, p. 169) refers to as "a continuity in the content of consecutive sessions." Over a series of psycholytic sessions, "the resolution of that matrix [i.e., the COEX system] occurs when the unconscious content is experienced consciously in its original form and full intensity."

What Grof refers to as *resolution* results in diminution, and perhaps complete "disappearance," of the COEX system. Procedural memories associated with these emotional memories (habitual behaviors such as avoidance, distorted perceptions, etc.) that may have been problematic are likely to persist for some time as habits. But without the persistent compelling force of painful emotional memories to drive them, they may in a sense wind down, becoming less compulsive, automatic, and nonconscious, to the

point at which an individual acquires a sense of awareness and agency, and a feeling of choice regarding whether or not to engage in such formerly automatic and nonconscious actions (Grigsby & Stevens, 2000). This may account in part for the fact that post-psychedelic session integration occurs over a period of days, weeks, or even months (Grof, 1980, p. 159).

Having gained access to consciousness in a psychedelic session, an emotional memory becomes an attractor that has a relatively high probability of activation depending on one's physiological–psychological state. Any given COEX system may dominate the content of a single psychedelic session, and often it recurs in some form across a series of such sessions. It may also affect an individual's psychological state "for an indefinite period of time" (Grof, 1976, p. 91) between sessions. Having experienced a COEX system memory directly, fully, and repeatedly, and the associated "enormous amount of affective energy that usually has to be discharged before the core experience is recovered, and the system extinguished and integrated" (p. 76), the emotional memory essentially disappears. Repeated reactivation of the memory, destabilization of the neural network that *is* the physiological substrate of the memory and experiencing of the emotion in the context of a relaxed, accepting attitude, may facilitate reorganization of the network and reconsolidation in an altered form. When a COEX system has been resolved, it no longer influences a person's behavior, or his or her self- and world-representations, and different emotional memories will become salient and begin to emerge. The important question is how the process of resolution occurs.

■ Memory Consolidation and Reconsolidation

Memory is an emergent property of a Hebbian type of learning that involves the formation and activation of neural networks distributed throughout the brain. Several anatomically and functionally distinct networks are specialized for the learning, retention, and recall of phenomena such as images, events, information, skills and habits, autonomic responses, and emotions. Certain of these functional systems facilitate the conscious acquisition of memories that are potentially accessible to awareness. These systems are referred to as involving *explicit* (or declarative) memory, and such memories include the recall of events and information. Other types of memories, frequently acquired without awareness and not readily expressible, are referred to as *implicit* memory systems. These include the implicit acquisition of habits, skills, emotion, and classically conditioned responses, the access to awareness of which is restricted.

In PTSD, for example, an individual may experience an overwhelming event that involves intense feelings of fear, anxiety, grief, hopelessness, and helplessness, often associated with classically conditioned hypervigilance, and sometimes with physical pain. Thinking about the event (i.e., activation of a declarative, episodic memory) may precipitate recall of the related emotional memories in an intense form by way of associations between the emotional and episodic memories, but the different memory systems are nevertheless relatively independent of one another. An individual may inadvertently or deliberately discover that certain habitual behaviors (e.g., interpersonal withdrawal, drug use, compulsive ritual, or superstitious actions) modulate or reduce the occurrence or the intensity of the emotional memory (or COEX system). These procedurally learned behaviors, which with repetition become habitual, automatic, and nonconscious, are similarly associated with the intense traumatic emotion, as may be classically conditioned hyperarousal or freezing. It is the intense traumatic emotion itself that people with PTSD find so aversive. Memories of the details of a traumatic episode per se are troublesome primarily because they are associated with and lead to the emotion. Further downstream, behavioral problems emerge that disrupt the individual's life (e.g., withdrawal, poorly modulated expression of anger).

Consolidation, the acquisition and storage of a memory, involves a series of processes dependent on alterations of the structure of the postsynaptic neural membrane that "entail changes in the excitability of the cell" (Fuster, 2009, p. 2061). The memory itself is "a cortical network, an array of connective links" that are formed between neurons as a result of experience (Fuster, 1994, p. 97). The processes of gene expression and associated protein synthesis involved in consolidation are distinct for each memory system, involving different patterns of gene expression over periods that may range from hours to weeks. Although a consolidated memory may persist indefinitely in a more or less unchanged form, it is not permanent and immutable, and both its storage and retrieval are dynamic processes.

The consolidation of memories is associated with a process of protein synthesis at synapses that are active in close temporal proximity at the time of an experience. It was formerly thought that after some period of time, these synaptic connections, and the neural networks of which they are components, became fixed and unchanging. However, it now appears that the neural network that "stores" a memory may be modified or "updated" in certain ways as a result of subsequent experience. One way in which a memory can change is by extinction, in which a learned behavior becomes less likely to occur when a previously rewarded behavior is no longer reinforced. This process of extinction represents new learning. The neural network that mediates an acquired behavior, for example, is inhibited—the memory still exists and could potentially be activated, but because of new learning, the probability of its activation has decreased.

Young, Andero, Ressler, and Howell (2015), for example, found that administering 3,4-methylenedioxymethamphetamine (MDMA) alleviated fear learning in a murine model of PTSD, via a brain-derived neurotrophic factor (BDNF)–dependent extinction mechanism. Similarly, Caitlow, Song, Paredes, Kirstein, and Sanchez-Ramos (2013) found that when fear-conditioned mice were administered low-dose psilocybin, extinction occurred, reducing the likelihood of a fearful response to stimuli related to the original conditioning. Extinction, however, does not eliminate the fear memory—it only makes its occurrence less likely. The fear is inhibited but could return rapidly under the right circumstances, a phenomenon referred to as *spontaneous recovery*. The neural network that mediates the memory remains intact, but the probability that it will be activated decreases. However, it has become evident that memory can be changed in a more durable way that differs considerably from extinction. In the process of *reconsolidation,* memories are not merely inhibited by new learning (which would leave them potentially accessible) but are instead modified significantly—a crucial distinction.

Physiologically, the neural network that represents a memory is *reactivated* when "the memory it represents is retrieved by the associative processes of recall or recognition" (Fuster, 1997, p. 455). Remembering (or recall) represents the emergent psychological aspect of this reactivation. An explicit memory, for example, is reactivated and enters awareness when one recollects what one ate for breakfast, or recalls that World War I began in 1914. An implicit memory acquired through the procedural learning system is reactivated during the performance of a learned skill or other process (e.g., dribbling a basketball). An emotional memory is reactivated when one feels the emotion directly (e.g., the sense of anxiety and helplessness one may have experienced during a traumatic event).

Upon reactivation, a network is destabilized, becoming malleable or *labile,* at which time it is amenable to reorganization associated with alteration of within-network synaptic efficacies, secondary to protein synthesis. A conscious, labile memory can be significantly modified in a way that is not possible when the network is inactive. It can be updated or revised. As noted by Nadel, Hupbach, Gomez, and Newman-Smith (2012, p. 1641), changes in such a reactivated neural network can involve "weakening or even erasure, strengthening, or alteration" of the memory.

What happens to the network that represents a memory is a function of what happens during the period of memory reactivation and lability. Perhaps most commonly, a reactivated network is simply restabilized. Having been transiently destabilized, it quickly returns to its original configuration when it passes out of awareness because nothing occurred that might modify it. This is *reconsolidation*. In different circumstances, something may happen that induces reconsolidation of the memory in an altered form—a disruption of reconsolidation. If the memory is for facts or information (a semantic memory), exposure to new or different information may lead to its storage in a differently organized neural network. Some research suggests that "reconsolidation may only take place when memory reactivation involves an experience that engages new learning (prediction error)" (Sevenster, Beckers, & Kindt, 2013, p. 830).

Reconsolidation also may modify emotional memories. This could occur, for example, when one is able to face, accept, and fully experience a traumatic emotional memory while in the psychedelic state. During recall of a strong emotional memory, the memory's neural network is activated, and the emotion is experienced as though it is happening again in the present. Depending on what takes place during the associated period of destabilization and lability, the emotional memory may or may not change. Most of the time, nothing happens, but under the right circumstances, the memory may be experienced differently than during acquisition, and has an increased likelihood of undergoing alteration of its intensity or nature. Hence, if a person is retraumatized, he or she may feel significantly worse, and this could intensity the recalled affect. This is why an intense, traumatic emotional state recalled in the course of *in vivo* exposure during a poorly handled psychotherapy session may induce a *reconsolidation* of the memory that further traumatizes a patient, intensifying the memory. The result is a "negative therapeutic reaction." In this way, emotional memories (COEX systems) may become more severe, enduring, or generalized over time in association with the repetition of a specific affective state, as with repeated physical abuse of a child. The strengthening of emotional memories resulting from multiple incidents of maltreatment represents a reconsolidation of the neural network, so that "the emotional charge involved [is] a summation product that resulted from a number of similar traumatic situations from different periods of life" (Grof, 1976, p. 70). This is how a COEX system forms and grows as a result of adverse life events.

Conversely, the process of reconsolidation may lead to a decrease in the intensity of an emotional memory during reactivation of its neural network. It has been found, for example, that a properly timed injection into the amygdala of a protein synthesis inhibitor such as anisomycin, or treatment with propranolol, has the potential to disrupt restabilization of the memory in its original form. Under such circumstances, a reorganization or disintegration of the neural network may reduce, or even eliminate, the fear memory that is experienced in association with the network's reactivation (Kindt, Soeter, & Vervliet, 2009; Schwabe, Nader, & Pruessner, 2014). In contrast to what takes place when an emotional memory undergoes extinction, disruption of reconsolidation seems to have the potential to eliminate or "erase" the memory by reorganizing its neural network. A crucial way in which this differs from extinction is that when the memory (namely, the underlying neural network) has been sufficiently disrupted and altered, there is no possibility of relapse because the emotional memory essentially no longer exists.

Whether reconsolidation is a therapeutic mechanism with LSD or psilocybin is as yet unknown; however the data regarding MDMA are interesting in this regard. While Young and colleagues (2015) reported that extinction plays a role in the effectiveness of MDMA in treating mice that had been exposed to a fear-learning experimental situation, in a more recent series of experiments using a rodent (rat) model of fear learning, a single administration of MDMA during the reactivation/reconsolidation phase disrupted persistent conditioned fear without the relapse often observed after extinction (Hake et al., 2019, p. 343). This suggests that "MDMA could augment psychotherapy by modifying fear memories during reconsolidation without necessarily enhancing their extinction." In other words, emotional memory reconsolidation with MDMA may facilitate the reduction or elimination of the neural network that *is* the emotional memory, by reconsolidating the network in a significantly reorganized configuration, altering synaptic efficacies within the neural array. Reconsolidation rather than extinction, as a mechanism for therapeutic change, is consistent with the large effect sizes, and with the rapid and enduring effects observed clinically when MDMA is used as an adjunct

to psychotherapy with PTSD (Mithoefer et al., 2013, 2019; Ot'alora et al., 2018).

Although reconsolidation has not yet been examined as a mechanism for the rapid and enduring therapeutic effects of the classic hallucinogens, the apparently similar efficacy of LSD, psilocybin, and MDMA makes this an attractive hypothesis. In addition, follow-up data for both MDMA at a mean of 12–16 months (Mithoefer et al., 2013; Ot'alora et al., 2018), and psilocybin at a mean of 14 months (Griffiths et al., 2008) or between 27 and 65 months (Agin-Liebes et al., 2020) showed consistent improvement at the long-term follow-up, with very few relapses. These findings likewise suggest that the effect may have been due to reconsolidation and not extinction.

Also of interest in this context is the description by Nichols and Nichols (Chapter 1, this volume) of LSD and the indoleamines as potent agonists at the 5-HT_{1A} receptor, as that receptor has been implicated in the reconsolidation of certain types of fear memories (Ögren et al., 2008; Pavlova & Ryaskova, 2018; Stiedl, Pappa, Konradsson-Geuken, & Ögren, 2015). The 5-HT_5, 5-HT_6, and 5-HT_7 receptors, which interact with the classic hallucinogens (Nichols, 2004; Vollenweider & Kometer, 2010), all appear to have some involvement in emotional memory reconsolidation (Schmidt et al., 2017). Finally, psilocybin is known to modulate the "major connectivity hubs of the amygdala" (Grimm, Kraehenmann, Preller, Seifritz, & Vollenweider, 2018), which plays a role in reconsolidation (Roesler, 2017).

Disruption of reconsolidation of emotional memories that enter awareness during a psychedelic session could account for the considerable importance of set and setting in hallucinogen-assisted therapy. If an individual can simply relax, breathe, and focus attention inwardly on his or her experience throughout a psychedelic session, with nonjudgmental awareness and acceptance of whatever emerges, the process of reconsolidation may "erase" painful emotional memories.

The biochemical cascade that occurs during a hallucinogen-assisted session appears to have a negligible effect on memory for the details of an autobiographical memory—their recall is, for the most part, unaffected.

As Beckers and Kindt (2017, p. 103) noted regarding their findings with propranolol, "the intervention does not make one forget what happened; rather it makes one less emotionally affected when remembering what happened, as if the emotional edge were removed from the memory." However, it may be that a therapeutic experience with LSD or psilocybin facilitates reconsolidation of the emotional memory—or COEX system—when one surrenders to the experience, engaging one's feelings fully and without avoidance.

Of considerable interest are research findings indicating that reconsolidation, rather than extinction, may be an effective approach to the treatment of addiction by interfering with craving. Schwabe, Nader, and Pruessner (2014, p. 277) posit that "targeting reconsolidation of the mechanisms that mediate drug wanting should increase the likelihood of long-term abstinence in humans," and there is support for this in animal models of craving and addiction (Lee, Di Ciano, Thomas, & Everitt, 2005; Taylor, Olausson, Quinn, & Torregrossa, 2009). These data have considerable relevance to research conducted with LSD and psilocybin as therapeutic interventions for addiction to alcohol, tobacco, and opioids (Bogenschutz & Johnson, 2016; Bogenschutz & Pommy, 2012; Bogenschutz et al., 2015; Bogenschutz & Ross, 2018; Johnson, Garcia-Romeu, Cosimano, & Griffiths, 2014). These investigators reported that one to three psilocybin or LSD sessions resulted in a persistently reduced craving for, and temptation to use, the addictive substance. The therapeutic approach to addiction with hallucinogens has generally used a variant of the psychedelic, rather than psycholytic, method, yet this decreased feeling of wanting or craving may be similar to the decreased intensity of emotional memories observed in psycholytic psychotherapy. Hence, memory reconsolidation may be a contributor to the effectiveness of psychedelics in treating substance dependency and addiction.

Reconsolidation of a traumatic emotional memory in the treatment of a relatively uncomplicated adult-onset case of PTSD might be completed in a short series of psychedelic sessions, as appears to happen with MDMA. Psycholytic psychotherapy, however, when the objective is personality change more extensive than the elimination of discrete symptoms (as in PTSD) or problematic behaviors (as in addiction) is likely to require repeated sessions—generally between 20 and 100 or so (Leuner, 1963, 1967; Sandison & Whitelaw, 1957)—to resolve multiple COEX systems that have accumulated and been reinforced over a lifetime. Hence, according to Grof (1976, p. 93), in the course of repeated psycholytic sessions,

> an emerging COEX system assumes a governing influence on all the aspects of the experience. Elements of a particular COEX constellation keep appearing in the sessions until the oldest memory, the core experience, is relived and integrated. Following this, such a system permanently loses its governing function and its derivatives never reappear in subsequent LSD sessions.

The observation that a thoroughly resolved COEX system permanently loses its strength, and that evidence of that emotional memory does not reappear in subsequent LSD sessions, is consistent with what would be expected if disruption of reconsolidation had "erased" the emotional memory. Spontaneous recovery, at least as Grof describes the therapeutic process of psycholytic therapy, does not appear to be a significant issue.

▓ Conclusion

Psycholytic and psychedelic psychotherapies are two very different approaches to the use of the classic hallucinogens. Psycholytic therapy typically utilized relatively low doses of LSD in the context of ongoing psychodynamic/psychoanalytic psychotherapy, two to four times a month, several dozen times. The LSD or psilocybin sessions were considered an adjunct to the psychotherapy that could accelerate a patient's progress. In psychedelic therapy, on the other hand, after a preparatory phase, patients underwent one to three high-dose LSD sessions. The goal was typically more circumscribed than was the case for psycholytic treatment—treatment of alcohol dependence, for example, or to improve quality of life in persons with late-stage cancer. In this case, the nondrug therapy was provided as an "integrative" adjunct to the LSD sessions. Most research in the 21st century has used psilocybin rather than LSD, typically using a variant of the psychedelic approach, and has demonstrated the efficacy of psilocybin for several different indications.

The two methods were adapted and integrated, influenced to some extent by the anaclitic approach, in the work of Stan Grof, who settled on the use of a moderately high dose of LSD over multiple sessions. Grof (1980) contends that LSD serves as a nonspecific amplifier of psychological processes, and that the state it induces permits access to very intense emotional memories that are typically inaccessible in ordinary waking consciousness. This increased accessibility of dissociated affect is most likely associated with the entropic connectivity that characterizes the state induced by the classic hallucinogens. Grof emphasized the importance of working through these emotional memories—or COEX systems in his terminology—as the primary therapeutic mechanism of LSD. Such emotional memories are of several distinct types (e.g., fear, self-loathing, shame, grief, anger, and sexual arousal, among others). They are relatively independent of one another, and their resolution usually involves sequentially revisiting them on multiple occasions, for much of the duration of each psychedelic session.

A moderately high dose of LSD or psilocybin, in the context of a carefully prepared set and setting, the use of eyeshades, and evocative music, are standard aspects of the contemporary psycholytic protocol for sessions using classic hallucinogens (Cosimano, Chapter 20, this volume). There are commonly (but not always) two guides (often called facilitators or sitters), the therapeutic approach of whom is generally nondirective. Their therapeutic activity is primarily oriented toward assisting the patient to focus attention inward, and to face and fully experience whatever emerges, without avoiding anything. The sitters' primary objective is thus to ameliorate or eliminate impediments to the patient's absorption in the COEX systems and related material.

In this setting, LSD and psilocybin induce a brain state characterized by alterations in the modular, self-organizing neurodynamics of the brain. The phenomenological and psychological manifestations of this state include some degree of what is commonly referred to as *ego dissolution*, which involves a loosening of, and sometimes a total loss of, one's sense of self as an individual (Richards, 2018, and Chapter 28, this volume). There is an interruption of habitual or routine connectivity between nodes in many neural networks, and notably in what is called the DMN. The DMN is often interpreted as the ego or self, or as some important aspect of ego/self. Whatever it is, the DMN is not a *thing*, but a self-organized, modular and heterarchically arranged set of higher-order processes, and the same is true of the self or ego.

The DMN seems to be relatively consistent in ordinary waking consciousness and may be involved in providing a sense of unity and continuity to our experience. The data suggest that the DMN may be significantly disrupted by the altered brain state catalyzed by the administration of LSD or other hallucinogens. The system becomes more deterministically chaotic and statistically random, and thoughts, perceptions, and memories that are typically inaccessible to awareness have a much higher probability of activation. This is what Carhart-Harris and his associates (2014) refer to as a state of increased entropy.

The emotional memories (or COEX systems) that one encounters during an LSD session are sometimes very disturbing and are commonly associated with some degree of anxiety. Given what appears to be a shift in brain state to a critical regime between highly ordered and chaotic dynamics, that state apparently increases the probability that emotional memories usually inaccessible to awareness will emerge. If a patient can relax and simply be aware of these feelings, experiencing them fully, then for that period of time, the emotion in its full intensity is in his or her awareness.

When an emotional memory gains access to awareness, the neural network that stores that memory becomes active, and whenever a memory is activated, the neural network representing it is susceptible to modification. This network lability means that when a memory that was previously consolidated is reactivated, it is amenable to change, and must go through a stage of protein synthesis to become restabilized. During the period

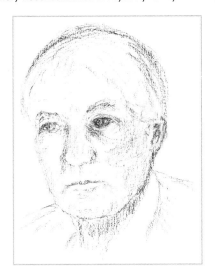

Timothy Leary

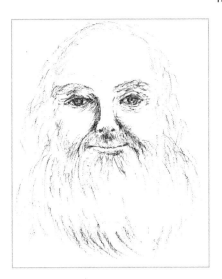

Ram Dass

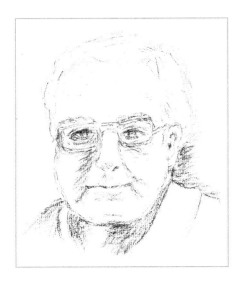

Ralph Metzner

of lability, the nature of one's experience at that time may update or revise a memory, affecting the way the memory is *reconsolidated*. Depending on what happens during the labile period, the memory may not change at all, it could be intensified (as in a so-called "bad trip"), or it could be weakened. Kindt and associates (2009), for example, reported that the reconsolidation of fear conditioning in humans could be disrupted, and the return of fear prevented, by oral administra-

tion of propranolol following reactivation of the specific emotional memory. Similarly, in a clinical trial of MDMA for treatment-resistant PTSD (Ot'alora et al., 2018), one participant's state of chronic hypervigilance, which had persisted for 6 years, was eliminated by the day following a session in which he was given what was considered a subtherapeutic comparator dose of 40 mg MDMA, with a 20 mg booster after onset. The participant's state of conditioned sympathetic arousal had not returned at the time of the 12-month follow-up, and he no longer had the associated persistent sleep disturbance.

If reconsolidation is a primary mechanism by which classic hallucinogens work, and assuming an individual remains patient and accepts whatever intense emotion he or she experiences as it moves through consciousness, the neural network that mediates a COEX system becomes labile and will reorganize itself. Afterward, it will be restabilized in a new configuration. The anticipated outcome would be a "weakened" or less intense emotional memory, as in the case of PTSD. Repetition of this process over a series of LSD sessions could potentially eliminate that memory.

There is evidence that reconsolidation of emotional memory is involved in the therapeutic efficacy of MDMA for the treatment of PTSD, and this may be the case with the classic hallucinogens as well. Rather than directly changing one's thoughts, LSD and psilocybin appear to act by eliminating or reducing the intensity of powerful and painful emotional memories. These memories color one's ordinary state, adding a negative affective valence to one's representations of oneself and of other people. If the COEX systems are resolved in a series of psychedelic-assisted sessions, this coloring of one's perceptions would consequently be changed, and the likelihood of activation of the neural networks that mediate these procedurally learned memories will decrease. Concomitantly, habitual patterns of procedurally learned "defensive" behavior acquired to help regulate the negative emotional memories lose the compelling affect that initially motivated them.

In association with reconsolidation of the COEX systems over a period of days or weeks following each session, these habitual behaviors will occur less frequently, weakening the synaptic efficacies of neurons within the procedurally learned networks (Grigsby & Stevens, 2000). Hence, changes in routine behavior are likely to follow the reorganization and diminished intensity of emotional memories. The phenomenon of insight into one's behavior likewise appears to occur following resolution of the emotional memories. Hence, insight may be a result rather than a cause of positive therapeutic change.

▓ Note

1. The term *metastability* refers to the fact that the brain's modular dynamical structure is only relatively stable across time. The various states (or attractors) that form in active neural networks are only transiently stable, the activity of their component nodes synchronous at times, but capable of shifting to another attractor that may be more or less ordered. According to Tognoli and Kelso (2014, p. 39), *metastability* means the system's components are able to influence one another, but they avoid "being trapped in a sustained state of synchronization, a collective state where no new information can be created."

▓ References

Abramson, H. A. (1955). Lysergic acid diethylamide (LSD-25): XIX. As an adjunct brief psychotherapy with special reference to ego enhancement. *Journal of Psychology, 41,* 199–229.

Abramson, H. A. (1956). Lysergic acid diethylamide (LSD-25): XXII. Effect on transference. *Journal of Psychology, 42,* 51–98.

Agin-Liebes, G., Malone, T., Mennenga, S., Yalch, M., Guss, J., Bossis, A. P., et al. (2020). Persistent effects of psilocybin therapy for psychiatric and existential distress in patients with life-threatening cancer: Long-term follow-up of randomized controlled trial. *Journal of Psychopharmacology, 34*(2), 155–166.

Atasoy, S., Roseman, L., Kaelen, M., Kringelbach, M. L., Deco, G., & Carhart-Harris, R. L. (2017). Connectome-harmonic decomposition of human brain activity reveals dynamical repertoire re-organization under LSD. *Scientific Reports, 7,* 17661.

Bak, P. (1996). *How nature works: The science of self-organized criticality.* New York: Copernicus.

Beckers, T., & Kindt, M. (2017). Memory reconsolidation interference as an emerging treatment for emotional disorders: Strengths, limitations, challenges, and opportunities. *Annual Review of Clinical Psychology, 13,* 99–121.

Bogenschutz, M. P., Forcehimes, A. A., Pommy, J. A., Wilcox, C. E., Barbosa, P. C., & Strassman, R. J. (2015). Psilocybin-assisted treatment for alcohol dependence: A proof-of-concept study. *Journal of Psychopharmacology, 29,* 289–299.

Bogenschutz, M. P., & Johnson, M. W. (2016). Classic hallucinogens in the treatment of addictions. *Progress in Neuro-Psychopharmacology and Biological Psychiatry, 64,* 250–258.

Bogenschutz, M. P., & Pommy, J. M. (2012).

Therapeutic mechanisms of classic hallucinogens in the treatment of addictions: From indirect evidence to testable hypotheses. *Drug Testing and Analysis, 4,* 543–555.

Bogenschutz, M. P., & Ross, S. (2018). Therapeutic applications of classic hallucinogens. *Current Topics in Behavioral Neurosciences, 36,* 361–391.

Brewer, J. A., Garrison, K. A., & Whitfield-Gabrieli, S. (2013). What about the "self" is processed in the posterior cingulate cortex? *Frontiers in Human Neuroscience, 7,* 647.

Busch, A. K., & Johnson, W. C. (1950). LSD-25 as an aid in psychotherapy: Preliminary report of a new drug. *Diseases of the Nervous System, 11,* 241–243.

Caitlow, B. J., Song, S., Paredes, D. A., Kirstein, C. L., & Sanchez-Ramos, J. (2013). Effects of psilocybin on hippocampal neurogenesis and extinction of trace fear conditioning. *Experimental Brain Research, 228,* 481–491.

Carhart-Harris, R. L. (2018). The entropic brain—revisited. *Neuropharmacology, 142,* 167–178.

Carhart-Harris, R. L. (2019). REBUS and the anarchic brain: Toward a united model of the brain action of psychedelics. *Pharmacological Reviews, 71,* 316–344.

Carhart-Harris, R. L., Erritzoe, D., Williams, T., Stone, J. M., Reed, L. J., Colasanti, A., et al. (2012). Neural correlates of the psychedelic state as determined by fMRI studies with psilocybin. *Proceedings of the National Academy of Sciences of the USA, 109,* 2138–2143.

Carhart-Harris, R. L., & Friston, K. J. (2010). The default-mode, ego-functions and free-energy: A neurobiological account of Freudian ideas. *Brain, 133,* 1265–1283.

Carhart-Harris, R. L., Leech, R., Hellyer, P. J., Shanahan, M., Feilding, A., Tagliazucchi, E., et al. (2014). The entropic brain: A theory of conscious states informed by neuroimaging research with psychedelic drugs. *Frontiers in Human Neuroscience, 8,* 20.

Carhart-Harris, R. L., Muthukumaraswamy, S., Roseman, L., Kaelen, M., Droog, W., Murphy, K., et al. (2016). Neural correlates of the LSD experience revealed by multimodal neuroimaging. *Proceedings of the National Academy of Sciences of the USA, 113,* 4853–4858.

Cohen, S. (1960). Lysergic acid diethylamide: Side effects and complications. *Journal or Nervous and Mental Disease, 130,* 30–40.

Eisner, B. G., & Cohen, S. (1958). Psychotherapy with lysergic acid diethylamide. *Journal of Nervous and Mental Disease, 127,* 528–539.

Frederking, W. (1955). Intoxicant drugs (LSD-25 and mescaline) in psychotherapy. *Journal of Nervous and Mental Disease, 121,* 263–266.

Freedman, D. X. (1984). LSD: The bridge from human to animal. In B. L. Jacobs (Ed.), *Hallucinogens: Neurochemical, behavioral, and clinical perspectives* (pp. 203–226). New York: Raven Press.

Freud, S. (1923). The ego and the id. In *Standard edition of the complete works of Sigmund Freud* (Vol. 19). London: Hogarth Press.

Fuster, J. M. (1994). *Memory in the cerebral cortex.* Cambridge, MA: Bradford Books/MIT Press.

Fuster, J. M. (1997). Network memory. *Trends in Neurosciences, 20,* 451–459.

Fuster, J. M. (2009). Cortex and memory: Emergence of a new paradigm. *Journal of Cognitive Neuroscience, 21,* 2047–2072.

Gallagher, S. (2000). Philosophical conceptions of the self: Implications for cognitive science. *Trends in Cognitive Sciences, 4,* 14–21.

Gallagher, S. (2005). *How the body shapes the mind.* Oxford, UK: Oxford University Press.

Griffiths, R. R., Johnson, M. W., Carducci, M. A., Umbricht, A., Richards, W. A., Cosimano, M. P., et al. (2016). Psilocybin produces substantial and sustained decreases in depression and anxiety in patients with life-threatening cancer: A randomized double-blind trial. *Journal of Psychopharmacology, 30,* 1181–1197.

Griffiths, R. R., Johnson, M. W., Richards, W. A., Richards, B. D., McCann, U., & Jesse, R. (2011). Psilocybin occasioned mystical-type experiences: Immediate and persisting dose-related effects. *Psychopharmacology, 218,* 649–665.

Griffiths, R. R., Richards, W. A., Johnson, M. W., McCann, U. D., & Jesse, R. (2008). Mystical-type experiences occasioned by psilocybin mediate the attribution of personal meaning and spiritual significance 14 months later. *Journal of Psychopharmacology, 22,* 621–632.

Griffiths, R. R., Richards, W. A., McCann, U., & Jesse, R. (2006). Psilocybin can occasion mystical-type experiences having substantial and sustained personal meaning and spiritual significance. *Psychopharmacology, 187,* 268–283.

Grigsby, J., & Stevens, D. W. (2000). *Neurodynamics of personality.* New York: Guilford Press.

Grimm, O., Kraehenmann, R., Preller, K. H., Seifritz, E., & Vollenweider, F. X. (2018). Psilocybin modulates functional connectivity of the amygdala during emotional face discrimination. *European Neuropsychopharacology, 26,* 691–700.

Grob, C. S., Danforth, A. L., Chopra, G. S., Hagerty, M., McKay, C. R., Halberstadt, L. A., et al. (2011). Pilot study of psilocybin treatment for anxiety in patients with advanced-stage cancer. *Archives of General Psychiatry, 68*, 71–78.

Grof, S. (1976). *Realms of the human unconscious: Observations from LSD psychotherapy.* New York: Dutton.

Grof, S. (1980). *LSD psychotherapy.* Pomona, CA: Hunter House.

Grof, S., Goodman, L. E., Richards, W. A., & Kurland, A. A. (1973). LSD-assisted psychotherapy in patients with terminal cancer. *International Pharmacopsychiatry, 8*, 129–144.

Hake, H. S., Sanchez, A., Loetz, E. C., Ostrovskyy, M., Wood, R. R., Oleson, E. B., et al. (2019). 3,4-methylenedioxymethamphetamine (MDMA) impairs the extinction and reconsolidation of fear memory in rats. *Physiology and Behavior, 199*, 343–350.

Hoffer, A. (1967). A program for treatment of alcoholism: LSD, malvaria, and nicotinic acid. In H. A. Abramson (Ed.), *The use of LSD in psychotherapy and alcoholism* (pp. 343–406). Indianapolis, IN: Bobbs-Merrill.

Jeannerod, M. (2006). *Motor cognition: What actions tell the self.* Oxford, UK: Oxford University Press.

Johnson, M. W., Garcia-Romeu, A., Cosimano, M. P., & Griffiths, R. R. (2014). Pilot study of the 5-HT$_{2A}$R agonist psilocybin in the treatment of tobacco addiction. *Journal of Psychopharmacology, 28*, 983–992.

Kast, E. (1966). LSD and the dying patient. *Chicago Medical School Quarterly, 26*, 80–87.

Kast, E. (1967). Attenuation of anticipation: A therapeutic use of lysergic acid diethylamide. *Psychiatric Quarterly, 41*, 646–657.

Katzenelbogen, S., & Fang, A. D. (1953). Narcosynthesis effects of sodium amytal, methedrine and LSD-25. *Diseases of the Nervous System, 14*, 85–88.

Kauffman, S. A. (1992). The sciences of complexity and "origins of order." In J. Mittenthal & A. Baskin (Eds.), *Principles of organization in organisms,* (Vol 13, pp. 303–319). Reading, MA: Addison-Wesley.

Kindt, M., Soeter, M., & Vervliet, B. (2009). Beyond extinction: Erasing human fear responses and preventing the return of fear. *Nature Neuroscience, 12*, 256–258.

Krebs, T. S., & Johansen, P. Ø. (2011). Lysergic acid diethylamide (LSD) for alcoholism: Meta-analysis of randomized controlled trials. *Journal of Psychopharmacology, 26*(7), 994–1002.

Leary, T., Litwin, G. H., & Metzner, R. (1963). Reactions to psilocybin administered in a supportive environment. *Journal of Nervous and Mental Disease, 137*, 561–573.

Lebedev, A. V., Lövden, M., Rosenthal, G., Feild-ing, A., Nutt, D. J., & Carhart-Harris, R. L. (2015). Finding the self by losing the self: Neural correlates of ego-dissolution under psilocybin. *Human Brain Mapping, 36*, 3137–3153.

Lee, J. L. C., Di Ciano, P., Thomas, K. L., & Everitt, B. J. (2005). Disrupting reconsolidation of drug memories reduces cocaine-seeking behavior. *Neuron, 47*, 795–801.

Leuner, H. (1963). Psychotherapy with hallucinogens: A clinical report with special reference to the revival of emotional phases of childhood. In R. W. Crocket, R. A. Sandison, & A. Walk (Eds.), *Hallucinogenic drugs and their psychotherapeutic use* (pp. 67–73). London: Lewis.

Leuner, H. (1967). Present state of psycholytic therapy and its possibilities. In H. A. Abramson (Ed.), *The use of LSD in psychotherapy and alcoholism* (pp. 101–116). Indianapolis, IN: Bobbs-Merrill.

Martin, A. J. (1957). L.S.D. (lysergic acid diethylamide) treatment of chronic psychoneurotic patients under day-hospital conditions. *International Journal of Social Psychiatry, 3*, 188–195.

Maslow, A. H. (1964). *Religions, values, and peak experiences.* London: Penguin Books.

McCririck, P. (n.d.). *The importance of fusion in therapy and maturation.* Unpublished mimeographed paper.

Mithoefer, M. C., Feduccia, A. A., Jerome, L., Mithoefer, A., Wagner, M., Walsh, Z., et al. (2019). MDMA-assisted psychotherapy for treatment of PTSD: Study design and rationale for phase 3 trials based on pooled analysis of six phase 2 randomized controlled trials. *Psychopharmacology (Berlin), 236*, 2735–2745.

Mithoefer, M. C., Wagner, M. T., Mithoefer, A. T., Jerome, L., Martin, S. F., Yazar-Klosinski, B., et al. (2013). Durability of improvement in posttraumatic stress disorder symptoms and absence of harmful effects or drug dependency after 3,4-methylenedioxymethamphetamine-assisted psychotherapy: A prospective long-term follow-up study. *Journal of Psychopharmacology, 27*, 28–39.

Nadel, L., Hupbach, A., Gomez, R., & Newman-Smith, K. (2012). Memory formation, consolidation and transformation. *Neuroscience and Biobehavioral Reviews, 36*, 1640–1645.

Nichols, D. E. (2004). Hallucinogens. *Pharmacology and Therapeutics, 101*, 131–181.

Nichols, D. E. (2016). Psychedelics. *Pharmacological Reviews, 68*, 264–355.

Northoff, G., Heinzel, A., De Greck, M., Bermpohl, F., Dobrowolny, H., & Panksepp, J. (2006). Self-referential processing in our brain—a meta-analysis of imaging studies on the self. *NeuroImage, 31*, 440–457.

Ögren, S. O., Eriksson, T. M., Elvander-Tottie, E., D'Addario, C., Ekström, J. C., Svenningsson, P., et al. (2008). The role of 5-HT$_{1A}$ receptors in learning and memory. *Behavioural Brain Research, 195,* 54–77.

Ot'alora, G. M., Grigsby, J., Poulter, B., Van Derveer, J. W., Giron, S. G., Jerome, I., et al. (2018). 3,4-methylenedioxymethamphetamine-assisted psychotherapy for treatment of chronic posttraumatic stress disorder: A randomized phase 2 controlled trial. *Journal of Psychopharmacology, 32,* 1295–1307.

Pahnke, W. N., Kurland, A. A., Goodman, L. E., & Richards, W. A. (1969). LSD-assisted psychotherapy with terminal cancer patients. *Current Psychiatric Therapies, 9,* 144–152.

Pahnke, W. N., & Richards, W. A. (1969). Implications of LSD and experimental mysticism. *Journal of Religion and Health, 5,* 175–208.

Pavlova, I. V., & Rysakova, M. P. (2018). Effects of administration of serotonin 5-HT$_{1A}$ receptor ligands into the amygdala on the behavior of rats with different manifestations of conditioned reflex fear. *Neuroscience and Behavioral Physiology, 48,* 267–278.

Preller, K. H., Burt, J. B., Ji, J. L., Schleifer, C. H., Adkinson, B. D., Stämpfli, P., et al. (2018). Changes in global and thalamic brain connectivity in LSD-induced altered states of consciousness are attributable to the 5-HT$_{2A}$ receptor. *eLife, 7,* e35082.

Preller, K. H., Razi, A., Zeidman, P., Stämpfli, P., Friston, K. J., & Vollenweider, F. X. (2019). Effective connectivity changes in LSD-induced altered states of consciousness in humans. *Proceedings of the National Academy of Sciences of the USA, 116,* 2743–2748.

Preller, K. H., & Vollenweider F. X. (2016). Phenomenology, structure, and dynamic of psychedelic states. In A. L. Halberstadt, F. X. Vollenweider, & D. E. Nichols (Eds.), *Behavioral neurobiology of psychedelic drugs* (pp. 221–256). Berlin: Springer.

Prigogine, I. (1980). *From being to becoming: Time and complexity in the physical sciences.* New York: Freeman.

Raichle, M. E. (2015). The brain's default mode network. *Annual Review of Neuroscience, 38,* 433–447.

Raichle, M. E., MacLeod, A. M., Snyder, A. Z., Powers, W. J., Gusnard, D. A., & Shulman, G. L. (2001). A default mode of brain function. *Proceedings of the National Academy of Sciences of the USA, 98,* 676–682.

Richards, W. A. (2018). *Sacred knowledge: Psychedelics and religious experiences.* New York: Columbia University Press.

Roesler, R. (2017). Molecular mechanisms controlling protein synthesis in memory reconsolidation. *Neurobiology of Learning and Memory, 142*(Pt. A), 30–40.

Ross, S., Bossis, A., Guss, J., Agin-Liebes, G., Malone, T., Cohen, B., et al. (2016). Rapid and sustained symptom reduction following psilocybin treatment for anxiety and depression in patients with life-threatening cancer: A randomized controlled trial. *Journal of Psychopharmacology, 30,* 1165–1180.

Rudy, J. W., & Morledge, P. (1994). Ontogeny of contextual fear conditioning in rats: Implications for consolidation, infantile amnesia, and hippocampal system function. *Behavioral Neuroscience, 108,* 227–234.

Sandison, R. A. (1954). Psychological aspects of the LSD treatment of the neuroses. *Journal of Mental Science, 100,* 508–515.

Sandison, R. A. (1963). Certainty and uncertainty in the LSD treatment of psychoneurosis. In R. Crocket, R. A. Sandison, & A. Walk (Eds.), *Hallucinogenic drugs and their psychotherapeutic use* (pp. 33–36). London: Lewis.

Sandison, R. A., & Whitelaw, J. D. A. (1957). Further studies in the therapeutic value of lysergic acid diethylamide in mental illness. *Journal of Mental Science, 103,* 332–343.

Savage, C., & McCabe, O. L. (1973). Residential psychedelic (LSD) therapy for the narcotic addict: A controlled study. *Archives of General Psychiatry, 28,* 808–814.

Schmid, Y., Enzier, F., Gasser, P., Grouzmann, E., Preller, K. H., Vollenweider, F. X., et al. (2015). Acute effects of lysergic acid diethylamide in healthy subjects. *Biological Psychiatry, 78,* 544–553.

Schmidt, S. D., Furini, C. R. G., Zinn, C. G., Cavalcante, L. E., Ferreira, F. F., Behling, J. A. K., et al. (2017). Modulation of the consolidation and reconsolidation of fear memory by three different serotonin receptors in hippocampus. *Neurobiology of Learning and Memory, 142*(Pt. A), 48–54.

Schwabe, L., Nader, K., & Pruessner, J. C. (2014). Reconsolidation of human memory: Brain mechanisms and clinical relevance. *Biological Psychiatry, 76,* 274–280.

Seitzman, B. A., Snyder, A. Z., Leuthardt, E. C., & Shimony, J. S. (2019). The state of resting networks. *Topics in Magnetic Resonance Imaging, 28,* 189–196.

Sevenster, D., Beckers, T., & Kindt, M. (2013). Prediction error governs pharmacologically induced amnesia for learned fear. *Science, 339,* 830–833.

Shannon, C. E. (1948). A mathematical theory of communication. *Bell System Technical Journal, 27,* 379–423, 623–656.

Skarda, C. A., & Freeman, W. J. (1987). How brains make chaos in order to make sense of the world. *Behavioral and Brain Sciences, 10,* 161–195.

Sporns, O. (2011). *Networks of the brain.* Cambridge, MA: MIT Press.

Stiedl, O., Pappa, E., Konradsson-Geuken, A., & Ögren, S. O. (2015). The role of the serotonin receptor subtypes 5-HT$_{1A}$ and 5-HT$_7$ and its interaction in emotional learning and memory. *Frontiers in Pharmacology, 6,* 162.

Tagliazucchi, E. (2014). Enhanced repertoire of brain dynamical states during the psychedelic experience. *Human Brain Mapping, 35,* 5442–5456.

Tagliazucchi, E., Roseman, L., Kaelen, M., Orban, C., Muthukumaraswamy, S. D., Murphy, K., et al. (2016). Increased global functional connectivity correlates with LSD-induced ego dissolution. *Current Biology, 26,* 1043–1050.

Taylor, J. R., Olausson, P., Quinn, J. J., & Torregrossa, M. M. (2009). Targeting extinction and reconsolidation mechanisms to combat the impact of drug cues on addiction. *Neuropharmacology, 56*(Suppl. 1), 186–195.

Tognoli, E., & Kelso, J. A. S. (2014). The metastable brain. *Neuron, 81,* 35–48.

Vollenweider, F. X., & Kometer, M. (2010). The neurobiology of psychedelic drugs: Implications for the treatment of mood disorders. *Nature Reviews Neuroscience, 11,* 642–651.

Young, M. D., Andero, R., Ressler, K. J., & Howell, L. L. (2015). 3,4-methylenedioxymethamphetamine facilitates fear extinction learning. *Translational Psychiatry, 5*(9), e634.

Zhang, G., & Stackman, R. W., Jr. (2015). The role of serotonin 5-HT2A receptors in memory and cognition. *Frontiers in Pharmacology, 6,* 225.

PART III

Individual Hallucinogens

CHAPTER 8

LSD

KRISTINE PANIK and DAVID E. PRESTI

▨ Introduction

Lysergic acid diethylamide (LSD) is one famous molecule—in many ways *the* archetypal psychedelic substance. Its fame is underscored by its wide recognition simply as "acid." Its potency, long duration of action, and penetration into society (especially in the United States) during the impassioned 1960s, has created for it an enduring legacy.

Psychedelic medicines are old, very old: peyote spirituality in ancient America, shamanic use of *Psilocybe* mushrooms, ayahuasca and other medicine plants of Amazonia, iboga in Africa, the mysterious *soma* of ancient central Asia, and the equally mysterious *kykeon* of the ancient Greek Eleusinian Mysteries. LSD is new. It has not been found—at least not yet—as a natural product created by plants or fungi, and it was not the first psychedelic chemical to be identified (this being mescaline, many years prior). Its psychoactive properties were discovered in 1943, and it burst onto the cultural scene in the second half of the 20th century via promising clinical investigation and large-scale popular use having far-flung ramifications to philosophical, musical, and artistic expression, and to social activism as well. While legally restricted at the highest

level for the past half-century—classified a Schedule I (One) controlled substance in the United States Controlled Substances Act of 1970 and the United Nations Single Convention of 1971—its popularity remains high. Lifetime prevalence of use (2010 survey data) in the United States is estimated to be around 23 million individuals, corresponding to 9% of the population over the age of 12 years (Krebs & Johansen, 2013a).

LSD and other psychedelics may be described as amplifiers or activators of mental processes, leading to heightened awareness of perceptions, thoughts, and feelings, as well as loosening of psychological defenses. This may reveal aspects of mind normally out of awareness and catalyze experiences that are powerfully novel and galvanizing. The complex effects of psychedelics have resulted in a variety of terms applied to describe them: *psychotomimetic* (mimicking the symptoms of psychosis), *hallucinogen* (generating hallucinations), *entheogen* (generating experiences of the divine), and *psychedelic* (mind revealing).

On the one hand, this manifesting or revealing of normally hidden aspects of the psyche may contribute to insight and creativity, catalyze transformative mystical or spiritual experiences, and provide a springboard for psychotherapeutic work. On the other hand, the same amplification of the psyche may contribute to acute anxiety and panic—a "bad trip"—and possibly ongoing psychological distress. LSD and other psychedelics, like all drugs, are *pharmakon*—the ancient Greek word from which the English words *pharmaceutical, pharmacy,* and *pharmacology* are derived. *Pharmakon* means "medicine" *and* "poison" at the same time—a profound notion, all too often forgotten.

The acute and long-term effects of LSD and other psychedelics are highly sensitive to *set* and *setting. Set* is used to describe what the user brings to the experience: intentions, expectations, prior experience (or the lack thereof), memories, personality, and current state of one's mind and body. *Setting* is the environment in which use takes place: alone, with others, with a therapist or guide, inside in a closed space, outside in a natural setting, and so forth.

The word *psychedelic* was coined in 1956 by psychiatrist Humphry Osmond (1917–2004). He sought to create a new term that better captured the uniquely powerful qualities of these substances. He shared some of his thoughts on this in correspondence with the author Aldous Huxley (1894–1963; 1977). After considering a number of possibilities, Osmond (1957) settled on *psychedelic* (Greek *psyche* = "soul, mind"; *deloun* = "make visible, reveal") because "it is clear, euphonious, and uncontaminated by other associations."

Osmond formally proposed the name in a paper he delivered at a 1956 meeting at the New York Academy of Sciences on the topic of "psychotomimetic drugs." After listing a small number of substances (including LSD) known at the time to be psychedelic, Osmond (1957, p. 419) remarked,

> What an array of substances for daring inquiry! What work for generations to come! . . . We know little enough about the most familiar of these agents, and there are only vague correlations between the physical and mental changes that they cause. Considering their interest in medicine alone, our lack of information is disquieting, but they are of more than medical significance. They reach out to psychology, sociology, philosophy, art, and even to religion. Surely we are woefully ignorant of these agents and this ignorance must be remedied.

Chemical and Pharmacological Properties of LSD

LSD is the diethylamide derivative of lysergic acid, the latter being the core structure of the ergot alkaloids, a group of chemicals produced by ergot fungus (*Claviceps purpurea*). The LSD molecule (see Figure 8.1) possesses two chiral centers at carbons 5 and 8; thus, there are four enantiomeric stereoisomers. Of these, only one—(5*R*,8*R*)-LSD—is known to have significant physiological activity. This isomer is dextrorotatory; thus, the physiologically active isomer is sometimes referred to as (+)-LSD or *d*-LSD. Hereafter, we will simply designate it as LSD. Inverting (reflecting) the chiral configuration at the 8-position gives (5*R*,8*S*)-*d*-iso-LSD. Inverting the configuration at the 5-position gives (5*S*,8*R*)-*l*-iso-LSD. And inverting the chiral configuration at both the 5v-position and the 8-position gives (5*S*,8*S*)-*l*-LSD (Nichols, 2018a). None of these enantiomers has shown any significant psychoactivity in humans (Shulgin & Shulgin, 1997).

Indeed, most chemical modifications of the LSD molecule result in substantial decreases in potency. A very small number of analogues have been found to have potency comparable to LSD in laboratory animal tests of drug discrimination: the dimethylazetidine derivative of the amide, and the N-6 replacements of methyl with either allyl or ethyl (Hoffman & Nichols, 1985; Nichols, 2018a, 2018b; Nichols, Frescas, Marona-Lewicka, & Kurrasch-Orbaugh, 2002). The N-6 allyl and ethyl analogues

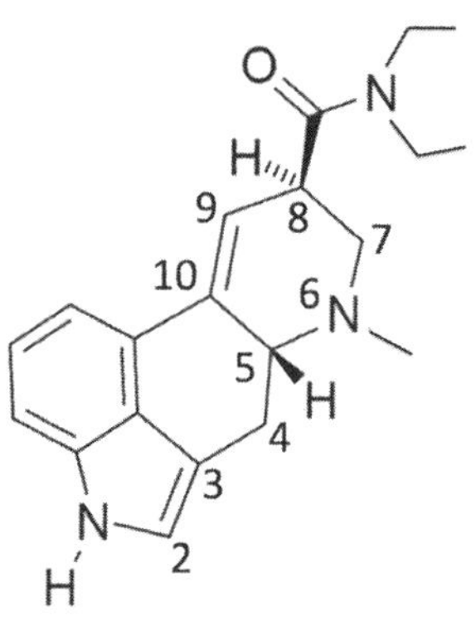

■ FIGURE 8.1. (5*R*,8*R*)-Lysergic acid diethylamide, or *d*-LSD.

have also been described as psychedelically active in humans, with potency comparable to that of LSD (Shulgin & Shulgin, 1997).

LSD is generally referenced as either the free base (molecular weight [MW] = 323.5) or the tartrate salt (MW = 398.5; ratio of two molecules of LSD to one molecule of tartrate). Sometimes in published work it is not stated whether reported quantities refer to the free base or tartrate salt; thus, there may be a degree of uncertainty as to the exact quantity of active drug employed. With respect to stability, renowned chemist Alexander Shulgin (1925–2014) has remarked that "LSD is an unusually fragile molecule, [though] as a salt, in water, cold, and free from air and light exposure, it is stable indefinitely" (Shulgin & Shulgin, 1997, p. 492).

At the time of its discovery, LSD was the most potent psychoactive substance known. Threshold psychoactive dose—the dose below which no alteration of mental state is generally discernable—is around 5–10 µg (0.005–0.01 mg). Fifty to 400 µg is generally considered the typical psychedelic dose range. Although higher doses can and have been administered, there have been no carefully controlled studies of doses outside of this typical range. There are, however, intriguing case reports suggesting that higher doses (e.g., 500–1,500 µg) may confer additional therapeutic benefit for some people (Grof, 1980/2001). An impressive self-report chronicling more than 70 personal LSD sessions using doses of 500–600 µg and conducted on a regular schedule over a period of 20 years described remarkable transpersonal and transcendental experiences of deep and lasting psychological value (Bache, 2019).

Human and rodent studies indicate that tolerance to the behavioral and psychological effects of LSD occurs rapidly, with substantial loss of effect after 2–3 days of repeated use. There is cross-tolerance with other "classical psychedelics"—mescaline and psilocybin. Tolerance also dissipates rapidly, after several days of cessation (Cholden, Kurland, & Savage, 1955; Gresch, Smith, Barrett, & Sanders-Bush, 2005; Hintzen & Passie, 2010; Isbell, Belleville, Fraser, Wikler, & Logan, 1956; Nichols, 2016).

LSD is efficiently absorbed via the oral-digestive route. Time of onset is around 30 minutes, with peak effects generally reached by 2–3 hours. Peak effects may be maintained for another 2–3 hours, and substantial effects may continue for 10–12 hours following administration (Dolder et al., 2017; Hintzen & Passie, 2010).

Following oral-digestive administration of 100 or 200 µg in healthy humans, plasma concentration peaks at approximately 1.3 ng/ml or 3.1 ng/ml, respectively. Peak is reached at about 1.5 hours and exhibits a half-life of 2.6 hours. LSD induces modest increases in blood pressure, with 100–200 µg doses producing peak systolic increases of 15–20 mm Hg and peak diastolic increases of 10 mm Hg. Heart rate increased by 10–15 beats per minute at peak, and body temperature by 0.5 degrees Celsius. Autonomic changes varied in proportion to plasma concentration of LSD (Dolder et al., 2017). The lag between peak plasma concentration and peak subjective effects may be attributable to movement of LSD from the blood circulation to active sites in the brain and/or other mechanisms of delay in cellular–molecular response pathways (Dolder et al., 2017).

Studies in a variety of animals since the 1950s indicate that LSD is metabolized by liver enzymes to structurally related, though physiologically inactive, derivatives (Passie, Halpern, Stichtenoth, Emrich, & Hintzen, 2008). A predominant metabolite is 2-oxo-3-hydroxy-LSD. Very little (~1%) LSD is eliminated in urine as unchanged drug (Dolder et al., 2017).

In the published research studies, LSD has been administered either via capsule by the oral-digestive route, or by intravenous injection. However, illicit LSD used in nonmedical settings is frequently self-administered via the oral-buccal route; that is, small dosage amounts and methods of illicit packaging (e.g., blotter paper, liquid, small tablet) are conducive to simply letting the drug be absorbed in the mouth. Because of hepatic metabolism, one would expect this to have greater bioavailability relative to that of oral-digestive absorption. However, to our knowledge, this comparison has not yet been carefully investigated.

With respect to the comparative effects of LSD administered by intravenous versus oral-digestive routes, it has been noted that an intravenous dose of 75 µg produced similar ratings on an altered state of consciousness assessment scale as an oral dose of 100 μg, and lower ratings than an oral dose of 200 μg (Liechti, 2017). It has also been noted that the comparative dose effects of LSD administered by intravenous versus oral-digestive routes are far more similar than the comparative dose effects of psilocybin administered by these two routes; psilocybin is approximately 10 times less potent by the oral route compared to the intravenous route (Carhart-Harris et al., 2015).

The Discovery of LSD by Albert Hofmann

The story of LSD's discovery as told by Albert Hofmann (1906–2008) is truly one of the great tales in the history of modern science. Hofmann (2013) relates the story eloquently in his autobiographical memoir, *LSD: My Problem Child*.

Following doctoral work at the University of Zurich investigating the chemistry of chitin, the structural material from which invertebrate exoskeleton is composed, Hofmann in 1929 went to work for Sandoz, a pharmaceutical company located in Basel, Switzerland. There he joined a project investigating cardioactive glycosides isolated from squill and foxglove plants. After completing work elucidating the chemical structures of these compounds, he transitioned in 1935 to work on ergot alkaloids.

Ergot (*Claviceps purpurea*) is a fungus that grows on cereal grains and wild grasses, especially rye. Extracts of ergot have been used by midwives for centuries as an aid to childbirth, promoting uterine contractions and facilitating difficult childbirth. Also possessing vasoconstrictive properties, ergot extracts were useful in reducing postpartum bleeding.

Outbreaks of ergot growth on cereal grains appear to have led to mass poisonings of entire villages in Europe during the Middle Ages. Symptoms of ergot toxicity include the central nervous system effects of seizures, mania, and psychosis, as well as painful gangrene resulting from peripheral vasoconstriction. Ergot poisoning was referred to as Saint Anthony's fire, referencing the fiery pain of the condition and the third-century Christian monk Anthony of Egypt (251–356), patron saint in the healing of skin conditions.

Ergot contains a diverse array of alkaloids, many of which are derivatives of lysergic acid. Arthur Stoll (1887–1971), Albert Hofmann's supervisor at Sandoz, had spent several years investigating the chemistry of the ergot alkaloids and had isolated and identified ergotamine several years prior to Hofmann's arrival at Sandoz. When Hofmann began work on ergot alkaloids, the intention was to develop chemical derivatives having beneficial medicinal properties, while perhaps also being less toxic. In 1938, Hofmann sought to produce a diethylamide derivative of lysergic acid, drawing inspiration from the commercial pharmaceutical agent Coramine, a respiratory and circulatory stimulant marketed by Ciba, another Basel pharmaceutical company. Coramine is nicotinic acid diethylamide, and Hofmann hoped that lysergic acid diethylamide might be a new and improved respiratory and circulatory stimulant.

Thus, in November 1938, Hofmann synthesized lysergic acid diethylamide (*Lysergsäure-diethylamid*), labeling it in his notes "LSD-25," because it was the 25th in a series of ergot alkaloid derivatives he had made. Hofmann passed the new chemical along to his colleagues in the pharmacological testing department of Sandoz, where it was found to have unremarkable effects in tests with laboratory animals and deemed not suitable for further exploration. Hofmann moved on to making other derivatives of ergotamine.

The following year, World War II began to consume Europe. Although Switzerland was a neutral country, it nonetheless maintained a small defensive army, and Hofmann spent time engaged in military activities during this period (Hagenbach & Werthmüller, 2011). He also had a growing family, and he and his wife Anita were parents of three young children by 1943. All the while, he continued his work on derivatives of ergot alkaloids. Two of his products of that era later became widely used medications: methylergometrine (Methergine) for stimulation of uterine contractions and reduction of postpartum bleeding, and dihydroergotoxine (Hydergine) to improve cognitive function, especially in elderly persons. And amid all this, Hofmann did not stop thinking about LSD. He had a feeling, an intuition, that this chemical was more interesting than what had been appreciated in the initial investigation of its properties.

And yet I could not forget the relatively "uninteresting" LSD-25. A peculiar presentiment—the feeling that this substance might possess properties beyond those established in the first pharmacological studies—induced me, five years after that first synthesis, again to produce LSD-25, so that a sample could be given to the pharmacological department for further tests. This was quite unusual; experimental substances, as a rule, were definitely stricken from the research program when once deemed to be lacking in pharmacological interest. (Hofmann, 2013, p. 18)

Thus, on April 16, 1943, Hofmann resynthesized his creation of 5 years earlier. During the final purification steps, he began to experience unusual sensations. Later, he submitted this description as part of a report to his supervisor:

Last Friday, 16 April 1943, I was forced to interrupt my work in the laboratory in the middle of the afternoon and to go home, being affected by a remarkable restlessness, combined with a slight dizziness. At home I lay down and sank into a not unpleasant, intoxicated-like condition, characterized by an extremely stimulated imagination. In a dream-like state with eyes closed (I found the daylight to be unpleasantly glaring), I perceived an uninterrupted stream of fantastic pictures, extraordinary shapes with an intense, kaleidoscopic play of colors. After some two hours this condition faded away. (Hofmann, 2013, p. 18)

Rather than simply dismiss his unusual Friday-afternoon experience, Hofmann surmised that perhaps it resulted from inadvertent absorption of a small amount of the novel chemical he had been synthesizing. He resolved to investigate this possibility the following Monday by intentionally ingesting a small measured amount of LSD. Thus, near the end of his day of work on April 19, 1943, Hofmann measured out a very small quantity of LSD—0.25 mg (250 µg)—an amount chosen to be at the lower limit of any presumed effectiveness of even a very potent ergot alkaloid or other natural product. At 5:00 P.M., 40 minutes after ingesting

the LSD, Hofmann recorded in his laboratory notebook:

"beginning dizziness, feeling of anxiety, visual distortions, symptoms of ataxia, desire to laugh." Here the notes in my laboratory journal cease. I was able to write the last words only with great difficulty. By then it was quite clear to me that LSD had been the cause of the remarkable experience of the previous Friday, for the altered perceptions were of the same type as before, only much more intense. I had to struggle to speak intelligently. I asked my laboratory assistant, who had been informed of my self-experiment, to escort me home. We went by bicycle, no automobile being available because of wartime restrictions on their use. On the way home, my condition began to assume threatening forms. Everything in my field of vision wavered and was distorted as if seen in a fun-house mirror. I also had the sensation of being unable to move from the spot. Nonetheless, my assistant later told me that we had bicycled quite rapidly. Finally, we arrived at home. (Hofmann, 2013, p. 19)

My surroundings had now transformed themselves in a most terrifying manner. Everything in the room spun around, and familiar objects and pieces of furniture assumed grotesque, threatening forms. . . . Even worse than these demonic transformations of the outer world were the alterations that I perceived within myself, in my inner being. Every exertion of my will, every attempt to put an end to the disintegration of the outer world and the dissolution of my ego, seemed so much wasted effort. A demon had invaded me, had taken possession of my body, mind, and soul. . . . My body seemed to be without sensation, lifeless, strange. Was I dying? (Hofmann, 2013, p. 20)

Albert Hofmann was inadvertently experiencing the world's first full-blown acid trip. He was unprepared for the experience, and it was not pleasant. The family physician was summoned, as was Hofmann's wife, Anita. She and their three children had traveled that day to visit her parents in another city. The physician indicated that there were no signs of a threatening illness, extremely dilated pupils being the only abnormal symptom present. After several hours, Hofmann's distress began to abate.

Slowly I returned from a weird, unfamiliar world to my reassuring, everyday reality. The horror softened and gave way to a feeling of great fortune and immense gratitude; more normal perceptions and thoughts returned, and I became more confident that the danger of insanity was decidedly past. Now, little by little, I could begin to *enjoy* the unprecedented colors and plays of shapes that persisted behind my closed eyes. Kaleidoscopic, fantastic images burst in upon me, alternating, variegated, opening and then closing themselves in circles and spirals, exploding in colored fountains, rearranging and hybridizing themselves in constant flux. It was particularly remarkable how every acoustic perception, such as the sound of a doorknob or of a passing automobile, became transformed into optical perceptions. Every sound generated a vividly changing image, with its own particular form and color. (Hofmann, 2013, p. 21; original emphasis)

Late in the evening Hofmann's wife arrived back home and, exhausted, he was finally able to sleep. Upon awakening the next morning, he was struck by how refreshed he felt.

A sensation of well-being and renewed life suffused me. My breakfast tasted delicious and gave me extraordinary pleasure. When I later walked out into the garden, in which the sun now shown after a springtime rain, everything glistened and sparkled in a fresh light. The world was as if newly created. All my senses vibrated in a state of utmost sensitivity, which lasted for the entire day. (Hofmann, 2013, p. 22)

Hofmann was impressed that his memory of the previous evening's experience of extreme intoxication was clear and vivid, and there were no negative "hangover" effects. He quickly appreciated that he had synthesized a truly amazing chemical—one that generated a novel constellation of powerful psychological effects, having potency unprecedented among known pharmaceuticals, and possibly low physiological toxicity as well. In 1943, there was little appreciation of the brain as a neurochemical system. The only known neurotransmitters at the time were acetylcholine and norepinephrine, and these were known via their actions in the peripheral autonomic and neuromuscular systems, not the brain. Yet here was a chemical—LSD—a very tiny quantity of which had a powerful impact on the psyche,

presumably because of some chemical interaction within the brain. Hofmann and his colleagues proposed that this could be of extraordinary utility as a therapeutic and research tool in psychiatry.

That same year, a report describing LSD's chemical properties was published by Arthur Stoll and Albert Hofmann (1943). In 1947, Werner Stoll, son of Arthur and a physician at the Psychiatric Clinic of the University of Zurich, described the effects of a series of LSD administrations on several dozen healthy individuals, as well as a number of patients suffering from various mental disorders (including schizophrenia). A U.S. patent for LSD as a therapeutic agent was filed in 1948. However, Sandoz believed that more research was needed to explore LSD's potential therapeutic utility. To facilitate this, beginning in the late 1940s (and continuing until 1966), Sandoz produced LSD under the brand name Delysid and made it available to physicians and psychologists for the purpose of conducting clinical and scientific research. The user's manual (package insert) for Delysid indicated the availability of two forms—a sugar-coated tablet (25 µg) and a liquid solution (100 µg)—and provided the following descriptive text (Hofmann, 2013, pp. 40–41):

INDICATIONS AND DOSAGE

Analytic psychotherapy, to elicit release of repressed material and provide mental relaxation, particularly in anxiety states and obsessional neuroses. The initial dose is 25 mcg. This dose is increased at each treatment by 25 mcg until the optimum dose (usually between 50 and 200 mcg) is found. The individual treatments are best given at intervals of one week.

Experimental studies on the nature of psychoses: By taking Delysid himself, the psychiatrist is able to gain an insight into the world of ideas and sensations of mental patients. Delysid can also be used to induce model psychoses of short duration in normal subjects, thus facilitating studies on the pathogenesis of mental disease. In normal subjects, doses of 25 to 75 mcg are generally sufficient to produce a hallucinatory psychosis.

Pathological mental conditions may be intensified by Delysid. . . . Delysid should only be administered under strict medical supervision. The supervision should not be discontinued until the effects of the drug have completely worn off.

Hofmann often stated that he did not find LSD, that rather, it found him—that it was a discovery the world needed and he was but the vehicle, a "little Swiss chemist." Hofmann's "scientific discoveries, his philosophical writings, his wisdom and the depth of his humanity, have established his reputation as one of the outstanding personalities of our era" (Feilding, 2008, p. v). LSD has had an enormous and extended impact on the modern world, and Hofmann's scientific work was of the kind deserving a Nobel Prize. However, due to the complex circumstances that followed the emergence of the use of psychedelic chemicals in the wider culture, such honors are not yet within the realm of consideration. Contemporary society is still working to achieve a balanced perspective on LSD.

■ LSD and the Origins of Biological Psychiatry and Neuropsychopharmacology

The early 1950s witnessed the beginnings of conceptualizing connections between brain function and behavior in terms of chemistry. In 1949, the lithium ion's calming effect on mania in psychiatric patients was reported from Australia. In 1952, in Paris, the antihistamine and sedative chlorpromazine was tested on psychiatric patients and found to have dramatic effects in reducing symptoms of mania and psychosis. Not long thereafter, the mood-elevating effects of antituberculosis drugs, later appreciated to be inhibitors of monoamine oxidase, were observed.

Also in 1952, a seminal paper proposing a relationship among brain chemistry, mental illness, and the psychotomimetic effects of mescaline was published by British psychiatrists Humphry Osmond and John Smythies (1922–2019). Another important event in this early trajectory was the 1952 discovery of the chemical serotonin (5-hydroxytryptamine [5-HT]) in the mammalian brain. This substance was known at the time to be present in the gut and in the blood and to affect smooth-muscle contraction and blood-vessel tone (Green, 2008; Twarog, 1988; Whitaker-Azmitia, 1999). The appreciation of serotonin's structural similarity to LSD then led to the proposal that "mental disturbances caused by lysergic acid diethylamide were to

be attributed to an interference with the action of serotonin in the brain" (Woolley & Shaw, 1954, p. 229; see also Green, 2008).

In the years that followed, biogenic amine theories of psychosis and depression came to dominate the emerging field of biological psychiatry, and dozens of medications to treat the symptoms associated with psychosis and depression were developed with these hypotheses in mind. This has continued unabated now for more than a half-century. The development of the contemporary disciplines of biological psychiatry, psychopharmacology, and neurochemistry owe a great deal to the discovery of LSD and the connecting of its powerful effects on the psyche to chemical interactions in the brain (Nichols & Nichols, 2008).

LSD has high affinity for many neurotransmitter receptors in the brain and body, in particular receptors for serotonin and dopamine (Nichols, 2016; Nichols et al., 2002). The major psychedelic effects of LSD, as well as other classical psychedelics (psilocybin, mescaline, DMT), have been largely associated with agonist actions at the serotonin type-2A (5-HT_{2A}) receptor (Nichols, 2016). Elegant studies have revealed elements of the complex molecular orchestrations activated by the binding of LSD (as well as other ligands—neurotransmitters and drugs both psychedelic and nonpsychedelic) to serotonin receptors (Kim et al., 2020; Wacker et al., 2013, 2017).

Additional support for the interaction between LSD and monoamine neurotransmitter systems comes from interview data assessing the impact of chronic use of several psychiatric medications on the magnitude of LSD's psychedelic effects. Use of tricyclic antidepressants or lithium was found to be associated with subjective increases in hallucinatory and psychological responses to LSD, while use of selective serotonin reuptake inhibitor or monoamine oxidase inhibitor antidepressants was found to decrease or even eliminate the subjective response to LSD (Bonson, Buckholtz, & Murphy, 1996; Bonson & Murphy, 1996).

Serotonin and multiple types of serotonin receptors are located throughout the body and brain, and serotonin is known to be involved in the regulation of numerous processes, including modulatory effects on mood, anxiety, arousal, sleep, sexual activity, appetite, memory, perception, and emotion (Nichols & Nichols, 2008).

While LSD's effects at 5-HT$_{2A}$ and other serotonin receptors is a key aspect of its interaction with human physiology, it is good to keep in mind our inclination to oversimplify the complexity of living organisms. We often seek straightforward explanatory pictures revolving around single identified neurotransmitters and receptors, and simplistic ways of thinking about brain circuits. However, the functioning of even a single living cell is well beyond our capacity to explain in detail, and certainly there are many pieces of the cellular and molecular story linking LSD and its psychedelic effects yet to be discovered.

■ The First Phase of Clinical Research: 1950s and 1960s

Throughout the 1950s and 1960s, there were numerous clinical studies of the therapeutic utility of LSD in diverse circumstances. Among these were facilitation of psychological exploration in analytic psychotherapy; production of "model psychoses" in order to investigate and appreciate experiences of psychotic patients (e.g., psychiatrists, other clinicians, and researchers working with psychoses could ingest the drug to induce a personal experience of the symptoms); treatment of anxiety and depression associated with terminal illness; treatment of alcoholism and other addictions; and treatment of chronic depression, manic–depression, and psychosis (schizophrenia).

Many of these studies were conducted rather informally in the clinics and offices of psychotherapists. And even when investigations were conducted in research institutions associated with medical centers and universities, they were conducted at a time that lacked today's standards of institutional oversight and scientific meticulousness. An excellent review of this era indicates that "the standards for scientific reporting on clinical studies were often much less rigorous than they are today and relied heavily on the judgment of clinical investigators (rather than on validated outcome measures). . . . Thus, the early studies with LSD are best understood as providing valuable pilot data on safety and efficacy, as well as testable hy-

potheses for future studies" (Bonson, 2018, pp. 592, 598).

The first human clinical study with LSD published in English appeared in 1950 and described the administration of LSD to 29 psychiatric patients, most of whom were diagnosed with schizophrenia and other severe conditions (Busch & Johnson, 1950). The study was intended to facilitate the expression of material that might be of use in analytic psychotherapy. While other clinical investigations of this era also administered LSD to patients having psychosis, it is often concluded that there is little evidence that it produced beneficial results in such cases (Bonson, 2018). Nonetheless, pioneer LSD clinical researcher and psychotherapist Stansilav Grof (born in 1931) describes examples of successful treatment of select psychotic individuals in highly structured, intensive inpatient settings (Grof, 1975, 1980/2001).

As a component of the psychotherapeutic treatment of anxiety and mood disorders, LSD was primarily explored in two different ways (Pahnke, Kurland, Unger, Savage, & Grof, 1970). So-called *psycholytic therapy* involved using smaller doses of LSD (e.g., 25–150 µg) on a periodic basis as a component of ongoing psychoanalytic therapy, to loosen psychological defenses and facilitate exploration and processing of emotionally charged material. *Psychedelic therapy* used larger doses (>200 µg) with the intention of producing ego dissolution and perhaps a full mystical experience. In this circumstance, LSD's transformative power is proposed to derive from some sort of dramatic reconfiguration of neural and psychological dynamics.

Another area of significant clinical research during the 1950s and 1960s was the treatment of alcohol addiction (Dyck, 2006, 2008; Grinspoon & Bakalar, 1979/1997; Liester, 2014; Mangini, 1998). While many of these projects claimed to be effective in reducing alcohol abuse, they suffer, like other investigations of that era, from lack of clear standards of outcome and well-designed controls (Bonson, 2018). Nonetheless, a meta-analysis of six published studies from the 1960s—all of which were conducted using randomized controls—showed efficacy of LSD in decreasing drinking behavior from a single high dose (210–800 µg) administered in the context of a therapeutic treatment program (Krebs & Johansen, 2012).

The initial investigation of alcoholism treatment in the early 1950s (Humphry Osmond and collaborators) operated from a hypothesis that a psychedelic-induced state of somatic and cognitive chaos might have similarities to the life-threatening delirium tremens (DTs) of alcohol withdrawal, and foster such a psychic shaking-up that sobriety would be a result. Later the hypothesis shifted away from any specific association with DTs and more toward the evocation of a transformative mystical experience, wherein the subject would experience illuminative insights that resulted in lasting changes of reduced self-destructive behavior (e.g., addictive use of alcohol).

These studies drew the attention of Bill Wilson (1895–1971), a recovering alcoholic who in the 1930s cofounded the very successful self-help network of Alcoholics Anonymous (AA). Wilson's own recovery from alcoholism had been catalyzed by a spiritual (mystical) experience he had while in treatment in 1934 (Alcoholics Anonymous, 1984). By the late 1950s, Wilson had been abstinent from alcohol for more than 20 years, but he was nonetheless interested in seeing what the LSD experience was about, and whether it would be something that AA ought to recommend to those who were still struggling with breaking free from the grip of alcohol dependence.

Between 1956 and 1958, Wilson traveled to California and engaged in several LSD psychotherapy sessions at the UCLA/LA Veterans Administration Medical Center with Drs. Sidney Cohen (1910–1987) and Betty Eisner (1915–2004). He found these experiences to be similar to the experience that propelled him into recovery years before and was thus optimistic that LSD might be of help to other alcoholics. However, the AA directorship was not supportive of the idea of recommending a psychoactive drug to individuals suffering from a drug (i.e., alcohol) addiction; thus the use of LSD as a therapeutic tool was not further discussed within the AA organization (Alcoholics Anonymous, 1984; Walsh & Grob, 2005).

Reviews of clinical work with LSD in those early decades, covering tens of thousands of drug administrations in controlled settings, describe wide-ranging results while speaking to valuable therapeutic potential and very low rates of adverse reactions (Cohen, 1960; Malleson, 1971; Pahnke et al., 1970). The early era of clinical research was ripe with promise and set the stage for further and more careful exploration of the complex effects of LSD on the psyche.

■ The Cultural Context of the 1960s

In parallel with the academic and clinical investigation of LSD in the 1950s, the U.S. government (the Central Intelligence Agency [CIA] and various components of the Department of Defense) sponsored secret programs of investigation that explored the use of LSD as a chemical weapon, one that could mentally incapacitate an enemy without killing them. Also of interest was the possibility that LSD might aid interrogation, placing individuals in a vulnerable state of mind more conducive to disclosing information. While some of the academic and clinical investigations taking place at legitimate research institutions received funding through these government programs, other programs were more covert and blatantly unethical, such as those that administered LSD and other intoxicating drugs to individuals without their knowledge or consent, in order to observe the effects. Although many of the records of these projects appear to have been destroyed or redacted, enough remains for journalists, using the U.S. Freedom of Information Act, to have produced several comprehensive exposés of the era (Kinzer, 2019; Lee & Shlain, 1985; Marks, 1991; Stevens, 1987). And at least one of the researchers has recalled and recorded events of that era as well (Ketchum, 2006).

Concern developed at the time regarding dependence on a foreign company (Sandoz in Switzerland) to supply LSD, prompting the CIA to ask an American pharmaceutical company to develop a means of syntheses that could be independently patented. Thus, a total synthesis of lysergic acid—one not requiring ergot fungus as the starting material—was published in 1956, and a patent was filed the same year (Kornfeld et al., 1956). Eventually the U.S. government abandoned these programs exploring the weaponization of LSD (Lee & Shlain, 1985).

By the end of the 1950s, information about psychedelic substances was penetrating popular American culture. The influential author Aldous Huxley (1954) had written *The Doors of Perception,* detailing his experience with mescaline, and R. Gordon Wasson (1898–1986) had authored an article in 1957 in the popular weekly magazine *Life* describing his experience with shamanic ceremonial use of hallucinogenic mushrooms in Mexico. Poet Allen Ginsberg (1926–1997) wrote in 1959 a 154-line poem on "Lysergic Acid" and another on "Mescaline" (Ginsberg, 1961), and the popular philosopher of Asian spiritual traditions Alan Watts (1915–1973) wrote glowingly of the psychological power and potential of LSD in 1960 and 1962.

For several years beginning in 1958, Ken Kesey (1935–2001) was affiliated with a postgraduate writing program at Stanford University in California. Nearby, at the Menlo Park Veterans Administration Hospital, government-funded research projects were taking place, administering LSD and other powerful psychoactive substances to volunteer subjects and recording their effects. Kesey, who previously had no appreciation of such substances, volunteered to ingest LSD and answer questions put to him about his experience. Around the same time, he also worked as a clinical aid in the psychiatric treatment unit at the same hospital. All this contributed to the creation of his highly acclaimed novel *One Flew Over the Cuckoo's Nest* (1962).

Kesey went on to become a public advocate of LSD, traveling far and wide in a wildly painted bus named *Further*—including a trip across the breadth of the United States in 1964. He and a group of friends, the "Merry Pranksters," orchestrated a series of West Coast LSD parties called "Acid Tests," with music provided by a new band, The Grateful Dead. At one point, the author Tom Wolfe (1930–2018) tagged along with the Pranksters for several weeks and subsequently birthed a widely read and highly acclaimed book describing the philosophy and adventures of Kesey and the Pranksters: *The Electric Kool-Aid Acid Test* (1968).

Meanwhile, on the East Coast at Harvard University, Timothy Leary (1920–1996) and Richard Alpert (1931–2019) began their Psilocybin Research Project in 1961. In 1963 they were dismissed from Harvard as a result of the psychic turmoil that can ensue with use of psychedelics (Dass, Metzner,

& Bravo, 2010; Lattin, 2010). Immediately after this, their focus of exploration shifted to LSD. They produced a classic guidebook of sorts—*The Psychedelic Experience: A Manual Based on the Tibetan Book of the Dead* (Leary, Metzner, & Alpert, 1964)—appreciated for its recommendations in use of the psychedelic experience as an opportunity for psychological and spiritual learning and growth.

Unfettered by the etiquette of the academy, Leary attracted a great deal of media attention with his flamboyant and provocative style. He gave numerous public lectures promoting personal experimentation with LSD and other psychedelics (Leary, 1983). Alpert journeyed to India in 1967 and came back as Ram Dass (Dass, 1971; Walsh & Grob, 2005). His writings and public lectures over the decades have contributed to the introduction of Asian spiritual philosophies into American culture. Ralph Metzner (1936–2019), a graduate student who worked with Leary and Alpert at Harvard, went on to become a pioneering scholar of consciousness and its transformations, academic educator, renowned shamanic teacher, and psychotherapist (Metzner, 1968, 2017).

There were multiple other foci of experimentation with LSD during the 1960s. A legendary and enigmatic character of the era, Al Hubbard (1901–1982), sometimes called the "Johnny Appleseed of LSD," introduced key individuals far and wide to its powerful experiential effects (Lee & Shlain, 1985; Fahey, 1991). And in the San Francisco region later known as Silicon Valley, a group of engineers and psychologists investigated LSD's potential to aid creative problem solving (Fadiman, 2011; Walsh & Grob, 2005).

As millions of doses of LSD were being ingested in a vast array of uncontrolled settings, adverse reactions to its powerful psychological effects may have been anticipated. The impressive safety record and positive outcomes of LSD used in controlled therapeutic and research settings did not necessarily extend to situations of uncontrolled and ill-prepared use, and the adverse events that did occur were often exaggerated by the media (Siff, 2015). By 1966 there were widely read magazine stories with headlines such as "LSD: The exploding threat of the mind drug that got out of control. Turmoil in a capsule: One dose of LSD is enough to set off a riot of vivid colors and insights—or of terror and convulsions" (*Life* magazine cover of March 25, 1966).

Research concluding that LSD produced chromosome damage and birth defects appeared in prominent scientific and medical journals and was repeated often in the popular press. While these findings were soon discredited, the additional negative contribution to LSD's reputation had been accomplished and there was no going back (Dishotsky, Loughman, Mogar, & Lipscomb, 1971; Presti & Beck, 2001).

Genetic damage was only one of many 1960s-era myths that sprang up around this powerful substance. Others were that users frequently "went crazy" and remained crazy: "Use LSD seven times and you are legally insane," went one such myth. Staring at the sun and going blind, thinking one can fly and jumping from a high place, and ingesting LSD often contaminated with additives such as strychnine and amphetamine were among other pervasive myths (Presti & Beck, 2001). The social discourse related to LSD very likely had substantial impact on how users interpreted their experiences: Was one dealing with the complexities of the psyche and the state of the world, or was one going permanently insane? The development of informed-user subcultures in the 1960s—peer groups that could educate and counsel one another—likely helped to modulate and reduce potential adverse reactions (Becker, 1967).

In 1966, Sandoz withdrew Delysid from the market. But it was clear already that Delysid (diverted from clinical and research projects) alone could not provide for the demand engendered by the growing popularity of LSD. Other sources were necessary; thus, there emerged a number of underground chemists who operated with an intention to synthesize LSD and make it widely available. This began in the United States and Europe in the early 1960s. Among these chemists who became publicly well known were Augustus Owsley Stanley (1935–2011), known as Owsley, who produced LSD between 1965 and 1967; Tim Scully (born in 1944), who produced LSD from 1966 to 1969; and Nicholas Sand (1941–2017), who produced LSD on and off between 1966 and 1996. All

were arrested at various times, and all spent periods in prison for manufacturing LSD. Tens of millions of doses were synthesized and distributed. And to this day, LSD continues to be available in the illicit market.

For at least some of these underground chemists, their mission was self-described as alchemical—a bow to the ancient discipline that preceded modern chemistry. Alchemy was concerned both with transformations of matter (here, the synthesis of LSD) and with transformations of the psyche (here, the belief held by the chemists that their work would shift and transform the collective human mindset) (for a beautiful exposition on alchemy and LSD, see Metzner, 2017). Quoting Nicholas Sand (2001, p. 39; Grimes, 2017): "This planet must be lovingly cared for or we are all doomed. We are the guardians of life and planetary harmony. This is where we are going. That is what I have seen in my visions, and that is what I have been working for all of my life. That is what I will continue to do until my last breath."

The high potency of LSD requires that small quantities be accurately partitioned into individual dosage units. Sandoz's Delysid came packaged as a tablet or liquid solution of precise concentration. The LSD produced by chemists such as Owsley and his contemporaries was primarily distributed in tablet or capsule form. Another method of dose packaging was called "windowpane"—LSD-impregnated gelatin. In the 1960s, the dosage unit of illicitly synthesized and distributed LSD was typically in the 200- to 333-µg range—a strong psychedelic dose. Sometime in the 1970s, "blotter" LSD began to appear, a mode of distribution that has remained a dominant form of illicit LSD for nearly five decades. Here, absorbent paper is saturated with LSD in solution, calibrated so that the quantity of LSD absorbed into a small measured area (one-fourth inch square) contains a one-unit dose of drug. The blotter paper is perforated, so that the dosage units can be easily divided and a sheet of blotter paper typically has 30 × 30 = 900 dosage units. In addition, over the decades, LSD blotter paper has been imprinted with an astounding panoply of colorful art. Beginning in the early 1970s, illicit LSD began to appear in reduced dosage: Rather than 200+ µg per dosage unit, a unit dose was found to often be in the 60 to 100 μg range (based on estimates determined from blotter acid confiscated by law enforcement).

Perhaps the single most important factor in bringing about the severe legal restrictions on LSD was its association with the 1960s counterculture, driven in large part by opposition to the war in Southeast Asia, but also very much opposing the growing military–corporate control of society in general. The impact of this association is difficult to overestimate in its import to the demonization of LSD and subsequent draconian legal control (also applied to other psychedelics, and to cannabis as well) (Lee & Shlain, 1985; Stevens, 1987).

The first laws against LSD were instituted in 1966, including U.S. federal prohibition of manufacture and sale (although not yet possession). An increasing set of legal restrictions at state and federal levels developed over the following years. In 1968, LSD possession was outlawed federally, and when the comprehensive Federal Controlled Substances Act was implemented in 1970, LSD (as well as other known psychedelic chemicals) were deemed Schedule I controlled substances—drugs lacking approved medical use and considered highly dangerous and prone to abuse as well. The following year, the United Nations Convention on Psychotropic Substances pronounced LSD to be Schedule I internationally. Once widely accepted for its therapeutic and research potential, LSD was now illegal at the highest level, worldwide.

While it has sometimes been convenient to place blame for this severe regulation as a response largely catalyzed by the activities of a few specific individuals—with the most frequently scapegoated individual by far being Timothy Leary—it seems highly likely the complex course of events of the 1950s and 1960s would have resulted in a similar outcome no matter what individuals with their unique personalities had been involved. LSD and other psychedelics are incredibly powerful, and contemporary Western society lacked the shamanic and spiritual infrastructure to guide and contain that power. It is important to remember this as we move forward with the benefits—such as they may be—of hindsight.

Adverse Effects and Toxicity

For LSD (and other psychedelic substances) the most significant adverse effects are acute anxiety and panic—the so-called "bad trip." Such adverse effects can be minimized or contained with appropriate attention to set and setting. Actually, in the context of a therapeutic process, such firsthand contact with difficult psychological material can be the springboard for significant positive shifts—a transformational antecedent rather than an adverse effect. This may be supported by a skilled therapist or guide, and also may happen within the course of one's own internal process. Any single experience with LSD may contain both positive and negative mood states. The longer-term takeaway from an experience depends altogether on how one relates to psychological material that emerges and, very importantly, how one then integrates the experience into one's life.

There are reports of individuals suffering long-term anxiety, depression, and psychosis in association with LSD use. Even so, reviews of clinical administrations of LSD during the 1950s and 1960s have documented very low rates of adverse effects (Cohen, 1960; Malleson, 1971). Moreover, the published literature from this era suggests that chronic adverse effects, when they do occur, are most often associated with psychological instability prior to exposure to LSD (Grinspoon & Bakalar, 1979/1997; Strassman, 1984). For example, persons with certain personality disorders, active bipolar or psychotic conditions, or latent mental disorders (e.g., a positive family history for schizophrenia, suggesting a possible genetic risk for developing psychosis) may have symptoms triggered from LSD use and suffer chronic problems thereafter. Such individuals would also be at risk from exposure to a variety of other environmental stressors.

More recently, assessments of LSD and other psychedelic use in uncontrolled nonmedical settings have been conducted by analyzing comprehensive survey data compiled annually in the United States via the National Survey of Drug Use and Health (NSDUH). Analyses of NSDUH data between 2001 and 2004 (Krebs & Johansen, 2013b) and between 2008 and 2012 (Hendricks, Thorne, Clark, Coombs, & Johnson, 2015; Johansen & Krebs, 2015) found no relationship between lifetime use of psychedelics (LSD, psilocybin-containing mushrooms, mescaline, peyote cactus) and any negative mental health outcomes—including symptoms characteristic of a variety of mood, anxiety, and psychotic disorders, other serious psychological distress, and engagement with mental-health treatment (inpatient, outpatient, psychiatric medication). One of these studies found an association between lifetime psychedelic use and reduced likelihood of psychological distress, suicidal ideation, and suicidal behavior (Hendricks et al., 2015). By way of contrast, lifetime prevalence of use of other illicit drugs (cocaine, stimulants, sedatives, opioids, cannabis) was associated with increased psychological distress and suicidal ideation, as well as suicide planning and attempts (Hendricks et al., 2015).

It is now generally agreed that LSD is physiologically safe, especially when moderate doses are used. Cardiovascular and other autonomic effects are modest. There has never been a documented death due to LSD use at typical recreational doses (Erowid, 2018a; Nichols & Grob, 2018). Moreover, there have been cases of individuals consuming massive doses and surviving without any reported residual effects. For example, eight individuals insufflated a very high dose of LSD, believing it to be cocaine (Klock, Boerner, & Becker, 1974; Nichols & Grob, 2018). They received emergency medical treatment 15 minutes after insufflating the drug, at which point five were comatose. Three required assisted ventilation. Tachycardia was also present, as well as hyperthermia and generalized bleeding in some of the patients. Blood analyses measured up to 26 ng/ml, and gastric analyses up to 7 mg/100 ml. There were no seizures reported, and none of the eight patients required supportive treatment extending past 12 hours. "Most did not remember being brought to the hospital; otherwise no apparent psychologic or physical ill effects were noted in a year of follow-up examinations of five patients" (Klock et al., 1974).

While there have been fatalities associated with engaging in dangerous behavior while intoxicated, there appear to be only a very small number of such reports involving LSD—impressively low when contrasted with the tens of millions of doses of LSD consumed over more than 50 years of widespread popular use. Other deaths initially associated with LSD were later ruled to be due to excessive restraint by police or to ingestion of drugs other than LSD (Nichols & Grob, 2018).

The advent of synthetic drugs unrelated to LSD but possessing substantial physiological activity at submilligram doses has given rise to a situation wherein blotter sold at festivals, concerts, and other venues and portrayed as "blotter acid" containing LSD actually may contain no LSD and rather, on a number of occasions, has been found to instead contain potent synthetic intoxicants that carry dangers not associated with LSD. One such substance, 25I-NBOMe (4-iodo-2,5-dimethoxy-*N*-[2-methoxybenzyl]-phenethylamine), is powerfully active at submilligram doses. Unlike LSD, the NBOMe substances can produce potentially lethal effects such as hyperthermia, hypertension, tachycardia, agitated delirium, seizure, and rhabdomyolysis (Erowid, 2018b; Gee, Schep, Jensen, Moore, & Barrington, 2016; Nichols, 2016; Nichols & Grob, 2018; Walterscheid et al., 2014).

Another possible adverse effect that is often associated with LSD, especially in popular discussion, is the notion of a *flashback*. This word was introduced in early 20th-century English to describe insertion into the temporal sequence of a narrative or film of events taking place at an earlier time. By 1970, it had appeared in the popular media in association with LSD (Linkletter & Bell, 1970) and soon thereafter was used in the clinical literature (Shick & Smith, 1970). Years later Timothy Leary (1983) would poetically use the word as the title for his autobiographic memoir. (The word has also been applied as a descriptor of dissociative reaction in the diagnostic criteria for posttraumatic stress disorder [PTSD], for example, in the *Diagnostic and Statistical Manual of Mental Disorders* [DSM]).

In their excellent discussion of the flashback notion applied to LSD and other psychedelics, Grinspoon and Bakalar (1979/1997, p. 159) have this to say:

Studies of flashbacks are hard to evaluate because the term has been used so loosely and variably. On the broadest definition, it means the transitory recurrence of emotions and perceptions originally experienced while under the influence of the drug. It can last seconds or hours; it can mimic any of the myriad aspects of a trip; and it can be blissful, interesting, annoying, or frightening. Most flashbacks are episodes of visual distortion, time distortion, physical symptoms, loss of ego boundaries, or relived intense emotion lasting a few seconds to a few minutes. Ordinarily they are only slightly disturbing, especially since the drug user usually recognizes them for what they are; they may even be regarded lightheartedly as "free trips." Occasionally they last longer, and in a small minority of cases they turn into frightening images or thoughts.

One way of conceptualizing flashbacks is that memories may be recorded more robustly in the psychedelic state and may subsequently be more prone to reactivation and recall. Another related conceptualization of flashbacks is psychodynamic, a reemergence of conflictual material encountered during the time of the drug action and not yet fully processed: "Sessions in which the drug activates areas of difficult emotional material and the individual tries to avoid facing them can lead to prolonged reactions, unsatisfactory integration, subsequent residual emotional or psychosomatic problems, or a precarious mental balance that becomes the basis for later 'flashbacks'" (Grof, 1980/2001, p. 134).

In the 1980s a small number of case reports detailing hallucinatory visual sensations persisting beyond the phase of acute intoxication with psychedelics led to the introduction of a new diagnostic category in DSM-III-R (American Psychiatric Association, 1987): posthallucinogen perception disorder. The diagnostic criteria were slightly modified in DSM-IV (American Psychiatric Association, 1994) and the diagnosis given a new name: hallucinogen persisting perception disorder (flashbacks). This condition is abbreviated as HPPD and has continued as a diagnosis (without the inclusion of the word *flashbacks*) in DSM-5 (American Psychiatric Association, 2013). There are claims that HPPD is more commonly associated with LSD than with other psychedelics.

Note that the early reviews of adverse effects associated with tens of thousands of administrations of LSD in clinical settings did not report any occurrence of persisting sensory disturbances or other flashback-type symptoms (Cohen, 1960; Malleson, 1971). Nor did the more recent analysis of NSDUH data reveal anything that looked like symptoms of HPPD or flashbacks (Krebs & Johansen, 2013b). Attempts to study the validity and prevalence of HPPD have concluded that while it may be a genuine, although uncommon, condition, and that symptoms may indeed develop in association with psychedelic use, it is perhaps more related to exacerbation of preexisting psychological and neurological conditions of anxiety and/or disturbances of visual processing (Baggott, Coyle, Erowid, Erowid, & Robertson, 2011; Halpern, Lerner, & Passie, 2018; Halpern & Pope, 2003).

Because of its legal classification as a Schedule I controlled substance, which, by definition, possesses a "high potential for abuse," LSD is often assumed to be addictive. However, LSD, like other classical psychedelics, has negligible addictive potential, and very low potential for people to use repeatedly and suffer adverse consequences as a result (Nichols, 2016).

▦ The Renewal of Human Research with LSD

The legal restrictions imposed on LSD beginning in the late 1960s resulted in virtually no formal human investigation for nearly 40 years. The emergence of the current phase of sanctioned clinical and scientific investigation with LSD began after human studies using other Schedule I psychedelic substances (DMT, 3,4-methylenedioxymethamphetamine [MDMA], and psilocybin) had paved the way.

Beginning in the first decade of the 21st century, survey research (> 500 persons) indicated that individuals suffering from painful cluster headaches reported shortening of headache duration and extended periods of remission from oral doses of self-administered LSD (or psilocybin, in the form of mushrooms), sometimes with doses that were infrequent and subpsychedelic (Schindler et al., 2015; Sewell, Halpern, & Pope, 2006). The therapeutic efficacy of LSD and psilocybin mushrooms in this regard was seen as comparable to or better than the best of the conventional available medical treatments. There has also been one small study (five patients) demonstrating therapeutic efficacy in cluster headache of the nonpsychoactive LSD analogue 2-bromo-LSD, a derivative originally synthesized by Hofmann and colleagues at Sandoz in the 1950s (Karst, Halpern, Bernateck, & Passie, 2010; Troxler & Hofmann, 1957).

One of the therapeutic indications for ergot-based pharmaceuticals produced by Sandoz since the early days has been treatment of migraines and cluster headaches. Ergotamine tartrate, sometimes used in conjunction with caffeine (Sandoz: Cafergot) has long been available. Another lysergic acid derivative is methysergide (1-methyl-D-lysergic acid butanolamide; Sandoz: Deseril and Sansert). The use of these ergot-derived pharmaceuticals has been largely eclipsed by the introduction of triptan medications, beginning with sumatriptan in the early 1990s. There has yet to be a controlled clinical study of LSD for the treatment of headaches.

The first controlled (randomized, double-blind, placebo-controlled) clinical study of LSD since circa 1970 was conducted in Switzerland and initial findings published by Gasser and colleagues (2014). Twelve patients with anxiety associated with life-threatening illness were treated with LSD-assisted psychotherapy using a moderate dose (200 µg) or an active placebo (20 µg). The participants who received the psychotherapy with the active dose showed a significant reduction in state, or short-term, anxiety at 2-month follow-up. A 12-month follow-up study reported sustained reductions in both short-term and long-term, or trait, anxiety and increases in quality of life, with no reported adverse effects (Gasser, Kirchner, & Passie, 2015).

A major aspect of the current human studies with psychedelics (LSD and, even more extensively, psilocybin) has been to revisit some of the themes that emerged from the first phase of human research (e.g., treatment of anxiety and depression associated with life-threatening illness, treatment of addiction, and capacity to occasion spiritual experience) now applying modern standards of rigorous controls and validated assessment instruments. Another major aspect is to bring to bear the technologies of functional brain imaging (functional magnetic resonance imaging [fMRI], electroencephalography [EEG], magnetoencephalography [MEG], etc.) and cellular and molecular biology to further elucidate physiological mechanisms associated with the actions of LSD and other psychedelics on the human brain and body.

Studies (double-blind, placebo-controlled) with healthy human subjects in Switzerland have resulted in a number of published reports commenting on phenomenology, physiology, and psychological effects, as well as data on neural correlates of LSD-induced states of mind (summarized in Liechti, 2017). These studies used either 100 or 200 µg of LSD orally. Various physiological and psychological changes are described, including increased happiness, closeness to others, openness, trust and empathy, and impaired recognition of fearful faces (Dolder, Schmid, Müller, Borgwardt, & Liechti, 2016; Schmid et al., 2015).

Several reports describe neural correlates related to perceptual, cognitive, and emotional experiences, and hypothesize relationships between regional brain activity and emotional processing, as well as neural network connectivity and subjective experiences (Mueller et al., 2017; Müller et al., 2017, 2018; Schmidt et al., 2018). Another study out of Switzerland linked LSD-induced effects, including induction of a dream-like state of consciousness and attributions of personal meaningfulness, to $5\text{-}HT_{2A}$ receptor agonism and also to activity in particular brain regions (Kraehenmann et al., 2017; Preller et al., 2017).

Studies in London (using intravenous doses of 40–80 µg LSD, found to be approximately equivalent to 100 µg by oral administration) looked at a number of psychological outcome measures, as well as measures of brain activity using fMRI and MEG. Researchers commented on imagination, mental imagery, synesthesia, psychosis-like symptoms, emotional response to music, heighted mood, and increases in optimism and trait openness (Carhart-Harris et al., 2015; Carhart-Harris, Kaelen, et al., 2016; Kaelen et al., 2015; Terhune et al., 2016).

Also described were increases in cortical and thalamic functional connectivity and its relationship with subjective reports of *ego dissolution* (defined as a lessening of a sense of a "self" or "ego" distinct from others and separate from the environment) (Carhart-Harris, Muthukumaraswamy, et al., 2016; Tagliazucchi et al., 2016).

The capacity of LSD-catalyzed experiences to have long-term (perhaps lifelong) impact on behavior suggests that LSD may have profound impact on neuronal connectivity and memory formation. At cellular and molecular levels, LSD and other psychedelics have been found (both *in vivo* and in cell culture) to enhance processes associated with synaptic plasticity, such as growth of dendritic spines and other neuronal processes (Ly et al., 2018). LSD has also been found to influence the expression of genes associated with transcription factors and other mediators of synaptic plasticity (Martin & Nichols, 2018; Nichols & Sanders-Bush, 2002).

■ Microdosing of LSD

Microdosing is a term used in pharmacology to describe administration of miniscule doses of a drug, well below the threshold for therapeutic activity (Passie, 2019). Lately it has been applied in reference to ingesting a small, subperceptual amount of a psychedelic substance—usually about one-tenth of a moderate dose generally used for a full psychedelic trip—and has reportedly grown in popularity over the past several years (Anderson et al., 2019; Passie, 2019). A commonly used microdose of LSD is in the range of 5–10 µg. However, it is important to bear in mind that contemporary information about microdosing of LSD comes primarily from users in informal settings who often do not know precisely what dose they are taking.

A study of the impact of small doses of LSD (4–20 µg) on 14 individuals was conducted in the 1950s (Greiner, Burch, & Edelberg, 1958). And the effects of subpsychedelic doses (e.g., 20–50 µg), although not generally subperceptual doses, were often researched in the early days of LSD clinical investigation (Passie, 2019). In addition, some of the pioneer investigators occasionally referenced the potential psychological value of lower (subpsychedelic) dosages. Albert Hofmann speculated in a 1970s interview that perhaps doses of circa 25 µg might be useful to investigate for potential antidepressant effects (Hofmann & Horowitz, 1976).

Contemporary interest in microdosing has been in part catalyzed by James Fadiman (born in 1939), a psychologist whose involvement in LSD research dates to the early 1960s (Walsh & Grob, 2005). Fadiman (2011) has offered a protocol to personally assess the effects of microdosing by taking the subperceptual dose on the morning of every fourth day for a period of perhaps 1 month, tracking and recording any perceived differences between these different days, all the while engaging in one's regular daily activities. This protocol avoids the buildup of tolerance, as well as provides opportunities to contrast one's experience of "on" versus "off" days. Accounts of individuals using this protocol describe things such as improvement in focus of attention and productivity, and sometimes improvement in mood. Reports were summed up as indicating that many respondents related "positive and valuable" experiences. A common denominator of several stories was offered—that these individuals reported functioning "a little better than normal" (Fadiman, 2011; Fadiman & Korb, 2019).

Currently, the number of published studies on the microdosing of LSD or other psychedelics is very small and largely uncontrolled. Internet-based surveys have addressed self-reported effects of respondents to microdosing of a variety of psychedelics (Johnstad, 2018) and personality differences between individuals who microdose versus nonmicrodosing controls (Anderson et al., 2019). An unblinded study in the Netherlands using microdoses of psilocybin-containing mushrooms found increases on several measures of creative thinking (Prochazkova et al., 2018). The first randomized, double-blind, placebo-controlled study of LSD microdosing (5, 10, and 20 µg), conducted in the United Kingdom, reported the only significant effect of small doses of LSD was overestimation of intervals of elapsed time by the participants (Yanakieva et al., 2019).

The question of therapeutic benefits aside, one may wonder whether the regular and frequent use—even if not daily use—of small doses of LSD or other psychedelic substances might result in subtle, or not-so-subtle, withdrawal symptoms when regular dosing is curtailed, as has been found to occur with antidepressant medications—so-called "antidepressant discontinuation syndrome" (Horowitz & Taylor, 2019). Given the role that serotonergic mechanisms likely have in withdrawal effects that occur after stopping daily antidepressant medications, one may surmise that analogous mechanisms could be operative with regular microdosing of LSD.

As other facets of human LSD research have been initiated or renewed within the last decade, we can expect more well-controlled and published investigations of microdosing in the near future. Such investigation should be able to establish more definitively the effects on human cognition and emotion of ingesting tiny doses of LSD. Until this is accomplished, it is impossible to say which and how much of the reported effects of subperceptual doses are due to specific pharmacological interaction of LSD with brain physiology, and how much may be attributed solely to belief and expectation—so-called "placebo effects." Such expectation effects might even be enhanced as a result of LSD's complex and colorful history; that is, how could something not be expected from such a remarkable substance? Placebo effects in pharmacology can be and often are substantial, and this alone is a profound statement about the power of the mind–body connection.

■ Coda: Shamans, Medicines, and the Nature of Mind

The most salient aspect of LSD and other classical psychedelics is the effect they can have on the psyche—shaking it up, opening it to new information and insight, even transforming one's worldview. Somehow this is related to interactions with brain physiology, although the details are likely to be more subtle and complex than what are presently envisioned. This metamorphic potential of LSD, used under suitable conditions, could transform the landscape of treatment for conditions of mental distress, such as depression and anxiety.

The discovery of LSD set Albert Hofmann on a lifelong path investigating the chemistry of plants and fungi used by indigenous cultures around the world in spiritual and healing ceremonies. All the while, he continued his work at Sandoz in pharmaceutical chemistry, going on to become the director of the department of natural products (Hagenbach & Werthmüller, 2011). Hofmann collaborated with mycologist-botanist Roger Heim (1900–1979) and ethnomycologist R. Gordon Wasson to investigate *Psilocybe* mushrooms used by Mazatec shamans of southern Mexico. Conducting extractions and separations, with subsequent testing on himself for psychoactive effects, Hofmann identified the molecules psilocybin and psilocin from *Psilocybe* mushrooms and established their psychedelic activity (Hofmann, 2013; Hofmann, Heim, Brack, & Kobel, 1958).

His work with *Psilocybe* mushrooms led Hofmann to investigate the chemical constituents of another shamanic substance from southern Mexico known as *ololiuhqui* in the ancient language of the region, the seeds of flowering morning glory plants: *Turbina (Rivea) corymbosa* and *Ipomoea violacea*. Here, he identified the surprising presence of lysergic acid amide and other related alkaloids similar to what had been previously identified in ergot. He furthermore concluded the psychoactive potency of lysergic acid amide to be at least 10 times less than that of LSD and far less interesting in its effects (Hofmann, 2013; Hofmann & Tscherter, 1960).

In 1962, Hofmann accompanied Wasson to Mexico to collect samples of a novel plant used in Mazatec healing ceremonies. Ritual use was documented, and plant samples were obtained and brought back for botanical and chemical investigation. Botanical identification established the plant as one not previously described, and it was given the name *Salvia divinorum*. Hofmann's attempt to identify the psychoactive chemical component was not successful, in that the material he carried back with him to Switzerland no longer retained psychoactivity. Twenty years later, the primary psychoactive chemical component was isolated and identified by Mexican scientists and named salvinorin A (Hofmann, 2013).

Hofmann collaborated with renowned ethnobotanist Richard Evans Schultes

(1915–2001) to write two books on psychoactive plants and fungi used by indigenous cultures for healing and shamanic rituals: *The Botany and Chemistry of Hallucinogens* (Schultes & Hofmann, 1980) and *Plants of the Gods: Origins of Hallucinogenic Use* (Schultes & Hofmann, 1979; later expanded in Schultes, Hofmann, & Rätsch, 2001). And he collaborated again with Wasson and with scholar of classics Carl Ruck (born in 1935) to propose that the *kykeon* beverage consumed by the participants in the sacred ritual of the Eleusinian Mysteries of ancient Greece may have contained hallucinogenic ergot alkaloids (Wasson, Hofmann, & Ruck, 1998).

Ancient and contemporary spiritual and shamanic traditions may hold wisdom about the nature of mind and world that modern biophysical science—and psychology, psychiatry, and medicine—is perhaps poised to receive and integrate into our evolving understanding of who we are as conscious beings and how we relate to the physical world. As Grof (1980/2001, p. 12) wrote in the reissue of his classic 1980 book *LSD Psychotherapy,* "It does not seem to be an exaggeration to say that psychedelics, used responsibly and with proper caution, would be for psychiatry what the microscope is for biology and medicine or the telescope is for astronomy. These tools make it possible to study important processes that under normal circumstances are not available for direct observation."

LSD and other psychedelics expand our capacity to probe mental states directly and open the psyche to far-reaching new kinds of experience. Let us be propelled by the inspiring winds of this venture, deepening our understanding of mind and allowing us to more clearly chart a course toward personal and societal healing and transformation.

■ References

Alcoholics Anonymous. (1984). *"Pass it on": The story of Bill Wilson and how the A.A. message reached the world.* New York: Alcoholic Anonymous World Services.

American Psychiatric Association. (1987). *Diagnostic and statistical manual of mental disorders* (3rd ed., rev.). Washington, DC: Author.

American Psychiatric Association. (1994). *Diagnostic and statistical manual of mental disorders* (4th ed.). Washington, DC: Author.

American Psychiatric Association. (2013). *Diagnostic and statistical manual of mental disorders* (5th ed.). Arlington, VA: Author.

Anderson, T., Petranker, R., Rosenbaum, D., Weisman, C. R., Dinh-Williams, L. A., Hui, K., et al. (2019). Microdosing psychedelics: Personality, mental health, and creativity differences in microdosers. *Psychopharmacology, 236,* 731–740.

Bache, C. M. (2019). *LSD and the mind of the universe: Diamonds from heaven.* Rochester, VT: Park Street Press.

Baggott, M. J., Coyle, J. R., Erowid, E., Erowid, F., & Robertson L. C. (2011). Abnormal visual experiences in individuals with histories of hallucinogen use: A web-based questionnaire. *Drug and Alcohol Dependence, 114,* 61–67.

Becker, H. S. (1967). History, culture and subjective experience: An exploration of the social bases of drug-induced experiences. *Journal of Health and Social Behavior, 8,* 163–176.

Bonson, K. R. (2018). Regulation of human research with LSD in the United States (1949–1987). *Psychopharmacology, 235,* 591–604.

Bonson, K. R., Buckholtz, J. W., & Murphy, D. L. (1996). Chronic administration of serotonergic antidepressants attenuates the subjective effects of LSD in humans. *Neuropsychopharmacology, 14,* 425–436.

Bonson, K. R., & Murphy, D. L. (1996). Alterations in responses to LSD in humans associated with chronic administration of tricyclic antidepressants, monoamine oxidase inhibitors or lithium. *Behavioural Brain Research, 73,* 229–233.

Busch, A. K., & Johnson, W. C. (1950). L.S.D. 25 as an aid to psychotherapy: Preliminary report of a new drug. *Diseases of the Nervous System, 11*(8), 241–243.

Carhart-Harris, R. L., Kaelen, M., Bolstridge, M., Williams, T. M., Williams, L. T., Underwood, R., et al. (2016). The paradoxical psychological effects of lysergic acid diethylamide (LSD). *Psychological Medicine, 46,* 1379–1390.

Carhart-Harris, R. L., Kaelen, M., Whalley, M. G., Bolstridge, M., Feilding, A., & Nutt, D. J. (2015). LSD enhances suggestibility in healthy volunteers. *Psychopharmacology, 232,* 785–794.

Carhart-Harris, R. L., Muthukumaraswamy, S., Roseman, L., Kaelen, M., Droog, W., Murphy, K., et al. (2016). Neural correlates of the LSD experience revealed by multi-modal neuroimaging. *Proceedings of the National Academy of Sciences of the USA, 113,* 4853–4858.

Cholden, L. S., Kurland, A., & Savage, C. (1955). Clinical reactions and tolerance to LSD in chronic schizophrenia. *Journal of Nervous and Mental Disease, 122,* 211–221.

Cohen, S. (1960). Lysergic acid diethylamide: Side effects and complications. *Journal of Nervous and Mental Disease, 130,* 30–40.

Dass, R. (1971). *Be here now.* San Cristobal, NM: Lama Foundation.

Dass, R., Metzner, R., & Bravo, G. (2010). *Birth of a psychedelic culture: Conversations about Leary, the Harvard experiments, Millbrook, and the Sixties.* Santa Fe, NM: Synergetic Press.

Dishotsky, N. I., Loughman, W. D., Mogar, R. E., & Lipscomb, W. R. (1971). LSD and genetic damage. *Science, 172,* 431–440.

Dolder, P. C., Schmid, Y., Müller, F., Borgwardt, S., & Liechti, M. E. (2016). LSD acutely impairs fear recognition and enhances emotional empathy and sociality. *Neuropsychopharmacology, 41,* 2638–2646.

Dolder, P. C., Schmid, Y., Steuer, A. E., Kraemer, T., Rentsch, K. M., Hammann, F., et al. (2017). Pharmacokinetics and pharmacodynamics of lysergic acid diethylamide in healthy subjects. *Clinical Pharmacokinetics, 56,* 1219–1230.

Dyck, E. (2006). "Hitting highs at rock bottom": LSD treatment for alcoholism, 1950–1970. *Social History of Medicine, 19,* 313–329.

Dyck, E. (2008). *Psychedelic psychiatry: LSD from clinic to campus.* Baltimore: Johns Hopkins University Press.

Erowid. (2018a). The vaults of Erowid: LSD (acid) fatalities/deaths. Retrieved April 19, 2019, from *erowid.org/chemicals/lsd/lsd_death.shtml.*

Erowid. (2018b). The vaults of Erowid: 25I-NBOMe. Retrieved April 19, 2019, from *erowid.org/chemicals/2ci_nbome.*

Fadiman, J. (2011). *The psychedelic explorer's guide: Safe, therapeutic, and sacred journeys.* Rochester, VT: Park Street Press.

Fadiman, J., & Korb, S. (2019). Might microdosing psychedelics be safe and beneficial?: An initial exploration. *Journal of Psychoactive Drugs, 51,* 118–122.

Fahey, T. B. (1991, November). The original Captain Trips. *High Times Magazine,* pp. 18–23.

Feilding, A. (Ed.). (2008). *Hofmann's elixir: LSD and the new Eleusis.* Oxford, UK: Beckley Foundation.

Gasser, P., Holstein, D., Michel, Y., Doblin, R., Yazar-Klosinski, B., Passie, T., et al. (2014). Safety and efficacy of lysergic acid diethylamide-assisted psychotherapy for anxiety associated with life-threatening diseases. *Journal of Nervous and Mental Disease, 202,* 513–520.

Gasser, P., Kirchner, K., & Passie, T. (2015). LSD-assisted psychotherapy for anxiety associated with a life-threatening disease: A qualitative study of acute and sustained subjective effects. *Journal of Psychopharmacology, 29,* 57–68.

Gee, P., Schep, L. J., Jensen, B. P., Moore, G., & Barrington, S. (2016). Case series: Toxicity from 25B-NBOMe—a cluster of N-bomb cases. *Clinical Toxicology, 54,* 141–146.

Ginsberg, A. (1961). *Kaddish and other poems: 1958–1960.* San Francisco: City Light Books.

Green, A. R. (2008). Gaddum and LSD: The birth and growth of experimental and clinical neuropharmacology research on 5-HT in the UK. *British Journal of Pharmacology, 154,* 1583–1599.

Greiner, T., Burch, N. R., & Edelberg, R. (1958). Psychopathology and psychophysiology of minimal LSD-25 dosage: A preliminary dosage–response spectrum. *AMA Archives of Neurology and Psychiatry, 79,* 208–210.

Gresch, P. J., Smith, R. L., Barrett, R. J., & Sanders-Bush, E. (2005). Behavioral tolerance to lysergic acid diethylamide is associated with reduced serotonin-2A receptor signaling in rat cortex. *Neuropsychopharmacology, 30,* 1693–1702.

Grimes, W. (2017, May 12). Nicholas Sand, chemist who sought to bring LSD to the world, dies at 75. *New York Times,* p. A24.

Grinspoon, L., & Bakalar, J. B. (1997). *Psychedelic drugs reconsidered.* New York: Lindesmith Center. (Original work published 1979)

Grof, S. (1975). *Realms of the human unconscious: Observations from LSD research.* New York: Viking Press.

Grof, S. (2001). *LSD psychotherapy* (3rd ed.). Sarasota FL: Multidisciplinary Association for Psychedelic Studies. (Original work published 1980)

Hagenbach, D., & Werthmüller, L. (2011). *Mystic chemist: The life of Albert Hofmann and his discovery of LSD.* Santa Fe, NM: Synergetic Press.

Halpern, J. H., Lerner, A. G., & Passie, T. (2018). A review of hallucinogen persisting perception disorder (HPPD) and an exploratory study of subjects claiming symptoms of HPPD. *Current Topics in Behavioral Neuroscience, 36,* 333–360.

Halpern, J. H., & Pope, H. G., Jr. (2003). Hallucinogen persisting perception disorder: What do we know after 50 years? *Drug and Alcohol Dependence, 69,* 109–119.

Hendricks, P. S., Thorne, C. B., Clark, C. B., Coombs, D. W., & Johnson, M. W. (2015). Classic psychedelic use is associated with reduced psychological distress and suicidality in the United States adult population. *Journal of Psychopharmacology, 29,* 280–288.

Hintzen, A., & Passie, T. (2010). *The pharmacology of LSD: A critical review.* Oxford, UK: Oxford University Press.

Hofmann, A. (2013). *LSD: My problem child* (J. Ott, Trans.). Oxford, UK: Oxford University Press. (Original German publication, *LSD: Mein Sorgenkind*, 1979; original English translation, 1980; new English translation, 2013)

Hofmann, A., Heim, R., Brack, A., & Kobel, H. (1958). Psilocybin, ein psychotroper Wirkstoff aus dem mexikanischen Rauschpilz *Psilocybe mexicana* Heim. *Experientia, 14,* 107–109.

Hofmann, A., & Horowitz, M. (1976, July). Interview with Albert Hofmann. *High Times Magazine,* 11.

Hoffman, A. J., & Nichols, D. E. (1985). Synthesis and LSD-like discriminative stimulus properties in a series of N(6)-alkyl norlysergic acid N,N-diethylamide derivatives. *Journal of Medicinal Chemistry, 28,* 1252–1255.

Hofmann, A., & Tscherter, H. (1960). Isolierung von Lysergsäure-Alkaloiden aus der mexikanischen Zauberdroge Ololiuqui (*Rivea corymbosa* (L.) Hall. f.). *Experientia, 16,* 414.

Horowitz, M. A., & Taylor, D. (2019). Tapering of SSRI treatment to mitigate withdrawal symptoms. *Lancet Psychiatry, 6*(7), 561–562.

Huxley, A. (1954). *The doors of perception.* New York: Harper & Brothers.

Huxley, A. (1977). *Moksha: Writings on psychedelics and the visionary experience (1931–1963)* (M. Horowitz & C. Palmer, Eds.). New York: Stonehill.

Isbell, H., Belleville, R. E., Fraser, H. F., Wikler, A., & Logan, C. R. (1956). Studies on lysergic acid diethylamide (LSD-25): I. Effects in former morphine addicts and development of tolerance during chronic intoxication. *AMA Archives of Neurology and Psychiatry, 76,* 468–478.

Johansen, P. Ø., & Krebs, T. S. (2015). Psychedelics not linked to mental health problems or suicidal behavior: A population study. *Journal of Psychopharmacology, 29,* 270–279.

Johnstad, P. G. (2018). Powerful substances in tiny amounts: An interview study of psychedelic microdosing. *Nordic Studies on Alcohol and Drugs, 35,* 39–51.

Kaelen, M., Barrett, F. S., Roseman, L., Lorenz, R., Family, N. Bolstridge, M., et al. (2015). LSD enhances the emotional response to music. *Psychopharmacology, 232,* 3607–3614.

Karst, M., Halpern, J. H., Bernateck, M., & Passie, T. (2010). The non-hallucinogen 2-bromo-lysergic acid diethylamide as preventative treatment for cluster headache: An open, non-randomized case series. *Cephalalgia, 30,* 1140–1144.

Kesey, K. (1962). *One flew over the cuckoo's nest.* New York: Viking Press.

Ketchum, J. S. (2006). *Chemical warfare: Secrets almost forgotten.* Santa Rosa, CA: ChemBooks.

Kim, K., Che, T., Panova, O., DiBerto, J. F., Lyu, J., Krumm, B. E., et al. (2020). Structure of a hallucinogen-activated Gq-coupled 5-HT$_{2A}$ serotonin receptor. *Cell, 182,* 1574–1588.

Kinzer, S. (2019). *Poisoner in chief: Sidney Gottlieb and the CIA search for mind control.* New York: Henry Holt.

Klock, J. C., Boerner, U., & Becker, C. E. (1974). Coma, hyperthermia, and bleeding associated with massive LSD overdose: A report of 8 cases. *Western Journal of Medicine, 120,* 183–188.

Kornfeld, E. C., Fornefeld, E. J., Kline, G. B., Mann, M. J., Morrison, D. E., Jones, R. G., et al. (1956). The total synthesis of lysergic acid. *Journal of the American Chemical Society, 78,* 3087–3114.

Kraehenmann, R., Pokorny, D., Vollenweider, L., Preller, K. H., Pokorny, T., Seifritz, E., et al. (2017). Dreamlike effects of LSD on waking imagery in humans depend on serotonin 2A receptor activation. *Psychopharmacology, 234,* 2031–2046.

Krebs, T. S., & Johansen, P. Ø. (2012). Lysergic acid diethylamide (LSD) for alcoholism: Meta-analysis of randomized controlled trials. *Journal of Psychopharmacology, 26,* 994–1002.

Krebs, T. S., & Johansen, P. Ø. (2013a). Over 30 million psychedelic users in the United States. *F1000 Research, 2,* 98.

Krebs, T. S., & Johansen, P. Ø. (2013b). Psychedelics and mental health: A population study. *PLOS ONE, 8*(8), e63972.

Latin, D. (2010). *The Harvard Psychedelic Club: How Timothy Leary, Ram Dass, Huston Smith, and Andrew Weil killed the fifties and ushered in a new age for America.* New York: HarperCollins.

Leary, T. (1983). *Flashbacks: An autobiography.* Los Angeles: Tarcher.

Leary, T., Metzner, R., & Alpert, R. (1964). *The psychedelic experience: A manual based on the Tibetan Book of the Dead.* New Hyde Park, NY: University Books.

Lee, M. A., & Shlain, B. (1985). *Acid dreams: The CIA, LSD, and the sixties rebellion.* New York: Grove Press.

Liechti, M. E. (2017). Modern clinical research on LSD. *Neuropsychopharmacology, 42,* 2114–2127.

Liester, M. B. (2014). A review of lysergic acid diethylamide (LSD) in the treatment of addictions: Historical perspectives and future prospects. *Current Drug Abuse Reviews, 7,* 146–156.

Linkletter, A., & Bell, J. N. (1970). We must declare war on drugs. *Good Housekeeping, 170*(4), 94–95, 158, 160–162.

LSD: The exploding threat of the mind drug. (1966, March 25). Retrieved from *www.psychedelic-library.org/magazines/lifelsd.htm*.

Ly, C., Greb, A. C., Cameron, L. P., Wong, J. M., Barragan, E. V., Wilson, P. C., et al. (2018). Psychedelics promote structural and functional neural plasticity. *Cell Reports, 23,* 3170–3182.

Malleson, N. (1971). Acute adverse reactions to LSD in clinical and experimental use in the United Kingdom. *British Journal of Psychiatry, 118,* 229–230.

Mangini, M. (1998). Treatment of alcoholism using psychedelic drugs: A review of the program of research. *Journal of Psychoactive Drugs, 30,* 381–418.

Marks, J. (1991). *The search for the "Manchurian candidate": The CIA and mind control: The secret history of the behavioral sciences* (rev. ed.). New York: Norton. (Original work published 1979)

Martin, D. A., & Nichols, C. D. (2018). The effects of hallucinogens on gene expression. *Current Topics in Behavioral Neuroscience, 36,* 137–158.

Metzner, R. (1968). *The ecstatic adventure.* New York: Macmillan.

Metzner, R. (2017). *Ecology of consciousness: The alchemy of personal, collective, and planetary transformation.* Oakland, CA: New Harbinger.

Mueller, F., Lenz, C., Dolder, P. C., Harder, S., Schmid, Y., Lang, U. E., et al. (2017). Acute effects of LSD on amygdala activity during processing of fearful stimuli in healthy subjects. *Translational Psychiatry, 7*(4), e1084.

Müller, F., Dolder, P. C., Schmidt, A., Liechti, M. E., & Borgwardt, S. (2018). Altered network hub connectivity after acute LSD administration. *NeuroImage: Clinical, 18,* 694–701.

Müller, F., Lenz, C., Dolder, P., Lang, U., Schmidt, A., Liechti, M., et al. (2017). Increased thalamic resting-state connectivity as a core driver of LSD-induced hallucinations. *Acta Psychiatrica Scandinavica, 136,* 648–657.

Nichols, C. D., & Sanders-Bush, E. (2002). A single dose of lysergic acid diethylamide influences gene expression patterns within the mammalian brain. *Neuropsychopharmacology, 26,* 634–642.

Nichols, D. E. (2016). Psychedelics. *Pharmacological Reviews, 68,* 264–355.

Nichols, D. E. (2018a). Chemistry and structure–activity relationships of psychedelics. *Current Topics in Behavioral Neuroscience, 36,* 1–43.

Nichols, D. E. (2018b). Dark classics in chemical neuroscience: Lysergic acid diethylamide (LSD). *ACS Chemical Neuroscience, 9,* 2331–2343.

Nichols, D. E., Frescas, S., Marona-Lewicka, D., & Kurrasch-Orbaugh, D. M. (2002). Lysergamides of isomeric 2,4-dimethylazetidines map the binding orientation of the diethylamide moiety in the potent hallucinogenic agent *N,N*-diethyllysergamide (LSD). *Journal of Medicinal Chemistry, 45,* 4344–4349.

Nichols, D. E., & Grob, C. S. (2018). Is LSD toxic? *Forensic Science International, 284,* 141–145.

Nichols, D. E., & Nichols, C. D. (2008). Serotonin receptors. *Chemical Reviews, 108,* 1614–1641.

Osmond, H. (1957). A review of the clinical effects of psychotomimetic agents. *Annals of the New York Academy of Science, 66,* 418–434.

Osmond, H., & Smythies, J. (1952). Schizophrenia: A new approach. *Journal of Mental Science (British Journal of Psychiatry), 98,* 309–315.

Pahnke, W. N., Kurland, A. A., Unger, S., Savage, C., & Grof, S. (1970). The experimental use of psychedelic (LSD) psychotherapy. *Journal of the American Medical Association, 212,* 1856–1863.

Passie, T. (2019). *The science of microdosing psychedelics.* London: Psychedelic Press.

Passie, T., Halpern, J. H., Stichtenoth, D. O., Emrich, H. M., & Hintzen, A. (2008). The pharmacology of lysergic acid diethylamide: A review. *CNS Neuroscience and Therapeutics, 14,* 295–314.

Preller, K. H., Herdener, M., Pokorny, T., Planzer, A., Kraehenmann, R., Philipp, S., et al. (2017). The fabric of meaning and subjective effects in LSD-induced states depend on serotonin 2A receptor activation. *Current Biology, 27,* 451–457.

Presti, D. E., & Beck, J. E. (2001). Strychnine and other enduring myths: Expert and user folklore surrounding LSD. In T. B. Roberts (Ed.), *Psychoactive sacramentals: Essays on entheogens and religion* (pp. 125–137). San Francisco: Council on Spiritual Practices.

Prochazkova, L., Lippelt, D. P., Colzato, L. S., Kuchar, M., Sjoerd, Z., & Homme, B. (2018). Exploring the effect of microdosing psychedelics on creativity in an open-label natural setting. *Psychopharmacology, 235,* 3401–3413.

Sand, N. (2001). Moving into the sacred world of DMT (Published under the pseudonym: ∞ Ayes). *Entheogen Review, 10*(1), 32–39.

Schindler, E. A. D., Gottschalk, C. H., Weil, M. J., Shapiro, R. E., Wright, D. A., & Sewell, R. A. (2015). Indoleamine hallucinogens in cluster headache: Results of the Clusterbusters medication use survey. *Journal of Psychoactive Drugs, 47,* 372–381.

Schmid, Y., Enzler, F., Gasser, P., Grouzmann, E., Preller, K. H., Vollenweider, F. X., et al.

(2015). Acute effects of lysergic acid diethylamide in healthy subjects. *Biological Psychiatry, 78,* 544–553.

Schmidt, A., Müller, F., Lenz, C., Dolder, P. C., Schmid, Y., Zanchi, D., et al. (2018). Acute LSD effects on response inhibition neuronal networks. *Psychological Medicine, 48,* 1464–1473.

Schultes, R. E., & Hofmann, A. (1979). *Plants of the gods: Origins of hallucinogenic use.* New York: McGraw-Hill.

Schultes, R. E., & Hofmann, A. (1980). *The botany and chemistry of the hallucinogens* (2nd ed.). Springfield IL: Charles C Thomas.

Schultes, R. E., Hofmann, A., & Rätsch, C. (2001). *Plants of the gods: Their sacred, healing, and hallucinogenic powers* (rev. & expanded ed.). Rochester, VT: Healing Arts Press.

Sewell, R. A., Halpern, J. H., & Pope, H. G., Jr. (2006). Response of cluster headache to psilocybin and LSD. *Neurology, 66,* 1920–1922.

Shick, J. F. E., & Smith, D. E. (1970). Analysis of the LSD flashback. *Journal of Psychedelic Drugs, 3*(1), 13–19.

Shulgin, A., & Shulgin, A. (1997). *TiHKAL: The continuation.* Berkeley, CA: Transform Press.

Siff, S. (2015). *Acid hype: American news media and the psychedelic experience.* Champaign: University of Illinois Press.

Stevens, J. (1987). *Storming heaven: LSD and the American dream.* New York: Grove Atlantic.

Stoll, A., & Hofmann, A. (1943). Partialsynthese von Alkaloiden von Typus des Ergobasins. *Helvetica Chimica Acta, 26,* 944–965.

Stoll, W. A. (1947). Lysergsäure-diäthylamid, ein Phantastikum aus der Mutterkorngruppe. *Schweizer Archiv für Neurologie und Psychiatrie, 60,* 279–323.

Strassman, R. J. (1984). Adverse reactions to psychedelic drugs: A review of the literature. *Journal of Nervous and Mental Disease, 172,* 577–595.

Tagliazucchi, E., Roseman, L., Kaelen, M., Orban, C., Muthukumaraswamy, S., Murphy, K., et al. (2016). Increased global functional connectivity correlates with LSD-induced ego dissolution. *Current Biology, 26,* 1043–1050.

Terhune, D. B., Luke, D. P., Kaelen, M., Bolstridge, M., Feilding, A., Nutt, D., et al. (2016). A placebo-controlled investigation of synaesthesia-like experiences under LSD. *Neuropsychologia, 88,* 28–34.

Troxler, F., & Hofmann, A. (1957). Substitutionen am Ringsystem der Lysergsäure: III. Halogenierung. 45. Mitteilung über Mutterkornalkaloide. *Helvetica Chimica Acta, 57,* 2160–2170.

Twarog, B. M. (1988). Serotonin: History of a discovery. *Comparative Biochemistry and Physiology, 91C,* 21–24.

Wacker, D., Wang, C., Katritch, V., Han, G. W., Huang, X. P., Vardy, E., et al. (2013). Structural features for functional selectivity at serotonin receptors. *Science, 340,* 615–619.

Wacker, D., Wang, S., McCorvy, J. D., Betz, R. M., Venkatakrishnan, A. J., Levit, A., et al. (2017). Crystal structure of an LSD-bound human serotonin receptor. *Cell, 168,* 377–389.

Walsh, R., & Grob, C. S. (Eds.). (2005). *Higher wisdom: Eminent elders explore the continuing impact of psychedelics.* Albany: State University of New York Press.

Walterscheid, J. P., Phillips, G. T., Lopez, A. E., Gonsoulin, M. L., Chen, H. H., & Sanchez, L. A. (2014). Pathological findings in 2 cases of fatal 25I-NBOMe toxicity. *American Journal of Forensic Medicine and Pathology, 35,* 20–25.

Wasson, R. G. (1957). Seeking the magic mushroom. *Life, 42*(19), 100–120.

Wasson, R. G., Hofmann, A., & Ruck, C. A. P. (1998). *The road to Eleusis: Unveiling the secret of the Mysteries.* Los Angeles: William Dailey Rare Books. (20th anniversary edition, original work published 1978)

Watts, A. W. (1960). *This is IT: And other essays on Zen and spiritual experience.* New York: Pantheon/Random House.

Watts, A. W. (1962). *The joyous cosmology: Adventures in the chemistry of consciousness.* New York: Pantheon/Random House.

Whitaker-Azmitia, P. M. (1999). The discovery of serotonin and its role in neuroscience. *Neuropsychopharmacology, 21*(Suppl. 2), 2S–8S.

Wolfe, T. (1968). *The electric kool-aid acid test.* New York: Farrar, Straus & Giroux.

Woolley, D. W., & Shaw, E. (1954). A biochemical and pharmacological suggestion about certain mental disorders. *Proceedings of the National Academy of Sciences of the USA, 40,* 228–231.

Yanakieva, S., Polychroni, N., Family, N., Williams, L. T., Luke, D. P., & Terhune, D. B. (2019). The effects of microdose LSD on time perception: A randomized, double-blind, placebo-controlled trial. *Psychopharmacology, 236,* 1159–1170.

CHAPTER 9

Psilocybin

STEPHEN ROSS, SILVIA FRANCO, COLLIN REIFF,
and GABRIELLE AGIN-LIEBES

▓ History, Anthropology, and Ethnobotany

Psilocybin-containing mushrooms are part of a polyphyletic division of Basidiomycota fungi and consist of more than 200 species distributed among the following genera in descending order of prevalence: *Psilocybe, Gymnopilus, Panaeolus, Copelandia, Hypholoma, Pluteus, Inocybe, Conocybe, Panaelina, Gerronema, Agrocybe, Galerina,* and *Mycena* (Guzmán, 2005; Stamets, 1996). Psilocybin-containing mushrooms are most abundant among the Psilocybe genus with approximately 144 species (Guzmán, 2005). The name *psilocybe* is derived from the Greek words *psilo*, meaning "bald," and *cybe*, meaning "head," which refer to the *Psilocybe cubensis* mushroom cap (McGraw, 2004). Psilocybin-containing mushrooms are found on all continents (with predominant concentrations in Latin America and 53 species found in Mexico alone) and grow in the subtropics and tropics, with the majority of species in subtropical humid forests; while *P. cubensis* is commonly found in the tropics and commonly used recreationally, *P. semilanceata* is the most widely distributed psilocybin mushroom in the world, although it is not found in Mexico (Guzmán, Allen, & Gartz, 1998). Psilocybin mushrooms contain psychedelic alkaloids (psilocybin, psilocin), and are known to occasion profound altered states of consciousness (Badham, 1984).

Prehistory

Throughout history, numerous civilizations have consumed psilocybin mushrooms and other psychedelic plants (Stamets, 1996). Prehistoric art from rock formations at the Tassili caves in Algeria (dating as far back as 9,000 years ago) suggest human use of *Psilocybe mairei*, and rock art found in Villar del Humo in Spain suggest use of *Psilocybe hispanica* in rituals dating back 6,000 years (Samorini, 1992). The earliest documented

Psilocybin and psilocin

report of human use of psilocybin-containing mushrooms was 1502, and involved the ritualistic coronation of Montezuma II, the last leader of the Aztecs (Del Pozo, 1975). The Aztecs referred to the mushroom as *teōnanācatl*, translated to "wondrous" or "sacred" mushroom or "God's flesh" (Singer & Smith, 1958). Evidence obtained from archaeological and ethnographic sources (throughout Mexico and parts of Central America, including modern-day Honduras, Guatemala, and El Salvador) revealed hundreds of stone-carved mushroom relics in pre-Colombian Mesoamerican cultures, including the Mayan, Aztecs, Sinus, and Mazatec, dating as far back as 3,500 years (Wasson & Wasson, 1957). It has been proposed that these icons are suggestive of the existence of a religious mushroom cult among these Latin American civilizations, particularly among Mayan and Aztec societies (Carod-Artal, 2015; Wasson, 1962). Yet only in Mexico are psilocybin mushrooms confirmed to have been consumed by humans as visionary sacraments used as part of indigenous religious practice (Badham, 1984).

Suppression of Indigenous Practice

The Spanish Inquisition waged a vigorous holy war against the indigenous use of the psilocybin mushroom, declaring such rituals as heresy and a form of devil worship (Del Pozo, 1975). As a result of the fierce condemnation by Spanish conquerors in the 16th century, Catholic missionaries and priests seized and destroyed artifacts and books in which mushrooms were depicted, and suppression of the practice of sacramental mushroom use included reports of the torture of indigenous practitioners and shamans (Austin, 1967). For the next four centuries, the Indians of Mesoamerica hid their practice of using psilocybin mushrooms for spiritual purposes from the Spanish conquerors. Even though only a handful of relics remain from which to ascertain these ancient practices and beliefs (Del Pozo, 1975), fungi were portrayed prominently in paintings and artifacts that survived the Spanish conquests (Wasson, 1980). Priests and friars accompanying Cortes on his expeditions documented descriptions of unusual ceremonies, many held underground in caves,

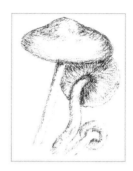

Psilocybe cubensis

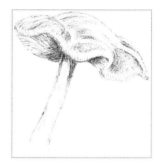

Psilocybe cyanescens

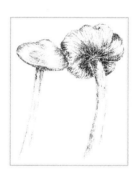

Psilocybe azurescens

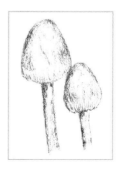

Psilocybe semilanceata

in which Mayan peoples would gather and consume mushrooms, often with honey, followed by periods of dancing, signing, and conversation (Del Pozo, 1975). The primary purpose of these ceremonies was to remedy sickness and to garner vital information from the spirit or underworld (Borhegyi, 1963). Often shamans would ingest the psychedelic fungi in order to acquire knowledge and insights to carry back into the material world (Carod-Artal, 2015).

First Report in the Medical Literature: 1799

The first reliable account in the medical literature describing intoxication with psychedelic mushrooms occurred in October 1799, and was reported by Dr. Everdad Brande, who visited and observed a British family in London whose members experienced visions and hysterical laughter after ingesting wild psilocybin-containing mushrooms, later identified as *P. semilanceata* (Wasson & Wasson, 1957).

Richard Evan Schultes's and the Wassons' Rediscovery of Psilocybin: 1930s–1950s

Nearly all mention of the psychedelic mushroom vanished from the literature until the late 1930s, when a young Harvard-based ethnobotany professor, Richard Evan Schultes, reignited contemporary scholarship in psilocybin mushrooms by conducting systematic anthropological research (Schultes & Farnsworth, 1980). Motivated to identify a unique mushroom specimen (passed onto him by an Austrian enthnobotanist, Blas Pablo Reko) and used by several Mexican Indian tribes, Schultes visited northern Oaxaca in 1938 with Reko. They collected three types of mushrooms on their quests; however, it was not until several years later that the sacred mushroom was correctly identified (Wasson, 1980).

In 1952, New York City–based amateur mycologists, R. Gordon Wasson (an investment banker) and his wife Dr. Valentina Pavlovna Wasson (a pediatrician), picked up where Shultes had left off. The couple received a letter from the poet Robert Graves with information about an enigmatic Mexican mushroom, suggesting the existence of a primitive mushroom cult in Mexico (Wasson, 1980). Motivated by an interest to understand the traditional use of mushrooms around the world, and having discovered the work of Schultes and references in 16th- and 17th-century literature (d'Olwer, 1952), the Wassons proceeded to make several trips to Mexico accompanied by the French mycologist Roger Heim. After two initial trips to Mexico in 1953 and 1954 with Valentina and Heim, Gordon Wasson returned in 1955 with his photographer and managed to obtain a large quantity of *Psilocybe mexicana* (Wasson, 1957). He was also introduced to the esteemed Mazatec shaman (or *curandero*), María Sabina, who agreed to guide Wasson and his photographer through a ceremony that same day, the first outside Westerner to ingest the sacred Mexican mushroom. Wasson reveled in the visionary effects of the mushroom, which seemed to explain why these fungi had been worshiped. Wasson returned again with Heim to participate in an additional ceremony with Sabina in 1955 with *Psilocybe mexicana*. In 1956, Heim identified the psychoactive mushroom that the Wassons discovered as a member of the *Psilocybe* genus, and in May of 1957, Wasson detailed his discovery of the visionary mushroom in an article in *Life* magazine, "Seeking the Magic Mushroom," sparking the public's interest and imagination (Wasson, 1957).

Albert Hofmann and Sandoz Pharmaceuticals: 1957–1965

In 1957, Heim returned home from Mexico with samples of various *Psilocybe* mushrooms, with the goal of extracting and analyzing the psychoactive compounds in their pure form in a laboratory (Wasson & Heim, 1958). After sending several specimens to laboratories in the United States and Paris that were unable to successfully isolate the active components, Heim sent the Swiss chemist Albert Hofmann a large quantity for chemical analysis at the Sandoz laboratories (Hofmann, Frey, Ott, & Troxler, 1958). Hofmann (who previously synthesized and serendipitously discovered the psychedelic properties of lysergic acid diethylamide [LSD]) agreed to take on the project, and Roger Heim sent Albert Hofmann 100 grams of dried mushrooms,

Psilocybe mexicana (Hofmann, 2005). Hofmann extracted two different kinds of crystals from the mushrooms. Through self-experimentation, he determined that these crystals were responsible for the "magical" experiences previously reported by Gordon Wasson. In 1958, Hofmann identified two compounds (psilocybin and psilocin) as the main psychoactive and psychedelic constituents of the mushroom, and in 1959 he first synthesized psilocybin (Hofmann, 1978). Shortly thereafter, the Sandoz laboratories began the synthetic chemical production of psilocybin, eliminating the previously required cultivation of mushrooms for psilocybin. Sandoz began manufacturing and distributing pure synthetic psilocybin pills (under the name Indocybin) to curious physicians and researchers around the world and would do so until recalling the drug in 1965 due to a growing political backlash in the United States (Hofmann, 2005). Sandoz also produced two synthetic drugs derived from mushroom-extracted psilocybin, CZ-74 (4-hydroxy-*N*,*N*-diethyltryptamine) and CEY-19 (4-phosphoryloxy-*N*,*N*-diethyltryptamine), both of which are shorter (approximately 3 hours in duration) acting than psilocybin (Baer, 1967). Interestingly, in 1962, Hofmann brought psilocybin he had synthesized to María Sabina in Oaxaca and according to Sabina, although this synthetic form was slower to become psychoactive, there was no perceptible difference between synthetic psilocybin and ingesting the mushrooms themselves (Hofmann, 1978).

■ Basic Pharmacology

Mode of Administration and Dosage

Psilocybin-containing mushrooms are generally consumed orally; however, intravenous administration of the extracted chemical, psilocybin, has occurred in research settings. The mushrooms can be eaten raw or dried, boiled in water to make tea, or cooked with other foods to cover its bitter flavor. The minimum amount of mushrooms needed to get the desired psychological effect is about 1 g of dried mushrooms or 10 g of fresh mushrooms. However, the dose generally used for recreational purposes is somewhat higher (between 1 and 5 g of dried mushrooms or 10–50 g for fresh mushrooms), with individual metabolism playing a role in determining a person's response to psilocybin (van Amsterdam, Opperhuizen, & van den Brink, 2011). Additionally, the concentration of psilocybin in the mushrooms varies, so dose ranges should be interpreted with caution. As a reference, psilocybin makes up roughly 1% of the weight of a dried *Psilocybe cubensis* mushroom (van Amsterdam et al., 2011). The average dose that induces hallucinogenic effects is 15 mg of oral psilocybin (Beck, Helander, Karlson-Stiber, & Stephansson, 1998; Hasler, Grimberg, Benz, Huber, & Vollenweider, 2004), or a plasma concentration of 4–6 ng/ml of the active metabolite psilocin (Hasler, Bourquin, Brenneisen, Bär, & Vollenweider, 1997). Safety guidelines define high but not medically dangerous doses of oral psilocybin as anything higher than 25 mg (Johnson, Richards, & Griffiths, 2008). In terms of relative potency, psilocybin is approximately 45 times less potent than LSD and 66 times more potent than mescaline (Isbell, 1959; Wolbach, Miner, & Isbell, 1962).

Pharmacokinetics

Psilocybin (4-phosphoryloxy-*N*,*N*-dimethyltryptamine) is a substituted indolealkylamine and belongs to the chemical group of hallucinogenic tryptamines. Psilocybin, considered a prodrug, is rapidly dephosphorylated to psilocin in the intestinal mucosa and liver (by alkaline phosphatase and a nonspecific esterase) before entering the systemic circulation and penetrating into the central nervous system (CNS). Competitive blockade of the dephosphorylation of psilocybin to psilocin abolishes the psychoactive effects of psilocybin (Horita, 1963), confirming that psilocin (*N*,*N*-dimetyltryptamine) is the main psychoactive metabolite and psychedelic substance in hallucinogenic mushrooms (Tyls, Palenicek, & Horacek, 2014). Psilocin is glucuronidated by endoplasmic enzymes uridine 5'-diphospho-glucuronosyltransferase (UDP)-glucuronosyltransferase (UGTs) to psilocin-*O*-glucuronide (Manevski et al., 2010), the main urinary metabolite (Dinis-Oliveira, 2017). Psilocin also undergoes oxidative metabolism with demethylation and deamination to 4-hydroxyindole-

3-yl-acetaldehyde (4-H1A), followed by oxidation to 4-hydroxyindole-3-acetic acid (4-HIAA) and 4-hydroxytryptophol (4-HT) (Hasler et al., 1997; Lindenblatt, Kramer, Holzmann-Erens, Gouzoulis-Mayfrank, & Kovar, 1998; Passie, Seifert, Schneider, & Emrich, 2002). Another potential metabolic pathway involves psilocin oxidation by hydroxyindol oxidases to produce a compound with an iminchinon or o-quinone structure (Kovacic, 2009).

Psilocin has a half-life of 2.5 hours in plasma, and following oral administration of psilocybin in humans, onset of psychoactive/psychedelic effects begin within 20–40 minutes (coinciding with detectable plasma levels of psilocin), with peak concentration and effects between 60 and 90 minutes, followed by an approximate 60-minute plateau before decreasing concentration, and within 6–8 hours, the main effects have mostly disappeared (Hasler et al., 2004). Psilocybin administered intravenously has a much shorter half-life (mean 74.1 ± 19.6 minutes) compared to oral administration and a much shorter duration of action (subjective effects lasting only 15–30 minutes) (Carhart-Harris et al., 2011; Hasler et al., 1997). The elimination of psilocin (mostly glucuronidated metabolites) as well as unaltered psilocybin (3–10%) occurs through the kidneys, with most of the psilocybin excreted within the first 3 hours following oral intake and completely within approximately 24 hours (Grieshaber, Moore, & Levine, 2001; Sticht & Kaferstein, 2000).

Pharmacodynamics, Molecular Effects, and Implications in Treatment

Serotonergic Effects

Psilocin, like all of the classical psychedelics, has a high affinity for serotonin receptors in the brain. It has predominant agonist activity on serotonin 5-HT$_{2A}$, 5-HT$_{2C}$, and 5-HT$_{1A}$ receptors. Preadministration of ketanserin, a 5-HT$_{2A}$ receptor antagonist, abolishes almost all of the psilocin-induced psychedelic effects, supporting the primacy of 5-HT$_{2A}$ receptor activation in mediating its subjective effects (Preller et al., 2016, 2017; Vollenweider, Vollenweider-Scherpenhuyzen, Babler, Vogel, & Hell, 1998). Ad-

ditionally, psilocin interacts to some degree with other serotonin receptors including 5-HT$_{1B}$, 5-HT$_{1D}$, 5-HT$_{1E}$, 5-HT$_{2B}$, 5-HT$_{5A}$, 5-HT$_6$, 5-HT$_7$ (Tyls et al., 2014). Interactions with serotonin receptors are clinically relevant for the treatment of psychiatric disorders. Patients with major depression have increased 5-HT$_{2A}$ receptor density in the prefrontal cortex, which can be reduced by chronic treatment with antidepressants, and the down-regulation of these receptors coincides with the onset of clinical efficacy (Van Oekelen, Luyten, & Leysen, 2003). Additionally fronto-limbic 5-HT$_{2A}$ receptor density is directly correlated with anxiety and difficulty coping with stress (Frokjaer et al., 2008). Various lines of evidence suggest that down-regulation of prefrontal 5-HT$_{2A}$ receptors might underlie some of the therapeutic effects of psilocybin in the treatment of depression and anxiety (Vollenweider & Kometer, 2010).

Dopaminergic Effects

Interactions with nonserotonergic receptors also contribute to the subjective and behavioral effects of psilocybin. One study indicated that psilocybin indirectly increases dopamine concentrations in the striatum, and this increase was correlated with depersonalization and euphoric effects (Vollenweider, Vontobel, Hell, & Leenders, 1999). However, the dopaminergic system contributes just partially to the psilocybin-induced psychological effects, as only about 30% of these symptoms are reduced by haloperidol, a nonselective dopamine receptor antagonist (Vollenweider et al., 1998). Unlike LSD, which binds to D$_2$-like dopamine receptors, psilocybin has no affinity for the dopamine D$_2$ receptors (Marona-Lewicka, Thisted, & Nichols, 2005; Vollenweider & Kometer, 2010). Despite the evidence that classic psychedelics can increase dopamine transmission in striatal areas in humans, they fail to significantly activate the nucleus accumbens in positron emission tomographic (PET) imaging studies, consistent with the lack of evidence linking classical psychedelics with addictive disorders syndromes (Bogenschutz & Ross, 2018; Geyer & Vollenweider, 2008; Vollenweider et al., 1998, 1999), (see the section "Addiction Liability" below).

Glutamatergic and Neurotrophic Effects

Psilocybin also appears to have glutamatergic mechanism of actions. Activation of postsynaptic 5-HT$_{2A}$ receptors located on a subpopulation of pyramidal cells in the deep layers of the prefrontal cortex leads to increase in glutamatergic recurrent network activity (Aghajanian, 2009; Beique, Imad, Mladenovic, Gingrich, & Andrade, 2007; Vollenweider & Kometer, 2010). The increase in glutamatergic synaptic activity engenders activation of α-amino-3-hydroxy-5-methyl-4-isoxazolepropionic acid (AMPA) and N-methyl-D-aspartate (NMDA) receptors on cortical pyramidal neurons, which ultimately leads to increased expression of brain-derived neurotrophic factor (BDNF) (Vollenweider & Kometer, 2010). Neurotrophic factors such as BDNF are molecules involved in neuronal growth and maturation, neuronal survival, synaptic plasticity, and the formation of long-lasting memories (Hardy & Spanos, 2002). Decreased blood levels of neurotrophic factors and reduced expression in the prefrontal cortex and hippocampus have been associated with stress and depression in addition to other mood disorders (Bathina & Das, 2015). Thus, drugs that target neuronal plasticity may offer a novel approach to mood disorder treatment (Vollenweider & Kometer, 2010).

Studies have shown that classical psychedelics are powerful inducers of neuroplasticity and enhance the expression of neurotrophic factors *in vitro* and in animal models (Vollenweider & Kometer, 2010). Similar effects occur with antidepressants, which increase the expression of neurotrophic factors in limbic structures, most notably the hippocampus (Russo-Neustadt, Beard, & Cotman, 1999). However, antidepressant effects by standard pharmacological medications (i.e., selective serotonin reuptake inhibitors [SSRIs]) occur several weeks after starting treatment. An exception to this is ketamine, a dissociative anesthetic that can lead to rapid antidepressant effects after administration (Machado-Vieira, Salvadore, Diazgranados, & Zarate, 2009). Similar to ketamine, there is some evidence that psilocybin may produce rapidly acting antidepressant effects in patients with depressive spectrum disorders (Carhart-Harris et al., 2016; Ross et al., 2016). Psilocybin and ketamine appear to share a common mechanism of action. Like psilocybin and other classical hallucinogens, ketamine modulates glutamatergic neurotransmission in the prefrontal–limbic circuitry, which leads to neuroplastic adaptations and may partially explain the shared rapid antidepressant effects observed in clinical studies with ketamine and psilocybin (Vollenweider & Kometer, 2010). However, unlike ketamine (whose antidepressant effects tend to last no longer than 1–2 weeks) (DeWilde, Levitch, Murrough, Mathew, & Iosifescu, 2015), there is some evidence that psilocybin may produce sustained antidepressant effects lasting several months after single dosing administration (Carhart-Harris et al., 2016; Griffiths et al., 2016; Grob et al., 2011; Ross et al., 2016).

▦ Range of Effects in Humans

Physiological Effects

Psilocybin causes a state of sympathetic arousal, causing mydriasis, increased deep tendon reflexes, and mild-to-moderate increases in respiratory rate, heart rate, blood pressure, and body temperature (Gouzoulis-Mayfrank et al., 1999; Griffiths et al., 2011; Griffiths, Richards, McCann, & Jesse, 2006; Isbell, 1959). In general, the physiological effects are not clinically significant but may cause headache, dizziness, tremors, weakness, yawning, nausea, anorexia, muscle aching, shivering, restlessness, arousal, sweating, abdominal pain, dry mouth or sleep disturbances, in addition to impaired motor coordination and working memory.

Psychological/Subjective Effects

The psychological and experiential effects of psilocybin include significant alterations in perception (i.e., visual and auditory illusions or hallucinations; synesthesia), cognition (i.e., tangential thought processes, dissociative phenomena), and affect (i.e., mood fluctuations ranging from euphoria to extreme anxiety) (Gouzoulis-Mayfrank et al., 1999; Hollister, 1961; Malitz, Esecover, Wilkens, & Hoch, 1960; Vollenweider et al., 1999). The psychological content and emotional tone of the experience with psilocybin can be unpredictable. Its effects are variable and can change rapidly during a single episode of use. The psilocybin-induced experience is greatly influenced by set (mental state, preparation, and intention of the person taking the drug), setting (environment in which the effects are experienced), dose, and route of administration (i.e., oral vs. intravenous) (Johnson et al., 2008). The sum total of the experience can range from positive spiritual or mystical-type experiences associated with enduring positive changes in affect, cognition or behavior, to very unpleasant experiences dominated by dysphoria, fear, and psychotic-like phenomena.

The mystical experience does not refer to supernatural or metaphysical ideas, but to a psychometrically validated description of the psychedelic experience. It is defined by several domains in the Pahnke and Richards Mystical Experience Questionnaire (MEQ), which is based on the classic descriptive work on mystical experiences by William James and the psychology of religion by Stace (1961; Pahnke, 1963, 1969). The MEQ measures core characteristics of the mystical experience: feelings of unity, transcendence of time and space (i.e., time and space have no meaning), noetic quality (sense of encountering ultimate reality that is more real than everyday reality), sacredness (a sense that what is encountered is holy or sacred), positive mood (joy, ecstasy, peace, bliss, tranquility, awe), ineffability (the experience is difficult to put into words), and paradoxicality (i.e., coexistence of mutually exclusive states or concepts). In a confirmatory factor analysis of the 30-item Mystical Experience Questionnaire (MEQ30) that analyzed 184 participants who received moderate to high oral doses of psilocybin (at least 20 mg/70 kg), four main factors were identified: mystical; positive mood; transcendence of time and space; and ineffability. The MEQ30 total score had the greatest predictive validity (compared to the individual factors) in terms of retrospective ratings of psilocybin experiences and persisting effects attributed to these experiences (Barrett, Johnson, & Griffiths, 2015). The MEQ is important to research because psilocybin-induced mystical experiences are associated with abrupt, substantial, and sustained positive changes

in attitudes and behavior (Griffiths et al., 2006, 2016; Griffiths, Richards, Johnson, McCann, & Jesse, 2008; Ross et al., 2016). The mystical experience (as measured by the MEQ) has been shown to partially mediate anxiolytic or antidepressant therapeutic effects of psilocybin in the treatment of patients with cancer-related psychiatric distress (Griffiths et al., 2016; Ross et al., 2016).

In addition to the MEQ, the APZ or Five-Dimensional Altered States of Consciousness Questionnaire (5D-ASC) questionnaire is another standardized scale that has been used to measure altered states of consciousness (ASCs) induced by psilocybin. The APZ comprises three primary dimensions: oceanic boundlessness (OBN), anxious ego dissolution (AED), and visionary restructuralization (VIR) (Dittrich, 1998). OBN reflects a highly pleasurable state of dissolution of self, oneness with the universe, and an experience of transcendence of space and time with emotions of bliss and ecstasy. High OBN scores are indicative of "mystical experiences" as defined by Stace (1961). AED reflects the negative experiences of depersonalization and derealization. It is characterized by disintegration of self, loss of self-control over one's autonomy, feelings of estrangement from the environment, anxiety, panic, and loss of thought and body control. High AED scores can reflect a highly disturbing emotional state, colloquially referred to as a "bad trip" (Preller & Vollenweider, 2018). VIR consists of visual illusions or, more rarely, frank hallucinations. Visions can range from abstract kaleidoscopic images to elaborate dream-like narratives, with vivid imagery often perceived with open and closed eyes. Additionally, this dimension includes synesthesias (the mixing of various sensory stimuli, e.g., hearing colors), changes in the meaning of perception, vivid recollection of memories, and facilitated imagination. Two additional secondary dimensions are acoustic alteration (AA) and vigilance reduction (VR). AA refers to distortions, illusions, and hallucinations in the acoustic sphere, which are usually described as accentuations of external stimuli (i.e., the music being more intensely felt and deeply influencing the experience) and VR depicts dreaminess, reduced alertness, and drowsiness (Preller & Vollenweider, 2018; Studerus, Gamma, & Vollenweider, 2010).

▣ Potential for Adverse Effects: Safety

Physiological Side Effects, Toxicity, and Lethality

Animal studies have demonstrated low levels of medical toxicity associated with psilocybin, with the LD50 in rodents approximately 2,000 to 3,000 times the typical human dose on a mg/kg basis (Efron & Usdin, 1972; Tyls et al., 2014). In expert reviews comparing relative acute toxicity, safety, and addictive potential of 20 psychoactive substances (i.e., opioids, sedative-hypnotics, alcohol, cocaine, tobacco, 3,4-methylenedioxymethamphetamine (MDMA), LSD, and psilocybin), heroin was at the extreme end of most harmful (highest levels of addictive potential and acute toxicity), while psilocybin occupied the least harmful end of the spectrum (Gable, 1993, 2004). Other expert consensus analyses of the relative harms (i.e., physical harm, social harm, addiction potential) of various psychoactive drugs are consistent in finding opioids (i.e., heroin) at the most harmful end of the spectrum and the serotonergic psychedelics toward the least harmful end of the spectrum (Morgan, Noronha, Muetzelfeldt, Feilding, & Curran, 2013; Nutt, King, Saulsbury, & Blakemore, 2007). Psilocybin is an extremely safe drug from the perspective of physiological toxicity when administered to humans and is not associated with major organ system damage (i.e., cardiac, neurological, hepatic, renal), carcinogenicity, teratogenicity, enduring neuropsychological deficits, or overdose deaths (Johnson et al., 2008). In healthy humans without preexisting medical conditions, cardiovascular effects of psilocybin are not expected to cause serious complications. However, transient increases in blood pressure and pulse may be a risk for those with serious cardiovascular conditions (i.e., malignant hypertension, tachyarrythmias). Individuals with serious cardiac comorbidities have been excluded from modern psilocybin clinical trials. Although psilocybin is not known to cause any direct neurological damage, clinical trials so far have excluded participants with CNS involvement (i.e.,

brain tumor), and there has never been a trial using psilocybin to treat a neurological disorder. However, there is no reason to believe that psilocybin is absolutely contraindicated in individuals with CNS pathology and it may be useful for various neuropsychiatric disorders (i.e., psychological distress associated with primary neurological illness). Johns Hopkins is planning a trial of psilocybin treatment in patients with anxiety associated with newly diagnosed Alzheimer's illness (R. Griffiths, personal communication, October 10, 2019).

In terms of overdose risk, the toxicity of psilocybin is extremely low (Johnson et al., 2008). Psilocybin makes up roughly 1% of the weight of *Psilocybe cubensis* mushrooms and nearly 1.7 kg of dried mushrooms (or 17 kg of fresh mushrooms) would be required for a 60-kg person to reach the 280 mg/kg lethal dose, 50% (LD50) rate of rats (van Amsterdam et al., 2011). Despite the low intrinsic toxicity, impaired judgment or reckless behavior may lead to severe and sometimes fatal accidents or legal trouble associated with psilocybin ingestion. A review of the potential harms of recreational psilocybin ingestion indicated that fatal accidents due to exposure to psilocybin are rare and often due to the combination with other drugs, mostly alcohol (van Amsterdam et al., 2011).

Psilocybin administration to carefully screened and monitored participants (ranging from normal volunteers to those with psychiatric disorders) in research settings has an excellent safety record. In the re-emergence of psychedelic research since the early 1990s, over 1,000 doses of psilocybin (ranging from low to high doses) have been administered safely in Europe and the United States at major academic medical centers (University Hospital of Psychiatry Zurich, Johns Hopkins University [JHU], New York University Langone Medical Center [NYULMC], UCLA, University of New Mexico, University of Arizona, Imperial College, University of Alabama, University of California, San Francisco [UCSF]) with no reports of any treatment-related serious adverse events (SAEs), including no reports of serious medical toxicity and no reported cases of prolonged psychosis or hallucinogen persisting perception disorder (HPPD) (see later sections on psychosis and HPPD) (Bogenschutz & Ross, 2018; Studerus, Kometer, Hasler, & Vollenweider, 2011). The key commonality among all these studies is the careful attention to screening (i.e., screening out individuals with psychotic spectrum illnesses or unstable medical conditions), set, setting for dosing sessions, dose, preparation, and integration.

Psychological Distress

Acute adverse psychological experiences ("bad trips") remain the biggest concern in psilocybin administration and typically include anxiety, panic, dysphoria, depersonalization, paranoia, agitation, fear that the experience will never end, or fear of losing one's mind. These negative experiences are more likely to occur in recreational settings, with poorly prepared individuals who use the substance in an uncontrolled setting and have psychological risk factors (e.g., severe mental illness, recent trauma) (Johnson et al., 2008). However, several clinical trials have noted that despite careful participant screening, preparation, and sessions being conducted in a comfortable, well-supervised setting, high doses of psilocybin (i.e., 30 mg/70 kg) can still cause transient episodes of anxiety/dysphoria, extreme fear, or psychotic-like reactions during the session (dos Santos, Bouso, Alcázar-Córcoles, & Hallak, 2018; Griffiths et al., 2006, 2011). During such adverse reactions, however, users usually retain insight into the fact that their symptoms are related to drug ingestion, and they are usually resolved by providing strong interpersonal support. Such difficult and challenging experiences can often have a positive therapeutic valence (Belser et al., 2017; Carbonaro, Johnson, Hurwitz, & Griffiths, 2018; Swift et al., 2017).

Psychosis

The classical psychedelics provide evidence implicating the serotonergic system in the pathophysiology of schizophrenia and related psychotic disorders (Halberstadt & Geyer, 2013; Murray, Paparelli, Morrison, Marconi, & Di Forti, 2013; Szara, 1956). Psilocybin administration can induce a psychotic-like state that mimics certain aspects

of acute and emerging stages of schizophrenia (i.e., paranoia, mood lability, disorganized thought patterns, and visual or auditory disturbances). A pooled analysis of experimental studies with data from 227 psilocybin administrations showed that despite careful preparation and selection of subjects in research studies, a small percentage of participants (about 7%) receiving high-dose psilocybin fulfill the criteria for strong, anxious ego dissolution measures (loss of self-control, thought disorder, arousal, or anxiety) which can be suggestive of acute psychotic reactions (Studerus et al., 2011). However, these reactions were confined to the acute phase of psilocybin administration and were readily managed by providing interpersonal support without psychopharmacological intervention. In that same study, follow-up questionnaires found no persisting perceptual disorders, prolonged psychotic reactions, precipitation of schizophrenia spectrum disorders or other long-term impairments of functioning in any of the subjects. An epidemiological study that analyzed data from 135,000 people, who took part in the U.S. National Survey on Drug Use and Health (NSDUH) from 2008 to 2011, Johansen and Krebs (2015) found that individuals with a lifetime use history of three classic psychedelics (LSD, psilocybin, or mescaline) were not at increased risk of developing 11 indicators of mental health problems including schizophrenia and other psychotic-spectrum disorders, as well as anxiety and depressive disorders and suicide attempts. Despite this, given that psilocybin and other classic psychedelics are known to exacerbate psychosis in individuals with psychotic spectrum illnesses, all modern human psychedelic clinical trials at academic medical centers have excluded individuals with psychotic spectrum illness (i.e., schizophrenia, schizoaffective disorder, bipolar I with psychotic features) or those with a known positive family history of psychotic or bipolar I illnesses (Bogenschutz & Ross, 2018).

HPPD

HPPD is an uncommon clinical disorder that occurs within a certain time frame after cessation of the use of a psychedelic or other drugs such as MDMA, ketamine, and cannabis (Lerner et al., 2002). It encompasses a range of perceptual disturbances, mostly visual, that are reminiscent of those generated by the use of hallucinogenic substances. Examples include geometric hallucinations, halos or auras surrounding objects, trails following objects in motion, illusion of movement in a static setting, intensified colors, macropsia, and micropsia. The symptoms can occur spontaneously or be triggered by stress, anxiety, exercise, fatigue, entering into a dark environment, or use of another drug (i.e., cannabis, alcohol) (Abraham, 1983). It is important to rule out other conditions with perceptual disturbances such as visual seizures (i.e., occipital or temporal–occipital lobe epilepsy), migraine with aura, brain tumor, head trauma, delirium, dementia, psychotic spectrum illnesses, and hypogognic or hypnopompic hallucinations. It appears that it is more likely to occur in individuals with chronic use of hallucinogens, use of other substances with hallucinogens (i.e., cannabis, MDMA, alcohol), or those with co-occurring psychiatric illness such as a panic disorder or major depressive disorder (Halpern & Pope, 2003; Johnson et al., 2008; Studerus et al., 2011).

There are two proposed types of HPPD, Type 1 and Type 2. Type 1 consists of brief reexperiences ("flashbacks") of changes in perception (usually involving the visual system), mood, or consciousness as previously experienced during psychedelic intoxication that can occur days to months after the psychedelic use (Halpern, Lerner, & Passie, 2018). The time course of the illness is typically self-limited with diminutions in duration, frequency and intensity of symptoms over time (Holland & Passie, 2011). Type 2 HPPD is a more chronic form of the illness with constant or near-constant distortions in the visual system, typically including halos (i.e., glow surrounding objects), trails (i.e., afterimages following sight of moving objects), visual snow (i.e., TV static-like graininess superimposed on the visual field), and palinopsia (i.e., persistent perception of a removed object). These chronic visual distortions tend to be experienced as disturbing, can adversely affect function and quality of life, and are often accompanied by depersonalization, derealization, depression, or anxiety (Holland & Passie, 2011).

It is important to note that HPPD is not a psychotic spectrum illness, and patients have intact reality testing and awareness that the illusions and hallucinations are not real (Bogenschutz & Ross, 2018). The exact prevalence of HPPD is unclear; however, it is thought to be a rare condition (especially Type 2) given the relatively few cases reported out of the tens of millions of doses of hallucinogens used over the last 50 years, and it appears to be significantly less common in research settings with careful screening and preparation (Halpern & Pope, 2003; Johnson et al., 2008; Studerus et al., 2011). In two recent Web-based surveys of psychedelic users, persisting visual distortions and illusions were commonly reported, but only 4–11% reported being distressed by these experiences (Baggott, Coyle, Erowid, Erowid, & Robertson, 2011; Carhart-Harris & Nutt, 2010). Data from a U.S. population study derived from the 2001–2004 NSDUH found no association between lifetime use of serotonergic hallucinogens and past-year visual phenomena consistent with HPPD (Krebs & Johansen, 2013).

The pathophysiology of HPPD is unclear. However, it has been proposed that HPPD represents a type of misbalance between excitatory and inhibitory input in the visual system at the cortical level, and that the various types of visual disturbances are due to increases in glutamatergic excitation, decreases in γ-aminobutyric acid (GABA)ergic inhibition, or some combination of the two (Kilpatrick & Ermentrout, 2012; Litjens, Brunt, Alderliefste, & Westerink, 2014). Abraham and Aldridge (1993) proposed that damage to inhibitory cortical interneurons in the occipital lobe (which expresses 5-HT_{2A} receptors and releases GABA upon activation) may play a role in HPPD symptoms due to a deficit in inhibitory functions.

Regarding treatments for HPPD, there is no established evidence-based pharmacological or psychosocial algorithm. Treatment recommendations are based almost entirely on noncontrolled studies of small patient populations or single-case reports (Orsolini et al., 2017). Supportive and cognitive-behavioral therapies (CBTs) are warranted to help individuals cope and adapt to their symptoms. Type 1 HPPD tends to remit without formal treatment or through brief supportive psychotherapy. Type 2 HPPD is typically treated with pharmacological interventions, in addition to supportive psychotherapy and CBT. However, there are no controlled trials of pharmacological or psychosocial treatments for HPPD, and there is no established best practices pharmacological treatment algorithm. In line with the proposed neurobiological mechanism of HPPD involving disturbances of excitatory and inhibitory function in the occipital cortex, medications that increase GABAergic tone and decrease glutamatergic hyperexcitability have been shown to be helpful pharmacological treatments. Benzodiazepines (GABA A agonists), both at low and high doses, have been shown to ameliorate some symptoms of HPPD without leading to disease remission (Lerner, Rudinski, & Bor, 2014; Lerner, Skladman, Kodesh, Sigal, & Shufman, 2001). Their efficacy may be related to their action at cortical serotonergic inhibitory interneurons with GABAergic outputs (Abraham, 2000). Additionally, the visual disturbances with sudden paroxysmal onset seen in patients with HPPD have been interpreted as akin to visual seizures and prompted the use of antiepileptic drugs as pharmacological treatments, especially if the visual disturbances are accompanied by co-occurring mood disorders (Martinotti et al., 2018). Lamotrigine (at 200–300 mg daily dosing) was shown to ameliorate HPPD symptomatology in a recent severe case of HPPD with some electroencephalographic (EEG) abnormalities (Anderson, Lake, & Walterfang, 2018), as well as a case of HPPD resistant to treatment with risperidone and antidepressants (Hermle, Simon, Ruchsow, & Geppert, 2012). Lamotrigine acts by blocking sodium and voltage-gated calcium channels and inhibiting glutamate-mediated excitatory neurotransmission, thereby suggesting its potential use in the treatment of HPPD (Hermle et al., 2012). There is some evidence that phenytoin (which in addition to inhibiting sodium channels also increases CNS GABA levels and potentiates GABA-mediated postsynaptic inhibition) decreases symptoms of HPPD; however, its side ef-

fect profile limits its use (Martinotti et al., 2018; Thurlow & Girvin, 1971). There is some evidence to suggest that levetiracetam (an antiepileptic drug) could reduce some visual symptoms as well as HPPD-related depersonalization and derealization (Casa & Bosio, 2005). Other antiepileptic drugs such as valproic acid, carbamazepine, oxcarbazepine, gabapentin, and topiramate may be useful (Martinotti et al., 2018).

There is some evidence supporting the use of first-generation antipsychotics in treating symptoms of HPPD, although adverse side effect profiles (i.e., tardive dyskinesia) limit their use, and exacerbation of flashbacks in the early phases of treatment with haloperidol may occur (Anderson & O'Malley, 1972; Lerner, 2017; Lerner et al., 2002; Moskowitz, 1971). The use of second-generation antipsychotics in patients with HPPD without comorbid psychotic disorders is debated. It was hypothesized that risperidone (a potent antagonist of postsynaptic 5-HT_2 and dopamine D_2 receptors) (Orsolini et al., 2016) might be efficacious in treating HPPD, as 5-HT_2 receptor antagonists are effective in treating hallucinations in schizophrenia. However, most studies report a worsening of HPPD symptomatology (particularly visual disturbances, as well as worsening anxiety), with symptoms returning to baseline after risperidone discontinuation (Lerner et al., 2014; Martinotti et al., 2018; Orsolini et al., 2017). A case report described an improvement in HPPD symptomatology with a combination of sertraline and risperidone (Espiard, Lecardeur, Abadie, Halbecq, & Dollfus, 2005).

The data on the utility of SSRIs to ameliorate symptoms of HPPD are mixed, with some data supporting their efficacy (Aldurra & Crayton, 2001; Young, 1997), and some suggesting a worsening of symptoms (Markel, Lee, Holmes, & Domino, 1994). Symptom alleviation has been reported in some patients treated with presynaptic α_2 adrenergic agonists such as clonidine, suggesting a possible role of sympathetic nervous system activation in the pathophysiology of HPPD (Lerner et al., 2002, 2014; Martinotti et al., 2018); however, one study reported clonidine to be ineffective (Hermle, Simon, Ruschow, Batra, & Geppert, 2013).

Addiction Liability

Although classical psychedelics (including psilocybin) are classified as Schedule 1 drugs (i.e., highest addictive liability), they are not typically considered drugs of addiction, as they are not capable of producing sufficient reinforcing effects to produce addiction (O'Brien, 2005; Ross & Peselow, 2012). They engender rapid tachyphylaxis, can produce unreliable experiences that may be profoundly unpleasant and frightening, are not associated with a known withdrawal syndrome, are rarely used on a daily basis, and do not normally lead to compulsive drug-seeking behavior (Fantegrossi, Murnane, & Reissig, 2008; Ross, 2012). Drugs capable of producing addiction tend to substantially increase extracellular dopamine (DA) levels in the nucleus accumbens (Baler & Volkow, 2006), and psilocybin lacks affinity for DA receptors or the DA transporter, and it does not directly affect dopaminergic transmission (Passie et al., 2002). Even though classic hallucinogens indirectly increase DA transmission in striatal areas in humans, they fail to significantly activate the nucleus accumbens in PET imaging studies, consistent with the lack of evidence linking classical hallucinogens with addiction syndromes (Bogenschutz & Ross, 2018; Ross, 2012). Animal models (i.e., self-administration, conditioned place preference) have also failed to reliably demonstrate clear rewarding potential of psychedelics, suggesting that they do not possess sufficient pharmacological properties to initiate or maintain addiction (Deneau, Yanagita, & Seevers, 1969; Fantegrossi et al., 2008; Passie et al., 2002; Ross, 2012). Pooled data from eight double-blind, placebo-controlled experimental studies conducted between 1999 and 2008, with a total of 110 healthy subjects who had received one to four oral doses of psilocybin (45–315 µg/kg body weight) showed that the administration of psilocybin to healthy volunteers within an experimental setting did not increase the risk for subsequent abuse of psilocybin or other illicit drugs (Studerus et al., 2011). In addition to the lack of biological evidence, epidemiological studies have also failed to reliably demonstrate support for psilocybin addiction or dependence syndromes (Bogenschutz & Ross, 2018; Ross, 2012).

▇ Early-Phase Clinical Research with Psilocybin: 1959–1977

Promising early-phase clinical research with serotonergic psychedelics (conducted from the late 1950s through the mid-1970s on over 40,000 participants and producing thousands of scientific papers) was halted before any definitive conclusions could be reached concerning the clinical efficacy of psychedelic therapy for any psychiatric disorder (Grinspoon & Bakalar, 1979). However, clinical research conducted in that era (mostly with LSD) strongly suggested therapeutic signals of psychedelic-assisted psychotherapy, with data strongest for the treatment of alcoholism and cancer-related psychological and existential distress (Bogenschutz & Ross, 2018).

In 1959, the first publications documenting the administration of psilocybin to animals (Delay, Pichot, Lempêrière, & Quetin, 1959), normal human volunteers (Isbell, 1959), and in clinical populations ("convulsive neurosis") (Delay et al., 1959) appeared in the medical literature. Early researchers with psilocybin studied the effects of the drug without understanding the important influences of set and setting (Hollister, 1961; Malitz et al., 1960). Over time, the importance of preparation, support during sessions with dyad therapy clinicians, the use of supportive environments (i.e., living-room-like setting), and integration was introduced and led to decreased adverse psychological reactions and reports of positively valued experiences (Metzner, Litwin, & Weil, 1965; Pahnke, 1969). From 1959 to 1977, psilocybin was studied to treat a variety of clinical populations in psychiatry, with some data suggesting positive effects in neurotic spectrum disorders (Grinspoon & Bakalar, 1979), as well as childhood treatment-resistant autism and schizophrenia (Fisher, 1970). Except for some studies (Duke & Keeler, 1968; Pahnke, 1969; Rynearson, Wilson, & Bickford, 1968), most of the clinical trials with psilocybin did not include a comparison or control group. Psilocybin (at low doses) was investigated (predominantly in Europe) as a means of facilitating psychotherapy ("psycholytic therapy"), especially combined with pychoanalytically oriented treatments (popular in the 1960s), to treat anxiety, depressive, and somatoform spectrum disorders (Leuner, 1962). Approximately 2,000 participants underwent psychedelic and psycholytic psychotherapy during this first phase of clinical research with psilocybin (Metzner, 2005).

The Harvard Psilocybin Project: 1960–1962

In 1960, after reading and being captivated by the Wassons' article in *Life* magazine, Timothy Leary (a professor of psychology at Harvard responsible for developing *The Interpersonal Diagnosis of Personality*) ingested psychedelic mushrooms he had purchased from a shaman in Toluca, Mexico (Greenfield, 2006; Hofmann, 2005). Inspired by what he described as the deepest religious experience of his life, he decided to devote his energy to investigating psilocybin and other hallucinogens. After returning to Harvard in 1960, Leary started the Harvard Psilocybin Project with his colleague, Richard Alpert (who later changed his name to Ram Dass after a spiritual journey to India), to study the psychological and spiritual properties of psilocybin and other psychedelic substances. Leary and Alpert began to receive synthetic psilocybin from Sandoz, and their work with psilocybin commenced (Hofmann, 2005). The two most significant trials with psilocybin conducted by the Harvard Psilocybin Project group were the Good Friday Experiment and the Concord Prison Experiment (see details below).

On March 28, 1962, *The Harvard Crimson* reported that George A. Michael, the deputy commissioner of the Massachusetts State Health Department, believed that psilocybin fell into the classification of drugs that must be administered by a physician (Greenfield, 2006). Michael started an inquiry into Leary and Alpert's psilocybin research. In an effort to learn more about psilocybin and recent events at Harvard, the state narcotics office, the U.S. Food and Drug Administration (FDA), and the Federal Bureau of Investigation (FBI) began interviewing Timothy Leary and Richard Alpert. In an effort to protect its faculty from a larger investigation, Harvard took matters into its own hand and created strict regulations for psilocybin research, including the prohibition of administering psychedelics to undergraduates at Harvard. Leary

agreed to hand over his remaining supply of psilocybin pills to Dr. Dana Farnsworth, a psychiatrist and head of Harvard University Health Services. Leary no longer had immediate access to psilocybin. However, he continued his research with psychedelics using compounds that were readily available: LSD and dimethyltryptamine (DMT). Following a series of disagreements with the Harvard administration (including reports of administration of psychedelics to undergraduates at Harvard), and after abandoning his classes for other endeavors, Timothy Leary was fired from Harvard's faculty in the Spring of 1963 (Greenfield, 2006). Leary moved to the Hitchcock Estate in Millbrook, New York, with his colleague Richard Alpert, and psilocybin gradually made its way from the research laboratory to the mainstream (Lee & Shlain, 1992). Psilocybin became heavily associated with LSD and the American counterculture movement.

Prohibition and the Controlled Substance Act of 1970

In response to concerns about an increase in recreational use and associated harms, the United States began to restrict the use of psilocybin by the general public. In 1966, U.S. laws were passed that prohibited the production, trade, and ingestion of psychedelic drugs, and in that same year Sandoz terminated production of psilocybin and LSD. Further backlash occurred against psychedelic drugs, leading Nixon to declare war on drugs and to declare Timothy Leary "the most dangerous man in America." In 1970, Congress passed the Controlled Substance Act (CSA) and all serotonergic psychedelics (including psilocybin) were classified in the most restrictive category as U.S. Drug Enforcement Administration (DEA) Schedule 1 drugs (by definition highest addictive liability and no known medical utility) (Bogenschutz & Ross, 2018). Due to legal restrictions and stigma, federal funding (mostly through the National Institute of Mental Health (NIMH), which had amounted to several million dollars funding psychedelic research in this first wave of research) ended for clinical research with psychedelics. Subsequently, scientists working in this area were marginalized and had to abandon their efforts.

Evidence-Based Clinical Applications for Psilocybin Therapy: A New Wave of Psychedelic Research

After a quiescent period of about two decades, human research with the classical psychedelics resumed in the early 1990s with Rick Strassman's studies of the subjective and physiological effects of intravenous DMT on normal volunteers. In the late 1990s, after almost three decades of minimal psilocybin research in humans, researchers in Europe (predominantly conducted by Franz Vollenweider at the University of Zurich in Switzerland) began conducting research with psilocybin on humans as a drug model for understanding part of the neurobiology of schizophrenia (Salomé, Boyer, & Fayol, 2000; Vollenweider et al., 1999). This slowly led to translational research projects that raised questions about the therapeutic potential of psychedelics within psychiatry (Griffiths et al., 2006; Hasler et al., 2004). Shortly after the turn of the 21st century, psilocybin once again entered therapeutic clinical trials and rekindled the flames of psychedelic research. In the past decade, clinical trials have resumed, investigating the effects of psilocybin in the treatment of various psychiatric illnesses (i.e., cancer-related psychiatric disorders, treatment-resistant depression, obsessive–compulsive disorder [OCD]) and addictive disorders (i.e., alcohol, nicotine, cocaine). The studies that have been completed to date are open-label or randomized controlled trials (RCTs) with small sample sizes, and although the results have been very promising, they are not sufficient to definitively establish treatment efficacy.

Cancer-Related Psychiatric and Existential Distress

In the past decade of clinical research with psilocybin, the most studied indication and the one with the most robust data from Phase II RCTs is the use of classic psychedelics to treat cancer-related psychiatric disorders. Two recently published review articles (Reiche et al., 2018; Ross, 2018) identified 10 peer-reviewed published clinical trials (N = 445) in which participants with advanced or terminal cancer-related psychiatric disorders were treated with a classical psychedelic (i.e., LSD, psilocybin, dipropyltryptamine [DPT]): six open-label trials (N = 341) published between 1964 and 1980, and four RCTs (N = 104) published between 2011 and 2016. Across the 10 trials, six examined the therapeutic use of LSD (N = 323) (Gasser et al., 2014; Grob et al., 2011; Kast, 1966, 1967; Kast & Collins, 1964; Pahnke, Kurland, Goodman, & Richards, 1969), three studied treatment with psilocybin (N = 92) (Griffiths et al., 2016; Grob et al., 2011; Ross et al., 2016), and one examined the use of DPT (N = 30) (Richards, 1980).

The RCTs examining psilocybin-assisted psychotherapy to treat psychological (e.g., depression, anxiety) and existential (e.g., demoralization) distress associated with advanced or terminal cancer have been conducted in the United States at University of California Los Angeles (UCLA), the New York University Langone Medical Center (NYULMC), and Johns Hopkins University (JHU) Medical Center. The three RCTs were similar in the following ways: (1) double-blind design methodology; (2) use of active placebo control; (3) use of validated outcome measures; (4) randomization among groups; (5) administration of single, moderate-to-high-dose oral psilocybin; (6) psychiatric exclusion criteria relating to major mental illness, in particular psychotic spectrum illnesses (e.g., schizophrenia, schizoaffective disorder, bipolar I disorder) or a family history of these disorders; (7) crossover methodology; (8) preparation for the experimental sessions by trained psychotherapists (as part of a dyad therapy team), including (9) a life review and review of their cancer diagnosis and its negative psychological and existential impact; (10) instruction set to participants designed to increase the likelihood of inducing mystical state (i.e., participants instructed to lie supine on a couch with eyeshades on to reduce external visual distractions, and to focus on their inner experiences while a preselected music program played throughout the medication session); (11) dosing sessions conducted in a comfortable living-room-like setting designed for maximal safety and comfort; and (12) postintegrative psychotherapy after the dosing sessions (Ross, 2018). The three trials differed in the following ways: (1) active control—niacin at NYU and UCLA versus low-dose psilocybin at JHU; (2) dose of psilocybin—UCLA (0.2 mg/kg) versus. JHU (0.31 mg/kg) and NYU (0.3 mg/kg); (3) inclusion of non-terminally ill cancer patients—at JHU and NYU versus only terminally ill cancer patients at UCLA; (4) typology of cancer-related psychiatric distress—mostly anxiety at UCLA and NYU versus mix of anxiety and depression at JHU.

The first RCT to assess the efficacy of psilocybin-assisted psychotherapy in patients with cancer-related psychological distress occurred at UCLA in a crossover trial that included 12 participants with terminal cancer and a DSM-IV diagnosis of adjustment disorder with anxiety, anxiety disorder due to cancer, acute stress disorder, or generalized anxiety disorder (Grob et al., 2011). Participants were administered two treatment sessions, one with psilocybin (0.2 mg/kg) and the other with placebo (niacin 250 mg) in random order, spaced 2 weeks apart (at which point the crossover occurred). The primary measures were the Beck Depression Inventory (BDI), the Profile of Mood States (POMS), and the State–Trait Anxiety Inventory (STAI) administered the day before each experimental session, at the conclusion of/1-day after/2 weeks after each experimental session, and subsequently at 1-month intervals after the final experimental session up to 6 months. Psilocybin produced mystical-type experiences with substantial subjective differences between the psilocybin and placebo experiences as measured by the 5D-ASC, particularly VIR ($F_{1,11}$ = 18.95; p = .001) and OB ($F_{1,11}$ = 33.12; p < .001). Although there were no statistically significant between-group differences prior to the crossover, there was a significant decrease in the self-report STAI Trait score for the entire 6-month follow-up that reached significance at 1 month (p = .001), and 3 months (p = .03) after the second treatment session. There was not a significant decrease in STAI State score at any time point. BDI scores dropped by almost 30% one month after the second treatment session (p = .05), a difference that was sustained and reached significance at 6-month follow-up (p = .03) (Grob et al., 2011). The failure to find between-group differences in anxiety and depression between the psilocybin and niacin groups prior to the crossover was likely a result of the study being underpowered in terms of dose and sample size.

The NYULMC trial (Ross et al., 2016) compared single-dose psilocybin (0.3 mg/kg) and single-dose niacin (250 mg), administered in conjunction with a psychotherapy platform that included elements of the following types of psychotherapies: supportive, cognitive-behavioral, psychodynamic, existential. The trial included a crossover design (at 7 weeks post dose 1) with the final outcome assessment at 6.5 months post dose 2 (i.e., after the crossover). It recruited 29 individuals with life-threatening cancers (with nearly two-thirds with advanced-stage cancer) with the following breakdown of psychiatric disorders: adjustment disorder with anxiety (N = 18, 62%); adjustment disorder with anxiety and depression (N = 8, 28%); and generalized anxiety disorder (N = 3, 10%). The main therapeutic outcome variables measuring cancer-related depression and anxiety were the following self-rated measures: Hospital Anxiety and Depression Scale (HADS), BDI, and STAI. There were no medical or psychiatric SAEs reported. The most scientifically rigorous findings were demonstrated prior to the crossover in comparing the psilocybin dose 1 to niacin dose 1 groups, where psilocybin produced rapid (e.g., measured from 1 day prior to 1 day postdosing), substantial (i.e., large effect sizes) and sustained (up to 7-weeks post single dosing) improvements in depressive and anxiety symptoms associated with cancer. These improvements were clinically significant. For instance, at 7 weeks post dose 1: 83% of subjects in the psilocybin dose 1 group (compared to 14% in the niacin dose 1 group) met criteria for antidepressant response (i.e., ≥50% decrease relative to baseline with the BDI) and 58% of participants in the psilocybin dose 1 group met criteria for an anxiolytic response (i.e., ≥50% decrease relative to baseline) using the HADS Anxiety subscale (compared to 14% in the niacin first group). Although it is not possible to attribute enduring clinical improvements in depression or anxiety to psilocybin after the crossover, this study reported anxiolytic or anti-depressant response rates of 60–80% at the 6.5-month final follow-up assessment. In terms of secondary outcome measures, prior to the crossover (at 2 weeks post dose 1), psilocybin produced statistically significant improvements in: cancer-related demoralization, hopelessness, quality of life, and spiritual well-being. At the final 6.5-month follow-up, in addition to sustained improvements in spiritual well-being, quality of life, and existential distress (demoralization, hopelessness), there was an improvement in a measure of attitudes toward death and dying (although there were no acute or longer-term improvements in a death anxiety measure). Participants rated the psilocybin experience as being one of the most significant events of their lives: 52 and 70% rated the experience as the singular or among the top 5 most spiritual or meaningful experience of their entire lives, respectively. Compared to the placebo group, psilocybin produced mystical-type experiences consistent with prior trials of psilocybin administration in normal volunteers (Griffiths et al., 2006, 2008, 2011) and terminally ill cancer patients (Grob et al., 2011). The psilocybin-induced mystical experience was found to both correlate with and partially mediate the anxiolytic and antidepressant effects of psilocybin (Ross et al., 2016).

From 2007 to 2014, Roland Griffiths at JHU Medical Center conducted a similar but larger study investigating the effects of psilocybin for the treatment of depression and anxiety in patients with life-threatening cancer ($N = 51$) who met DSM-IV criteria for a mood or anxiety disorder (Griffiths et al., 2016). The study design was a double-blind, randomized crossover that comprised two psilocybin sessions, one high dose (22 or 30 mg/70 kg), and one low dose (1 or 3 mg/70 kg) active-control session. Crossover from high dose to low dose, and vice versa, occurred 5 weeks after the first session. The primary outcome measures were the GRID-HAMD-17, and the Hamilton Anxiety Rating Scale (HAM-A) conducted at baseline, 5 weeks after each session and 6 months after the second session. Included were 51 participants with life-threatening cancers and the following psychiatric disorders: major depressive disorder (MDD; $N = 14$; 27%); adjustment disorder with anxiety ($N = 11$, 22%); adjustment disorder with anxiety and depression ($N = 11$, 22%); generalized anxiety disorder (GAD; $N = 5$, 9.8%); MDD and GAD ($N = 4$, 7.8%); and GAD and dysthymic disorder ($N = 1$, 1.9%). Similar to the UCLA and NYULMC trials, there were no medical or psychiatric SAEs in this trial attributable to psilocybin, further demonstrating the safety of administering psilocybin to a population of patients with advanced or life-threatening cancers. The most rigorous findings (prior to the crossover at 5 weeks) were that high-dose psilocybin produced substantial (i.e., large effect sizes) and sustained (up to 5 weeks post single dosing) improvements in cancer-related anxiety and depressive symptoms. These improvements were of considerable clinically significant. For instance, at 5 weeks postsession-1, 76% of participants in the high-dose-group 1 met criteria for a clinically significant anxiolytic response rate (as measured with the HAM-A) compared to 24% in the low-dose-group 1, and 92% of participants in the high-dose-group 1 demonstrated a clinically significant antidepressant response (i.e., ≥50% improvement relative to baseline scores) on the GRID-HAMD-17 compared to a 32% response rate in the low-dose-group 1. At the final 6-month follow-up assessment, collapsed across the two dose sequence groups, the overall clinical response rate for depression and anxiety and depression was 78% and 83%, respectively, and the overall rates of symptom remission for depression and anxiety and depression were 65% and 57%, respectively. Moreover, the trial reported that prior to the crossover (at 5 weeks), high-dose psilocybin produced improvements in death acceptance, life meaning, optimism, and quality of life, all of which were sustained at the final 6-month follow-up assessment. Subjects rated the psilocybin experience as being one of the most significant events of their lives: 70% and 67% rated the experience as the singular or top five most spiritually significant or personally meaningful experience of their entire lives, respectively. Similar to the NYULMC trial, the psilocybin-induced mystical experience was found to both correlate with and to partially mediate the antidepressant and anxiolytic effects of psilocybin (Griffiths et al., 2016).

Addiction

Tobacco

Starting in 2007, Matthew Johnson at JHU began the first ever investigation of psilocybin-assisted psychotherapy (with a CBT platform) for the treatment of tobacco use disorder in individuals with an intention to quit smoking (N = 15). The study design was open-label and included participants being administered moderate and high doses of psilocybin (20mg/70 kg or 30mg/70 kg) over two or three sessions during a 15-week combination treatment that comprised four weekly preparatory meetings integrating CBT, elements of mindfulness training, and guided imagery for smoking cessation (Johnson, Garcia-Romeu, Cosimano, & Griffiths, 2014). The moderate dose of psilocybin was given in the fifth week of treatment, and the high dose of psilocybin was given approximately 2 weeks after the moderate dose. Before each psilocybin session, participants repeated their brief motivational statement for smoking cessation. Abstinence was biologically verified with exhaled carbon monoxide and urinary cotinine levels. At the 6-month follow-up, 12/15 (80%) participants were abstinent; at the 12-month follow-up, 10/15 (67%) participants were abstinent; and at the 2.5-year follow-up, 9/12 (75%) participants were abstinent (Johnson et al., 2014, 2017). This success rate far exceeds those seen in clinical trials of any currently available medications for tobacco addiction. Psilocybin-induced mystical experiences, as well measures of personal meaning and spiritual significance attributed to the sessions were significantly correlated with positive smoking outcomes (Garcia-Romeu et al., 2014). Based on these very promising results, a comparative efficacy trial (psilocybin vs. nicotine replacement) is now being conducted at the JHU School of Medicine (NCT01943994) that will include 95 participants and is estimated to be completed December 2022. will likely be completed by December 2022 (M. Johnson, personal communication, 2018). The trial includes a functional magnetic resonance imaging (fMRI) neuroimaging component to assess functional and structural changes that may be induced by psilocybin and that may correlate with clinical outcomes.

Alcohol

From the 1950s to the early 1970s, alcoholism was the most studied disease utilizing psychedelic therapy, with thousands of patients treated in clinical settings and over 30 publications reported in the medical literature of LSD treatment for alcoholism (Abuzzahab & Anderson, 1971; Dyck, 2006; Grinspoon & Bakalar, 1979; Halpern, 1996; Mangini, 1998). The results were mixed, and a clear treatment effect was not established. However, in a contemporary meta-analysis, Krebs and Johansen (2012) examined six RCTs (Hollister, Shelton, & Krieger, 1969; Ludwig & Levine, 1965; Pahnke, Kurland, Unger, Savage, & Grof, 1971; Smart, Storm, Baker, & Solursh, 1966; Tomsovic & Edwards, 1970) of single-dose LSD therapy versus single-dose placebo for alcoholism that reported on alcohol drinking outcomes. The meta-analysis reported that treatment effects were significant at the first posttreatment follow-up period: 59% of the LSD-treated group was significantly improved compared to 38% of the control group (odds ratio 1.96; p = .0003), and these effects remained significant until the 6-month follow-up point.

This historical and positive data suggesting efficacy of LSD-assisted therapy for alcoholism set the stage for the reemergence of research using psychedelic therapy to treat alcohol use disorders. In 2015, Michael Bogenschutz and colleagues (at the University of New Mexico) published the first trial investigating the efficacy of psilocybin coupled with a psychosocial intervention (motivational interviewing) for the treatment of alcohol use disorder in patients who met DSM-IV criteria for alcohol dependence with at least two heavy drinking days in the past 30 days (N = 10). The open-label study design included 14 sessions: seven sessions of motivational enhancement therapy (MET), two psilocybin sessions, three preparation sessions, and two debriefing session. The first psilocybin session (0.3 mg/kg) occurred after the fourth psychosocial session (at week 4 of the trial), and the second psilocybin session (0.4 mg/kg) occurred four sessions after the first psilocybin session. Pre–post significant improvements in abstinence occurred acutely after receiving the first dose of psilocybin (p < .05), and these improvements were maintained at final follow-up at 36 weeks. The intensity of the first psilocybin session correlated with decreases in cravings, increases in abstinence self-efficacy during week 5, and decreased drinking between weeks 5 and 8 (Bogenschutz et al., 2015). There were no psilocybin-related serious adverse events reported.

Based on these promising findings, a double-blind RCT is being led by Michael Bogenschutz and Stephen Ross at the NYULMC comparing two oral doses of psilocybin to two oral doses of active control (diphenhydramine), both delivered in the context of a motivational interviewing therapy platform. The study (NCT#02061293), has completed enrollment of 96 participants with expected publication in early 2021 (M. Bogenschutz, personal communication, 2020) and includes an fMRI neuroimaging component to assess functional and structural changes that may be induced by psilocybin and may correlate with clinical outcomes.

Cocaine

An RCT (NCT02037126) is currently being conducted by Peter Hendricks at the University of Alabama in the first ever trial examining psilocybin-assisted treatment for cocaine addiction. The parallel-design RCT will recruit 40 participants and compare single-dose oral psilocybin (0.36 mg/kg) and single-dose oral active control (diphenhydramine 100 mg) in a cohort of patients with cocaine use disorder. The trial will include fMRI assessments, as well as measurements to detect abnormalities in brain glutamate levels in the anterior cingulate cortex and hippocampus. The trial is nearing completion, and the sample so far has been predominantly African Americans (men more than women) from impoverished socioeconomic backgrounds, with crack cocaine as the most common form of cocaine used (P. Hendricks, personal communication, 2020). A preliminary planned analysis of the first 10 participants suggests a treatment effect of psilocybin (vs. placebo) in terms of reduction of cocaine use and reduction of cocaine-related functional impairment (Hendricks presentation at the Horizons Conference, October 6, 2018). It is vital to develop pharmacotherapies for cocaine use disorders, especially given the considerable prevalence and public health impact of cocaine addiction and the fact that there are currently no FDA-approved medications for this type of addiction.

Opioids

Clinical trials investigating the use of psilocybin to treat opioid use disorders are beginning or planned at multiple academic medical centers in the United States, with the first trial underway at University of Wisconsin–Madison led by Randy Brown (personal communication, November 13, 2019) to explore the safety and potential efficacy of psilocybin administration to patients with opioid use disorders maintained on buprenorphine. It will be important to conduct research with psilocybin treatment models for opioid use disorders given the current opioid epidemic and the need for new and effective pharmacotherapies.

MDD

In 2015, Robin Carhart-Harris at Imperial College London conducted an open-label pilot study with patients diagnosed with moderate to severe treatment-resistant depression (TRD), defined as a score on the Hamilton Rating Scale for Depression (HAM-D) > 17, who had failed two adequate trials of antidepressant medication (N = 12) (Carhart-Harris et al., 2016). Patients were given two oral doses of psilocybin, one low dose (10 mg) followed by one higher dose (25 mg) 7 days later. Baseline fMRI scans were performed prior to any psychological or pharmacological interventions, and the day after the high dose psilocybin-assisted psychotherapy session for an adjacent imaging study. The primary outcome measure for antidepressant efficacy was the 16-item Quick Inventory for Depressive Symptoms (QIDS-16). All measures were performed at baseline, 1 week and 3 months after the higher dose psilocybin session. No SAEs were reported in this trial. Pre–post depression scores were significantly decreased from baseline to 1-week (mean QIDS difference: 11.8, 95% confidence interval [CI], –9.15 to –14.25, p + .002, Hedges's g = 3.1) and 3-months (mean QIDS difference: 9.2, 95% CI, –5.69 to –12.71, p = .003, Hedges's g = 2) post high-dose psilocybin treatment (Carhart-Harris et al., 2016). The improvements in depressive scores was maintained at 6-month follow-up (Carhart-Harris et al., 2018). As a follow-up to the above trial, in 2018, Carhart-Harris plans to start a randomized controlled comparative efficacy trial at Imperial College comparing single-dose psilocybin to 6 weeks of daily treatment with escitalopram in the treatment of MDD. This trial will include an fMRI assessment component.

The first RCT of psilocybin treatment for MDD (NCT03181529) is being conducted at the JHU School of Medicine. It is a parallel group design with 24 participants randomized to an immediate versus delayed group. There is no active pharmacological control employed in this trial. Participants will receive two moderate to high doses of psilocybin. The trial is expected to be completed by the end of 2020.

OCD

From 2001 to 2004, Francisco Moreno conducted a double-blind clinical trial investigating the safety, tolerability, and efficacy of psilocybin for the treatment of OCD. The study enrolled nine participants who met DSM-IV criteria for OCD and gave each participant three doses of psilocybin: low (100 µg/kg), medium (200 µg/kg), and high (300 µg/kg) in consecutive order. A subthreshold dose of (25 µg/kg) was given randomly after the first dosage. At 0, 4, 8, and 24 hours after psilocybin ingestion, the participants were administered the Yale–Brown Obsessive–Compulsive Scale (Y-BOCS) and a visual analogue scale measuring symptom severity. The trial reported 23–100% decreases in Y-BOCS scores across all doses, including the subthreshold dose of psilocybin (Moreno, Wiegand, Taitano, & Delgado, 2006). While psilocybin may be efficacious for the treatment of OCD at a wide range of doses, the findings can also be interpreted as a result of the placebo effect (Nichols, Johnson, & Nichols, 2017).

There are currently two randomized controlled Phase 1 studies investigating psilocybin's potential therapeutic effects on OCD. One study (NCT03356483), which is being led by Benjamin Kelmendi at the Yale School of Medicine is an RCT using a parallel design, with the goal of recruiting 30 participants with OCD who will receive a single dose of psilocybin at .25 mg/kg or a single dose of niacin. In addition to acute outcome measures at 24 and 48 hours postdosing, longer-term clinical outcomes will be assessed at 1-week, 2-weeks, 1-month, 3-months, and 6-months postdosing. The trial is expected to be complete by July 2022 and will include an fMRI assessment component. The other trial (NCT 03300947), which is being led by Francisco Moreno at the University of Arizona, will be an RCT that recruits 15 participants with OCD randomized to three arms: low dose (0.1 mg/kg) psilocybin, high dose (0.3 mg/kg) psilocybin, and an active control lorazepam (1 mg). In each of the arms, participants will receive study medication once per week over an 8-week treatment period. The primary efficacy outcome will be acute effects (first 8 hours postdosing and 1 week postdosing) on OCD symptom severity, and secondary efficacy outcomes will be assessed every month postdosing for 3 months, then at final 6-month follow-up. This trial will also include an fMRI assessment component and is expected to be completed by July 2021.

Cluster Headaches

One published case series (N = 53) of individuals with cluster headaches suggests that psilocybin-containing mushrooms (as well as LSD) may possess therapeutic efficacy in acutely treating and longitudinally preventing cluster headaches (Sewell, Halpern, & Pope, 2006). As a follow-up to this case series, Emmanuelle Schindler of Yale University School of Medicine is conducting an RCT (NCT02981173) with a crossover design, with the goal of treating 24 participants with cluster headaches assigned to three groups: mild- to moderate-dose psilocybin (0.143 mg/kg) versus low-dose psilocybin (0.0143 mg/kg) vs inactive placebo. All treatment arms will include drug administration daily over a 3-day treatment period. The primary outcome measures will include time to first cluster headache attack after completion of treatment period, time to last attack after completion of treatment period, as well as changes in frequency, intensity, and duration of attacks longitudinally.

Psilocybin-Assisted Group Therapy for Demoralization in Long-Term AIDS Survivors

Brian Anderson and Joshua Woolley at the UCSF School of Medicine have recently (August 2020) published the first-ever trial utilizing psilocybin-assisted group therapy to treat demoralization in older long-term AIDS survivor men (Anderson et al., 2020). The study utilized an open-label design and recruited 18 participants who received a single-dose (either 0.3 mg/kg or 0.36 mg/kg) psilocybin administration session in combination with 8–10 group therapy integration sessions. The trial reported on safety (no SAEs), feasibility of recruitment, and preliminary efficacy of a clinically significant improvement in demoralization as measured from baseline to 3-month follow-up (mean difference –5.78 [SD 6.01]; within group effect size 0.47; 90% CI 0.21–0.60). A next step would be to conduct randomized, placebo-controlled trials in this population to determine efficacy. If psilocybin were to be found to treat psychiatric and existential distress in AIDS patients, it could have enormous public health benefits in treating the mental health sequelae of this long-standing epidemic.

Psilocybin-Assisted Treatment for Antisocial Behavior and Criminal Recidivism

The Concord Prison Psilocybin Experiment: 1961–1963

Timothy Leary, Ralph Metzner, and Gunther Weil conducted the Concord Prison Experiment, an open-label, nonrandomized trial investigating the efficacy of psilocybin administration in group psychotherapy sessions for reducing rates of recidivism in prison inmates (Leary & Metzner, 1968; Timothy et al., 1965). The hypothesis was that psilocybin would lead to reductions in prison recidivism by diminishing antisocial behavior. The study was conducted at the maximum security Concord State Prison for young offenders in Concord, Massachusetts, from 1961 to 1963. The study enrolled inmates ($N = 32$) who underwent two psilocybin-facilitated group therapy sessions (with doses ranging from 20 mg to 70 mg, depending on the choice of the prisoner), followed by integration therapy sessions. Interestingly, as a means of establishing trust and rapport, and providing emotional support to participants, one of the group leaders would self-administer psilocybin during the group therapy sessions (Doblin, 1998). The primary outcome was to compare recidivism rates

in the psilocybin-treated group with the mean base recidivism rate for other Concord prison inmates (generated by calculating the recidivism rate of all 311 prisoners freed or paroled from Concord Prison in 1959).

Leary initially reported that the recidivism rate in the psilocybin group (measured January 1963 in 28 out of 32 participants released from Concord, with an average of 10 months postrelease [range 1–18 months]) was 32% and significantly less than the recidivism base rate of 56%, which led Leary to claim, "We had kept twice as many convicts out on the street as the expected number" (Leary & Metzner, 1968). However, Leary compared apples and oranges by calculating the base recidivism rate at 30 months postrelease rather than 10 months postrelease, which would have made it comparable to the average postrelease assessment time point in the experimental group. If he had used 10 months instead of 30 months to calculate the base recidivism rate, it would have been 34.3%, which is not significantly different than the 32% rate calculated for the experimental group (Doblin, 1998). A longer follow-up period included data gathered as of July 1964 (with 27 participants evaluated 18 to 26 months postrelease) and reported that 59% in the experimental group had been reincarcerated, a rate not statistically different from the base rate of 56% (Timothy et al., 1965). Despite these negative findings, Leary continued to claim positive benefits from the experimental group by reporting on lower than expected rates of new crimes committed in the experimental versus control groups (Doblin, 1998).

Doblin's 34-Year Follow-Up to the Concord Prison Experiment

A 34-year follow-up to the Concord Prison Experiment was conducted by Rick Doblin, by evaluating the effect of the experimental treatment on recidivism rates for both parole violations and new crimes at 2.5 years postrelease, which was the longest point in time that the base recidivism rates at Concord had been collected and were available for comparison. Of 21 participants who had records at 2.5 years postrelease, the recidivism rate at 2.5 years (30 months) was 71%, higher than the base rate of 56% at 2.5 years postrelease, although not statistically significant (Doblin, 1998). Even though Doblin determined that Leary's claims of a positive treatment effect for the experimental group were false, he concludes by stating, "Whether a new program of psilocybin-assisted group psychotherapy and post-release programs would significantly reduce recidivism rates is an empirical question that deserves to be addressed within the context of a new experiment."

Epidemiological Associations between Serotonergic Psychedelic Use and Criminal Recidivism: 2013–2018

In the modern era, Peter Hendricks, a research psychologist at the University of Alabama, has picked up the baton in terms of assessing the potential of psychedelic therapy to reduce antisocial behavior and criminal recidivism. In a longitudinal naturalistic trial, data were collected on 25,622 individuals (2002–2007) in the southeastern United States charged with a felony, and monitored under community corrections supervision as part of Treatment Accountability for Safer Communities (TASC) program. The main findings from this trial were that serotonergic hallucinogen use (including psilocybin) predicted a reduced likelihood of supervision failure (i.e., noncompliance with legal requirements including alcohol and drug use), whereas most other drugs of abuse (alcohol, cocaine, cannabis, amphetamine) were associated with an increased probability of supervision failure (Hendricks, Clark, Johnson, Fontaine, & Cropsey, 2014). Furthermore, Hendricks and colleagues (2018) examined the relationships between the use of a variety of drugs of abuse and criminal behavior by examining over 480,000 U.S. adult respondents pooled from the NSDUH (a yearly cross-sectional survey conducted by the Substance Abuse and Mental Health Services Administration) from 2002 to 2014. Lifetime use of serotonergic hallucinogens (including psilocybin) was associated with reduced odds of past-year theft, assault, arrest for property crime, and arrest for a violent crime, whereas lifetime illicit use of most other drugs was associated with increased odds of a variety of criminal behavior events. Together, these results sug-

gest that psilocybin may have protective or therapeutic effects relative to criminal behavior and provide a compelling rationale to reinitiate clinical research using psilocybin-assisted therapy to treat antisocial behavior and criminal recidivism.

■ Issues Related to Nonmedical Use

Although the vast majority of clinical research with psilocybin has focused on treating ailments, anecdotal and preliminary empirical evidence suggest that psilocybin and classic psychedelics also support the enrichment of healthy individuals (Elsey, 2017). Motivations for self-experimentation outside of medical settings include creativity enhancement and problem solving, as well as spiritual and philosophical exploration (Grof, 1973). The historical contexts in which psychedelics have been administered provide informative models for understanding responsible methods for consumption. Such historical frameworks have served to inform the guidelines for conducting contemporary clinical trials (Johnson et al., 2008). Indigenous cultures have restricted the usage of psychedelics to ceremonial contexts such as rites of passage and religious rituals (Carod-Artal, 2015). Some modern examples of the use of psychedelics as part of organized religious (i.e., Christian) practice include the use of peyote in the Native American Church or ayahuasca in the Santo Daime and União do Vegetal religions (Santos, Landeira-Fernandez, Strassman, Motta, & Cruz, 2007). The highly structured and ritualized contexts are believed to minimize the likelihood of adverse reactions (Harding & Zinberg, 1977). The safeguards developed in these practices include regimented preparation, restricted access to the medicine, guidance and supervision by more experienced practitioners, and a societal appreciation for the powerful properties of the medicines (Harding & Zinberg, 1977).

Recreational Use

There are a number of risks associated with psilocybin use in nonmedical and nonritualized settings. In nonmedical settings, individuals are generally less inclined to appreciate the importance of set and setting and may not appreciate or prepare to mitigate the risks associated with use (Grof, 1973).

In a medical or treatment context, there is adequate preparation, monitoring, and safeguards, with appropriately trained clinicians to manage any medical or psychiatric adverse events that may occur. When pursuing a psilocybin experience for nontreatment purposes, it is unlikely that the treatment will occur with a trained mental health or medical professional and more likely to occur with a lay neoshaman or shaman (Halpern & Pope, 2003). Recreational users are also less likely to be screened for psychiatric disorders, which could potentially predispose individuals to traumatic psychedelic experiences (Halpern & Pope, 2003). Psilocybin, obtained in recreational settings or from the street, carries a higher likelihood of chemical impurities and contaminations (including amphetamines and phencyclidine), and it is common to combine multiple drugs of abuse during a single use occasion (Grof, 1973). This type of use may result in unpredictable effects, increasing the risk of a medical or psychiatric crisis episode (Johnson et al., 2008). Despite the relatively low rates of acute and prolonged adverse psychiatric and medical effects of psilocybin compared to other substances of abuse (i.e., alcohol, opioids, amphetamines), these incidents are nontrivial. Case reports have captured transient episodes of fear (van Amsterdam et al., 2011), delusional experiences, paranoid ideation (Strassman, 1984), depression, cognitive disturbances (e.g., disorientation, loosening of self-boundaries, depersonalization, and dissociative reactions), and physiological symptoms such as increases in blood pressure and nausea (Frecska & Luna, 2006; Johnson et al., 2008; McCabe, 1977). Episodes of dangerous behavior including suicide and violence toward others have been reported with individuals under the influence of psychedelics, especially when used in unsafe and recreational settings (Schwartz & Smith, 1988; van Amsterdam et al., 2011).

Two Web-based survey studies targeting recreational drug users in naturalistic settings have captured descriptive rates of adverse events and phenomenological patterns of individuals' experiences with psilocybin (Carbonaro et al., 2016; Carhart-Harris & Nutt, 2010). Carbonaro and colleagues (2016) recruited 1,993 individuals who had endorsed experiencing a difficult psilocybin mushroom session at some point in their lives. Survey findings revealed that difficult experiences were commonly reported (with 39% of respondents rating their psilocybin experience as being among the top five most difficult experiences of their lives) and 11% endorsed items related to putting themselves or others in potential physical danger. Furthermore, 84% reported that despite the difficult nature of their psilocybin experiences, they experienced meaningful benefits from these experiences. These paradoxical results may appear counterintuitive when interpretations are made outside of the context of a psychotherapeutic process. The authors noted that the duration of the difficult experience (not necessarily the peak difficulty) was negatively associated with persistent reports of well-being, suggesting that one of the important roles of a clinical setting is as a container to manage the duration of difficult experiences (Carbonaro et al., 2016). Analyses also revealed that the resolution of psychologically challenging material often yields meaningful insights and should not be overlooked. There can be a narrow margin separating positive experiences from highly adverse ones. These experiences are multifaceted and have the potential to trigger personal crises, as well as to initiate personal growth. However, it appears that if variables related to set and setting are optimized, the occurrence of acute and persistent crises and adverse events connected to psilocybin usage can be well managed and minimized. Carhart-Harris and Nutt (2010) investigated the perceived benefits and harms associated with individuals' use of popular recreational substances. Participants ($N = 626$) were specifically queried about their use of psilocybin, LSD, ketamine, MDMA, cannabis, and alcohol. Of the total respondents, 503 endorsed having used psilocybin. Psilocybin was the drug least associated with causing or exacerbating mental health or physical problems; however, 13% of psilocybin users reporting that psilocybin had "definitely" (2%) or "probably" (11%) caused or worsened mental health or physical problems. In this survey, psilocybin and LSD were reported as having the greatest positive effect on mental or physical well-being. Even though psilocybin was not reported to be associated with dangerous behavior causing injury while intoxicated or prolonged psychosis, four (0.8%) of the participants reported symptoms suggestive of HPPD (Carhart-Harris & Nutt, 2010).

Psilocybin, Religion, and Spirituality

The Good Friday Experiment: 1962

In 1962, Walter Pahnke conducted the Marsh Chapel Experiment, also known as "The Good Friday Experiment." Pahnke (a Harvard trained psychiatrist and minister) designed the experiment as part of his PhD thesis in Religion and Society at the Harvard Divinity School, and was supervised by Timothy Leary. Pahkne was investigating whether psilocybin could reliably occasion mystical experiences in religiously oriented trainees and what enduring positive or negative effects the experiences would have on attitudes and behaviors (Pahnke, 1963). Pahnke (1963) recruited 20 white male Protestant divinity students at the same theological program in Boston ($N = 20$) for a randomized (1:1), double-blind, placebo-controlled trial in which participants were administered single high-dose oral psilocybin (30 mg) or oral placebo (niacin) in the basement of the Marsh Chapel at Boston University and exposed to the broadcasting of a 2½-hour live religious sermon. Similar to the Concord Prison experiment, as a means of establishing rapport and providing emotional support to participants, Leary insisted (over Pahnke's objection) that some of the group leaders self-administer psilocybin during the group therapy sessions (Doblin, 1991). The primary outcome measure was an eight-category typology of MEQ based on the work of William James and Walter Stace (1961). A 147-item version of the MEQ was administered 1–2 days after receiving the study drug and a 100-item version of the MEQ was administered 6 months postdosing. Pahnke's main finding was that acutely (i.e., 1–2 days postdosing) those participants who received psilocybin had increased scores on all eight categories of the MEQ, compared to placebo (Pahnke, 1967). At 6-month follow-up, the participants in the psilocybin group continued to report mystical-type experiences and demonstrated statistically significant improvements in persistence of positive changes in attitude and behavior, compared to the control group (Doblin, 1991). In summary, Pahnke's pilot study strongly suggested that in religiously oriented divinity students, psilocybin could occasion mystical-type experiences that were highly religious and meaningful, and associated with enduring positive changes in attitudes and behavior. Interestingly, Huston Smith (the famous religious scholar; 2000) was a participant in the Good Friday Experiment and described his experience as "the most power cosmic homecoming I have ever experienced."

Doblin conducted a long-term follow-up to the Good Friday Experiment approximately 25 years after the initial experiment. Of the original 20 participants, 16 were available for the follow-up and the 100-item MEQ was readministered. The main findings were that at 25-year follow-up, the participants in the psilocybin group continued to retrospectively report mystical-type experiences from the dosing session and continued to report significant improvements in persisting positive changes in attitude and behavior, compared to the control group (Doblin, 1991).

The JHU Replication of the Good Friday Experiment: 2002–2006

From 2002 until 2006, a more rigorously designed version of the Good Friday Experiment was conducted at the JHU School of Medicine and led by Roland Griffiths (Griffiths et al., 2006). The randomized, active placebo-controlled crossover study recruited psychologically and medically healthy normal volunteers who were hallucinogen naive and reported regular participation in religious or spiritual practices, with 56% of the volunteers ($N = 20$) reporting daily practice of spiritual or religiously oriented activities. Thirty participants received high-dose psilocybin (30 mg/70 kg) and an active control (methylphenidate at 40 mg/70 kg) in counterbalanced order. Psilocybin acutely induced mystical-type experiences and at 2-month follow-up (at the time of the crossover), the psilocybin group (relative to the placebo group) reported improvements in the following domains: positive attitudes about life and/or self; positive mood changes; increased altruism; and positive behavioral changes. The psilocybin experiences were rated as substantially significant in terms of being highly meaningful and spiritual and remarkably 67% of participants rating the psilocybin experience as the singular or top five most meaningful experiences of their entire lives (Griffiths et al., 2006). The positive cognitive and behavioral changes reported by participants and attributed to psilocybin were confirmed by ratings of community observers. At the 14-month follow-up to this trial, participants continued to report that the psilocybin experience was highly meaningful and spiritual (58 and 67%, respectively, rated the experience as among the five most personally meaningful and among the five most spiritually significant experiences of their lives); a majority (64%) attributed improvements in life satisfaction and well-being to the psilocybin experience, and the acute mystical experience was strongly associated with follow-up high ratings of personal meaning and spiritual significance (Griffiths et al., 2008).

The JHU and NYU Religious Professional Study: 2015–Ongoing

As a follow-up to both the Good Friday Experiment and the JHU replication of the Good Friday Experiment, the Psilocybin Religious Professional Project is a joint collaboration between the JHU School of Medicine (NCT02243813), led by Roland Griffiths, and NYULMC (NCT02421263), led by Stephen Ross. It is a pilot (N = 24), randomized, wait-list-controlled trial of the effects and possible benefit of psilocybin-facilitated experiences on professional religious leaders. Participants receive 2 doses of high-dose psilocybin (20 mg/70 kg, 30 mg/70 kg) delivered under supportive conditions. A primary objective of this study is to characterize the phenomenology of psilocybin-induced mystical experiences in professional religious leaders following psilocybin experiences by assessing psychological functioning, spirituality, health, well-being, and prosocial attitudes and behaviors. A secondary objective is to determine whether participants who report having had the strongest mystical-type effects during psilocybin sessions will show the largest positive enduring changes in attitudes and behavior. This study will provide new information about how psilocybin experiences in religious professionals affect subsequent attitudes and behaviors in daily life, including meditation and prayer practices, religious perspectives, and interpersonal relationships. Another goal of the trial is to better understand the mechanism of action behind the mystical experience and psilocybin-facilitated spiritual and mystical states. A hypothesis is that religious professionals, given their interests, training, and life experience, will be able to make nuanced discriminations of their psilocybin experiences, thus contributing to the scientific understanding of mystical-type experience and possibly informing the design of therapeutic clinical trials. It will be important to determine whether and how religious professionals find these experiences to be of value in their vocation and whether their moods, attitudes, and behaviors are changed positively or negatively. This trial is nearing completion and is scheduled to be completed June 2021.

It would be interesting to consider how psilocybin experiences might change the nature of religious training or religious practice. Psilocybin-facilitated experiences might allow religious trainees or practitioners to have direct access to spiritual or mystical states of consciousness, and this could have significant effects on their understanding and practice of their religion.

■ Potential Clinical Applications in the Future

Advanced-Phase Research (the Future): Phase II/III Clinical Trials

Phase II/III Psilocybin Treatment for MDD

The open-label trial suggesting acute and sustained antidepressant effect of psilocybin in patients with TRD (Carhart-Harris, 2016), in conjunction with the three RCTs (Griffiths et al., 2016; Grob et al., 2011; Ross et al., 2016) of single-dose psilocybin for cancer-related anxiety and depression (which together suggested rapid, robust, and sustained antidepressant effects of psilocybin), have formed the justification for pharma entities to start working with the FDA and the European Medicines Agency (EMA) to move forward with Phase II/III trials of psilocybin treatment for MDD. The most mature of these initiatives is led by Compass Pathways, a for-profit newly established pharmaceutical company that was formed to conduct clinical trials of psilocybin treatment for MDD. In August 2018, Compass received approval from the FDA for a Phase 2b dose-finding study of psilocybin treatment for TRD that would be conducted in approximately 12 to 15 sites throughout the United Kingdom and North America. If the results of this phase 2b trial are successful, Compass could transition to pivotal Phase III trials of psilocybin treatment for TRD. In October 2018, the FDA granted Compass breakthrough status, which has the potential to quicken the drug development process. On a parallel track, the Usona Institute (a 501(c)(3) nonprofit medical research organization with the mission of supporting and conducting preclinical and clinical research of the therapeutic effects of psilocybin treatment) is currently in discussion with the FDA for a Phase II trial of psilocybin treatment for MDD that would be conducted at seven sites in the United States (including NYULMC, JHU, Yale, UCSF, University of Wisconsin). It is likely that Usona will also apply for breakthrough status with the FDA to study psilocybin treatment for MDD. Having a medication that can work rapidly for MDD (TRD or non-TRD), and lead to sustained antidepressant effects lasting weeks to months, would be a game changer in the pharmacotherapy of MDD. It would represent the second antidepressant after ketamine that works rapidly and has sustained effects. However, given that ketamine has abuse liability and its antidepressant effects tend to degrade after 1–2 weeks (DeWilde et al., 2015), psilocybin would be a clear advantage over ketamine in terms of both decreased addictive potential and sustained clinical improvements.

Phase III Psilocybin Treatment for Cancer-Related Psychiatric Distress

The three FDA Phase II trials in the United States that examined single-dose psilocybin treatment for cancer-related psychiatric distress included a total cohort of 92 participants (Griffiths et al., 2016; Grob et al., 2011; Ross et al., 2016). Combined, these trials strongly suggest that psilocybin-assisted therapy for patients with cancer-related psychiatric illness produces rapid, robust (e.g., large effect sizes, large antidepressant and anxiolytic response and remission rates), and sustained improvements (e.g., up to several months) in cancer-related anxiety and depression, as well as improvements in existential distress (e.g., demoralization, hopelessness, death- and dying-related distress) and quality of life. Given that these trials had relatively small sample sizes, they are liable to various biases (i.e., selection), the possibility of type I errors, and lack of external validity. It is therefore important as a next step to proceed to larger clinical trials with the goal of replicating the findings. Such a trial would likely be a multicenter trial that would include a nationally representative sample of patients with cancer-related psychiatric distress. It could include a sample size of 100–200, and it would be important to design the trial optimally to replicate some of the most novel and interesting findings from the three Phase II trials (i.e., rapidity of onset of psilocybin and sustained clinical benefits). One such design might be single-dose psilocybin at 0.3 mg/kg versus niacin, with psychological and existential distress measured at baseline, the day before dosing, the day after dosing, and up to 6 months postdosing. Existential measures might include death anxiety, demoralization, and hopelessness. Such a multicenter trial could be funded through a public–private partnership, such as a combination of funding from the National Institutes of Health (NIH; possibly a joint National Institute of Mental Health/National Cancer Institute [NIMH/NCI] collaboration) plus private philanthropy or through pharma. If cosponsored by a pharma entity for the purpose of drug development, such a large trial could represent a pivotal Phase III trial that could go toward rescheduling of psilocybin for cancer-related psychiatric and existential distress.

The availability of psilocybin-assisted therapy could provide a novel and groundbreaking treatment model for patients with cancer-related psychological and existential distress in several ways:

1. *Rapidity of therapeutic effect.* A medication that can work immediately for cancer-related depression would have considerable benefits for patients given the delay

(e.g., weeks) for typical antidepressants to exert antidepressant effects and given the increased risk of suicidal thinking and behaviors associated with cancer-related psychological and existential distress.

2. *The use of psilocybin early in a cancer diagnosis when psychological and existential symptoms start to manifest.* This could have the potential benefit of preventing progression to more severe psychological symptoms (i.e., anxiety, depression, hastened desire for death) and could protect against suicide and even protect against cancer disease progression (Ross, 2018).

3. *Sustained antidepressant and anxiolytic clinical effects from single dosing* (e.g., up to 7 weeks in the Ross et al. [2016] trial and up to 5 weeks in the Griffiths et al. [2016] trial). The benefits could include minimization of side effects related to having to take an anxiolytic or antidepressant on a chronic basis. Further research is needed to validate the length of therapeutic benefit of single-dose psilocybin and test the potential need for booster dosing intervention models.

4. *Providing a pharmacological–psychosocial intervention for existential distress in cancer patients.* Existential distress is underrecognized and undertreated in cancer patients within Western medicine; there are no established medications with efficacy for this type of distress, and having an intervention that can decrease the fear associated with the dying process could have enormous benefit for patients as they approach death. The application of psilocybin treatment in the terminally ill could be especially useful for patients in outpatient or inpatient hospice settings, and could aid the process of dying with dignity to help occasion a "good" death, in contrast to the current poor state of existential and end-of-life care of the dying in the United States and worldwide (Meier et al., 2016).

Phase II/III Psilocybin Treatment for Alcoholism and Tobacco Addiction

Both the Phase II trials of psilocybin treatment for alcoholism and tobacco addiction are nearing completion, with the trial for alcoholism finished with enrollment and likely publication in early 2021 (M. Bogenschutz, personal communication) and the trial for tobacco addiction to be completed by approximately December 2022 (M. Johnson, personal communication). If these Phase II trials produce positive therapeutic effects of psilocybin treatment, these findings would need to be replicated in larger multicenter trials and (similar to the case mentioned for psilocybin treatment for cancer-related psychiatric distress) they could be funded through a public–private partnership such as a combination of funding from NIH (i.e., National Institute on Alcohol Abuse and Alcoholism [NIAAA], National Institute on Drug Abuse [NIDA]) plus private philanthropy or through pharma. If sponsored by pharma, these larger trials could represent pivotal Phase III trials that could go toward rescheduling of psilocybin for alcoholism, tobacco addiction, or both. Whether NIAAA or NIDA is ready to fund such trials is still very uncertain.

Phase III Trials, Compassionate Use, Rescheduling, and Licensed Psychedelic Treatment Clinics

If Phase III trials of psilocybin treatment occur for various psychiatric indications, it is possible that the FDA would allow contemporaneous "compassionate use" (also known as expanded access) to be conducted alongside the Phase III trials, which would allow a greater cohort of the treatment population to potentially benefit from psilocybin treatment in a more expedited manner. The success of any Phase III pivotal trials of psilocybin treatment (i.e., MDD, cancer-related psychiatric distress, alcoholism, tobacco addiction) could potentially set the stage for the rescheduling of psilocybin out of Schedule 1 (the most restrictive category, in which it is currently not available for clinical use in humans) to another category in which it could become available for therapeutic use in clinical populations (e.g., in the United States, rescheduling from Schedule 1 to 2 or 3). This would make psilocybin available as a prescription medication, to be used in conjunction with preparatory and integrative psychotherapy. It could be used to treat the particular psychiatric disorder that generated the positive Phase III results. The FDA would likely require the use of psilocybin to be monitored through its Risk Evaluation and Mitigation Strategy (REMS) program, which can require drug manufacturers to ensure that the benefits of a drug product outweigh its risks. The REMS program is essentially a safety strategy to manage known or potentially serious risks associated with a new drug product and to enable patients to have access to the medication while maintaining safety of the drug. Given that psilocybin has known serious adverse psychological risks (i.e., chronic psychosis in individuals predisposed to psychotic illness, Type 2 HPPD, potential for dangerous behavior to self or others when used in uncontrolled settings), it is likely that FDA would require that its use be managed through an REMS mechanism. Given the known risks of psilocybin administration in uncontrolled settings administered without supervision by trained professionals, psilocybin would likely be dispensed and administered only in specially designated and certified psychedelic treatment clinics. In addition to providing psychedelic treatments (i.e., psilocybin, MDMA, ketamine), such clinics could provide a variety of traditional evidence-based psychiatric treatment modalities (i.e., standard pharmacotherapies; individual, group, family, and couple therapy) and nontraditional treatment approaches (i.e., yoga, meditation, reiki, pet therapy, music and art therapies, drama therapy, flotation tanks). Training of therapists and fidelity to treatment models would have to be considered, and it would be important to establish specific psychedelic therapy training programs given the unique nature of this type of therapy. Regulatory oversight, drug accountability (e.g., protecting against drug diversion), quality control management, and protocols to optimize treatment efficacy and patient safety would have to be key components of managing psychedelic treatment clinics. If psilocybin were approved for a particular psychiatric indication (i.e., MDD), off-label use of psilocybin for other psychiatric indications might be allowed by appropriate state regulatory agencies or be restricted to disease conditions that have data supporting efficacy from clinical trials (i.e., cancer-related psychiatric distress given the strength of the data from the combined Phase II trials). If psilocybin were rescheduled for cancer-related psychiatric or existential distress, its use off-label might include psychological and existential distress occurring in other serious general medical conditions (e.g., end-stage pulmonary disease, AIDS).

Other Potential Clinical Applications of Psilocybin Treatment

There is a dizzying array of potential clinical applications of psilocybin-assisted psychotherapies for a variety of psychiatric and addictive disorders. In addition to being actively studied for alcohol, tobacco, cocaine, and opioid use disorders, psilocybin could be explored to treat other drugs of abuse (i.e., methamphetamine, tetrahydrocannabinol [THC] addiction) or behavioral addictions (i.e., gambling, overeating, gaming, sex). There have never been any clinical trials of psilocybin to treat eating disorders, and psilocybin treatment for anorexia would be particularly important to pursue given that anorexia is the most lethal psychiatric disorder and there are no approved pharmacotherapies to treat the disorder (Chesney, Goodwin, & Fazel, 2014). JHU has begun the first clinical trial (first enrollment August 2019), using an open-label design, of psilocybin treatment for anorexia nervosa. Personality disorders represent another group of disorders that might benefit from studies of psilocybin-assisted psychotherapies. Given that psilocybin is known to increase the personality trait of openness (MacLean, Johnson, & Griffiths, 2011), it could potentially be beneficial for personality disorders marked by rigid defenses (i.e., obsessive–compulsive personality disorder [OCPD], narcissistic personality disorder) and given that psilocybin is associated with increases in altruism (Griffiths et al., 2008, 2016; Ross et al., 2016), it could be potentially helpful for personality disorders marked by deficits in empathy (i.e., narcissistic personality disorder, antisocial personality disorder [ASPD]). It is also worth exploring psilocybin treatment for posttraumatic stress disorder (PTSD), although one would have to be careful about challenging experiences that could lead to retraumatization or worsening of traumatic memories.

References

Abraham, H. (1983). Visual phenomenology of the LSD flashback. *Archives of General Psychiatry, 40,* 884–889.

Abraham, H. D. (2000). Hallucinogen related disorders. In H. Kaplan & B. Sadock (Eds.), *Comprehensive textbook of psychiatry* (7th ed.). Philadelphia: Lippincott Williams & Wilkins.

Abraham, H. D., & Aldridge, A. M. (1993). Adverse consequences of lysergic acid diethylamide. *Addiction, 88*(10), 1327–1334.

Abuzzahab, F., & Anderson, B. (1971). A review of LSD treatment in alcoholism. *International Pharmacopsychiatry, 6*, 223–235.

Aghajanian, G. K. (2009). Modeling "psychosis" in vitro by inducing disordered neuronal network activity in cortical brain slices. *Psychopharmacology (Berlin), 206*(4), 575–585.

Aldurra, G., & Crayton, J. W. (2001). Improvement of hallucinogen persisting perception disorder by treatment with a combination of fluoxetine and olanzapine: Case report. *Journal of Clinical Psychopharmacology, 21*(21), 343–344.

Anderson, B. T., Danforth, A., Daroff, R., Stauffer, C., Ekman, E., Agin-Liebes, G., et al. (2020). Psilocybin-assisted group therapy for demoralized older long-term AIDS survivor men: An open-label safety and feasibility pilot study. *EClinical Medicine.* [Epub ahead of print]

Anderson, L., Lake, H., & Walterfang, M. (2018). The trip of a lifetime: Hallucinogen persisting perceptual disorder. *Australas Psychiatry, 26*(1), 11–12.

Anderson, W. H., & O'Malley, J. E. (1972). Trifluoperazine for the "trailing" phenomenon. *Journal of the American Medical Association, 220*(9), 1244–1245.

Austin, A. L. (1967). Términos del nahuallatolli. *Historia Mexicana, 17*(1), 1–36.

Badham, E. R. (1984). Ethnobotany of psilocybin mushrooms, especially *Psilocybe cubensis. Journal of Ethnopharmacology, 10*(2), 249–254.

Baer, G. (1967). Statistical results on reactions of normal subjects to the psilocybin derivatives CEY 19 and CZ 74. In H. Brill (Ed.), *Neuropsycho-pharmacology* (pp. 400–404). Amsterdam: Excerpta Medica.

Baggott, M. J., Coyle, J. R., Erowid, E., Erowid, F., & Robertson, L. C. (2011). Abnormal visual experiences in individuals with histories of hallucinogen use: A web-based questionnaire. *Drug and Alcohol Dependence, 114*(1), 61–67.

Baler, R. D., & Volkow, N. D. (2006). Drug addiction: The neurobiology of disrupted self-control. *Trends in Molecular Medicine, 12*(12), 559–566.

Barrett, F., Johnson, M., & Griffiths, R. (2015). Validation of the revised Mystical Experience Questionnaire in experimental sessions with psilocybin. *Journal of Psychopharmacology, 29*(11), 1182–1190.

Bathina, S., & Das, U. N. (2015). Brain-derived neurotrophic factor and its clinical implications. *Archives of Medical Science, 11*(6), 1164–1178.

Beck, O., Helander, A., Karlson-Stiber, C., & Stephansson, N. (1998). Presence of phenylethylamine in hallucinogenic Psilocybe mushroom: Possible role in adverse reactions. *Journal of Analytical Toxicology, 22*(1), 45–49.

Beique, J. C., Imad, M., Mladenovic, L., Gingrich, J. A., & Andrade, R. (2007). Mechanism of the 5-hydroxytryptamine 2A receptor-mediated facilitation of synaptic activity in prefrontal cortex. *Proceedings of the National Academy of Sciences of the USA, 104*(23), 9870–9875.

Belser, A. B., Agin-Liebes, G., Swift, T. C., Terrana, S., Devenot, N., Friedman, H. L., et al. (2017). Patient experiences of psilocybin-assisted psychotherapy: An interpretative phenomenological analysis. *Journal of Humanistic Psychology, 57*(4), 354–388.

Bogenschutz, M. P., Forcehimes, A. A., Pommy, J. A., Wilcox, C. E., Barbosa, P. C. R., & Strassman, R. J. (2015). Psilocybin-assisted treatment for alcohol dependence: A proof-of-concept study. *Journal of Psychopharmacology, 29*(3), 289–299.

Bogenschutz, M. P., & Ross, S. (2018). Therapeutic applications of classic hallucinogens. *Current Topics in Behavioral Neuroscience, 36*, 361–391.

Borhegyi, S. (1963). Pre-Columbian pottery mushrooms from Mesoamerica. *American Antiquity 28*, 328–338.

Carbonaro, T., Bradstreet, M., Barrett, F., MacLean, K., Jesse, R., Johnson, M., & Griffiths, R. (2016). Survey study of challenging experiences after ingesting psilocybin mushrooms: Acute and enduring positive and negative consequences. *Journal of Psychopharmacology, 30*(12), 1268–1278.

Carbonaro, T., Johnson, M., Hurwitz, E., & Griffiths, R. (2018). Double-blind comparison of the two hallucinogens psilocybin and dextromethorphan: Similarities and differences in subjective experiences. *Psychopharmacology (Berlin), 235*(2), 521–534.

Carhart-Harris, R., Bolstridge, M., Day, C., Rucker, J., Watts, R., Erritzoe, D., et al. (2018). Psilocybin with psychological support for treatment-resistant depression: Six-month follow-up. *Psychopharmacology, 235*(2), 399–408.

Carhart-Harris, R. L., Bolstridge, M., Rucker, J., Day, C. M., Erritzoe, D., Kaelen, M., et al. (2016). Psilocybin with psychological support for treatment-resistant depression: An open-label feasibility study. *Lancet Psychiatry, 3*(7), 619–627.

Carhart-Harris, R. L., & Nutt, D. (2010). User perceptions of the benefits and harms of hallucinogenic drug use: A web-based questionnaire study. *Journal of Substance Use, 15*(4), 283–300.

Carhart-Harris, R. L., Williams, T. M., Sessa, B., Tyacke, R. J., Rich, A. S., Feilding, A., et al. (2011). The administration of psilocybin to healthy, hallucinogen-experienced volunteers in a mock-functional magnetic resonance imaging environment: A preliminary investigation of tolerability. *Journal of Psychopharmacology, 25*(11), 1562–1567.

Carod-Artal, F. (2015). Hallucinogenic drugs in pre-Columbian Mesoamerican cultures. *Neurología (English Edition), 30*(1), 42–49.

Casa, B., & Bosio, A. (2005). Levetiracetam efficacy in hallucinogen persisting perception disorders: A prospective study. *Journal of Neurological Science, 238*, S504.

Chesney, E., Goodwin, G. M., & Fazel, S. (2014). Risks of all-cause and suicide mortality in mental disorders: A meta-review. *World Psychiatry, 13*(2), 153–160.

Del Pozo, E. C. (1975). Las Fuentes historicas de las drogas vegetales mexicanas. *Cuademos Cientificos (CEMEF), 4*, 3–16.

Delay, J., Pichot, P., Lempêrière, T., & Quetin, A. (1959). *Therapeutic effect of psilocybin on convulsive neurosis.* Paper presented at the Annales Medico-Psychologiques.

Deneau, G., Yanagita, T., & Seevers, M. H. (1969). Self-administration of psychoactive substances by the monkey. *Psychopharmacologia, 16*(1), 30–48.

DeWilde, K. E., Levitch, C. F., Murrough, J. W., Mathew, S. J., & Iosifescu, D. V. (2015). The promise of ketamine for treatment-resistant depression: Current evidence and future directions. *Annals of the New York Academy of Sciences, 1345*(1), 47–58.

Dinis-Oliveira, R. J. (2017). Metabolism of psilocybin and psilocin: Clinical and forensic toxicological relevance. *Drug Metabolism Reviews, 49*(1), 84–91.

Dittrich, A. (1998). The standardized psychometric assessment of altered states of consciousness (ASCs) in humans. *Pharmacopsychiatry, 31*(Suppl. 2), 80–84.

Doblin, R. (1991). Pahnke's "Good Friday experiment": A long-term follow-up and methodological critique. *Journal of Transpersonal Psychology, 23*(1), 1–28.

Doblin, R. (1998). Dr. Leary's Concord Prison Experiment: A 34-year follow-up study. *Journal of Psychoactive Drugs, 30*(4), 419–426.

d'Olwer, L. N. (1952). *Fray Bernardino de Sahagún, 1499–1590* (Vol. 40). Mexico City: Instituto Panamericano de Geografía e Historia.

dos Santos, R. G., Bouso, J. C., Alcázar-Córcoles, M. Á., & Hallak, J. E. (2018). Efficacy, tolerability, and safety of serotonergic psychedelics for the management of mood, anxiety, and substance-use disorders: A systematic review of systematic reviews. *Expert Review of Clinical Pharmacology, 11*(9), 889–902.

Duke, R. B., & Keeler, M. H. (1968). The effects of psilocybin, dextro-amphetamine and placebo on performance of the trail making test. *Journal of Clinical Psychology, 24*(3), 316–317.

Dyck, E. (2006). "Hitting highs at rock bottom": LSD treatment for alcoholism, 1950–1970. *Social History of Medicine, 19*(2), 313–329.

Efron, D. H., & Usdin, D. (1972). *Psychotropic drugs and related compounds.* Bethesda, MD: National Institute of Mental Health.

Elsey, J. W. (2017). Psychedelic drug use in healthy individuals: A review of benefits, costs, and implications for drug policy. *Drug Science, Policy and Law, 3*, 1–11.

Espiard, M. L., Lecardeur, L., Abadie, P., Halbecq, I., & Dollfus, S. (2005). Hallucinogen persisting perception disorder after psilocybin consumption: A case study. *European Psychiatry, 20*(5–6), 458–460.

Fantegrossi, W. E., Murnane, K. S., & Reissig, C. J. (2008). The behavioral pharmacology of hallucinogens. *Biochemical Pharmacology, 75*(1), 17–33.

Fisher, G. (1970). The psycholytic treatment of a childhood schizophrenic girl. *International Journal of Social Psychiatry, 16*(2), 112–130.

Frecska, E., & Luna, L. E. (2006). Neuro-ontological interpretation of spiritual experiences. *Neuropsychopharmacologia Hungarica, 8*(3), 143–153.

Frokjaer, V. G., Mortensen, E. L., Nielsen, F. A., Haugbol, S., Pinborg, L. H., Adams, K. H., et al. (2008). Frontolimbic serotonin 2A receptor binding in healthy subjects is associated with personality risk factors for affective disorder. *Biological Psychiatry, 63*(6), 569–576.

Gable, R. S. (1993). Toward a comparative overview of dependence potential and acute toxicity of psychoactive substances used nonmedically. *American Journal of Drug and Alcohol Abuse, 19*(3), 263–281.

Gable, R. S. (2004). Comparison of acute lethal toxicity of commonly abused psychoactive substances. *Addiction, 99*(6), 686–696.

Garcia-Romeu, A., Griffiths, R., & Johnson, M. (2014). Psilocybin-occasioned mystical experiences in the treatment of tobacco addiction. *Current Drug Abuse Reviews, 7*(3), 157–164.

Gasser, P., Holstein, D., Michel, Y., Doblin, R., Yazar-Klosinski, B., Passie, T., et al. (2014). Safety and efficacy of lysergic acid diethylamide-assisted psychotherapy for anxiety associated with life-threatening diseases. *Journal of Nervous and Mental Disease, 202*(7), 513–520.

Geyer, M. A., & Vollenweider, F. X. (2008). Serotonin research: Contributions to understanding psychoses. *Trends in Pharmacological Sciences, 29*(9), 445–453.

Gouzoulis-Mayfrank, E., Thelen, B., Habermeyer, E., Kunert, H., Kovar, K.-A., Lindenblatt, H., et al. (1999). Psychopathological, neuroendocrine and autonomic effects of 3, 4-methylenedioxyethylamphetamine (MDE), psilocybin and d-methamphetamine in healthy volunteers: Results of an experimental double-blind placebo-controlled study. *Psychopharmacology, 142*(1), 41–50.

Greenfield, R. (2006). *Timothy Leary: A biography.* New York: Houghton Mifflin/Harcourt.

Grieshaber, A. F., Moore, K. A., & Levine, B. (2001). The detection of psilocin in human urine. *Journal of Forensic Science, 46*(3), 627–630.

Griffiths, R., Johnson, M., Carducci, M., Umbricht, A., Richards, W., Richards, B., et al. (2016). Psilocybin produces substantial and sustained decreases in depression and anxiety in patients with life-threatening cancer: A randomized double-blind trial. *Journal of Psychopharmacology, 30*(12), 1181–1197.

Griffiths, R., Johnson, M., Richards, W., Richards, B., McCann, U., & Jesse, R. (2011). Psilocybin occasioned mystical-type experiences: Immediate and persisting dose-related effects. *Psychopharmacology (Berlin), 218*(4), 649–665.

Griffiths, R., Richards, W., Johnson, M., McCann, U., & Jesse, R. (2008). Mystical-type experiences occasioned by psilocybin mediate the attribution of personal meaning and spiritual significance 14 months later. *Journal of Psychopharmacology, 22*(6), 621–632.

Griffiths, R., Richards, W., McCann, U., & Jesse, R. (2006). Psilocybin can occasion mystical-type experiences having substantial and sustained personal meaning and spiritual significance. *Psychopharmacology (Berlin), 187*(3), 268–283; discussion 284–292.

Grinspoon, L., & Bakalar, J. B. (1979). *Psychedelic drugs reconsidered.* New York: Basic Books.

Grob, C. S., Danforth, A. L., Chopra, G. S., Hagerty, M., McKay, C. R., Halberstadt, A. L., et al. (2011). Pilot study of psilocybin treatment for anxiety in patients with advanced-stage cancer. *Archives of General Psychiatry, 68*(1), 71–78.

Grof, S. (1973). Theoretical and empirical basis of transpersonal psychology and psychothera-

py: Observations from LSD research. *Journal of Transpersonal Psychology, 5*(1), 15–53.

Guzmán, G. (2005). Species diversity in the genus *Psilocybe* (Basidiomycotina, Agaricales, Strophariaceae) of world mycobiota, with special attention to hallucinogenic properties. *International Journal of Medicinal Mushrooms, 7*(1/2), 305–331.

Guzmán, G., Allen, J., & Gartz, J. (1998). A worldwide geographical distribution of the neurotropic fungi, an analysis and discussion. *Annali Museo Civico Rovereto, 14,* 189–280.

Halberstadt, A. L., & Geyer, M. A. (2013). Serotonergic hallucinogens as translational models relevant to schizophrenia. *International Journal of Neuropsychopharmacology, 16*(10), 2165–2180.

Halpern, J. H. (1996). The use of hallucinogens in the treatment of addiction. *Addiction Research, 4*(2), 177–189.

Halpern, J. H., Lerner, A. G., & Passie, T. (2018). A review of hallucinogen persisting perception disorder (HPPD) and an exploratory study of subjects claiming symptoms of HPPD. *Behavioral Neurobiology of Psychedelic Drugs, 36,* 333–360.

Halpern, J. H., & Pope, H. G., Jr. (2003). Hallucinogen persisting perception disorder: What do we know after 50 years? *Drug and Alcohol Dependence, 69*(2), 109–119.

Harding, W. M., & Zinberg, N. E. (1977). The effectiveness of the subculture in developing rituals and social sanctions for controlled drug use. In B. M. DuToit (Ed.), *Drugs, rituals, and altered states of consciousness* (pp. 111–133). Rotterdam, the Netherlands: A. A. Balkema.

Hardy, K., & Spanos, S. (2002). Growth factor expression and function in the human and mouse preimplantation embryo. *Journal of Endocrinology, 172*(2), 221–236.

Hasler, F., Bourquin, D., Brenneisen, R., Bär, T., & Vollenweider, F. (1997). Determination of psilocin and 4-hydroxyindole-3-acetic acid in plasma by HPLC-ECD and pharmacokinetic profiles of oral and intravenous psilocybin in man. *Pharmaceutica Acta Helvetiae, 72*(3), 175–184.

Hasler, F., Grimberg, U., Benz, M. A., Huber, T., & Vollenweider, F. X. (2004). Acute psychological and physiological effects of psilocybin in healthy humans: A double-blind, placebo-controlled dose–effect study. *Psychopharmacology, 172*(2), 145–156.

Hendricks, P. S., Clark, C. B., Johnson, M. W., Fontaine, K. R., & Cropsey, K. L. (2014). Hallucinogen use predicts reduced recidivism among substance-involved offenders under community corrections supervision. *Journal of Psychopharmacology, 28*(1), 62–66.

Hendricks, P. S., Crawford, M. S., Cropsey, K. L., Copes, H., Sweat, N. W., Walsh, Z., et al. (2018). The relationships of classic psychedelic use with criminal behavior in the United States adult population. *Journal of Psychopharmacology, 32*(1), 37–48.

Hermle, L., Simon, M., Ruchsow, M., Batra, A., & Geppert, M. (2013). Hallucinogen persisting perception disorder (HPPD) and flashback—are they identical? *Journal of Alcohol and Drug Dependence, 1,* 4.

Hermle, L., Simon, M., Ruchsow, M., & Geppert, M. (2012). Hallucinogen-persisting perception disorder. *Therapeutic Advances in Psychopharmacology, 2*(5), 199–205.

Hofmann, A. (1978). History of the basic chemical investigation on the sacred mushrooms of Mexico. In J. Ott & J. Bigwood (Eds.), *Teonandcatl: Hallucinogenic mushrooms of North America* (pp. 47–61). Seattle, WA: Madrona.

Hofmann, A. (2005). *LSD: My problem child: Reflections on sacred drugs, mysticism, and science.* Sarasota, FL: MAPS. (Original work published 1979)

Hofmann, A., Frey, A., Ott, H., & Troxler, F. (1958). Elucidation of the structure and the synthesis of psilocybin. *Experientia, 14*(11), 397–399.

Holland, D., & Passie, T. (2011). *Flashback-Phänomene als Nachwirkung von Halluzinogeneinnahme: Eine kritische Untersuchung zu klinischen und ätiologischen Aspekten.* Berlin: Verlag für Wissenschaft und Bildung.

Hollister, L. E. (1961). Clinical, biochemical and psychologic effects of psilocybin. *Archives Internationales de Pharmacodynamie et de Therapie, 130,* 42–52.

Hollister, L. E., Shelton, J., & Krieger, G. (1969). A controlled comparison of lysergic acid diethylamide (LSD) and dextroamphetamine in alcoholics. *American Journal of Psychiatry, 125*(10), 1352–1357.

Horita, A. (1963). Some biochemical studies on psilocybin and psilocin. *Journal of Neuropsychiatry, 4,* 270–273.

Isbell, H. (1959). Comparison of the reactions induced by psilocybin and LSD-25 in man. *Psychopharmacologia, 1,* 29–38.

Johansen, P. O., & Krebs, T. S. (2015). Psychedelics not linked to mental health problems or suicidal behavior: A population study. *Journal of Psychopharmacology, 29*(3), 270–279.

Johnson, M., Garcia-Romeu, A., Cosimano, M., & Griffiths, R. (2014). Pilot study of the 5-HT2AR agonist psilocybin in the treatment of tobacco addiction. *Journal of Psychopharmacology, 28*(11), 983–992.

Johnson, M., Garcia-Romeu, A., & Griffiths, R. (2017). Long-term follow-up of psilocybin-facilitated smoking cessation. *American Journal of Drug and Alcohol Abuse, 43*(1), 55–60.

Johnson, M., Richards, W., & Griffiths, R. (2008). Human hallucinogen research: Guidelines for safety. *Journal of Psychopharmacology, 22*(6), 603–620.

Kast, E. (1966). LSD and the dying patient. *Chicago Medical School Quarterly, 26*(2), 80–87.

Kast, E. (1967). Attenuation of anticipation: A therapeutic use of lysergic acid diethylamide. *Psychiatric Quarterly, 41*(4), 646–657.

Kast, E. C., & Collins, V. J. (1964). Study of lysergic acid diethylamide as an analgesic agent. *Anesthesia and Analgesia, 43*(3), 285–291.

Kilpatrick, Z. P., & Ermentrout, G. B. (2012). Hallucinogen persisting perception disorder in neuronal networks with adaptation. *Journal of Computational Neuroscience, 32*(1), 25–53.

Kovacic, P. (2009). Unifying electron transfer mechanism for psilocybin and psilocin. *Medical Hypotheses, 73*(4), 626.

Krebs, T. S., & Johansen, P.-Ø. (2012). Lysergic acid diethylamide (LSD) for alcoholism: Meta-analysis of randomized controlled trials. *Journal of Psychopharmacology, 26*(7), 994–1002.

Krebs, T. S., & Johansen, P.-Ø. (2013). Over 30 million psychedelic users in the United States. *F1000Research, 2,* 98.

Leary, T., & Metzner, R. (1968). Use of psychedelic drugs in prisoner rehabilitation. *British Journal of Social Psychiatry, 2,* 27–51.

Lee, M. A., & Shlain, B. (1992). *Acid dreams: The complete social history of LSD: The CIA, the sixties, and beyond.* New York: Grove Press.

Lerner, A. G. F. (2017, March 23). *Flashbacks and hallucinogenic persisting perception disorder: Clinical aspects and pharmacological treatment.* Presentation at the First World Congress of the World Association on Dual Disorders, Madrid, Spain.

Lerner, A. G., Gelkopf, M., Skladman, I., Oyffe, I., Finkel, B., Sigal, M., et al. (2002). Flashback and hallucinogen persisting perception disorder: Clinical aspects and pharmacological treatment approach. *Israel Journal of Psychiatry and Related Sciences, 39*(2), 92–99.

Lerner, A. G., Rudinski, D., & Bor, O. (2014). Flashbacks and HPPD: A clinical-oriented concise review. *Israel Journal of Psychiatry and Related Sciences, 51*(4), 296–301.

Lerner, A. G., Skladman, I., Kodesh, A., Sigal, M., & Shufman, E. (2001). LSD-induced hallucinogen persisting perception disorder treated with clonazepam: Two case reports. *Israel Journal of Psychiatry and Related Sciences, 38*(2), 133–136.

Leuner, H. (1962). *Die experimentelle Psychose.* Berlin: Springer.

Lindenblatt, H., Kramer, E., Holzmann-Erens, P., Gouzoulis-Mayfrank, E., & Kovar, K. A. (1998). Quantitation of psilocin in human plasma by high-performance liquid chromatography and electrochemical detection: Comparison of liquid–liquid extraction with automated on-line solid-phase extraction. *Journal of Chromatography B: Biomedical Sciences and Applications, 709*(2), 255–263.

Litjens, R. P., Brunt, T. M., Alderliefste, G. J., & Westerink, R. H. (2014). Hallucinogen persisting perception disorder and the serotonergic system: A comprehensive review including new MDMA-related clinical cases. *Journal of the European College of Neuropsychopharmacology, 24*(8), 1309–1323.

Ludwig, A. M., & Levine, J. (1965). A controlled comparison of five brief treatment techniques employing LSD, hypnosis, and psychotherapy. *American Journal of Psychotherapy, 19*(3), 417–435.

Machado-Vieira, R., Salvadore, G., Diazgranados, N., & Zarate, C. A., Jr. (2009). Ketamine and the next generation of antidepressants with a rapid onset of action. *Pharmacology and Therapeutics, 123*(2), 143–150.

MacLean, K., Johnson, M., & Griffiths, R. (2011). Mystical experiences occasioned by the hallucinogen psilocybin lead to increases in the personality domain of openness. *Journal of Psychopharmacology, 25*(11), 1453–1461.

Malitz, S., Esecover, H., Wilkens, B., & Hoch, P. H. (1960). Some observations on psilocybin, a new hallucinogen, in volunteer subjects. *Comprehensive Psychiatry, 1,* 8–17.

Manevski, N., Kurkela, M., Höglund, C., Mauriala, T., Yli-Kauhaluoma, J., & Finel, M. (2010). Glucuronidation of psilocin and 4-hydroxyindole by the human UDP-glucuronosyltransferases. *Drug Metabolism and Disposition, 38*(3), 386–395.

Mangini, M. (1998). Treatment of alcoholism using psychedelic drugs: A review of the program of research. *Journal of Psychoactive Drugs, 30*(4), 381–418.

Markel, H., Lee, A., Holmes, R. D., & Domino, E. F. (1994). LSD flashback syndrome exacerbated by selective serotonin reuptake inhibitor antidepressants in adolescents. *Journa of Pediatrics, 125*(5, Pt. 1), 817–819.

Marona-Lewicka, D., Thisted, R. A., & Nichols, D. E. (2005). Distinct temporal phases in the behavioral pharmacology of LSD: Dopamine D2 receptor-mediated effects in the rat and implications for psychosis. *Psychopharmacology (Berlin), 180*(3), 427–435.

Martinotti, G., Santacroce, R., Pettorruso, M.,

Montemitro, C., Spano, M. C., Lorusso, M., et al. (2018). Hallucinogen persisting perception disorder: Etiology, clinical features, and therapeutic perspectives. *Brain Science, 8*(3), 47.

McCabe, O. L. (1977). Psychedelic drug crises: Toxicity and therapeutics. *Journal of Psychedelic Drugs, 9*(2), 107–121.

McGraw, J. J. (2004). *Brain and belief: An exploration of the human soul.* Del Mar, CA: Aegis Press.

Meier, E. A., Gallegos, J. V., Thomas, L. P. M., Depp, C. A., Irwin, S. A., & Jeste, D. V. (2016). Defining a good death (successful dying): Literature review and a call for research and public dialogue. *American Journal of Geriatric Psychiatry, 24*(4), 261–271.

Metzner, R. (2005). *Sacred mushroom of visions: Teonanacatl: A sourcebook on the psilocybin mushroom.* New York: Simon & Schuster.

Metzner, R., Litwin, G., & Weil, G. (1965). The relation of expectation and mood to psilocybin reactions: A questionnaire study. *Psychedelic Review, 5,* 3–13.

Moreno, F. A., Wiegand, C. B., Taitano, E. K., & Delgado, P. L. (2006). Safety, tolerability, and efficacy of psilocybin in 9 patients with obsessive–compulsive disorder. *Journal of Clinical Psychiatry, 67*(11), 1735–1740.

Morgan, C. J., Noronha, L. A., Muetzelfeldt, M., Feilding, A., & Curran, H. V. (2013). Harms and benefits associated with psychoactive drugs: Findings of an international survey of active drug users. *Journal of Psychopharmacology, 27*(6), 497–506.

Moskowitz, D. (1971). Use of haloperidol to reduce LSD flashbacks. *Military Medicine, 136*(9), 754–756.

Murray, R. M., Paparelli, A., Morrison, P. D., Marconi, A., & Di Forti, M. (2013). What can we learn about schizophrenia from studying the human model, drug-induced psychosis? *American Journal of Medical Genetics B: Neuropsychiatric Genetics, 162*(7), 661–670.

Nichols, D. E., Johnson, M. W., & Nichols, C. D. (2017). Psychedelics as medicines: An emerging new paradigm. *Clinical Pharmacology and Therapeutics, 101*(2), 209–219.

Nutt, D., King, L. A., Saulsbury, W., & Blakemore, C. (2007). Development of a rational scale to assess the harm of drugs of potential misuse. *Lancet, 369,* 1047–1053.

O'Brien, C. P. (2005). Drug addiction and drug abuse. In L. L. Brunton, J. S. Lazo, & K. L. Parker (Eds.), *Goodman and Gilman's the pharmacological basis of therapeutics* (pp. 607–627). New York: McGraw-Hill.

Orsolini, L., Papanti, G. D., De Berardis, D., Guirguis, A., Corkery, J. M., & Schifano, F. (2017). The "endless trip" among the NPS users: Psychopathology and psychopharmacology in the hallucinogen-persisting perception disorder: A systematic review. *Frontiers in Psychiatry, 8,* 240.

Orsolini, L., Tomasetti, C., Valchera, A., Vecchiotti, R., Matarazzo, I., Vellante, F., et al. (2016). An update of safety of clinically used atypical antipsychotics. *Expert Opinion on Drug Safety, 15*(10), 1329–1347.

Pahnke, W. N. (1963). *Drugs and mysticism: An analysis of the relationship between psychedelic drugs and the mystical consciousness.* Cambridge, MA: Harvard University Press.

Pahnke, W. N. (1967). LSD and religious experience. In R. C. DeBold & R. C. Leaf (Eds.), *LSD, man and society* (pp. 60–85). Middletown, CT: Wesleyan University Press.

Pahnke, W. N. (1969). Psychedelic drugs and mystical experience. *International Journal of Psychiatry in Clinical Practice, 5*(4), 149–162.

Pahnke, W. N., Kurland, A. A., Goodman, L. E., & Richards, W. A. (1969). LSD-assisted psychotherapy with terminal cancer patients. *Current Psychiatric Therapies, 9,* 144–152.

Pahnke, W., Kurland, A., Unger, S., Savage, C., & Grof, S. (1971). The experimental use of psychedelic (LSD) psychotherapy. *International Journal of Clinical Pharmacology, Therapy, and Toxicology, 4*(4), 446–454.

Passie, T., Seifert, J., Schneider, U., & Emrich, H. M. (2002). The pharmacology of psilocybin. *Addiction Biology, 7*(4), 357–364.

Preller, K. H., Herdener, M., Pokorny, T., Planzer, A., Kraehenmann, R., Stampfli, P., et al. (2017). The fabric of meaning and subjective effects in LSD-induced states depend on serotonin 2A receptor activation. *Current Biology, 27*(3), 451–457.

Preller, K. H., Pokorny, T., Hock, A., Kraehenmann, R., Stampfli, P., Seifritz, E., et al. (2016). Effects of serotonin 2A/1A receptor stimulation on social exclusion processing. *Proceedings of the National Academy of Sciences of the USA, 113*(18), 5119–5124.

Preller, K. H., & Vollenweider, F. X. (2018). Phenomenology, structure, and dynamic of psychedelic states. *Current Topics in Behavioral Neurosciences, 36,* 221–256.

Reiche, S., Hermle, L., Gutwinski, S., Jungaberle, H., Gasser, P., & Majić, T. (2018). Serotonergic hallucinogens in the treatment of anxiety and depression in patients suffering from a life-threatening disease: A systematic review. *Progress in Neuro-Psychopharmacology and Biological Psychiatry, 81,* 1–10.

Richards, W. A. (1980). Psychedelic drug-assisted psychotherapy with persons suffering from terminal cancer. *Journal of Altered States of Consciousness, 5*(4), 309–319.

Ross, S. (2012). Serotonergic hallucinogens and emerging targets for addiction pharmacotherapies. *Psychiatric Clinics, 35*(2), 357–374.

Ross, S. (2018). Therapeutic use of classic psychedelics to treat cancer-related psychiatric distress. *International Review of Psychiatry, 30,* 317–330.

Ross, S., Bossis, A., Guss, J., Agin-Liebes, G., Malone, T., Cohen, B., et al. (2016). Rapid and sustained symptom reduction following psilocybin treatment for anxiety and depression in patients with life-threatening cancer: A randomized controlled trial. *Journal of Psychopharmacology, 30*(12), 1165–1180.

Ross, S., & Peselow, E. (2012). Co-occurring psychotic and addictive disorders: Neurobiology and diagnosis. *Clinical Neuropharmacology, 35*(5), 235–243.

Russo-Neustadt, A., Beard, R. C., & Cotman, C. W. (1999). Exercise, antidepressant medications, and enhanced brain derived neurotrophic factor expression. *Neuropsychopharmacology, 21*(5), 679–682.

Rynearson, R., Wilson, M., Jr., & Bickford, R. (1968). Psilocybin-induced changes in psychologic function, electroencephalogram, and light-evoked potentials in human subjects. *Mayo Clinic Proceedings, 43,* 191–204.

Salomé, F., Boyer, P., & Fayol, M. (2000). The effects of psychoactive drugs and neuroleptics on language in normal subjects and schizophrenic patients: A review. *European Psychiatry, 15*(8), 461–469.

Samorini, G. (1992). The oldest representations of hallucinogenic mushrooms in the world (Sahara Desert, 9000–7000 B.P.). *Integration, 2*(3), 69–78.

Santos, R. D., Landeira-Fernandez, J., Strassman, R., Motta, V., & Cruz, A. (2007). Effects of ayahuasca on psychometric measures of anxiety, panic-like and hopelessness in Santo Daime members. *Journal of Ethnopharmacology, 112*(3), 507–513.

Schultes, R. E., & Farnsworth, N. R. (1980). Ethnomedical, botanical and phytochemical aspects of natural hallucinogens. *Botanical Museum Leaflets, 128,* 123–214.

Schwartz, R. H., & Smith, D. E. (1988). Hallucinogenic mushrooms. *Clinical Pediatrics, 27*(2), 70–73.

Sewell, R. A., Halpern, J. H., & Pope, H. G. (2006). Response of cluster headache to psilocybin and LSD. *Neurology, 66*(12), 1920–1922.

Singer, R., & Smith, A. (1958). Mycological investigations on teonanácatl, the Mexican hallucinogenic mushroom: Part II. A taxonomic monograph of Psilocybe, section Caerulescentes. *Mycologia, 50,* 262–303.

Smart, R. G., Storm, T., Baker, E. F., & Solursh, L. (1966). A controlled study of lysergide in the treatment of alcoholism: I. The effects on drinking behavior. *Quarterly Journal of Studies on Alcohol, 27,* 469–482.

Smith, H. (2000). *Cleansing the doors of perception: The religious significance of entheogenic plants and chemicals.* New York: Tarcher.

Stace, W. T. (1960). *The teachings of the mystics.* New York/Scarborough: New American Library.

Stace, W. T. (1961). *Mysticism and philosophy.* London: Macmillan.

Stamets, P. (1996). *Psilocybin mushrooms of the world.* Berkeley, CA: Ten Speed Press.

Sticht, G., & Kaferstein, H. (2000). Detection of psilocin in body fluids. *Forensic Science International, 113*(1–3), 403–407.

Strassman, R. J. (1984). Adverse reactions to psychedelic drugs: A review of the literature. *Journal of Nervous and Mental Disease, 172*(10), 577–595.

Studerus, E., Gamma, A., & Vollenweider, F. X. (2010). Psychometric evaluation of the altered states of consciousness rating scale (OAV). *PLOS ONE, 5*(8), e12412.

Studerus, E., Kometer, M., Hasler, F., & Vollenweider, F. X. (2011). Acute, subacute and long-term subjective effects of psilocybin in healthy humans: A pooled analysis of experimental studies. *Journal of Psychopharmacology, 25*(11), 1434–1452.

Swift, T. C., Belser, A. B., Agin-Liebes, G., Devenot, N., Terrana, S., Friedman, H. L., et al. (2017). Cancer at the dinner table: Experiences of psilocybin-assisted psychotherapy for the treatment of cancer-related distress. *Journal of Humanistic Psychology, 57*(5), 488–519.

Szara, S. (1956). Dimethyltryptamin: Its metabolism in man: The relation to its psychotic effect to the serotonin metabolism. *Experientia, 12*(11), 441–442.

Thurlow, H. J., & Girvin, J. P. (1971). Use of antiepileptic medication in treating "flashbacks" from hallucinogenic drugs. *Canadian Medical Association Journal, 105*(9), 947–948.

Timothy, L., Ralph, M., Madison, P., Gunther, W., Ralph, S., & Sara, K. (1965). A new behavior change program using psilocybin. *Psychotherapy: Theory, Research and Practice, 2*(2), 61–72.

Tomsovic, M., & Edwards, R. (1970). Lysergide treatment of schizophrenic and nonschizophrenic alcoholics: A controlled evaluation. *Quarterly Journal of Studies on Alcohol, 31*(4), 932–949.

Tyls, F., Palenicek, T., & Horacek, J. (2014). Psilocybin—summary of knowledge and new perspectives. *European Neuropsychopharmacology, 24*(3), 342–356.

van Amsterdam, J., Opperhuizen, A., & van den Brink, W. (2011). Harm potential of magic mushroom use: A review. *Regulatory Toxicology and Pharmacology, 59*(3), 423–429.

Van Oekelen, D., Luyten, W. H., & Leysen, J. E. (2003). 5-HT2A and 5-HT2C receptors and their atypical regulation properties. *Life Science, 72*(22), 2429–2449.

Vollenweider, F. X., & Kometer, M. (2010). The neurobiology of psychedelic drugs: Implications for the treatment of mood disorders. *Nature Reviews Neuroscience, 11*(9), 642–651.

Vollenweider, F. X., Vollenweider-Scherpenhuyzen, M. F., Babler, A., Vogel, H., & Hell, D. (1998). Psilocybin induces schizophrenia-like psychosis in humans via a serotonin-2 agonist action. *NeuroReport, 9*(17), 3897–3902.

Vollenweider, F. X., Vontobel, P., Hell, D., & Leenders, K. L. (1999). 5-HT modulation of dopamine release in basal ganglia in psilocybin-induced psychosis in man—a PET study with [^{11}C]raclopride. *Neuropsychopharmacology, 20*(5), 424–433.

Wasson, R. (1957). Seeking the magic mushroom. *Life, 42*(19), 100–120.

Wasson, R. (1962). A new Mexican psychotropic drug from the mint family. *Botanical Museum Leaflets, 20*(3), 77–84.

Wasson, R. (1980). *The wondrous mushroom: Mycolatry in Mesoamerica.* McGraw-Hill.

Wasson, R., & Heim, R. (1958). Les champignons hallucinogènes du Mexique-Etudes ethnologiques, taxinomiques, biologiques, physiologiques et chimiques. *Archives du Muséum national d'Histoire naturelle, 7ème série, 6,* 1–445.

Wasson, V., & Wasson, R. (1957). *Mushrooms: Russia and history.* Pantheon Books.

Wolbach, A. B., Jr., Miner, E. J., & Isbell, H. (1962). Comparison of psilocin with psilocybin, mescaline and LSD-25. *Psychopharmacologia, 3,* 219–223.

Young, C. R. (1997). Sertraline treatment of hallucinogen persisting perception disorder. *Journal of Clinical Psychiatry, 58*(2), 85–85.

CHAPTER 10

Therapeutic Potential of Fast-Acting Synthetic Tryptamines

RAFAEL LANCELOTTA and ALAN K. DAVIS

▓ Introduction

Research has shown the promise of psychedelics used as an adjunct to psychotherapy in the treatment of various mental health disorders, including posttraumatic stress disorder (PTSD), treatment-resistant depression, and anxiety-related disorders (Barone et al., 2019; Carhart-Harris et al., 2018; Garcia-Romeu, Kersgaard, & Addy, 2016; Griffiths et al., 2016; Ot'alora et al., 2018; Ross et al., 2016). Psychedelics such as O-phosphoryl-4-hydroxy-N,N-dimethyltryptamine (4-PO-DMT; commonly known as psilocybin), and psychedelic-like drugs such as 3,4-methylenedioxymethamphetamine (MDMA) may be approved for medical use by the U.S. Food and Drug Administration and the European Medicines Agency in the coming years. However, their long duration of psychoactive effects (4–6 hours for psilocybin, approximately 4 hours for MDMA) increases the clinical and infrastructure resources needed for daylong treatment sessions, thus likely to result in high costs associated with these treatments. Such high costs could limit the accessibility of psilocybin- and MDMA-assisted psychotherapy to many people who

could benefit from this type of treatment, especially those from vulnerable populations such as people of color, sexual and gender minorities, and military veterans. In order to decrease the fiscal burden of these treatments, psychedelics such as N,N-dimethyltryptamine (DMT), 5-methoxy-N,N-dimethyltryptamine (5-MeO-DMT), and N,N-dipropyltryptamine (DPT), used as an adjunct to psychotherapy, may provide a more cost-effective alternative due to their quick onset and short duration of acute effects. Although all three of these substituted tryptamines have similar molecular structures, each has slightly different profiles of acute effects that could show promise for clinical indications. In this chapter, we review the current literature on the history, basic pharmacology, and acute phenomenol-

N,N-Dimethyltryptamine (DMT)

ogy of DMT, 5-MeO-DMT, and DPT, and explain the therapeutic potential by presenting evidence of their potential to alleviate symptoms associated with various mental health conditions.

DMT

DMT is a psychoactive compound found naturally in a variety of plants and animals (Christian et al., 1977; Halpern, 2004) and has been used by humans as a recreational and ceremonial drug, with some anthropological and archaeological evidence suggesting that it may have been used for more than 1,000 years (Miller et al., 2019; Palamar & Le, 2018; Sand, 2001; Torres, 2019). When consumed orally, DMT is rapidly metabolized through oxidative deamination by gastrointestinal monoamine oxidase A enzymes (Carbonaro & Gatch, 2016), thus making it inactive. However, it is found in trace amounts in traditional plant-based snuffs and in larger concentrations in various plants that are used in combination with the *Banisteriopsis caapi* vine to produce ayahuasca (Barker, 2018; Beyer, 2010), which confers intense psychoactive effects (Cott & Rock, 2008; Hancock, 2007; Kjellgren et al., 2009; McKenna, 2004). DMT was first synthesized in 1931 (Manske, 1931), but the psychoactive effects of DMT went undocumented in the scientific literature until 1956, when acute effects were reported following consumption. In Szára's (1957) own words:

> In the third or fourth minute after the injection vegetative symptoms appeared, such as tingling sensation, trembling, slight nausea, mydriasis, elevation of the blood pressure and increase of the pulse rate. At the same time eidetic phenomena, optical illusions, pseudo-hallucinations, and later real hallucinations, appeared. The hallucinations consisted of moving, brilliantly coloured oriental motifs, and later I saw wonderful scenes altering very rapidly. The faces of the people seemed to be masks. My emotional state was elevated sometimes up to euphoria. At the highest point I had compulsive athetoid movements in my left hand. My consciousness was completely filled by hallucinations, and my attention was firmly bound to them; therefore I could not give an account of the events happening around me.

> After 3/4–1 hour the symptoms disappeared, and I was able to describe what had happened.

At present, synthetic DMT is most frequently consumed via inhalation (i.e., smoking or vaporizing; Winstock et al., 2014), among people who consume a variety of other psychedelic substances primarily for recreational purposes (i.e., curiosity and interest in psychedelic drugs), or for a potential therapeutic experience (Cakic et al., 2010; Sand, 2001). Pharmacologically, DMT is derived from tryptophan and the enzyme responsible for its endogenous synthesis from tryptamine, indolethylamine-N-methyltransferase, is distributed throughout mammalian tissues (Carbonaro & Gatch, 2016). A variety of receptors potentially mediate the effects of DMT, including serotonin (e.g., affinity for $5\text{-HT}_{7, 6, 5A, 2C, 2B, 2A, 1D, \& 1B}$), σ-1, trace amine-associated and adrenergic receptors, glutamate, and dopamine (Carbonaro & Gatch, 2016; Ray, 2010). This complex set of interactions may contribute to DMT's subjective effect profile (Winkleman, 2018). Few published studies have systematically examined the acute effects of DMT in humans. When injected, synthetic DMT elicits psychedelic effects characterized by a rapid onset and short duration of action, with peak effects within 2–5 minutes and acute effects having largely dissipated by 20–30 minutes (Strassman, 1995; Strassman & Qualls, 1994). In a laboratory assessment, Strassman and Qualls administered four doses (0.05, 0.1, 0.2, and 0.4 mg/kg) of intravenous DMT to 11 subjects, demonstrating dose-dependent acute subjective effects related to intensity of psychoactive effects, increase in maximum heart rate and blood pressure, somesthesia, and changes in perception, volition, affect, and cognition.

More recently, large cross-sectional survey studies are further elucidating the acute

Tryptamine

effects of DMT, showing that many people report encountering seemingly autonomous entities (Davis et al., 2020), sometimes described as "God" or "God of one's understanding (Griffiths et al., 2019), and other times referred to as "spirits," "beings," or an "alien" or "angel" (Davis et al., 2020). Furthermore, large proportions of participants in these studies report that these DMT effects are one of the top five or single most personally meaningful, spiritually significant, and psychological insightful experiences of their lives. Unpublished qualitative reports of these entity encounters reveal experiences such as the following:

"The first time I broke through was also the time I am most sure that I met a seemingly autonomous being(s). I went through a sort of tunnel and when I emerged to the other side it felt like I had skipped over to a different dimension. There was this woman-like shape, but not a woman in front of me. She was surrounded by other figures and she was dancing around the room and came towards me. She definitely spoke to me, but without words. The other entities present in that other 'dimension' were looking at me and felt very real. The woman was more of a pink light shape that danced around with arms that seemed to beckon me—like a Siren. When I heard my friends voices back on Earth, I knew I was slipping away from the dimension. I remember reaching out towards the ceiling and the entities, including the Siren, crowded around me and said goodbye to me. That experience has led me to question my atheism."

"I was escorted out of reality as we know it and shown the entire structure of the Universe. It looked like a large iris, like a large living human eye laying horizontally. I was told that this was all of existence as I knew it, and that everything is a game. The entire reality I know is only a game. I asked if I could stay, I was enamored and didn't really want to come back. They said that the only way I could stay was if I died. I said that would be fine, . . . but they told me I had to come back."

DMT users have also reported that these entity encounters often confer specific messages, tasks, insights, and predictions about the future:

"I learned that when I resist uncomfortable emotions, I am selling myself short of the possibility to learn and grow."

"It was on a personal level as I had been struggling with addiction of opiates at the time. She basically told me that I really needed to cut it out of my life because all it will bring is pain. I had not previously thought negatively about my use of opiates before this encounter."

"This experience was them showing me that we are all connected, all one."

"There was an indescribably powerful notion that this dimension in which the entity and I convened was infinitely more 'real' than the consensus reality I usually inhabit. It felt truer than anything else I'd ever experienced."

"I was shown the way my life was heading into further depression and potential suicide and how it would impact my family and I was going to be alone unless I made some changes."

"The main future prediction was concerning my consciousness. That it will continue on after I die."

Due to its endogenous production in humans (Barker, 2018), DMT has also been theorized to be associated with several non-drug-occasioned, non-ordinary states of consciousness such as dreaming, spiritual and mystical experiences, encounters with nonhuman intelligence (e.g., alien and UFO encounters), psychosis, and parapsychological phenomena such as out-of-body experiences, extrasensory perception, and near-death experiences (Gallimore, 2013; Hernandez et al., 2018; Luke, 2008, 2011, 2012; Luke & Kittenis, 2005; Ring, 1992; St. John, 2016; Strassman, 2001, 2008; Timmerman et al., 2018). Indeed, recent evidence has shown that the rodent brain is capable of producing and releasing DMT at concentrations similar to other neurotransmitters in the visual cortex, and that DMT production is increased after a cardiac arrest (Dean et al., 2019). However, there has been much debate regarding the role of endogenous DMT in humans (Barker, 2018; Christiansen et al., 1977; Rodrigues, Almeida, & Vieira-Coelho, 2019; Strassman, 2008; Szabo, 2015), and critiques of the endogenous role of DMT suggest that there are not sufficient quantities of endogenous DMT to substantially alter brain function during birth, death, or a near-death experiences (Nichols, 2018).

Although more research is needed, the combination of physiological and psycholog-

5-Methoxy-*N*,*N*-dimethyltryptamine (5-MeO-DMT)

ical effects of DMT, and anecdotal reports from users, suggests therapeutic potential (Rodrigues et al., 2019; Szara, 2009). For example, preclinical studies have described physiological mechanisms by which DMT could be therapeutic, such as a catalyst of immunomodulatory and inflammatory processes that have been linked to depression and Alzheimer's disease (Szabo, 2015). Furthermore, although the acute effects are shorter in duration compared to other psychedelics (e.g., psilocybin), several acute effects and enduring beliefs about such experiences are similar. For example, Griffiths and colleagues (2019) reported that rates of the intensity of mystical experiences, and the proportion endorsing the experience of gaining psychological insight, are similar between people who use psilocybin and those who use DMT. Given that the mystical and insightful experiences have been associated with the therapeutic outcomes of psilocybin administration in samples of cancer patients, people with substance use disorder, and people with depression/anxiety (Davis et al., 2020; Garcia-Romeu et al., 2019; Griffiths et al., 2016), it is possible that DMT may also confer such therapeutic effects when administered with psychological support. Although not yet fully understood, the combination of physiological and psychological effects of DMT suggest potential therapeutic value.

5-MeO-DMT

5-MeO-DMT, a potent, fast-acting, psychoactive compound, is found in the venom of *Incilius alvarius* toads (also known as *Bufo alvarius*), in various plants, and in humans

(e.g., lung, brain, blood, cerebrospinal fluid, liver, and heart), and it has also been made by synthetic preparation (Agurell et al., 1969; Lyttle et al., 1996; McKenna & Towers, 1984; Ott, 2001; Pachter et al., 1959; Shen et al., 2010; Szabo et al., 2014; Torres & Repke, 2006; Weil & Davis, 1994; Yu, 2008). The documented history of human contact with exogenous 5-MeO-DMT includes evidence of spiritual and recreational use in the form of snuffs derived from *Virola theiodora* resin or *Anadenanthera peregrina* seeds (Agurell et al., 1969; McKenna et al., 1984a, 1984b; Schultes, 1984; Torres & Repke, 2006; Trout, 2015). For example, reports dating as far back as 100 years detail use of *Anadenanthera peregrina* seeds in snuff preparations by the Taíno Indians of the Greater Antilles (Torres & Repke, 2006). Analysis of these seed preparations have shown that DMT and bufotenin (5-HO-DMT) are primary constituents, with 5-MeO-DMT content varying from 0.11 to 1% of total alkaloids found (Trout, 2007). The snuffs produced from *Virola theiodora* resin by the Waikás tribe have been reported to contain higher concentrations of 5-MeO-DMT, with ranges of 514.8 mg to 9,680 mg per 100 g of snuff (Agurell et al., 1969). Although some reports suggest that toad venom containing 5-MeO-DMT may have been used historically by indigenous cultures (Weil & Davis, 1994), there does not appear to be much evidence supporting this claim (Viceland, 2017). In recent years, the discovery of high concentrations of 5-MeO-DMT in *Incilius alvarius* toad venom secretions has led to an increase in reported recreational and spiritual use (Davis et al., 2018; Uthaug et al., 2019; Weil & Davis, 1994). Reasons for this may include recent evidence showing that concentrations of 5-MeO-DMT in toad venom secretions varies between 20 and 30% of total dry weight, that is to say, approximately 200–300 mg 5-MeO-DMT per dried gram (Uthaug et al., 2019), substantially higher concentrations compared to 5-MeO-DMT found in plant-derived preparations.

5-MeO-DMT was first synthesized by Hoshino and Shimodaira (1936), and in animal models, acts as a nonselective 5-HT agonist (e.g., $_{1A}$ and $_{2A}$ receptors; Jiang et al., 2016; Shen et al., 2011), appears to have a higher affinity for the 5-HT$_{1A}$ receptor subtype (Alhaider et al., 1993; Spencer et al., 1987), and inhibits the reuptake of 5-HT (Nagai et al., 2007). This pattern of neurotransmitter binding affinity is similar to that of structurally similar psychedelic tryptamines (e.g., DMT; Fantegrossi et al., 2006; Rabin et al., 2002; Sadzot et al., 1989; Winter, 2009), and somewhat different from tryptamines with stronger affinity for the 5-HT$_{2A}$ receptor (e.g., psilocybin; McKenna et al., 1990; Winter et al., 2000). Furthermore, Szabo and colleagues (2014) found that 5-MeO-DMT inhibited production of proinflammatory cytokines and increased the production of anti-inflammatory cytokines, suggesting that 5-MeO-DMT may play a role in endogenous immune system homeostasis via its activity at the σ-1 receptor.

The synthetic form of 5-MeO-DMT is reportedly ingested via several routes of administration, including inhalation, insufflation, or injection (Davis et al., 2018; Ott, 2001; Sexton et al., 2019). Davis and colleagues (2018) found that inhalation (e.g., smoking or vaporizing) is the most common route of consumption (81%), and prior evidence suggests that initial onset of effects occurs within 60 seconds and peak total duration of effect between 5 and 20 minutes after inhalation (Erowid, 1999). Published studies describe a range of subjective effects of 5-MeO-DMT: intense emotional experiences; auditory, visual, and time perception distortions; memory impairment (Ott, 2001; Shulgin & Shulgin, 1997); mystical experiences, and minimal challenging physical or psychological effects (Davis et al., 2018), with peak effects between 35 and 40 minutes after insufflation or within seconds-to-minutes when inhaled or injected intravenously (Ott, 2001; Shulgin & Shulgin, 1997). Unpublished qualitative reports from large survey studies (Davis et al., 2018, 2019) elucidate these acute effects:

> "Removes the veil between our perceived reality and ultimate reality."

> "My hypothesis of death became something more like an understanding."

> "Imbued me with . . . confidence to look at my trauma and grief and heal it."

> "Experience bliss . . . peace and tranquility . . . feeling connection to the love and beauty that surrounds us all."

> "Very intensely pleasurable body high."

> "The self-realization and increased awareness that remain for some time while working on oneself."

Despite these perceived positive acute effects, challenging experiences are also reported:

> "Extremely jarring . . . too much information/revelation to know what to do with."

> "Physical danger . . . due to involuntary/unaware bodily movements."

> "Inability to regulate the intensity."

Anecdotally, people have also reported a "reactivation" phenomenon in which the effects of 5-MeO-DMT are reexperienced after the acute effects have worn off, typically as someone is falling asleep or attempting to meditate (5 Hive, 2019). Interestingly, recent analyses of unpublished data from three survey studies (Davis et al., 2018, 2019; Uthaug et al., 2020) found that approximately one-fourth and sometimes as high as three-fourths of 5-MeO-DMT users report having a reactivation. Interestingly, unpublished data from Davis and colleagues (2018, 2019) showed that despite many people reporting a reactivation, the vast majority of these individuals (95–97%) believed that the reactivation was a "neutral" or "positive" experience.

The scientific evidence regarding the psychotherapeutic potential of 5-MeO-DMT is limited to preclinical studies (Szabo, 2015), cross-sectional survey studies of recreational and ceremonial users (Barsuglia, Davis, et al., 2018; Davis et al., 2018, 2019; Lancelotta & Davis, 2020), and emerging observational studies using a prospective design in the natural environment (Uthaug et al., 2020). For example, preclinical studies have shown potent anti-inflammatory effects of 5-MeO-DMT (Dakic et al., 2017; Szabo, 2015), and cross-sectional survey studies have found reported reductions in depression and anxiety among a sample of people who reported using 5-MeO-DMT in a ceremonial context (Davis et al., 2019; Sepeda et al., 2019), and that people in the general population report improvement in several mental health conditions postconsumption, including improvements in depression, anxiety, PTSD, and addiction (Cox, Lancelotta, Barsuglia, & Davis, 2018; Cox, Moshman, Barsuglia, Lancelotta, & Davis, 2018; Davis et al., 2019). Furthermore, high ratings of personal meaning and spiritual significance, and moderate-to-strong acute mystical effects, associated with 5-MeO-DMT consumption have been reported (Davis et al., 2018, 2019), and recent prospective studies conducted in the natural environment have shown that 5-MeO-DMT administration is related to a decrease in depression and anxiety, as well as increases in satisfaction with life (Uthaug et al., 2019).

Evidence also suggests that mystical experiences occasioned by vaporized 5-MeO-DMT in a psychologically supported environment are similar in intensity to moderately high doses of oral psilocybin administered in the laboratory (Barsuglia, Polanco, et al., 2018), and are associated with naturalistic improvement in depression and anxiety after 5-MeO-DMT use (Davis et al., 2019). However, some have argued for differing routes of 5-MeO-DMT administration (e.g., intramuscular injection, insufflation) in order to capitalize on a more gradual onset and sustained plateau of acute effects (HumbleVoyager, 2017; Metzner, 2013; Uthaug et al., 2020). Although more research is needed to determine the optimal route of administration for 5-MeO-DMT, it is possible that 5-MeO-DMT may eventually be shown to confer psychotherapeutic effects when administered in a clinical laboratory setting.

N,N-Dipropyltryptamine (DPT)

DPT

DPT is a synthetically produced psychoactive compound and a close structural homologue of DMT (Fantegrossi et al., 2008; Soskin, 1975). Though DPT has been used in various clinical populations, there are few published studies about its origins. The first synthesis of DPT was reported by Speeter and Anthony (1954) under the name 3-(2-n-propylaminoethyl)-indole (International Union of Pure and Applied Chemistry [IUPAC] nomenclature standards had not yet been established). The study described a novel route of tryptamine synthesis and the potential for psychoactive activity through the administration of various tryptamine compounds (including DPT) (Speeter & Anthony, 1954). In animal studies, DPT demonstrated relative potency in various tissues (Bertaccini & Zamboni, 1961) and evidence for 5-HT$_{1A}$ and 5-HT$_{2A}$ receptor agonism and binding affinities (Li et al., 2007; Thiagaraj et al., 2005).

In terms of acute effects, DPT has been administered by intramuscular injection at doses of 15–165 mg with effects lasting approximately 2 hours at smaller doses (15–30 mg) and up to 6 hours at larger doses (75–165 mg) with no reported adverse physical effects (Soskin, 1975). DPT is commonly found as a hydrochloride salt and can be ingested via several routes of administration, including oral, insufflation, or vaporization of the freebase (Tittarelli et al., 2015). Although DPT has been found to be effective via these varied routes of administration, original research conducted with this compound was done with the assumption that DPT is not orally active and has best clinical effects when administered intramuscularly (Soskin, 1975). Published studies report visionary, visual, dream-like effects that are often emotional and, at higher doses, mystical in nature (Shulgin & Shulgin, 1997). A description of characteristics of a DPT experience session can be found in Shulgin and Shulgin (1997): "[with 100 mg intramuscularly] I was being led by the hand of a wise old man who I know was God, and we went off to the front of the synagogue. I was handed a Torah for me to carry as a sign that I had been accepted, and forgiven, and that I had come home."

Other descriptions of the DPT experience can be found on Erowid (InnerExplorer, 2016) that highlight the ability for this compound to occasion mystical experiences:

"[with 20 mg intramuscularly] Flowing visuals around the sides of vision . . . Lose concept/track of time entirely, seemed to be falling through a series of fractal realities. Was shown how humans are an amazingly complex and evolutionarily advanced design. Essentially human beings together comprise a huge brain (fractal reality of each individual). Each human being has 'free will' in order to facilitate a greater array of possible novel ideas generated. There was a great feeling that this experience is one of the most significant of life itself, right up there with birth and death. There were several moments where it felt like the whole 'veil' of reality had been lifted. There were also several moments where I felt like it was on the edge of being 'too much' but with deep breaths I was able to keep pressing on. The only way out is through. I felt an incredible emotional release as well, crying at several points as I processed various emotions I had been holding on to the past few days. As during other high-ish doses of tryptamines, my body felt compelled to move around . . . Definitely not something to be taken recreationally. . . . it is a quite intense experience which feels as significant as being born or dying. . . . I could also not 'escape' the experience, as sense of self dissolves quite readily within the first few minutes. All I could do was let go and flow with the experience. . . . I think if someone were trying to 'reboot' their personality, this might be a good choice for a peak experience."

The earliest human study with DPT was conducted in a hospital setting with a sample of individuals diagnosed with an alcohol use disorder. Patients were administered intramuscular injections of *N,N*-diethyltryptamine (DET), DPT, and 6-fluorodiethyltryptamine (6-FDET) (Faillace et al., 1967). The study did not show efficacy in the treatment of alcohol use disorder but demonstrated that DPT was a psychoactive and potent short-acting psychedelic drug (Faillace et al., 1967). Other experiments using DPT in clinical settings were conducted in the 1970s, particularly in the treatment of alcohol use disorder and anxiety secondary to terminal illness in cancer patients. In these studies, DPT was shown to catalyze "peak" experiences that were associated

N,N-Diethyltryptamine (DET)

with positive change in mental health problems (Rhead et al., 1977; Richards et al., 1977). At low doses, DPT has also shown promise as a tool for deepening the efficacy of talk therapy (Soskin et al., 1973). Indeed, Soskin created a manual for DPT-assisted talk therapy, wherein he postulated that it could be a good alternative to LSD-assisted psychotherapy due to DPT's short duration of effects (Soskin, 1975). Accordingly, DPT was used at the Maryland Psychiatric Research Center to treat over 100 patients with evidence for positive outcomes (Grof et al., 1973; Soskin, 1975; Soskin et al., 1973). Similar to the reasoning for why DMT and 5-MeO-DMT may confer psychotherapeutic effects, it could be that the "peak" or mystical and insightful experiences occasioned by DPT-assisted psychotherapy could show promise in the treatment of a variety of mental health problems.

Conclusions and Future Directions

Each of these fast-acting tryptamines, when administered as an adjunct to psychotherapy, could catalyze a process of cognitive, emotional, and behavioral changes associated with improvements in mental health functioning and life satisfaction. Additionally, they might provide a more cost-effective approach to treatment of mental health problems such as depression, anxiety, addiction, or PTSD given their quick onset and short duration of action. That DMT, 5-MeO-DMT, and DPT appear to occasion rapid and robust mystical and insightful experiences suggests that their effects could show promise in different clinical settings with limited resources to catalyze healing (e.g., opioid detoxification units, emergency departments, psychiatric inpatient units), for people with co-occurring mental health diagnoses (e.g., alcohol use disorder and depression; PTSD and substance use disorder) or to treat the associated sequela of high-risk mental health problems (e.g., acute suicidality or other self-harm behavior). However, before such hypotheses can be empirically tested, more research is needed to determine the feasibility, safety, pharmacokinetics, and acute subjective effects of these synthetic drugs among healthy human volunteers. If these studies provide evidence supporting the safe administration of these compounds in laboratory settings, then future research should investigate whether they occasion positive clinical outcomes when tested as part of a randomized controlled trial in clinical populations.

■ References

5 Hive. (2019). The reactivations thread. Retrieved September 10, 2020, from *https://forums. 5meodmt.org/index.php?topic=50940.0.*

Agurell, S., Holmstedt, B., Lindgren, J. E., & Schultes, R. E. (1969). Alkaloids in certain species of *Virola* and other South American plants of ethnopharmacologic interest. *Acta Chemica Scandinavica, 23*(3), 903–916.

Alhaider, A. A., Hamon, M., & Wilcox, G. L. (1993). Intrathecal 5-methoxy-N,N-dimethyltryptamine in mice modulates 5-HT1 and 5-HT3 receptors. *European Journal of Pharmacology, 249*(2), 151–160.

Barker, S. A. (2018). N,N-Dimethyltryptamine (DMT), an endogenous hallucinogen: Past, present, and future research to determine its role and function. *Frontiers in Neuroscience, 12,* 536.

Barone, W., Beck, J., Mitsunaga-Whitten, M., & Perl, P. (2019). Perceived benefits of MDMA-assisted psychotherapy beyond symptom reduction: Qualitative follow-up study of a clinical trial for individuals with treatment-resistant PTSD. *Journal of Psychoactive Drugs, 51*(2), 199–208.

Barsuglia, J., Davis, A. K., Palmer, R., Lancelotta, R., Windham-Herman, A.-M., Peterson, K., et al. (2018). Intensity of mystical experiences occasioned by 5-MeO-DMT and comparison with a prior psilocybin study. *Frontiers in Psychology, 9,* 2459.

Barsuglia, J. P., Polanco, M., Palmer, R., Mal-
colm, B. J., Kelmendi, B., & Calvey, T. (2018). A case report SPECT study and theoretical rationale for the sequential administration of ibogaine and 5-MeO-DMT in the treatment of alcohol use disorder. *Progress in Brain Research, 242,* 121–158.

Bertaccini, G., & Zamboni, P. (1961). The relative potency of 5-hydroxytryptamine like substances. *Archives Internationales De Pharmacodynamie Et De Therapie, 133,* 138–156.

Beyer, S. V. (2010). *Singing to the plants: A guide to mestizo shamanism in the upper Amazon.* Albuquerque: University of New Mexico Press.

Cakic, V., Potkonyak, J., & Marshall, A. (2010). Dimethyltryptamine (DMT): Subjective effects and patterns of use among Australian recreational users. *Drug and Alcohol Dependence, 111*(1), 30–37.

Carbonaro, T. M., & Gatch, M. B. (2016). Neuropharmacology of N,N-Dimethyltryptamine. *Brain Research Bulletin, 126*(Pt. 1), 74–88.

Carhart-Harris, R. L., Bolstridge, M., Day, C. M. J., Rucker, J., Watts, R., Erritzoe, D. E., et al. (2018). Psilocybin with psychological support for treatment-resistant depression: Six-month follow-up. *Psychopharmacology, 235*(2), 399–408.

Christian, S. T., Harrison, R., Quayle, E., Pagel, J., & Monti, J. (1977). The in vitro identification of dimethyltryptamine (DMT) in mammalian brain and its characterization as a possible endogenous neuroregulatory agent. *Biochemical Medicine, 18*(2), 164–183.

Cott, C., & Rock, A. (2008). Phenomenology of N,N-dimethyltryptamine use: A thematic analysis. *Journal of Scientific Exploration, 22*(3), 359–370.

Cox, K., Lancelotta, R., Barsuglia, J., & Davis, A. (2018, November). *5-MeO-DMT and subjective improvements in post-traumatic stress disorder.* Presented at the annual conference of the Maryland Psychological Association, Baltimore, MD.

Cox, K., Moshman, S., Barsuglia, J., Lancelotta, R., & Davis, A. (2018, July). *Subjective improvements in substance use problems following 5-MeO-DMT use in an international sample.* Paper presented at the BPRU Poster Symposium, Baltimore, MD.

Dakic, V., Nascimento, J. M., Sartore, R. C., Maciel, R. de M., de Araujo, D. B., Ribeiro, S., et al. (2017). Short term changes in the proteome of human cerebral organoids induced by 5-MeO-DMT. *Scientific Reports, 7*(1), 1–13.

Davis, A. K., Barsuglia, J. P., Lancelotta, R., Grant, R. M., & Renn, E. (2018). The epidemiology of 5-methoxy-N,N-dimethyltryptamine (5-MeO-DMT) use: Benefits, consequences, patterns of use, subjective effects, and reasons for consumption. *Journal of Psychopharmacology (Oxford), 32*(7), 779–792.

Davis, A. K., Clifton, J. M., Weaver, E. G., Hurwitz, E. S., Johnson, M. W., & Griffiths, R. R. (2020). Entity encounter experiences occasioned by inhaled *N,N*-dimethyltryptamine (DMT): Phenomenology, interpretation, and enduring effects. *Journal of Psychopharmacology, 34*(9), 1008–1020.

Davis, A. K., So, S., Lancelotta, R., Barsuglia, J. P., & Griffiths, R. R. (2019). 5-Methoxy-*N,N*-dimethyltryptamine (5-MeO-DMT) used in a naturalistic group setting is associated with unintended improvements in depression and anxiety. *American Journal of Drug and Alcohol Abuse, 45*(2), 161–169.

Dean, J. G., Liu, T., Huff, S., Sheler, B., Barker, S. A., Strassman, R. J., et al. (2019). Biosynthesis and extracellular concentrations of *N,N*-dimethyltryptamine (DMT) in mammalian brain. *Scientific Reports, 9*(1), Article No. 9333.

Erowid. (1999, May 7). Erowid 5-MeO-DMT vault: Effects. Retrieved August 5, 2019, from *https://erowid.org/chemicals/5meo_dmt/5meo_dmt_effects.shtml.*

Faillace, L. A., Vourlekis, A., & Szara, S. (1967). Clinical evaluation of some hallucinogenic tryptamine derivatives. *Journal of Nervous and Mental Disease, 145*(4), 306–313.

Fantegrossi, W. E., Harrington, A. W., Kiessel, C. L., Eckler, J. R., Rabin, R. A., Winter, J. C., et al. (2006). Hallucinogen-like actions of 5-methoxy-*N,N*-diisopropyltryptamine in mice and rats. *Pharmacology Biochemistry and Behavior, 83*(1), 122–129.

Fantegrossi, W. E., Reissig, C. J., Katz, E. B., Yarosh, H. L., Rice, K. C., & Winter, J. C. (2008). Hallucinogen-like effects of *N,N*-dipropyltryptamine (DPT): Possible mediation by serotonin 5-HT1A and 5-HT2A receptors in rodents. *Pharmacology, Biochemistry, and Behavior, 88*(3), 358–365.

Gallimore, A. (2013). Building alien worlds—the neuropsychological and evolutionary implications of the astonishing psychoactive effects of *N,N*-dimethyltryptamine (DMT). *Journal of Scientific Exploration, 27*(3), 455–503.

Garcia-Romeu, A., Davis, A. K., Erowid, F., Erowid, E., Griffiths, R. R., & Johnson, M. W. (2019). Cessation and reduction in alcohol consumption and misuse after psychedelic use. *Journal of Psychopharmacology, 33*(9), 1088–1101.

Garcia-Romeu, A., Kersgaard, B., & Addy, P. H. (2016). Clinical applications of hallucinogens: A review. *Experimental and Clinical Psychopharmacology, 24*(4), 229–268.

Griffiths, R. R., Hurwitz, E. S., Davis, A. K., Johnson, M. W., & Jesse, R. (2019). Survey of subjective "God encounter experiences": Comparisons among naturally occurring experiences and those occasioned by the classic psychedelics psilocybin, LSD, ayahuasca, or DMT. *PLOS ONE, 14*(4), e0214377.

Griffiths, R. R., Johnson, M. W., Carducci, M. A., Umbricht, A., Richards, W. A., Richards, B. D., et al. (2016). Psilocybin produces substantial and sustained decreases in depression and anxiety in patients with life-threatening cancer: A randomized double-blind trial. *Journal of Psychopharmacology (Oxford), 30*(12), 1181–1197.

Grof, S., Soskin, R. A., Richards, W. A., & Kurland, A. A. (1973). DPT as an adjunct in psychotherapy of alcoholics. *International Pharmacopsychiatry, 8*(1), 104–115.

Halpern, J. H. (2004). Hallucinogens and dissociative agents naturally growing in the United States. *Pharmacology and Therapeutics, 102*(2), 131–138.

Hancock, G. (2007). *Supernatural: Meetings with the ancient teachers of mankind* (rev. ed.). New York: Disinformation Company.

Hernandez, R., Klimo, J., & Schild, R. (2018). A report on Phase I and II of FREE's Experiencer Research Study: The results of a quantitative study. In R. Hernandez, J. Klimo, & R. Schild (Eds.), *Beyond UFOs: The science of consciousness and contact with non-human intelligence* (pp. 1–121). Orlando, FL: FREE.

Hoshino, T., & Shimodaira, K. (1936). Über die synthese des bufotenin-methyl-äthers (5-methoxy-n-dimethyl-tryptamin) und bufotenins (synthesen in der indol-gruppe. XV). *Bulletin of the Chemical Society of Japan, 11*(3), 221–224.

HumbleVoyager. (2017, September 30). So you want to intramuscularly administer 5-MeO-DMT HCl (or other salt) [Forum]. Retrieved August 20, 2019, from *https://forums.5meodmt.org/index.php?topic=50533.0.*

InnerExplorer. (2016, March 30). Erowid Experience Vaults—"A fractal zoom out: DPT." Retrieved August 21, 2019, from *https://erowid.org/experiences/exp.php?id=108204.*

Jiang, X.-L., Shen, H.-W., & Yu, A.-M. (2016). Modification of 5-methoxy-*N,N*-dimethyltryptamine-induced hyperactivity by monoamine oxidase A inhibitor harmaline in mice and the underlying serotonergic mechanisms. *Pharmacological Reports, 68*(3), 608–615.

Kjellgren, A., Eriksson, A., & Norlander, T. (2009). Experiences of encounters with ayahuasca—"the vine of the soul." *Journal of Psychoactive Drugs, 41*(4), 309–315.

Lee, M. A., & Shlain, B. (2007). *Acid dreams:*

The complete social history of LSD. New York: Grove Press.

Li, J.-X., Rice, K. C., & France, C. P. (2007). Behavioral effects of dipropyltryptamine in rats: Evidence for 5-HT1A and 5-HT2A agonist activity. *Behavioural Pharmacology, 18*(4), 283–288.

Luke, D. (2008). Psychedelic substances and paranormal phenomena: A review of the research. *Journal of Parapsychology, 72,* 77–107.

Luke, D. (2011). Discarnate entities and dimethyltryptamine (DMT): Psychopharmacology, phenomenology and ontology. *Journal of the Society for Psychical Research, 75*(902), 26–42.

Luke, D. (2012). Psychoactive substances and paranormal phenomena: A comprehensive review. *International Journal of Transpersonal Studies, 31*(1), 97–156.

Luke, D., & Kittenis, M. D. (2005). A preliminary survey of paranormal experiences with psychoactive drugs. *Journal of Parapsychology, 69*(2), 305–327.

Lyttle, T., Goldstein, D., & Gartz, J. (1996). Bufo toads and bufotenine: Fact and fiction surrounding an alleged psychedelic. *Journal of Psychoactive Drugs, 28*(3), 267–290.

Manske, R. H. F. (1931). A synthesis of the methyltryptamines and some derivatives. *Canadian Journal of Research, 5*(5), 592–600.

McKenna, D. J. (2004). Clinical investigations of the therapeutic potential of ayahuasca: Rationale and regulatory challenges. *Pharmacology and Therapeutics, 102*(2), 111–129.

McKenna, D. J., Repke, D. B., Lo, L., & Peroutka, S. J. (1990). Differential interactions of indolealkylamines with 5-hydroxytryptamine receptor subtypes. *Neuropharmacology, 29*(3), 193–198.

McKenna, D. J., & Towers, G. H. N. (1984). Biochemistry and pharmacology of tryptamines and β-carbolines: A minireview. *Journal of Psychoactive Drugs, 16*(4), 347–358.

McKenna, D. J., Towers, G. H. N., & Abbott, F. (1984a). Monoamine oxidase inhibitors in South American hallucinogenic plants: Tryptamine and β-carboline constituents of ayahuasca. *Journal of Ethnopharmacology, 10*(2), 195–223.

McKenna, D. J., Towers, G. H. N., & Abbott, F. S. (1984b). Monoamine oxidase inhibitors in South American hallucinogenic plants: Part 2. Constituents of orally-active Myristicaceous hallucinogens. *Journal of Ethnopharmacology, 12*(2), 179–211.

Metzner, R. (2013). *The toad and the jaguar: A field report of underground research on a visionary medicine: Bufo alvarius and 5-me-thoxy-dimethyltryptamine.* Berkeley, CA: Regent Press.

Miller, M. J., Albarracin-Jordan, J., Moore, C., & Capriles, J. M. (2019). Chemical evidence for the use of multiple psychotropic plants in a 1,000-year-old ritual bundle from South America. *Proceedings of the National Academy of Sciences of the USA, 116*(23), 11207–11212.

Nagai, F., Nonaka, R., & Satoh Hisashi Kamimura, K. (2007). The effects of non-medically used psychoactive drugs on monoamine neurotransmission in rat brain. *European Journal of Pharmacology, 559*(2–3), 132–137.

Nichols, D. E. (2018). N,N-dimethyltryptamine and the pineal gland: Separating fact from myth. *Journal of Psychopharmacology, 32*(1), 30–36.

Ot'alora, G. M., Grigsby, J., Poulter, B., Van Derveer, J. W., Giron, S. G., Jerome, L., et al. (2018). 3,4-methylenedioxymethamphetamine-assisted psychotherapy for treatment of chronic posttraumatic stress disorder: A randomized Phase 2 controlled trial. *Journal of Psychopharmacology (Oxford), 32*(12), 1295–1307.

Ott, J. (2001). Pharmepéna-Psychonautics: Human intranasal, sublingual and oral pharmacology of 5-methoxy-N,N-dimethyl-tryptamine. *Journal of Psychoactive Drugs, 33*(4), 403–407.

Pachter, I. J., Zacharias, D. E., & Ribeiro, O. (1959). Indole alkaloids of *Acer saccharinum* (the silver maple), *Dictyoloma incanescens, Piptadenia colubrina,* and *Mimosa hostilis. Journal of Organic Chemistry, 24*(9), 1285–1287.

Palamar, J. J., & Le, A. (2018). Trends in DMT and other tryptamine use among young adults in the United States. *American Journal on Addictions, 27*(7), 578–585.

Rabin, R. A., Regina, M., Doat, M., & Winter, J. C. (2002). 5-HT2A receptor-stimulated phosphoinositide hydrolysis in the stimulus effects of hallucinogens. *Pharmacology, Biochemistry and Behavior, 72*(1–2), 29–37.

Ray, T. S. (2010). Psychedelics and the human receptorome. *PLOS ONE, 5*(2), e1909.

Rhead, J. C., Soskin, R. A., Turek, I., Richards, W. A., Yensen, R., Kurland, A. A., et al. (1977). Psychedelic drug (DPT)-assisted psychotherapy with alcoholics: A controlled study. *Journal of Psychedelic Drugs, 9*(4), 287–300.

Richards, W. A., Rhead, J. C., Dileo, F. B., Yensen, R., & Kurland, A. A. (1977). The peak experience variable in DPT-assisted psychotherapy with cancer patients. *Journal of Psychedelic Drugs, 9*(1), 1–10.

Ring, K. (1992). *The Omega Project: Near death*

experiences, UFO encounters, and mind at large. New York: Morrow.

Rodrigues, A. V., Almeida, F. J., & Vieira-Coelho, M. A. (2019). Dimethyltryptamine: Endogenous role and therapeutic potential. *Journal of Psychoactive Drugs, 51*, 299–310.

Ross, S., Bossis, A., Guss, J., Agin-Liebes, G., Malone, T., Cohen, B., et al. (2016). Rapid and sustained symptom reduction following psilocybin treatment for anxiety and depression in patients with life-threatening cancer: A randomized controlled trial. *Journal of Psychopharmacology (Oxford), 30*(12), 1165–1180.

Sadzot, B., Baraban, J. M., Glennon, R. A., Lyon, R. A., Leonhardt, S., Jan, C.-R., et al. (1989). Hallucinogenic drug interactions at human brain 5-HT2 receptors: Implications for treating LSD-induced hallucinogenesis. *Psychopharmacology, 98*(4), 495–499.

Sand, N. (2001). Moving into the sacred world of DMT. *Entheogen Review, 10*(1), 32–39.

Schultes, R. E. (1984). Fifteen years of study of psychoactive snuffs of South America: 1967–1982—a review. *Journal of Ethnopharmacology, 11*(1), 17–32.

Sepeda, N., Doyle, L., Clifton, J., Barsuglia, J., Lancelotta, R., Griffiths, R., et al. (n.d.). The influence of set and setting on the acute subjective effects of 5-MeO-DMT. Retrieved from *https://doi.org/10.13140/RG.2.2.36752.46085.*

Sexton, J. D., Crawford, M. S., Sweat, N. W., Varley, A., Green, E. E., & Hendricks, P. S. (2019). Prevalence and epidemiological associates of novel psychedelic use in the United States adult population. *Journal of Psychopharmacology (Oxford), 33*, 1058–1067.

Shen, H.-W., Jiang, X.-L., Winter, J. C., & Yu, A.-M. (2010). Psychedelic 5-methoxy-N,N-dimethyltryptamine: Metabolism, pharmacokinetics, drug interactions, and pharmacological actions. *Current Drug Metabolism, 11*(8), 659–666.

Shen, H.-W., Jiang, X.-L., & Yu, A.-M. (2011). Nonlinear pharmacokinetics of 5-methoxy-N,N-dimethyltryptamine in mice. *Drug Metabolism and Disposition, 39*(7), 1227–1234.

Shulgin, A., & Shulgin, A. (1997). *TiHKAL: The continuation.* Berkeley, CA: Transform Press.

Soskin, R. A. (1975). Dipropyltryptamine in psychotherapy. *Current Psychiatric Therapies, 15*, 147–156.

Soskin, R. A., Grof, S., & Richards, W. A. (1973). Low doses of dipropyltryptamine in psychotherapy. *Archives of General Psychiatry, 28*(6), 817–821.

Speeter, M. E., & Anthony, W. C. (1954). The action of oxalyl chloride on indoles: A new approach to tryptamines. *Journal of the American Chemical Society, 76*(23), 6208–6210.

Spencer, D. G., Glaser, T., & Traber, J. (1987). Serotonin receptor subtype mediation of the interoceptive discriminative stimuli induced by 5-methoxy-N,N-dimethyltryptamine. *Psychopharmacology, 93*(2), 158–166.

St. John, G. (2016). The DMT gland: The pineal, the spirit molecule, and popular culture. *International Journal for the Study of New Religions, 7*(2), 153–174.

Strassman, R. J. (1995). Human psychopharmacology of N,N-dimethyltryptamine. *Behavioural Brain Research, 73*(1), 121–124.

Strassman, R. (2001). DMT: The spirit molecule: A doctor's revolutionary research into the biology of near-death and mystical experiences. Retrieved from *www.myilibrary.com?id=260342.*

Strassman, R. (Ed.). (2008). *Inner paths to outer space: Journeys to alien worlds through psychedelics and other spiritual technologies.* Rochester, VT: Park Street Press.

Strassman, R. J., & Qualls, C. R. (1994). Dose–response study of N,N-dimethyltryptamine in humans: I. Neuroendocrine, autonomic, and cardiovascular effects. *Archives of General Psychiatry, 51*(2), 85–97.

Szabo, A. (2015). Psychedelics and immunomodulation: Novel approaches and therapeutic opportunities. *Frontiers in Immunology, 6*, 358.

Szabo, A., Kovacs, A., Frecska, E., & Rajnavolgyi, E. (2014). Psychedelic N,N-dimethyltryptamine and 5-methoxy-N,N-dimethyltryptamine modulate innate and adaptive inflammatory responses through the sigma-1 receptor of human monocyte-derived dendritic cells. *PLOS ONE, 9*(8), e106533.

Szára, S. (1957). The comparison of the psychotic effect of tryptamine derivatives with the effects of mescaline and LSD-25 in self-experiments. In S. Garattini & V. Ghetti (Eds.), *Psychotropic drugs* (pp. 460–467). Amsterdam: Elsevier.

Szára, S. (2009). *DMT (N,N-dimethyltryptamine) and homologues: Clinical and pharmacological considerations.* Washington, DC: Section on Psychopharmacology, Division of Special Mental Health Research, National Institute of Mental Health, St. Elizabeths Hospital.

Thiagaraj, H. V., Russo, E. B., Burnett, A., Goldstein, E., Thompson, C. M., & Parker, K. K. (2005). Binding properties of dipropyltryptamine at the human 5-HT1a receptor. *Pharmacology, 74*(4), 193–199.

Timmermann, C., Roseman, L., Williams, L., Erritzoe, D., Martial, C., Cassol, H., et al.

(2018). DMT models the near-death experience. *Frontiers in Psychology, 9*, 1424.

Tittarelli, R., Mannocchi, G., Pantano, F., & Romolo, F. S. (2015). Recreational use, analysis and toxicity of tryptamines. *Current Neuropharmacology, 13*(1), 26–46.

Torres, C. M. (2019). The use of psychoactive plants by ancient indigenous populations of the North Andes. *Journal of Psychedelic Studies, 3*, 198–211.

Torres, C. M., & Repke, D. B. (2006). *Anadenanthera: Visionary plant of ancient South America*. New York: Haworth Herbal Press.

Trout, K. (2007). Some simple tryptamines (2nd ed.). Retrieved from *https://troutsnotes.com/pdf/SomeSimpleTryptamines_2ndEd_2007_with_addendum.pdf*.

Trout, K. (2015, February 10). Ayahuasca: Alkaloids, plants, and analogs. Retrieved August 5, 2019, from *https://erowid.org/library/books_online/ayahuasca_apa/aya_sec3_part2_anadenanthera_analysis.shtml*.

Uthaug, M. V., Lancelotta, R., Bernal, A. M. O., Davis, A. K., & Ramaekers, J. G. (2020). A comparison of reactivation experiences following vaporization and intramuscular injection (IM) of synthetic 5-methoxy-N,N-dimethyltryptamine (5-MeO-DMT) in a naturalistic setting. *Journal of Psychedelic Studies, 4*(2), 104–113.

Uthaug, M. V., Lancelotta, R., van Oorsouw, K., Kuypers, K. P. C., Mason, N., Rak, J., et al. (2019). A single inhalation of vapor from dried toad secretion containing 5-methoxy-N,N-dimethyltryptamine (5-MeO-DMT) in a naturalistic setting is related to sustained enhancement of satisfaction with life, mindfulness-related capacities, and a decrement of psychopathological symptoms. *Psychopharmacology (Berlin), 236*, 2653–2666.

Viceland. (2017). Hamilton Morris learns about the toad ceremonies of the Yaqui Tribe. Retrieved from *www.youtube.com/watch?v=m5u9d7y5er4*.

Weil, A. T., & Davis, W. (1994). Bufo alvarius: A potent hallucinogen of animal origin. *Journal of Ethnopharmacology, 41*(1–2), 1–8.

Winkelman, M. J. (2018). An ontology of psychedelic entity experiences in evolutionary psychology and neurophenomenology. *Journal of Psychedelic Studies, 2*(1), 5–23.

Winstock, A. R., Kaar, S., & Borschmann, R. (2014). Dimethyltryptamine (DMT): Prevalence, user characteristics and abuse liability in a large global sample. *Journal of Psychopharmacology (Oxford), 28*(1), 49–54.

Winter, J. C. (2009). Hallucinogens as discriminative stimuli in animals: LSD, phenethylamines, and tryptamines. *Psychopharmacology, 203*(2), 251–263.

Winter, J. C., Filipink, R. A., Timineri, D., Helsley, S. E., & Rabin, R. A. (2000). The paradox of 5-methoxy-N,N-dimethyltryptamine. *Pharmacology, Biochemistry, and Behavior, 65*(1), 75–82.

Yu, A.-M. (2008). Indolealkylamines: Biotransformations and potential drug–drug interactions. *AAPS Journal, 10*(2), 242–253.

CHAPTER 11

Mescaline

WILL VAN DERVEER

■ Background

Mescaline (3,4,5-trimethoxy-phenethylamine), one of the classical hallucinogens, occupies a unique place in the history of indigenous human spiritual practice, and for the past 120 years, in psychedelic research. Although few investigations of mescaline have occurred in the past 50 years, its significance is not to be underestimated.

In ceremonial use among Native American and other indigenous groups for thousands of years throughout South, Central, and North America, mescaline is the psychoactive compound found in several spe-

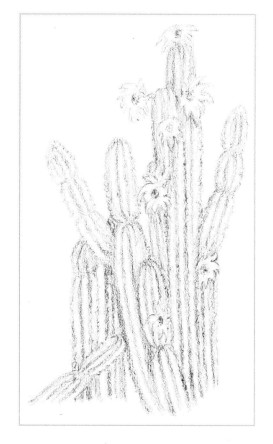

San Pedro cactus

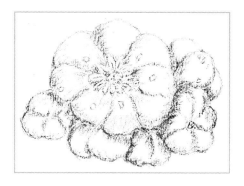

Peyote cactus

cies of cactus, including, most prominently, peyote (*Lophophora williamsii*) and San Pedro (*Echinopsis pachanoi*). Sixteenth-century Franciscan friar Bernadino de Sagahún chronicled widespread ritualized use of peyote by Aztecs in northern Mexico in *The Florentine Codex* (1970). El Seedi and colleagues (2005) carbon-dated a sample of peyote cactus found in an archeological site in Rio Grande, Texas, to 5,700 years ago.

Religious use of peyote continues to this day by the Native American Church, whose members enjoy some legal protection for its use. The San Pedro cactus has been used in indigenous ceremonies in the highlands of Peru, in an uninterrupted tradition, since at least 1300 B.C.E.

Early Research

Early German pharmacologist Arthur Heffter first isolated mescaline from peyote cactus (Heffter, 1896). This was the first time in history that a naturally occurring psychedelic alkaloid had been isolated by a scientist. Prior to Albert Hofmann's synthesis of lysergic acid diethylamide (LSD) in 1938 (and his discovery of its psychedelic properties in 1943), mescaline was investigated for its potential applications, both in a medical setting and for military purposes. In the medical setting, mescaline intoxication was used to as a model for studying symptoms of psychosis.

In the 1920s, Heinrich Kluver investigated the effects of mescaline on normal volunteers, hypothesizing that the blurring of the boundary between subjective and objective experience on mescaline was similar to the experience of schizophrenics.

American and Nazi military research occurred in the 1940s, in an effort to develop a "truth drug" that could be used to gather intelligence from unwilling war prisoners, prior to extensive LSD research by the CIA in the 1950s (Passie et al., 2017).

The 1954 publication of *The Doors of Perception* by Aldous Huxley ushered in the popularity of mescaline due to its description of the author's personal experience with the drug. The term "psychedelic" (meaning "mind-manifesting") was born out of an exchange of letters between Aldous Huxley

and Humphrey Osmond, after Osmond's treatment of Huxley with mescaline (Osmond 1957).

By the end of the 1950s, interest in mescaline was shifting toward interest in LSD. Since the 1950s, there has been very little new research on clinical applications for mescaline.

Pharmacology of Mescaline

The "traditional psychedelics" are compounds that act as agonists at the serotonin 5-HT_{2A} receptor and produce subjective psychedelic experiences such as hallucinations. "Psychedelics" are further categorized by similarity of molecular structure as follows (Nichols, 2004):

- Tryptamines: psilocin; bufotenin; dimethyltryptamine (DMT)
- Ergolines: LSD; ergot mold
- Phenylethylamines (PEAs): mescaline; (–)-2,5-dimethoxy-4-iodoamphetamine hydrochloride (DOI); 1-(2,5-dimethoxy-4-methylphenyl)-2-aminopropane (DOM); 2,5-dimethoxy-4-bromophenethylamine (2C-B)

Receptors

It is now well accepted that the primary behavioral and physiological effects of tryptamine (psilocin and DMT), ergoline (LSD), and phenethylamine (mescaline) hallucinogens are mediated primarily by 5-HT_{2A} receptors. Not all compounds affecting 5-HT_{2A} are psychedelic, however. As well, there are other receptors involved in the mechanisms of these compounds, including 5-HT_{1A}, as well as dopamine receptor D_2 and α_1 adrenergic receptors. Members of the PEA structural family generally have lower affinity for the 5-HT_{1A} receptor than LSD (Hanks & González-Maeso, 2016). Included in the PEA structural family are derivatives of mescaline such as DOI, DOM, and 1-(2,5-dimethoxy-4-bromophenyl)-2-aminopropane (DOB) (Hanks & González-Maeso, 2016).

The 5-HT_{2A} receptor is considered to be the primary target for all traditional psychedelic molecules, including mescaline, LSD, psilocybin, and DMT. Mescaline binds this receptor at a much lower binding affinity than does LSD, perhaps explaining the much higher doses needed for mescaline to have effects similar to a few micrograms of the high-affinity 5-HT_{2A} ligand LSD.

Structure

The structure of mescaline (3,4,5-trimethoxy-β-phenylethylamine) is the best described as a PEA. Figures 11.1, 11.2, and 11.3 illustrate, respectively, the chemical structures of the PEAs mescaline, DOI, and DOM. Figures 11.4, 11.5, 11.6, and 11.7 illustrate, respectively, the chemical structures of the tryptamines serotonin (5-hydroxytryptamine [5-HT]), psilocin, bufotenin, and DMT.

Potency

In terms of its potency,

mescaline shows an extremely low potency, with effective oral doses in the range of 200–400 mg in humans and 10–20 mg/kg in mice. Nevertheless, its hallucinogenic efficacy is well known, and this compound served as a backbone for the development of other PEA

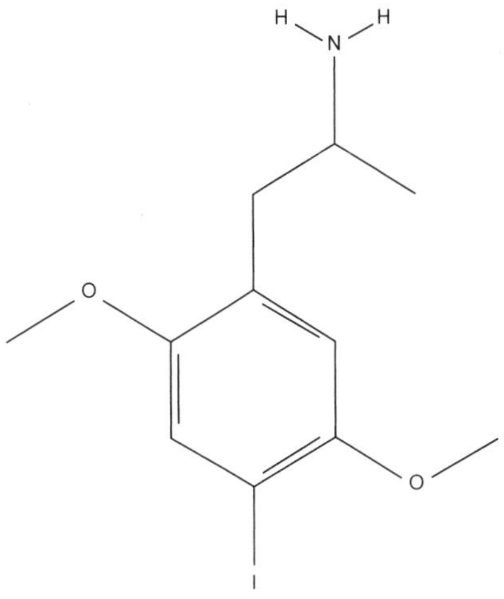

■ FIGURE 11.2. Chemical structure of DOI.

hallucinogens such as DOI, DOM, and DOB. (Hanks & González-Maeso, 2016).

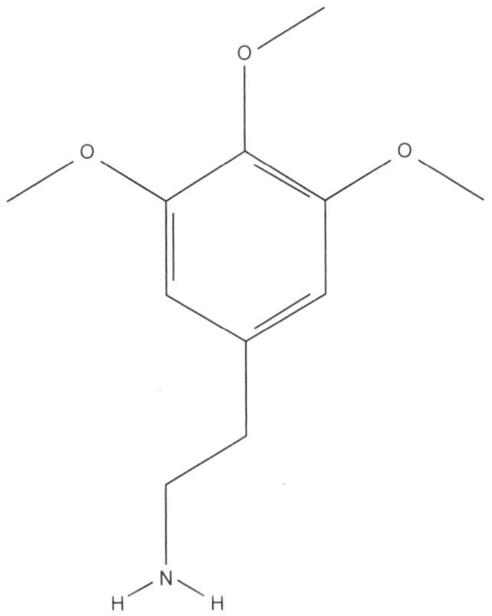

The typical oral dose of mescaline in humans is between 300 and 500 mg, and its effects last 6–8 hours (Halberstadt, 2015). Because of poor lipid solubility, mescaline does not easily pass the blood–brain barrier, contributing to its low-potency and its substantial physical side effects, most notably nausea and vomiting. These side effects are posited to account for the eclipse of mescaline research by LSD in the 1950s (Deniker, 1957).

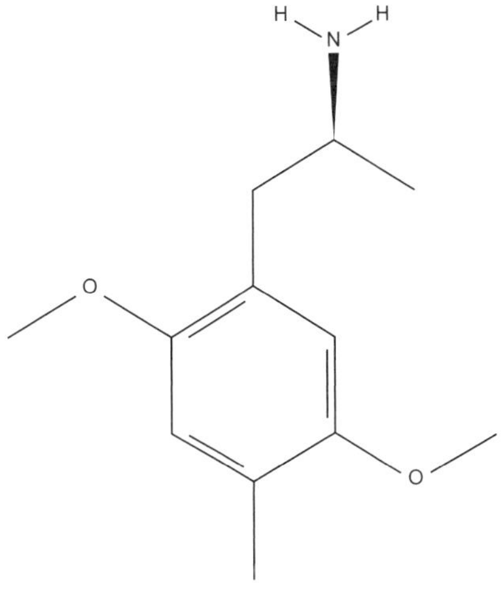

■ FIGURE 11.1. Chemical structure of mescaline.

■ FIGURE 11.3. Chemical structure of DOM.

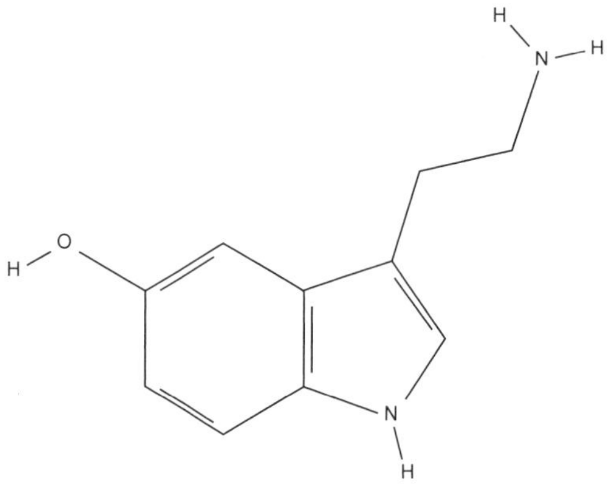

FIGURE 11.4. Chemical structure of serotonin.

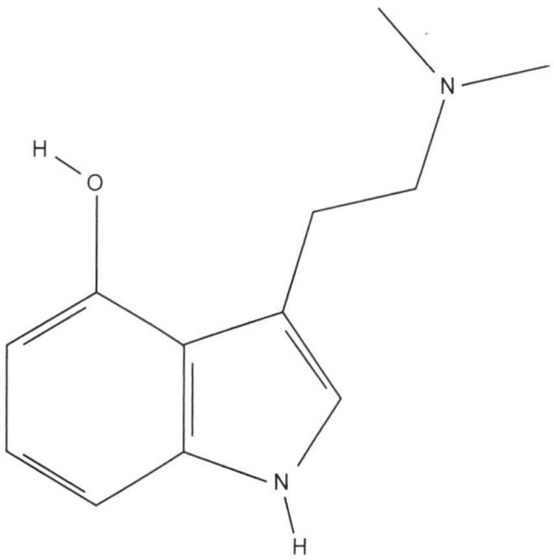

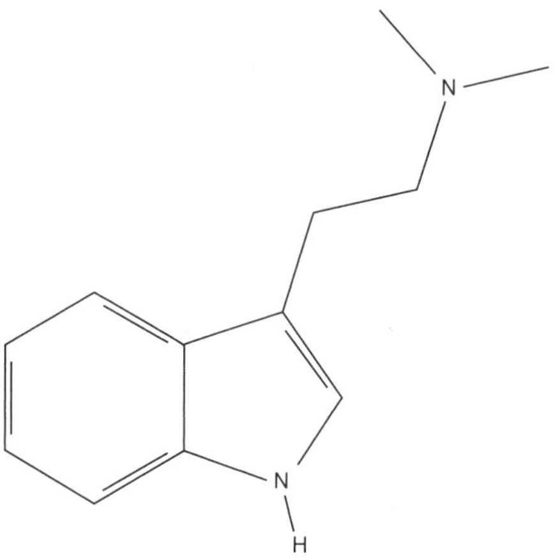

FIGURE 11.7. Chemical structure of DMT.

FIGURE 11.5. Chemical structure of psilocin.

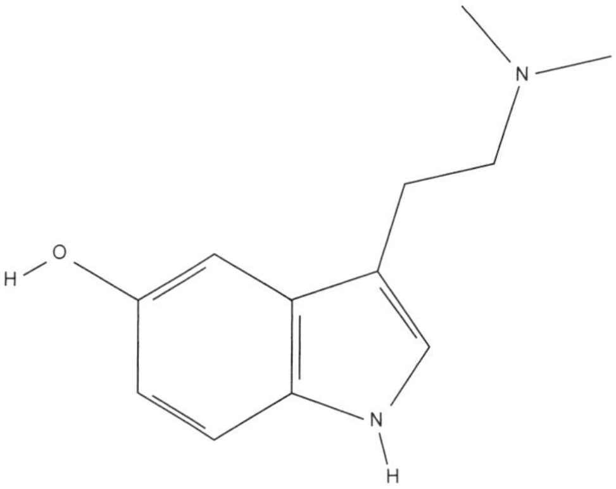

Toxicity and Safety

The lethal dose, 50% (LD50) for mescaline in rats is 132 mg/kg, and for the monkey, *Macaca mulatta*, it is 130 (Hardman et al., 1973). If the human LD50 is around 130 mg/kg, then mescaline ranks, alongside LSD, marijuana, and psilocybin, as one of the safer drugs due to a large window of tolerability. Not surprisingly, then, it is difficult to find a case report of death by mescaline, since it may require upwards of 9,000 mg to cause death in a 75-kg human. Mescaline's emetic effects may provide some additional measure of safety following accidental overdoses.

Elimination of Mescaline

The half-life of mescaline in humans is 6 hours. Although mescaline is subject to liver metabolism, approximately 87% of the dose passes through the kidneys within 24 hours, and 92% is excreted by 48 hours. Some mescaline is metabolized by O-demethylation, N-acetylation, and amine oxidation, but all metabolites are inactive (Dasgupta, 2017).

Effects of Mescaline on the Brain

In the early years, a number of groups studied mescaline as a chemically induced model for the hallucinating state, or acute psycho-

FIGURE 11.6. Chemical structure of bufotenin.

sis. For example, Hollister (1968) showed that, similar to acute schizophrenia, mescaline causes striato-limbic hyperactivity in the right hemisphere. Later studies using modern single-photon emission computed tomography (SPECT) scans showed hyperfrontality during mescaline intoxication (Hermle et al., 1992), helping to overturn the "hypofrontality" theory of schizophrenia that had been proposed in the 1970s as an explanation for the cognitive impairments seen in schizophrenia.

More recently, Carhart-Harris and Nutt at the Imperial College of London have reported significant effects of the classic psychedelics (LSD, psilocybin, and DMT) on specific components of the default mode network (DMN), measured by functional magnetic resonance imaging (fMRI). Specifically, fMRI shows significantly reduced α activity in the posterior cingulate cortex (PCC)/hippocampus medial, effectively decoupling the DMN from the medial temporal lobe network (MTL). This neurophysiological observation, which has been replicated in several studies, correlates highly ($p = .00016$) with the subjective experience of ego disintegration (Carhart-Harris et al., 2014).

Contemporary Clinical Applications

Several groups (Albaugh & Anderson, 1974; Bergman, 1971; Garrity, 2000; Prue, 2013) have studied the safety and efficacy of peyote in the treatment of alcoholism, in naturalistic observational studies with members of the Native American Church. More recently, Halpern and colleagues (2005) evaluated cognitive effects and quality-of-life effects of peyote on Native Americans in three groups: long-term peyote users (mean 300 lifetime exposures to peyote) who use few other drugs ($n = 61$), nondrug user controls ($n = 79$), and alcohol abusers ($n = 36$). Long-term users of peyote showed no cognitive deficits compared to nondrug user controls and reported significantly better overall well-being than controls.

Although mescaline has been relatively ignored in recent years, further clinical research could uncover new clinical applications for this plant-derived alkaloid, which has been continuously used traditionally for as long as any known ceremonial compound. In a rare recent study, Hendricks and colleagues (2017) reported that use of LSD, psilocybin, and peyote is associated with decreased criminal behavior. Mescaline enjoys a well-established safety record and an important role in the history of spiritual traditions, and its clinical applications for the rising rates of modern psychiatric conditions remain mostly unexplored.

References

Albaugh, B. J., & Anderson, P. O. (1974). Peyote in the treatment of alcoholism among American Indians. *American Journal of Psychiatry, 131*(11), 1247–1250.

Bergman, R. (1971). Navajo peyote use: Its apparent safety. *American Journal of Psychiatry, 128*(6), 695–699.

Carhart-Harris, R. L., et al. (2014). The entropic brain: A theory of conscious states informed by neuroimaging research with psychedelic drugs. *Frontiers in Human Neuroscience, 8,* 20.

Dasgupta, A. (2017). Challenges in laboratory detection of unusual substance abuse: Issues with magic mushroom, peyote cactus, khat, and solvent abuse. *Advances in Clinical Chemistry, 78,* 163–186.

de Sagahún, B. (1970). *The Florentine codex: General history of the things of new Spain* (C. E. Anderson & A. J. Dibble, Trans.). Salt Lake City: University of Utah Press.

Deniker, P. (1957). Biological changes in man following intravenous administration of mescaline. *Journal of Nervous and Mental Disease, 125,* 427–431.

El-Seedi, H. R., et al. (2005). Prehistoric peyote use: Alkaloid analysis and radiocarbon dating of archaeological specimens of *Lophophora* from Texas. *Journal of Ethnopharmacology, 101,* 238–242.

Garrity, J. F. (2000). Jesus, peyote, and the holy people: Alcohol abuse and the ethos of power in Navajo healing. *Medical Anthropology Quarterly, 14,* 521–542.

Halberstadt, A. L. (2015). Recent advances in the neuropsychopharmacology of serotonergic hallucinogens. *Behavioural Brain Research, 277,* 99–120.

Halpern, J. H., et al. (2005). Psychological and cognitive effects of long-term peyote use among Native Americans. *Biological Psychiatry, 58,* 624–631.

Hanks, J. B., & González-Maeso, J. (2016). Molecular and cellular basis of hallucinogen action. In V. R. Preedy (Ed.), *Neuropathology of drug addictions and substance misuse* (Vol. 2). Cambridge, MA: Elsevier.

Hardman, H. F., et al. (1973). Relationship of the structure of mescaline and seven analogs to toxicity and behavior in five species of laboratory animals. *Toxicology and Applied Pharmacology, 25,* 299–309.

Heffter, A. (1896). Ueber cacteenalkaloïde. *Berichte der Deutschen Chemischen Gesellschaft, 29,* 216–227.

Hendricks, P. S., et al. (2017). The relationships of classic psychedelic use with criminal behavior in the United States adult population. *Journal of Psychopharmacology, 32*(1), 37–48.

Hermle, L., et al. (1992). Mescaline-induced psychopathological, neuropsychological, and neurometabolic effects in normal subjects: Experimental psychosis as a tool for psychiatric research. *Biological Psychiatry, 32*(11), 976–991.

Hollister, L. E. (1968). *Chemical psychoses: LSD and related drugs.* Springfield, IL: Charles C Thomas.

Nichols, D. E. (2004). Hallucinogens. *Pharmacology and Therapeutics, 101,* 131–181.

Nichols, D. E. (2016). Psychedelics. *Pharmacological Reviews, 68,* 264–355.

Osmond, H. (1957). A review of the clinical effects of psychotomimetic agents. *Annals of the New York Academy of Sciences, 66,* 418–434.

Passie, T., et al. (2017). MDA, MDMA, and other "mescaline-like" substances in the US military's search for a truth drug (1940s to 1960s): Review. *Drug Testing and Analysis, 10,* 72–80.

Prue, B. (2013). Indigenous supports for recovery from alcoholism and drug abuse: The Native American Church. *Journal of Ethnic and Cultural Diversity in Social Work, 22,* 271–287.

CHAPTER 12

MDMA

MICHAEL MITHOEFER and ANNIE MITHOEFER

▓ Introduction

There is growing evidence that 3,4-methylenedioxymethamphetamine (MDMA) and other psychedelic drugs have the potential to powerfully catalyze psychological healing if they are used wisely. Data to support this hypothesis are now available from rigorously designed and conducted clinical research. Clinical trials using MDMA are not simply drug trials in the usual sense; they are designed to test MDMA in combination with psychotherapy. This approach, using a drug as a catalyst during psychotherapy sessions, indicates a new direction in psychiatry. Interest in such an approach arose in the 1950s with lysergic acid diethylamide (LSD) and other psychedelics, but despite promising results published in respected journals, clinical psychedelic research was virtually abandoned for more than 20 years because of regulatory and political opposition beginning in the 1970s (Tupper, Wood, Yensen, & Johnson, 2015).

The medical use of psychedelics does have historical precedent in ancient practices by indigenous cultures using psychedelic plants as tools for healing, spirituality, and community life (Alrashedy & Molina, 2016), but has not yet been incorporated into current Western medical practice. Fortunately, careful exploration of this drug-assisted therapeutic approach was taken up again in the 1990s, primarily with studies of psilocybin and MDMA as therapeutic tools. Data from six Phase II clinical trials of MDMA-assisted psychotherapy sponsored by the Multidisciplinary Association for Psychedelic Studies (MAPS) was presented to the U.S. Food and Drug Administration (FDA) in 2016. These data were the basis upon which the FDA granted Breakthrough Therapy designation to MDMA-assisted psychotherapy for posttraumatic stress disorder (PTSD) in order to expedite Phase III clinical trials that were then begun in November 2018. If the results of these trials confirm the levels of safety and efficacy demonstrated in Phase II studies, regulatory approval of MDMA for clinical use should follow. This treatment has the potential to save lives and reduce suffering for millions of people for whom existing treatments are inadequate.

We present in this chapter quantitative data regarding treatment effects and discuss some of what is understood about therapeutic mechanisms of MDMA-assisted psychotherapy. In addition, we present observations from clinical research in descriptive form, aimed at conveying the richness of the therapeutic process that can be catalyzed by MDMA and the questions it raises about the nature of human healing. These descriptive observations are offered in the interest of avoiding premature conclusions or reductionist explanations for complex phenomena that our current conceptual models do not adequately explain. Researchers exploring treatments using the combination of psychedelics and psychotherapy are confronted with the challenge of understanding and facilitating complex interactions among at least three factors: (1) drug effects, (2) the psychotherapeutic method, and (3) influences of the relationship with the therapists. Making therapeutic use of and attempting to understand this interaction challenges our current limited understanding of psychological injury and the mechanisms by which it is healed. In addition to direct physiological effects of MDMA, it is hypothesized that MDMA can increase access to an intrinsic healing potential within the psyche.

▧ History of MDMA Prior to Controlled Clinical Trials

Ongoing clinical trials of MDMA-assisted psychotherapy fall under an investigational new drug (IND) application number granted by the FDA to MAPS. This IND for MDMA is unusual in two respects: (1) MAPS, as a 501c3 organization is engaged in not-for-profit drug development and (2) MDMA is not a new drug. It is relatively new in terms of the FDA drug development evaluation process, but it has been taken by millions of individuals over more than 40 years under names such as "Adam," "Ecstasy," or "Molly" (National Institute on Drug Abuse [NIDA], 2018). A detailed description of this unique and interesting history is beyond the scope of this chapter, but well-researched accounts providing more detail are available, and this section has relied heavily on information from these sources, where primary references can be found (Holland, 2001; Passie, 2018; Passie & Benzenhöfer, 2016).

MDMA was first synthesized in 1912 and patented in 1914 by the German pharmaceutical company Merk as a possible hemostatic drug. Animal testing was subsequently conducted but use of the drug was not pursued further by the company. Some additional animal studies were conducted at the University of Michigan for the U.S. Army, but were kept secret, and no human studies were conducted until the 1970s, the same period when the first seizures of MDMA were made by U.S. and Canadian law enforcement. By the late 1970s, MDMA use had begun to spread, following two different tracks: use by psychotherapists as a tool to catalyze psychotherapy, and so-called "recreational use," which presumably included a range of activities from thoughtful use for self-exploration, interpersonal communication and connection with other people, to more careless and risky use in uncontrolled settings and in conjunction with other drugs.

While not the first chemist to synthesize MDMA in the 1960s and 1970s, Alexander Shulgin was instrumental in setting it onto the therapeutic track in 1977 by giving a sample to Leo Zeff, a therapist who had previously used other psychedelics in psychotherapy. Zeff's enthusiasm for MDMA as an adjunct to psychotherapy reportedly led him to postpone retirement in order to teach other therapists about it (Stolaroff, 2004). Ann Shulgin, Alexander Shulgin's wife, was one of the people who became involved in this work on the West Coast, and she influenced other therapists by developing guidelines for conducting MDMA sessions. At about the same time, another group on the East Coast, sometimes referred to as "The Boston Group," was also exploring MDMA in conjunction with psychotherapy (Passie, 2018). At this point MDMA, while not an approved drug, was not illegal to possess, and it is estimated that several hundred therapists in the United States used it in their practices until it became illegal to do so in 1985. Although there were no controlled trials conducted during this time, there were published series and case reports by psychiatrists describing the therapeutic effects of MDMA in well-supported psychotherapy sessions (Downing, 1986; Greer & Tolbert, 1986). It is important to note that these therapists focused on the therapeutic potential of MDMA and were exploring approaches to make safe and effective use of this potential (Adamson & Metzner, 1988; Greer & Tolbert, 1998). Much of what they learned from clinical experience informed the therapeutic approaches and dosages used subsequently in more formal research. We discuss these therapeutic approaches later in the chapter.

Therapeutic work with MDMA during the late 1970s and early 1980s was intentionally carried out with relatively little publicity because therapists were concerned that widespread use could lead to criminalization. Despite these precautions, less controlled, "recreational" use was steadily increasing, and by 1983 had come to the attention of the U.S. Drug Enforcement Administration (DEA). In July 1984, the DEA (n.d.) recommended that MDMA be placed in Schedule 1 of the Controlled Substances Act, the criteria for which are defined as "drugs with no currently accepted medical use and a high potential for abuse."

A month later, an organization called Earth Metabolic Design Laboratories (EMDL) requested a hearing on the proposed scheduling, a request that the DEA was required to grant. EMDL had been formed by a group that included many of the psychiatrists and others who had an interest in preserving access to MDMA as a therapeutic tool and in raising money for MDMA research. One of the founders was Rick Doblin, who later went on to found MAPS, which has been the sponsor of all recent and current clinical trials of MDMA-assisted psychotherapy. At the DEA hearings, testimony was given by experts in the field, including prominent physicians and scientists who argued that MDMA has therapeutic potential and can be used safely. The conclusion of the administrative law judge conducting the hearings was that MDMA did not fit the criteria for Schedule 1 and should be placed in Schedule 3. Despite this conclusion based on medical and scientific testimony, the DEA did not follow the judge's recommendation, and MDMA was placed in Schedule 1. This decision stopped all legal therapeutic use and made clinical research much more difficult because of added regulatory requirements and scarcity of funding sources, while "recreational use" continued to increase dramatically. NIDA (2020) reports that in 2017 the prevalence of using Ecstasy or Molly (purported to be MDMA) in the United States was 12% in 18- 25-year-olds and 7% in people over 25.

Another striking result of the DEA decision to criminalize MDMA was that a number of therapists, probably several hundred in the United States and Europe, continued to treat patients with MDMA-assisted therapy in secret or "underground." One estimate is that between 1985 and 2017, more than 60,000 patients were treated underground with MDMA-assisted therapy (Passie, 2018). No doubt, there was a wide range of motivations for this among the therapists, but for people with professional training and licenses to risk the loss of their livelihoods and even criminal prosecution, one must assume that the decision was not taken lightly. The implication is that there must have been something very compelling about the experience of using MDMA in psychotherapy, both to the therapists and to the thousands of patients who elected to have this treatment underground.

An interesting exception to the criminalization of MDMA occurred in Switzerland, when, between 1988 and 1993, a group of five psychiatrists, who had formed the Swiss Medical Society for Psycholytic Therapy (SÄPT), were granted government permission to use MDMA and LSD to treat patients (Gasser, 1996). No formal research was done, but a good safety record was reported, and in a follow-up survey, patients generally reported benefit (Gasser, 1994). Several SÄPT members later conducted MAPS-sponsored Phase II clinical trials in Switzerland: Peter Oehen and Verena Widmer with MDMA and Peter Gasser with LSD.

■ Subjective Effects

MDMA is administered orally, typically on an empty stomach to avoid a delay in absorption. Subjective effects are usually noticed in 30–60 minutes after administration, though in treatment trials, onset between 60 and 90 minutes has been observed. Peak effects occur at 90–120 minutes and last from 3 to 6 hours (Vollenweider, Gamma, Liechti, & Huber, 1998). The elimination half-life is 8–9 hours (de la Torre et al., 2000).

MDMA is often referred to as a psychedelic or hallucinogen, but it is quite different in many respects from classic psychedelics such as LSD or psilocybin. MDMA rarely causes hallucinations and has less tendency to be disorienting or frightening than many psychedelics. People taking MDMA are usually more inclined and better able to engage in verbal interaction than those taking classic psychedelics. Other terms that have been suggested for MDMA and similar compounds are "empathogen" (Metzner, 1983), referring to the tendency of MDMA to increase empathy for self and other, and "entactogen" (Nichols, 1986), referring to the increased self-awareness or ability to "touch within" that is often stimulated.

Therapists who administered MDMA before it was placed in Schedule 1 described the effects as follows:

- MDMA "reduced defensiveness and fear of emotional injury, thereby facilitating more direct expression of feelings and opinions, and enabling people to receive both praise and criticism with more acceptance than usual" (Greer, 1985).
- MDMA can cause "artificial sanity, a temporary anesthesia of the neurotic self" (Naranjo, 1989).
- "It produces no images or hallucinations. It does produce a general sense of well-being . . . feelings of fear and anxiety lift. One feels that one can examine both one's motives and actions, and those of others, calmly and objectively, with acceptance and compassion. . . . Depending on the material contained in the unconscious, the patient will deal with any situation, from childhood traumas to long-felt adult insecurities, to deeply repressed emotions" (Downing, 1985).
- "The psychological problem-solving that occurs is . . . most frequently a shift in perspective, a reframing of the belief that may also be healing" (Adamson & Metzner, 1988).

Observations from clinical trials of MDMA-assisted psychotherapy have been largely consistent with these early reports; however, it has been noted that, especially in individuals with severe PTSD, significant anxiety and feelings of loss of control can occur, especially as the effects of MDMA are beginning. In addition, processing traumatic memories in MDMA-assisted psycho-therapy is often challenging and painful, even with the helpful effects of MDMA described earlier (Mithoefer, Mithoefer, Feduccia, et al., 2018). Several participants in the PTSD studies remarked, "I don't know why they call this 'ecstasy.'" They reported that MDMA allowed them to revisit traumatic experiences without being overwhelmed by anxiety or becoming emotionally numb as they had in therapy without MDMA, but it was still a painful process (Mithoefer, 2018). Later in this chapter examples from MDMA-assisted sessions further illustrate the subjective effects.

■ Neurophysiological Effects

MDMA stimulates release and inhibits reuptake of the monoamines serotonin, dopamine, and norepinephrine, with most potent effects on serotonin (de la Torre et al., 2000), and has affinity for 5-HT_{2A} receptors (Simmler, Rickli, Hoener, & Liechti, 2014). Pretreatment with a serotonin reuptake inhibitor attenuates most physiological and psychological effects (Liechti, Baumann, Gamma, & Vollenweider, 2000; Liechti & Vollenweider, 2000). Coadministration with a monoamine oxidase inhibitor could cause dangerous serotonin syndrome and is contraindicated (Gillman, 2005). Interestingly, MDMA has self-limiting subjective and physiological effects with frequent repeated administration because it inhibits activity on tryptophan hydroxylase that prevents further serotonin production and release (Bonkale & Austin, 2008; Schenk, Abraham, Aronsen, Colussi-Mas, & Do, 2013).

Other neurobiological effects of MDMA include increased serum levels of oxytocin and arginine vasopressin (AVP) (Dumont et al., 2009; Hysek et al., 2014). Some studies suggest that MDMA increases interpersonal trust and decreases reactivity to threatening cues such as angry faces, an effect thought to be partially associated with oxytocin release as well as monoamine receptor activation (Bedi, Hyman, & de Wit, 2010; Dumont et al., 2009), though the role of oxytocin in MDMA-induced increases in empathy is in doubt (Kuypers et al., 2014). It is likely that these combined effects contribute to improving the therapeutic alliance in MD-MA-assisted psychotherapy, particularly in patients with PTSD, who may have difficulty trusting and may be hypervigilant about perceived anger or disapproval in therapists' expressions or behavior.

Neuroimaging with MDMA and psychedelics is a rapidly evolving area of research. In several studies, MDMA has been shown to decrease cerebral blood flow (CBF) in the amygdala and hippocampus and increase CBF in prefrontal cortex, among other effects (Carhart-Harris et al., 2015; Gamma et al., 2000). The changes in CBF correlates with the intensity of the drug effect. This fits well with clinical observations during treatment trials that participants are often able to approach traumatic memories with a capacity for introspection and cognitive clarity, without being overwhelmed by fear or anxiety, and without the sedation or memory impairment that occurs with most anxiolytics. This state has been referred to in publications about other therapeutic methods as the "optimal arousal zone" or "window of tolerance": the level of arousal at which effective therapeutic processing can occur (Ogden, Minton, & Pain, 2006).

Also reported in the Carhart-Harris and colleagues (2015) study were decreases in resting-state functional connectivity (RSFC) between midline cortical regions, the ventromedial prefrontal cortex (vmPFC), and medial temporal lobe regions, including the posterior cingulate cortex (PCC), as well as increases in connectivity between the amygdala and hippocampus. There were trend-level correlations between these effects and ratings of intense and positive subjective effects. The authors note that

> decreased vmPFC–PCC RSFC has also been found with psilocybin (Carhart-Harris et al., 2012), a nonselective $5\text{-}HT_{2A}$ receptor agonist with potent consciousness-altering properties. Psilocybin produces an unconstrained style of cognition that is the inverse of the constrained, ruminative style of thinking that is characteristic of depression. Participants described a similar liberation of cognition and imagination after MDMA administration and vmPFC–PCC coupling was decreased after administration of MDMA. (Carhart-Harris et al., 2015)

This "unconstrained style of cognition" and "liberation of . . . imagination" is consistent with observations that MDMA-assisted psychotherapy sessions often afford striking shifts in perspective and understanding for individuals who have been at the mercy of the negatively skewed thinking typical of PTSD (Mithoefer et al., 2013). To describe the therapeutic significance of these brain changes, Mendel Kaelen, a neuroscientist in Carhart-Harris's lab, uses the analogy that habitual thought patterns and information flow in the brain are like sleds going down a snowy hill; the more they take the same track, the harder it is to deviate from that deepening track. Perhaps MDMA and classic psychedelics temporarily flatten the snow so new and more adaptive routes can be explored (Kaelen, 2017a, 2017b).

▨ Cardiovascular Effects

MDMA reliably produces sympathomimetic effects including elevation of heart rate and blood pressure (BP) (Downing, 1986; Lester et al., 2000), primarily due to norepinephrine release (Hysek, Schmid, Rickli, & Liechti, 2013). Greater elevations have been seen in individuals with certain catechol-O-methyltransferase (COMPT) or serotonin reuptake transporter (SERT) genotypes, but the degree of increase does not suggest a contraindication in these groups (Pardo-Lozano et al., 2012). In subjects with PTSD in Phase II clinical trials, the percentage who reached systolic BP values of 160 mmHg or greater was 44.8% for those receiving 125 mg of MDMA compared to 16.7% for those receiving 40 mg, and 0% for lower doses. The maximum systolic BP reached for any subject receiving MDMA was 200 mmHg. Diastolic BP elevations above 110 mmHg occurred in 10.3% of subjects receiving 125 mg of MDMA, with the maximum value reached being 135 mmHg. Heart rate exceeded 110 beats per minute in 50% of subjects with 125 mg, and the maximum rate observed was 160 beats per minute. All values returned to baseline without need for medical intervention (MAPS, 2017); however, it should be noted that these were carefully screened and relatively medically healthy research subjects. Anyone with known underlying cardiovascular disease or cerebrovascular disease was excluded from enrollment. Some individuals with well-controlled chronic hypertension were enrolled but only after additional screening with a nuclear or echo exercise test and carotid ultrasound. The only drug-related serious adverse event in six Phase II studies with a total of 105 participants was one subject, who had an increase in frequency of preexisting ventricular premature beats (VPBs) after receiving 125 mg MDMA. There were no ill effects, but because frequent VPBs persisted into the evening, the subject was admitted to the hospital overnight for monitoring and further evaluation. The extra systoles returned to baseline, and workup did not reveal cardiac ischemia or structural abnormalities. He was discharged after one night in the hospital without sequelae (Mithoefer, Mithoefer, Feduccia, et al., 2018).

▧ Other Physiological Effects

Thermoregulatory Effects

In studies of healthy volunteers, MDMA was found to produce a mean elevation in body temperature of 0.6°C that was not affected by ambient temperature (Freedman, Johanson, & Tancer, 2005). In Phase II trials of patients with PTSD, the increases were greater than 1°C in 50% of subjects receiving any dose of MDMA, compared to 20% (2 of 10) receiving inactive placebo. The maximum temperature observed was 38.7°C, and there were no related complications or need for medical intervention (MAPS, 2017). These thermoregulatory effects of MDMA are distinct from the possibility of rare events such as malignant hyperthermia or serotonin syndrome, and the moderate doses of known purity and controlled setting are distinct from settings in which ecstasy is used in conjunction with physical exertion, variable hydration, and sometimes concurrently with other drugs. There have been reports of deaths from complications of rhabdomyolysis and hyperthermia outside of research or clinical settings (Eede, Montenij, Touw, & Norris, 2012; Gowing, Henry-Edwards, Irvine, & Ali, 2002; Henry, Jeffreys, & Dawling, 1992).

Osmoregulatory Effects

Associated with an acute rise in AVP following MDMA ingestion, a small decrease in serum sodium has been observed (Forsling et al., 2001). This effect has not been clinically significant in clinical trials, but there are reports of fatal cerebral edema after ecstasy ingestion, probably related to an AVP-mediated decrease in free water clearance combined with excessive water intake. In one reported case, several gallons of water were consumed in a short time in an attempt to avoid dehydration (Ghatol & Kazory, 2012).

Immunological Effects

An oral dose of 100 mg of MDMA has been shown to have modest immunosuppressive and anti-inflammatory effects that are diminishing but still detectable 24 hours later (Pacifici et al., 2001). This effect is attenuated by administration of paroxetine, a serotonin reuptake inhibitor (Pacifici et al., 2004). This degree of immunosuppression is unlikely to be clinically significant in healthy individuals beyond the possibility of transient increased susceptibility to infections.

Hepatic Effects

Some degree of hepatotoxicity was reported in approximately 16% of 199 case reports of adverse events in ecstasy users, and was thought to be influenced by a number of factors, including polydrug use, temperature, and other environmental factors (Carvalho, Pontes, Remião, Bastos, & Carvalho, 2010). Acute liver failure has been reported after ingestion of as little as one ecstasy tablet (Ellis, Wendon, Portmann, & Williams, 1996). In contrast, standard toxicity studies in rats or dogs failed to find liver damage after 28 days of MDMA exposure, and a study in 166, mostly MDMA-naive, healthy volunteers failed to detect any changes in liver function following MDMA administration (Vizeli & Liechti, 2017). In Phase II trials with patients with PTSD there were no liver-related adverse events, and in the two trials that measured alanine aminotransferase (ALT), there were no significant changes after MDMA exposure (MAPS, 2017).

Acute Cognitive Effects

MDMA has been shown to decrease perfor-mance acutely on some measures of psycho-motor speed, visual memory, and attention to digital symbol substitution (Cami et al., 2000), but not on tasks requiring attention and response to visual stimuli or visually presented words (Vollenweider et al., 1998). MDMA also acutely impaired performance in learning and remembering lists of words and recalling object position, but not in spotting scene changes, and it reduced weav-ing in a driving simulation (Kuypers & Ra-maekers, 2005, 2007).

Mood Effects

Some reports indicate an association be-tween ecstasy use and mild depressive symp-toms (MacInnes, Handley, & Harding, 2001); however, a recent Phase II trial com-paring Beck Depression Inventory (BDI-II) scores before and after two administrations of MDMA found a statistically significant improvement in the group receiving 125 mg of MDMA compared to the compara-tor group receiving 30 mg of MDMA (–24.6 vs. –4.6, *p* = .0003) and a trend toward improvement in the group receiving 75 mg compared to that receiving 30 mg (–15.4 vs. –4.6, p = .052) (Mithoefer, Mithoefer, Fe-duccia, et al., 2018).

▨ Possible Chronic Toxicity

Concern about possible chronic neurotox-icity was originally raised in animal stud-ies showing that repeated or high doses of MDMA in rats or monkeys reduce brain serotonin production for 2 weeks or longer (Mechan et al., 2006), but do not increase markers of neurotoxicity associated with neurodegeneration (Wang, Baumann, Xu, Morales, & Rothman, 2005). Monkeys self-administering MDMA over 18 months had slight reductions in brain serotonin but no chemical markers of neuronal injury (Fan-tegrossi et al., 2004; MAPS, 2017). Some studies in rodents and primates using repeat-ed high doses showed damage to serotonin axons (Green, Mechan, Elliott, O'Shea, & Colado, 2003; Slikker et al., 1989); however,

it appears that doses used in most of these studies were too high to be comparable to clinical doses used in humans (Baumann et al., 2009; Mueller et al., 2009).

Because of concerns raised by animal studies, researchers in many countries have conducted neuropsychological studies of ec-stasy users. Interpretation of these results is difficult because studies are often conflict-ing, and almost all are retrospective, so that premorbid functioning is not known, the ec-stasy taken is of unknown purity, and often polydrug use and other lifestyle factors are possible confounds. A retrospective study with a relatively pure sample of ecstasy users and a control group matched for lifestyle concluded that "in a study designed to mini-mize limitations found in many prior inves-tigations, we failed to demonstrate marked residual cognitive effects in ecstasy users. This finding contrasts with many previous findings—including our own—and em-phasizes the need for continued caution in interpreting field studies of cognitive func-tion in illicit ecstasy users" (Halpern et al., 2011). One of the only prospective studies of cognitive function before and after initia-tion of ecstasy use did find an association between ecstasy use and verbal memory, but not attention or working memory. All scores were within the normal range, and the dif-ference was that the people not reporting ecstasy use had greater improvement on the second assessment. As the authors point out, the groups were similar at baseline in most respects, but the ecstasy users had more baseline cannabis use and higher baseline scores associated with attention seeking, so it is possible that they had less patience with repeating tedious and demanding cognitive tests (Schilt et al., 2007). Considering these preclinical and nonclinical studies together, there is still some uncertainty about whether repeated heavy ecstasy use could cause some adverse effects on memory, but there is little reason to think that the doses and frequency under study for psychiatric treatment pose a significant risk in this regard.

More germane to the risk–benefit assess-ment of clinical use of MDMA are prospec-tive data from controlled clinical trials. In two of the U.S. Phase II trials of MDMA-assisted psychotherapy for PTSD, neuropsy-chological testing was performed at baseline and after two MDMA or placebo sessions using the Repeatable Battery for Assessment of Neuropsychological Status (RBANS) (Randolph, Tierney, Mohr, & Chase, 1998) and the Paced Auditory Serial Addition Task (PASAT) (Gronwall, 1977). There was no significant pre-post difference in either test (Mithoefer et al., 2019; see Figures 12.1 and 12.2).

▦ Acute, Self-Limited Side Effects in Clinical Trials

Side effects in Phase II clinical trials of MD-MA-assisted psychotherapy for PTSD were common but self-limited. Table 12.1 shows the most common treatment emergent reactions during 8-hour psychotherapy sessions, with control groups receiving either inactive placebo, low-dose MDMA as an active comparator, or active dose of MDMA (75 mg, 100 mg, or 125 mg), each dose followed by an optional supplemental dose of half the original dose 90–150 minutes later.

Anxiety, the most common side effect during MDMA sessions, often occurs initially as participants first notice the effects of the drug. The sympathomimetic effects can simulate past experiences of anxiety or panic, and the sense of shifting consciousness can raise fears of loss of control. This early anxiety generally responds best to reassurance and techniques such as diaphragmatic breathing to aid in relaxation. Later in the session, anxiety is more likely related to specific content that is coming up, and the approach is to encourage participants to experience, express, and explore the feelings as much as possible. Anxiety was treated with a medication only once in more than 300 sessions in the six Phase II studies. That occurred in the second half of a 30-mg session at the insistence of a participant who had tapered off chronic benzodiazepine use during the enrollment period as required by the protocol. She later tolerated three 125-mg sessions without requesting treatment for anxiety.

For more details about MDMA effects, a comprehensive review of the MDMA literature that is updated regularly can be found in the Investigator's Brochure at *maps.org* (MAPS, 2017).

▦ Regulatory Challenges with MDMA Clinical Research

Unlike most drugs in development as potential treatments, MDMA, while proceeding through the FDA regulatory process as an IND, continues to be widely ingested around the world (NIDA, 2018). Another unusual feature of the MDMA drug development process is the series of regulatory challenges and delays that have marked, and often impeded, the course of legal MDMA research. Fortunately, over time, these obstacles have been overcome, and MDMA is proceeding into Phase III trials much as any other drug with promising Phase II data. One remaining distinctive feature of MDMA clinical research is that it is sponsored by a small not-for-profit organization without government or pharmaceutical industry funding. Now that the research has reached this stage of the process, science will prevail; if Phase III results are statistically significant, there is no reason to think that MDMA will not receive an FDA indication for use as a legal treatment. However, to understand the science in context, it is worth remembering that nonscientific factors have played a major role in causing a 40-year delay between reports of promising clinical use and the start of Phase III trials of MDMA. It is important to remember this history and strive to avoid repeating it because undue delay in investigating new treatments for people who are suffering and dying is not consistent with the ethical values of healing professions or with the quest for scientifically based treatment approaches.

In 1985, when it became clear that MDMA would be placed in Schedule 1, EMDL, later to become MAPS, contracted with Purdue University chemist, David Nichols to produce 1 kg of MDMA to be registered with FDA and used for legal research purposes. This batch of MDMA has remained remarkably stable and was used for all MAPS studies prior to Phase III trials, as well as being donated for other research. Securing a legal source of highly pure MDMA was an important first step in Rick Doblin's determined efforts toward making MDMA into a legal medicine.

Before human research can begin with any drug, preclinical research in animals is

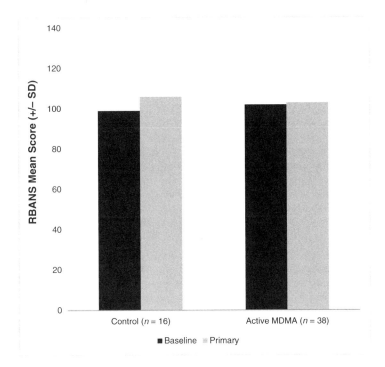

■ FIGURE 12.1. Repeatable Battery for the Assessment of Neuropsychological Status (RBANS) total scores at baseline and the primary endpoint for control group (MDMA 0–40 mg) and active group (MDMA 100–125 mg).

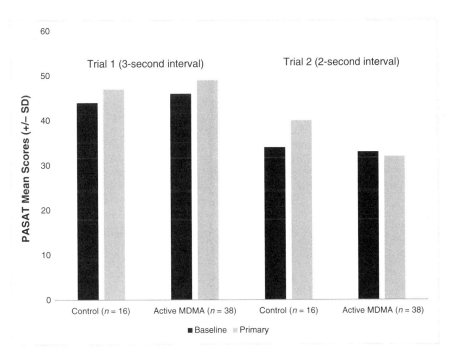

■ FIGURE 12.2. Paced Auditory Serial Addition Task (PASAT) total scores at baseline and the primary endpoint for control group (MDMA 0–40 mg) and active group (MDMA 100–125 mg).

TABLE 12.1. Treatment-Emergent Adverse Events and Expected Reactions during Two Blinded MDMA Sessions and 7 Days Following

	Control (n = 31)	Active MDMA (n = 72)	Total (n = 103)
Top reactions during experimental sessions, No. (%)[a]			
Anxiety	15 (48.39)	52 (72.22)	67 (65.05)
Dizziness	6 (19.35)	29 (40.28)	35 (34.00)
Fatigue	18 (58.06)	35 (48.61)	53 (51.46)
Headache	22 (70.97)	38 (52.78)	60 (58.25)
Jaw clenching, tight jaw	6 (19.35)	46 (63.89)	52 (50.49)
Lack of appetite	7 (22.58)	35 (48.61)	42 (40.78)
Nausea	6 (19.35)	29 (40.28)	35 (33.98)
Psychiatric TEAEs, No. (%)[b]			
Anxiety	3 (9.7)	17 (23.6)	20 (19.4)
Depressed mood	1 (3.2)	6 (8.3)	7 (6.8)
Irritability	0	3 (5.6)	3 (2.9)
Panic attack	0	3 (5.6)	3 (2.9)

Note. TEAEs, treatment-emergent adverse events.

[a]Frequency of subjects who reported an expected, spontaneously reported reaction collected during and 7 days following blinded experimental Sessions 1 and 2 (only reactions reported by ≥40% of participants in any group are displayed, see supplemental for full list of reactions).

[b]Frequency of subjects who self-reported psychiatric adverse events after first drug administration until the day before experimental Session 3 (only AEs reported by three or more subjects in either group displayed).

required. Although MAPS did fund some preclinical research, one of the few advantages stemming from the widespread illegal use of MDMA is that governments around the world have funded a large number of preclinical MDMA studies. There was no need to repeat these already published studies, which saved MAPS millions of dollars. The first MAPS-sponsored clinical trial, and the first FDA-approved human administration of MDMA was a Phase I trial in healthy volunteers conducted by Charles Grob, Division Chief and Professor of Psychiatry and Pediatrics at Harbor UCLA Medical Center (Grob, 1998; Grob, Poland, Chang, & Ernst, 1996). Two other U.S. Phase I trials followed (Harris et al., 2002; Tancer & Johanson, 2001), paving the way for Phase II trials. Grob later considered resubmitting to the FDA a Phase II protocol to study MDMA for treating anxiety in cancer patients; however, in part because of a politicized climate around published research claiming that MDMA caused neurotoxicity,

he decided to proceed with a similar protocol using psilocybin instead of MDMA. Grob had been very critical of the methodology and conclusions of MDMA research, including the failure to publish data demonstrating a no-effect dose of MDMA (Grob, 2000; Grob, Bravo, & Walsh, 1990). This is an example of the course of research being influenced by obstacles arising from attitudes toward a drug rather than investigators' objective scientific conclusions based on reliable data.

In early 2000, Doblin was able to obtain necessary approvals for a Phase II trial in Spain designed to study MDMA in conjunction with psychotherapy for treating PTSD. Unfortunately, because of political pressures, not scientific or medical concerns, the study was shut down 2 years later after only seven subjects were treated with relatively low doses of MDMA (Bouso, Doblin, Farré, Alcázar, & Gómez-Jarabo, 2008). Meanwhile in the United States, Doblin and Mithoefer had agreed to develop a similar protocol to submit to the FDA, which they did in October 2001 (Wagner, Mithoefer, & Doblin, 2019). The fact that this application was approved by the FDA 1 month later demonstrates the objectivity of the FDA scientific review process, as well as the merits of the protocol and careful preparation of the application. The fact that final Institutional Review Board (IRB) and DEA approval were not obtained until March 2004 is an example of a lack of objectivity leading to regulatory delays not based on reliable scientific data. A more detailed account of these delays is available elsewhere (Wagner et al., 2019), so here we provide only a brief outline based on that paper. The original FDA-approved protocol had listed the study site as the General Clinical Research Center at the Medical University of South Carolina (MUSC), where Mithoefer held a clinical faculty appointment.

Shortly following FDA approval, there was a national media article about the study, and it immediately became clear that there was resistance at the medical school to being involved in MDMA research because of its controversial nature. After 6 months of unsuccessful attempts to have the protocol reviewed by the MUSC IRB, a protocol amendment was submitted to the FDA requesting a change of the study location to Mithoefer's private office. He was later told by the acting chairman of the MUSC Department of Psychiatry that the University had been concerned that the government might perform a "punitive audit" of all their federally funded research if they got involved in MDMA studies. After 3 months of negotiation about equipment and personnel to provide emergency medical backup at the office, the amended protocol was approved by the FDA. A short time later, approval was obtained from the Western IRB, a freestanding review board.

With FDA and IRB approval in hand, the only additional approvals needed for research with a Schedule 1 drug were from the DEA and the State Bureau of Drug Control. Unfortunately, less than 2 months later, the IRB reversed its decision and withdrew approval, saying that their executive committee had decided not to get involved in "this kind of research." It turned out that the decision was prompted by a paper by George Ricaurte, a prominent NIDA-funded researcher, that had been accepted for publication in the prestigious journal *Science*. The paper claimed to have demonstrated that MDMA, at doses claimed to be equivalent to typical human recreational or clinical doses, caused toxicity to dopamine neurons, causing severe illness and death in the primates studied (Ricaurte et al., 2002).

A letter from the MAPS researchers published in response to the Ricaurte paper was met with a dismissive response by the authors (Mithoefer, Jerome, Doblin, & Ricaurte, 2003). Because of concerns raised by this paper, all attempts to gain approval from a different IRB were unsuccessful until, almost exactly 1 year after the Western IRB withdrawal letter, Ricaurte and colleagues (2002) retracted their paper, stating that they had discovered that the bottle labeled as MDMA was mislabeled. They had inadvertently administered methamphetamine not MDMA to the primates (Ricaurte, 2003). After a year's delay caused by Ricaurte's paper, the MAPS protocol was promptly approved by the Copernicus IRB.

Approval by the DEA was not to be forthcoming until February 24, 2004, 19 months after the initial DEA application, and this occurred only after many e-mails, letters, and phone calls between the investigators and the DEA, and after Mithoefer appealed to U.S. Senator Fritz Hollings to ask for a more timely response from the DEA.

It is easy to understand why these undue regulatory delays, along with absence of government or industry funding, would have discouraged many researchers from doing clinical studies with MDMA or other Schedule 1 compounds. It is encouraging to report that subsequent MAPS MDMA protocols have been handled much more expeditiously by the DEA, while FDA and IRB reviews have continued to be rigorous but efficient.

▨ Phase II Clinical Trials

Between 1994 and 2018, nine MAPS-sponsored Phase II clinical trials of MDMA-assisted psychotherapy were completed at seven different sites in four different countries. Six of these studies treated individuals with PTSD and are the basis upon which the FDA has granted permission for Phase III trials under the Breakthrough Therapy designation. We discuss these studies first and mention the studies of other indications later in the section.

Study Design

After informed consent and careful screening, including baseline measures administered by an independent rater, participants were enrolled and had three 90-minute preparatory sessions with a male–female therapy team. They were then randomized to receive either active doses of MDMA, inactive placebo, or low dose MDMA as a comparator, depending on the particular study protocol, which varied somewhat among the six studies. MDMA or comparator was administered in two 8-hour therapy sessions 1 month apart, referred to as "experimental sessions." Each session was followed by an overnight stay in the clinic (with a night attendant on duty) and a follow-up 90-minute "integration session" with the therapists the next morning, then daily phone check-in for 7 days. Two or three more integration sessions occurred over the next several weeks before the next experimental session, which was followed by the same schedule of overnight stay, integration sessions, and phone follow-up.

Approximately 1 month after the second experimental session, outcome measures were administered by the independent rater, the primary outcome measure being the Clinician-Administered PTSD Scale, DSM-IV version (CAPS-IV). Following the outcome measures, the blind was broken and people who had received full doses of MDMA (125 mg followed by an optional supplemental dose of 62.5 mg) received a third full dose in an open-label continuation. Participants who had received placebo or low-dose comparator could elect to enter an open-label crossover protocol with three full-dose sessions accompanied by the same schedule of integration sessions. Outcome measures were repeated 2 months and 1 year or more after the last MDMA session. Figure 12.3 illustrates the general design used in Phase II trials. The full protocols can be found at maps.org.

Results of MAPS-Sponsored Phase II Clinical Trials

Analysis of pooled data from the six Phase II trials showed a large between-group Cohen's d effect size of 0.8. When the group randomized to receive psychotherapy with comparator drug (inactive placebo or low-dose MDMA, depending on the study), crossed over to receive psychotherapy with MDMA, the response was comparable to that of the original active-dose group. Gains were maintained by most participants, with mean CAPS scores 12 months or more after the last MDMA session for both groups (see Figure 12.4; Mithoefer et al., 2019).

Secondary Measures in Phase II Studies

The BDI-II was administered in four of the six trials. Depression symptom improvement on the BDI-II was greatest for the active-dose group, estimated mean standard error (SE) change active –12.4 (1.84) versus control group –6.5 (2.69), with the difference between groups trending toward significance [t(61) = –1.97, p = .053] (Mithoefer et al., 2019).

Sleep quality was measured in two studies with the Pittsburg Sleep Quality Index (PSQI). In the first of these studies, the two active-dose groups showed statistically significant improvements compared to the low-dose comparator group (analysis of variance [ANOVA] for mean change in PSQI scores p = .029), and t-tests indicated superiority in the 75 mg (p = .014) and 125 mg (p = .022) groups compared with the 30-mg group (Mithoefer et al., 2018a). In the second study using the PSQI the mean (standard deviation [SD]) change in PSQI total scores was –0.8 (2.5) for 40 mg, –3.6 (6.2) for 100 mg, and –2.0 (4.7) for 125 mg, indicating some improvement in sleep quality for all groups, yet this failed to reach significance ($F2,26$ = .583, p = .57) (Ot'alora et al., 2018).

In two studies in which personality factors were assessed with the Neuroticism–Extroversion–Openness Personality Inventory—Revised (NEO-PI-R), one showed statistically significant increased openness (p = .032) and decreased neuroticism (p = .003) when comparing baseline personality traits with long-term follow-up traits. Only the increased openness correlated with improvement in CAPS scores. In the other

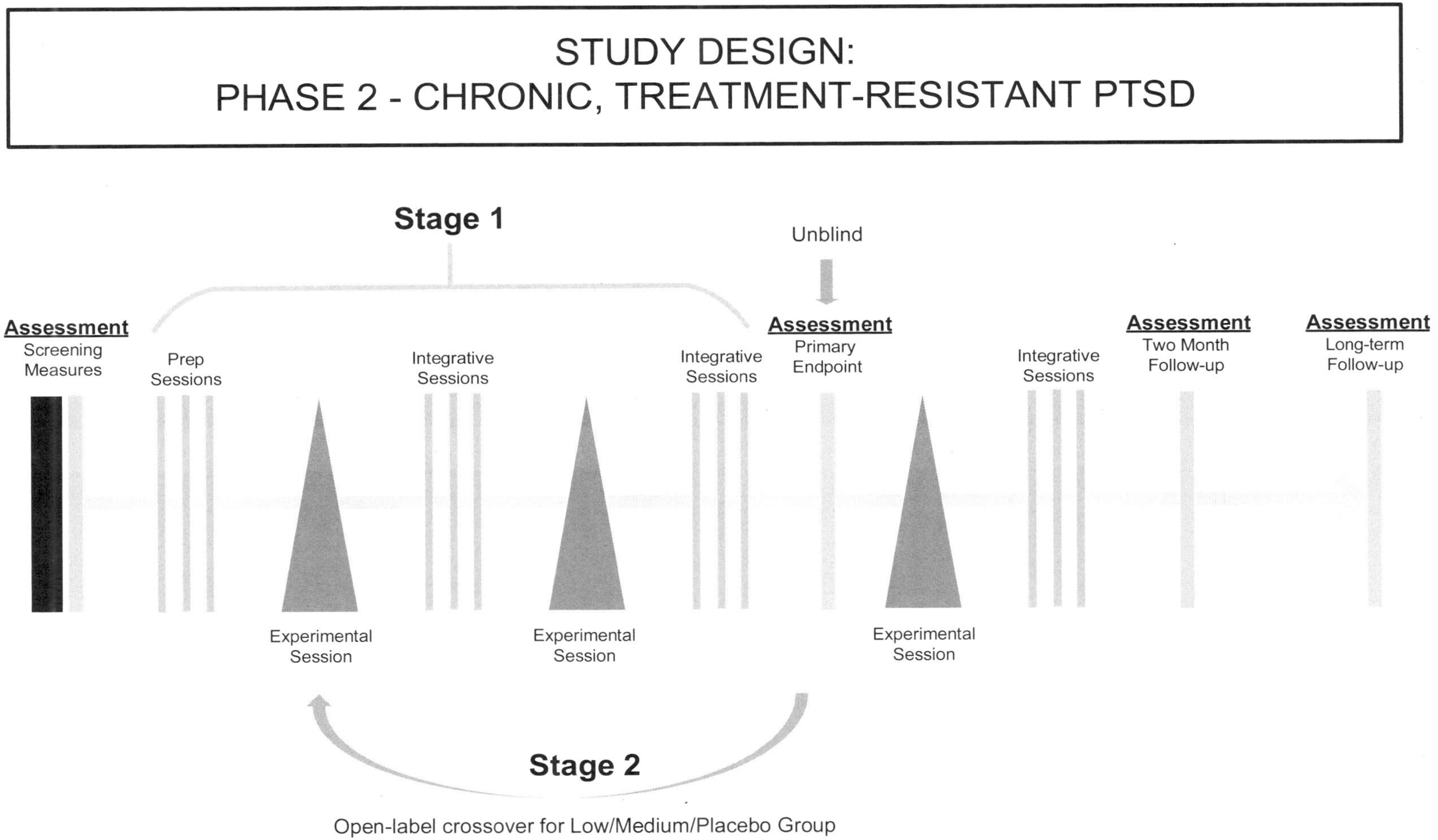

STUDY DESIGN:
PHASE 2 - CHRONIC, TREATMENT-RESISTANT PTSD

FIGURE 12.3. MDMA-assisted psychotherapy Phase II study design.

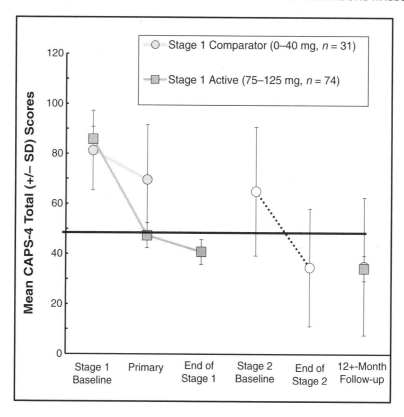

■ FIGURE 12.4. Pooled CAPS data from six Phase II studies.

study, the group receiving 75 mg of MDMA had a greater increase in openness than the 30-mg comparator group ($p = .02$)

Results of four of the six completed Phase II trials have been published (Mithoefer et al., 2011; Mithoefer, Mithoefer, Feduccia, et al., 2018; Oehen, Traber, Widmer, & Schnyder, 2013; Ot'alora et al., 2018). Of note is the fact that the same treatment approach was effective for both for victims of crime such as childhood physical or sexual abuse or adult rape or assault (Mithoefer et al., 2011) and for military veterans, firefighters and police officers with PTSD from their service (Mithoefer, Mithoefer, Feduccia, et al., 2018).

■ Phase III Study Design and the Challenge of Study Blinding

A challenge inherent in studying psychoactive drugs is that it is very difficult to maintain an effective double blind. In the first

of the six Phase II studies, two participants who received inactive placebo thought they has received MDMA in their first blinded session only, but all the rest guessed correctly. The therapists, while not always certain, always guessed the condition correctly. It was judged that an "active placebo" such as niacin or an amphetamine would not significantly improve the blinding and could have unknown effects on the therapy. In subsequent Phase II trials, various low doses of MDMA, ranging from 25 mg to 75 mg, were used as active comparators in hopes of producing a more effective blind or finding a dose escalation effect.

There were two discoveries in these studies that informed the Phase III design:

1. There is a threshold dose below which the blind is not significantly improved and above which the blind is improved but the treatment is effective, so there is no inactive comparator and no dose esca-

lation effect at higher doses. The threshold dose is in the neighborhood of 75 mg, which was found to be even more effective than 125 mg in one study (Mithoefer, Mithoefer, Feduccia, et al., 2018).

2. Doses of 50 mg and below appear to interfere with the psychotherapy by increasing anxiety without being helpful, so lower doses are not valid comparators because, by interfering with the effect of the psychotherapy, they could make the active doses appear more effective than they actually are.

At one study site the improvement in CAPS scores with psychotherapy plus inactive placebo was 20.5 points (Mithoefer et al., 2011), and in a separate study with the same therapist team the CAPS improvement with 30 mg MDMA (followed by a 15-mg supplemental dose) was 11.4 points (Mithoefer, Mithoefer, Feduccia, et al., 2018). The conclusion from Phase II was that there is no valid and effective way to maintain a strong double blind in studies of MDMA-assisted psychotherapy, much as there is no effective blind in psychotherapy studies without drug administration.

In meetings with FDA at the end of Phase II, it was agreed that valid Phase III studies could be done comparing active doses of MDMA to inactive placebo combined with the same therapy as long as the outcome measures were conducted by well-blinded independent raters. In current Phase III trials, there is a centralized pool of experienced CAPS raters administering the measures remotely by telemedicine who never rate the same participant twice and are blind not only to condition but to which study visit they are rating. No subject will be unblinded until all subjects at all sites have completed the study.

A MAPS-sponsored Phase III trial has recently been completed at 13 sites in the United States, two sites in Canada (results pending), and two sites in Israel comparing inactive placebo with active doses of MDMA, each administered during three 8-hour psychotherapy sessions at monthly intervals with accompanying preparatory and integration sessions. The doses of MDMA are 80 mg in the first session, with the option to either stay at 80 mg or increase to 120 mg in the second and third sessions (each initial dose is followed by an optional supplemental dose 90–120 minutes later).

■ Pilot Studies of Other Indications

Most MDMA treatment research to date has focused on individuals with PTSD in support of a future FDA New Drug Application (NDA) for that indication; however, MAPS has also sponsored exploratory studies for three other indications, all of which have produced promising data calling for further studies in the future.

MDMA-Assisted Therapy for the Treatment of Social Anxiety in Adults with Autism

In a study by Danforth and colleagues (2018) at UCLA, 12 adults with autism were randomized to receive either MDMA (75–125 mg) or inactive placebo in two 8-hour psychotherapy sessions 1 month apart. Improvement in the primary outcome measure, the Leibowitz Social Anxiety Scale (LSAS), from baseline to the primary endpoint was significantly greater for the MDMA group compared to the placebo group ($p = .037$), as was the improvement at 6-month follow-up ($p = .036$). The placebo-subtracted Cohen's d effect size was large at both time points ($d = 1.4$ and 1.2, respectively) (Danforth et al., 2018).

MDMA-Assisted Psychotherapy for Anxiety Associated with Life-Threatening Illness

Wolfson (2020) recently completed a study in which 18 participants with anxiety from a life-threatening illness were randomized in a double-blind study to receive MDMA (125 mg, $n = 13$) or placebo ($n = 5$) during two 8-hour psychotherapy sessions. The primary outcome was change from baseline in State–Trait Anxiety Inventory (STAI) Trait scores at 1 month post the second experimental session. The MDMA group had the largest mean drop in STAI, indicating less anxiety compared to the placebo group, with group differences trending toward significance, a large effect size, and good safety record.

MDMA-Assisted Cognitive-Behavioral Conjoint Therapy

Therapeutic use of MDMA before scheduling in 1985 included use in couple therapy, and it was reported to be very helpful for that purpose because couples who took MDMA together in a therapeutic setting "experienced more closeness and/or enhanced communication, and found it easier to receive compliments or criticism" (Greer & Tolbert, 1998). After MDMA was placed in Schedule 1, there was not a clear path to studying this formally because it would involve testing the effects of a drug when administered to two people simultaneously, for which there had been no FDA precedent. In late 2013 and early 2014, there were two meetings between MAPS representatives and leading researchers in the National PTSD Center, which directs PTSD research and treatment in the U.S. Department of Veterans Affairs (VA). Rick Doblin, PhD, Richard Rockefeller, MD, and Michael Mithoefer, MD, had requested the meetings to discuss the possibility of starting MDMA research in the VA system. The National Center was represented by Matthew Friedman, MD, PhD, Director; Paula Schnurr, PhD (now director); John Krystal, MD, Director, Clinical Neurosciences; and Candice Monson, PhD, a leading VA PTSD researcher and developer of cognitive-behavioral conjoint therapy (CBCT). The meetings did not lead to any research within the VA, but the group decided that this was a worthwhile area to explore through a MAPS-funded study, and suggested that Monson and Mithoefer might do a study together combining CBCT with MDMA-assisted psychotherapy. Monson, whose method was focused on treating the couple rather than the individual, had published outcome data demonstrating that CBCT for couples in which one person had PTSD significantly improved both CAPS scores of PTSD symptoms and measures of relationship satisfaction. This was the rationale for submitting and obtaining regulatory approval for an open-label treatment development study embedding two sessions of MDMA-assisted psychotherapy within a compressed course of CBCT lasting 6 weeks (Monson et al., in press). Six dyads were treated with very encouraging results, and

the treatment protocol was refined at several points during the study as experience was gained with combining the methods. Because there was no control group, the study was not designed to separate the effects of MDMA from the effects of CBCT; however, the results provided a basis for designing larger, controlled trials in the future. The researchers' impression was that MDMA helped the couples overcome obstacles to communication and mutual empathy, and CBCT provided valuable skills and structure for integrating the MDMA experiences and maintaining the gains over time (Monson, Wagner, & Macdonald, 2015; Wagner, Mithoefer, Mithoefer, & Monson, 2017).

■ The Therapeutic Method in MAPS-Sponsored MDMA Clinical Trials

Note that all quotes in italics are from participants in clinical trials conducted by Michael and Annie Mithoefer as recorded in their notes or in audio recordings. Most are verbatim, but some are paraphrased.

The therapeutic method used in these clinical trials is described in detail in the MAPS MDMA-Assisted Psychotherapy Training Manual (Mithoefer, Mithoefer, Jerome, et al., 2018). In Phase II MDMA clinical trials the therapy has been delivered by two cotherapists, usually a male and female, in aesthetically pleasing rooms with a futon or sofa that allows participants either to sit leaning against pillows or lie down comfortably. MDMA sessions last 8 hours, and participants in most studies spend the night at the office with a night attendant on site. Figure 12.5 shows one of the research sites.

Undoubtedly there are other methods that could be equally or more effective, and it is our hope that the future will bring continued exploration and innovation. What is known is that this approach has been effective in a series of Phase II clinical trials and is now being further tested in Phase III trials using trained adherence raters to verify fidelity to the method across sites and treatment conditions.

The most direct influence on the therapeutic method presented here and in the manual came from Stanislav Grof and other trainers

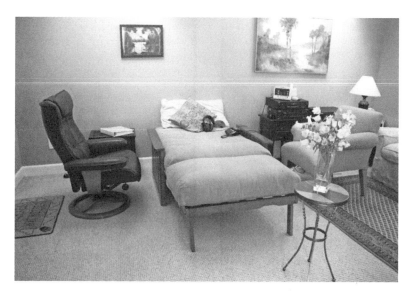

■ FIGURE 12.5. MDMA research site. *Photo:* Hunter McRae.

who worked with him in the Grof Transpersonal Training Program for Holotropic Breathwork facilitators. Holotropic Breathwork is a nondrug method based largely on Grof's experience treating patients with LSD and other psychedelics in therapeutic settings when these drugs were still legal (Grof, 2019, 2001). Other important influences, both through published work and personal communications, come from therapists who had experience with the therapeutic use of MDMA or other psychedelics before they became illegal. This group includes George Greer and Requa Tolbert (1998), Ralph Metzner (Adamson & Metzner, 1988), Claudio Naranjo (Naranjo & Holland, 2001), Anne Shulgin (Shulgun & Shulgin, 1991), William Richards (Naranjo & Holland, 2001; Richards, 2015), James Fadiman (2011), and others. An overarching, less direct, influence on the field comes from the many indigenous cultures that have used psychedelic plants such as peyote, psilocybin mushrooms, ayahuasca teas, ibogaine, and others as tools for healing and spiritual practices. Over centuries, these cultures learned to respect these tools and to develop practices for using them wisely and safely (Nichols, 2016).

Our observations, and the observations of other therapists conducting clinical trials (Ot'alora et al., 2018), are consistent with early reports of the use of MDMA in conjunction with psychotherapy. The basic premise of this treatment approach is that the therapeutic effect is not due simply to the physiological effects of the medicine; rather, it is the result of an interaction among the effects of the medicine, the therapeutic setting, and the mindsets of the participant and the therapists. MDMA produces an experience that appears to temporarily reduce fear, increase the range of positive emotions toward self and others, and increase interpersonal trust without clouding the sensorium or preventing access to emotions. MDMA may catalyze therapeutic processing by allowing participants to stay emotionally engaged while revisiting traumatic experiences, without being overwhelmed by anxiety or other painful emotions. Frequently, participants are able to experience and express fear, anger, and grief as part of the therapeutic process, with less likelihood of either feeling overwhelmed by these emotions or avoiding them by dissociation or emotional numbing. As study participants have described this effect,

"Maybe one of the things the drug does is let your mind relax and get out of the way because the mind is so protective about the injury."

"I felt deeply connected to painful feelings of the traumas as I saw them go by in spheres, but it didn't cause anxiety. I felt deep sadness in my heart [crying] but also deep happiness that I was healing it and letting it go."

"It's like, every time I go inside I see flowers and I pick one, and that's the thing to work on next. And there are things that are hard to take, but each time I move through them it feels so much better."

In addition, MDMA can enable a heightened state of empathic rapport that facilitates the therapeutic alliance and allows for a corrective experience of secure attachment and collaboration with the therapists. Often at some point during the MDMA experience, feelings of empathy, love, and deep appreciation emerge in conjunction with a clearer perspective of the trauma as a past event and a heightened awareness of the support and safety that exist in the present.

"I had never before felt what I felt today in terms of loving connection. I'm not sure I can reach it again without MDMA but I'm not without hope that it's possible. Maybe it's like having an aerial map so now I know there's a trail."

Research participants have said that being able to successfully process painful emotions during MDMA-assisted psychotherapy without being overwhelmed, while still painful, has given them a template for feeling and expressing pain that has changed their relationship to their emotions.

"I have respect for my emotions now (rather than fear of them). What's most comforting is knowing now I can handle difficult feelings without being overwhelmed. I realize feeling the fear and anger is not nearly as big a deal as I thought it would be."

In addition to these salutary effects on the therapeutic relationship and on trauma processing, MDMA-assisted psychotherapy sessions conducted in the relatively nondirective manner described in this manual invariably go beyond a focus on trauma to include exploration and processing of other life experiences, including family and relationship dynamics. MDMA may also catalyze access to meaningful spiritual and other transpersonal experiences, release of tensions in the body, and a sense of healing

on a nonverbal level. Though incompletely understood from a scientific viewpoint, these experiences are considered important by many participants.

"It wasn't an easy experience, but it was so worth it. It was a very spiritual experience, very expansive. I feel a sense of calm and stability now."

"I see huge white doors with beautiful white glass, so huge and heavy, but a master has engineered them so you can open them with one hand. It's only without the fear that the doors are so light. How interesting! If I go up to them with all the fears, it makes me weak. I'm taking those fears out of different parts of my body, looking at them and saying, 'It's OK but I'm leaving you here.' The fear served me well at one time, but not now for going through these doors."

In MDMA studies that formally tracked spiritual experiences (n = 33) using the States of Consciousness Questionnaire (SOCQ; Griffiths, Richards, McCann, & Jesse, 2006), approximately one-third of participants reached the threshold for a "full blown mystical experience." For the subset of individuals who had them, these powerful spiritual or mystical experiences appeared to be important aspects of their process, and likely contributed to their therapeutic outcome; however, in the group as a whole, there was no significant correlation between improvement on CAPS and whether there was a mystical experience. This points to the individual variation in participants' therapeutic process that is consistently observed across studies and supports the rationale for a relatively nondirective approach that does not make assumptions in advance about what kind of experience is most helpful for any given person. In psilocybin studies, not surprisingly, the incidence of mystical experience was greater, but in contrast to MDMA studies, the therapeutic outcome was mediated by the occurrence of drug-induced mystical experiences (Griffiths et al., 2016; Ross et al., 2016).

Perhaps the most important core principle of the approach described in the manual is that the potential benefits of MDMA are mediated through access to each individual's innate healing capacity. This capacity can be most fully expressed when the therapists' goal is to support each individual's spontaneously arising and unique therapeutic process rather than to direct the therapy sessions according to some preconceived concept or agenda. The therapists' role can be described as relatively *nondirective*. This term does apply in many ways to the stance of the therapists; however, it can mislead by suggesting that there are not situations in which therapists do give direction.

From the perspective of the patient or research participant, the approach can be described as "inner directed," pointing to the fact that direction ideally comes primarily from within the individual, either through cognitive realizations or on a nonverbal level of images, emotions, or physical sensations. A corollary is that while therapists' knowledge and training are important, they often find that their own instincts and felt sense are the most reliable guides to engagement with their clients in MDMA-assisted sessions. One of the greatest cognitive challenges for many therapists is to remember that beyond providing a conducive therapeutic set and setting, and compassionate, attuned presence, in most circumstances they are not called on to figure out what the participant needs next or how to make it happen. Agendas are replaced by engaged curiosity about where the person's process will go next.

On the other hand, direction from the therapists can be very helpful at times, and is consistent with this method as long as it is in response to the participant's unfolding process, and is proposed only after ample time and encouragement have been given for the process to take its own direction, and as long as any direction is offered as a choice that the participant is free to decline rather than as an instruction. As Mendel Kaelen's earlier analogy vividly points out, MDMA can allow for a new and unexpected track down the mind's snowy hill, a chance to escape the restriction of following established ruts of either the participant or the therapists. As Irvin Yalom (2007) has said of his approach to psychotherapy, "The therapist must strive to create a new therapy for each patient." In MDMA-assisted psychotherapy this might be extended to say, "The therapists must strive to allow and encourage each patient to create a new therapy for themselves." An example of the benefit of this approach is as follows:

A veteran of the Iraq war had been suffering with severe PTSD for 10 years when he enrolled in a Phase II MDMA study. His first MDMA session (125 mg) was spent almost entirely focused inward with eyeshades and headphones, and he spoke to the therapists only briefly once an hour, when they checked in with him and took his vital signs. Each time he indicated he was doing well and had no need to talk further. At one check-in he said, "When I check inside to see if I need to talk about it my body says, 'No, lets keep going deeper.'"

Consistent with the therapeutic approach, since he reported that he was handling the experience well, the therapists validated his decision and did not ask him to tell them more about his experience, either during the session or at the end of the day. That night he wrote extensively about his experience and read it to the therapists during the follow-up session the next morning. During his MDMA session, he had confronted the one of his many war traumas that bothered him the most and about which he felt tremendous guilt, when a friend was hit by a mortar blast and died in front of him. In the session he had a vivid experience of meeting his friend's soul and being forgiven.

"The explosion hit. Seconds later I'm standing over him, he looks at me for salvation. I'm frozen in fear. Suddenly everything stops; he stands up and walks to me and tells me it's OK. There was never anything I could have done. As I'm writing this, I still imagine that we are hugging in eternity, a moment fixated in time, an embrace of forgiveness not just by (my friend) but for myself to allow me to let go, understanding that I did what I could . . . and there is no reason to hold onto something that cannot be changed. [My friend] would want that. He wouldn't want his death to inspire pain for years and years to come, but rather love and forgiveness. I salute you (my friend) and I will never forget."

Later he added:

"It was such a surreal, spiritual experience. Almost like a rebirth. It was Christ-like in the sense that my ego was crucified and rose again with a softer, more open-minded and new spiritual consciousness. . . . I felt alive, fulfilled by God . . . finally detached from a past that has kept me a prisoner. . . . I'm confident again, ready to take on whatever comes."

Years of psychotherapy had not gotten him to this perspective and this self-forgiveness. The study therapists had no way of knowing in advance that this direct experience of making peace with his friend would be a crucial element in his therapy. Too much direction or even much more interaction on their part might have interfered. He said later that the presence of the therapists was very important in helping him trust that he could surrender to whatever experience came, and that their noninterference was equally important. His global CAPS-IV score at baseline was 79; after two MDMA sessions, it was 9, and at 1 year, it was 2.

In keeping with this approach, we have been struck by how readily most people recognize the experience catalyzed by MDMA as their own creation rather than as something created by the drug. When asked their perspectives about the MDMA sessions, it is rare for participants to dismiss them as simply the artificial effects of the drug. They often say things such as the following:

> "It was a real experience. It was my own experience. The drug made it possible, but it was my experience."

> "I got a glimpse of more of what I'm capable of growing into. . . . I'm motivated to keep practicing openness until it gets more developed."

> "I know this is part of the drug, but when I ask myself, 'Am I going to be able to hold onto this understanding, this wisdom, this knowledge I have now?' I feel like it's so profound that I don't think I could really forget it."

The Importance of Preparation

In addition to addressing any of the participants' questions or concerns and developing an effective therapeutic alliance as one would in any psychotherapy, it is important to prepare participants for the possible effects of MDMA and the inner-directed approach to the sessions. To ensure adequate informed consent, as well as effective preparation, individuals should understand that unlike most psychiatric drugs that are intended to directly reduce symptoms,

MDMA is intended to catalyze processing of the underlying cause of the symptoms, and as that is happening, symptoms may become more pronounced before they improve. The participant should be encouraged to cultivate an attitude of curiosity and openness toward whatever occurs during the MDMA-facilitated experience, remembering that the deepest, most effective healing experiences often take a course that is quite different from what might be predicted by the participant's or the therapists' rational minds. The participant is encouraged to welcome difficult emotions as much as possible rather than to suppress them, operating from the assumption that whatever arises is being presented at that moment as an opportunity for healing. Fully feeling, exploring, and expressing whatever emotions, memories, images, or body sensations arise can make best therapeutic use of the session.

The format of the sessions should be discussed, including the encouragement of participants to spend periods of time focused inward without talking (using eyeshades and listening to music through headphones if they are comfortable doing so), alternating with periods of time talking to the therapists. Careful agreements should be made about whether the participant is open to the possibility of nurturing touch from the therapists such as hand holding, a hand on the shoulder or a hug. It should be explicitly stated that there will be no sexual touch and the participants boundaries will be scrupulously respected. The same ethical guidelines and importance of boundaries in any therapy apply to MDMA-assisted psychotherapy, and therapists should be aware that the intensity of working with drugs that stimulate shifts in consciousness can present particular challenges in this regard (Taylor, 2017).

The Importance of Integration

The importance of integration is discussed during the introductory therapy sessions, when the participant and therapists discuss the likely trajectory of the therapeutic process, emphasizing that the MDMA sessions catalyze a process that will continue to unfold over time. It helps participants to know there will undoubtedly be issues left unresolved and symptoms that persist at the end of the session, but they can expect that with proper intention and support, the therapeutic process stimulated by the MDMA will continue long after the MDMA has worn off. As we often say, "It's not about just what happens during the MDMA sessions." Knowing this, participants are encouraged to make time every day to attend to their inner experience and to reach out for support if needed.

The challenges during the integration stage are to facilitate continued emotional processing and address any difficulties that arise as the experience from the session continues to unfold, and at the same time to help the participant apply to daily life any benefits gained in the MDMA-assisted sessions. These benefits are likely to include valuable insights and perspectives, a broader emotional range, greater resilience, and deepened interpersonal skills.

Since it is hard to predict how much difficulty a given participant will have during the integration process, it is important to be alert to possible problems, such as shame and self-judgment about having revealed secrets, or challenging shifts in relationships and family systems as the participant heals and changes. Conversely, the therapists should be open to the possibility of an easy integration that requires minimal intervention beyond empathic listening and sharing appreciation for the participant's healing and growth. The therapists should therefore remain flexible in their response to each participant's particular experiences. Some illustrative participants' comments during integration sessions follow:

"Now that the medicine has worn off, I sometimes feel guilty for saying the things I did about my parents not being emotionally available. I know it wasn't about blame, but there's still that judging voice that says we don't talk about any of this."

"The anger feels like a volcano. I'm afraid of being a one-man wrecking crew. I feel such sadness, loneliness, nausea."

"Since I've realized how shut down I had been, I don't ever want to go back to being that way, so I'm having a hard time in business situations or with my father, knowing when not to say everything I'm feeling."

"After all these years of not talking about it, was it really safe to reveal that I felt physi-cal pleasure along with horror when I was abused?"

"I don't have my defense mechanisms anymore. . . . I opened a door that I'd kept locked." With support in integration sessions and reminders that opening doors is part of the healing process, he came to realize, "I don't know what I was thinking, that I could clean the house out and not touch some of the stuff in the attic!"

"As interesting as the sessions are, I know from experience now that it's even more interesting what happens after the sessions when you're making connections."

Phase II trials of MDMA-assisted psychotherapy have enrolled people with a history of suicidal thoughts and some who have attempted suicide quite recently. For some people, suicidal thoughts have become more pronounced at the end of MDMA sessions or in the course of therapy afterward. In one study, a participant randomized initially to receive 30 mg MDMA was hospitalized for 6 days for suicidal thoughts that increased 13 days after a low-dose MDMA session, but was able to continue in the study and receive the full dose in the open-label crossover. Suicidal thoughts and behavior were tracked using the Columbia Suicide Severity Rating Scale (CSSRS), and results were that "at all posttreatment endpoints, the percentage of participants reporting suicidal ideation and behavior was reduced compared with baseline lifetime and pretreatment report" (Mithoefer, Mithoefer, Feduccia, et al., 2018). Across six Phase II trials there was no suicidal behavior during the treatment period after dosing (Mithoefer et al., 2019), however, without proper attention to follow-up integration and support, suicide could be a risk.

■ How Different Is This from Other Methods of Psychotherapy?

Some features of MDMA-assisted psychotherapy are dramatically different from most methods of psychotherapy: 8-hour sessions, two cotherapists, periods of time listening to music with eyeshades and headphones, using a drug to shift consciousness, and a taking a largely inner-directed approach.

At the same time, much of what occurs in MDMA sessions would be recognizable to most therapists as familiar elements of other therapeutic approaches (Mithoefer, 2013). Some examples follow.

Imaginal Exposure

A core element of one of the most widespread trauma-focused treatments, *prolonged exposure*, in which clients are directed to repeatedly talk about their "index trauma" in order to overcome avoidance and decrease distress associated with the memories (Foa, Keane, Friedman, & Cohen, 2008), is referred to as *imaginal exposure*. In MDMA sessions participants are not directed to do imaginal exposure, but at some point they almost always do it spontaneously. For some people, this happens almost immediately; for others, it occurs after other aspects of their lives or suffering are encountered first.

For example, a middle-aged married woman who had been raped 7 years previously and had severe PTSD despite treatment with psychotherapy and psychopharmacology, was enrolled in a Phase II clinical trial. She told the research therapists during preparation sessions that she knew she had a lot to feel good about in her life now, but she was unable to feel any of those good feelings. Along with many other PTSD symptoms, this feeling of disconnection from love and support added to her suffering. Early in her first MDMA session (125 mg) she had a profound experience of feeling love, safety, and gratitude for her current life. She spent little time in that first session revisiting the rape, and after the session she remarked, "Now I feel like I have a better platform to operate from, so maybe next time I'll be able to go more into the rape, now I have a map of the battlefield."

During her second MDMA session, without prompting, she processed the rape intensely and in great detail. Her CAPS-IV score went from 103 at baseline to 6, 2 months after the second session.

A military veteran who had served two tours in the war in Iraq enrolled in a Phase II trial because his PTSD had not responded to treatment at the VA clinics. During preparation sessions, he said the symptom that troubled him most was the sudden rage that would erupt and be verbally directed toward his wife. He described an image of a monster in his chest that was constantly trying to come out, so he was trying to choke it to prevent that, as the monster was stabbing him in the side. In his first MDMA session, approximately 2 hours after receiving MDMA (75 mg + 37.5 mg 90 minutes later), he took off his eyeshades and headphones and talked about what he had just been experiencing:

> "I tried thinking about that aspect of me that's really rageful. . . . I had an image of it in a jail cell, like I have that part of me locked up in jail. I felt like I had put it there, and I went to it and opened the door. . . . I stopped trying to choke it and really embraced it. . . . I visualized both of us taking apart the jail cell and really becoming friends. I realized I was keeping him locked up because I was so afraid of him . . . because I think in Iraq I saw what he was capable of. By putting him in that cell and keeping him locked up I was making it worse for him. Of course, when he gets out he's going to be mean and hurtful. . . . It would be more beneficial if we worked together; I mean I know it's me but I just describe it that way. . . . I get this amazing sense of just, I guess wisdom. I feel so much more at peace with everything.

Later in that session and in subsequent sessions, he revisited traumatic experiences from Iraq and described them in great detail with better recall than ever before: "When I got blown up myself, I see it completely different now, I can really go back and visualize. I've never been able to visualize it so hard before and really feel what it was like." Later, when tears of grief came, he said, "I don't let myself feel sometime how much it hurts."

His CAPS-IV score at baseline was 75; a month after two MDMA sessions, it was 6; and at 12-month follow-up, it was 19.

These two examples illustrate one of the advantages of a relatively nondirective approach. For both these people, vivid imaginal exposure was an important part of the therapeutic process. The other experiences that spontaneously occurred first were obviously healing for them and appeared to give them "a better platform to work from" when revisiting the trauma. If there had been an agenda to direct them toward exposure earlier, the opportunity for these other experiences might have been missed.

For these two study participants, as for most others, imaginal exposure did not require the frequent repetition used in prolonged exposure therapy. This may be, at least in part, because they were better prepared to benefit from imaginal exposure after the other healing experiences that spontaneously arose first. There is also evidence from animal studies that the pharmacological effect of MDMA can enhance fear extinction (Young, Andero, Ressler, & Howell, 2015; Young et al., 2017), and there is an ongoing human study testing this hypothesis in healthy volunteers (*clinicaltrials.gov*; Identifier: NCT03181763). A study by the same investigators is planned to test prolonged exposure combined with MDMA administration (Williams, 2017).

Cognitive Restructuring

Cognitive restructuring—identifying and correcting cognitive distortions—is a focus of cognitive-behavioral therapy that is approached in a structured way directed by the therapist. In MDMA-assisted psychotherapy, it happens frequently without direction from the therapists: "I said things I'd never thought before. It's not like I'd remember something cognitively and then say it; I'd just say it and then say 'Wow, where'd that come from?'"

Attention to Transference and Countertransference

In preparation sessions of MDMA-assisted psychodynamic psychotherapy, the therapists discuss transference and countertransference as normal phenomena that provide an opportunity for discovering and processing previously unconscious material in the present moment. Participants taking MDMA can be exquisitely sensitive to verbal and nonverbal expression from the therapists, and the therapists encourage honesty and openness about any feelings that arise. MDMA may make the unconscious conscious quite rapidly, while also increasing the participant's capacity to acknowledge and discuss transference issues and to tolerate and benefit from this faster rate of change. At the same time, the therapists are challenged to be aware of their own reactions and to be honestly and empathically engaged with the participant from moment to moment. An example illustrates that with MDMA, therapists rarely need to point out or interpret the transference because the participants usually do it spontaneously.

A woman who had been severely sexually abused as a child was also neglected and sent to grade school with dirty clothes and messy hair. At one point during an MDMA session (125 mg), she spent approximately 30 minutes in deep conversation with the female therapist, with her back turned toward the male therapists. At the end of that time, she asked the female therapist, "Will you brush my hair?" The female therapist spent time brushing her long hair, with the male therapist looking on in appreciation for this very touching interaction. At the end of that time, the participant thanked the female therapist, lay down in silence for a few minutes, then turned to the male therapist and said:

> "OK, I'm ready to talk to you now. Have you noticed that every time I've talked to you before I've tried to impress you with how smart I am? That's what I did with my father because he was smart and wasn't around much. Now I'm ready to have a real conversation with you."

This example also illustrates the fact that MDMA often fosters an experience of corrective secure attachment for participants who have suffered early attachment injury.

The Multiplicity of the Psyche

The multiplicity of the psyche, while problematic at the extreme, is recognized as a normal phenomenon by several models of psychotherapy that provide specific methods for working with it therapeutically. These models include psychosynthesis, voice dialogue, and internal family systems (IFS) therapy. In our experience, MDMA in a therapeutic setting often raises awareness of different "parts" of the psyche and simultaneously brings forth more of the awareness referred to in IFS as "self energy," allowing exploration of the parts with greater compassion and clarity. In one Phase II trial of MDMA-assisted psychotherapy, the frequency with which parts were discussed was tracked with an exploratory, unvalidated, instrument. In the sessions with active-dose MDMA (75, 100, or 125 mg) discussion of parts occurred in over 75% of sessions compared to less than 30% of sessions with a low-dose comparator (30 mg). In 68% of these sessions, participants brought the subject up spontaneously, and in the other sessions, the therapists mentioned it only in response to the participant's indirectly referring to the phenomenon.

> "I realize that part of me is not a monster, he's a warrior, a valuable part of me, and he needs healing too."

> "I have a sense of much greater connection with a wise inner voice, inner knowing. It used to happen occasionally over the years, but now since the MDMA sessions it's very common."

Attention to Somatic Manifestations of Trauma

Somatic manifestations of trauma are directly addressed in a number of therapeutic approaches such as sensorimotor psychotherapy, somatic experiencing, Holotropic Breathwork, Hakomi and others. In *The Body Keeps the Score,* Bessel van der Kolk (2015 discusses the importance of "bottom-up" processing and of "allowing the body to have experiences that deeply and viscerally contradict the helplessness, rage or collapse that result from trauma." Awareness of somatic manifestations of past experience is often amplified in MDMA sessions. The primary approach to working with them is for the therapists to inquire about body sensations and encourage participants to bring attention to the body and allow the free expression of movements or sounds. If the therapists have training in working directly with the body, it can occasionally be helpful for them to provide some direct work with the body in the form of offering resistance for the body to push or move against. This is only done with explicit permission from the participant and clear agreements about respecting boundaries (Mithoefer, Mithoefer, Jerome, et al., 2018).

The variety of experiences that occur during MDMA-assisted sessions using this inner-directed approach may raise the question, "Is this therapy standardized enough across different sessions and study sites for valid research?" In one way, it is less standardized than most manualized therapies, such as prolonged exposure or cognitive processing therapy, which have specific instructions about what should be addressed in each session. Our observations suggest that the inner-directed approach is standardized in another way. In the MDMA studies, what happens in each session is primarily directed by that individual's spontaneous process. If one accepts the premise that there is a capacity to heal within each person, and that MDMA helps to remove obstacles to the realization of that capacity, then it follows that this approach is standardized to provide each person with access to his or her own particular healing process. Observations from clinical trials suggest that this may be the optimal way to arrive at whichever type of therapeutic experience is most appropriate and effective for a given individual at a given time. At any given time that may or may not be imaginal exposure, cognitive restructuring, or whatever technique might have been dictated by a more structured therapeutic approach. A reductionist approach that limits treatment to focusing on only one aspect of healing, such as fear extinction or cognitive restructuring, may miss the opportunity for a broader and richer range of healing experiences than an individual would have the capacity to access under the right circumstances.

An Unexplained Feature of MDMA-Assisted Psychotherapy

Often in their first MDMA sessions, well before they have processed their trauma or experienced an improvement in their symptoms, participants become convinced that they will be able to heal. An example of this is a woman with a history of sexual assault who was referred by her clinical psychologist after several years of psychotherapy, along with treatment by a psychiatrist with a series of drugs. During one of three non-drug preparatory sessions prior to her first MDMA-assisted session, she said to the therapists, "I never thought I would consider taking a drug like MDMA, but nothing else has worked and I'm desperate so I'll do anything to get better; I'll even go to Tibet if I have to!"

The following day, about an hour after taking 125 mg of MDMA, she took off her eyeshades and, with a smile, the first thing she said was, "I guess I won't have to go to Tibet." How is it that suddenly, after 7 years of suffering, and years of unsuccessful treatment, she knew she could heal? She had not yet healed; it would take some painful hours of processing the trauma and its aftermath in subsequent MDMA-assisted sessions for her PTSD symptoms to remit, but she knew from that moment she could do it. It is no surprise that a drug could make someone suddenly more hopeful, regardless of how unrealistic his or her expectations might be, and we may well discover the neurophysiological correlate to accessing this hope, or this sense of knowing. So one possible explanation is simply that MDMA made her feel more hopeful, and she also went on to recover from PTSD, so her prediction happened to be correct. Perhaps being hopeful contributed to her willingness and ability to engage in the treatment, but she had no way of knowing what the outcome would be. The danger of insisting on this explanation, simply because it fits with our current limited understanding of the psyche and our theories of trauma recovery, is that we might miss a clue pointing to new discoveries and a deeper understanding.

What she and others actually reported was not just feeling hopeful, it was an experience of knowing, of having apprehended something fundamental about themselves and perhaps the nature of the psyche and its ability to heal. For clinical as well as scientific reasons we should remain intensely curious about this phenomenon.

Risk Evaluation and Management Strategy

If ongoing Phase III clinical trials lead to FDA approval of an NDA that makes MDMA available for clinical use, the FDA (n.d.) is likely to require a Risk Evaluation and Mitigation Strategy (REMS), requirements designed "to ensure that the benefits of a drug or biological product outweigh its risks." The details of the REMS for MDMA will not be determined until after the NDA is submitted, which is expected in 2021 (Doblin, 2018). Based on scientific advice meetings with the European Medicines Agency in preparation for planned European trials, it appears likely that a comparable REMS will be required in Europe. MAPS is in favor of having an appropriate REMS, and, during meetings with FDA, has tentatively recommend that the following requirements be included in the REMS for MDMA:

1. Only prescribed by certified therapists with specific specialized training
2. Only administered in certified clinics
3. Defined safety screening for specified patient population
4. Driving prohibited for five half-lives of MDMA
5. Shipped directly from manufacturer to the prescriber for dispensing at a certified clinic.

Training Program

MAPS has developed a therapist training program in the method described in the manual (Mithoefer, Mithoefer, Jerome, et al., 2018). This training has been required for all Phase II and Phase III therapists (in parallel, there is a training program for adherence raters who verify fidelity to the method by watching video recordings of research sessions). This program is being extended and expanded in order to provide the specialized training required for additional MDMA therapists who will be needed. The FDA has approved limited use of MDMA-assisted psychotherapy prior to the completion of Phase 3 trials through an Expanded Access Program (compassionate use). This protocol will initially include treatment of 50 patients with PTSD and is scheduled to start in 2021. Many more therapists are expected to be needed postapproval, which may occur in 2023. The training is in five parts: (1) an online training module, (2) 6-day in-person training that includes watching and discussing videos from research sessions, (3) individual activities to expand skills, such as workshops in Holotropic Breathwork or somatic therapy trainings, (4) role play with cotherapists at each site, and (5) supervision of at least one participant's course of treatment via supervisors watching session video and providing feedback in videoconferencing meetings.

After completing the program, therapists have the option to enroll in an open Phase I protocol administering MDMA to healthy volunteers using the same setting and method as is used in clinical trials. Enrollment is limited to therapists who have gone through MAPS training and is an opportunity for firsthand experience receiving MDMA in a therapeutic setting in preparation for administering it to study participants or patients. More than 75 therapists have completed this study to date and have uniformly reported it to be valuable preparation for their role as MDMA therapists.

■ Conclusion

MDMA administered in conjunction with psychotherapy shows promise as a new treatment for PTSD and perhaps other psychiatric indications. This is strongly supported by data from Phase II Clinical Trials leading to FDA Breakthrough Therapy designation and is now being more definitively tested in international Phase III trials. If these trials are successful in demonstrating safety and efficacy, MDMA could become available for clinical use as early as 2022. In addition to the promise MDMA holds for treating specific conditions, recent research with MDMA and other psychedelics is presenting the possibility of a much-needed new direction in psychiatry and psychology that bridges the gap between psychopharmacology and psychotherapy. Over 50 years ago, LSD served as a clue to understanding the role of serotonin in the brain (Woolley & Shaw, 1954). MDMA and other psychedelics are now giving us clues to a deeper understanding of the nature of the psyche and how we can more effectively access the potential within each individual for psychological healing and growth.

■ References

Adamson, S., & Metzner, R. (1988). The nature of the MDMA experience and its role in healing, psychotherapy, and spiritual practice. *Re-Vision, 10*(4), 59–72.

Alrashedy, N. A., & Molina, J. (2016). The ethnobotany of psychoactive plant use: A phylogenetic perspective. *PeerJ, 4*, e2546.

Baumann, M. H., Zolkowska, D., Kim, I., Scheidweiler, K. B., Rothman, R. B., & Huestis, M. A. (2009). Effects of dose and route of administration on pharmacokinetics of (+ or −)-3,4-methylenedioxymethamphetamine in the rat. *Drug Metabolism and Disposition, 37*(11), 2163–2170.

Bedi, G., Hyman, D., & de Wit, H. (2010). Is ecstasy an "empathogen"?: Effects of ±3,4-methylenedioxymethamphetamine on prosocial feelings and identification of emotional states in others. *Biological Psychiatry, 68*(12), 1134–1140.

Bonkale, W. L., & Austin, M. C. (2008). 3,4-methylenedioxymethamphetamine induces differential regulation of tryptophan hydroxylase 2 protein and mRNA levels in the rat dorsal raphe nucleus. *Neuroscience, 155*(1), 270–276.

Bouso, J. C., Doblin, R., Farré, M., Alcázar, M. A., & Gómez-Jarabo, G. (2008). MDMA-assisted psychotherapy using low doses in a small sample of women with chronic posttraumatic stress disorder. *Journal of Psychoactive Drugs, 40*(3), 225–236.

Cami, J., Farré, M., Mas, M., Roset, P. N., Poudevida, S., Mas, A., et al. (2000). Human pharmacology of 3,4-methylenedioxymethamphetamine ("Ecstasy"): Psychomotor performance and subjective effects. *Journal of Clinical Psychopharmacology, 20*(4), 455–466.

Carhart-Harris, R. L., Erritzoe, D., Williams, T., Stone, J. M., Reed, L. J., Colasanti, A., et al. (2012). Neural correlates of the psychedelic state as determined by fMRI studies with psilocybin. *Proceedings of the National Academy of Sciences of the USA, 109*(6), 2138–2143.

Carhart-Harris, R. L., Murphy, K., Leech, R., Erritzoe, D., Wall, M. B., Ferguson, B., et al. (2015). The effects of acutely administered 3,4-methylenedioxymethamphetamine on spontaneous brain function in healthy volunteers measured with arterial spin labeling and blood oxygen level-dependent resting state functional connectivity. *Biological Psychiatry, 78*(8), 554–562.

Carvalho, M., Pontes, H., Remião, F., Bastos, M. L., & Carvalho, F. (2010). Mechanisms underlying the hepatotoxic effects of ecstasy. *Current Pharmaceutical Biotechnology, 11*(5), 476–495.

Danforth, A. L., Grob, C. S., Struble, C., Feduccia, A. A., Walker, N., Jerome, L., et al. (2018). Reduction in social anxiety after MDMA-assisted psychotherapy with autistic adults: A randomized, double-blind, placebo-controlled pilot study. *Psychopharmacology, 235*(11), 3137–3148.

de la Torre, R., Farré, M., Ortuño, J., Mas, M.,

Brenneisen, R., Roset, P. N., et al. (2000). Non-linear pharmacokinetics of MDMA ("Ecstasy") in humans. *British Journal of Clinical Pharmacology, 49*(2), 104–109.

Doblin, R. (2018, Summer). From the Desk of Rick Doblin, Ph.D. Retrieved from *https://maps.org/news/bulletin/articles/430-maps-bulletin-summer-2018-vol-28-no-2-research-edition/7333-from-the-desk-of-rick-doblin,-ph-d-summer-2018.*

Downing, J. (1985). Testimony of Joseph J. Downing, M.D. In the Matter of MDMA Scheduling. Docket No. 84-48. United States Department of Justice, Drug Enforcement Administration. Retrieved from *www.maps.org/research-archive/dea-mdma/pdf/0015.pdf.*

Downing, J. (1986). The psychological and physiological effects of MDMA on normal volunteers. *Journal of Psychoactive Drugs, 18*(4), 335–340.

Dumont, G. J. H., Sweep, F. C. G. J., van der Steen, R., Hermsen, R., Donders, A. R. T., Touw, D. J., et al. (2009). Increased oxytocin concentrations and prosocial feelings in humans after ecstasy (3,4-methylenedioxymethamphetamine) administration. *Social Neuroscience, 4*(4), 359–366.

Eede, H. V., Montenij, L. J., Touw, D. J., & Norris, E. M. (2012). Rhabdomyolysis in MDMA intoxication: A rapid and underestimated killer: "Clean" ecstasy, a safe party drug? *Journal of Emergency Medicine, 42*(6), 655–658.

Ellis, A. J., Wendon, J. A., Portmann, B., & Williams, R. (1996). Acute liver damage and ecstasy ingestion. *Gut, 38*(3), 454–458.

Fadiman, J. (2011). *The psychedelic explorer's guide: Safe, therapeutic, and sacred journeys.* Rochester, VT: Park Street Press.

Fantegrossi, W. E., Kiessel, C. L., Leach, P. T., Van Martin, C., Karabenick, R. L., Chen, X., et al. (2004). Nantenine: An antagonist of the behavioral and physiological effects of MDMA in mice. *Psychopharmacology, 173*(3–4), 270–277.

Foa, E. B., Keane, T. M., Friedman, M. J., & Cohen, J. A. (Eds.). (2008). *Effective treatments for PTSD: Practice guidelines from the International Society for Traumatic Stress Studies* (2nd ed.). New York: Guilford Press.

Forsling, M., Fallon, J. K., Kicman, A. T., Hutt, A. J., Cowan, D. A., & Henry, J. A. (2001). Arginine vasopressin release in response to the administration of 3,4-methylenedioxymethamphetamine ("ecstasy"): Is metabolism a contributory factor? *Journal of Pharmacy and Pharmacology, 53*(10), 1357–1363.

Freedman, R. R., Johanson, C.-E., & Tancer, M. E. (2005). Thermoregulatory effects of 3,4-methylenedioxymethamphetamine (MDMA) in humans. *Psychopharmacology, 183*(2), 248–256.

Gamma, A., Buck, A., Berthold, T., Liechti, M. E., Vollenweider, F. X., & Hell, D. (2000). 3,4-methylenedioxymethamphetamine (MDMA) modulates cortical and limbic brain activity as measured by [H(2)(15)O]-PET in healthy humans. *Neuropsychopharmacology, 23*(4), 388–395.

Gasser, P. (1994). Psycholytic therapy with MDMA and LSD in Switzerland. *MAPS Bulletin, 5*(3), 3–7.

Gasser, P. (1996). The psycholytic psychotherapy in Switzerland from 1988–1993. *Swiss Archives of Neurology and Psychiatry, 147*(2), 59–65.

Ghatol, A., & Kazory, A. (2012). Ecstasy-associated acute severe hyponatremia and cerebral edema: A role for osmotic diuresis? *Journal of Emergency Medicine, 42*(6), e137–e140.

Gillman, P. K. (2005). Monoamine oxidase inhibitors, opioid analgesics and serotonin toxicity. *British Journal of Anaesthesia, 95*(4), 434–441.

Gowing, L. R., Henry-Edwards, S. M., Irvine, R. J., & Ali, R. L. (2002). The health effects of ecstasy: A literature review. *Drug and Alcohol Review, 21*(1), 53–63.

Green, A. R., Mechan, A. O., Elliott, J. M., O'Shea, E., & Colado, M. I. (2003). The pharmacology and clinical pharmacology of 3,4-methylenedioxymethamphetamine (MDMA, "ecstasy"). *Pharmacological Reviews, 55*(3), 463–508.

Greer, G. (1985). Using MDMA in psychotherapy. *Advances, 2*(2), 57–59.

Greer, G., & Tolbert, R. (1986). Subjective reports of the effects of MDMA in a clinical setting. *Journal of Psychoactive Drugs, 18*(4), 319–327.

Greer, G. R., & Tolbert, R. (1998). A method of conducting therapeutic sessions with MDMA. *Journal of Psychoactive Drugs, 30*(4), 371–379.

Griffiths, R. R., Johnson, M. W., Carducci, M. A., Umbricht, A., Richards, W. A., Richards, B. D., et al. (2016). Psilocybin produces substantial and sustained decreases in depression and anxiety in patients with life-threatening cancer: A randomized double-blind trial. *Journal of Psychopharmacology (Oxford), 30*(12), 1181–1197.

Griffiths, R. R., Richards, W. A., McCann, U., & Jesse, R. (2006). Psilocybin can occasion mystical-type experiences having substantial and sustained personal meaning and spiritual significance. *Psychopharmacology, 187*(3), 268–283.

Grob, C. (1998). MDMA research: Preliminary

investigations with human subjects. *International Journal of Drug Policy, 9,* 119–124.

Grob, C. S. (2000). Deconstructing ecstasy: The politics of MDMA research. *Addiction Research, 8*(6), 549–588.

Grob, C. S., Bravo, G., & Walsh, R. (1990). Second thoughts on 3,4-methylenedioxymethamphetamine (MDMA) neurotoxicity. *Archives of General Psychiatry, 47,* 288–289.

Grob, C. S., Poland, R. E., Chang, L., & Ernst, T. (1996). Psychobiologic effects of 3,4-methylenedioxymethamphetamine in humans: Methodological considerations and preliminary observations. *Behavioural Brain Research, 73*(1–2), 103–107.

Grof, S. (2001). *LSD psychotherapy.* Sarasota, FL: Multidisciplinary Association for Psychedelic Studies.

Grof, S. (2019). *The way of the psychonaut.* Santa Cruz, CA: Multidisciplinary Association for Psychedelic Studies.

Gronwall, D. M. (1977). Paced auditory serial-addition task: A measure of recovery from concussion. *Perceptual and Motor Skills, 44*(2), 367–373.

Halpern, J. H., Sherwood, A. R., Hudson, J. I., Gruber, S., Kozin, D., & Pope, H. G. (2011). Residual neurocognitive features of long-term ecstasy users with minimal exposure to other drugs. *Addiction, 106*(4), 777–786.

Harris, D. S., Baggott, M., Mendelson, J. H., Mendelson, J. E., & Jones, R. T. (2002). Subjective and hormonal effects of 3,4-methylenedioxymethamphetamine (MDMA) in humans. *Psychopharmacology, 162*(4), 396–405.

Henry, J. A., Jeffreys, K. J., & Dawling, S. (1992). Toxicity and deaths from 3,4-methylenedioxymethamphetamine ("ecstasy"). *Lancet, 340*(8816), 384–387.

Holland, J. (2001). *Ecstasy: The complete guide: A comprehensive look at the risks and benefits of MDMA.* Rochester, VT: Inner Traditions/Bear & Company.

Hysek, C. M., Schmid, Y., Rickli, A., & Liechti, M. E. (2013). Carvedilol inhibits the cardiostimulant and thermogenic effects of MDMA in humans: Lost in translation. *British Journal of Pharmacology, 170*(6), 1273–1275.

Hysek, C. M., Schmid, Y., Simmler, L. D., Domes, G., Heinrichs, M., Eisenegger, C., et al. (2014). MDMA enhances emotional empathy and prosocial behavior. *Social Cognitive and Affective Neuroscience, 9*(11), 1645–1652.

Kaelen, M. (2017a, July). *The psychedelic future of mental health care.* Cambridge, UK: Cambridge University, TedX Talk. Retrieved from *www.youtube.com/watch?v=ehi0cfm4dqm&t=1s.*

Kaelen, M. (2017b, April). *The psychological and neurophysiological effects of music in combination with psychedelics.* Unpublished doctoral thesis, Imperial College, London, UK.

Kuypers, K. P. C., de la Torre, R., Farre, M., Yubero-Lahoz, S., Dziobek, I., Van den Bos, W., et al. (2014). No evidence that MDMA-induced enhancement of emotional empathy is related to peripheral oxytocin levels or 5-HT1A receptor activation. *PLOS ONE, 9*(6), e100719.

Kuypers, K. P. C., & Ramaekers, J. G. (2005). Transient memory impairment after acute dose of 75mg 3.4-methylene-dioxymethamphetamine. *Journal of Psychopharmacology (Oxford), 19*(6), 633–639.

Kuypers, K. P. C., & Ramaekers, J. G. (2007). Acute dose of MDMA (75 mg) impairs spatial memory for location but leaves contextual processing of visuospatial information unaffected. *Psychopharmacology, 189*(4), 557–563.

Lester, S. J., Baggott, M., Welm, S., Schiller, N. B., Jones, R. T., Foster, E., et al. (2000). Cardiovascular effects of 3,4-methylenedioxymethamphetamine: A double-blind, placebo-controlled trial. *Annals of Internal Medicine, 133*(12), 969–973.

Liechti, M. E., Baumann, C., Gamma, A., & Vollenweider, F. X. (2000). Acute psychological effects of 3,4-methylenedioxymethamphetamine (MDMA, "Ecstasy") are attenuated by the serotonin uptake inhibitor citalopram. *Neuropsychopharmacology, 22*(5), 513–521.

Liechti, M. E., & Vollenweider, F. X. (2000). The serotonin uptake inhibitor citalopram reduces acute cardiovascular and vegetative effects of 3,4-methylenedioxymethamphetamine ("Ecstasy") in healthy volunteers. *Journal of Psychopharmacology, 14*(3), 269–274.

MacInnes, N., Handley, S. L., & Harding, G. F. (2001). Former chronic methylenedioxymethamphetamine (MDMA or ecstasy) users report mild depressive symptoms. *Journal of Psychopharmacology (Oxford), 15*(3), 181–186.

Mechan, A., Yuan, J., Hatzidimitriou, G., Irvine, R. J., McCann, U. D., & Ricaurte, G. A. (2006). Pharmacokinetic profile of single and repeated oral doses of MDMA in squirrel monkeys: Relationship to lasting effects on brain serotonin neurons. *Neuropsychopharmacology, 31*(2), 339–350.

Metzner, R. (1983, May). *Psychedelics and spirituality.* Lecture presented at Psychedelics and Spirituality, Santa Barbara, CA.

Mithoefer, M. (2013, Spring). MDMA-assisted psychotherapy—how different is it from other psychotherapy? *MAPS Bulletin, 23*(1), 110–114.

Mithoefer, M. C. (2018, April). *I don't know why they call this "Ecstasy": What's going on in MDMA-assisted psychotherapy for PTSD?* Presented at the Royal College of Psychiatrists, Faculty of Medical Psychotherapy annual conference, Cardiff, Wales.

Mithoefer, M., Feduccia, A. A., Jerome, L., Mithoefer, A. T., Wagner, M., Walsh, Z., et al. (2019). MDMA-assisted psychotherapy for treatment of PTSD: Study design and rationale for Phase 3 trials based on pooled analysis of six Phase 2 randomized controlled trials. *Pschopharmacology (Berlin), 236,* 2735–2745.

Mithoefer, M., Jerome, L., Doblin, R., & Ricaurte, G. A. (2003). MDMA ("ecstasy") and neurotoxicity. *Science, 300,* 1504–1505.

Mithoefer, M., Mithoefer, A., Feduccia, A., Jerome, L., Wagner, M., Wymer, J., et al. (2018). 3,4-methylenedioxymethamphetamine (MDMA)-assisted psychotherapy for posttraumatic stress disorder in military veterans, firefighters, and police officers: A randomised, double-blind, dose–response, Phase 2 clinical trial. *Lancet Psychiatry, 5*(6), 486–497.

Mithoefer, M., Mithoefer, A., Jerome, L., Ruse, J., Doblin, R., Ot'alora, M., & Sola, E. (2018). *A manual for MDMA-assisted psychotherapy in the treatment of PTSD* (9th ed.). Retrieved from *https://maps.org/research/mdma/mdma-research-timeline/4887-a-manual-for-mdma-assisted-psychotherapy-in-the-treatment-of-ptsd.*

Mithoefer, M. C., Wagner, M. T., Mithoefer, A. T., Jerome, L., & Doblin, R. (2011). The safety and efficacy of 3,4-methylenedioxymethamphetamine-assisted psychotherapy in subjects with chronic, treatment-resistant posttraumatic stress disorder: The first randomized controlled pilot study. *Journal of Psychopharmacology, 25*(4), 439–452.

Mithoefer, M., Wagner, M., Mithoefer, A., Jerome, L., Martin, S., Yazar-Klosinski, B., et al. (2013). Durability of improvement in posttraumatic stress disorder symptoms and absence of harmful effects or drug dependency after 3,4-methylenedioxymethamphetamine-assisted psychotherapy: A prospective long-term follow-up study. *Journal of Psychopharmacology, 27*(1), 28–39.

Monson, C., Wagner, A., & Macdonald, A. (2015, August). *MDMA-facilitated cognitive-behavioral conjoint therapy for PTSD. In cognitive-behavioral conjoint therapy for PTSD: Delivery Alternatives, Outcomes and Dissemination.* Presented at the American Psychological Association, Toronto, Canada.

Monson, C. M., Wagner, A. C., Mithoefer, A. T., Liebman, R. E., Feduccia, A. A., Jerome, L. I., et al. (in press). MDMA-facilitated cognitive-behavioral conjoint therapy for posttraumatic stress disorder: An uncontrolled trial. *European Journal of Psychotraumatology.*

Mueller, M., Kolbrich, E. A., Peters, F. T., Maurer, H. H., McCann, U. D., Huestis, M. A., et al. (2009). Direct Comparison of (±) 3,4-methylenedioxymethamphetamine ("Ecstasy") disposition and metabolism in squirrel monkeys and humans. *Therapeutic Drug Monitoring, 31*(3), 367–373.

Multidisciplinary Association for Psychedelic Studies. (2017, May 21). MDMA Investigator's Brochure and FDA Annual Report. Retrieved October 26, 2018, from *https://maps.org/research/mdma/mdma-research-timeline/104-other-mdma-resources/5400-mdma-investigator-s-brochure-and-fda-annual-report&Itemid=485.*

Naranjo, C. (1989). MDMA in group therapy. In B. Eisner (Ed.), *Ecstasy: The MDMA story* (pp. 107–111). Berkeley, CA: Ronin.

Naranjo, C., & Holland, J. (Eds.). (2001). Experience with the interpersonal psychedelics. In *Ecstasy: The complete guide* (pp. 208–221). Rochester, VT: Park Street Press.

National Institute on Drug Abuse. (2018). MDMA (Ecstasy/Molly). Retrieved October 25, 2018, from *www.drugabuse.gov/drugs-abuse/mdma-ecstasymolly.*

National Institute on Drug Abuse (NIDA). (2020). *What is the scope of MDMA use in the United States?* Retrieved September 8, 2020, from *www.drugabuse.gov/publications/research-reports/mdma-ecstasy-abuse/what-is-the-scope-of-mdma-use-in-the-united-states.*

Nichols, D. E. (1986). Differences between the mechanism of action of MDMA, MBDB, and the classic hallucinogens: Identification of a new therapeutic class: Entactogens. *Journal of Psychoactive Drugs, 18*(4), 305–313.

Nichols, D. E. (2016). Psychedelics. *Pharmacological Reviews, 68*(2), 264–355.

Oehen, P., Traber, R., Widmer, V., & Schnyder, U. (2013). A randomized, controlled pilot study of MDMA (± 3,4-methylenedioxymethamphetamine)-assisted psychotherapy for treatment of resistant, chronic posttraumatic stress disorder (PTSD). *Journal of Psychopharmacology (Oxford), 27*(1), 40–52.

Ogden, P., Minton, K., & Pain, C. (2006). *Trauma and the body: A sensorimotor approach to psychotherapy.* New York: Norton.

Ot'alora G, M., Grigsby, J., Poulter, B., Van Derveer, J. W., Giron, S. G., Jerome, L., et al. (2018). 3,4-methylenedioxymethamphetamine-assisted psychotherapy for treatment of chronic posttraumatic stress disorder: A randomized Phase 2 controlled trial. *Journal of Psychopharmacology (Oxford),* 1295–1307.

Pacifici, R., Pichini, S., Zuccaro, P., Farré, M., Segura, M., Ortuño, J., et al. (2004). Paroxetine inhibits acute effects of 3,4-methylenedioxymethamphetamine on the immune system in humans. *Journal of Pharmacology and Experimental Therapeutics, 309*(1), 285–292.

Pacifici, R., Zuccaro, P., López, C. H., Pichini, S., Carlo, S. D., Farré, M., et al. (2001). Acute effects of 3,4-methylenedioxymethamphetamine alone and in combination with ethanol on the immune system in humans. *Journal of Pharmacology and Experimental Therapeutics, 296*(1), 207–215.

Pardo-Lozano, R., Farré, M., Yubero-Lahoz, S., O'Mathúna, B., Torrens, M., Mustata, C., et al. (2012). Clinical pharmacology of 3,4-methylenedioxymethamphetamine (MDMA, "Ecstasy"): The influence of gender and genetics (CYP2D6, COMT, 5-HTT). *PLOS ONE, 7*(10), e47599.

Passie, T. (2018). The early use of MDMA ("Ecstasy") in psychotherapy (1977–1985). *Drug Science, Policy and Law, 4*, 2–12.

Passie, T., & Benzenhöfer, U. (2016). The history of MDMA as an underground drug in the United States, 1960–1979. *Journal of Psychoactive Drugs, 48*(2), 67–75.

Randolph, C., Tierney, M. C., Mohr, E., & Chase, T. N. (1998). The Repeatable Battery for the Assessment of Neuropsychological Status (RBANS): Preliminary clinical validity. *Journal of Clinical and Experimental Neuropsychology, 20*(3), 310–319.

Ricaurte, G. A. (2003). Retraction. *Science, 301*(5639), 1479.

Ricaurte, G. A., Yuan, J., Hatzidimitriou, G., Cord, B. J., & McCann, U. D. (2002). Severe dopaminergic neurotoxicity in primates after a common recreational dose regimen of MDMA ("ecstasy"). *Science, 297*(5590), 2260–2263.

Richards, W. A. (2015). *Sacred knowledge: Psychedelics and religious experiences.* New York: Columbia University Press.

Ross, S., Bossis, A., Guss, J., Agin-Liebes, G., Malone, T., Cohen, B., et al. (2016). Rapid and sustained symptom reduction following psilocybin treatment for anxiety and depression in patients with life-threatening cancer: A randomized controlled trial. *Journal of Psychopharmacology (Oxford), 30*(12), 1165–1180.

Schenk, S., Abraham, B., Aronsen, D., Colussi-Mas, J., & Do, J. (2013). Effects of repeated exposure to MDMA on 5HT1a autoreceptor function: Behavioral and neurochemical responses to 8-OHDPAT. *Psychopharmacology, 227*(2), 355–361.

Schilt, T., de Win, M. M. L., Koeter, M., Jager, G., Korf, D. J., van den Brink, W., et al. (2007). Cognition in novice ecstasy users with minimal exposure to other drugs: A prospective cohort study. *Archives of General Psychiatry, 64*(6), 728–736.

Shulgun, A., & Shulgin, A. (1991). *Phikal.* Berkeley, CA: Transform Press.

Simmler, L. D., Rickli, A., Hoener, M. C., & Liechti, M. E. (2014). Monoamine transporter and receptor interaction profiles of a new series of designer cathinones. *Neuropharmacology, 79*, 152–160.

Slikker, J. W., Holson, R. R., Ali, S. F., Kolta, M. G., Paule, M. G., Scallet, A. C., et al. (1989). Behavioral and neurochemical effects of orally administered MDMA in the rodent and nonhuman primate. *Neurotoxicology, 10*(3), 529–542.

Stolaroff, M. J. (2004). *The secret chief revealed.* Sarasota, FL: Multidisciplinary Association for Psychedelic Studies.

Tancer, M. E., & Johanson, C. E. (2001). The subjective effects of MDMA and mCPP in moderate MDMA users. *Drug and Alcohol Dependence, 65*(1), 97–101.

Taylor, K. (2017). *The ethics of caring: Finding right relationship with clients: For profound, transformative work in professional healing relationships* (3rd ed.). Santa Cruz, CA: Hanford Mead.

Tupper, K. W., Wood, E., Yensen, R., & Johnson, M. W. (2015). Psychedelic medicine: A re-emerging therapeutic paradigm. *Canadian Medical Association Journal, 187*(14), 1054–1059.

U.S. Drug Enforcement Administration. (n.d.). Drug scheduling. Retrieved October 25, 2018, from *www.dea.gov/drug-scheduling.*

U.S. Food and Drug Administration. (n.d.). Risk Evaluation and Mitigation Strategies (REMS). Retrieved November 4, 2018, from *www.fda.gov/drugs/drugsafety/rems/default.htm.*

van der Kolk, B. J. (2015). *The body keeps the score.* New York: Penguin Books.

Vizeli, P., & Liechti, M. E. (2017). Safety pharmacology of acute MDMA administration in healthy subjects. *Journal of Psychopharmacology (Oxford), 31*(5), 576–588.

Vollenweider, F. X., Gamma, A., Liechti, M., & Huber, T. (1998). Psychological and cardiovascular effects and short-term sequelae of MDMA ("ecstasy") in MDMA-naive healthy volunteers. *Neuropsychopharmacology, 19*(4), 241–251.

Wagner, A., Mithoefer, M., & Doblin, R. (2019). Bringing psychedelics and entactogens into mainstream pharmaceuticals: A focus on MDMA. In M. Winkleman & B. Sessa (Eds.), *Advances in psychedelic medicine* (Vol. 3, pp. 336–357). Santa Barbara, CA: ABC-CLIO.

Wagner, A. C., Mithoefer, M. C., Mithoefer, A. T., & Monson, C. M. (2019). Combining cognitive-behavioral conjoint therapy for PTSD with 3,4-methylenedioxymethamphetamine (MDMA): A case example. *Journal of Psychoactive Drugs, 51*(2), 166–173.

Wang, X., Baumann, M. H., Xu, H., Morales, M., & Rothman, R. B. (2005). (±)-3,4-methylenedioxymethamphetamine administration to rats does not decrease levels of the serotonin transporter protein or alter its distribution between endosomes and the plasma membrane. *Journal of Pharmacology and Experimental Therapeutics, 314*(3), 1002–1012.

Williams, E. (2017, Spring). Towards breakthrough healing: A history and overview of clinical MDMA research. Retrieved from *https://maps.org/news/bulletin/articles/420-bulletin-spring-2017/6618-towards-breakthrough-healing-a-history-and-overview-of-clinical-mdma-research.*

Wolfson, P. (2020). *MDMA-assisted psychotherapy for treatment of anxiety related to life-threatening illnesses: A double-blind, randomized clinical trial with an open-label crossover.* Manuscript submitted for publication.

Woolley, D. W., & Shaw, E. (1954). A biochemical and pharmacological suggestion about certain mental disorders. *Proceedings of the National Academy of Sciences of the USA, 40*(4), 228–231.

Yalom, I. D. (2007). The gift of therapy: An open letter to a new generation of therapists and their patients. Retrieved from *http://search.ebscohost.com/login.aspx?direct=true&scope=site&db=nlebk&db=nlabk&AN=204877.*

Young, M. B., Andero, R., Ressler, K. J., & Howell, L. L. (2015). 3,4-methylenedioxymethamphetamine facilitates fear extinction learning. *Translational Psychiatry, 5*, e634.

Young, M. B., Norrholm, S. D., Khoury, L. M., Jovanovic, T., Rauch, S. A. M., Reiff, C. M., et al. (2017). Inhibition of serotonin transporters disrupts the enhancement of fear memory extinction by 3,4-methylenedioxymethamphetamine (MDMA). *Psychopharmacology, 234*(19), 2883–2895.

CHAPTER 13

Therapeutic and Social Uses of MDMA

SCOTT SHANNON, ROB COLBERT, and SHANNON HUGHES

▦ Introduction

We are witnessing a societal and professional shift in our orientation to the psyche, moving from a suppressive model to an evocative model of mental health. Suppressive models of psychopharmacology (antipsychotics, benzodiazepines, antidepressants, etc.) have been dominant in mental health for the last 60 years. Psychiatry by and large has become a specialty based on symptomatic suppression by medications that never cure. These medications often cloud consciousness and prevent deeper psychological processing or effective access to emotions. The medical profession now considers daily pharmacological intervention as a necessity to manage the darker realms of the psyche and keep unwanted emotional and behavioral expressions at bay. New paradigms from outside the medical model have emerged that honor the psyche and the innate power to heal. The applications outlined in this chapter reflect this new perspective, specifically highlighting MDMA as a catalyst to healing through deeper exploration of the psyche. These applications appreciate the intrinsic wholeness of our body–mind–spirit and a new respect for our inner world. MDMA-assisted psychotherapy will play a critical role in bringing greater awareness to this new style of care.

The chemical 3,4-methylenedioxy-methamphetamine (MDMA) was created over 100 years ago. However, only in the last 50 years or so have mental health professionals recognized some of the outsized potential for this chemical. While MDMA shows great promise in the treatment of posttraumatic stress disorder (PTSD) (see Mithoefer & Mithoefer, Chapter 12), the usefulness of MDMA goes well beyond this single diagnosis. In this chapter we consider novel potential applications of this medicine, including a discussion of its complex psychodynamic and psychotherapeutic effects. With an entire subculture having adopted MDMA use in social and recreational contexts, this chapter further questions whether the broader value and implications of MDMA use are necessarily limited to clinical applications only. Through exploring its history, range, and contexts of use, and emerging philosophies of mental health care, this chapter provides a broad overview of the shifting landscape and the possibilities ahead for this medicine.

History and Range of Use

The psychedelic pioneers of the late 20th century (Adamson & Metzner, 1988; Downing, 1985; Grob, Bravo, & Walsh, 1990; Ingrasci, 1985; Nichols, 1986; Shulgin & Nichols, 1978) and numerous unnamed others, explored MDMA's ability to increase empathy, emotional connectedness, and sensations of euphoria, as well as the implications of these effects for personal discovery and self-healing (Greer & Tolbert, 1986). These pioneers recognized the enhanced self-exploration facilitated by MDMA in an individual therapeutic process, and created structures and processes for the accomplishment of this inner-directed work.

Ann Shulgin (1980) began by helping close friends work on personal issues, later accepting referred clients, and eventually distributing a pamphlet to networks of therapists and others working with MDMA in the early 1980s. The pamphlet described two methods for facilitating MDMA group sessions. The first is an isolated, inner-directed experience using eyeshades and music, with group processing at the end of the journey. The second and preferred method involves the group leader also consuming MDMA, with all group members interacting freely throughout the medicine session.

Leo Zeff further organized weekend retreat-type settings for "group tripping," which he believed maximized the potential benefit of MDMA and psychedelic substances such as lysergic acid diethylamide (LSD), *Psilocybe cubensis* mushrooms, and mescaline (Stolaroff, 2004). Guidelines for "group tripping" were developed to lay out specific safety measures and rules, including no sexual contact, no leaving before the end of the weekend, and an agreement to follow the instructions of sober guides at all times. While intentions regarding the desired outcomes from tripping that weekend were shared as a group, the focus of the sessions again was on the individual's own personal experience and inner discovery. Following the first method described by Shulgin, reconnecting with the rest of the group occurred only later in the session, or perhaps the next day.

A second camp of practitioners posited that MDMA could facilitate insight during an individual guided session and improve interpersonal relationships. Claudio Naranjo (2001) explored the value of MDMA for growth within "groups of people who had ongoing relationships with one another," and for "clearing away the garbage so as to keep the relationship healthy." These practitioners explored MDMA for its expressive qualities by encouraging individuals not only to utilize the time spent under the influence of MDMA for intimate connection and expression, but also to continue to integrate those encounters to transform their relationships afterward.

After prohibition in 1985, small groups and communities continued to use MDMA in ways that community members often perceived as beneficial. In the late 1980s, MDMA helped spark the development of the rave scene in New York, which began during a tumultuous time of turf wars, crack epidemics, AIDS, and racial tensions throughout the city (Wender, 2015). The Peace, Love, Unity, and Respect (PLUR) movement was born from underground recreational use of MDMA when the rave community began to organize with the values of PLUR as the underlying tenet of its culture (Bort, 2015). The values and guiding principles laid down by psychotherapists and unconventional practitioners using psychedelics for individual growth and relationship transformation prior to the criminalization of MDMA began to take on their own deeper meaning for underground rave communities in the postscheduling era. The rise of the PLUR social movement reflects the values of MDMA as a transformational substance, albeit in an unregulated and loosely managed grassroots context.

In the decades following prohibition, media and political focus on the dangers associated with recreational MDMA use drove the public narrative. This was based on the assumption that users were inherently at risk and were using this substance for mere escapism, similar to alcohol and other street drugs. On the one hand, the dominant narrative of criminalized, recreational MDMA use painted a picture of hedonistic partygoers having wild, risky sex and dancing for hours. This was a narrative intended to cultivate fear and panic regarding illicit use in underground rave culture, without fair media representation that considered how or why MDMA provided value to communities of recreational users.

On the other hand, ethnographic research during this time demonstrated community patterns that aimed to reduce the harms individuals experienced from frequent recreational exposure to MDMA and other drugs. One study of MDMA users revealed that young people involved with the illicit sale and distribution of the drug rejected the identity of "drug dealers," largely due to their belief that MDMA should not be illegal in the first place, and that the groups of friends to whom they provided the drug benefited from taking it (Jacinto, Duterte, Sales, & Murphy, 2008). Klitzman (2006) discussed the term "suicide Tuesday," by which communities of MDMA users referred to a feeling of depletion and depression in the days following a weekend of use. Klitzman's investigation, similar to other studies of recreational users, demonstrated how communities of users have a period of initiation, in which social networks raise awareness of potential adverse effects to protect each other from the negative consequences of taking MDMA or other substances. Today, similar information sharing and community safety planning is found on the Internet, such as the online archive Erowid.

Repeated MDMA use in recreational contexts created a new set of needs for ensuring the safety of users. Because policies that criminalize substances place liability on not only users but also venue owners, promoters, and organizers of events at which illicit drugs might be used, nonprofits and grassroots community organizers have responded with harm reduction measures. Prohibition of MDMA forced its manufacture, production, and distribution into unregulated, clandestine laboratories where the illegal chain of exchange makes adulterating or substituting MDMA with other chemicals much more likely. Organizations such as Dance Safe and Bunk Police have responded by educating partygoers about these risks and providing testing kits to help people identify the substances they use. Policies that criminalize drug use also put recreational users at risk for ingesting unknown and potentially excessive doses of MDMA, with associated bad trips or intense negative effects. Organizations such as the Zendo project and Kosmicare have recognized the importance of providing support to people at venues where recreational users might congregate (e.g., music festivals) and experience these types of crises. This harm reduction work aims to support people through intense psychedelic experiences and crisis states, while avoiding more drastic medical interventions such as tranquilizers and restraints, or law enforcement measures such as arrest and incarceration.

Prohibition, however, failed to eliminate psychotherapeutic exploration of MDMA completely. Michael Pollan's 2018 book, *How to Change Your Mind,* arguably ignited the imagination and curiosity of the broader public about underground practitioner networks for exploring the transformational qualities of psychedelics in an illicit therapeutic context. Underground networks of professionals and practitioners reportedly use MDMA and other psychedelic substances with clients to treat a variety of clinical problems, including depression, anxiety, trauma, PTSD, childhood abuse, alcoholism, and opioid addiction (Pollan, 2018). Many times, as in the Swiss case of Friederike Meckel and Konrad Fischer, practitioners of underground networks are only exposed when a client experiences a grievance, which in turn alerts law enforcement agencies of the purported illicit use (Sessa & Fischer, 2015).

The portrayal of risky recreational use in the era of criminalization is now balanced by the more recent therapeutic narrative that heralds MDMA as a major advance in the treatment of severe PTSD. Presently, a resurgent perspective posits that MDMA not only aids individual healing in strictly therapeutic contexts but also can facilitate positive change in human relationships when used in a range of therapeutic and social contexts.

■ Effects

The inherent value of this or any chemical compound in mental health radiates from both the specific neurochemistry and the neurological localization of these induced effects. Single-dose administration of MDMA triggers a release of monoamines, especially serotonin and norepinephrine (Nichols, Lloyd, Hoffman, Nichols, & Yim, 1982; Piercey, Lum, & Palmer, 1990). MDMA also reduces the effectiveness of the monoamine oxidase enzymes for both serotonin and dopamine, thus enhancing their effective transmission (Steuer, Boxler, Stock, & Kraemer, 2016). This, in turn, creates a linked release of other neuroendocrine molecules, including vasopressin, prolactin, and oxytocin (Forsling et al., 2002; Thompson, Callaghan, Hunt, Cornish, & McGregor, 2007). Serotonin is known to reduce anxiety and enhance mood (Kraus, Castrén, Kasper & Lanzenberger, 2017), dopamine supports motivation and reward (Volkow, Wise, & Baler, 2017), while norepinephrine enhances cognitive arousal (España, Schmeichel, & Berridge, 2016). Oxytocin and vasopressin are linked with love, bonding, trust and prolong social memory (Stoop, Hegoburu, & van den Burg, 2015). These molecules significantly enhance the communication between the amygdala fear center and the hippocampus in humans (Carhart-Harris et al., 2015). This may indicate the enhanced processing of fear memory. MDMA also targets the hypothalamic–pituitary–adrenal (HPA) axis (Parrott et al., 2014; Wetherell & Montgomery, 2013), which is dysregulated in both trauma and chronic stress (Agorastos, Pervanidou, Chrousos, & Kolaitis, 2018). Recently, functional magnetic resonance imaging (fMRI) data have suggested the occurrence of alterations in the insula and salience network that may drive trait anxiety features (Walpola et al., 2017).

Moving from the chemistry and anatomy of these effects to the psychological relevance is challenging. Taken as a whole, the biochemical activity of MDMA typically induces a profound state of calm, clarity, and safety. MDMA can also frequently create an atmosphere of openness and trust that can promote introspection and self-examination (Grinspoon & Bakalar, 1986). It should be noted that MDMA appears to enhance the access of repressed trauma memories and as such can unleash a firestorm of painful experience. This negative reexperiencing is one of the hallmarks of work with traumatized patients in MDMA-assisted psychotherapy.

In both animal and human models, MDMA appears to enhance prosocial and empathic responses, while decreasing aggression (Kamilar-Britt & Bedi, 2015). Significantly, it also enhances fear memory extinction (Young et al., 2017). A survey of psychiatrists who had significant personal experience with MDMA in the 1970s and 1980s reported a number of common effects (seen by half or more). These included enhanced ability to be open; decreased defensiveness, fear, and aggression; and heightened awareness of emotions and less aggression (Liester, Grob, Bravo, & Walsh, 1992). Taken as a whole, these effects begin to characterize the complex effects of MDMA administration.

In summary, one can begin to construct a speculative psychological profile of this tool. It enhances the sense of connection between individuals. It makes it easier to look at one's behavior and one's self in a safe and less threatening manner. It reduces the excessive fear that is linked to past traumatic events. It enhances interpersonal bonding and the expression of deeper feelings of affection. MDMA may decrease the level of aggression triggered in communication. It also appears to improve our ability to forgive others and ourselves for imperfections and past failures. While speculative, the picture painted is quite different from any commonly used agent in psychiatry, one with a broad range of prospective applications.

▨ Potential Applications

The array of potential applications is wide-ranging but fundamentally built on a model of episodic growth and facilitation. None of these applications involves daily use to suppress and minimize distressing thinking, mood, or behavior. Rather, all of these proposed applications flow from a model based on MDMA as a catalyst to enhance inter- and intrapersonal growth. This discussion is divided into three main categories: (1) professional training and facilitation, (2) interpersonal process, and (3) individual inner process.

Professional Training and Facilitation

MDMA has the potential to catalyze the inner growth and development of practitioners. Practitioner training experiences enhanced with MDMA could facilitate therapists' ability to bond more deeply with clients, and to create a sense of safety, alignment, and trust that has been shown to constitute the foundation of psychotherapy ("the nonspecific effects") (Palpacuer et al., 2017). MDMA typically creates a profound sense of calm and acceptance that reflects the unconditional positive regard of Carl Rogers (and Fred Rogers). As an *empathogen* (i.e., drugs that produce emotional communion with others) or *entactogen* (i.e., drugs that allow one to "touch within") (Nichols, 1986), MDMA can help to increase a practitioner's self-awareness and responsiveness in the process of learning psychotherapy.

In the Phase III MDMA-assisted psychotherapy study for severe PTSD sponsored by the Multidisciplinary Association for Psychedelic Studies (MAPS), the sponsors felt strongly about the need for a personal experience of the medicine and provided a fully facilitated MDMA experience for each of the therapists involved in the study. This inner work also enhances therapists' ability to recognize and process their own personal blind spots and shadow elements. In the psychoanalytic and psychodynamic framework, personal psychotherapy is recognized as an integral facet of the training process. With the rise of interest in psychedelic-assisted models of personal growth and mental health care, MDMA-facilitated psychotherapy training has the potential to help practitioners involved in this new model of care to better assess their inner landscape and relational patterns.

Interpersonal Process

MDMA holds potential for cultivating intimacy, open communication, and interpersonal healing in human relationships. Quite simply, MDMA opens the heart. This might sound unscientific and ill-defined, but consider the process. MDMA often creates a calm, confident, and sensitive clarity that allows an individual to plumb strong emotions without the typical distortions so common to our intrapsychic world. These distortions are associated with one's attachment concerns, trauma history, and critical inner narrative. With these distortions removed, one's true affections, concerns, and connections are better available for communication to others. Freed of one's neurotic filters, one can share one's love with an honesty and directness that is often lacking in typical dialogue. With these barriers to communication and appreciation removed, interpersonal conflicts, relationship work, and marital therapy may be expedited and deepened. This is not a false euphoria that an individual regrets the next day. Rather, one is typically left with the feeling that the MDMA experience is somehow a truer, deeper revelation of one's inner self. Some amount of sadness frequently wells up in the aftermath, with remorse over why this deep interchange occurs only while under the influence.

One of us (S. S.) had the opportunity to work extensively with MDMA professionally in the early 1980s, prior to U.S. Drug Enforcement Administration (DEA) scheduling. Most of this MDMA-assisted psychotherapy centered on couple work and interpersonal growth. Participants commonly observed that the psychotherapy with this agent vastly outpaced their prior psychotherapeutic work. One Jungian-oriented physician remarked that two sessions of work with MDMA accomplished more for him than 2 years of intensive analysis (C. Harter, personal communication, April 12, 1985). Often, couples that work with MDMA feel so resourced and enhanced that the professional is mainly there to create ritual and a therapeutic container.

In a similar vein, MAPS (2018) has expanded clinical trial testing of MDMA as an adjunct to psychotherapy with marital dyads, one member of which is diagnosed with PTSD. In these trials, both partners receive MDMA in sessions together. This, of course, also echoes early use of MDMA for patients with cancer and their significant others (Grob, 1995).

Recent qualitative investigations with recreational users document how dyads in a committed relationship used MDMA independently, in the absence of a therapist (Anderson, Reavey, & Boden, 2018). These authors found that MDMA allowed partners to do a rebalancing of what they describe as affective inequality. This stems from the tendency for men to be socialized to dampen or hide emotional expressions, while women are socialized in the opposite manner. In this study, MDMA was described as creating a space between intimate partners in which they can openly share and empathically connect, feel a sense of closeness with each other, and reconfigure gender-based social norms around communication and expression of emotion.

Colbert (2018) offered a cognitive-relational model of MDMA use based on an investigation into how adult couples use MDMA recreationally in ways they perceive as beneficial to their intimate partnership. Couples reported that MDMA use added depth to their relationship and provided insights and lessons that they integrate into their everyday relationship patterns. This model of recreational MDMA use posits that adults can acquire information and make healthful choices about MDMA consumption. Couples operating within this model expect their use to result in durable changes to their intimate relationship and to other relationships in their lives. While this model of MDMA use is unlikely to receive U.S. Food and Drug Administration (FDA) approval, it reflects another real-world context that contradicts prohibition narratives of reckless or risky recreational users. As researchers continue to document such nonclinical applications of safe MDMA use, the body of evidence might serve advocates who (1) question the legal status of MDMA as medical-only use and (2) foresee decriminalization or full legalization as its future trajectory.

Individual Inner Process

Given the profile of MDMA presented earlier in this chapter, many different psychiatric disorders might respond to MDMA-facilitated psychotherapy. Bulimia, for example, is often associated with a deep sense of shame and loss of personal control that might respond to the enhanced personal acceptance and forgiveness often found in this

work. Addictions could be addressed by the enhanced insight and personal honesty intrinsic to these MDMA-assisted states. This was suggested by the findings of George Greer, who used MDMA clinically in the early 1980s. He noted that 14 of 29 patients reported a decreased desire for alcohol, cannabis or caffeine after MDMA-assisted psychotherapy (Greer & Tolbert, 1986).

The efficacy of MDMA-assisted psychotherapy in alcohol use disorders (AUDs) is currently under investigation by British psychiatrist Ben Sessa (2017a). The early history of psychedelic research was marked by a number of positive studies exploring the efficacy of LSD in the treatment of alcoholism. More recent reviews include a positive summary of this early work (Bogenschutz & Johnson, 2016; Bogenschutz & Ross, 2018), applying a similar model to MDMA-assisted psychotherapy for AUDs. Panic, agoraphobia, and chronic anxiety also may have potential for healing given the increased insight and reduced fear found with the MDMA experience.

One recent study found very significant benefit (effect size of 1.4) in the use of MDMA-assisted psychotherapy for social anxiety in a small group of adults diagnosed with autism and severe social anxiety (Danforth et al., 2018). MDMA relational therapy might represent an approach to the alleviation of domestic violence by deepening insight and interpersonal conflict resolution, while supporting more processing of personal trauma history. The chronic suicidality found in severe depression might respond well to this enhanced insight and self-acceptance, or some other yet-to-be-identified characteristic of this medicine. MDMA typically provides an inner experience that is free of the self-loathing so common to these states.

Child and Adolescent Mental Health

Many clinical presentations in child and adolescent psychiatry occur because of issues of fit between parent and child. In these cases, the power differential, cognitive discrepancy, and inherent family dynamics make direct facilitation of these issues challenging. Most family therapy sessions aim to improve communication, solve problems, and improve respect, but often struggle to shift parental awareness. A single, individual session with a parent could facilitate a shift in parental awareness. Interestingly, a nationally representative survey of adolescents found substantially increased suicide risk for those who have used MDMA (Kim, Fan, Liu, Kerner, & Wu, 2011).

Trauma, as exemplified by PTSD, adverse childhood experiences (ACEs), and chronic stress reactions, represents a massively undertreated and underappreciated foundation for chronic mental illness in modern society. Current forms of treatment (cognitive-behavioral therapy [CBT], eye movement desensitization and reprocessing [EMDR], and selective serotonin reuptake inhibitors [SSRIs]) have been found wanting in their effectiveness for those with severe or chronic illness. This prompted the FDA to award MDMA breakthrough status based on the Phase II results in August 2017.

The biggest potential boon for MDMA in child and adolescent psychiatry lies in its potential to address trauma, abuse, and neglect decades before it leads to poverty, addiction, and chronic medical and mental illness. Witness the predictive utility of the simple ACEs scale that measures potential early traumatic experiences (Anda et al., 2006). Sessa (2017b) makes a strong argument for the use of MDMA in children and adolescents to mitigate the lifelong impact of early trauma given the significant shortfalls of our current treatment options. Imagine if we could positively treat and reduce the burden of trauma early in life. Perhaps no single public health intervention (aside from preventing the actual incidence of trauma, abuse, or neglect in childhood) could cause a more dramatic reduction in the suffering in our population and the long-term cost to our society If MDMA reaches FDA approval based on the Phase III study now in process, the FDA will mandate a Phase IV study in a pediatric population. This is as least 4 years out. The potential utility of MDMA-assisted psychotherapy to address trauma in child and adolescent psychiatry is so significant that it is hard to enumerate.

Similarly, MDMA has the potential to address attachment failures that arise early in life. This work can be done with conventional psychotherapy, but it moves a glacial pace. One of us (S. S.) recently had experience working with attachment issues using MDMA-assisted psychotherapy in a Phase II subject, and found that while the response was much slower than the resolution found in PTSD, this treatment modality appears to be very helpful to address attachment issues. One can speculate that attachment issues constitute a deeper and more foundational layer in the psyche (often occurring in a pre-verbal relational failure) and benefit from a more powerful method to access and repair this relational wound.

■ Safety Issues

MDMA has a long track record given its extensive use over the last 30+ years. The number of doses taken is likely to number in the hundreds of millions. The vast majority of that use is in a recreational, festival, or underground scenes. In this illegal scenario, the use is poorly supervised, if at all. In the absence of medical/psychiatric guidance, instruction tends to spread mainly by word of mouth, informal tradition, and popular Internet forums (Hearne & Van Hout, 2016). Heavy use in festivals and raves is often complicated by excessive or repetitive dosing, alcohol, cannabis, dehydration from dancing, lack of sleep, poor nutrition, and hyperthermia from dancing and mixing other drugs such as psychedelics. Beyond this, the purity of the compound as delivered is likely suspect and inconsistent. Many of these dangers, however, are linked to MDMA's legal status more than the inherent risks of the drug itself. Nevertheless, the reported morbidity and mortality statistics take on a different perspective.

According to the Substance Abuse and Mental Health Services Administration (SAMHSA; 2013) bulletin (last updated in 2017), about 22,000 MDMA emergency department mentions were reported on yearly average over the last decade by the Drug Abuse Warning Network. This peaked in 2009, then plateaued. This pattern is concerning, but to add perspective, cannabis had over 450,000 mentions and antidepressants had over 100,000 mentions in the same year. One study estimated that about 50 deaths occurred each year from MDMA

(Rogers et al., 2009) and, by comparison, over-the-counter acetaminophen (Tylenol, etc.) causes over 450 deaths in the United States each year. This is not to minimize the safety concerns related to MDMA, but merely to put them into perspective.

One critical review of MDMA psychotherapy posits that while MDMA may have psychotherapeutic benefits, some real concerns exist (Parrott, 2014). Those concerns are relevant and should be considered. The first concern is that MDMA is not selective in the thoughts or emotions that it solicits. This observation is true and actually underlies the nature of its value in psychotherapy. At times, MDMA can bring up repressed traumas, deep psychological wounds, or dissociated sensations. This unpredictability and nonselective nature forms one key facet of its value in dealing with repressed and dissociated elements of our being.

Parrott (2014) then mentions that MDMA has powerful neurohormonal effects, including the release of cortisol. Traumatic memories are created in the context of the release of cortisol and other stress hormones. The phenomena of state-dependent memory dictates enhanced access to traumatic memories created with the influence of cortisol in this state (Berridge & Waterhouse, 2003; Morey et al., 2015). This cortisol state is not inherently dangerous in an acute setting, but takes on true toxicity when it occurs over the lifetime of someone afflicted with PTSD who is constantly flooded with cortisol. An elevated cortisol level will likely enhance therapeutic recall (Henckens, Hermans, Pu, Joels, & Fernandez, 2009). MDMA administration causes a significant release of neurochemicals and is followed by a recovery period. Parrott (2014) has concerns that this may create problems for the user on days 2, 3, and 4 postingestion. In the Phase II study with MDMA, this concern was not documented (M. Mithoefer, personal communication, June 2018).

Parrott (2014) further notes that regular use may be associated with memory problems, serotonergic neurotoxicity, and "other psychobiologic problems." The format and design of current treatment protocols eliminate most of that concern, as individuals in treatment are only administered MDMA two or three times total, with a month separation between treatment sessions. Nothing documented in the existing scientific literature on the application of MDMA in a clinical setting reinforces these wide-ranging concerns.

In the context of recreational or illicit social use, studies on neurotoxicity and harms have been critiqued for methodological shortcomings, such as the reliability and validity of neuroimaging measurement tools, retrospective designs that prohibit implying causal links, and the persistent problem of confounding polydrug use (Gouzoulis-Mayfrank & Daumann, 2006; Kish, 2002; Reneman, de Win, van den Brink, Booji, & den Heeten, 2006). For example, of 106 MDMA-related fatalities identified over a 6-year period in Australia, 41% involved the concomitant use of MDMA with another drug (Pilgrim, Gerostamoulos, & Drummer, 2011) Other reviews note how fatal adverse reactions to MDMA generally do not appear to be dose-related, with no acknowledged median lethal dose for orally administered MDMA in humans (Cole, 2014).

In a recent review of 33 animal and human molecular imaging studies, heavy users in particular showed significant effects on the serotonin receptor (5-HT) system, potentially (but not necessarily) reflecting 5-HT neurotoxicity (Vegting, Reneman, & Booij, 2016). Significant recovery of 5-HT transporter binding occurred over time (40–200 days) among abstinent users. No significant effects of MDMA use were found on the dopamine system. Recovery of 5-HT transporter binding was also found in a prospective longitudinal study of heavy users, leading the authors to posit that reduced 5-HT transporter availability might be a transient effect of heavy use (Thomasius et al., 2006).

Regular underground therapists and recreational users often employ supplements strategies with agents such as 5-hydroxy-tryptophan (5-HTP; the precursor of serotonin) that may address some of these concerns. Other studies have noted MDMA's apparent impact on cognitive deficits, particularly verbal memory, and negative mood. However, confounding factors cannot be ruled out. Psychopathology scores related to depression and impulsivity do not appear related to MDMA specifically, but rather to polydrug use generally (Schilt et al., 2010).

Negative impacts of MDMA use on mood appear to be mediated by sleep disruptions (Pirona & Morgan, 2010). After controlling for sleep quality among regular polydrug MDMA users, subacute effects on working memory and decision making were minimal in the days following MDMA use compared to a similar polydrug control group that chose to abstain (Pirona & Morgan, 2010).

The most relevant statistic on safety comes from the Phase II studies of MDMA-assisted psychotherapy for the treatment of PTSD: In hundreds of administrations of this medication in a controlled and monitored setting, there has not been a single serious adverse effect (Vizeli & Liechti, 2017). This summary article summarized the safety of MDMA by stating that "MDMA administration was overall safe in physically and psychiatrically healthy subjects and in a medical setting." Michael reported that the MAPS Phase II study had one serious adverse event that was drug related (an increase in premature ventricular contractions [PVCs]), and this is acknowledged in the study design as a risk.

MDMA is a potent agent with significant physiological and psychological effects and, as with all psychoactive drugs, comes with risks. Our best current data in a medicalized setting demonstrate a favorable benefit-to-risk ratio, with no serious adverse events. Past uses and abuses of MDMA in unsupervised nonmedical settings are not the same, as the drug's legal status creates problems with quality and purity. It is difficult to separate polydrug use and exposure to adulterants in underground markets from the inherent risks of MDMA. Some critics further argue that the overarching "ecstasy" research program of today stems from prohibition narratives of inherently risky recreational use and biases the research toward producing evidence to demonstrate MDMA is dangerous (Cole, 2014). Despite decades of research, however, evidence fails to clearly show MDMA's damaging impacts on users. While the immediate future of MDMA will be medically driven, recreational and underground use of MDMA is likely to continue. Ensuring the safety of users via harm reduction strategies, dissemination of good information, and policies appropriate to the actual degree of risk involved with MDMA are warranted.

Conclusion

MDMA synergizes and connects the two disparate wings of modern mental health care: psychotherapy and psychopharmacology. Both of these poles have some value on their own merit but are typically separated by a professional and practical divide that often places the two different professionals providing care to the typical mental health client at odds and speaking a different language. These polarities find union in the model of MDMA-assisted psychotherapy currently being studied by MAPS in the FDA Phase III trial. MDMA speeds and enhances the benefits of psychotherapy. This moves the entire mental health profession closer to a fully shared perspective.

Within the therapeutic context, MDMA might also represent a movement from an external expert, found in the psychotherapist/psychiatrist, to the inner expert. The work with MDMA in the MAPS study recognizes the presence of an inner healer and terms the process *inner-directed therapy*. This model challenges the long-standing bias that professionals, even with little knowledge of the client's experience and inner world, know more than the client in his or her lived experience. With MDMA we move to a collaborative model in which the dyad of client and professional work together as partners. Ostensibly, this assumption already underlies many psychodynamic psychotherapies, but it represents a major shift in the practice of psychiatry at large.

Even more broadly, MDMA typically provides individuals with a sense of calm, confident clarity that is often quite novel but extremely helpful to explore the deeper realms of the psyche and relationships. This medicine appears to reduce the negative self-talk, insecurity, and fear that limit true introspection. Sometimes MDMA brings up trauma and negative elements found in the psyche, but this emotional pain may be in the service of healing. The experience is not always easy or predictable. However, the evidence supports it functioning as a catalyst for trauma resolution.

Many communities and subcultures have built on these qualities and utilize MDMA to facilitate their own inner growth and healing without professionals in attendance.

This self-healing process partially grew out of a recreational culture found in raves and all-night dance celebrations based on values of the PLUR movement. MDMA has also lent itself to a more reflective process, individually and in interpersonal relationships, that honors the therapeutic, healing, and sacred qualities inherent in this medicine.

The development of a separate subculture that honors inner growth and wisdom facilitated by a medicine is not limited to MDMA, but it does form a classic example of this evolving and rapidly growing element in our society. Books such as Michael Pollan's (2018) *How to Change Your Mind* reflect this hunger for deeper and more sacred experiences. This pattern in our society challenges the need for professional curation of this process and perhaps eliminates the superfluous roles ossified in the practitioner–client polarity. Psychedelic psychotherapy brings a new model, exemplified by the role of the sitter, that provides a nondirective container for the inner explorations brought on by the psychoactive agent.

Safety concerns related to MDMA recreational use with chronic or excessive administration do exist. MDMA is a potent agent with significant physiological and psychological effects, and its use should be based on access to good information and the appropriate management of risks. This is arguably one of the values of the practitioner role in MDMA-assisted therapy that can be absent with recreational use. Despite the legal status of MDMA compounding inherent drug risks with problems of quality, purity, and access to useful supports, recreational use is unlikely to go away and should be part of the larger conversation about power and access to healing medicines.

MDMA and other agents (psychedelics, ketamine, etc.) allow us to mine more fully the depths of the psyche. The broader implications of this for how we use medicines both therapeutically and socially are profound. The rising gravitas and popularity of this work reflect a fundamental shift in our society and the mental health profession. The mental health field is a prime example of a culturally driven system that evolves over time and place. As Thomas Kuhn pointed out in *The Structure of Scientific Revolutions* (1962), science is more culturally and socially driven than we wish to consider, and nowhere is that more relevant than in mental health.

Our mental health system is in crisis. Seventy-seven percent of the counties in the United States express a mental health crisis with unmet behavioral health needs, and 55% report having no mental care providers available (Levin, 2017; SAMHSA, 2014). According to the National Institute of Mental Health (2020), the suicide rate has risen 35% over the last 20 years in spite of broad attempts to reduce it. The vast majority of children with a serious mental health issue never find treatment (Merikangas et al., 2011). Psychotherapy is in the decline in terms of *per capita* use, and our psychiatric medications have come under more severe scrutiny for issues related both to efficacy and safety (Whitaker, 2010). In the United States, we have fully medicalized mental illness and its treatment. Clearly, these statistics and others indicate that our current model is failing us.

MDMA is a simple chemical compound, yet it may present us with a new paradigm and eventually usher in a new system of mental health care. It could help to move us away from a system in which we have medicalized the suppression of the psyche (and in ways, the greater community also). The model of MDMA-assisted psychotherapy and growth may transform our entire mental health system. This new model values both chemistry and relationship in the support of enhanced growth and well-being. It is both ironic and only fitting that our journey toward a more evocative and spiritually grounded perspective may be launched by a pharmaceutical compound.

■ **References**

Adamson, S., & Metzner, R. (1988). The nature of the MDMA experience and its role in healing, psychotherapy and spiritual practice. *ReVision, 10*(4), 59–72.

Agorastos, A., Pervanidou, P., Chrousos, G. P., & Kolaitis, G. (2018). Early life stress and trauma: Developmental neuroendocrine aspects of prolonged stress system dysregulation. *Hormones (Athens), 17,* 507–520.

Anda, R. F., Felitti, V. J., Bremner, J. D., Walker, J. D., Whitfield, C., Perry, B. D., et al. (2006).

The enduring effects of abuse and related adverse experiences in childhood: A convergence of evidence from neurobiology and epidemiology. *European Archives of Psychiatry and Clinical Neuroscience, 256*(3), 174–186.

Anderson, K., Reavey, P., & Boden, Z. (2018). An affective (re)balancing act?: The liminal possibilities for heterosexual partners on MDMA. In T. Juvonen & M. Kolehmainen (Ed.), *Affective inequalities in intimate relationships*. London: Routledge.

Berridge, C. W., & Waterhouse, B. D. (2003). The locus coeruleus–noradrenergic system: Modulation of behavioral state and state-dependent cognitive processes. *Brain Research Reviews, 42*(1), 33–84.

Bogenschutz, M. P., & Johnson, M. W. (2016). Classic hallucinogens in the treatment of addictions. *Progress in Neuro-Psychopharmacology and Biological Psychiatry, 64,* 250–258.

Bogenschutz, M. P., & Ross, S. (2018). Therapeutic applications of classic hallucinogens. *Current Top Behavioral Neuroscience, 36,* 361–391.

Bort, C. (2015). PLUR isn't just a moment, it's a lifestyle: Peace, love, unity, and respect. Retrieved from *www.theodysseyonline.com/plur-lifestyle*.

Carhart-Harris, R. L., Murphy, K., Leech, R., Erritzoe, D., Wall, M. B., Ferguson, B., et al. (2015). The effects of acutely administered 3,4-methylenedioxymethamphetamine on spontaneous brain function in healthy volunteers measured with arterial spin labeling and blood oxygen level-dependent resting state functional connectivity. *Biological Psychiatry, 78*(8), 554–562.

Colbert, R. (2018). *Evenings with Molly: A grounded theory discovery with adult couples who use MDMA recreationally.* Doctoral dissertation, California Institute of Integral Studies, San Francisco, CA.

Cole, J. (2014). MDMA and the "ecstasy paradigm." *Journal of Psychoactive Drugs, 46*(1), 44–56.

Danforth, A. L., Grob, C. S., Struble, C., Feduccia, A. A., Walker, N., Jerome, L., et al. (2018). Reduction in social anxiety after MDMA-assisted psychotherapy with autistic adults: A randomized, double-blind, placebo-controlled pilot study. *Psychopharmacology (Berlin), 235*(11), 3137–3148.

Downing, J. (1985). Testimony of Joseph J. Downing, M.D.: In the matter of MDMA Scheduling Docket No 84-48. Retrieved from *https://maps.org/research-archive/dea-mdma/pdf/0045.PDF*.

España, R. A., Schmeichel, B. E., & Berridge, C. W. (2016). Norepinephrine at the nexus of arousal, motivation and relapse. *Brain Research, 164*(Pt. B), 207–216.

Forsling, M. L., Fallon, J. K., Shah, D., Tilbrook, G. S., Cowan, D. A., Kicman, A. T., et al. (2002). The effect of 3,4-methylenedioxymethamphetamine (MDMA, "ecstasy") and its metabolites on neurohypophysial hormone release from the isolated rate hypothalamus. *British Journal of Pharmacology, 135*(3), 649–656.

Gouzoulis-Mayfrank, E., & Daumann, J. (2006). The counfounding problem of polydrug use in recreational ecstasy/MDMA users: A brief overview. *Journal of Psychopharmacology, 20*(2), 188–193.

Greer, G., & Tolbert, R. (1986). Subjective reports of the effects of MDMA in a clinical setting. *Journal of Psychoactive Drugs, 18*(4), 319–327.

Grinspoon, L., & Bakalar, J. B. (1986). Can drugs be used to enhance the psychotherapeutic process? *American Journal of Psychotherapy, 40*(3), 393–404.

Grob, C. (1995). A dose/response human pilot study: Safety and efficacy of 3,4-methylenedioxymethamphetamine (MDMA) in modification of physical pain and psychological distress in end-stage cancer patients. Retrieved from *https://maps.org/mdma-cancer/5523*.

Grob, C., Bravo, G., & Walsh, R. (1990). Second thoughts on 3,4-methylenedioxymethamphetamine (MDMA) neurotoxicity. *Archives of General Psychiatry, 47*(3), 288–289.

Hearne, E., & Van Hout, M. C. (2016). "Trip-Sitting" in the black hole: A netnographic study of dissociation and indigenous harm reduction. *Journal of Psychoactive Drugs, 48*(4), 233–242.

Henckens, M. J., Hermans, E. J., Pu, Z., Joels, M., & Fernandez, G. (2009). Stressed memories: How acute stress affects memory formation in humans. *Journal of Neuroscience, 29*(32), 10111–10119.

Ingrasci, R. (1985). Testimony for MDMA hearing submitted by Richard Ingrasci, MD, MPH: In the matter of MDMA scheduling. Retrieved from *https://maps.org/research-archive/dea-mdma/pdf/0011.PDF*.

Jacinto, C., Duterte, M., Sales, P., & Murphy, S. (2008). "I'm not a real dealer": The identity process of ecstasy sellers. *Journal of Drug Issues, 38*(2), 419–444.

Kamilar-Britt, P., & Bedi, G. (2015). The prosocial effects of 3,4-methylenedioxymethamphetamine (MDMA): Controlled studies in humans and laboratory animals. *Neuroscience Biobehavioral Review, 57,* 433–446.

Kim, J., Fan, B., Liu, X., Kerner, N., & Wu,

P. (2011). Ecstasy use and suicidal behavior among adolescents: Findings from a national survey. *Suicide and Life Threatening Behavior, 41*(4), 435–444.

Kish, S. (2002). How strong is the evidence that brain serotonin neurons are damaged in human users of ecstasy? *Pharmacology Biochemistry and Behavior, 71*(4), 845–855.

Klitzman, R. (2006). From "male bonding rituals" to "suicide Tuesday": A qualitative study of issues faced by gay male ecstasy (MDMA) users. *Journal of Homosexuality, 51*(3), 7–32.

Kraus, C., Castrén, E., Kasper, S., & Lanzenberger, R. (2017). Serotonin and neuroplasticity—Links between molecular, functional and structural pathophysiology in depression. *Neuroscience and Biobehavioral Reviews, 77,* 317–326.

Kuhn, T. (1962). *The structure of scientific revolutions.* Chicago: University of Chicago Press.

Levin, A. (2017). Report details national shortage of psychiatrists and possible solutions. *Psychiatric News.* {Epub ahead of print]

Liester, M. B., Grob, C. S., Bravo, G. L., & Walsh, R. N. (1992). Phenomenology and sequelae of 3,4-methylenedioxymethamphetamine use. *Journal of Nervous and Mental Disease, 180*(6), 345–352.

Merikangas, K., He, J., Burstein, M., Swendsen, J., Avenevoli, S., Case, B., et al. (2011). Service utilization for lifetime mental disorders in U.S. adolescents: Results of the National Comorbidity Survey–Adolescent Supplement (NCS-A). *Journal of the American Academy of Child and Adolescent Psychiatry, 50*(1), 32–45.

Morey, R. A., Dunsmoor, J. E., Haswell, C. C., Brown, V. M., Vora, A., Weiner, J., et al. (2015). Fear learning circuitry is biased toward generalization of fear associations in posttraumatic stress disorder. *Translational Psychiatry, 5,* e700.

Multidisciplinary Association for Psychedelic Studies. (2018). MDMA-assisted psychotherapy for PTSD (cognitive-behavioral conjoint therapy). Retrieved from *https://maps.org/research/mdma/ptsd/conjoint-therapy.*

Naranjo, C. (2001). Experience with the interpersonal psychedelics. In J. Holland (Ed.), *Ecstasy: The complete guide.* Rochester, VT: Park Street Press.

National Institute of Mental Health. (2020). Suicide. Retrieved from *www.nimh.nih.gov/health/statistics/suicide.shtml.*

Nichols, D. E. (1986). Differences between the mechanism of action of MDMA, MBDB, and the classic hallucinogens: Identification of a new therapeutic class: Entactogens. *Journal of Psychoactive Drugs, 18*(4), 305–313.

Nichols, D. E., Lloyd, D. H., Hoffman, A. J., Nichols, M. B., & Yim, G. K. (1982). Effects of certain hallucinogenic amphetamine analogues on the release of [3H]serotonin from rat brain synaptosomes. *Journal of Medicinal Chemistry, 25*(5), 530–535.

Palpacuer, C., Gallet, L., Drapier, D., Reymann, J. M., Falissard, B., & Naudet, F. (2017). Specific and non-specific effects of psychotherapeutic interventions for depression: Results from a meta-analysis of 84 studies. *Journal of Psychiatric Research, 87,* 95–104.

Parrott, A. C. (2014). The potential dangers of using MDMA for psychotherapy. *Journal of Psychoactive Drugs, 46*(1), 37–43.

Parrott, A. C., Montgomery, C., Wetherell, M., Downey, L., Stough, C., & Scholey, A. (2014). MDMA, cortisol, and heightened stress in recreational ecstasy users. *Behavioral Pharmacology, 25*(5–6), 458–472.

Piercey, M. F., Lum, J. T., & Palmer, J. R. (1990). Effects of MDMA ("ecstasy") on firing rates of serotonergic, dopaminergic, and noradrenergic neurons in the rat. *Brain Research, 526*(2), 203–206.

Pilgrim, J., Gerostamoulos, D., & Drummer, O. (2011). Deaths involving MDMA and the concomitant use of pharmaceutical drugs. *Journal of Analytical Toxicology, 35*(4), 219–226.

Pirona, A., & Morgan, M. (2010). An investigation of the subacute effects of ecstasy on neuropsychological performance, sleep, and mood in regular ecstasy users. *Journal of Psychopharmacology, 24*(2), 175–185.

Pollan, M. (2018). *How to change your mind: What the new science of psychedelics teaches us about consciousness, dying, addiction, depression, and transcendence.* New York: Penguin Press.

Reneman, L., de Win, M., van den Brink, W., Booij, J., & den Heeten, G. (2006). Neuroimaging findings with MDMA/ecstasy: Technical aspects, conceptual issues and future prospects. *Journal of Psychopharmacology, 20*(2), 164–175.

Rogers, G., Elston, J., Garside, R., Roome, C., Taylor, R., Younger, P., et al. (2009). The harmful health effects of recreational ecstasy: A systematic review of observational evidence. *Health Technology Assessment, 13*(6), iii–iv, ix–xii, 1–315.

Schilt, T., Koeter, M., Smal, H., Gouwetor, M., van den Brink, W., & Schmand, B. (2010). Long-term neuropsychological effects of ecstasy in middle-aged ecstasy/polydrug users. *Psychopharmacology, 207,* 583–591.

Sessa, B. (2017a). Why MDMA therapy for alcohol use disorder?: And why now? *Neuropharmacology, 142,* 83–88.

Sessa, B. (2017b). Why psychiatry needs 3,4-methylenedioxymethamphetamine: A child psychiatrist's perspective. *Neurotherapeutics, 14*(3), 741–749.

Sessa, B., & Fischer, F. M. (2015). Underground MDMA-, LSD- and 2-CB-assisted individual and group psychotherapy in Zurich: Outcomes, implications and commentary. *Drug Science, Policy and Law, 2*, 1–8.

Shulgin, A. (1980). MDMA: General information. Retrieved from *https://erowid.org/chemicals/mdma/mdma_info12.shtml*.

Shulgin, A. T., & Nichols, D. E. (1978). Characterization of three new psychotomimetics: The pharmacology of hallucinogens. In R. C. Stillman & R. E. Willette (Eds.), *The psychopharmacology of hallucinogens*. New York: Pergamon Press.

Steuer, A. E., Boxler, M. I., Stock, L., & Kraemer, T. (2016). Inhibition potential of 3,4-methylenedioxymethamphetamine (MDMA) and its metabolites on the in vitro monoamine oxidase (MAO)-catalyzed deamination of the neurotransmitters serotonin and dopamine. *Toxicology Letters, 243*, 48–55.

Stolaroff, M. J. (2004). *The secret chief revealed: Conversations with a pioneer of the underground psychedelic therapy movement*. Sarasota, FL: Multidisciplinary Association for Psychedelic Studies.

Stoop, R., Hegoburu, C., & van den Burg, E. (2015). New opportunities in vasopressin and oxytocin research: A perspective from the amygdala. *Annual Review of Neuroscience, 38*, 369–388.

Substance Abuse and Mental Health Services Administration. (2013). *Drug abuse warning network, 2011: National estimates of drug-related emergency department visits*. Rockville, MD: Author.

Substance Abuse and Mental Health Services Administration. (2014). Building the behavioral health workforce. Retrieved from *www.samhsa.gov/samhsanewsletter/volume_22_number_4/building_the_behavioral_health_workforce*.

Thomasius, R., Zapletalova, P., Peterson, K., Buchert, R., Andresen, B., Wartberg, L., et al. (2006). Mood, cognition, and serotonin transporter availability in current and former ecstasy (MDMA) users: The longitudinal perspective. *Journal of Psychopharmacology, 20*(2), 211–225.

Thompson, M. R., Callaghan, P. D., Hunt, G. E., Cornish, J. L., & McGregor, I. S. (2007). A role for oxytocin and 5-HT(1A) receptors in the prosocial effects of 3,4 methylenedioxymethamphetamine ("ecstasy"). *Neuroscience, 146*(2), 509–514.

Vegting, Y., Reneman, L., & Booij, J. (2016). The effects of ecstasy on neurotransmitter systems: A review on the findings of molecular imaging studies. *Psychopharmacology, 233*, 3473–3501.

Vizeli, P., & Liechti, M. (2017). Safety pharmacology of acute MDMA administration in healthy adults. *Journal of Psychopharmacology, 31*(5), 576–588.

Volkow, N. D., Wise, R. A., & Baler, R. (2017). The dopamine motive system: Implications for drug and food addiction. *Nature Reviews Neuroscience, 18*(12), 741–752.

Walpola, I. C., Nest, T., Roseman, L., Erritzoe, D., Feilding, A., Nutt, D. J., et al. (2017). Altered insula connectivity under MDMA. *Neuropsychopharmacology, 42*(11), 2152–2162.

Wender, D. (2015). How Frankie Bones' Storm Rave birthed the PLUR movement. Retrieved from *https://thump.vice.com/en_us/article/pg8d4g/how-frankie-bones-storm-rave-birthed-the-plur-movement*.

Wetherell, M., & Montgomery, C. (2013). Basal functioning of the hypothalamic–pituitary–adrenal (HPA) axis and psychological distress in recreational ecstasy polydrug users. *Psychopharmacology, 231*(7), 1365–1375.

Whitaker, R. (2010). *Anatomy of an epidemic: Magic bullets, psychiatric drugs, and the astonishing rise of mental illness in America*. New York: Crown.

Young, M. B., Norrholm, S. D., Khoury, L. M., Jovanovic, T., Rauch, S. A. M., Reiff, C. M., et al. (2017). Inhibition of serotonin transporters disrupts the enhancement of fear memory extinction by 3,4-methylenedioxymethamphetamine (MDMA). *Psychopharmacology (Berlin), 234*(19), 2883–2895.

CHAPTER 14

Biological and Psychological Mechanisms Underlying the Therapeutic Use of Ayahuasca

DRÁULIO BARROS DE ARAÚJO, LUÍS FERNANDO TÓFOLI,
STEVENS REHEN, and SIDARTA RIBEIRO

▓ A Brief History of Ayahuasca

The Quechua word *ayahuasca* stems from the composition of *aya* (spirit/ancestor/dead person) and *waska* (vine/rope), to mean "the vine of the spirits."[1] Ayahuasca is a psychedelic brew with various formulations that always include the vine *Banisteriopsis caapi*, a liana with a thick stem that typically twines up to the treetops on the river banks of the Amazon basin and Andean valleys (Wallace & Spruce, 1908). There are several indigenous names for *Banisteriopsis caapi* including *yajé, yagé, natema, nepe,* and *kaji* (Luna, 2011). In Brazil, *Banisteriopsis caapi* is known as *mariri* or *jagube* (Dos Santos et al., 2016). In the Tupi Amerindian linguistic family, *Banisteriopsis caapi* is called *caapi,* and among the Tucanos it is called *cadána-píra,* both meaning "thin leaf." On the Andes it is known as *ayahuasca* (Wallace & Spruce, 1908).

Ayahuasca was first brought to scientific attention in the mid-19th century by Western ethnographers dedicated to the exploration of the New World (Metzner, 2005). Despite the growing mythology surrounding ayahuasca, to date there is no solid archeological evidence to support its ancient use by Amerindian populations, neither in the form of specific iconography nor of preserved plant specimens (Naranjo, 1979). The single piece of evidence available comes from a gas chromatography/mass spectrometry study of hair samples of Andean mummies, which

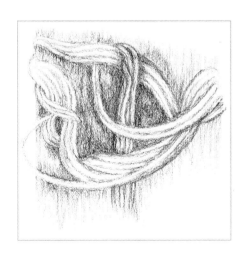

Banistereopsis caapi

contain harmine—an alkaloid contained in ayahuasca—dated between 500 and 1,000 C.E. (Ogalde et al., 2009).

The earliest reports on the use of ayahuasca by Amerindian populations were produced in the 18th century by Jesuit missionaries traveling along the Napo River that traverses Ecuador, Peru, and Brazil. The first detailed account of ayahuasca use was only published a century later by Ecuadorian geographer Manuel Villavicencio (1958), who drank the brew among the Zaparos and described a typical ayahuasca inebriation. During the same period, the English botanist Richard Spruce was gathering plant specimens for taxonomic identification during his expedition to the Amazon and the Andes (1849–1864). Spruce also recorded a detailed description of their use by various Amerindian groups. One of these plants was *B. caapi*, described by Spruce as follows:

> "I regret being unable to tell what is the peculiar narcotic principle that produces such extraordinary effects. Opium and hemp are its most obvious analogs, but *caapi* would seem to operate on the nervous system far more rapidly and violently than either. Some traveler who may follow my steps, with greater resources at his command, will, it is to be hoped, be able to bring away materials adequate for the complete analysis of this curious plant." (Wallace & Spruce, 1908)

Eventually it became clear that most ayahuasca preparations include plants other than *B. caapi* to enhance its psychoactive properties (Pinkley, 1969). The plants most

commonly used are *Psychotria viridis* (chacruna) and *Diplopterys cabrerana* (chaliponga) (Rivier & Lindgren, 1972). The preparation of ayahuasca involves the stems of *Banisteriopsis caapi* and leaves of *Psychotria spp.*, which are cooked in water for hours—most typically days.

There are records of ayahuasca use among dozens of Amerindian ethnic groups within Brazil, Peru, Colombia, Ecuador, Venezuela, Bolivia, Paraguai, Panamá and Argentina, including the Airo-Pai, Ashaninka, Achuar, Avá Guaraní, Baniuas, Barasanas, Boras, Campas, Camsás, Canamaris, Catuquinas, Cubeos, Chama, Caxinauás, Culinas, Culinas-Madirrás, Culinas-Pano, Cofán, Colorado, Coreguage, Cayapas, Callawaya, Desana, Emberá, Guahibo, Huaorani, Hupdás, Huni Kuin, Ingano, Kamsá, Macus, Matises, Matsés, Machigenguas, Muísca, Macuna, Marubos, Noanama, Piaroa, Piros Yines, Salibas, Sharanahua, Siona, Secoya, Shipibo-Conibo, Ticuna, Tucanos, Tuyukas Tucanos, Tarianas, Uitotos, Yagua, Yekuana, Yaminawá, Yawanawá, and Zaparos Napurunas (Bolsanello, 1995; Labate & Jungaberle, 2011; Steward, 1963; Taussig, 1987).

Between the 19th and 20th centuries, the arrival of rubber tappers to the Amazon region—mostly migrants from the Northeast of Brazil—greatly increased the contact between Amerindian ayahuasca users and Portuguese-speaking Brazilians of Christians. This social exchange expanded the traditional use of ayahuasca by indigenous groups into a sacrament of different syncretic religions, such as the *Santo Daime* founded in 1930, the *Barquinha* from 1945, and the *União do Vegetal* (UDV), from 1961 (Labate & MacRae, 2016). Over the years these religions spread throughout Brazil, South America, and beyond. In 1987, after years of political pressure from these religions (most notably the UDV), the Brazilian government provisionally removed ayahuasca from the list of prohibited substances. In 2006, this decision was made permanent by the Brazilian National Council on Drug Policies, and in 2010, the use of ayahuasca was regulated for religious purposes. In 2008, ayahuasca was declared part of the cultural heritage of Peru. In 2006, the U.S. Supreme Court allowed the ritual use of ayahuasca by a UDV

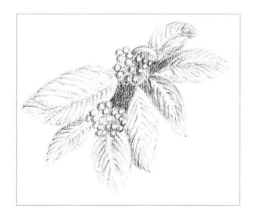

Psychotria viridis

center in the state of New Mexico. a ruling that extended to other groups on the basis of the legal religious use of peyote by the Native American Church. Ayahuasca use is increasing worldwide, in great part due to the expansion of ayahuasca religions (Labate & Jungaberle, 2011).

Pharmacology of Ayahuasca

The color of ayahuasca is brownish-green, and its taste can be sweet, sour, or bitter depending on the specific preparation and conditions of storage. Ayahuasca is a very complex brew with no exact composition and a plethora of traditional uses (Labate et al., 2014). The most typical ayahuasca preparation comprises *P. viridis* and *B. caapi*, which provide, respectively, *N,N*-dimethyltryptamine (*N,N*-DMT) and β-carboline alkaloids such as harmine and tetrahydroharmine (THH), with harmaline in lower concentrations (Callaway et al., 1999; McKenna et al., 1984; Rivier & Lindgren, 1972). In isolation, each and every one of these substances has psychoactive properties, but their complex combination in a single brew leads to very powerful effects, with unique pharmacodynamics (McKenna et al., 1998; Riba et al., 2003). It is likely that their unique combinations in different preparations correspond to clinically relevant synergistic actions akin to the concept of *entourage effect,* coined to refer to the cooperative effects of the multiple compounds present in cannabis, which may potentiate clinical efficacy while attenuating side effects (Ben-Shabat et al., 1998).

N,N-DMT is a tryptamine isolated for the first time from the *Mimosa tenuiflora* tree, by the Brazilian chemist Oswaldo de Lima (1946). *N,N*-DMT occurs naturally

Harmine

in different plants, and in animals such as rats and humans (Barker et al., 2013). It has a high affinity for serotonin (5-HT) receptors but also acts on glutamate, dopamine, acetylcholine, trace amine-associated receptor (TAAR), and ε-1 receptors (Carbonaro & Gatch, 2016). *N,N*-DMT is considered a classic psychedelic. Its psychoactive effects are transitory and begin almost immediately after intravenous (IV) administration or after being smoked. Its peak effects occur within the first minutes and lasts for about 30 minutes (Strassman et al., 1994; Szára, 2007). *N,N*-DMT is orally inactive, however, even at massive doses of 100 mg/kg (~1,000 mg). The presence of monoamine oxidase (MAO) enzymes in the gut degrades *N,N*-DMT before it gets to the circulatory system. However, the β-carboline alkaloids present is ayahuasca, particularly harmine and harmaline, are all powerful reversible inhibitors of monoamine oxidase-A (MAOIs), and therefore protect *N,N*-DMT from deamination, allowing its effects on the central nervous systems (Callaway et al., 1999; McKenna et al., 1984).

Besides protecting *N,N*-DMT, these β-carboline alkaloids have their own psychoactive effects. The effects of harmine peaks after 2 hours and subsides after 4–8 hours. At low dose, drowsiness is observed, with intermittent drowsiness and sleep at higher doses, with the first phase of excitation giving place to body numbness at later stages (Pennes & Hoch, 1957; Sanchez-Ramos, 1991).

Short-Term Effects of Ayahuasca on Human Subjects

The effects of ayahuasca begin to be felt between 20 and 40 minutes after ingestion, peak between 1 and 2 hours, and subside

Harmaline

gradually for 4 hours. During this period, most individuals remain quiet and immobile, are able to communicate coherently, remain aware of the environment and of what they are doing, and that they are under the influence of ayahuasca. At early stages, the effects include the perception of changes in body temperature, numbness, body lightness, and yawning. Nausea and vomiting are frequently seen, and diarrhea less often.

Blood pressure, body temperature, and heart and respiratory rates are mildly affected by ayahuasca (Callaway et al., 1999; Dos Santos et al., 2011, 2012; Riba et al., 2003). Systolic and diastolic blood pressures increase slightly, from typical 120/80 mmHg to 130/90 mmHg (Callaway et al., 1999; Dos Santos et al., 2011). Transient tremor and nystagmus are also observed (Callaway et al., 1999), together with increased pupil diameter (Callaway et al., 1999; Dos Santos et al., 2011).

Visual phenomena also occur quite frequently and happen mainly with the eyes closed (de Araujo et al., 2012; Callaway et al., 1999; Palhano-Fontes et al., 2019; Riba et al., 2003; Shanon, 2002). Some traditions give a special name to such a visual change and call it miração.[2] During a miração, imagery can be vivid as reality, yet completely fantastic, with the presence of deep, colorful, and bright entities that incorporate and often mix people, animals, plants, and all kinds of objects to convey messages deemed to be of major importance by ayahuasca drinkers. The visions often comprise reports of encounters with ancestors, spirits, and deities able to guide and heal when the substance, set, and setting are properly combined. Typically, contact with these entities is full of symbolism and deeply meaningful. In fact, the whole experience of miração is often compared to very vivid dreaming (Kraehenmann, 2017) or lucid dreaming (Sanz & Tagliazucchi, 2018).

A wide range of other subjective effects is frequently described, such as increased introspection (the ability to observe one's own thoughts and emotions), transient anxiety, transient dissociation and depersonalization, and distortions in the sense of time and space (de Araujo et al., 2012; Palhano-Fontes et al., 2019; Riba et al., 2003; Shanon, 2002). Mystical experiences are fre-

quently observed, even in laboratory settings (Griffiths et al., 2006; MacLean et al., 2011; Palhano-Fontes et al., 2019). The psychological properties that characterize this experience include ineffability, transcendence of time and space, positive mood, internal unity, external unity, noetic quality, and sacredness (Barrett et al., 2015; MacLean et al., 2012; Pahnke, 1963, 1969). The Mystical Experience Questionnaire (MEQ) has been adapted and validated to Brazilian Portuguese (Schenberg et al., 2017).

At the psychological level, the effects of ayahuasca have been explored with neuropsychological evaluation. One study compared the performance of occasional and experienced users under a single dose of ayahuasca in three neuropsychological assessments: the Stroop task, the Sternberg task, and the Tower of London (Bouso et al., 2013). With respect to baseline, the number of errors increased in both groups in the Sternberg task and decreased in reaction time and maintenance of accuracy in the Stroop task. In the Tower of London there was a significant increase in execution times, resolution, and number of movements performed by inexperienced volunteers, but not inexperienced volunteers. In addition, an inverse correlation was observed between the worsening of performance in the Tower of London and time of use of ayahuasca; that is, the more experienced, the lower the degradation of the response (Bouso et al., 2013).

Ayahuasca is often used as a tool for self-knowledge. During its peculiar state, individuals seem able to detach themselves from more defensive patterns of behavior. This operation may not be as easy and blissful as described here. Though sometimes insights just come in a very gentle fashion, ayahuasca drinkers frequently report that they may also undergo a lot of mental distress before they are able to detect what may have caused their distress and find ways of dealing with it. Just as a dream analysis brings insight to the dreamer, ayahuasca visions offer a rich material for psychotherapy, even when their interpretation is not obvious (Diament et al., in press).

For moments, ayahuasca leads to a state where advice is offered to the individual, often coming as a thought, sometimes a vivid thought, or less commonly as a voice that is heard. Although it seems to be a psychotic experience, the individual is aware that whatever his or her state, it is due to the brew, and that he or she is going to come back. These experiences are so common that the ayahuasca traditions have incorporated them, and have specific ways to symbolize them. It is often believed that the ayahuasca experience is being under the control not of oneself, but of the spirit of the plant, and it is the spirit of the plant that is counseling one (Diament et al., in press).

The purgative effects of the brew are considered a fundamental aspect of the experience for many groups. A ritual with more purging may represent a stronger experience of cleansing one's own feelings and thoughts (Diament et al., in press). After vomiting, ayahuasca drinkers usually feel better and commonly are aware of what their suffering and purging is related to. Such realization commonly arrives as a certainty or strong personal truth, something different from the conclusions that come from rational thinking, much like a *catharsis*, a term that is used in psychoanalysis and literally means "purification." Insights about the changing of the drinker's behavior and the actual behavioral change are not uncommon after these purging events (Diament et al., in press). These challenging experiences may also occur without physical purging (e.g., vomiting, diarrhea) and be similar to the classic psychedelic "bad trip" (Barrett et al., 2017).

■ Neurological Basis of the Short-Term Effects on Human Subjects

The search for the neural basis of the trance induced by ayahuasca took off with laboratory-based electroencephalographic (EEG) recordings performed before and after the ingestion of ayahuasca (Barbanoj et al., 2006; Riba et al., 2002, 2004). In a pioneering placebo-controlled study, Dr. Jordi Riba and collaborators showed that the ingestion of lyophilized ayahuasca administered in pills leads to a significant decrease in absolute EEG power across all frequency bands for a DMT dose of 0.85 mg/kg^{-1}, but not at lower doses (0.6 mg/kg^{-1}) (Riba et al., 2002). The effects of ayahuasca on the nervous system must not be attributed exclusively to the presence of DMT but to the full-fledged entourage effect of all ayahuasca psychoactive ingredients. In fact, it has been reported that the EEG power in the α band (8–13 Hz) decreases 50 minutes after ingestion, while increase the γ band (40–100 Hz) 75–125 minutes after ingestion (Schenberg et al., 2015).

Ayahuasca also leads to changes in cerebral blood flow (CBF) at specific parts of the brain. Using single-photon emission computed tomography (SPECT) during the acute effects of ayahuasca, Riba and colleagues (2006) found significantly increased CBF in the anterior insula, the right anterior cingulate cortex (ACC)/medial prefrontal cortex (mPFC), and the left amygdala/parahippocampal gyrus. All these brain areas have been implicated somehow with the attention, emotion, and interoception.

We explored the influence of ayahuasca on the human visual system using functional magnetic resonance imaging (fMRI; de Araujo et al., 2012). We compared the activity of different brain areas when experienced ayahuasca users (members of the Santo Daime) were asked to imagine different scenes with their eyes closed, while under the influence of ayahuasca. These periods were compared to periods when participants were asked to look at visual scenes (pictures). We observed that great parts of the visual system were just as active during perceiving as they were during imagining. This effect was found in parts of the primary Brodmann area [BA] 17 and higher visual cortices (BAs 18 and 19), besides other areas involved in memory, metacognition (Fleming & Dolan, 2012) and lucid dreaming (Dresler et al., 2012), such as the fusiform gyrus (BA 37), parahippocampal gyrus (BA 30), and frontopolar cortex (BA 10) (de Araujo et al., 2012).

A remarkable increase in introspection is at the core of the ayahuasca experience. Consistent with this idea, we found that ayahuasca leads to a significant decrease in the activity of the default mode network (DMN), a set of brain regions consistently implicated in self-oriented mental activity and to the stream of thoughts. For instance, increased DMN activity has been found to be related to rumination, a pattern of recurrent negative thoughts typically seen in depression (Rood et al., 2009; Sheline et al., 2009). On the opposite end of the spectrum, we found reduced activity of the DMN, which is compatible with what has been observed in studies with meditation (Hasenkamp et al., 2012), psilocybin (Carhart-Harris et al., 2012) and lysergic acid diethylamide (LSD) (Carhart-Harris et al., 2016). These findings are consistent with the notion that the experience with ayahuasca requires elevated mental effort and concentration, increasing the ability to observe one's own thoughts and emotion.

We also explored the way that ayahuasca influences how different parts of the brain are connected to each other. Using resting-state fMRI and complex network techniques, we observed increased entropy of node degree distribution during the acute effects of ayahuasca and found a local increased, but global decreased, network integration (Viol et al., 2017). One possible interpretation of these findings might reflect a variation in the modular structure of the network, characterized by the existence of reasonably well-defined subnetworks in which internal connections are denser than connections between distinct subnetworks (Viol et al., 2017). This is consistent with the hypothesis that the mental state induced by ayahuasca, and other psychedelics, increases the distribution of features of brain organization, compared to the ordinary waking state, leading to a wider spectrum of experiences (Carhart-Harris, 2018; Viol et al., 2017). In this sense, ordinary consciousness can be thought of as a more constrained state consciousness (Watts, 2011).

Middle-Term Effects of Ayahuasca on Human Subjects

The middle-term, or subacute effects of ayahuasca, are usually assessed between 24 and 48 hours after drinking. Studies of this nature are sparser but have indicated that these changes are not negligible in a number of dimensions, from creativity to depression and anxiety (Dos Santos et al., 2016).

There is evidence that ayahuasca affects the structure and dynamics of thoughts. For instance, it has been found that ayahuasca

leads to increased creative divergent thinking. The picture concept test (PCT) was used to assess both divergent thinking and convergent thinking, during acute inebriation (Kuypers et al., 2016). Divergent thinking represents a spontaneous pattern of thoughts whereby new ideas flow freely and randomly, allowing unexpected connections to be drawn. It is a flexible style of thinking, from which flexible and creative psychological strategies might emerge, allowing new cognitive, emotional, and behavioral insights, and creating an appropriate window for psychotherapy (Frecska et al., 2016; Winkelman, 2014).

Changes in thought processes linger, at least partially, into the subacute phase. A recent study revealed that ayahuasca leads to changes in visual creativity. Using the visual parts of the Torrance Tests of Creative Thinking at baseline and between 24 and 48 hours after an ayahuasca session, Frecska and colleagues (2012) found a significantly increased number of original solutions, which suggests an increase in visual creativity.

Convergent thinking, on the other hand, refers to a much more rigid pattern of thinking that follows a specific set of logical steps to arrive at one particular solution. It also serves as a way to organize and structure ideas and concepts that emerge during the process of divergent thinking. While it has been observed that convergent thinking is decreased during the acute effects of ayahuasca (Kuypers et al., 2016), another study suggests its moderate increase one day after the session, reaching significance after 4 weeks (Uthaug et al., 2018). Divergent thinking, on the other hand, did not changed either 1 day or 4 weeks after the ayahuasca session (Uthaug et al., 2018).

Changing thought processes might also be responsible for the observed significant increase in mindfulness traces after ayahuasca. The word *mindfulness* refers to a state of mind in which attention is directed to the present moment-by-moment experience of the individual, nonjudgmentally. Different psychometric scales have been developed to assess traits and states of mindfulness, among which is the Five Facet Mindfulness Questionnaire (FFMQ; Baer et al., 2006).

Two out of the five FFMQ factors were significantly changed 24 hours after the ayahuasca section, with decreased judgmental processing and reduced reactivity, as well as increased decentering, in the same direction observed after meditative practices (Soler et al., 2016). The mid-term impact of ayahuasca in these mindful traces (no-judge, no-react, *decentering*) have been monitored with magnetic resonance spectroscopy and functional connectivity 24 hours after the session. With respect to the baseline, the study reports significant changes in glutamate/glutamine metabolite concentration, and changes in functional connectivity between the posterior cingulate cortex (PCC) and the ACC, and between the ACC and limbic structures (Sampedro et al., 2017).

Anecdotal reports and an increased number of scientific studies suggest that ayahuasca reduces depression and stress at subacute stages after the session (Osório et al., 2015; Palhano-Fontes et al., 2019; Sanches et al., 2016; Uthaug et al., 2018). Recent clinical trials with ayahuasca suggest an antidepressant effect of ayahuasca, particularly at the subacute phases (Osório et al., 2015; Palhano-Fontes et al., 2018; Sanches et al., 2016). Two clinical trials were carried out, one open-label trial (Sanches et al., 2016) and a subsequent randomized controlled trial (RCT) with ayahuasca for treatment-resistant depression (Palhano-Fontes et al., 2019). In the first trial, 17 naive patients participated in a single ayahuasca session in a university hospital, and their depressive symptoms were monitored for 21 days. Depressive severity was assessed with two clinical scales (Hamilton Rating Scale for Depression [HAM-D] and Montgomery–Åsberg Depression Rating Scale [MADRS) at baseline (1 day before), and at 1, 2, and 7 days after the session (Osório et al., 2015; Sanches et al., 2016). We found significantly reduced depressive symptoms 24 hours after the session, which lasted for 21 days (Osório et al., 2015; Sanches et al., 2016). In the follow-up placebo-controlled RCT, 29 patients with severe depression were randomly assigned to participate in a single dosing session with either ayahuasca or placebo. The antidepressant effect of ayahuasca was superior to that of the placebo (Palhano-Fontes

et al., 2019). Our results are comparable with trials that used ketamine, although the dynamic is different. While ketamine effect size is largest 1 day after the session (Cohen's $d = 0.89$) and reduces toward 1 week after the session (Cohen's $d = 0.41$), the effect sizes observed for ayahuasca is smallest and compatible to ketamine at day 1 (Cohen's $d = 0.84$), and it increases and is largest 7 days after the session (Cohen's $d = 1.49$) (Palhano-Fontes et al., 2019).

Some of these changes have been monitored using neuroimaging techniques. In our open-label trial, we used SPECT 8 hours after the session to access subacute changes in blood perfusion. Patients showed increased CBF in the left nucleus accumbens, right insula, and left subgenual cortices, all of which are implicated in the regulation of mood and emotions (Sanches et al., 2016).

Subacute effects of ayahuasca also impact other biological dimensions, such as sleep (Barbanoj et al., 2008). Quality of sleep was assessed in the night following a single diurnal session with ayahuasca. Results indicated that ayahuasca inhibits rapid eye movement (REM) sleep, decreasing its duration, with a trend toward increased REM latency. The opposite, increased REM and reduced REM latency are often observed in depression (Minkel et al., 2017).

In our RCT with ayahuasca, a few biologically relevant substances were dosed 24 hours before and 36 hours after the session. Our patients showed decreased cortisol levels (hypocortisolemia) and blunted awakening salivary cortisol response at baseline. Patients treated with ayahuasca, but not with placebo, stabilized their awakening salivary cortisol response to the same level found in the healthy control group (Galvão et al., 2018). We also explored changes in serum brain-derived neurotrophic factor (BDNF) levels in healthy controls and patients and observed higher BDNF levels in both patients and controls who ingested ayahuasca, when compared to placebo (de Almeida et al., 2019). Moreover, just patients treated with ayahuasca, and not those treated with placebo, presented a significant negative correlation between serum BDNF levels and depressive symptoms (de Almeida et al., 2019). A possible mediator of these changes are the σ-1 receptors, as they upregulate neurotrophic factors such as BDNF (Cai et al., 2015).

Long-Term Effects of Ayahuasca on Human Subjects

Early studies suggest no sign of psychopathological, personality, or cognitive deteriorations in long-term members of Brazilian religions (Barbosa et al., 2009, 2018; Bouso et al., 2012; Grob et al., 1996). A 6-month longitudinal study followed up 23 individuals after their first ayahuasca experience and reported general improvements in mental health and minor psychiatric symptoms (Barbosa et al., 2009).

There is no evidence that ayahuasca is addictive or that it produces the negative psychosocial repercussions that often characterize the problematic use of other psychoactive substances (Fábregas et al., 2010; Grob et al., 1996). A study of two consecutive doses of ayahuasca with a 4-hour interval detected no signs of sensitization or acute tolerance with regard to the psychological effects (Dos Santos et al., 2012).

There is some evidence of long-term personality changes, most with members of ayahuasca religions (Barbosa et al., 2009, 2018; Grob et al., 1996; Halpern et al., 2008). In the largest and best-controlled study on the subject, ayahuasca users showed higher reward dependence and self-transcendence personality traits when compared to controls, and lower harm avoidance and self-directedness. Users scored significantly lower on all psychopathology measures (Bouso et al., 2012). So far, the overall conclusion is that deleterious effects of ayahuasca on personality have not been demonstrated; however, more studies are needed on the subject (Bouso & Riba, 2011).

Magnetic resonance imaging (MRI) was also used to assess eventual neuroanatomical changes in long-term ayahuasca users (Bouso et al., 2015). Compared to controls, long-term users showed increased cortical thickness (CT) in the mPFC and reduced CT in the PCC/precuneus. In addition, there was a significant correlation between the CT of the PCC/precuneus cluster and *openness*,

from the Big Five Personality Test[3] (Bouso et al., 2015).

From observational studies and anecdotal reports, ayahuasca shows promise as a tool in the treatment for substance use disorders (Nunes et al., 2016). Adolescents who drink ayahuasca regularly presented lower past month and past year alcohol use compared to matched controls (Doering-Silveira et al., 2005). Members of a Santo Daime church in the United States presented higher remission rates of drug/alcohol misuse compared to the general U.S. population (Halpern et al., 2008), a finding that is consistent with previous studies of members of ayahuasca communities (Fábregas et al., 2010; Loiza-ga-Velder & Verres, 2014). U.S. UDV members had greater past alcohol misuse but lower recent use when compared to controls, members of other Christian churches (Barbosa et al., 2016). In a large survey sample, past use of alcohol and tobacco was higher among Brazilian UDV members, but current use was significantly lower (Barbosa et al., 2018). Also, the Global Drug Survey ($N = 96,901$) presented increased well-being and reduced alcohol use among those who had taken ayahuasca when compared to both users of other psychedelics and nonpsychedelic users (Lawn et al., 2017). There is a single open-label observational study with 12 participants who attended an ayahuasca retreat and reported decreased cocaine, tobacco, and alcohol use (Thomas et al., 2013).

Animal Studies Relevant to Toxicity and Risk Groups

The use of animal models to investigate acute or chronic ayahuasca effects is important to disambiguate substance-related effects from setting-related effects. Animal models are of utmost importance to optimize the therapeutic benefits and to evaluate the potential toxicological risks of ayahuasca intake. Some animal studies have corroborated the notion that ayahuasca consumption is safe for most adults. For instance, female rats acutely treated with ayahuasca doses equivalent to 30–50 times a typical ritual dose (up to 15.1 mg/kg of DMT) showed only a moderate locomotion decrease in comparison to controls, of the same magnitude of that induced by fluoxetine. In the forced swimming test, ayahuasca-treated animals swam more than both controls and the fluoxetine-treated group (Pic-Taylor et al., 2015). In another study, daily oral doses of up to 480 mg/kg of freeze-dried ayahuasca were given to male rats, and performance on the spatial navigation and fear conditioning tasks was assessed. The performance was unchanged in all groups, with the exception of an increase in contextual fear conditioning in the group treated with the lowest dose tested (Favaro et al., 2015). Longer experiments corroborate these findings: Adult mice chronically treated with ayahuasca (3.1 mg/kg of DMT, orally) twice a week for 12 months were no different from control animals treated with water when tested in the Morris water maze, open field, and elevated plus maze task (Correa-Netto et al., 2017).

Since ayahuasca intake produces moderate cardiovascular effects, research on the cardiovascular function of chronic ayahuasca consumers is a necessity. An investigation of the acute and chronic effects of ayahuasca in the rat aorta observed flattening and stretching of vascular smooth muscle cells and changes in the arrangement and distribution of collagen and elastic fibers. Chronic treatment with the higher dose significantly increased media thickness and the ratio of media thickness to lumen diameter (Pitol et al., 2015). This single study suggests that individuals with a cardiopathy may be a risk group for ayahuasca consumption.

A few developmental studies of ayahuasca recommend caution (Dos Santos, 2013). A study of the effects of ayahuasca on zebrafish larvae found that exposure to high concentrations may cause developmental anomalies, including hatching delay, loss of equilibrium, edema, accumulation of red blood cells, and decreased locomotor activity (Andrade et al., 2018). The lethal concentration, 50% (LC50) after 96 hours corresponded to 0.02 mg/mL DMT, 0.017 mg/mL harmaline, and 0.22 mg/mL harmine. Also, chronic daily regimen of ayahuasca for pregnant Wistar rats caused visceral and skeletal abnormalities in fetuses and, in higher doses (4.2 mg/mL DMT, 13.7 mg/mL harmine, and 6.2 mg/mL harmaline), a decrease in

weight in fetuses and in weight gain in dams (Oliveira et al., 2010). Though the relevance of these results for pregnant women, who use ayahuasca more sporadically in ritual contexts, has been contested (Dos Santos, 2010), a cautionary note should remain about ayahuasca and fetal development. Moreover, ayahuasca was considered mutagenic in the Salmonella/microsome assay, which is usually the first line of the mutagenicity evaluation of products intended for therapeutic use. This effect seems to be partially explained by the presence of harmaline (Kummrow et al., 2019).

Animal Studies Relevant to the Acute and Long-Term Effects of Ayahuasca

If the acute effects of ayahuasca are proportional to its long-term effects (i.e., if the magnitude of the psychedelic experience is proportional to the clinical benefits days, weeks or years later), then it is very important to understand the neurophysiological mechanisms that underlie both short- and long-term effects ayahuasca. A pioneering electrophysiological study of the effects of N,N-DMT showed facilitation of firing in septal and hippocampal neurons (DeFrance et al., 1975). In contrast, serotonergic neurons recorded from raphe nuclei in freely behaving animals respond to 5-methoxy-N,N-dimethyltryptamine (5-MeO-DMT) with a major decrease in unit activity (Fornal et al., 1985; Rebec & Curtis, 1983; Trulson & Jacobs, 1979). 5-MeO-DMT, a more powerful analogue of N,N-DMT, causes a dose-related inhibition of the firing of midline medullary 5-HT neurons, nearly identical to that observed for dorsal raphe 5-HT neurons (Clement & McCall, 1991). Experiments with specific agonists showed that the phenomenon is not dependent on the 5-HT$_2$ receptor, but rather on the α1-adrenergic receptor (Clement & McCall, 1991). More recently, a neurophysiological study on the effects of 5-MeO-DMT on cortical activity assessed in rats by single-unit recordings and blood oxygen level-dependent (BOLD) fMRI found that the compound modified mPFC activity, both increasing and decreasing the firing rates of 51 and 35% of the recorded pyramidal neurons, respectively. 5-MeO-DMT also reduced the power of slow cortical oscillations in the δ band (<4 Hz). This effect depended on 5-HT_{1A} and 5-HT_{2A} receptors and was reversed by haloperidol, clozapine, risperidone, and the metabolic glutamate (mGlu2/3) agonist LY379268. 5-MeO-DMT also decreased BOLD responses in the visual cortex (V1) and the mPFC (Riga et al., 2014). Given that the changes in cortical activity produced by 5-MeO-DMT are similar to those produced by other serotonergic drugs, and that the same antipsychotic drugs antagonize these effects, it is likely that the neurophysiological changes induced by 5-MeO-DMT are indeed part of the mechanistic framework that underlies the effect of N,N-DMT in the ayahuasca visions and perhaps even dreaming (Riga et al., 2014).

Interestingly, long-term (1 month) daily oral administration of ayahuasca improved contextual fear conditioning in rats at the lowest dose tested (Favaro et al., 2015). The fact that this process is hippocampal dependent suggests that this brain region could be involved in the effects of ayahuasca on learning (Dos Santos & Hallak, 2017). High doses seem to have detrimental effects for learning, as suggested by a study about the effects of ayahuasca on the ability of adult zebrafish to discriminate objects in a one-trial learning task. The study showed impairment after chronic treatment but not acutely, except at the highest dose, which hindered locomotion (Lobao-Soares et al., 2018).

The use of animal models has also allowed for steady exploration of the therapeutic uses of ayahuasca. Studies of harmine and N,N-DMT in animal models of depression have shown that these constituents of ayahuasca decrease behaviors that indicate anxiety and depression (Cameron et al., 2018; Fortunato et al., 2010a, 2010b). Quite recently, the antidepressant effects of ayahuasca were assessed on a model of depression: young marmosets subjected to social isolation for 1 month [da Silva et al., 2019]. The results showed that a single dose of ayahuasca reduced the frequency of behaviors associated with depression, such as scratching, and promoted a homeostatic regulation of cortisol levels following 2 months of social isolation. Marmosets treated with ayahuasca showed faster effects than animals treated with the antidepressant nortriptyline (da Silva et al., 2019).

It has been theorized that β-carbolines may prove useful in treating opioid addiction, as harmine has been reported to reduce the symptoms of morphine withdrawal in rats (Aricioglu-Kartal et al., 2003). A study in mice found that ayahuasca attenuated ethanol-induced behavioral sensitization at all doses tested without affecting spontaneous locomotor activity. Importantly, ayahuasca inhibited the early behaviors associated with ethanol addiction and reversed some of its long-term effects (Oliveira-Lima et al., 2015).

▨ Potential Molecular Mechanisms: Insight from *In Vitro* Studies

Changes at the cellular and systemic levels have only recently began to unravel. Some fundamental insight came recently from the development of new ways to study the human nervous system *in vitro*. Beyond bidimensional models comprising neural cells on a dish, novel techniques now allow the evaluation of cerebral organoids (i.e., artificially grown miniature organs resembling the human brain in some key aspects). Recently, we used large-scale screening systems applied to human neural cells and cerebral organoids derived from stem cells to characterize—at the cellular and molecular levels—the effects of harmine (Dakic et al., 2016) and 5-MeO-DMT (Dakic et al., 2017). While the latter cannot simply be extrapolated to N,N-DMT, as we discuss below, these experiments represent an important early step toward dissecting the effects of ayahuasca in the human nervous system.

Harmine increased the pool of neural cells, which could help explain the antidepressant effects of ayahuasca (Dakic et al., 2016). This proliferative effect is caused by inhibition of an enzyme called DYRK1A (dual-specificity tyrosine phosphorylated and regulated kinase 1A). Our results suggest that harmine induces neurogenesis by driving the differentiation of neural stem cells into radial glial cells, the major source of neuronal and glial cells in the developing brain (Götz & Barde, 2005). Besides, harmine, tetrahydroharmine, and harmaline stimulate neural stem cell proliferation, migration, and differentiation into adult neurons in neurospheres derived from brain progenitor cells obtained from adult mice (Morales-García et al., 2017).

Analyses of global protein expression in brain organoids exposed to 5-MeO-DMT revealed changes in proteins pertaining a range of functional activities, such as cellular protrusion formation, microtubule dynamics, and cytoskeletal reorganization (Dakic et al., 2017), which are correlated to novel dendritic spine formation, neuronal plasticity, and memory. This conclusion goes along with the hypothesis suggesting that the indirect activation of glutamate networks by classical hallucinogens enhances neuroplasticity (Vollenweider & Kometer, 2010). Interestingly, fast antidepressants also have a strong effect on synaptic plasticity, reversing functional and structural synaptic deficits caused by stress (Duman et al., 2016). Recently, 5-MeO-DMT was also shown to induce proliferation and accelerate maturation of newborn neurons in the ventral dentate gyrus of adult mice. A single dose of 5-MeO-DMT was able to promote an increase the dendritic complexity and alter the electrophysiological pattern in hippocampal newborn neurons (Lima da Cruz et al., 2018). Based on our molecular data from human brain organoids and recent mice studies, it is very likely that 5-MeO-DMT regulates neural plasticity and synaptogenesis, as recently shown for other classic psychedelics (Ly et al., 2018).

5-MeO-DMT modulates proteins that participate in LTP (long-term potentiation), memory, and formation and maturation of novel dendritic spines (Dakic et al., 2017). This pattern points to robust actions on synaptic plasticity, which is a mechanism characteristic of fast antidepressants. The proteomic analysis also highlighted the potential anti-inflammatory properties of 5-MeO-DMT (Dakic et al., 2017). Psychedelics have been reported to repress inflammation in low doses, probably by blocking the inflammatory cascade through serotonin receptors signaling (Flanagan & Nichols, 2018). Many neuropsychiatric disorders, including depression, may be explained based on inflammation, in which exacerbated immune responses contributes to its etiology and symptomatology (Szabo & Frecska, 2016). In this context, the σ-1 receptor has been pointed out as a mediator of anti-inflammatory effects of both N,N-DMT and 5-MeO-DMT (Frecska et al., 2016). These compounds have been demonstrated to boost anti-inflammatory interleukins production, while inhibiting the production of inflammatory interleukins, chemokines, and the crosstalk between innate and adaptive immunity (Szabo et al., 2014).

■ Conclusion

Ayahuasca is a traditional indigenous brew that is used in Amerindian shamanism, neoshamanic traditions, and Brazilian churches for ritual and mystical purposes. During the last three decades, the scientific scrutiny of the brew and its effects has provided insights about its biological mechanisms, potential therapeutic applications, and safety limits. So far, the evidence reviewed in this chapter supports the notion that ayahuasca could have therapeutic uses for Parkinson's disease, substance use disorders, and depression. Perception, emotion, memory, attention, and spontaneous thought processes and their physiological mechanisms in the brain are affected by ayahuasca effects. The mental and symbolic processes elicited by these acute and subacute effects may also provide psychological responses that could help to alleviate symptoms caused by depression, anxiety, and addiction.

Other potential therapeutic applications for ayahuasca and its constituents are currently being studied. They include posttraumatic stress disorder, autoimmune diseases, cancer, Alzheimer's disease, eating disorders, and obsessive–compulsive disorders. These perspectives come mostly from surveys, pharmacological rationale, psychological rationale, and also from anecdotal reports from therapeutic centers (see Domínguez-Clavé et al., 2016; Frecska et al., 2016; Labate & Cavnar, 2014; Renelli et al., 2020; Winkelman, 2014). However, robust scientific evidence—from bench to bedside—is still lacking to support these claims and explore what has already been discovered. Thus, ayahuasca is a promising subject for further scientific inquiry in neuroscience, psychiatry, psychology and the health sciences in general.

Notes

1. Quechua corresponds to a family of languages spoken primarily by indigenous populations of the Andes in South America.

2. Translated from Brazilian Portuguese as "mirage," "seeing," or "vision."

3. The five-factor model (Big Five) dissects personality in five major dimensions: Openness, Conscientiousness, Agreeableness, Extraversion, and Neuroticism.

References

Andrade, T. S., de Oliveira, R., da Silva, M. L., Von Zuben, M. V., Grisolia, C. K., Domingues, I., et al. (2018). Exposure to ayahuasca induces developmental and behavioral alterations on early life stages of zebrafish. *Chem Biol Interact, 293*, 133–140.

Aricioglu-Kartal, F., Kayir, H., & Tayfun Uzbay, I. (2003). Effects of harman and harmine on naloxone-precipitated withdrawal syndrome in morphine-dependent rats. *Life Sci, 73*, 2363–2371.

Baer, R. A., Smith, G. T., Hopkins, J., Krietemeyer, J., & Toney, L. (2006). Using self-report assessment methods to explore facets of mindfulness. *Assessment, 13*, 27–45.

Barbanoj, M. J., Riba, J., Clos, S., Giménez, S., Grasa, E., & Romero, S. (2006). Increased sleep pressure, as measured by EEG slow wave activity, following daytime administration of ayahuasca, the Amazonian hallucinogen. *J Sleep Res, 15*, 193.

Barbanoj, M. J., Riba, J., Clos, S., Giménez, S., Grasa, E., & Romero, S. (2008). Daytime ayahuasca administration modulates REM and slow-wave sleep in healthy volunteers. *Psychopharmacology, 196*, 315–326.

Barbosa, P. C. R., Cazorla, I. M., Giglio, J. S., & Strassman, R. (2009). A six-month prospective evaluation of personality traits, psychiatric symptoms and quality of life in ayahuasca-naive subjects. *J Psychoactive Drugs, 41*, 205–212.

Barbosa, P. C., Strassman, R. J., da Silveira, D. X., Areco, K., Hoy, R., Pommy, J., et al. (2016). Psychological and neuropsychological assessment of regular hoasca users. *Compr Psychiatry, 71*, 95–105.

Barbosa, P. C., Tofoli, L. F., Bogenschutz, M. P., Hoy, R., Berro, L. F., Marinho, E. A. V., et al. (2018). Assessment of alcohol and tobacco use disorders among religious users of ayahuasca. *Front Psychiatry, 9*, 136.

Barker, S. A., Borjigin, J., Lomnicka, I., & Strassman, R. (2013). LC/MS/MS analysis of the endogenous dimethyltryptamine hallucinogens, their precursors, and major metabolites in rat pineal gland microdialysate. *Biomed Chromatogr, 27*, 1690–1700.

Barrett, F. S., Johnson, M. W., & Griffiths, R. R. (2015). Validation of the revised Mystical Experience Questionnaire in experimental sessions with psilocybin. *J Psychopharmacol, 29*, 1182–1190.

Barrett, F. S., Johnson, M. W., & Griffiths, R. R. (2017). Neuroticism is associated with challenging experiences with psilocybin mushrooms. *Pers Individ Dif, 117*, 155–160.

Ben-Shabat, S., Fride, E., Sheskin, T., Tamiri, T., Rhee, M. H., Vogel, Z., et al. (1998). An entourage effect: Inactive endogenous fatty acid glycerol esters enhance 2-arachidonoyl-glycerol cannabinoid activity. *Eur J Pharmacol, 353*, 23–31.

Bolsanello, D. P. (1995). *Busca do Graal brasileiro: A doutrina do Santo Daime*. Rio de Janeiro: Bertrand Brasil.

Bouso, J. C., Fábregas, J. M., Antonijoan, R. M., Rodríguez-Fornells, A., & Riba, J. (2013). Acute effects of ayahuasca on neuropsychological performance: Differences in executive function between experienced and occasional users. *Psychopharmacology, 230*, 415–424.

Bouso, J. C., González, D., Fondevila, S., Cutchet, M., Fernández, X., Ribeiro Barbosa, P. C., et al. (2012). Personality, psychopathology, life attitudes and neuropsychological performance among ritual users of ayahuasca: A longitudinal study. *PLOS ONE, 7*, e42421.

Bouso, J. C., Palhano-Fontes, F., Rodríguez-Fornells, A., Ribeiro, S., Sanches, R., Crippa, J. A. S., et al. (2015). Long-term use of psychedelic drugs is associated with differences in brain structure and personality in humans. *Eur Neuropsychopharmacol 25*, 483–492.

Bouso, J. C., & Riba, J. (2011). An overview of the literature on the pharmacology and neuropsychiatric long term effects of ayahuasca. In R. G. Dos Santos (Ed.), *The ethnopharmacol-*

ogy of ayahuasca (pp. 55–63). Kerala, India: Transworld Research Network.

Cai, S., Huang, S., & Hao, W. (2015). New hypothesis and treatment targets of depression: An integrated view of key findings. *Neurosci Bull, 31,* 61–74.

Callaway, J. C., McKenna, D. J., Grob, C. S., Brito, G. S., Raymon, L. P., Poland, R. E., et al. (1999). Pharmacokinetics of Hoasca alkaloids in healthy humans. *J Ethnopharmacol, 65,* 243–256.

Cameron, L. P., Benson, C. J., Dunlap, L. E., & Olson, D. E. (2018). Effects of N,N-dimethyltryptamine on rat behaviors relevant to anxiety and depression. *ACS Chem Neurosci, 9,* 1582–1590.

Carbonaro, T. M., & Gatch, M. B. (2016). Neuropharmacology of N,N-dimethyltryptamine. *Brain Res Bull, 126,* 74–88.

Carhart-Harris, R. L. (2018). The entropic brain—revisited. *Neuropharmacology, 142,* 167–178.

Carhart-Harris, R. L., Erritzoe, D., Williams, T., Stone, J. M., Reed, L. J., Colasanti, A., et al. (2012). Neural correlates of the psychedelic state as determined by fMRI studies with psilocybin. *Proc Natl Acad Sci USA, 109,* 2138–2143.

Carhart-Harris, R. L., Muthukumaraswamy, S., Roseman, L., Kaelen, M., Droog, W., Murphy, K., et al. (2016). Neural correlates of the LSD experience revealed by multimodal neuroimaging. *Proc Natl Acad Sci USA, 113,* 4853–4858.

Clement, M. E., & McCall, R. B. (1991). Pharmacological characterization of medullary serotonin neurons. *Brain Res, 542,* 205–211.

Correa-Netto, N. F., Coelho, L. S., Galfano, G. S., Nishide, F., Tamura, F., Shimizu, M. K., et al. (2017). Chronic intermittent exposure to ayahuasca during aging does not affect memory in mice. *Braz J Med Biol Res, 50,* e6037.

da Silva, F. S., Silva, E. A. S., de Sousa, G. M., Jr., Maia-de-Oliveira, J. P., Soares-Rachetti, V. de P., de Araujo, D. B., et al. (2019). Acute effects of ayahuasca in a juvenile non-human primate model of depression. *Braz J Psychiatr, 41,* 280–288.

Dakic, V., Maciel, R. de M., Drummond, H., Nascimento, J. M., Trindade, P., & Rehen, S. K. (2016). Harmine stimulates proliferation of human neural progenitors. *PeerJ, 4,* e2727.

Dakic, V., Minardi Nascimento, J., Costa Sartore, R., Maciel, R de M., de Araujo, D. B., Ribeiro, S., et al. (2017). Short term changes in the proteome of human cerebral organoids induced by 5-MeO-DMT. *Sci Rep, 7,* 12863.

de Almeida, R. N., de Menezes Galvão, A. C., da Silva, F. S., dos Santos Silva, E. A., Palh-ano-Fontes, F., Maia-de-Oliveira, J. P., et al. (2019). Modulation of serum brain-derived neurotrophic factor by a single dose of ayahuasca: Observation from a randomized controlled trial. *Front Psychol, 10,* 1234.

de Araujo, D. B., Ribeiro, S., Cecchi, G. A., Carvalho, F. M., Sanchez, T. A., Pinto, J. P., et al. (2012). Seeing with the eyes shut: Neural basis of enhanced imagery following Ayahuasca ingestion. *Hum Brain Mapp, 33,* 2550–2560.

de Lima, O. G. (1946). Observações sobre o "vinho da Jurema" utilizado pelos indios Pancaru de Tacaratu (Pernambuco). *Separata de Archivos do I.P.A., 4,* 45–80.

DeFrance, J. F., McCrea, R. A., & Yoshihara, H. (1975). Effects of certain indoleamines in the hippocampal-septal circuit. *Exp Neurol, 48,* 352–377.

Diament, M., Gomer, B. R., & Tófoli, L. F. (in press). Ayahuasca and psychotherapy: Beyond integration. In C. C. Beatriz Labate (Ed.), *Ayahuasca healing and science.* Cham, Switzerland: Springer.

Doering-Silveira, E., Grob, C. S., de Rios, M. D., Lopez, E., Alonso, L. K., Tacla, C., et al. (2005). Report on psychoactive drug use among adolescents using ayahuasca within a religious context. *J Psychoactive Drugs, 37,* 141–144.

Domínguez-Clavé, E., Soler, J., Elices, M., Pascual, J. C., Álvarez, E., de la Fuente Revenga, M., et al. (2016). Ayahuasca: Pharmacology, neuroscience and therapeutic potential. *Brain Res Bull, 126,* 89–101.

Dos Santos, R. G. (2010). Toxicity of chronic ayahuasca administration to the pregnant rat: How relevant it is regarding the human, ritual use of ayahuasca? *Birth Defects Res B Dev Reprod Toxicol, 89,* 533–535.

Dos Santos, R. G. (2013). Safety and side effects of ayahuasca in humans—an overview focusing on developmental toxicology. *J Psychoactive Drugs, 45,* 68–78.

Dos Santos, R. G., Balthazar, F. M., Bouso, J. C., & Hallak, J. E. (2016). The current state of research on ayahuasca: A systematic review of human studies assessing psychiatric symptoms, neuropsychological functioning, and neuroimaging. *J Psychopharmacol, 30,* 1230–1247.

Dos Santos, R. G., Grasa, E., Valle, M., Ballester, M. R., Bouso, J. C., Nomdedéu, J. F., et al. (2012). Pharmacology of ayahuasca administered in two repeated doses. *Psychopharmacology, 219,* 1039–1053.

Dos Santos, R. G., & Hallak, J. E. C. (2017). Effects of the natural β-carboline alkaloid harmine, a main constituent of ayahuasca, in memory and in the hippocampus: A systematic literature review of preclinical studies. *J Psychoactive Drugs, 49*, 1–10.

Dos Santos, R. G., Valle, M., Bouso, J. C., Nomdedéu, J. F., Rodríguez-Espinosa, J., McIlhenny, E. H., et al. (2011). Autonomic, neuroendocrine, and immunological effects of ayahuasca: A comparative study with d-amphetamine. *J Clin Psychopharmacol, 31*, 717–726.

Dresler, M., Wehrle, R., Spoormaker, V. I., Koch, S. P., Holsboer, F., Steiger, A., et al. (2012). Neural correlates of dream lucidity obtained from contrasting lucid versus non-lucid REM sleep: A combined EEG/fMRI case study. *Sleep, 35*, 1017–1020.

Duman, R. S., Aghajanian, G. K., Sanacora, G., & Krystal, J. H. (2016). Synaptic plasticity and depression: new insights from stress and rapid-acting antidepressants. *Nat Med, 22*, 238–249.

Fábregas, J. M., González, D., Fondevila, S., Cutchet, M., Fernández, X., Barbosa, P. C. R., et al. (2010). Assessment of addiction severity among ritual users of ayahuasca. *Drug Alcohol Depend, 111*, 257–261.

Favaro, V. M., Yonamine, M., Soares, J. C. K., & Oliveira, M. G. M. (2015). Effects of long-term ayahuasca administration on memory and anxiety in rats. *PLOS ONE, 10*, e0145840.

Flanagan, T. W., & Nichols, C. D. (2018). Psychedelics as anti-inflammatory agents. *Int Rev Psychiatry*, 1–13.

Fleming, S. M., & Dolan, R. J. (2012). Review: Neural basis of metacognition. *Philos Trans R Soc Lond B Biol Sci, 367*, 1338–1349.

Fornal, C., Auerbach, S., & Jacobs, B. L. (1985). Activity of serotonin-containing neurons in nucleus raphe magnus in freely moving cats. *Exp Neurol, 88*, 590–608.

Fortunato, J. J., Réus, G. Z., Kirsch, T. R., Stringari, R. B., Fries, G. R., Kapczinski, F., et al. (2010a). Chronic administration of harmine elicits antidepressant-like effects and increases BDNF levels in rat hippocampus. *J Neural Transm, 117*, 1131–1137.

Fortunato, J. J., Réus, G. Z., Kirsch, T. R., Stringari, R. B., Fries, G. R., Kapczinski, F., et al. (2010b). Effects of beta-carboline harmine on behavioral and physiological parameters observed in the chronic mild stress model: Further evidence of antidepressant properties. *Brain Res Bull, 81*, 491–496.

Frecska, E., Bokor, P., & Winkelman, M. (2016). The therapeutic potentials of ayahuasca: Possible effects against various diseases of civilization. *Front Pharmacol, 7*, 35.

Frecska, E., Móré, C. E., Vargha, A., & Luna, L. E. (2012). Enhancement of creative expression and entoptic phenomena as after-effects of repeated ayahuasca ceremonies. *J Psychoactive Drugs, 44*, 191–199.

Galvão, A. C., de Almeida, R. N., Silva, E. A. D. S., Freire, F. A. M., Palhano-Fontes, F., Onias H., et al. (2018). Cortisol modulation by ayahuasca in patients with treatment resistant depression and healthy controls. *Front Psychiatry, 9*, 185.

Götz, M., & Barde, Y.-A. (2005). Radial glial cells: Defined and major intermediates between embryonic stem cells and CNS neurons. *Neuron, 46*, 369–372.

Griffiths, R. R., Richards, W. A., McCann, U., & Jesse, R. (2006). Psilocybin can occasion mystical-type experiences having substantial and sustained personal meaning and spiritual significance. *Psychopharmacology, 187*, 268–283.

Grob, C. S., McKenna, D. J., Callaway, J. C., Brito, G. S., Neves, E. S., Oberlaender, G, et al. (1996). Human psychopharmacology of hoasca, a plant hallucinogen used in ritual context in Brazil. *J Nerv Ment Dis, 184*, 86–94.

Halpern, J. H., Sherwood, A. R., Passie, T., Blackwell, K. C., & Ruttenber, A. J. (2008). Evidence of health and safety in American members of a religion who use a hallucinogenic sacrament. *Med Sci Monit, 14*, SR15–SR22.

Hasenkamp W., Wilson-Mendenhall, C. D., Duncan, E., & Barsalou, L. W. (2012). Mind wandering and attention during focused meditation: A fine-grained temporal analysis of fluctuating cognitive states. *NeuroImage, 59*, 750–760.

Kraehenmann, R. (2017). Dreams and psychedelics: Neurophenomenological comparison and therapeutic implications. *Curr Neuropharmacol, 15*, 1032–1042.

Kummrow, F., Maselli, B. S., Lanaro, R., Costa, J. L., Umbuzeiro, G. A., & Linardi, A. (2019). Mutagenicity of ayahuasca and their constituents to the salmonella/microsome assay. *Environ Mol Mutagen, 60*, 269–276.

Kuypers, K. P. C., Riba, J., de la Fuente Revenga, M., Barker, S., Theunissen, E. L., & Ramaekers, J. G. (2016). Ayahuasca enhances creative divergent thinking while decreasing conventional convergent thinking. *Psychopharmacology, 233*, 3395–3403.

Labate, B. C., & Cavnar, C. (Eds.). (2014). *The therapeutic use of ayahuasca*. Berlin/Heidelberg: Springer.

Labate, B. C., Cavnar, C., & Freedman, F. B. (2014). Notes on the expansion and reinvention of ayahuasca shamanism. In B. C. Labate & C. Cavnar (Eds.), *Ayahuasca shamanism in the Amazon and beyond* (pp. 3–15). New York: Oxford University Press.

Labate, B. C., & Jungaberle, H. (2011). *The in-*

ternationalization of Ayahuasca. Münster, Germany: LIT Verlag.

Labate, B. C., & MacRae, E. (2016). *Ayahuasca, ritual and religion in Brazil*. New York: Routledge.

Lawn, W., Hallak, J. E., Crippa, J. A., Dos Santos, R., Porffy, L., Barratt, M. J., et al. (2017). Well-being, problematic alcohol consumption and acute subjective drug effects in past-year ayahuasca users: A large, international, self-selecting online survey. *Sci Rep 7*, 15201.

Lima da Cruz, R. V., Moulin, T. C., Petiz, L. L., & Leão, R. N. (2018). A single dose of 5-MeO-DMT stimulates cell proliferation, neuronal survivability, morphological and functional changes in adult mice ventral dentate gyrus. *Front Mol Neurosci, 11*, 312.

Lobao-Soares, B., Eduardo-da-Silva, P., Amarilha, H., Pinheiro-da-Silva, J., Silva, P. F., & Luchiari, A. C. (2018). It's tea time: Interference of Ayahuasca brew on discriminative learning in zebrafish. *Front Behav Neurosci, 12*, 190.

Loizaga-Velder, A., & Verres, R. (2014). Therapeutic effects of ritual ayahuasca use in the treatment of substance dependence—qualitative results. *J Psychoactive Drugs, 46*, 63–72.

Luna, L. E. (2011). Indigenous and mestizo use of ayahuasca: An overview. In R. G. Dos Santos (Ed.), *The ethnopharmacology of ayahuasca* (pp. 1–21). Kerala, India: Transworld Research Network.

Ly, C., Greb, A. C., Cameron, L. P., Wong, J. M., Barragan, E. V., Wilson, P. C., et al. (2018). Psychedelics promote structural and functional neural plasticity. *Cell Rep, 23*, 3170–3182.

MacLean, K. A., Johnson, M. W., & Griffiths, R. R. (2011). Mystical experiences occasioned by the hallucinogen psilocybin lead to increases in the personality domain of openness. *J Psychopharmacol, 25*, 1453–1461.

MacLean, K. A., Leoutsakos, J.-M. S., Johnson, M. W., & Griffiths, R. R. (2012). Factor analysis of the Mystical Experience Questionnaire: A study of experiences occasioned by the hallucinogen psilocybin. *J Sci Study Relig, 51*, 721–737.

McKenna, D. J. (2004). Clinical investigations of the therapeutic potential of ayahuasca: Rationale and regulatory challenges. *Pharmacol Ther, 102*, 111–129.

McKenna, D. J., Callaway, J. C., & Grob, C. S. (1998). The scientific investigation of ayahuasca: A review of past and current research. In D. E. Nichols (Ed.), *The Heffter review of psychedelic research* (Vol. 1, pp. 195–223). Santa Fe, NM: Hefftner Research Institute.

McKenna, D. J., Towers, G. H., & Abbott, F. (1984). Monoamine oxidase inhibitors in South American hallucinogenic plants: Tryptamine and beta-carboline constituents of ayahuasca. *J Ethnopharmacol, 10*, 195–223.

Metzner, R. (2005). *Sacred vine of spirits: Ayahuasca*. Rochester, VT: Inner Traditions/Bear & Company.

Minkel, J. D., Krystal, A. D., & Benca, R. M. (2017). Unipolar major depression. In M. Kryger, T. Roth, & W. C. Dement (Eds.), *Principles and practice of sleep medicine* (6th ed., pp. 1352–1362). Philadelphia: Elsevier.

Morales-García, J. A., de la Fuente Revenga, M., Alonso-Gil, S., Rodríguez-Franco, M. I., Feilding, A., Perez-Castillo, A., et al. (2017). The alkaloids of *Banisteriopsis caapi*, the plant source of the Amazonian hallucinogen ayahuasca, stimulate adult neurogenesis in vitro. *Sci Rep, 7*, 5309.

Naranjo, P. (1979). Hallucinogenic plant use and related indigenous belief systems in the Ecuadorian Amazon. *J Ethnopharmacol, 1*, 121–145.

Nunes, A. A., Dos Santos, R. G., Osório, F. L., Sanches, R. F., Crippa, J. A. S., & Hallak, J. E. C. (2016). Effects of ayahuasca and its alkaloids on drug dependence: A systematic literature review of quantitative studies in animals and humans. *J Psychoact Drugs, 48*, 195–205.

Ogalde, J. P., Arriaza, B. T., & Soto, E. C. (2009). Identification of psychoactive alkaloids in ancient Andean human hair by gas chromatography/mass spectrometry. *J Archaeol Sci, 36*, 467–472.

Oliveira, C. D. R., Moreira, C. Q., de Sá, L. R. M., de Spinosa, H, & Yonamine, M. (2010). Maternal and developmental toxicity of ayahuasca in Wistar rats. *Birth Defects Res B Dev Reprod Toxicol, 89*, 207–212.

Oliveira-Lima, A. J., Santos, R., Hollais, A. W., Gerardi-Junior, C. A., Baldaia, M. A., Wuo-Silva, R., et al. (2015). Effects of ayahuasca on the development of ethanol-induced behavioral sensitization and on a post-sensitization treatment in mice. *Physiol Behav, 142*, 28–36.

Osório, F. de L., Sanches, R. F., Macedo, L. R., Dos Santos, R. G., Maia-de-Oliveira, J. P., Wichert-Ana, L., et al. (2015). Antidepressant effects of a single dose of ayahuasca in patients with recurrent depression: A preliminary report. *Rev Bras Psiquiatr, 37*, 13–20.

Pahnke, W. N. (1963). *Drugs and mysticism: An analysis of the relationship between psychedelic drugs and the mystical consciousness: A thesis*. Doctoral dissertation, Harvard University, Cambridge, MA.

Pahnke, W. N. (1969). Psychedelic drugs and mystical experience. *Int Psychiatry Clin, 5*, 149–162.

Palhano-Fontes, F., Barreto, D., Onias, H., Andrade, K. C., Novaes, M. M., Pessoa, J. A., et al. (2019). Rapid antidepressant effects of the psychedelic ayahuasca in treatment-resistant depression: A randomized placebo-controlled trial. *Psychol Med, 49,* 655–663.

Pennes, H. H., & Hoch, P. H. (1957). Psychoto-mimetics, clinical and theoretical consider-ations: Harmine, Win-2299 and nalline. *Am J Psychiatry, 113,* 887–892.

Pic-Taylor, A., da Motta, L. G., de Morais, J. A., Junior, W. M., Santos, A. de F. A., Campos, L. A., et al. (2015). Behavioural and neurotoxic effects of ayahuasca infusion (*Banisteriopsis caapi* and *Psychotria viridis*) in female Wistar rat. *Behav Processes, 118,* 102–110.

Pinkley, H. V. (1969). Plant admixtures to aya-huasca, the South American hallucinogenic drink. *Lloydia, 32,* 305–314.

Pitol, D. L., Siéssere, S., Dos Santos, R. G., Rosa, M. L. N. M., Hallak, J. E. C., Scalize, P. H., et al. (2015). Ayahuasca alters structural param-eters of the rat aorta. *J Cardiovasc Pharmacol, 66,* 58–62.

Rebec, G. V., & Curtis, S. D. (1983). Recipro-cal changes in the firing rate of neostriatal and dorsal raphe neurons following local infusions or systemic injections of D-amphetamine: Evi-dence for neostriatal heterogeneity. *J Neuro-sci, 3,* 2240–2250.

Renelli, M., Fletcher, J., Tupper, K. W., Files, N., Loizaga-Velder, A., & Lafrance, A. (2020). An exploratory study of experiences with conven-tional eating disorder treatment and ceremo-nial ayahuasca for the healing of eating disor-ders. *Eat Weight Disord, 25,* 437–444.

Riba, J., Anderer, P., Jané, F., Saletu, B., & Barbanoj, M. J. (2004). Effects of the South American psychoactive beverage ayahuasca on regional brain electrical activity in humans: A functional neuroimaging study using low-res-olution electromagnetic tomography. *Neuro-psychobiology 50,* 89–101.

Riba, J., Anderer, P., Morte, A., Urbano, G., Jané, F., Saletu, B., et al. (2002). Topographic pharmaco-EEG mapping of the effects of the South American psychoactive beverage aya-huasca in healthy volunteers. *Br J Clin Phar-macol, 53,* 613–628.

Riba, J., Romero, S., Grasa, E., Mena, E., Car-rió, I., & Barbanoj, M. J. (2006). Increased frontal and paralimbic activation following ayahuasca, the pan-Amazonian inebriant. *Psychopharmacology, 186,* 93–98.

Riba, J., Valle, M., Urbano, G., Yritia, M., Morte, A., & Barbanoj, M. J. (2003). Human pharmacology of ayahuasca: Subjective and cardiovascular effects, monoamine metabolite excretion, and pharmacokinetics. *J Pharmacol Exp Ther, 306,* 73–83.

Riga, M. S., Soria, G., Tudela, R., Artigas, F., & Celada, P. (2014). The natural hallucino-gen 5-MeO-DMT, component of ayahuasca, disrupts cortical function in rats: Reversal by antipsychotic drugs. *Int J Neuropsychophar-macol, 17,* 1269–1282.

Rivier, L., & Lindgren, J.-E. (1972). "Ayahuas-ca," the South American hallucinogenic drink: An ethnobotanical and chemical investiga-tion. *Econ Bot, 26,* 101–129.

Rood, L., Roelofs, J., Bögels, S. M., Nolen-Hoeksema, S., & Schouten, E. (2009). The influence of emotion-focused rumination and distraction on depressive symptoms in non-clinical youth: A meta-analytic review. *Clin Psychol Rev, 29,* 607–616.

Sampedro, F., de la Fuente Revenga, M., Valle, M., Roberto, N., Domínguez-Clavé, E., Eli-ces, M., et al. (2017). Assessing the psychedel-ic "after-glow" in ayahuasca users: Post-acute neurometabolic and functional connectivity changes are associated with enhanced mind-fulness capacities. *Int J Neuropsychopharma-col, 20,* 698–711.

Sanches, R. F., de Lima Osório, F., Dos Santos, R. G., Macedo, L. R. H., Maia-de-Oliveira, J. P., Wichert-Ana, L., et al. (2016). Antidepres-sant effects of a single dose of ayahuasca in patients with recurrent depression: A SPECT study. *J Clin Psychopharmacol, 36,* 77–81.

Sanchez-Ramos, J. R. (1991). Banisterine and Parkinson's disease. *Clin Neuropharmacol, 14,* 391–402.

Sanz, C., & Tagliazucchi, E. (2018). The expe-rience elicited by hallucinogens presents the highest similarity to dreaming within a large database of psychoactive substance reports. *Front Neurosci, 12,* 7.

Schenberg, E. E., Alexandre, J. F. M., Filev, R., Cravo, A. M., Sato, J. R., Muthukumaraswa-my, S. D., et al. (2015). Acute biphasic effects of ayahuasca. *PLOS ONE, 10,* e0137202.

Schenberg, E. E., Tófoli, L. F., Rezinovsky, D., & Silveira, D. X. D. A. (2017). Translation and cultural adaptation of the States of Conscious-ness Questionnaire (SOCQ) and statistical validation of the Mystical Experience Ques-tionnaire (MEQ30) in Brazilian Portuguese. *Arch Clin Psychiatry (São Paulo), 44,* 1–5.

Shanon, B. (2002). *The antipodes of the mind: Charting the phenomenology of the ayahuas-ca experience.* Oxford, UK: Oxford University Press.

Sheline, Y. I., Barch, D. M., Price, J. L., Rundle, M. M., Vaishnavi, S. N., Snyder, A. Z., et al. (2009). The default mode network and self-referential processes in depression. *Proc Natl Acad Sci USA, 106,* 1942–1947.

Soler, J., Elices, M., Franquesa, A., Barker, S.,

Friedlander, P., Feilding, A., et al. (2016). Exploring the therapeutic potential of Ayahuasca: Acute intake increases mindfulness-related capacities. *Psychopharmacology, 233,* 823–829.

Steward, J. H. (1963). *Handbook of South American Indians: The comparative ethnology of South American Indians* (Vol. 143). New York: Cooper Square.

Strassman, R. J., Qualls, C. R., Uhlenhuth, E. H., & Kellner, R. (1994). Dose–response study of *N,N*-dimethyltryptamine in humans: II. Subjective effects and preliminary results of a new rating scale. *Arch Gen Psychiatry, 51,* 98–108.

Szabo, A., & Frecska, E. (2016). Dimethyltryptamine (DMT): A biochemical Swiss Army knife in neuroinflammation and neuroprotection? *Neural Regeneration Res, 11,* 396–397.

Szabo, A., Kovacs, A., Frecska, E., & Rajnavolgyi, E. (2014). Psychedelic *N,N*-dimethyltryptamine and 5-methoxy-*N,N*-dimethyltryptamine modulate innate and adaptive inflammatory responses through the sigma-1 receptor of human monocyte-derived dendritic cells. *PLOS ONE, 9,* e106533.

Szára, S. (2007). DMT at fifty. *Neuropsychopharmacol Hung, 9,* 201–205.

Taussig, M. T. (1987). *Xamanismo, colonialismo e o homem selvagem: Um estudo sobre o terror e a cura.* Rio de Janeiro, Brazil: Paz e Terra.

Thomas, G., Lucas, P., Capler, N. R., Tupper, K. W., & Martin, G. (2013). Ayahuasca-assisted therapy for addiction: Results from a preliminary observational study in Canada. *Curr Drug Abuse Rev, 6,* 30–42.

Trulson, M. E., & Jacobs, B. L. (1979). Effects of 5-methoxy-*N,N*-dimethyltryptamine on behavior and raphe unit activity in freely moving cats. *Eur J Pharmacol, 54,* 43–50.

Uthaug, M. V., van Oorsouw, K., Kuypers, K. P. C., van Boxtel, M., Broers, N. J., Mason, N. L., et al. (2018). Sub-acute and long-term effects of ayahuasca on affect and cognitive thinking style and their association with ego dissolution. *Psychopharmacology, 235,* 2979–2989.

Villavicencio, M. (1858). *Geografía de la república del Ecuador.* New York: Imprenta de Robert Craighead.

Viol, A., Palhano-Fontes, F., Onias, H., de Araujo, D. B., & Viswanathan, G. M. (2017). Shannon entropy of brain functional complex networks under the influence of the psychedelic Ayahuasca. *Sci Rep, 7,* 7388.

Vollenweider, F. X., & Kometer, M. (2010). The neurobiology of psychedelic drugs: Implications for the treatment of mood disorders. *Nat Rev Neurosci, 11,* 642–651.

Wallace, A. R., & Spruce, R. (1908). *Notes of a botanist on the Amazon and Andes.* London: Macmillan.

Watts, A. (2011). *The wisdom of insecurity: A message for an age of anxiety.* New York: Vintage Books.

Winkelman, M. J. (2014). Therapeutic applications of ayahuasca and other sacred medicines. In B. C. Labate & C. Cavnar (Eds.), *The therapeutic use of ayahuasca* (pp. 1–21). Berlin: Springer.

CHAPTER 15

The Ibogaine Project
Urban Ethnomedicine for Opioid Use Disorder

KENNETH ALPER

History

Ibogaine is a monoterpene indole alkaloid that occurs in the root bark of *Tabernanthe iboga Baill*. As a small molecule with apparent clinical effects in the alleviation of opioid withdrawal and diminution of drug self-administration, and an unknown and apparently novel mechanism of action, ibogaine offers an interesting prototype for drug discovery and neurobiological investigation.

In Gabon and elsewhere in West Central Africa, ibogaine has been ingested in the form of *eboga*, scrapings of *Tabernanthe iboga* root bark, as a psychoactive sacrament in the Bwiti religion for several centuries, and likely among Pygmies in much earlier times (Fernandez, 1982). The ritual aim of eating eboga has been conceptualized

Ibogaine

as "binding" across time through "the work of the ancestors," and across space, socially on the basis of a common experience of a distinctive consciousness (Fernandez & Fernandez, 2001). In the colonial era, Bwiti offered a dignified realm of spiritual endeavor that supported psychological resistance to the anomie and dislocation imposed by the colonial presence and became constellated with Gabonese national identity.

Outside of Africa, ibogaine has been used most frequently for the treatment of substance use disorders, specifically for detoxification from opioids. Ibogaine has a storied past and an association with controversy, and the medical and nonmedical settings that have been collectively designated as a "vast uncontrolled experiment" (Vastag, 2005) or "medical subculture" (Alper et al., 2008). Ibogaine has been classified as a hallucinogen and as illegal in the United States since 1967 and is similarly scheduled in nine of the 27 countries presently in the European Union. As of this writing ibogaine is unregulated (i.e., it is neither officially approved nor illegal in much of the rest of the world). New Zealand, Canada, Brazil, and South Africa have classified ibogaine as a pharmaceutical substance and restrict its use to licensed medical practitioners. In Australia and Canada ibogaine is unapproved but is classified as a pharmaceutical compound that may be prescribed by a physician who obtains a specific regulatory exemption on the basis of medical need. Apparently no physician in either country has sought to prescribe ibogaine utilizing this regulatory mechanism to date. A systematic survey and description of the known settings of ibogaine use as of 2006 indicated that approximately 3,400 individuals had taken ibogaine, 68% of whom did so for the treatment of a substance-related disorder, 53% specifically for opioid detoxification (Alper et al., 2008). Now, over a decade later the total number treated has likely increased severalfold.

The ethnopharmacological paradigm of drug discovery begins with observational evidence of a clinical effect in an indigenous context of use, followed by subsequent identification and isolation of the active agent, or possible synthesis of derivatives as candidates for development. With regard to ibogaine in the treatment of addiction, the indigenous context of this urban ethnomedicine is distinct from the use of *T. iboga* as a religious sacrament in Africa. The majority of participants in the ibogaine medical subculture are dependent on opioids. The sacramental alkaloid is used in the hydrochloride form, the ritual aim is opioid detoxification, and ritual space is a clinic outside the United States, or an apartment or hotel room.

In June 1962, in Brooklyn (the exact date is not recalled), Howard Lotsof, a 19-year-old heroin-dependent lay drug experimenter in an era in which hallucinogens had not yet been regulated, serendipitously experienced the resolution of withdrawal following the use of ibogaine (Alper et al., 2001; Lotsof, 1985). Lotsof, an engaging and intrepid provocateur of scientific curiosity, credentialed only with a New York University film degree, was eventually able to convince the National Institute on Drug Abuse (NIDA) to support a project of research on ibogaine, with a total of approximately 2 million USD in direct cost support. During its existence from 1991 to 1996, the NIDA ibogaine project supported preclinical contract work, including toxicology and pharmacokinetics that enabled a privately funded Phase I study

of single dosages of ibogaine for cocaine dependence that was approved by the U.S. Food and Drug Administration (FDA) in 1993. This study ended in contractual and intellectual property disputes (Mash, 1997) and dosages of 1 and 2mg/kg were without reported adverse events (Mash, Kovera, et al., 1998). Data from that study regarding a possible effect of ibogaine on drug use is apparently unavailable. NIDA eventually terminated its ibogaine research program in 1996, and no subsequent clinical research with ibogaine has been conducted in the United States.

Beginning in 2012, NIDA has committed a total of over 6 million USD for the development of 18-methoxycoronaridine (18-MC), an apparently safer structural analogue discovered by rational design (National Institutes of Health, 2012). 18-MC differs from ibogaine at three of the 21 positions on the ibogamine skeleton that define the iboga alkaloid class (Figure 15.1) (Le Men & Taylor, 1965). NIDA has supported preclinical toxicology, pharmacokinetics, and chemical manufacturing and control work, which now enables a Phase I/II study, the next developmental step at the present time.

■ Ibogaine Treatment

Dosing and Monitoring

Ibogaine is used most frequently for detoxification from opioids, typically administered in the HCl form in a range of approximately 94–98% purity according to certificates of analyses. Crude extracts of *T. iboga* root bark vary with regarded to estimated total alkaloid content, which is typically between 15 and 50%, about 25–50% of which might be expected to be ibogaine (Alper et al., 2008; Alper, Stajic, & Gill, 2012). Other iboga alkaloids co-occurring with ibogaine in *T. iboga* root bark include ibogamine, ibogaline, tabernanthine and voacangine (Bartlett et al., 1958), and are present to a variable extent in extracts (see Figure 15.1).

As described in an observational study (Brown & Alper, 2018), the "test–flood–booster" opioid detoxification protocol presently in common use begins with a "test" dose of ibogaine on the order of approximately 3 mg/kg, typically administered

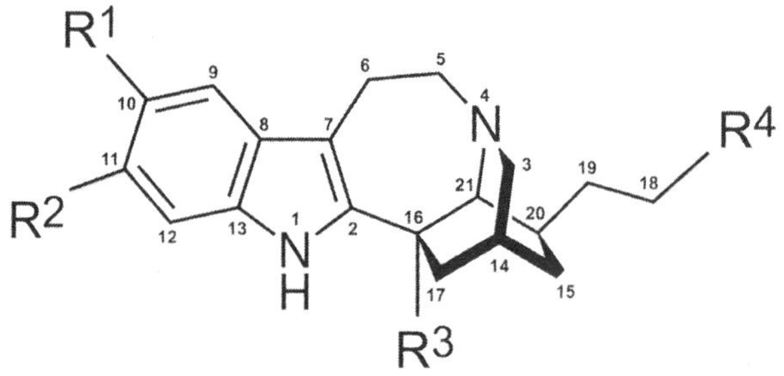

Compound	R^1	R^2	R^3	R^4
Ibogamine	H	H	H	H
Ibogaine	OCH$_3$	H	H	H
Noribogaine	OH	H	H	H
Ibogaline	OCH$_3$	OCH$_3$	H	H
Tabernanthine	H	OCH$_3$	H	H
Voacangine	OCH$_3$	H	CO$_2$CH$_3$	H
Coronaridine	H	H	CO$_2$CH$_3$	H
18-Methoxycoronaridine	H	H	CO$_2$CH$_3$	OCH$_3$

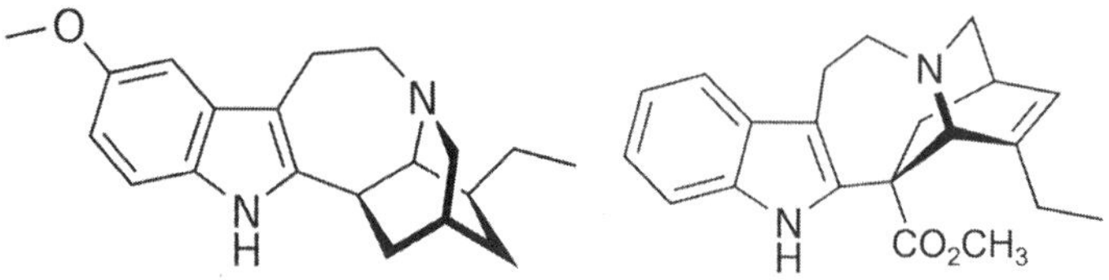

Ibogaine   Catharanthine

■ FIGURE 15.1. (A) Ibogaine and other iboga alkaloids and structural analogues numbered using the Le Men and Taylor (1965) system. Ibogamine is the parent iboga alkaloid structural skeleton. Ibogamine, ibogaline, tabernanthine, voacangine co-occur with ibogaine in *T. iboga*. Noribogaine is ibogaine's major metabolite. Coronaridine also occurs naturally. 18-Methoxycoronaridine (18-MC) is a synthetic congener. (B) Ibogaine and catharanthine, another iboga alkaloid of pharmacological importance belonging to an opposite optical series.

in the morning after a subjects has abstained from opioid use overnight, and begins to exhibit some initial signs of withdrawal. The providers appear to view the response to the test dose, which typically has some effect of reducing withdrawal signs, as providing some indication of the degree of physical dependence on opioids. A "flood" ibogaine dose, typically four times the test dose, is given 2–12 hours following the test dose. Additional "booster" dosages of ibogaine of 3–5 mg/kg may follow the flood dose at intervals in a range from 1 to 16 hours, with the intention either to alleviate residual or reemergent withdrawal symptoms, or to increase the intensity of the psychoactive experience.

The total dosages of ibogaine administered in recent observational studies (Brown & Alper, 2018; Noller et al., 2018) are very similar to those used in prior treatments in the United States in the 1960s and the Netherlands in the late 1980s (Alper et al., 1999), even though subjects in the present era use larger amounts of heroin that is of substantially greater purity (U.S. Drug Enforcement Administration, 2016). In the earlier era, nearly all of the total ibogaine dosage was administered at once. The test–flood–booster approach appears to be an adaptation intended toward maximizing dose efficiency in the face of severe levels of physiological dependence, and suggests that contemporary treatment providers perceive a dose ceiling, possibly due to a greater awareness of medical risk (Alper, Stajic, & Gill, 2012; Dickinson et al., 2016).

A set of clinical guidelines for detoxification from opioids with ibogaine has been developed by the Global Ibogaine Therapy Alliance (GITA), a group of physicians and lay ibogaine treatment providers (Dickinson et al., 2016). Briefly, the guidelines recommend pretreatment evaluation that includes a medical history, electrocardiogram (EKG), and electrolyte and liver function tests. Intravenous access, continuous pulse oximetry and three-lead EKG, and monitoring of blood pressure are recommended throughout the treatment, with a medical professional (MD, nurse, or paramedic) certified in Advanced Cardiac Life Support (ACLS) present for at least the first 24 hours of the treatment. While the guidelines are unfortunately not followed across all of the varied settings in which ibogaine treatment is available, the emergence of an organized attempt by providers themselves to develop standards for ibogaine treatment is notable. A GITA conference in 2016 featured a training course in ACLS certification led by credentialed instructors.

Clinical Evidence of Efficacy

Ibogaine has been administered most often for opioid detoxification (Alper et al., 2008). A substantive ibogaine treatment effect is reported in two early case series. In a series of 33 opioid detoxification treatment episodes in nonmedical settings with single mean dosages of 19.3 mg/kg, full resolution of opioid withdrawal signs and symptoms without drug-seeking behavior over a 72-hour post-treatment interval was observed in 25 of 33 patients. Another study of 32 patients treated in a medical setting for the indication of opioid detoxification with fixed dosages of 800 mg reported the resolution of withdrawal of opioid withdrawal signs as indicated by physician-rated structured instruments at 24 hours, with sustained reductions in subjective ratings of withdrawal symptoms during the week following treatment (Mash et al., 2001).

In two unpublished case series, ibogaine appeared effective in opioid detoxification, and about one-third of subjects reported abstinence from opioids for periods of 6 months or longer following treatment. In a series of 52 outcomes assessed by interview following single dosages of ibogaine that became a basis for NIDA's decision to undertake its ibogaine project from 1991 to 1995, individuals reported cessation of use of the substances for which ibogaine treatment had been sought for 2–6 months in 30 cases (57%), and over 6 months in 17 cases (32%) (Alper, 2001). The other series, summarized in an academic thesis, is 21 subjects who responded to a Web-based questionnaire adapted from the European Addiction Severity Index at a mean interval of 21.8 months following treatment with ibogaine (Bastiaans, 2004). Of the 17 of 21 patients (81%) who identified opioids as the primary substance for which they had sought treatment, five reported abstinence from all substances, and another nine reported abstinence from their primary substance of dependence while continuing to use alcohol or cannabis after treatment with ibogaine.

A prospective observational study reported on 1-year follow-up of 30 individuals treated with ibogaine for opioid detoxification with mean amount total of $1,540 \pm 920$ mg ibogaine HCl administered according to a test–flood–booster dosing scheme (Brown & Alper, 2018). The subjects in this study were heavy opioid users with histories of failure with conventional treatment. The subjects used mainly oxycodone ($n = 21$; 70%) and/or heroin ($n = 18$; 60%) in respective amounts of 250 ± 180 mg/day and 1.3 ± 0.94 g/day, with a mean of 3.1 ± 2.6 prior previous episodes of treatment for opioid dependence. The Subjective Opioid Withdrawal Scale (SOWS; Handelsman et al., 1987) was used to assess detoxification outcome, and Addiction Severity Index Composite (ASIC) scores (McGahan et al., 1986) were used to assess posttreatment effects at 1, 3, 6, 9, and 12 months.

Assessed just prior to the test ibogaine dose, the pretreatment baseline SOWS score decreased a mean of 17 points, from 31.0 to 14.0 at 76.5 ± 30 hours following the initiation of treatment. This clinical effect of ibogaine on acute withdrawal symptoms appeared consistent with prior results and to be of a comparable order of magnitude to that of methadone reported in the original study

that described the development and validation of the SOWS (Handelsman et al., 1987).
In that study, subjects were administered the
SOWS following 2 days of methadone stabilization. SOWS decreased by a mean of 18.7
points (from 24.3 to 5.6) in subjects who
used opioid exclusively, and 8.7 points (from
23.1 to 14.4) in subjects who additionally
abused other, nonopioid substances.

The numbers of subjects who reported no
opioid use during the previous 30 days at
respective posttreatment time intervals of 1
and 3 months were 15 (50%) and 10 (33%).
This appears to be a substantive treatment
effect in comparison to those reported in
the published literature. For example, recent systematic reviews of studies of opioid
detoxification without subsequent maintenance treatment found rates of abstaining
from illicit opioid use of 18% at 4 weeks following detoxification with buprenorphine
(Bentzley et al., 2015), and 26% at 6 weeks
following detoxification with methadone
(Amato et al., 2013). Figure 15.2 plots individual trajectories of the ASIC Drug Use
score from pretreatment baseline to 1, 3, 6,
9, and 12 months. The figure indicates an
apparently sustained posttreatment effect on
opioid use in a subset of subjects, evident as
trajectories characterized by large decreases

from baseline to 1 month that are sustained
at subsequent time points.

Other relatively recent work, conducted in
New Zealand with a design similar to that
discussed earlier but on a smaller subject
population (n = 14) reported comparable
outcomes regarding SOWS ASIC Drug Use
scores in subjects followed up for 1 year
(Noller et al., 2018). The study also included
assessment with the Beck Depression Inventory, which indicated progressive improvement throughout the interval of follow-up.

Reported studies on ibogaine as treatment
for substance use disorders have been uncontrolled and reliant on self-report, without
laboratory verification. While laboratory
verification will be a necessary feature in future efforts to develop ibogaine or its structural derivatives, self-reporting in clinical
research on substance use disorders can be
accurate (Darke, 1998), particularly when
there are no negative consequences to the
subject for reporting use. Reported detoxification outcomes appear valid. The clinical expression of acute opioid withdrawal
evolves acutely over a limited time frame,
tends to be robust in its expression, and can
be assessed accurately by lay providers in the
settings in which ibogaine is administered
(Alper et al., 2008). Patient self-reports also

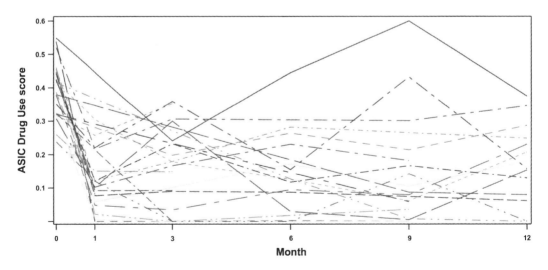

■ FIGURE 15.2. Individual trajectories of the Addiction Severity Index Composite Drug Use score in
patients at 1-, 3-, 6-, 9-, and 12-month follow-up after opioid detoxification with ibogaine (Brown
& Alper, 2017) (n = 30).

suggest a substantive, pharmacologically mediated effect of ibogaine, especially in view of the lack of a significant effect of placebo in opioid detoxification (Amato et al., 2013; Gowing et al., 2016, 2017).

Preclinical Evidence of Efficacy

There are more than 50 published studies of ibogaine or its structural analogues 18-MC or noribogaine in animal models of drug self-administration or opiate withdrawal. Consistent with its apparent effect in opioid detoxification in humans, ibogaine administered intraperitoneally or intracerebrally to animals reduces naloxone- or naltrexone-precipitated opioid withdrawal signs in rats (Cappendijk et al., 1994; Dzoljic et al., 1988; Glick et al., 1992; Parker et al., 2002), mice (Frances et al., 1992; Layer et al., 1996; Leal et al., 2003; Popik et al., 1995), and primates (Aceto et al., 1992; Koja et al., 1996). Single dosages of ibogaine administered to rodents diminish self-administration of multiple abused substances, including morphine (Belgers et al., 2016; Glick et al., 1991, 1994, 1996), heroin (Dworkin et al., 1995), cocaine (Cappendijk & Dzoljic, 1993; Glick et al., 1994, 1996; Maisonneuve & Glick, 1992; Sershen et al., 1994), amphetamine (Maisonneuve, Keller, & Glick, 1992), and alcohol (Rezvani et al., 1995), with normal responding for water. A meta-analysis of 30 animal studies of the effect of ibogaine on drug self-administration of morphine, alcohol, or cocaine found a significant effect on drug self-administration across studies that was greatest at 24 hours but persisted for > 72 hours (Belgers et al., 2016). Sustained effects on morphine self-administration for even longer time intervals have been observed in individual animals (Glick et al., 1991).

Both ibogaine and 18-MC diminish an experimental pharmacological correlate of drug salience, the sensitized response of dopamine efflux in the nucleus accumbens in response to morphine (Maisonneuve & Glick, 1999; Maisonneuve et al., 1991) and nicotine (Glick et al., 1998; Maisonneuve et al., 1997). Ibogaine has had no significance on conditioned place preference, an animal behavioral model of drug craving (Belgers et al., 2016).

Subjective Effects: Phenomenology, Neurophysiology, and Ibogaine as a Psychotherapeutic Adjunct

Historically, the use of ibogaine in the medical model began in the 1950s, when clinicians and researchers viewed ibogaine much as they did other compounds classified as hallucinogens. Some, such as Jan Bastiaans, MD (Snelders & Kaplan, 2002), Leo Zeff, PhD (Stolaroff, 2004), and Claudio Naranjo, MD (1973), were interested in ibogaine as an adjunct to psychotherapy. Ibogaine, like other hallucinogens, was of interest as an experimental model of psychosis (Fabing, 1956; Salmoiraghi & Page, 1957; Schneider & Sigg, 1957; Turner et al., 1955). As with other hallucinogens, ibogaine may have also been investigated for military or intelligence purposes as a "truth serum," or a means of "brainwashing" or incapacitating an adversary, which was the focus the U.S. Central Intelligence Agency project MKULTRA (Isbell, 1955; U.S. Senate, 1977).

French chemist Robert Goutarel hypothesized that ibogaine produces a state with functional aspects shared by the brain states of rapid eye movement (REM) sleep (Goutarel et al., 1993). Descriptions of subjective experiences associated with ibogaine have been designated as "oneiric" and likened to a "waking dream," with interrogatory verbal exchanges involving ancestral and archetypal beings, and movement and navigation within visual landscapes. Another frequently described experience is *panoramic memory*, the recall of a rapid, dense succession of vivid autobiographical visual memories, which has been termed "the slide show." Mechanistically, these subjective experiences associated with ibogaine possibly suggest functional muscarinic cholinergic effects, which are prominent in the mechanisms of dreaming and memory (Cantero et al., 2003).

Ibogaine is reported to enhance spatial memory retrieval in animals (Helsley et al., 1997; Popik, 1996), and produces an atropine-sensitive electroencephalographic (EEG) rhythm (Depoortere, 1987; Schneider & Sigg, 1957). The atropine-sensitive EEG rhythm is regarded as an animal model of REM sleep and attributed to muscarinic cholinergic input from the ascending reticular activating system (ARAS; Leung, 1998), and has been suggested to involve the inhibition of acetylcholinesterase (AChE) by ibogaine (Schneider & Sigg, 1957). More recent work indicates that ibogaine does not inhibit AChE (Alper, Reith, & Sershen, 2012), suggesting the possibility that functional muscarinic cholinergic effect may be mediated by modulation of signaling downstream from the receptor itself.

Individuals who have taken ibogaine frequently report that memories and other mental representations that have previously been associated with troubling emotions such as fear, or shame, or anger are experienced with equanimity, allowing a reevaluation and reprocessing of their content (Heink et al., 2017). As memorably expressed by one individual reflecting on her ibogaine treatment for dependence on opioids, "It's as if all information in your brain file cabinet is shaken out of its drawers on to one big pile, looked at 'objectively' and put back in, untwisted from emotional trauma" (Lotsof & Alexander, 2001). Equanimity is also a prevalent theme in Bwiti. Ritual outcomes and transactions with ancestors involving the use of eboga are described (utilizing Fernandez's translations) with terms such as "evenhandedness," "tranquilheartedness," or "oneheartedness." The quality of equanimity attributed to ancestral contact is evident in a Fang Bwiti poem (Fernandez, 1982), "Joy, the ancestors give joyful welcome and hear the news. The troubled life of the born ones is finished. . . . All the misfortunes are shorn away. They leave. Everything clean. All is new. All is bright. I have seen the dead and I do not fear."

Narratives of individuals treated with ibogaine appear consonant with themes of "oneheartedness" and "binding" to family and ancestors represented in Bwiti. A study that utilized ASIC scores found that Family/Social the most improved ASI composite factor apart from Drug Use (Brown & Alper, 2018). Lotsof provides a descriptive example of the clinical phenomenon of delayed benefit with ibogaine (Lotsof & Alexander, 2001), and suggests the interval of delay might correspond to the ongoing processing and behavioral integration of the psychoactive experience produced by ibogaine.

◼ Toxicology

Cardiotoxicity

Ibogaine has been associated with fatalities (Alper, Stajic, & Gill, 2012; Koenig & Hilber, 2015). Ibogaine and its major metabolite noribogaine prolong the QT interval of the EKG. The QT interval corresponds to ventricular repolarization between cardiac contractions, during which the electrical potential of the cardiac myocyte becomes more negative, inhibiting cell firing. With depolarization, the electrical potential in the cardiac myocyte becomes more positive and excitatory, resulting in cell firing and the action potential that underlies ventricular contraction. With prolongation of the QT interval, cardiac myocytes may escape control of the cardiac conduction system and depolarize spontaneously. QT prolongation is viewed as a correlate of cardiac instability, a loss of "repolarization reserve" (Roden & Yang, 2005), and is associated with polymorphic ventricular tachycardia (PVT), including torsades de pointes (TdP), a morphologically distinctive type of PVT that can progress to ventricular fibrillation and death (Kannankeril et al., 2010).

Repolarization of the cardiac myocyte depends importantly on the movement of positively charged potassium ions out of the cell through voltage-gated cardiac potassium channels. The protein that constitutes the pore of the channel is encoded by the human ether-a-go-go-related gene (hERG), hence the term hERG channel, and hERG blockade is the major cause of drug-induced QT prolongation and TdP (Kannankeril et al., 2010). Ibogaine and its major metabolite noribogaine block the hERG channel with comparable potency (Alper et al., 2016; Koenig & Hilber, 2015). Reported half-maximal inhibitory concentration (IC$_{50}$) values for 99.5% ibogaine produced by semisynthesis via voacangine, 95% ibogaine produced from extraction of T. iboga and noribogaine are 4.09 μM, 3.53 μM, and 2.86 μM, respectively. 18-MC produces substantially less hERG blockade (IC$_{50}$ > 50 μM) (Alper et al., 2016).

The reported values for IC$_{50}$ for hERG blockade by ibogaine and noribogaine appear clinically relevant. The half-life ($T_{1/2}$) of ibogaine in humans is estimated to be 4–7 hours (Kontrimaviĉiūtė et al., 2006; Mash et al., 2001), and the $T_{1/2}$ of noribogaine is apparently considerably longer than that of the parent compound, possibly on the order of days (Glue et al., 2015). In a sample of 24 subjects who were orally administered ibogaine dosages of 10mg/kg, mean peak blood levels for ibogaine and noribogaine, respectively, were 2.4 µM and 3.2 µM (Mash et al., 2001). From a postmortem series of 19 fatalities, the subset of 10 cases in which blood ibogaine levels were available, the mean was 7.6 µM (range 0.77–30 µM), and in the two cases for which they were available, noribogaine levels were 13.4 and 18.8 µM (Alper, Stajic, & Gill, 2012). Although the interpretation of levels from postmortem studies may be complicated by redistribution and taking into account that ibogaine is 65% protein-bound (Koenig et al., 2013), ibogaine or noribogaine may produce significant *hERG* channel blockade at clinically relevant concentrations (Koenig et al., 2013).

Bradycardia heightens the risk for fatal cardiac arrhythmia, including TdP (Cubeddu, 2009) and has been observed following administration of ibogaine in medical (Mash, Allen-Ferdinand, et al., 1998) and nonmedical (Samorini, 1998) settings, and in preclinical studies (Binienda et al., 1998; Dhahir, 1971; Glick et al., 1999; Schneider & Rinehart, 1957). Both laboratory models and multiple clinical case reports indicate that hypokalemia is a particularly important factor in the genesis of arrhythmia associated with ibogaine (Koenig & Hilber, 2015). A case of TdP in the setting of severe depletion of potassium from serum and tissue stores due to the aggressive use of cathartics prior to ibogaine treatment, in which lengthening of the QT interval, bradycardia, and ventricular tachydysrhythmias appeared to track potassium levels over an interval of 7 days illustrates the importance of potassium in ibogaine-related cardiac arrhythmia, as well as the idiosyncratic hazards associated with the unconventional settings in which ibogaine is often administered (Shawn et al., 2012).

Drug-induced TdP is typically multifactorial, involving multiple determinants of cardiac rhythm instability in addition to *hERG* blockade (Kannankeril et al., 2010), which

has been generally been the case with regard to fatalities temporally related to ingestion of ibogaine. Preexisting cardiovascular medical comorbidities appear to have been particularly prominent in deaths temporally associated with the administration of ibogaine (Alper, Stajic, & Gill, 2012). The role of preexisting advanced medical comorbidities as contributing causes in ibogaine-related deaths may also be paralleling a general association of risk of fatal overdose with systemic disease (Darke et al., 2006). For example, ibogaine-related fatalities have been associated with cardiac hypertrophy and atherosclerotic disease (Alper, Stajic, & Gill, 2012), which are associated with chronic methamphetamine and cocaine use (Kaye et al., 2007; Knuepfer, 2003). Additional factors that commonly contribute to cardiac instability in chronic substance-related disorders include various co-ingestants, systemic medical conditions, such as liver or respiratory disease, seizures, hypomagnesemia, or withdrawal from cocaine or alcohol (Cubeddu, 2009; Kannankeril et al., 2010; Levin et al., 2008; Otero-Anton et al., 1997).

Neurotoxicity

Degeneration of cerebellar Purkinje cells were observed in rats given substantially larger dosages of ibogaine than those used to study drug self-administration and withdrawal (O'Hearn & Molliver, 1993). Ibogaine activates the release of glutamate by neurons in the inferior olive, resulting in degeneration of the Purkinje cells in the cerebellum, which are vulnerable to excitotoxic injury due to the redundancy of inputs to cerebellar Purkinje cells, an effect that may be potentiated by ibogaine's [σιγμα]$_2$ agonist activity (Bowen, 2001; O'Hearn & Molliver, 1997). Subsequent research found no evidence of neurotoxicity in the primate (Mash, Kovera, et al., 1998) or mouse (Scallet et al., 1996) at dosages that produced cerebellar degeneration in the rat, or in the rat at dosages used in studies of drug self-administration and withdrawal (Molinari et al., 1996). The FDA was aware of the work that indicated the neurotoxic effect of high dosages of ibogaine in the rat at the time it approved a Phase I study in which humans received ibogaine (Alper, 2001). Clinical or postmortem evidence does not appear to suggest a characteristic syndrome of neurotoxicity (Alper, Stajic, & Gill, 2012).

Mechanism of Action

Distinct from Medications Known to Have Clinical Effects in Opioid Use Disorder

The mechanism of action of ibogaine is unknown and apparently novel and unexplained by actions of medications known to have clinical effects in opioid tolerance or withdrawal. Clinical observations suggest that ibogaine is not acting as a μ-opioid receptor (MOR) agonist. Doses of ibogaine sufficient to detoxify individuals with severe physical dependence do not produce signs of overdose in opioid-naive individuals (Alper et al., 2008). If ibogaine were acting as an opioid agonist, it would not be tolerated by opioid-naive individuals because the methadone dosage of 60–100 mg per day that is used to stabilize withdrawal symptoms in the maintenance treatment of opioid-dependent patients (Fareed et al., 2010) substantially exceeds the estimated the lethal dose, 50% (LD_{50}) of 40–50 mg in humans who are not pharmacologically tolerant to opioids (Corkery et al., 2004).

Although ibogaine, its major metabolite noribogaine, and 18-MC bind with low micromolar affinity to the MOR, they are neither orthosteric nor allosteric MOR agonists assessed by guanosine-5′-O-(γ-thio)-triphosphate ([^{35}S]GTPγS)-binding in cells expressing the MOR (Antonio et al., 2013). The potentiation of morphine analgesia by ibogaine in the animal model, without producing analgesia when administered alone, also suggests that ibogaine may alter signaling through opioid receptors but is not itself an orthosteric agonist (Bagal et al., 1996; Bhargava et al., 1997; Cao & Bhargava, 1997; Frances et al., 1992; Schneider, 1957; Schneider & McArthur, 1956; Sunder Sharma & Bhargava, 1998). Although the potentiation of morphine without analgesia when administered alone might be consistent with an effect as allosteric MOR agonist, these compounds do not potentiate the activation of G proteins by morphine or DAMGO (Antonio et al., 2013), indicating they do not act as allosteric MOR agonists.

Some evidence suggests that ibogaine might possibly modify neuroadaptations associated with chronic exposure to opioids, such as the apparent reversal of analgesic tolerance to chronic morphine by ibogaine (Pearl et al., 1995; Schneider, 1957; Sunder Sharma & Bhargava, 1998). Ibogaine and noribogaine diminish tolerance in morphine-tolerant mice (Bhargava & Cao, 1997; Cao & Bhargava, 1997; Sunder Sharma & Bhargava, 1998), and dose-dependently potentiate the antinociceptive effect of morphine in morphine-tolerant but not in morphine-naive mice (Sunder Sharma & Bhargava, 1998). Ibogaine has relatively selective effects on decreasing dopamine efflux in the nucleus accumbens (Pearl et al., 1996) and locomotor activity (Maisonneuve, Rossman, et al., 1992; Pearl et al., 1995) in morphine-tolerant versus nontolerant rats. Ibogaine's clinical effect of opioid detoxification without causing opioid overdose in nontolerant individuals also suggests selectivity for neuroadaptations associated with prior exposure.

Ibogaine is an N-methyl-D-aspartate (NMDA) receptor antagonist (Popik et al., 1995; Skolnick, 2001), and NMDA antagonists such as memantine diminish signs of opioid withdrawal in preclinical models (Trujillo & Akil, 1994) and humans (Bisaga et al., 2001). However, 18-MC, which lacks significant affinity for the NMDA receptor, is equally effective as ibogaine in animal models of opioid withdrawal (Cappendijk et al., 1994; Dzoljic et al., 1988; Glick et al., 1992, 2001; Panchal et al., 2005; Parker et al., 2002; Rho & Glick, 1998). Ibogaine has no significant affinity for the α_2 adrenergic receptor (Deecher et al., 1992; Sweetnam et al., 1995) or imidazoline I_2 site (MacInnes & Handley, 2002), indicating that it does not act as an imidazoline α_2 adrenergic receptor agonist such as clonidine.

Distinct from Other Compounds Designated as "Psychedelic"

Although ibogaine is designated as a hallucinogen and subsumed under the rubric of "psychedelics," it is pharmacologically distinct from the classical hallucinogens such as lysergic acid diethylamide (LSD), mescaline, or psilocybin, which are thought to act by binding as agonists to the serotonin type 2A (5-HT$_{2A}$) receptor (Nichols, 2016). The 5-HT$_{2A}$ receptor is nonessential for recognition of the ibogaine stimulus in drug discrimination studies (Helsley et al., 1998). Serotonin agonist or releasing activity does not appear to explain ibogaine's effects in opioid withdrawal (Glick et al., 2001; Wei et al., 1998). There appears to be no clinical evidence of the apparent effect of classical hallucinogens in opioid detoxification, and in the animal model ablation of 90% of the raphe, the major serotonergic nucleus of the brain does not significantly affect the expression of opioid withdrawal (Caille et al., 2002).

Although harmine does have an effect of diminution of antagonist-precipitated opioid withdrawal in rats, this effect is apparently due to its action of imidazoline I$_2$ receptor agonist (Aricioglu-Kartal et al., 2003). Ibogaine, in contrast, has no affinity at the I$_2$ receptor. In contrast to harmine, ibogaine does not inhibit monoamine oxidase A (MAOA) (Nelson et al., 1979).

The α3β4 Nicotinic Acetylcholine Receptor (nAChR), Neurotrophins

The enhanced expression of glial-derived neurotrophic factor (GDNF) has been proposed to account for ibogaine's effect on drug self-administration (He et al., 2005). Ibogaine increases GDNF expression *in vivo* and in cultured cells, and 18-MC reportedly does not (Carnicella et al., 2010), but both compounds are equally effective in animal models of drug self-administration (Glick et al., 2001). Ibogaine's action as an allosteric antagonist of the α3β4 nAChR is suggested to mediate its effect on drug self-administration (Glick et al., 2002), but does not appear to readily explain the prolonged effects that appear to persist beyond pharmacokinetic elimination (Pearl et al., 1997). Ibogaine's major metabolite, noribogaine has a longer half-life than the parent compound (Baumann et al., 2001; Glue et al., 2015), and has been suggested to account for persistence of effects on drug self-administration and withdrawal (Mash et al., 2016), although in the animal model, the effect of ibogaine in reducing drug self-administration appears to persist beyond the elimination of ibogaine

and noribogaine from serum or brain tissue (Pearl et al., 1997).

Adenylate Cyclase

Ibogaine may act downstream from receptor-coupled G protein activation to mediate effects on opioid withdrawal that are unexplained in view of the its lack of agonist activity at the MOR. Adenylate cyclase (AC) is one plausible target of ibogaine. The MOR is negatively coupled to AC via Gαi, and the inhibition of AC is a cardinal opioid agonist signaling effect, as is the AC "superactivation" or "overshoot" of increased production of cyclic adenosine monophosphate (cAMP) in opioid withdrawal (Christie, 2008; Nestler, 2001; Sharma et al., 1975). Ibogaine potentiates the inhibition of AC by morphine (Rabin & Winter, 1996), which may be consistent with its observed clinical effect in opioid withdrawal. The potentiation of morphine analgesia by ibogaine and noribogaine without analgesia when administered alone is also consistent with a possible effect of inhibition of AC in view of the upregulation of AC in pain sensitization associated with opioid withdrawal (Bie et al., 2005) and the analgesic effects of drugs that inhibit AC (Pierre et al., 2009; Zhuo, 2012). A hypothesis that iboga alkaloids could inhibit AC might explain why ibogaine does not itself produce signs of opioid overdose but potentiates the toxicity of coadministered opioids (Alper, Stajic, & Gill, 2012; Bhargava & Cao, 1997; Dhahir, 1971; MPI Research, 1996; Schneider & McArthur, 1956).

■ What Is Ibogaine Doing in the Plant?

The Iboga Class of Monoterpene Indole Alkaloids

Although there is some discussion regarding the precise criteria for the term *alkaloid*, core attributes include containing a basic nitrogen as an electron donor in a ring or ring system. The term *true alkaloid* has been used to designate those alkaloids that derive from amino acid and share a heterocyclic ring with nitrogen (Aniszewski, 2015). Indole alkaloids are true alkaloids and particularly well adapted structurally for noncovalent interactions, including cation-π interactions involving the ring system, and hydrogen bonds involving the nitrogen atom. G protein-coupled receptors (GPCRs) are typical targets of alkaloids, often involving aromatic side chains. Receptor binding tends to be diverse, with "off-target" and toxic effects.

Alkaloids are formed in plants from pathways of synthesis of amino acids, and extend on amino acid scaffolds, as do neurotransmitters. The monoamine neurotransmitters may be regarded as alkaloids, just as tryptamine is an alkaloid; so is 5-HT (5-hydroxytryptamine, serotonin), as is auxin, an important plant hormone with a close structural relationship to 5-HT. Morphine, nicotine, cocaine, amphetamine, and the major classical hallucinogens are alkaloids.

Alkaloids were historically initially viewed as "secondary metabolites"—chemical detritus, the by-product of primary metabolic processes such as photosynthesis or energy metabolism. The term *secondary metabolites* has been retained as generally synonymic with plant natural products; however, alkaloids are now recognized as serving ecological aims mediating between the plant and its environment, such as chemical defenses against herbivores or pathogens, or attractants for pollenating insects (Hartmann, 2007). The ecological view is well validated; however, an emerging view is that alkaloids may also serve functions within the plant itself as modulators of signaling pathways or gene expression (Aniszewski, 2015; Heinze et al., 2015; Neilson et al., 2013).

The phylogenetic lineage of many alkaloids tends to be narrow, as is the case with ibogaine, possibly due to evolutionary selection pressure for chemodiversity. The total number of all plant secondary metabolites is estimated on the order of 200,000 compounds (Neilson et al., 2013), with estimates of total number of alkaloids on the order of 20,000, occurring in quantities $\geq 0.01\%$ of the dry plant weight in approximately 20% (Seigler, 1998) of the 405 families of flowering plants (The Plant List, 2013). Ibogaine is a monoterpene indole alkaloid (MIA), a pharmacologically important class of compounds formed by the condensation of the alkaloid tryptamine and the monoterpene secologanin. Estimates of the number of MIAs are in the range of approximately 2,000 to 3,000 compounds, occurring predominantly in three plant families: Apocynaceae, Loganiaceae, and Rubiacea (O'Connor & Maresh, 2006; Szabó, 2008). The iboga class of MIAs consists of about 100 compounds (Lavaud & Massiot, 2017) apparently limited to five of 410 genera within the Apocynaceae family (The Plant List, 2013): *Tabernaemontana, Tabernanthe, Catharanthus, Voacanga,* and *Melodinus.*

Cross-Kingdom Commonality: Plant and Animal Homology

Plants lack many of the proteins targeted by drugs that are psychoactive in humans. Most approved psychopharmacological agents in clinical use (e.g., antidepressants, antipsychotics, some anxiolytics) as well as many drugs of abuse target GPCRs or monoamine transporters. Plants lack canonical GPCRs (Urano & Jones, 2014) such as opioid, dopamine, 5-HT, or cannabinoid receptors, they lack monoamine transporters (Hoglund et al., 2005) at which cocaine or amphetamine act, and they do not have pentameric ligand-gated ion channels (Jaiteh et al., 2016)—the targets of nicotine, benzodiazepines, or ketamine.

Plants do share remarkable homologies regarding G proteins and effectors that are conserved in plants and metazoans. Figure 15.3 presents two examples of downstream signaling elements homologously present in plants and linked in humans to GPCRs that activate cardinal signaling pathways of psychoactive substances. In the case of the MOR, the respective transducer, effector, and second messengers present in both plants and animals are Gα, adenylate cyclase, and cyclic AMP. In case of the 5-HT$_{2A}$R, they are Gα, phospholipase A$_2$ and C, arachidonic acid, and inositol 1,4,5-trisphosphate. Clinical psychopharmacology does not generally target transducers and effectors, but plant alkaloids apparently do, and the identification of their targets may provide an interesting paradigm for drug discovery and neurobiological investigation.

A recent study provides an example of an endogenous plant alkaloid as a specific modulator of an effector in the plant itself (Heinze et al., 2015). *Eschscholzia californi-*

Signaling Element	Opioids	Classical hallucinogens
Receptor (GPCR)	μ-opioid receptor (MOR)[*]	Serotonin 2A receptor (5-HT2A)[*]
Transducer (G proteins)	Gα[†]	Gα[†]
Effector (enzymes)	Adenylate cyclase[†]	Phospholipase A₂[†], C[†]
Second messenger (cyclic nucleotides, lipids/phospholipids)	Cyclic adenosine monophosphate (cAMP)[†]	Arachidonic acid (AA)[†], inositol 1,4,5-trisphosphate (IP3)[†]

[*]*occurs in animals, not in plants*
[†]*occurs in both plants animals*

■ FIGURE 15.3. Signaling elements linked to two mammalian GPCRs, the MOR and 5-HTAR. Plants lack G-protein coupled receptors, but some downstream G proteins, effectors and second messengers are conserved in plants and metazoans.

ca (Papaveraceae) and *Catharanthus roseus* (Apocynaceae) express alkaloids that function as phytoalexins, compounds with antimicrobial activity against fungi and bacteria that are produced and accumulated by plants in response to infection. Microbial elicitors added to cultured cells from either plant increase the production of alkaloids by Gα-dependent activation of phospholipase A₂ (PLA₂) to generate signaling molecules that code for the induction of biosynthetic enzymes downstream. The respective alkaloids in both of these evolutionary distant plants exert negative feedback to prevent their own overexpression by specifically targeting and inhibiting PLA₂. PLA₂ is present in metazoans and is an important downstream effector in the action of the classical hallucinogens, linked to the 5-HT$_A$R (Nichols, 2016), suggesting the possibility of a widely conserved, phylogenetically ancient signaling motif. Of note with regard to this present review, catharanthine (Figure 15.1), which occurs in *C. roseus* and inhibited *C. roseus* PLA₂ in the study discussed above (Heinze et al., 2015), is an iboga alkaloid of pharmacological importance (van der Heijden et al., 2004).

Plant Intelligence

Plants have extraordinary capacities to sense and respond to their environment, but should they be regarded as intelligent? Intelligence is the capacity for learning, which involves the modification of programs of behavior or thought on the basis of prior experience (Trewavas, 2017). Learning is shaped by reinforcement in individuals within that individual's lifetime. Habituation may be viewed as an elementary form of learning, but is limited to adaptations to manage the gain of environmental signals, and is shaped by repeated exposure to a habituating stimulus, such as leaf folding in response to mechanical disturbance (Gagliano et al., 2014). Intelligence differs from instinct, which is reinforced at the level of populations by adaptation and fitness over time spans of generations and may be exemplified in plants as epigenetic memory in clonal plants (Latzel et al., 2016). Intelligence is distinct from consciousness, which has been defined as "global subjective awareness" (John, 2005), and may only be inferred and not directly observed by the research investigator.

The example of the climbing behavior of *Passiflora caerulea L.,* an experimental paradigm favored by Charles Darwin, provides an example of plant intelligence that illustrates the capacity of plants to learn (Baillaud, 1962; Trewavas, 2005). The plant is presented with a support, which the tendril locates by circumnutation, a plant behavioral program of helical movement common in climbing plants that allows triangulation utilizing variations in light intensity registered by the moving tendril. The tendril finds the support each time it is moved to a new location. Locating the support requires some form of memory of the variations in light intensity over the trajectory of the circumnutatory movements (Trewavas, 2017). The tendrils appear to modify their search strategy with the progression of the experiment, and after the support is finally taken away altogether the plant appears to approach the last previous location of the support prior to it being removed.

Not only is the *Passiflora caerulea* plant itself apparently capable spatial learning, but *Passiflora incarnata L.* enhances spatial learning when ingested by rats (Jawna-Zboinska et al., 2016). Both *P. caerulea* and *P. incarnata* contain multiple harmala alkaloids, including harmine (Frye & Haustein, 2008). Harmine and ibogaine both enhance spatial learning in the rat (Dos Santos & Hallak, 2017; Helsley et al., 1997; Popik, 1996). Alkaloids frequently accumulate most heavily in the parts of the plant that are growing, such as root tips. This has been viewed as consistent with a hypothesis of alkaloids as chemodefenses, which are deployed more extensively in valuable, young growing plant tissue (McCall & Fordyce, 2010). However, in the root system, which navigates, senses, and responds to its environment, the accumulation of alkaloids in growing tissue might also reflect a role of alkaloids of endogenous modulators of plant signaling in programs of behavior or growth and development.

■ Conclusion

The iboga alkaloid structural skeleton appears to be a *privileged scaffold*, a term of medicinal chemistry for a basic molecular framework prototypical of a class of compounds on which systematic substitutions can be utilized to modulate therapeutic and toxic effects (Welsch et al., 2010). The effect of 18-MC in animal models of drug self-administration and opioid withdrawal is apparently equivalent to that of ibogaine (Maisonneuve & Glick, 2003), although its *hERG* blockade is much less (Alper et al., 2016), indicating the potential for isolating ibogaine's therapeutic effect from its cardiotoxicity. With an unknown and likely novel mechanism of action, and a structure that evidently accommodates rational drug design, ibogaine may provide an interesting prototype for discovery and development of fundamentally innovative pharmacotherapy.

When a growing root tip meets a rock that it cannot move, it revises its behavioral

program. In this instance, plants may output behavioral responses more intelligently than humans, who are prone to rigidly overdetermined repetitive behavior. It appears possible that a restricted subset of plant alkaloids interacts with an evolutionarily ancient commonality, shared across signaling pathways in both plant and animal kingdoms that may mediate programs of plant adaptive behavior, growth, or development in one kingdom, and modify the pathological neuroadaptations of opioid dependence and linkages of motivational states to drug-related memories, representations, or environmental cues. True intention, equanimity, distinct from the constraints of obsession and the pathological overattribution of salience, is both a cardinal spiritual goal and a desired outcome of pharmacological treatment of addiction. Recovery from addiction is often, typically, viewed by patients in spiritual terms. It is not entirely unexpected that a plant alkaloid used in an indigenous sacramental context may provide a valuable lead for discovery of pharmacotherapy for addiction.

■ Acknowledgment

This chapter was previously published in G. Prance, D. J. McKenna, B. DeLoenen, and W. Davis (Eds.), *Ethnopharmacologic Search for Psychoactive Drugs* (Vol. II). Santa Fe, NM: Synergetic Press, 2017. It is reproduced here with permission from the publisher and author.

■ References

Aceto, M. D., Bowman, E. R., Harris, L. S., & May, E. L. (1992). Dependence studies of new compounds in the rhesus monkey and mouse (1991). *NIDA Res Monogr, 119,* 513–558.

Alper, K. (2001). Ibogaine: A review. *Alkaloids Chem Biol, 56,* 1–38.

Alper, K., Bai, R., Liu, N., Fowler, S. J., Huang, X. P., Priori, S. G., et al. (2016). hERG blockade by iboga alkaloids. *Cardiovasc Toxicol, 16*(1), 14–22.

Alper, K., Beal, D., & Kaplan, C. D. (2001). A contemporary history of ibogaine in the United States and Europe. *Alkaloids Chem Biol, 56,* 249–281.

Alper, K., Lotsof, H. S., Frenken, G. M., Luciano, D. J., & Bastiaans, J. (1999). Treatment of acute opioid withdrawal with ibogaine. *Am J Addict, 8*(3), 234–242.

Alper, K., Lotsof, H. S., & Kaplan, C. D. (2008). The ibogaine medical subculture. *J Ethnopharmacol, 115*(1), 9–24.

Alper, K., Reith, M. E. A., & Sershen, H. (2012). Ibogaine and the inhibition of acetylcholinesterase. *J Ethnopharmacol, 139*(3), 879–882.

Alper, K., Stajic, M., & Gill, J. R. (2012. Fatalities temporally associated with the ingestion of ibogaine. *J Forensic Sci, 57*(2), 398–412.

Amato, L., Davoli, M., Minozzi, S., Ferroni, E., Ali, R., & Ferri, M. (2013). Methadone at tapered doses for the management of opioid withdrawal. *Cochrane Database Syst Rev, 2,* CD003409.

Aniszewski, T. (2015). Definition, typology, and occurrence of alkaloids. In *Alkaloids* (2nd ed., pp. 1–97). Boston: Elsevier.

Antonio, T., Childers, S. R., Rothman, R. B., Dersch, C. M., King, C., Kuehne, M., et al. (2013). Effect of iboga alkaloids on μ-opioid receptor-coupled G protein activation. *PLOS ONE, 8*(10), e77262.

Aricioglu-Kartal, F., Kayır, H., & Tayfun Uzbay, I. (2003). Effects of harman and harmine on naloxone-precipitated withdrawal syndrome in morphine-dependent rats. *Life Sci, 73*(18), 2363–2371.

Bagal, A. A., Hough, L. B., Nalwalk, J. W., & Glick, S. D. (1996). Modulation of morphine-induced antinociception by ibogaine and noribogaine. *Brain Res, 741*(1–2), 258–262.

Baillaud, L. (1962). Mouvements autonomes des tiges, vrilles et autres organes à l'exception des organes volubiles et des feuilles. In W. Ruhland (Ed.), *Handbuch der Pflanzenphysiologie* (Vol. 17, Part 2, pp. 562–634). Berlin: Springer-Verlag.

Bartlett, M. F., Dickel, D. F., & Taylor, W. I. (1958). The alkaloids of *Tabernanthe-Iboga*: Part VI. The structures of ibogamine, ibogaine, tabernanthine and voacangine. *J Am Chem Soc, 80*(1), 126–136.

Bastiaans, E. (2004). *Life after ibogaine: An exploratory study of the long-term effects of ibogaine treatment on drug addicts.* Doctorandus thesis Faculty of Medicine Vrije Universiteit Amsterdam, the Netherlands. Retrieved September 21, 2017, from *www.iceers.org/docs/science/iboga/bastiaans e_life_after_ibogaine.pdf.*

Baumann, M. H., Rothman, R. B., Pablo, J. P., & Mash, D. C. (2001). *In vivo* neurobiological effects of ibogaine and its O-desmethyl metabolite, 12-hydroxyibogamine (noribogaine), in rats. *J Pharmacol Exp Ther, 297*(2), 531–539.

Belgers, M., Leenaars, M., Homberg, J. R., Ritskes-Hoitinga, M., Schellekens, A. F., &

Hooijmans, C. R. (2016). Ibogaine and addiction in the animal model: A systematic review and meta-analysis. *Transl Psychiatry, 6*(5), e826.

Bentzley, B. S., Barth, K. S., Back, S. E., & Book, S. W. (2015). Discontinuation of buprenorphine maintenance therapy: Perspectives and outcomes. *J Subst Abuse Treat, 52,* 48–57.

Bhargava, H. N., & Cao, Y. J. (1997). Effects of noribogaine on the development of tolerance to antinociceptive action of morphine in mice. *Brain Res, 771*(2), 343–346.

Bhargava, H. N., Cao, Y. J., & Zhao, G. M. (1997). Effects of ibogaine and noribogaine on the antinociceptive action of mu-, delta- and kappa-opioid receptor agonists in mice. *Brain Res, 752*(1–2), 234–238.

Bie, B., Peng, Y., Zhang, Y., & Pan, Z. Z. (2005). cAMP-mediated mechanisms for pain sensitization during opioid withdrawal. *J Neurosci, 25*(15), 3824–3832.

Binienda, Z., Beaudoin, M. A., Thorn, B. T., Prapurna, D. R., Johnson, J. R., Fogle, C. M., et al. (1998). Alteration of electroencephalogram and monoamine concentrations in rat brain following ibogaine treatment. *Ann NY Acad Sci, 844,* 265–273.

Bisaga, A., Comer, S., Ward, A., Popik, P., Kleber, H., & Fischman, M. (2001). The NMDA antagonist memantine attenuates the expression of opioid physical dependence in humans. *Psychopharmacology (Berl), 157*(1), 1–10.

Bowen, W. D. (2001). Sigma receptors and *iboga* alkaloids. *Alkaloids Chem Biol, 56,* 173–191.

Brown, T. K., & Alper, K. (2018). Treatment of opioid use disorder with ibogaine: Detoxification and drug use outcomes. *Am J Drug Alcohol Abuse, 44,* 24–36.

Caille, S., Espejo, E. F., Koob, G. F., & Stinus, L. (2002). Dorsal and median raphe serotonergic system lesion does not alter the opiate withdrawal syndrome. *Pharmacol Biochem Behav, 72*(4), 979–986.

Cantero, J. L., Atienza, M., Stickgold, R., Kahana, M. J., Madsen, J. R., & Kocsis, B. (2003). Sleep-dependent theta oscillations in the human hippocampus and neocortex. *J Neurosci, 23*(34), 10897–10903.

Cao, Y. J., & Bhargava, H. N. (1997). Effects of ibogaine on the development of tolerance to antinociceptive action of mu-, delta- and kappa-opioid receptor agonists in mice. *Brain Res, 752*(1–2), 250–254.

Cappendijk, S. L., & Dzoljic, M. R. (1993). Inhibitory effects of ibogaine on cocaine self-administration in rats. *Eur J Pharmacol, 241*(2–3), 261–265.

Cappendijk, S. L., Fekkes, D., & Dzoljic, M. R. (1994). The inhibitory effect of norharman on morphine withdrawal syndrome in rats: Comparison with ibogaine. *Behav Brain Res, 65*(1), 117–119.

Carnicella, S., He, D. Y., Yowell, Q. V., Glick, S. D., & Ron, D. (2010). Noribogaine, but not 18-MC, exhibits similar actions as ibogaine on GDNF expression and ethanol self-administration. *Addict Biol, 15*(4), 424–433.

Christie, M. J. (2008). Cellular neuroadaptations to chronic opioids: Tolerance, withdrawal and addiction. *Br J Pharmacol, 154*(2), 384–396.

Corkery, J. M., Schifano, F., Ghodse, A. H., & Oyefeso, A. (2004). The effects of methadone and its role in fatalities. *Hum Psychopharmacol, 19*(8), 565–576.

Cubeddu, L. X. (2009). Iatrogenic QT abnormalities and fatal arrhythmias: Mechanisms and clinical significance. *Curr Cardiol Rev, 5*(3), 166–176.

Darke, S. (1998). Self-report among injecting drug users: A review. *Drug Alcohol Depend, 51*(3), 253–263.

Darke, S., Kaye, S., & Duflou, J. (2006). Systemic disease among cases of fatal opioid toxicity. *Addiction, 101*(9), 1299–1305.

Deecher, D. C., Teitler, M., Soderlund, D. M., Bornmann, W. G., Kuehne, M. E., & Glick, S. D. (1992). Mechanisms of action of ibogaine and harmaline congeners based on radioligand binding studies. *Brain Res, 571*(2), 242–247.

Depoortere, H. (1987). Neocortical rhythmic slow activity during wakefulness and paradoxical sleep in rats. *Neuropsychobiology, 18*(3), 160–168.

Dhahir, H. I. (1971). *A comparative study on the toxicity of ibogaine and serotonin.* Doctoral dissertation, Department of Pharmacology and Toxicology, Indiana University, Bloomington, IN.

Dickinson, J., McAlpin, J., Wilkins, C., Fitzsimmons, C., Guion, P., Paterson, T., et al. (2016). Clinical guidelines for Ibogaine-Assisted Detoxification (Version 1.1). Retrieved September 21, 2017, from *www.ibogainealliance.org/guidelines*.

Dos Santos, R. G., & Hallak, J. E. (2017). Effects of the natural beta-carboline alkaloid harmine, a main constituent of ayahuasca, in memory and in the hippocampus: A systematic literature review of preclinical studies. *J Psychoactive Drugs, 49*(1), 1–10.

Drug Enforcement Administration. (2016). National Heroin Threat Assessment Summary—Updated. Retrieved from *www.dea.gov/sites/default/files/2018-07/hq062716_attach.pdf*.

Dworkin, S. I., Gleeson, S., Meloni, D., Koves, T. R., & Martin, T. J. (1995). Effects of ibogaine on responding maintained by food, cocaine

and heroin reinforcement in rats. *Psychopharmacology (Berl), 117*(3), 257–261.

Dzoljic, E. D., Kaplan, C. D., & Dzoljic, M. R. (1988). Effect of ibogaine on naloxone-precipitated withdrawal syndrome in chronic morphine-dependent rats. *Arch Int Pharmacodyn Ther, 294,* 64–70.

Fabing, H. (1956). Trends in biological research in schizophrenia. *J Nerv Ment Dis, 124*(1), 1–7.

Fareed, A., Casarella, J., Amar, R., Vayalapalli, S., & Drexler, K. (2010). Methadone maintenance dosing guideline for opioid dependence, a literature review. *J Addict Dis, 29*(1), 1–14.

Fernandez, J. W. (1982). *Bwiti: An ethnography of religious imagination in Africa.* Princeton, NJ: Princeton University Press.

Fernandez, J. W., & Fernandez, R. L. (2001). "Returning to the path": The use of iboga[ine] in an equatorial African ritual context and the binding of time, space, and social relationships. *Alkaloids Chem Biol, 56,* 235–247.

Frances, B., Gout, R., Cros, J., & Zajac, J. M. (1992). Effects of ibogaine on naloxone-precipitated withdrawal in morphine-dependent mice. *Fundam Clin Pharmacol, 6*(8–9), 327–332.

Frye, A., & Haustein, C. (2008). Extraction, identification, and quantification of harmala alkaloids in three species of *Passiflora. Am J Undergrad Res, 6*(3), 19–26.

Gagliano, M., Renton, M., Depczynski, M., & Mancuso, S. (2014). Experience teaches plants to learn faster and forget slower in environments where it matters. *Oecologia, 175*(1), 63–72.

Glick, S. D., Kuehne, M. E., Raucci, J., Wilson, T. E., Larson, D., Keller, R. W., Jr., et al. (1994). Effects of iboga alkaloids on morphine and cocaine self-administration in rats: Relationship to tremorigenic effects and to effects on dopamine release in nucleus accumbens and striatum. *Brain Res, 657*(1–2), 14–22.

Glick, S. D., Maisonneuve, I. M., Hough, L. B., Kuehne, M. E., & Bandarage, U. K. (1999). (±)-18-Methoxycoronaridine: A novel iboga alkaloid congener having potential anti-addictive efficacy. *CNS Drug Rev, 5*(1), 27–42.

Glick, S. D., Maisonneuve, I. M., Kitchen, B. A., & Fleck, M. W. (2002). Antagonism of α3β4 nicotinic receptors as a strategy to reduce opioid and stimulant self-administration. *Eur J Pharmacol, 438*(1–2), 99–105.

Glick, S. D., Maisonneuve, I. M., & Szumlinski, K. K. (2001). Mechanisms of action of ibogaine: Relevance to putative therapeutic effects and development of a safer *iboga* alkaloid congener. *Alkaloids Chem Biol, 56,* 39–53.

Glick, S. D., Maisonneuve, I. M., Visker, K. E.,

Fritz, K. A., Bandarage, U. K., & Kuehne, M. E. (1998). 18-Methoxycoronardine attenuates nicotine-induced dopamine release and nicotine preferences in rats. *Psychopharmacology (Berl), 139*(3), 274–280.

Glick, S. D., Pearl, S. M., Cai, J., & Maisonneuve, I. M. (1996). Ibogaine-like effects of noribogaine in rats. *Brain Res, 713*(1–2), 294–297.

Glick, S. D., Rossman, K., Rao, N. C., Maisonneuve, I. M., & Carlson, J. N. (1992). Effects of ibogaine on acute signs of morphine-withdrawal in rats: Independence from tremor. *Neuropharmacology, 31*(5), 497–500.

Glick, S. D., Rossman, K., Steindorf, S., Maisonneuve, I. M., & Carlson, J. N. (1991). Effects and aftereffects of ibogaine on morphine self-administration in rats. *Eur J Pharmacol, 195*(3), 341–345.

Glue, P., Lockhart, M., Lam, F., Hung, N., Hung, C. T., & Friedhoff, L. (2015). Ascending-dose study of noribogaine in healthy volunteers: Pharmacokinetics, pharmacodynamics, safety, and tolerability. *J Clin Pharmacol, 55*(2), 189–194.

Goutarel, R., Gollnhofer, O., & Sillans, R. (1993). Pharmacodynamics and therapeutic applications of iboga and ibogaine. *Psychedelic Monogr Essays, 6*, 71–111.

Gowing, L., Ali, R., White, J. M., & Mbewe, D. (2017). Buprenorphine for managing opioid withdrawal. *Cochrane Database Syst Rev, 2*, CD002025.

Gowing, L., Farrell, M., Ali, R., & White, J. M. (2016). Alpha(2)-adrenergic agonists for the management of opioid withdrawal. *Cochrane Database Syst Rev, 5*, CD002024.

Handelsman, L., Cochrane, K. J., Aronson, M. J., Ness, R., Rubinstein, K. J., & Kanof, P. D. (1987). Two new rating-scales for opiate withdrawal. *Am J Drug Alcohol Abuse, 13*(3), 293–308.

Hartmann, T. (2007). From waste products to ecochemicals: Fifty years research of plant secondary metabolism. *Phytochemistry, 68*(22–24), 2831–2846.

He, D. Y., McGough, N. N. H., Ravindranathan, A., Jeanblanc, J., Logrip, M. L., Phamluong, K., et al. (2005). Glial cell line-derived neurotrophic factor mediates the desirable actions of the anti-addiction drug ibogaine against alcohol consumption. *J Neurosci, 25*(3), 619–628.

Heink, A., Katsikas, S., & Lange-Altman, T. (2017). Examination of the phenomenology of the ibogaine treatment experience: Role of altered states of consciousness and psychedelic experiences. *J Psychoactive Drugs, 49*, 201–208.

Heinze, M., Brandt, W., Marillonnet, S., & Roos, W. (2015). "Self" and "non-self" in the control of phytoalexin biosynthesis: Plant phospholipases A2 with alkaloid-specific molecular fingerprints. *Plant Cell, 27*(2), 448–462.

Helsley, S., Fiorella, D., Rabin, R. A., & Winter, J. C. (1997). Effects of ibogaine on performance in the 8-arm radial maze. *Pharmacol Biochem Behav, 58*(1), 37–41.

Helsley, S., Fiorella, D., Rabin, R. A., & Winter, J. C. (1998). Behavioral and biochemical evidence for a nonessential 5-HT2A component of the ibogaine-induced discriminative stimulus. *Pharmacol Biochem Behav, 59*(2), 419–425.

Hoglund, P. J., Adzic, D., Scicluna, S. J., Lindblom, J., & Fredriksson, R. (2005). The repertoire of solute carriers of family 6: Identification of new human and rodent genes. *Biochem Biophys Res Commun, 336*(1), 175–189.

Isbell, H. (1955). Letter from Harris Isbell to Ciba-Geigy Pharmaceutical Products dated 11-29-55 (Ciba Document No. AB0491-492410).

Jaiteh, M., Taly, A., & Henin, J. (2016). Evolution of pentameric ligand-gated ion channels: Pro-loop receptors. *PLOS ONE, 11*(3), e0151934.

Jawna-Zboinska, K., Blecharz-Klin, K., Joniec-Maciejak, I., Wawer, A., Pyrzanowska, J., Piechal, A., et al. (2016). *Passiflora incarnata L.* improves spatial memory, reduces stress, and affects neurotransmission in rats. *Phytother Res, 30*(5), 781–789.

John, E. R. (2005). From synchronous neuronal discharges to subjective awareness? *Prog Brain Res, 150*, 143–171, 593.

Kannankeril, P., Roden, D. M., & Darbar, D. (2010). Drug-induced long QT syndrome. *Pharmacol Rev, 62*(4), 760–781.

Kaye, S., McKetin, R., Duflou, J., & Darke, S. (2007). Methamphetamine and cardiovascular pathology: A review of the evidence. *Addiction, 102*(8), 1204–1211.

Knuepfer, M. M. (2003). Cardiovascular disorders associated with cocaine use: Myths and truths. *Pharmacol Ther, 97*(3), 181–222.

Koenig, X., & Hilber, K. (2015). The anti-addiction drug ibogaine and the heart: A delicate relation. *Molecules, 20*(2), 2208–2228.

Koenig, X., Kovar, M., Rubi, L., Mike, A. K., Lukacs, P., Gawali, V. S., et al. (2013). Anti-addiction drug ibogaine inhibits voltage-gated ionic currents: A study to assess the drug's cardiac ion channel profile. *Toxicol Appl Pharmacol, 273*(2), 259–268.

Koja, T., Fukuzaki, K., Kamenosono, T., Nishimura, A., Nagata, R., & Lukas, S. E. (1996, March 20–23). Inhibition of opioid abstinent phenomena by Ibogaine (69th annual meeting of the Japanese Pharmacological Society). *Jpn J Pharmacol, 71*(Suppl. 1), 89.

Kontrimavičiūtė, V., Mathieu, O., Mathieu-Daudé, J. C., Vainauskas, P., Casper, T., Baccino, E., et al. (2006). Distribution of ibogaine and noribogaine in a man following a poisoning involving root bark of the *Tabernanthe iboga* shrub. *J Anal Toxicol, 30*(7), 434–440.

Latzel, V., Gonzalez, A. P. R., & Rosenthal, J. (2016). Epigenetic memory as a basis for intelligent behavior in clonal plants. *Front Plant Sci, 7*, 1354.

Lavaud, C., & Massiot, G. (2017). The iboga alkaloids. *Prog Chem Org Nat Prod, 105*, 89–136.

Layer, R. T., Skolnick, P., Bertha, C. M., Bandarage, U. K., Kuehne, M. E., & Popik, P. (1996). Structurally modified ibogaine analogs exhibit differing affinities for NMDA receptors. *Eur J Pharmacol, 309*(2), 159–165.

Le Men, L., & Taylor, W. I. (1965). A uniform numbering system for indole alkaloids. *Experientia, 21*(9), 508–510.

Leal, M. B., Michelin, K., Souza, D. O., & Elisabetsky, E. (2003). Ibogaine attenuation of morphine withdrawal in mice: Role of glutamate N-methyl-D-aspartate receptors. *Prog Neuropsychopharmacol Biol Psychiatry, 27*(5), 781–785.

Leung, L. S. (1998). Generation of theta and gamma rhythms in the hippocampus. *Neurosci Biobehav Rev, 22*(2), 275–290.

Levin, K. H., Copersino, M. L., Epstein, D., Boyd, S. J., & Gorelick, D. A. (2008). Longitudinal ECG changes in cocaine users during extended abstinence. *Drug Alcohol Depend, 95*(1–2), 160–163.

Lotsof, H. S. (1985). Rapid method for interrupting the narcotic addiction syndrome. US Patent number 4,499,096. Retrieved from *https://patents.google.com/patent/us4499096a/en*.

Lotsof, H. S., Alexander, N. E. (2001). Case studies of ibogaine treatment: Implications for patient management strategies. *Alkaloids Chem Biol, 56*, 293–313.

MacInnes, N., & Handley, S. L. (2002). Characterization of the discriminable stimulus produced by 2-BFI: Effects of imidazoline I(2)-site ligands, MAOIs, beta-carbolines, agmatine and ibogaine. *Br J Pharmacol, 135*(5), 1227–1234.

Maisonneuve, I. M., & Glick, S. D. (1992). Interactions between ibogaine and cocaine in rats: *In vivo* microdialysis and motor behavior. *Eur J Pharmacol, 212*(2–3), 263–266.

Maisonneuve, I. M., & Glick, S. D. (1999). Attenuation of the reinforcing efficacy of morphine by 18-methoxycoronaridine. *Eur J Pharmacol, 383*(1), 15–21.

Maisonneuve, I. M., & Glick, S. D. (2003). Anti-addictive actions of an iboga alkaloid congener: A novel mechanism for a novel treatment. *Pharmacol Biochem Behav, 75*(3), 607–618.

Maisonneuve, I. M., Keller, R. W., Jr., & Glick, S. D. (1991). Interactions between ibogaine, a potential anti-addictive agent, and morphine: An *in vivo* microdialysis study. *Eur J Pharmacol, 199*(1), 35–42.

Maisonneuve, I. M., Keller, R. W., Jr., & Glick, S. D. (1992). Interactions of ibogaine and D-amphetamine: *In vivo* microdialysis and motor behavior in rats. *Brain Res, 579*(1), 87–92.

Maisonneuve, I. M., Mann, G. L., Deibel, C. R., & Glick, S. D. (1997). Ibogaine and the dopaminergic response to nicotine. *Psychopharmacology (Berl), 129*(3), 249–256.

Maisonneuve, I. M., Rossman, K. L., Keller, R. W., Jr., & Glick, S. D. (1992). Acute and prolonged effects of ibogaine on brain dopamine metabolism and morphine-induced locomotor activity in rats. *Brain Res, 575*(1), 69–73.

Mash, D. (1997). Deborah Mash v. NDA International, Inc., Case No. 96-3712-CIV-Moreno, Amended Complaint. Retrieved September 21, 2017, from *http://puzzlepiece.org/ibogaine/011198.html*.

Mash, D. C., Allen-Ferdinand, K., Mayor, M., Kovera, C. A., Ayafor, J. F., Williams, I. C., et al. (1998). Ibogaine: Clinical observations of safety after single oral dose administrations. In L. S. Harris (Ed.), *Problems of Drug Dependence 1998: Proceedings of the 60th annual meeting of the College on Problems of Drug Dependence* (p. 294). Scottsdale, AZ.

Mash, D. C., Ameer, B., Prou, D., Howes, J. F., & Maillet, E. L. (2016). Oral noribogaine shows high brain uptake and anti-withdrawal effects not associated with place preference in rodents. *J Psychopharmacol, 30*(7), 688–697.

Mash, D. C., Kovera, C. A., Buck, B. E., Norenberg, M. D., Shapshak, P., Hearn, W. L., et al. (1998). Medication development of ibogaine as a pharmacotherapy for drug dependence. *Ann NY Acad Sci, 844*, 274–292.

Mash, D. C., Kovera, C. A., Pablo, J., Tyndale, R., Ervin, F. R., Kamlet, J. D., et al. (2001). Ibogaine in the treatment of heroin withdrawal. *Alkaloids Chem Biol, 56*, 155–171.

McCall, A. C., & Fordyce, J. A. (2010). Can optimal defence theory be used to predict the distribution of plant chemical defences? *J Ecol, 98*(5), 985–992.

McGahan, P. L., Griffith, J. A., Parente, R., & McLellan, A. T. (1986). *Addiction Severity Index composite scores manual*. Philadelphia: University of Pennsylvania/Veterans Administration Center for Studies of Addiction.

Molinari, H. H., Maisonneuve, I. M., & Glick,

S. D. (1996). Ibogaine neurotoxicity: A re-evaluation. *Brain Res, 737*(1–2), 255–262.

MPI Research. (1996). *Determination of the acute interaction of combined ibogaine and morphine in rats* (MPI Research Identification: 693-082. Ibogaine Drug Master File Vol. 8). Bethesda, MD: National Institute on Drug Abuse.

Naranjo, C. (1973). *The healing journey: New approaches to consciousness*. New York: Pantheon, Random House.

National Institutes of Health. (2012). IND-Enabling studies and GMP scale-up of 18-Methoxycoronaridine Hydrochloride (18 MC) Project Number: 1U01DA034986-01. Retrieved September 21, 2017, from *https://projectreporter.nih.gov/project_info_description.cfm?aid=8448461&icde=16047111&ddparam=&ddvalue=&ddsub=&cr=41&csb=default&cs=asc.*

Neilson, E. H., Goodger, J. Q., Woodrow, I. E., & Moller, B. L. (2013). Plant chemical defense: At what cost? *Trends Plant Sci, 18*(5), 250–258.

Nelson, D. L., Herbet, A., Petillot, Y., Pichat, L., Glowinski, J., & Hamon, M. (1979). [^{3}H] Harmaline as a specific ligand of MAO-I: Properties of the active site of MAO A from rat and bovine brains. *J Neurochem, 32*(6), 1817–1827.

Nestler, E. J. (2001). Molecular neurobiology of addiction. *Am J Addict, 10*(3), 201–217.

Nichols, D. E. (2016). Psychedelics. *Pharmacol Rev, 68*(2), 264–355.

Noller, G. E., Frampton, C. M., & Yazar-Klosinski, B. (2018). Ibogaine treatment outcomes for opioid dependence from a twelve-month follow-up observational study. *Am J Drug Alcohol Abuse, 44,* 37–46.

O'Connor, S. E., & Maresh, J. J. (2006). Chemistry and biology of monoterpene indole alkaloid biosynthesis. *Nat Prod Rep 23*(4), 532–547.

O'Hearn, E., & Molliver, M. E. (1993). Degeneration of Purkinje cells in parasagittal zones of the cerebellar vermis after treatment with ibogaine or harmaline. *Neuroscience 55*(2), 303–310.

O'Hearn, E., & Molliver, M. E. (1997). The olivocerebellar projection mediates ibogaine-induced degeneration of Purkinje cells: A model of indirect, trans-synaptic excitotoxicity. *J Neurosci, 17*(22), 8828–8841.

Otero-Anton, E., Gonzalez-Quintela, A., Saborido, J., Torre, J. A., Virgos, A., & Barrio, E. (1997). Prolongation of the QTc interval during alcohol withdrawal syndrome. *Acta Cardiol, 52*(3), 285–294.

Panchal, V., Taraschenko, O. D., Maisonneuve,

I. M., & Glick, S. D. (2005). Attenuation of morphine withdrawal signs by intracerebral administration of 18-methoxycoronaridine. *Eur J Pharmacol, 525*(1–3), 98–104.

Parker, L. A., Burton, P., McDonald, R. V., Kim, J. A., & Siegel, S. (2002). Ibogaine interferes with motivational and somatic effects of naloxone-precipitated withdrawal from acutely administered morphine. *Prog Neuropsychopharmacol Biol Psychiatry, 26*(2), 293–297.

Pearl, S. M., Hough, L. B., Boyd, D. L., & Glick, S. D. (1997). Sex differences in ibogaine antagonism of morphine-induced locomotor activity and in ibogaine brain levels and metabolism. *Pharmacol Biochem Behav, 57*(4), 809–815.

Pearl, S. M., Johnson, D. W., & Glick, S. D. (1995). Prior morphine exposure enhances ibogaine antagonism of morphine-induced locomotor stimulation. *Psychopharmacology (Berl), 121*(4), 470–475.

Pearl, S. M., Maisonneuve, I. M., & Glick, S. D. (1996). Prior morphine exposure enhances ibogaine antagonism of morphine-induced dopamine release in rats. *Neuropharmacology 35*(12), 1779–1784.

Pierre, S., Eschenhagen, T., Geisslinger, G., & Scholich, K. (2009). Capturing adenylyl cyclases as potential drug targets. *Nat Rev Drug Discov, 8*(4), 321–335.

Popik, P. (1996). Facilitation of memory retrieval by the "anti-addictive" alkaloid, ibogaine. *Life Sci, 59*(24), PL379–PL385.

Popik, P., Layer, R. T., Fossom, L. H., Benveniste, M., Geterdouglass, B., Witkin, J. M., et al. (1995). NMDA antagonist properties of the putative antiaddictive drug, ibogaine. *J Pharmacol Exp Ther, 275*(2), 753–760.

Rabin, R. A., & Winter, J. C. (1996). Ibogaine and noribogaine potentiate the inhibition of adenylyl cyclase activity by opioid and 5-HT receptors. *Eur J Pharmacol, 316*(2–3), 343–348.

Rezvani, A. H., Overstreet, D. H., & Lee, Y. W. (1995). Attenuation of alcohol intake by ibogaine in three strains of alcohol-preferring rats. *Pharmacol Biochem Behav, 52*(3), 615–620.

Rho, B., & Glick, S. D. (1998). Effects of 18-methoxycoronaridine on acute signs of morphine withdrawal in rats. *NeuroReport, 9*(7), 1283–1285.

Roden, D. M., & Yang, T. (2005). Protecting the heart against arrhythmias: Potassium current physiology and repolarization reserve. *Circulation, 112*(10), 1376–1378.

Salmoiraghi, G. C., & Page, I. H. (1957). Effects of LSD 25, BOL 148, bufotenine, mescaline and ibogaine on the potentiation of hexobarbital hypnosis produced by serotonin and reserpine. *J Pharmacol Exp Ther, 120*(1), 20–25.

Samorini, G. (1998). The initiation rite in the Bwiti Religion (Ndea Narizanga Sect, Gabon). *Jahrbuch Ethnomedizin, 6–7*, 39–56.

Scallet, A. C., Ye, X., Rountree, R., Nony, P., & Ali, S. F. (1996). Ibogaine produces neurodegeneration in rat, but not mouse, cerebellum: Neurohistological biomarkers of Purkinje cell loss. *Ann NY Acad Sci, 801*, 217–226.

Schneider, J. A. (1957). Tabernanthine, ibogaine containing analgesic compositions. U.S. Patent No. 2,817,623. Retrieved from *https://patents.google.com/patent/us2817623a/en*.

Schneider, J. A., & McArthur, M. (1956). Potentiation action of ibogaine (Bogadin™) on morphine analgesia. *Experientia, 12*(8), 323–324.

Schneider, J. A., & Rinehart, R. K. (1957). Analysis of the cardiovascular action of ibogaine hydrochloride. *Arch Int Pharmacodyn Ther, 110*(1), 92–102.

Schneider, J. A., & Sigg, E. B. (1957). Neuropharmacological studies on ibogaine, an indole alkaloid with central-stimulant properties. *Ann NY Acad Sci, 66*(3), 765–776.

Seigler, D. S. (1998). *Plant secondary metabolism*. New York: Springer Science + Business Media.

Sershen, H., Hashim, A., & Lajtha, A. (1994). Ibogaine reduces preference for cocaine consumption in C57BL/6By mice. *Pharmacol Biochem Behav 47*(1), 13–19.

Sharma, S. K., Klee, W. A., & Nirenberg, M. (1975). Dual regulation of adenylate cyclase accounts for narcotic dependence and tolerance. *Proc Natl Acad Sci USA, 72*(8), 3092–3096.

Shawn, L. K., Alper, K., Desai, S. P., Stephenson, K., Olgun, A. M., Nelson, L. S., et al. (2012). Pause-dependent ventricular tachycardia and torsades de pointes after ibogaine ingestion (2012 annual meeting of the North American Congress of Clinical Toxicology [NACCT]). *Clin Toxicol, 50*, 654.

Skolnick, P. (2001). Ibogaine as a glutamate antagonist: Relevance to its putative antiaddictive properties. *Alkaloids Chem Biol, 56*, 55–62.

Snelders, S., & Kaplan, C. (2002). LSD therapy in Dutch psychiatry: Changing socio-political settings and medical sets. *Med Hist, 46*(2), 221–240.

Stolaroff, M. (2004). *The secret chief revealed*. Sarasota, FL: Multidisciplinary Association for Psychedelic Studies (MAPS).

Sunder Sharma, S., & Bhargava, H. N. (1998). Enhancement of morphine antinociception by ibogaine and noribogaine in morphine-tolerant mice. *Pharmacology 57*(5), 229–232.

Sweetnam, P. M., Lancaster, J., Snowman, A., Collins, J. L., Perschke, S., Bauer, C., et al. (1995). Receptor binding profile suggests multiple mechanisms of action are responsible for ibogaine's putative anti-addictive activity. *Psychopharmacology (Berl), 118*(4), 369–376.

Szabó, L. F. (2008). Rigorous biogenetic network for a group of indole alkaloids derived from strictosidine. *Molecules, 13*(8), 1875–1896.

The Plant List. (2013). Version 1.1. Retrieved September 21, 2017, from *www.theplantlist.org*.

Trewavas, A. (2005). Green plants as intelligent organisms. *Trends Plant Sci, 10*(9), 413–419.

Trewavas, A. (2017). The foundations of plant intelligence. *Interface Focus, 7*(3), 20160098.

Trujillo, K. A., & Akil, H. (1994). Inhibition of opiate tolerance by non-competitive N-methyl-D-aspartate receptor antagonists. *Brain Res, 633*(1–2), 178–188.

Turner, W. J., Merlis, S., & Carl, A. (1955). Concerning theories of indoles in schizophrenigenesis. *Am J Psychiatry, 112*(6), 466–467.

Urano, D., & Jones, A. M. (2014). Heterotrimeric G protein-coupled signaling in plants. *Annu Rev Plant Biol, 65*, 365–384.

U.S. Senate. (1977). *Project MKULTRA, The CIA's Program of Research In Behavioral Modification, Joint Hearing before the U.S. Senate Select Committee on Intelligence and the Subcommittee on Health and Scientific Research of the Committee on Human Resources* (p. 244). Washington, DC: U.S. Government Printing Office.

van der Heijden, R., Jacobs, D. I., Snoeijer, W., Hallared, D., & Verpoorte, R. (2004). The Catharanthus alkaloids: Pharmacognosy and biotechnology. *Curr Med Chem 11*(5), 607–628.

Vastag, B. (2005). Addiction research: Ibogaine therapy: A "vast, uncontrolled experiment." *Science 308*(5720), 345–346.

Wei, D., Maisonneuve, I. M., Kuehne, M. E., & Glick, S. D. (1998). Acute *iboga* alkaloid effects on extracellular serotonin (5-HT) levels in nucleus accumbens and striatum in rats. *Brain Res, 800*(2), 260–268.

Welsch, M. E., Snyder, S. A., & Stockwell, B. R. (2010). Privileged scaffolds for library design and drug discovery. *Curr Opin Chem Biol, 14*(3), 347–361.

Zhuo, M. (2012). Targeting neuronal adenylyl cyclase for the treatment of chronic pain. *Drug Discov Today, 17*(11–12), 573–582.

CHAPTER 16

Salvia divinorum

ANA ELDA MAQUEDA

Historical Context

Botanical Description and Geographical Distribution of *Salvia divinorum*

Salvia divinorum is certainly the most unique and mysterious herb of the more than 1,000 species of *Salvia* that inhabit the world. The genus name *Salvia* is derived from the Latin *salvare*, meaning "to heal" or "to save," because of the medicinal properties of this species. *S. divinorum* is a perennial and hydrophyte plant belonging to the mint family (Lamiaceae), and it has a height about 1 and 1.5 meters. It has a square and hollow stem, with decumbent secondary stems that enables the plant to reproduce vegetatively, and to regrow from senescent stems. The velvety leaves are arranged in opposite pairs, and their shape is between oval and lanceolate with dentate edges. The flowers have a slightly sigmoid hairy white corolla, surrounded by a violet chalice with distinctive upper lips of three veins (see Figures 16.1a and 16.1b).

Mexican biologist and botanist Arturo Gómez Pompa (1957) was the first to classify *S. divinorum* as belonging to the *Salvia* genus, but no flowering material was available, so he could not identify the plant further. The first flowering specimens of *S. divinorum* were collected by Robert Gordon Wasson (1962) and Albert Hofmann. In the original identification and description of the plant (Epling & Jativa-M, 1962), *S. divinorum* was classified within the section *Dusenostachys*. Many years later, in a study using a molecular phylogenetic approach by DNA sequencing (Jenks, Walker, & Kim, 2010), no evidence was found to include *S. divinorum* in the *Dusenostachys* section or to consider it a hybrid. Epling and Jativa-M

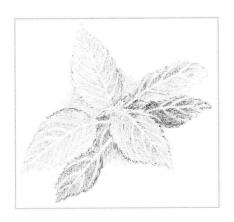

S. divinorum

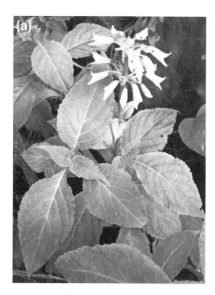
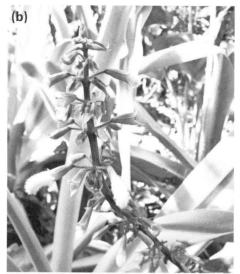

■ FIGURE 16.1. (a) The *Salvia divinorum* plant. (b) The *S. divinorum* flower. *Photos:* Ana Elda Maqueda.

(1962) also described the flowers with blue chalice and corolla, an error that persisted in the literature including in Richard Evan Schultes's *Hallucinogenic Plants* (1976), among others. The official description was corrected by Aaron S. Reisfield in 1993. Although the exact origin of *S. divinorum* remains a mystery, the results of the 2010 phylogenetic study suggest that *Salvia venulosa*, a rare perennial plant native to a small region of the Colombian Andes, is the closest relative of *S. divinorum*.

The native distribution of *S. divinorum* seems to be limited to the Mazatec Sierra, a mountainous area of tropical forests within in the Sierra Madre Oriental of Oaxaca, Mexico. *S. divinorum* prefers to grow near streams in extremely humid and semidark areas. The first specimens of living and flowering *S. divinorum* that came out of Mexico were collected at the Mazatec Sierra by psychiatrist and naturalist Sterling Bunnell, who introduced them to the United States in 1962. Therefore, the most common variety of *S. divinorum* commercially distributed around the world today is the "Bunnell strain," not the "Wasson and Hofmann strain," which in fact does not exist: The specimens that they collected were dried and pressed, remaining in Mexico (Siebert, 2003).

Ethnobotany of *S. divinorum:* Review of the Traditional and Nontraditional Uses

In 1939, anthropologist Jean Basset Johnson discovered that the Mazatec used the juice of the leaves of a plant called *hierba de María* for divination, in what constitutes the first academic report on the existence of *S. divinorum*. Johnson also noted that the Mazatec employed *semillas de la Virgen* ("seeds of the Virgin") in their ceremonies, which were later identified as seeds of the plant *ololiuhqui*, or "morning glory," *Turbina corymbosa*. These seeds contain ergine (LSA), an alkaloid similar in structure to lysergic acid diethylamide (LSD) (Hofmann & Tscherter, 1960). The Mazatec people, who have been using *S. divinorum* for its medicinal and psychoactive properties for hundreds of years, know the plant in their language as *ska pastora* [*sic*]. As the Mazatec language is a tonal one, the word *ska* (meaning "herb" or "leaf") has been reproduced in the literature as it sounds. However, it seems that a more appropriate form of writing herb in Mazatec, closest to the actual sound of the word, would be *xkà* (Maqueda, 2018). The Mazatec also refer to this plant with names in Spanish, such as *hojas de la pastora* ("shepherdess's leaves"). The names are related to the Virgin Mary, who they believe is incarnated in the plant. The lack of an indigenous name and the fact that some Mazatec have stated that the plant is foreign to their region (Wasson, 1962), suggest that *S. divinorum* could be a postcolonial introduction, or that the original name in Mazatec could have been modified by Christian influence (Ott, 1995).

In 1945, anthropologist Blas Pablo Reko mentioned the use by the Mazatec and the Cuicatec of a "divination leaf," which probably was *S. divinorum*. In 1952, Robert J. Weitlaner reported the therapeutic and divinatory use among the Mazatec of Jalapa de Díaz of a potion made by rubbing in water between 50 and 100 leaves of *hierba de María*, the highest dose being used for alcohol addicts. In addition to curing, Weitlaner (1952) observed that the leaves were employed to guess where an animal or person had been lost, or who had committed a robbery. For ceremonies, the leaves of *S. divinorum* are well chewed and swallowed, or the mixture of crushed leaves with water is drunk for a softer effect. Before and after the ritual, both healer and patient must refrain from eating certain foods, drinking alcohol and cold beverages, and from having sex for a period ranging from several days to several weeks. The ceremonies last for about 5 hours and take place in front of an altar at night in complete darkness. The effects are felt after 20 minutes and last for about an hour, but more leaves could be consumed if the healer consider it needed. After the ceremony, the healer prepares an amulet of plant leaves for the patient in order to complete the ritual.

Since the 1960s, the spread of *S. divinorum* worldwide has led to the development of new methods to consume the leaves. These new forms of administration include (1) the sublingual route using tinctures, which provides the most similar experience to that of the traditional method; (2) vaporization of the dried leaves; (3) vaporization of dry leaves potentiated with the active principle, salvinorin A; and (4) vaporization of concentrated extracts. The latter two methods are the most effective way of attaining strong psychedelic effects. The labeling of the concentrated extracts, which are commercialized online or in smart shops, roughly indicates the potency of the products, ranging from the lowest ("3×," "5×"), to the highest potencies ("50×," "100×"). Some research-

Salvinorin A.

ers who have analyzed these products have found a high variability in the concentration of the active principle (Wolowich, Perkins, & Cienki, 2006). Baggott, Erowid, and Erowid (2004) carried out the first survey to know the patterns of use of *S. divinorum*. Most participants were male (93%) from the United States (77.4%), and the average age was 23.4 years old. The researchers found that of the 500 respondents, 61.4% of them vaporized concentrated extracts, and 37.3% vaporized dried leaf. Commonly expressed reasons for *S. divinorum* use were to explore consciousness (86.2%), to satisfy curiosity (76.6%), to have a spiritual experience (74.0%), to pursue personal growth/self-understanding (69.2%), and for contemplation/meditation (52.0%). The survey showed that most users regarded the *S. divinorum* experience as very different from cannabis and classical hallucinogens, and from most other inebriants, reporting it to be unique and intense. The main effects that lingered after the consumption were increased insight, improved mood, calmness, increased connection with the Universe or Nature, or weird thoughts, among others. The researchers did not find persistent adverse effects.

▨ Bioactive Compounds Present in *S. divinorum*

Salvinorin A: Chemical Structure and Biological Targets

S. divinorum owes its psychoactive properties to its active ingredient, the diterpene salvinorin A (SA). SA was isolated and identified for the first time in 1982 in Mexico by Alfredo Ortega and his group, and shortly thereafter by Valdés and collaborators (Ortega, Blount, & Manchand, 1982; Valdés, Butler, Hatfield, Paul, & Koreeda, 1984). Daniel Siebert (1994) was the first researcher to study SA in humans. SA is very lipophilic, so it is easily soluble in organic solvents such as acetone, acetonitrile, chloroform, and methanol, but it is practically insoluble in water.

Thanks to receptor binding studies, it has been possible to determine that SA has a highly and selective affinity for the κ opioid receptor (KOR), exerting an agonist action at this receptor (Roth et al., 2002). The involvement of KORs in the effects of SA in humans has been recently confirmed (Maqueda et al., 2016). On the other hand, it differs from other compounds capable of modifying perception, the so-called "classic" hallucinogens, such as psilocybin (a psychoactive component in many species of fungi) or LSD. The latter are alkaloids (nitrogen compounds) and have affinity for serotonin 5-HT_{1A} and 5-HT_{2A} receptors.

The endogenous agonist of KOR is a family of peptides known as *dynorphins,* widely distributed throughout the central and peripheral nervous system. The KOR/dynorphin system is found in the spinal cord, in neurons that transmit nociceptive signals, and in the cerebellum. It is also present in the prefrontal and insular cortex, and in various subcortical areas. Thus, this system participates in the regulation of physiological functions essential for life, such as breathing, wakefulness, and cardiovascular functions. It also regulates neuroendocrine functions among which are the modulation of pain/analgesia, and acute and chronic stress. The KOR/dynorphin system also modulates high cognitive functions such as perception, cognition, behavior, and memory. There is a high density of KORs in brain circuits involved in the control of motivation, anxiety, and the hedonic and aversive responses mediated by the reward system to natural and chemical stimuli. KORs also modulate mood by means of projections to limbic areas, although they have received much less attention than the monoamine systems, with which they interact directly. In the case of drugs of abuse, the activation of the μ opioid receptor (MOR)/endorphins system induces euphoria in humans and produces reinforcement in animals, by increasing the release of the neurotransmitter dopamine (DA). On the contrary, the activation of the KOR/dynorphin system by endogenous or exogenous agonists produces dysphoria in humans and aversion in animals, antagonizing the actions mediated by the activation of MORs, by reducing the release of DA in structures innervated by the mesolimbic pathway. In this manner, the KOR/dynorphins system exerts a direct and complementary modulation on the reward system. In the specific case of SA, this compound regulates DA neurotransmission by two different mechanisms: (1) inhibiting its release in the dorsal striatum (Gehrke, Chefer, & Shippenberg, 2008), and in the nucleus accumbens (Carlezon et al., 2006) and (2) up-regulating the expression of its transporter. The final result of this second mechanism is an increase in the reuptake of the neurotransmitter (Kivell, Ewald, & Prisinzano, 2014).

Despite the great relevance and potential clinical application that κ-agonists would have in view of the previous discussion, these compounds have undesired side effects that have greatly restricted their clinical use. However, there are important differences between the actions of synthetic κ-agonists and SA, and it has been found that SA has effects on behavior other than those caused by synthetic κ-agonists (Wang et al., 2005). Additionally, the dose of SA plays a key role in the final profile of effects: While at high doses (3.2 mg/kg) it triggers some of the adverse effects of traditional κ-agonists, at lower doses no such effects are observed. Specifically, the anti-addiction, antireward, antidepressant, and anxiolytic effects of SA are observed at moderate doses, and when it is administered acutely and not chronically (Braida, Capurro, & Zani, 2009).

The activation of KORs transmits not only inhibitory signals but also excitatory ones, modulating the release of several neurotransmitters. SA facilitates the exocytosis of noradrenaline, and inhibits the release of serotonin (Grilli et al., 2009). It also acts as an allosteric modulator of MORs, and the similarity between the receptor binding profiles of SA and ketamine (KOR and N-methyl-D-aspartate [NMDA], respectively), could imply that SA has some interaction with glutamate (Rothman et al., 2007). It has been described an indirect action of SA on cannabinoid receptors, specifically on CB1 (Braida et al., 2007). An *in vitro* experiment suggested that SA binds to DA D_2 receptor with high affinity (Seeman, Guan, & Hirbec, 2009).

About the brain targets of SA, different studies in animals have shown that the compound is distributed throughout the brain in areas with a high KORs density, among them, in the cerebellum, involved in the integration of sensory perception and motor control, and in the visual cortex, probably due to the hallucinogenic properties of SA. Other SA targets are regions involved in the modulation of pain, in the regulation of the response to stress and anxiety, in visual perception, in addiction and motivation, in proprioception, in areas involved in mood and motivated behaviors, in emotional processes, and in areas responsible for cognition, executive functions, and the perception of the self (Chartoff et al., 2008; Hooker et al., 2008; Hooker, Patel, Kothari, & Schiffer, 2009). Some regions with very few KORs also showed activation, so it cannot be ruled out that SA may also exert its actions through the activation of one or more molecular targets not yet discovered. Another brain target of SA is the insular cortex (Coffeen et al., 2018), which is densely populated by KORs and believed perhaps to be involved in consciousness. It has an important role in cognitive processes and is involved in emotional processes such as compassion and empathy, and interpersonal experience. In particular, the insula modulates interoception, that is, body awareness: the perception of what happens in our bodies and the sensation of owning a body. The subjective effects observed in human studies may reflect this influence of SA in the insula, since high doses of the compound modify body awareness powerfully or directly suppress it. In contrast, low and medium doses of SA led to acute increases in body awareness and body-listening skills (Maqueda et al., 2015). Stiefel, Merrifield, and Holcombe (2014) have suggested that the disruption in consciousness observed in humans taking high doses of SA may be due to an inhibition of the role of the claustrum as a conductor of consciousness.

In laboratory animals, no changes in heart rate, body temperature, or the galvanic skin response have been observed after chronic administration of SA at high doses. Analyses of the organs did not reveal histological changes. The data from this study suggest that the toxicity of SA is very low, even at doses much higher than those that a human could ever consume (Mowry, Mosher, & Briner, 2003). The neoclerodane nucleus of SA provides an excellent structural template from which to synthesize structural derivatives and analogues. To date, there are more than 600 compounds analogous to SA (for a review, see Roach & Shenvi, 2018).

Other Terpenes Present in *S. divinorum*

The initial phytochemical investigation of *S. divinorum* identified SA and salvinorin B (SB). In the subsequent work carried out by several different groups of researchers (see the review of Casselman, Nock, Wohlmuth, Weatherby, & Heinrich, 2014), other diterpenes were isolated, such as salvinorins C–J, salvidivins A–D, divinatorins A–F, and salvinicins A and B, whose role in the pharmacological effects is not yet elucidated. The leaves of *S. divinorum* also contain loliolide (a potent ant-repellent), and hardwickiic acid and (E)-phytol, both with antimicrobial and antibacterial properties (*Staphylococcus aureus* and *Candida albicans*), and nepetoidin B, with antifungal properties.

▦ Pharmacological Effects in Humans

Subjective Effects

The available literature indicates two effective administration routes: through the oral mucosa, and through inhalation. There are marked differences between these two methods regarding the subjective effects and the final experience attained.

Through oral consumption, the leaves of *S. divinorum* must be well chewed and retained in contact with the inner part of the mouth and with the gums for at least 10 minutes to effectively obtain the effects. If the plant material is ingested, the active principle is rapidly degraded in the gut. It has been reported little or no effects on the first attempts consuming the leaves, which could be explained due to personal sensitivity or to genetic differences in KOR distribution. However, it seems that on consecutive attempts, there is an increased awareness of the plant's effects, followed by a gradual inversed tolerance if the leaves are consumed frequently. Buccal consumption of *S. divinorum* provides a gradual onset of the experience (starting at 10 minutes) and it has a duration of about an hour. The subjective effects can be interrupted by sounds or touch. Some of them include sensations of floating and of movement; changes in temperature and dysphoric effects; the feeling that one is becoming a plant; amplified sound perception; dream-like states; organic visions of animals and the forest, and inorganic visions of ornamented buildings or machinery; contact with entities that speak and interact with oneself; increased understanding of personal problems or insights about the nature of reality; and sensations of calm and relax (Aardvark, 2002; Bücheler, Gleiter, Schwoerer, & Gaertner, 2005; Díaz, 2013; Siebert, 1994; Valdés, Díaz, & Paul, 1983; Valdés, Hatfield, Koreeda, & Paul, 1987). Interestingly, it has been found that the sublingual route is not effective for pure SA at doses of up to 4.0 milligrams (Mendelson et al., 2011). This suggests that oral absorption requires a larger surface area, such as that offered by the inside of the cheek, or that there are other compounds present in the leaf that help with the absorption of SA.

Through inhalation of the vapors of pure SA or concentrated extracts, the peak effects are attained very fast, in less than a minute, and last 15–20 minutes (Addy, 2012). The subjective effects of pure SA are blocked by prior administration of the κ-antagonist naltrexone (Maqueda et al., 2016). Taking into account individual sensitivity to the substance, this could elicit more robust or weaker effects; with a low dose of 0.25 mg of pure SA, the subjective effects include increased connection with the body, relaxation, calm, closed-eye visions, and changes in bodily sensations. With a medium dose (0.50 mg), there is an increased interoceptive awareness, closed-eye visual imagery including carnival or fantasy scenes and kaleidoscopic or fractal visions, and somatic-dysphoric effects. Some of the

somatic effects consist of changes in temperature and tingling; sensations of being pulled or twisted by forces; sensations of being glued to a side of reality while trying to join another reality with the other half of the body; and visual-proprioceptive synesthesia that consists of merging with the objects present in the surroundings or in the mind. This special type of synesthesia is very rare compared with other psychedelics, and the perception of auditory phenomena is another peculiar feature of SA. It is interesting to note that the somatic effects are usually felt starting from the left side of the body, or they seem to come from a particular side of reality, affecting the body, then passing through it like a wave; this lateralization of the effects is another unique characteristic of SA inebriation (Maqueda et al., 2015). And with a high dose (1 mg), depersonalization, dissociation, and out-of-body experiences are much more common and a typical hallmark of high doses of SA. Volunteers report a profound immersion in the experience, not being able to stay present on consensus reality, which usually folds and creases at the beginning of the experience. Subjects describe their bodies as being pushed by forces or by entities, as being twisted, folded, or unzipped while passing through narrow conducts, before being thrown to other dimensions, where they no longer have a physical body. On those other dimensions, they describe the sensation of being pure mind, pure consciousness or energy. Once the experience has ended, as abruptly as it started, some volunteers report vague memories of the trip other than it being extremely weird, scary or difficult to explain scenarios that seemed to be repeated endlessly, and that it did not obey the laws of physics to which we are typically accustomed. On the other hand, other subjects can detail having visited remote and wondrous universes and having spoken with entities and achieved new and valuable personal or philosophical insights, all wrapped in a dream-like sensation. Volunteers universally affirm that SA experience is unique, intense, and difficult to compare with other psychedelics. The first human to experiment with pure SA, the pioneer researcher Daniel Siebert, vaporized for the first time 2.6 mg of the compound and related his experience as "tearing apart the fabric of reality":

> Then quite suddenly I found myself in a confused, fast moving state of consciousness with absolutely no idea where my body or for that matter my universe had gone. . . . Suddenly I realized that I had no memory of ever having lived in another state of consciousness, but in the disembodied condition in which I was at that moment. In this state, all points of time in my personal history coexisted. None preceded the next. (in Turner, 1996)

In his classical study with volunteers, Siebert (1994) reported other SA themes: (1) uncontrollable hysterical laughter; (2) visions of various two-dimensional surfaces, films and membranes; (3) revisiting places of the past, especially childhood; and (4) overlapping realities, the perception that one is in several locations at once.

Pharmacokinetics

After being vaporized, SA is transported through the blood–brain barrier with relative ease and accumulates in the central nervous system (CNS). The compound is metabolized at the intestinal and hepatic levels and excreted by the kidneys. The original product is hydrolyzed, which results in the formation of SB, which would be the main inactive metabolite of SA. That SA is rapidly metabolized is supported by the finding that only approximately 0.8% of a 0.5-mg dose of the compound was extracted from urine in human volunteers (Pichini et al., 2005). SA metabolism seems to depend on gender, being slower for females than for males, which may be the reason why females experience less dysphoric effects with KOR agonists (Russell et al., 2014). The perceived intensity of the subjective effects is correlated with the plasmatic concentration of the compound (Johnson, MacLean, Caspers, Prisinzano, & Griffiths, 2016; Johnson, MacLean, Reissig, Prisinzano, & Griffiths, 2011; Maqueda et al., 2016).

Cardiovascular and Autonomic Effects

In the study of Maqueda and collaborators (2016), at the 1-mg dose, SA elicited a short-lived increase in systolic blood pressure. No other significant effects have been found in cardiovascular measures in other human studies. However, the differences between the studies, such as the number of participants (Johnson et al., 2011, 2016; MacLean, Johnson, Reissig, Prisinzano, & Griffiths, 2013), the time between measurements (Addy, 2012), and the differences in the method of vaporization employed (Ranganathan et al., 2012), could imply different absorption and levels of the compound in plasma.

Neuroendocrine Effects

KORs regulate hormonal processes. There are sex differences in terms of distribution and KOR levels. SA increased plasma concentrations of prolactin and cortisol 5 minutes after inhalation, peaked at minute 15, and gradually decreased after 90 minutes (Johnson et al., 2016; Maqueda et al., 2016). However, these studies showed variations in individual measures, which could be explained due to the different responses of men and women to SA. Some participants did not show any cortisol response at all (Johnson et al., 2016).

Psychophysiology

Ranganathan and colleagues (2012) performed an electroencephalographic (EEG) analysis of the eight volunteers of their study. They found that inhalation of SA decreased β frequency in both high doses (8 and 12 mg), and θ frequency also showed a decrease with a tendency toward statistical significance. These results of very high doses of SA would be indicative of a reduction in the waking state, similar to deep sleep or a state of sedation. In our laboratory (Valle et al., 2016) we also measured EEG before and after the vaporization of 1 mg of SA. The results showed that SA suppressed α rhythm and markedly increased slow δ activity. Less prominent effects included increases in θ and low γ bands. While SA shares with serotonergic psychedelics the α-suppressing action, its main neurophysiological signature is an atypical enhancement of slow δ activity, associated with non-rapid eye movement (NREM) sleep.

▧ Adverse Reactions

In regard to laboratory studies, the literature shows that inhaled doses of up to 12 mg of pure SA are safe in terms of physiological measures. Of the 112 subjects in total, summing all the participants of the controlled studies performed until today, carried out in six laboratories in six different countries, no adverse reactions have been found in volunteers. In the case of the recreational use of potentiated extracts of *S. divinorum,* several published anecdotal reports suggest that SA could occasionally produce psychotic symptoms that required treatment by emergency care personnel. In one of these reports, the patient reported that the psychotic symptoms began after smoking a cannabis cigarette, to which material from a *S. divinorum* extract had been added without her knowledge (Paulzen & Gründer, 2008). However, relative to subjects of the reports, their prior psychiatric status, their personal and family background, or whether there was concomitant use of other drugs were not reported. In general, the side effects induced by the vaporization of *S. divinorum,* if produced, do not elicit excessive discomfort. These somatic–dysphoric effects include subjective changes in body temperature, sensations of electricity and tingling in the body, heaviness of head, and tiredness, which are transient and similar to those of classic hallucinogens.

Respecting harm reduction, it is very important to have an attentive and sober sitter to maintain safety of the user during the trip, and to start with low doses, until the individual's personal sensitivity to the compound is known. The intensity of the experience can be overwhelming, and the person may lose touch with reality. The effects of *S. divinorum* are exceptionally sensitive to context. Because of the particular synesthesia with the material world that this compound may induce, to be in a pleasing and comfortable context is recommended. A recent survey on wise-salvia users who smoked extracts remarked on the existing synergy between the substance, the context, and the sitter or guide (Hutton, Kivell, & Boyle, 2016). The respondents of the survey preferred to be at home or in isolated outdoor settings and accompanied by friends. The management of these considerations help in tackling unhelpful stigma surrounding this plant.

In the case of buccal consumption of *S. divinorum,* users have 10 minutes before feeling any effects, which allows a progressive adaptation to them. In fact, the effects have a very subtle onset, so they may even be missed if the user is distracted, or in a noisy or too luminous environment.

▧ Other Short- and Long-Term Psychological Effects

At the present moment there are no studies on the effects of long-term consumption of *S. divinorum.* One reason may be the low number of users who employ the plant repeatedly. Several surveys have revealed that nontraditional use of *S. divinorum* is sporadic due to unrewarding effects for the typical recreational consumption, and because many users find the effects too intense or unpleasant (Baggott, Erowid, Erowid, Galloway, & Mendelson, 2010). In a retrospective survey of recurrent recreational users of the plant, 13 respondents claimed to have gained a greater connection with others, and to have increased creativity and connection with nature, as well as a greater understanding about the nature of reality (Nygård, 2007). MacLean and his group (2013) carried out a 1-month follow-up of their study, finding no evidence of lasting negative effects such as depression, anxiety, psychiatric symptoms, or visual disturbances. Four of the eight participants reported specific positive changes that they attributed to the experiences on the day of the session, including greater self-confidence, a feeling of greater physical comfort and calmness, less emotional reactivity, improvements in interpersonal relationships, and renewed interest in daily responsibilities. There is a report of a young man who chewed or smoked dry leaves of the plant twice a week for 6 months, without reporting any detrimental effects on his health or social or academic life (Bücheler et al., 2005). The Mazatec have been consuming the leaves of *S. divinorum* for centuries. For them, this herb is a key piece of their culture and a sacred medicine that can be consumed for extended periods without any harmful effects on their mental or physical health. In fact, *S. divinorum* is the initiation plant or training herb for the future healer because it is considered the plant that is easiest to handle, with the least psychoactive power, followed by morning glory seeds, and finally, by the management of hallucinogenic mushrooms.

▪ Therapeutic Potential of *S. divinorum* and SA

Neither *S. divinorum* nor its active constituent has yet been approved for medical use in the United States. Currently, *S. divinorum* is controlled in 22 U.S. states and listed as a "drug of concern" by the U.S. Drug Enforcement Administration (2017). As reviewed in this chapter, *S. divinorum* is a nontoxic, non-addictive plant with multiple medicinal applications. There is no scientific justification based on research or on any public health concern to maintain this herb's criminalized status. Instead, a smarter approach is to keep *S. divinorum* legal while establishing age-control restrictions and other regulations. Outright prohibition of *S. divinorum* deters scientists from studying its medical benefits, and replaces a legal market that can be strictly and sensibly be regulated with an underground economy. Still, *S. divinorum* is legally and commercially available in many states and countries, so it could be possible to have a safe medicine and a Master Plant at home. Cuttings are relatively easy to cultivate, and dry leaves, tinctures, and concentrated extracts can be bought online.

▪ Therapeutic Potential of *S. divinorum*

As with many psychoactive plants, there is scarce research about the mental and behavioral effects of *S. divinorum*, but there are much more detailed data about its active principle. Fortunately, we have the centenary knowledge of the Mazatec to guide us in the use of this wonderful herb. I have created a nonprofit, the Center for Research and Ethnobotanical Conservation of *Salvia divinorum* (*xkapastora*.org), to compile and divulge the traditional uses of Salvia of the Mazatec. From articles published by the researchers who visited the Mazatec Sierra and participated in ceremonies with *S. divinorum*, we know that the Mazatec use the plant as a treatment for arthritis and inflammation, headaches, gastrointestinal problems, elimination dysfunctions, and as general relief or tonic for the sick, anemic, or the dying. During my own fieldwork conducted with the Mazatec (Maqueda, 2018), I learned that the leaves of *S. divinorum* are applied in poultices to treat insect bites, eczema, fungi, candidiasis and other vaginal diseases, and that the leaves are eaten to treat cystitis, menstrual cramps, bronchitis, and fever. For the treatment of pain, back contractions, water retention, and inflammation, the juice of 40 leaves or more is drunk right before going to sleep. The users that I interviewed reported vivid dreams, and a significant and lasting remission of the symptoms. For the treatment of addictions, the early literature has reported on use of the leaves for the treatment of alcoholics. I lived with a traditional healer and his family, whose older son had been addicted to inhalants and cocaine. The father treated his son successfully using *S. divinorum* in ceremonies, as well as with the administration of fresh leaves on alternate days for 1 month (Addy & Maqueda, 2015). I know, too, that *S. divinorum* is employed for treating symptoms of low mood, by eating a small pair of fresh leaves in the morning until the symptoms disappear. Hanes (2001) presented the clinical case of a 26-year-old woman with treatment-resistant depression, who showed improvement after taking subpsychoactive oral doses of *S. divinorum*. The patient chewed and kept in her mouth from 0.5 to 0.75 g of dried leaf for 15–30 minutes, two or three times a week, and also claimed to benefit from occasional psychoactive doses consisting of 2–4 g of leaves. Dr. Hanes reported on the total remission of depressive symptoms of the patient in the last 6 months, as well as a considerable improvement in self-esteem and psychospiritual development. Later, Hanes (2003) published a follow-up report on six additional patients who achieved a complete remission of the symptoms of treatment-resistant depression using the leaves. A growing body of research indicates that the endogenous opioid system is directly involved in the regulation of mood and is dysregulated in mayor depressive disorder. This involvement of the endogenous opioid system may underlie the disproportionate use of opioids among patients with mood disorders. The use of the leaves of *S. divinorum* for mood disorders could provide safe and nonaddictive treatment, instead of the highly addictive opioid medicines massively prescribed today. This would help to alleviate the opioid crisis that the United States is currently facing. *S. divinorum* produces a state of increased self-awareness. For this reason, some psychotherapists use it in tincture form as an adjuvant to psychotherapy, and some people use it as an aid to meditation, contemplation, and spiritual reflection (Soutar & Strassman, 2000). Future research could explore the profile of effects in humans and the potential of *S. divinorum* for psychotherapy. In animal research, only one study has explored the administration of a hydroponic extract of *S. divinorum* (Simón-Arceo et al., 2017). The authors found that the extract significantly reduced nociceptive and inflammatory processes.

▪ Therapeutic Potential of SA

The medicinal applications of the Mazatec using the leaves of *S. divinorum* are well supported by recent pharmacological findings with SA.

1. *Medications for addictions.* As previously mentioned, κ-agonists modulate dopaminergic activity. These compounds have been shown to decrease opioid withdrawal in both animals and humans, to decrease cocaine-, amphetamine-, and heroin-induced DA release, to decrease many behavioral effects of nicotine, and to attenuate self-administration of cocaine, morphine, and heroin, all of which supports the role of κ-agonists as pharmacotherapeutics for treating addictions (Morani, Kivell, Prisinzano, & Schenk, 2009). The compound SA has been shown to inhibit the hyperlocomotive activity, the rewarding effects, the reestablishment of self-administration, and the altered expression of genes induced by cocaine. The reduced profile of side effects compared to κ-agonists makes SA a compound of high therapeutic promise in treating drug abuse (Dos Santos, Crippa, Machado-de-Sousa, &

Hallak, 2014). Regarding the low addictive potential of *S. divinorum*, demonstrated by animal research (Serra et al., 2015), we have seen that the stimulation of KORs causes dysphoria, the opposite effect of the euphoria that entails the typical drug of abuse. As described earlier, dysphoria implies a detachment of one's own bodily sensations, an annoying or unpleasant sensation, that lies at the opposite pole of a pleasant sensation or one with addictive potential.

2. *Antidepressants.* Animal studies have demonstrated the antidepressant properties of SA (Braida et al., 2009), and it has been proposed as a candidate for the treatment of major depressive disorder (Taylor & Manzella, 2016).

3. *Medications for perceptive and cognitive disorders.* Due to its acute action on KORs, compounds derived from SA could offer new treatments for disorders that manifest alterations in perception and cognitive dysfunctions, such as schizophrenia, bipolar disorder, and Alzheimer's disease (Butelman & Kreek, 2015).

4. *Safe and nonaddictive analgesics.* Some of the analgesics employed in the current medical practice produce dependence (e.g., morphine). To find an opioid-strength analgesic devoid of side effects, especially addiction, has eluded pain researchers. Research supports the use of SA as a therapeutic alternative for the relief of chronic pain without addictive properties (Guida et al., 2012).

5. *Anti-inflammatories.* SA has ultrapotent effects on macrophages via KORs (Aviello et al., 2011), and it exerts an important attenuation of inflammation and intestinal motility in irritable bowel syndrome (Capasso et al., 2008). SA also inhibits the inflammatory response mediated by leukotrienes, which are crucial in various autoimmune and inflammatory conditions such as bronchial asthma, allergic rhinitis, urticaria, and cardiovascular problems (Rossi et al., 2016).

6. *Medications to treat different types of cancer.* When there are tumors in the brain, one of the difficulties of therapeutics is to get the drugs through the blood–brain barrier and reach the tumor. The terpene SA is able to cross the blood–brain barrier and

reach the brain and structures of the CNS in less than a minute. SA analogues have demonstrated antiproliferative properties that inhibit the growth of 77–86% of tumors in the MCF7 breast cancer cell line (Vasiljevik, Groer, Lehner, Navarro, & Prisinzano, 2014).

7. Assisting psychotherapy. SA has several properties that would make it effective as an adjunct to psychotherapy. In low doses, it helps to increase body awareness and awareness of the interconnectedness of the body, emotions, and mental states. It also produces a state of deep introspection, facilitates the recall of biographical episodes, and offers access to areas of the psyche that are not easily attainable ordinarily. I have received several personal communications from psychotherapists and patients about the extraordinary potential of vaporizing low doses of SA for psychological healing.

Other promising medications are neuroprotectors for acute brain pathologies (Sun et al., 2018), and short-term anesthetics that do not depress breathing (McCurdy, Sufka, Smith, Warnick, & Nieto, 2006).

▓ References

Aardvark, D. (Ed.). (2002). Salvia divinorum and salvinorin A. In K. Trout (Ed.), *The best of Entheogen Review 1992–2000* (2nd ed.). Sacramento, CA: Entheogen Review.

Addy, P. H. (2012). Acute and post-acute behavioral and psychological effects of salvinorin A in humans. *Psychopharmacology (Berlin), 220,* 195–204.

Addy, P. H., & Maqueda, A. E. (2015, August 11). Traditional medicine from southern Mexico offers help with addiction. Retrieved from *www.scientificamerican.com/article/traditional-medicine-from-southern-mexico-offers-help-with-addiction*.

Aviello, G., Borrelli, F., Guida, F., Romano, B., Lewellyn, K., De Chiaro, M., et al. (2011). Ultrapotent effects of salvinorin A, a hallucinogenic compound from Salvia divinorum, on LPS-stimulated murine macrophages and its anti-inflammatory action *in vivo*. *Journal of Molecular Medicine (Berlin), 89*(9), 891–902.

Baggott, M., Erowid, E., & Erowid, F. (2004). A survey of *Salvia divinorum* users. *Erowid Extracts, 6,* 12–14.

Baggott, M. J., Erowid, E., Erowid, F., Galloway, G. P., & Mendelson, J. (2010). Use patterns and self-reported effects of *Salvia divinorum:* An internet-based survey. *Drug and Alcohol Dependence, 111,* 250–256.

Braida, D., Capurro, V., & Zani, A. (2009). Potential anxiolytic and antidepressant-like effects of salvinorin A, the main active ingredient of *Salvia divinorum*, in rodents. *British Journal of Pharmacology, 157,* 844–853.

Braida, D., Limonta, V., Pegorini, S., Zani, A., Guerini-Rocco, C., & Gori, E. (2007). Hallucinatory and rewarding effect of salvinorin A in zebrafish: κ-opioid and CB_1-cannabinoid receptor involvement. *Psychopharmacology (Berlin), 190*(4), 441–448.

Bücheler, R., Gleiter, C. H., Schwoerer, P., & Gaertner, I. (2005). Use of nonprohibited hallucinogenic plants: Increasing relevance for public health?: A case report and literature review on the consumption of *Salvia divinorum* (diviner's sage). *Pharmacopsychiatry, 38,* 1–5.

Butelman, E. R., & Kreek, M. J. (2015). Salvinorin A, a kappa-opioid receptor agonist hallucinogen: Pharmacology and potential template for novel pharmacotherapeutic agents in neuropsychiatric disorders. *Frontiers in Pharmacology, 6,* 190.

Capasso, R., Borrelli, F., Zjawiony, J., Kutrzeba, L., Aviello, G., Sarnelli, G., et al. (2008). The hallucinogenic herb *Salvia divinorum* and its active ingredient salvinorin A reduce inflammation-induced hypermotility in mice. *Neurogastroenterology and Motility, 20,* 142–148.

Carlezon, W. A., Beguin, C., DiNieri, J. A., Baumann, M. H., Richards, M. R., & Todtenkopf, M. S. (2006). Depressive-like effects of the μ-opioid receptor agonist salvinorin A on behavior and neurochemistry in rats. *Journal of Pharmacology and Experimental Therapeutics, 316*(1), 440–447.

Casselman, I., Nock, C. J., Wohlmuth, H., Weatherby, R. P., & Heinrich, M. (2014). From local to global—fifty years of research on Salvia divinorum. *Journal of Ethnopharmacology, 151*(2), 768–783.

Chartoff, E. H., Potter, D., Damez-Werno, D., Cohen, B. M., & Carlezon, W. A. (2008). Exposure to the selective μ-opioid receptor agonist salvinorin A nodulates the behavioral and molecular effects of cocaine in rats. *Journal of Neuropsychopharmacology, 33*(11), 2676–2687.

Coffeen, U., Canseco, A., Simón-Arceo, K., Almanza, A., Mercado, F., Leon-Olea, M., et al. (2018). Salvinorin A reduces neuropathic nociception in the insular cortex of the rat. *European Journal of Pain, 22,* 311–318.

Díaz, J. L. (2013). *Salvia divinorum:* A psychopharmacological riddle and a mind–body prospect. *Current Drug Abuse Reviews, 6,* 43–53.

Dos Santos, R. G., Crippa, J. A., Machado-de-Sousa, J. P., & Hallak, J. E. (2014). Salvinorin A and related compounds as therapeutic drugs for psychostimulant-related disorders. *Current Drug Abuse Reviews, 7*(2), 128–132.

Epling, C., & Játiva-M, C. D. (1962). A new species of Salvia from Mexico. *Botanical Museum Leaflets, Harvard University, 20*(3), 75–76.

Gehrke, B. J., Chefer, V. I., & Shippenberg, T. S. (2008). Effects of acute and repeated administration of salvinorin A on dopamine function in the rat dorsal striatum. *Psychopharmacology (Berlin), 197,* 509–517.

Gómez Pompa, A. (1957). *Salvia divinorum* herbarium sheets, A. Gómez Pompa 87556 and 93216. Mexico, D.F.: National Herbarium (UNAM).

Grilli, M., Neri, E., Zappettini, S., Massa, F., Bisio, A., Romussi, G., et al. (2009). Salvinorin A exerts opposite presynaptic controls on neurotransmitter exocytosis from mouse brain nerve terminals. *Neuropharmacology, 57,* 523–530.

Guida, F., Luongo, L., Aviello, G., Palazzo, E., De Chiaro, M., Gatta, L., et al. (2012). Salvinorin A reduces mechanical allodynia and spinal neuronal hyperexcitability induced by peripheral formalin injection. *Molecular Pain, 8,* 60.

Hanes, K. R. (2001). Antidepressant effects of the herb *Salvia divinorum:* A case report. *Journal of Clinical Psychopharmacology, 21,* 634–635.

Hanes, K. R. (2003). *Salvia divinorum:* Clinical and research potential. *MAPS Bulletin, 13*(1), 18–20.

Hofmann, A., & Tscherter, H. (1960). Isolation of lysergic acid alkaloids from the Mexican drug ololiuqui (Rivea corymbosa (L.) Hall.f.) *Experientia, 16,* 414.

Hooker, J. M., Patel, V., Kothari, S., & Schiffer, W. K. (2009). Metabolic changes in the rodent brain after acute administration of salvinorin A. *Molecular Imaging and Biology, 11,* 137–143.

Hooker, J. M., Xu, Y., Schiffer, W., Shea, C., Carter, P., & Fowler, J. S. (2008). Pharmacokinetics of the potent hallucinogen, salvinorin A in primates parallels the rapid onset and short duration of effects in humans. *NeuroImage, 41,* 1044–1050.

Hutton, F., Kivell, B., & Boyle, O. (2016). "Quite a profoundly strange experience": An analysis of the experiences of *Salvia divinorum* users. *Journal of Psychoactive Drugs, 3,* 206–213.

Jenks, A. A., Walker, J. B., & Kim, S. C. (2010).

Evolution and origins of the Mazatec hallucinogenic sage, *Salvia divinorum* (Lamiaceae): A molecular phylogenetic approach. *Journal of Plant Research, 124*(5), 593–600.

Johnson, J. B. (1939). The elements of Mazatec witchcraft. *Göteborgs Etnografiska Museum, Etnologiska Studier, 9,* 119–149.

Johnson, M. W., MacLean, K. A., Caspers, M. J., Prisinzano, T. E., & Griffiths, R. R. (2016). Time course of pharmacokinetic and hormonal effects of inhaled high-dose salvinorin A in humans. *Journal of Psychopharmacology, 30,* 323–329.

Johnson, M. W., MacLean, K. A., Reissig, C. J., Prisinzano, T. E., & Griffiths, R. R. (2011). Human psychopharmacology and dose-effects of salvinorin A, a kappa opioid agonist hallucinogen present in the plant *Salvia divinorum. Drug and Alcohol Dependence, 115,* 150–155.

Kivell, B. M., Ewald, A. W. M., & Prisinzano, T. E. (2014). Salvinorin A analogs and other kappa-opioid receptor compounds as treatments for cocaine abuse. *Advances in Pharmacology, 69,* 481–511.

MacLean, K. A., Johnson, M. W., Reissig, C. J., Prisinzano, T. E., & Griffiths, R. R. (2013). Dose-related effects of salvinorin A in humans: Dissociative, hallucinogenic, and memory effects. *Psychopharmacology (Berlin), 226,* 381–392.

Maqueda, A. E. (2018). The use of *Salvia divinorum* from a Mazatec perspective. In B. C. Labate & C. Cavnar (Eds.), *Plant medicines, healing and psychedelic science: Cultural perspectives* (pp. 55–67). Cham, Switzerland: Springer.

Maqueda, A. E., Valle, M., Addy, P. H., Antonijoan, R. M., Puntes, M., Coimbra, J., et al. (2015). Salvinorin-A induces intense dissociative effects, blocking external sensory perception and modulating interoception and sense of body ownership in humans. *International Journal of Neuropsychopharmacology, 18,* pyv065.

Maqueda, A. E., Valle, M., Addy, P. H., Antonijoan, R. M., Puntes, M., Coimbra, J., et al. (2016). Naltrexone but not ketanserin antagonizes the subjective, cardiovascular, and neuroendocrine effects of salvinorin-A in humans. *International Journal of Neuropsychopharmacology, 19*(7), 1–13.

McCurdy, C. R., Sufka, K. J., Smith, G. H., Warnick, J. E., & Nieto, M. J. (2006). Antinociceptive profile of salvinorin A: A structurally unique kappa opioid receptor agonist. *Pharmacology, Biochemistry, and Behavior, 83*(1), 109–113.

Mendelson, J. E., Coyle, J. R., Lopez, J. C., Baggott, M. J., Flower, K., Everhart, E., et al. (2011). Lack of effect of sublingual salvinorin A, a naturally occurring kappa opioid, in humans: A placebo-controlled trial. *Psychopharmacology (Berlin), 214*, 933–939.

Morani, A. S., Kivell, B., Prisinzano, T. E., & Schenk, S. (2009). Effect of kappa-opioid receptor agonists U69593, U50488H, spiradoline and salvinorin A on cocaine-induced drug-seeking in rats. *Pharmacology Biochemistry and Behavior, 94*, 244–249.

Mowry, M., Mosher, M., & Briner, W. (2003). Acute physiologic and chronic histologic changes in rats and mice exposed to the unique hallucinogen salvinorin A. *Journal of Psychoactive Drugs, 35*, 379–382.

Nygård, E. A. (2007). *Listening to the sage: The experience of learning from the Salvia divinorum altered state*. Unpublished doctoral dissertation, Institute of Transpersonal Psychology, Palo Alto, CA.

Ortega, A., Blount, J. F., & Manchand, P. S. (1982). Salvinorin, a new trans-neoclerodane diterpene from *Salvia divinorum* (Labiatae). *Journal of the Chemical Society: Perkin Transactions, 1*, 2505–2508.

Ott, J. (1995). Ethnopharmacognosy and human pharmacology of *Salvia divinorum* and salvinorin A. *Curare, 18*, 103–129.

Paulzen, M., & Gründer, G. (2008). Toxic psychosis after intake of the hallucinogen salvinorin A. *Journal of Clinical Psychiatry, 69*, 1501–1502.

Pichini, S., Abanades, S., Farre, M., Pellegrini, M., Marchei, E., & Pacifici, R. (2005). Quantification of the plant-derived hallucinogen salvinorin A in conventional and non-conventional biological fluids by gas chromatography/mass spectrometry after *Salvia divinorum* smoking. *Rapid Communications in Mass Spectrometry, 19*, 1649–1656.

Ranganathan, M., Schnakenberg, A., Skosnik, P. D., Cohen, B. M., Pittman, B., Sewell, R. A., et al. (2012). Dose-related behavioral, subjective, endocrine, and psychophysiological effects of the μ opioid agonist Salvinorin A in humans. *Biological Psychiatry, 72*, 871–879.

Reisfield, A. S. (1993). The botany of *Salvia divinorum* (Labiatae). *SIDA, 15*(3), 349–366.

Reko, B. P. (1945). *Mitobotanica Zapoteca*. Tacubaya, Mexico: Private Printing,

Roach, J. J., & Shenvi, R. A. (2018). A review of salvinorin analogs and their kappa opioid receptor activity. *Bioorganic and Medicinal Chemistry Letters, 28*(9), 1436–1445.

Rossi, A., Pace, S., Tedesco, F., Pagano, E., Guerra, G., Troisi, F., et al. (2016). The hallucinogenic diterpene salvinorin A inhibits leukotriene synthesis in experimental models of inflammation. *Pharmacological Research Journal, 106*, 64–71.

Roth, B. L., Baner, K., Westkaemper, R., Siebert, D., Rice, K. C., Steinberg, S., et al. (2002). Salvinorin A: A potent naturally occurring nonnitrogenous kappa opioid selective agonist. *Proceedings of the National Academy of Sciences of the USA, 99*, 11934–11939.

Rothman, R. B., Murphy, D. L., Xu, H., Godin, J. A., Dersch, C. M., Partilla, J. S., et al. (2007). Salvinorin A: Allosteric interactions at the mu-opioid receptor. *Journal of Pharmacology and Experimental Therapeutics, 320*(2), 801–810.

Russell, S. E., Rachlin, A. B., Smith, K. L., Muschamp, J., Berry, L., Zhao, Z., et al. (2014). Sex differences in sensitivity to the depressive-like effects of the kappa opioid receptor agonist U-50488 in rats. *Biological Psychiatry, 76*(3), 213–222.

Schultes, R. E. (1976). *Hallucinogenic plants* (E. W. Smith, Illus.). New York: Golden Press.

Seeman, P., Guan, H., & Hirbec, H. (2009). Dopamine D2 receptors stimulated by phencyclidines, lysergic acid diethylamide, salvinorin A, and modafinil. *Synapse, 63*, 698–704.

Serra, V., Fattore, L., Scherma, M., Collu, R., Spano, M. S., Fratta, W., et al. (2015). Behavioral and neurochemical assessment of salvinorin A abuse potential in the rat. *Psychopharmacology, 232*(1), 91–100.

Siebert, D. J. (1994). *Salvia divinorum* and salvinorin A: New pharmacologic findings. *Journal of Ethnopharmacology, 43*(1), 53–56.

Siebert, D. J. (2003). The history of the first *Salvia divinorum* plants cultivated outside of Mexico. *Entheogen Review, 12*(4), 117–118.

Simón-Arceo, K., González-Trujano, M. E., Coffeen, U., Fernández-Mas, R., Mercado, F., Almanza, A., et al. (2017). Neuropathic and inflammatory antinociceptive effects and electrocortical changes produced by *Salvia divinorum* in rats. *Journal of Ethnopharmacology, 206*, 115–124.

Soutar, I., & Strassman, R. (2000). Meditation with *Salvia divinorum*/salvinorin A. Retrieved from *www.maps.org/researcharchive/salvia/sdmeditation.html*.

Stiefel, K. M., Merrifield, A., & Holcombe, A. O. (2014). The claustrum's proposed role in consciousness is supported by the effect and target localization of *Salvia divinorum*. *Frontiers in Integrative Neuroscience, 8*, 20.

Sun, J., Zhang, Y., Lu, J., Zhang, W., Yan, J., Yang, L., et al. (2018). Salvinorin A ameliorates cerebral vasospasm through activation of endothelial nitric oxide synthase in a rat model of subarachnoid hemorrhage. *Microcirculation, 25*, Article e12442.

Taylor, G. T., & Manzella, F. (2016). Kappa opioids, salvinorin A and major depressive disorder. *Current Neuropharmacology Journal, 14*(2), 165–176.

Turner, D. M. (1996). *Salvinorin: The psychedelic essence of Salvia Divinorum,* Matewan, NJ: Panther Press.

U.S. Drug Enforcement Administration. (2017). Salva divinorum. Retrieved from *www.dea.gov/factsheets/salvia-divinorum.*

Valdés, J. L., III, Butler, W. M., Hatfield, G. M., Paul, A. G., & Koreeda, M. (1984). Divinorin A, a psychotropic terpenoid, and divinorin B from the hallucinogenic Mexican mint *Salvia divinorum. Journal of Organic Chemistry, 49,* 4716–4720.

Valdés, J. L., III, Diaz, J. L., & Paul, A. G. (1983). Ethnopharmacology of ska Maria Pastora (*Salvia divinorum* Epling and Jativa-M.). *Journal of Ethnopharmacology, 7*(3), 287–312.

Valdés, J. L., III, Hatfield, G. M., Koreeda, M., & Paul, A. G. (1987). Studies of *Salvia divinorum* (Lamiaceae): A hallucinogenic mint from the Sierra Mazateca in Oaxaca, Central Mexico. *Economic Botany, 41*(2), 283–291.

Valle, M., Maqueda, A. E., Romero, S., Mañanas, M. A., Barker, S., & Riba, J. (2016, October). *Salvinorin-A induces a unique pattern of neurophyciological effects in humans characterized by alpha suppression and widespread increases in cortical delta activity.* Paper presented at congress 19th biennial IPEG meeting, Nijmegen, the Netherlands.

Vasiljevik, T., Groer, C. E., Lehner, K., Navarro, H., & Prisinzano, T. E. (2014). Studies toward the development of antiproliferative neoclerodanes from salvinorin A. *Journal of Natural Products, 77*(8), 1817–1824.

Wang, Y., Tang, K., Inan, S., Siebert, D., Holzgrabe, U., & Lee, D. Y. W. (2005). Comparison of pharmacological activities of three distinct k ligands (salvinorin A, TRK-820 and 3FLB) on k opioid receptors in vitro and their antipruritic and antinociceptive activities *in vivo. Journal of Pharmacology and Experimental Therapeutics, 312*(1), 220–230.

Wasson, R. G. (1962). A new Mexican psychotropic drug from the mint family. *Botanical Museum Leaflets, Harvard University, 20*(3), 77–84.

Weitlaner, R. J. (1952). Curaciones mazatecas. *Anales del Instituto Nacional de Antropologia e Historia, 4,* 279–285.

Wolowich, W. R., Perkins, A. M., & Cienki, J. J. (2006). Analysis of the psychoactive terpenoid salvinorin A content in five *Salvia divinorum* herbal products. *Pharmacotherapy, 26*(9), 1268–1272.

CHAPTER 17

Ketamine

GARY BRAVO, ROBERT GRANT, and RAQUEL BENNETT

Introduction

One of the most startling developments in 21st-century psychiatry has been the discovery of the antidepressant action of the anesthetic drug ketamine. The remarkable efficacy of ketamine in alleviating treatment-resistant depression (TRD) and suicidal ideation, particularly its rapid mechanism of action, and the resulting implications for the study of novel mechanisms for treating depression, have sent jolts of excitement throughout the neuroscientific and psychiatric communities. One prominent neuroscientist has noted that this discovery "might be the most important breakthrough in antidepressant treatment in decades" (Insel, 2014).

Although chemically distinct, ketamine has often been classified with the psychedelic drugs because, at subanesthetic doses that are six to 10 times less than those used for general anesthesia, it produces a profound alteration in consciousness, with psychoactive effects similar to psychedelics. Ketamine also has a history of being used as both an adjunct to psychotherapy with classic psychedelics (Wolfson, 2016b) and a primary psychedelic for psychotherapy (Krupitsky & Grinenko, 1997).

Despite its reputation as a "club drug" and as having abuse potential, ketamine is the only psychedelic medicine that is not classified by the Drug Enforcement Administration (DEA) as Schedule 1 (of high abuse potential and no medical use). Ketamine is a Schedule 3 drug, allowing clinical use and an easier path to research, without the constraints that hinder investigation of all other psychedelics.

In the decade since Zarate and colleagues (2006) published a seminal paper showing ketamine to be a rapid and robust treatment for TRD, there have been over 2,000 scientific papers on the use of ketamine for psychiatric conditions. However, the prevailing treatment paradigm has viewed ketamine strictly as a chemotherapeutic agent and does not include psychoactive or psychedelic effects as contributing to the therapeutic outcomes. In this view, the psychoactivity of ketamine, variously viewed as dissociative, deliriant, or psychotomimetic, is seen as an undesired and problematic side effect that needs to be avoided and sometimes medicated. However, other researchers and clinical practitioners, including many proponents of the newly reemergent field of psychedelic psychotherapy, have reported that ketamine-assisted psychotherapy (KAP), following treatment models that combine elements of psycholytic (ego-loosening) and psychedelic (ego-dissolving) methods, may enhance treatment outcomes for their patients by fostering a greater access to the unconscious, and greater self-acceptance, self-transcendence, and sense of meaning (Wolfson, 2016a).

In this chapter, we review the history, chemistry, and pharmacology of ketamine as a psychedelic agent; its burgeoning use as a psychiatric medicine, including its potential range of clinical effects; and finally, its role as a legal agent in psychedelic-assisted psychotherapy. We present the different paradigms of treatment, along with the challenges, controversies, and potential risks and dangers involved in this nascent field.

History

Ketamine is a member of a class of compounds called arylcyclohexylamines, developed by the Parke-Davis pharmaceutical company as anesthetic agents. The first compound in this class was phencyclidine (PCP), first synthesized in 1926 and patented in 1953, and used as an anesthetic agent for humans and animals until the mid-1960s, when it was abandoned for human use due to its extended postoperative psychotic-like effects, called "emergence delirium." Ketamine, with a chemical structure very similar to PCP, was first synthesized in 1962 by Calvin Stevens at Parke-Davis in the search for safer and more predictable anesthetic medications. The unique pharmacological effects of PCP and ketamine, including stimulation at lower doses and sedation at higher doses, lack of pulmonary or cardiac suppression, seeming indifference to pain, and dream-like imagery, led this class of chemicals to be labeled "dissociative anesthetics" (Domino, 2010). Unlike most other psychedelics, arylcyclohexylamines or their analogues have not as yet been discovered in the human body or anywhere else in nature.

Ketamine is U.S. Food and Drug Administration (FDA) approved for anesthesia and widely used for painful surgical procedures that do not require skeletal relaxation, or for patients who are hemodynamically compromised, such as victims of trauma (Chang et

al., 2016). It continues to be an anesthetic of choice for surgeries involving children, elderly adults, burn patients, cesarean sections, and procedural sedation both in emergency rooms and increasingly in the field for trauma victims. Subanesthetic doses of ketamine have also been utilized in pain medicine for decades (Visser & Schug, 2006).

Early on, there were reports, mostly outside of the United States, of ketamine being useful for psychiatric conditions (Khorramzadeh & Lofty, 1973). Ketamine's psychedelic effects were introduced to the psychedelic research program at the Maryland Psychiatric Research Institute in the early 1970s by a Mexican psychiatrist, Salvador Roquet, who used it primarily as an adjunct to psychedelic psychotherapy (Wolfson, 2016b).

The characterization of ketamine as a psychedelic with psychologically addictive potential became publicized with the release of a couple of books by high-profile authors, who appeared to use it excessively for the exploration of consciousness but ended up with severe adverse consequences. John Lilly (1978), a prominent research physician and neuroscientist, pioneer of human–dolphin communication, inventor of the isolation tank, and explorer of lysergic acid diethylamide (LSD), experienced several psychotic delusional states, presumably due to ketamine addiction. Marsha Moore, an author of New Age books, wrote of her spiritual explorations of ketamine in *Journeys into the Bright World* (Moore & Alltounian, 1978). However, she died under mysterious circumstances in 1979, presumably, but not certainly, while under the influence of ketamine.

Nonetheless, ketamine continued to be explored by the psychedelic community throughout the 1980s and 1990s. It gained a notorious reputation as a club drug and date-rape drug, and there were reports of addiction and dependency (Jansen & Darracot-Cankovic, 2001). In some parts of the world, especially East and Southeast Asia, ketamine addiction has become a major problem (Rao et al., 2015). These issues led to ketamine being placed in Schedule 3 by the DEA in 1999.

In the 1990s, ketamine was used in a psychedelic psychotherapy paradigm to research and treat alcohol addiction and neurosis in Russia (Krupitsky, 1993/1994), which led to further clinical work in the U.S. (Kolp et al., 2006). The first awakening of interest in ketamine by academic psychiatry (as opposed to anesthesiology), was by those who saw ketamine, because of its close structural relationship to PCP, as a potential ideal chemical means to produce a model schizophrenic state (Krystal et al., 2013). When administered to humans with no history of psychosis, ketamine produced effects of concrete thinking, loose associations, and disconnection with external reality, all partial features of schizophrenia (Vollenweider, Leenders, Scharfetter, et al., 1997), and especially negative symptoms of schizophrenia (Gouzoulis-Mayfrank et al., 2005). This led to the glutamate-mediated model of schizophrenia, which although of intense interest to biological psychiatrists, has not yet yielded a clinical application.

However, the group at Yale studying ketamine's effects as a psychotomimetic agent led to the surprising discovery that ketamine seemed to provide rapid relief from depression (Berman et al., 2000). But interest in ketamine's effects on depression did not really take off until a follow-up study (Zarate et al., 2006). The evidence has been robust for ketamine's antidepressant response for TRD (see Ryan et al., 2016, for a comprehensive review). Between 2000 and 2015, nine randomized controlled clinical trials were performed using ketamine for TRD. The control arms were a placebo or midazolam, a benzodiazepine. These studies generally followed the standard protocol developed by the National Institute of Mental Health (NIMH), which was infusing 0.5 mg/kg of ketamine intravenously over 40 minutes. This dose was designed to keep subjects conscious and responsive and minimize hallucinations. The studies using this protocol typically yielded remissions of depression in 60–70% of people who were previously treatment resistant (McGirr et al., 2015). However, such remissions were frequently short-lived, with about 10% of participants still in remission after 10 days.

To prolong the benefits of ketamine, further protocols were developed to allow repeated dosing, two or three times per week for several weeks, to induce remission of depression (aan het Rot et al., 2010; Cusin et al., 2017; Diamond et al., 2014; Ghasemi et al., 2014; Murrough et al., 2013; Rasmussen et al., 2013; Shiroma, Johns, et al., 2014; Singh et al., 2016). These studies generally found increasing response rates with repeated dosing, and this model has generally become the standard of care in clinical practices that utilize ketamine without psychotherapy.

But the use of ketamine to treat mood disorders continued to surprise clinicians, as it was discovered that ketamine, in addition to its antidepressant effect, also rapidly relieved suicidal ideation (Murrough, Soleimani, et al., 2015; Zhan et al., 2019). Wilkinson and colleagues' (2018) review of 10 studies using ketamine showed that 24 hours after a single infusion of ketamine, 54.9% of subjects were free of suicidal ideation, and 60% remained free after 1 week. This antisuicidal effect was partially independent of ketamine's effects on mood. A recent randomized controlled study, using midazolam as the control, showed that after 24 hours, ketamine significantly reduced measures of suicidal ideation, compared to the controls, again, partially independent of the reduction in depression scores (Grunebaum et al., 2018).

Despite the robust evidence for its rapid antidepressant and antisuicidal properties, ketamine's reputation as a psychedelic and a drug of abuse has led to a cautious acceptance by mainstream psychiatry. This has not stopped many physicians, including not only psychiatrists but also anesthesiologists and emergency physicians, from using ketamine off-label for TRD in clinical practice, often in specialized ketamine infusion centers, and interest in its clinical use for a wide variety of psychiatric conditions has continued to expand.

In 2017, representing the view of orthodox psychiatry, a research task force of the American Psychiatric Association published a consensus statement on the use of ketamine for the treatment of mood disorders (Sanacora et al., 2017). This statement highlighted the limited existing evidence-based knowledge about this treatment, citing relatively small sample sizes of studies, lack of longer-term data on efficacy, and limited data on safety. The statement stressed the importance of careful diagnosis, medical and psychiatric screening, history taking, pre- and postsymptom measurement, informed consent, need for adequate follow-up, and access to adjunctive therapies for physicians offering this therapy.

As ketamine had long been available as an inexpensive generic medication, there was little interest on the part of pharmaceutical companies to go through the rigorous approval process to get FDA approval for the treatment of TRD. However, Johnson and Johnson developed esketamine, the S-enantiomer of racemic ketamine, as a patented nasal spray product for the treatment of TRD, and esketamine was approved by the FDA on March 5, 2019, under the brand name Spravato, as the first FDA-approved rapid-acting treatment for depression. In addition, intense interest has been generated in the search for other glutaminergic agents that may not have the perceived adverse psychological effects of ketamine or esketamine (Krystal et al., 2013).

As all physicians, nurse practitioners, and physician assistants who have DEA licenses can prescribe ketamine, there is a large diversity of clinical practices with ketamine, many of which have been presented at conferences. The first conference devoted to the clinical use of ketamine to treat psychiatric conditions was the KRIYA Conference, a 2-day gathering of experienced ketamine practitioners who have met annually since 2015 (*www.kriyainstitute.com*). Other international conferences were held in 2018 at Oxford University in England, and in 2018 in Austin, Texas, and 2019 in Aurora, Colorado, the latter two sponsored by the American Society of Ketamine Physicians (*www.askp.org*). A PubMed search conducted on July 15, 2018 using the terms "ketamine" and "depression" or "anxiety" yielded 2,212 publications in the peer-reviewed literature. In addition, books that compile rich information that may guide clinical practice are *Ketamine: Dreams and Realities* (Jansen, 2004), *Ketamine for Depression* (Hyde, 2015), and *The Ketamine Papers* (Wolfson & Hartelius, 2016).

Many questions remain to be answered about ketamine therapy for depression and other psychiatric disorders. The effects, although often immediate, are temporary, lasting days, with a single administration, to several weeks, with multiple administrations. There are questions about optimal dose, frequency, and route of administration, the importance of the setting of the ketamine treatment, and who is qualified to administer ketamine to psychiatric patients. There are concerns about adverse medical and psychological side effects, both short and long term, and about its abuse and addictive potential (Loo, 2018).

Despite this widespread caution and skepticism in the medical community about ketamine as a treatment for psychiatric disorders, its use by physicians and mental health professionals continues to grow. Increasingly, many psychiatrists are starting to use ketamine, administered intravenously, sublingually, or intramuscularly in their offices, often combining it with psychotherapy, or partnering with therapists who provide talk therapy. The potential for ketamine to provide a legally available treatment as a form of psychedelic psychotherapy has largely been ignored by researchers in academic psychiatry, but it has been embraced by proponents of the reemerging field of psychedelic medicine (Schenberg, 2018; Wolfson, 2016a).

▨ Chemistry and Pharmacology

Ketamine is a racemic mixture containing equal parts of R-ketamine and S-ketamine. Both stereoisomers have antidepressant effects in animal models, although R-ketamine appears to have less psychotomimetic effects, a more prolonged antidepressant action, and greater synaptogenesis (Yang et al., 2015). S-ketamine has approximately fivefold greater affinity for the N-methyl-D-aspartate (NMDA) receptor and a commensurate increase in its anesthetic potency (Vollenweider, Leenders, Oye, et al., 1997).

Ketamine has several properties that contribute to its safe use in an appropriate setting. Unlike many other anesthetics, ketamine does not depress respiratory drive or suppress circulation, except at very high doses. The medication has a relatively rapid onset of action and short elimination half-life, making the level of sedation easier to titrate and recovery times less than most other anesthetics. The medication is soluble

Ketamine

in water, and there is no injection site irritation. Given this outstanding safety profile, the medication was initially dispensed to Army medics during the Vietnam War to assist with the transport of wounded soldiers to surgical centers. Indeed, it continues to be considered the best agent available for these situations. The popular term "K-hole," referring to a dissociated and immobile state, may have originated from the practice of nestling wounded soldiers safely into the ground after a ketamine injection while they awaited transport, according to a Vietnam veteran speaking with one of the authors (R. M. G.).

Ketamine has many potential routes of administration. While the majority of clinical trials have utilized intravenous (IV) dosing, ketamine is well tolerated by intramuscular injection (IM), intranasal insufflation of powder or an aqueous solution spray, buccal (or sublingual) lozenges, rectal suppositories, and oral dosing. The bioavailability of oral ketamine swallowed and taken into the alimentary tract is only 16% (Clements et al., 1982), due to a high rate of first-pass metabolism (Hijazi & Boulieu, 2002), whereas the bioavailability of ketamine absorbed sublingually is 35–50%. Ketamine given IV and IM is similar—97 and 93%, respectively.

▪ Mechanisms of Action

As with all antidepressant drugs, the mechanism by which ketamine exerts its antidepressant effect is a mystery. Considerable interest has been stirred by the rapidity of its action, which eliminates the 3- to 6-week wait for therapeutic effects of all other antidepressants. What is known is that ketamine is a partial antagonist of the NMDA gluta-

mate receptor, which has multiple functions in the brain. Ketamine, either through the NMDA or other neuroreceptors in the central nervous system, appears to affect glutaminergic function and initiates a number of cellular effects in neurons on signaling pathways, with downstream action that increases dendritic connections between neurons, resulting in new synaptogenesis. This neural plasticity is thought to be the basis for the antidepressant response (Galvez et al., 2017). Ketamine is also active at a number of other neuroreceptors in the brain, including opioid, dopamine, and muscarinic and nicotinic acetylcholine receptors, and attention has been given to various ketamine metabolites (Hashimoto, 2019), but the contribution of these possible targets for ketamine's myriad effects remains mysterious and controversial.

In a recent small study, Williams and colleagues (2018) reported that subjects pretreated with naltrexone, an opioid blocker, did not get an antidepressant response, although they experienced the full dissociative effects, therefore indicating that ketamine's antidepressant effects are possibly mediated through the opioid receptor and separate from the dissociative effects. Although this finding has been disputed (Wang & Kaplin, 2019; Yoon et al., 2019), it has raised concerns about an epidemic of iatrogenic addiction through ketamine treatment, similar to the opiate addiction crisis (George, 2018).

When viewed through the psychedelic paradigm, ketamine has more to offer than just as a chemotherapeutic agent. Ketamine can bring people into nonordinary states of consciousness that have the potential to disrupt rigid and maladaptive mental structures, reorient self-narratives, loosen defense mechanisms, and increase opportunities for personally meaningful experiences. Most research to date has not focused on the subjective experience of ketamine intoxication, but there is some evidence to indicate that the dissociative and psychedelic effects of ketamine are correlated with more robust therapeutic outcomes (Dakwar, Anerella, et al., 2014; Luckenbaugh et al., 2014; Mathai et al., 2018; Niciu et al., 2018; Pennybaker et al., 2017; Sos et al., 2013).

Ketamine has important effects on regional cerebral blood flow (rCBF) in regions of the brain that are extensively implicated in psychiatric illness and addiction (Rowland et al., 2010). Ketamine promotes blood flow elevations in anterior cingulate, orbitofrontal, and dorsal frontal lobes (Breier et al., 1997; Holcomb et al., 2001; Rowland et al., 2005; Vollenweider, Leenders, Oye, et al.,1997).

Vollenweider and Kometer (2010) have hypothesized that ketamine, acting primarily at NMDA receptors through a series of downstream effects, ultimately increases glutaminergic activity in the prefrontal cortex (PFC), and strengthens the connection between the PFC and the amygdala, thus allowing more executive control over emotional reactivity. Interestingly, they theorize that serotonergic hallucinogens, acting on 5-hydroxytryptamine (5-HT$_{2A}$) receptors, also have the same downstream effects, and this common therapeutic endpoint explains how ketamine and classic psychedelics relieve depression, obsessive–compulsive disorder (OCD), pain, and other psychiatric disorders.

■ Effects on Consciousness

What effects does ketamine have on consciousness? Like other psychedelics, there seem to be a few levels to the experience. The first level is mild sedation. Beyond that, the patient gets dreamy and the mind starts to float, followed at a higher dose by vivid imagery and hallucinations. At a still higher dose, awareness of the outside environment is lost. The subject has awareness of a psychedelic nature but cannot respond to outside stimuli and appears to be in a coma. Finally, when the dose goes high enough, the patient is both unresponsive and amnestic. This "dissociation" and coma-like state is in marked contrast with experiences provided by the classic psychedelics, such as LSD, psilocybin, and mescaline.

Here are some first-person accounts of ketamine-induced experiences, both from patients being treated for depression and those in higher-dose psychedelic sessions:

"I felt like I traveled far away from my body and had a different perspective about my life and my problems, and it was all right."

"I felt things snapped into place, all my issues and priorities."

"I saw my life from what seemed like a higher perspective, and that everything was perfect and I could tolerate my pain."

"It's so hard to describe in words, but I felt like my whole system was rebooted. I feel bright and clean."

"It is as if it is the space of death. If there is existence of consciousness after death of the physical body, this could be it—something like this."

"It was as if I completely understood the interconnectedness or oneness of all things at that very moment with my whole being. On returning to my body there was an overwhelming sense of peace, as if I now understood the answers to the ultimate questions."

"I was drifting way out there and I felt that my sense of self was an illusion. At first I was disturbed by this, and then I decided to go with it, and it was OK."

"I was aware, and yet felt I could not grasp any concepts. There was nothing to hold onto and everything seemed to be continually changing. This went on and on for what seemed like an eternity and appeared to be the true state of affairs."

Kolp and colleagues (2016, and talk given at the 2019 KRIYA Conference), have postulated four stages of ketamine dissociative states, also called *nonordinary states of consciousness*, with approximate dosage ranges that induce these states. It should be noted that there is much individual variation in the subjective response to ketamine, based on the subject's physical and mental condition and preparation. The first state, which Kolp labels the "mild dissociative state," with intravenous dosing of 0.25–0.5 mg/kg, or intramuscular dosing ranging from 25 to 50 mg, he calls "empathogenic," meaning "generating a state of empathy" or "heart-opening." This is a state of bodily and mental relaxation, often felt as pleasurable. The *ego*, defined here as the sense of individual identity and orientation, is preserved, but its defenses are significantly lessened. This state is akin to the psycholytic psychotherapy of the more traditional psychedelics. The subject, being in a detached yet positive state of consciousness, is verbally responsive and can work on unresolved trauma and other issues.

The second stage of ketamine intoxication, or "intermediate dissociative state," according to Kolp, is characterized by the out-of-body experience, typically brought on by 0.75–1.5 mg/kg (IV) or 75–125 mg (IM) of ketamine. Here the subject experiences feelings of separation from the body, and the self traveling through space, having transpersonal experiences typical of a psychedelic journey, such as intense visions, and meeting noncorporeal and archetypal beings. The ego structures are still intact but tenuous.

The third stage of nonordinary state of consciousness brought on by ketamine, or "severe dissociative state," at 2.0–3.0 mg/kg or 150–250 mg IM, is the near-death experience (NDE), in which the subject's ego totally dissolves and there is a loss of identity and a strong feeling that one is dead or in a state similar to death, yet a sense of awareness remains. There may be other aspects similar to an NDE, such as moving through a tunnel, and reviewing one's life with a moral inventory.

Kolp calls the fourth level of ketamine intoxication the "profound dissociative state," or the ego-dissolving transcendental experience, generally brought on by high doses similar to the third stage, but actually experienced only by a very few, in which the subject has a classic mystical experience of feeling at one with the universe, becoming white light, having a sense of identification with "God" or a divinity, and an accompanying deep sense of sacredness, ineffability, transcendence of time and space, peace, and joy. This state is the goal of many psychedelic therapies, and in Krupitsky's studies of alcoholics and opiate addicts, those who had a transcendental experience had better clinical outcomes, including significantly reduced relapse rates (Krupitsky & Grinenko, 1997; Krupitsky et al., 2002).

It was pointed out early on that a high-dose psychedelic ketamine experience provided the closest drug-induced correlate of the NDE, even more so than other psychedelics (Jansen, 1995). These similarities include dissolution of the ego, a compelling sense of being dead, sensations of moving through a tunnel, a life review, meeting people who are already dead, visits to nonphysical realities, encounters with noncorporeal entities, an experience of the void, and an experience of rebirth of the ego (Kolp et al., 2016). These experiences have been used in some types of "ego death–rebirth" psychotherapy (Krupitsky & Grinenko, 1997; Kungurtsev, 1991).

Other classic psychedelics at high doses can produce ego-death experiences, and two short-acting tryptamines, in particular, dimethyltryptamine (DMT) and 5-hydroxydimethyltryptamine (5-MeO-DMT) can reliably do this (Metzner, 2013). Martial and colleagues (2019) recently examined semantic similarities between anecdotal accounts of drug-induced ego-death experiences and NDEs, and found that ketamine was the psychedelic most similar to the NDE. Relying on the well-established preclinical literature that ketamine can slow down neuronal death after brain injury, this paper "suggests that ketamine could be used as a safe and reversible experimental model for NDE phenomenology, and supports the speculation that endogenous NMDA antagonists with neuroprotective properties may be released in the proximity of death."

The subjective experiences induced by ketamine are similar to those produced by the classic psychedelics. The sense of travel through space and time, through inner–outer landscapes both familiar and alien, encounters and identification with known and unknown beings, the sense of the numinous, being out of one's body, ego dissolution, sense of oneness, and identification with the divine are familiar to those who, under a conducive set and setting, ingest high enough or potent enough doses of classic psychedelics.

What distinguishes ketamine from the classic psychedelics? Ketamine is much more reliable at inducing dose-dependent dissociation in subjects, leading to, from an external vantage point, a catatonic and coma-like state, and from an internal point of view, an out-of-body, NDE, or transcendental experience. In addition, the anxiety or fear reactions that are often produced by all psychedelics seem to be attenuated, and often absent, with ketamine, especially if attention is given to careful preparation and a safe and comfortable setting.

■ Psychiatric Use

In addition to depression and suicidal ideation, ketamine has been investigated for treatment of a variety of other psychiatric disorders. Rodriguez and colleagues (2011, 2013) found that IV ketamine significantly reduced obsessions in patients with OCD. There is some indication that ketamine intentionally combined with cognitive-behavioral psychotherapy in open-label studies appeared to be associated with a more prolonged benefit in OCD and depression (Rodriguez et al., 2016; Wilkinson et al., 2017).

Given preclinical evidence of anxiolytic effects of ketamine in rodents (Zhang et al., 2015), it is not surprising that anxiety disorders have been targeted for treatment with ketamine. Feder and colleagues (2014) ran a double-blind, placebo-controlled study with 41 subjects who suffered from chronic posttraumatic stress disorder (PTSD), and found that ketamine produced significant reductions in symptoms, as measured by the Impact of Events Scale—Revised (IES-R). Glue and colleagues (2018), in an open-label trial, studied the impact of subcutaneous ketamine injections (1 mg/kg) weekly or twice a week on subjects with generalized and social anxiety disorders, and found significant reduction in fear and anxiety, and that the treatment was safe and well tolerated.

Other conditions for which ketamine has shown some indication of promise are eating disorders (Mills et al., 1998), autism (Wink et al., 2014), and substance use disorders, the latter of which we review in a later section.

The dose and route of administration for psychiatric disorders have not been optimized. Most randomized clinical trials of ketamine for depression have used racemic ketamine 0.5 mg/kg IV given over 40 minutes. One of the first multicenter studies exploring IV dose ranges for depression (Fava et al., 2020), found that one-time IV infusions of 0.5 mg/kg and 1.0 mg/kg of ketamine were superior to active placebo (midazolam) in measures of depression, and were more efficacious than doses of 0.1 mg/kg and 0.2 mg/kg of ketamine on short-term assessment of depressed mood. However, in a further study from this group, Ionescu and colleagues (2019) found that those with severe and chronic TRD who received six infusions over 3 weeks of the standard IV dose of 0.5 mg/kg did not respond robustly or do better than those receiving placebo after 3 weeks. The authors hypothesized that one potential explanation for this finding is that 0.5 mg/kg is not a sufficient dose for this severe and chronic population.

Doses higher than 1.0 mg/kg (IV or IM) are used in some clinical practices, and are reported to be safe provided that patients are prepared for the greater psychedelic effects, but systematic evaluations of these practices are not yet available.

There are several considerations when selecting a dose of ketamine. First, the majority of evidence derives from trials using 0.5 mg/kg (IV), so this approach is commonly used as an initial dose for depression. Advantages of this dose are that the level of sedation is typically no more than light (defined as "responsiveness to verbal command"). This dose is less likely to produce psychedelic effects, which minimizes preparation requirements and psychological distress among clients who are not prepared for these effects. The small dose also wears off quickly, allowing visits to be accomplished in a 90-minute period, although some clients want to rest for longer periods of time.

Doses of ketamine between 1.0 and 1.5 mg/kg (IM) are being used in clinical practice, typically with an intention to induce psychedelic experiences and facilitate psychotherapy. These doses are often sufficient to induce a dissociation from bodily sensations, which can provide powerful relief for clients who have chronic pain or who carry bodily sensations related to prior trauma. Ketamine at 1.25 mg/kg (IM) is typically psychedelic, and subjects experience perceptions of abstract shapes, images, and a sense of spaciousness.

Ego dissolution (sometimes called a "nondual" or "mystical experience") can occur at this dose in clients who are prepared for this to occur and feel safe in the setting, and is more likely to occur at a dose of ketamine of 1.5 mg/kg. Such mystical experiences have been found to be important for the therapeutic benefits of psilocybin, and similarly to psilocybin, there is some evidence that when ketamine is associated with mystical experiences, the benefits are more durable

(Dakwar et al., 2018; Mathai et al., 2018). From a client perspective, mystical experiences can be transformative and blissful, as a profound sense of belonging within something large and immutable is fostered. Without adequate preparation, or in settings that are not safe for deep psychological work, such mystical experiences can be terrifying, as the ego will vehemently resist dissolution in such situations.

Doses of ketamine greater than 1.5–2.0 mg/kg (IM) are generally not recommended, except for a few clients who have tolerated lower doses well and have had suboptimal responses. The ketamine experience above 1.5 mg/kg is typically not fully conscious (nonordinary or otherwise), not well remembered, involves less rich perceptions, and the incidence of moderate or deep sedation, headache, nausea, and prolonged fatigue are more common.

The recent FDA approval of esketamine, the S-enantiomer of racemic ketamine, in the form of a patented nasal spray product, has been hailed as a breakthrough in the treatment of depression, being the first rapid-acting antidepressant and glutaminergic agent. The drug manufacturer submitted evidence from Phase III trials, two of which showed statistically significant evidence of superior antidepressant response compared to placebo (FDA, 2019). One trial showed a mean lower depression score after 4 weeks administration of a new oral antidepressant combined with intranasal ketamine compared with a new oral antidepressant combined with placebo. The benefit of 4 points on the Montgomery–Åsberg Depression Rating Scale (MADRS) scale was modest, although statistically significant (Daly et al., 2018; Papova et al., 2019). The second trial that showed esketamine benefit was one that randomized people who had previously responded to esketamine therapy (plus a new oral antidepressant) to receive continued esketamine versus being withdrawn from esketamine. Those who continued esketamine had a significantly delayed time to relapse (Daly et al., 2019). Two other randomized clinical trials of esketamine plus a new oral antidepressant did not show statistically significant benefit at day 28 (Schatzberg, 2019).

The esketamine manufacturer recommends that it be administered intranasally twice a week for an initial 4 weeks, in addition to a newly initiated oral antidepressant (the induction phase). The FDA approval came with the proviso that patients be administered the nasal spray only in a medical office and be observed for 2 hours after the treatment, with monitoring of patients' blood pressure, heart rate, and signs of any other psychological or physiological adverse reactions (Mattingly & Anderson, 2019). The proposed initial adult esketamine dose is 28–56 mg intranasally at each administration, which can then be titrated to 84 mg by week 2. The manufacturer recommends treatment on a weekly basis for an additional 4 weeks, then weekly or every other week during an ongoing maintenance phase. The proposed utilization does not require combination of esketamine with psychotherapy. As such, esketamine is intended to be used as an antidepressant drug that is continued indefinitely in contrast to other psychedelic medicines that seek transformational change in a setting that includes psychotherapy for preparation and integration of insights from the psychedelic experience.

Researchers have just begun to study ketamine in special populations. A promising area for ketamine use is in palliative care, as the potential for pain and depression relief, combined with psychedelically derived insights, may help those who are facing death (Goldman et al., 2019; Iglewicz et al., 2015; Kolp et al., 2007).

KAP

Clinical practitioners have reported that KAP, following treatment models that combine elements of psychedelic (ego-dissolving) and psycholytic (ego-loosening) methods, may enhance treatment outcomes by fostering greater access to the unconscious, self-awareness, self-transcendence, and a greater sense of meaning. In addition, KAP may encourage personality transformation, relief from obsessions and trauma, and reduction of existential anxiety by providing the subject an experience of being intimately connected with a world larger than him- or herself (Wolfson, 2016a). Ketamine's fostering of immediate synaptogenesis may help explain why, of all the antidepressants, ketamine may be particularly suited for combination with psychotherapy (Hasler, 2020). Many of the initial published studies of KAP have focused on the treatment of substance abuse (Ivan Ezquerra-Romano et al., 2018; Kolp et al., 2009).

Evgeny Krupitsky, working in St. Petersburg, Russia, over two decades ago, found that a transcendental experience with IM ketamine correlated with a higher percentage of abstinence from alcohol (Krupitsky & Grinenko, 1997). Krupitsky's study of ketamine psychedelic therapy (KPT) with heroin-addicted patients used both low dose (0.2 mg/kg) and high dose (2.0 mg/kg) ketamine in a double-blind randomized clinical trial. The higher dose produced a significantly greater rate of abstinence within the first 2 years of follow-up, a greater and longer-lasting reduction in craving for heroin, and a greater positive change in nonverbal unconscious emotional attitudes than did low-dose KPT. Interestingly, the low-dose treatment elicited "subpsychedelic" experiences, enhancing guided imagery. The high dose elicited a full psychedelic experience as assessed by the Hallucinogen Rating Scale (Krupitsky et al., 2002).

In a more recent study of cocaine users, Dakwar, Levin, and colleagues (2014) found that there was a positive correlation between ketamine-induced mystical-type experiences and diminished craving for cocaine. It is hypothesized that the neuroplasticity component of low-dose ketamine treatment may lower cue-induced craving for cocaine (Dakwar, Levin, et al., 2014, 2017). Dakwar and colleagues (2019) also found that a single ketamine infusion combined with mindfulness-based behavioral modification in cocaine-dependent subjects led to significantly increased abstinence from cocaine, diminished craving, and reduced risk of relapse after 5 weeks.

There has been little published in the newly emerging field of office-based KAP. A recent compilation (Dore et al., 2019) of demographic and clinical outcome data of 235 patients treated with KAP in three psychiatry practices, using sublingual or IM routes of administration, showed significantly reduced depression, dropping an average of 11.24 points on the Beck Depression Inventory, and also improved measures of anxiety, dropping an average of 5.5 points on the Hamilton Anxiety Rating Scale. These averages were affected by poor responders and nonresponders and included a variety of diagnoses other than TRD. Patients with more severe symptoms experienced the most improvement. The most frequent adverse reactions were nausea (~13–14%), vomiting (~2%) and agitation (~2%). Although the data in this study are preliminary, they indicate that office-based KAP, as increasingly practiced in psychiatry offices, can be a safe and effective treatment for a number of psychiatric disorders. Nevertheless, further studies are needed to evaluate the parameters and efficacy of KAP.

▧ Adverse Effects

There has been much concern about the potential adverse effects of ketamine treatment for TRD and other psychiatric conditions. The main concerns have to do with dissociative effects, potential long-term effects with repeated doses, including uropathy and cognitive damage, and addiction.

The term *dissociative* in regard to ketamine is sometimes used interchangeably with *psychotomimetic*. This concern goes back to the use of ketamine in anesthesia and the "emergence reaction," with patients, especially those not psychologically prepared beforehand, waking up after undergoing a surgical procedure with a time-limited, delirium-like state characterized by agitation, visual hallucinations, and delusions. As mentioned earlier, the initial interest in ketamine's effects by academic psychiatry was as a potential psychotomimetic agent, as it was with the classic psychedelics.

However, the psychoactive side effects of ketamine have also been viewed through the lens of a psychedelic paradigm. Proponents of KAP believe these psychoactive effects are important to the therapy. Most research into ketamine treatment for depression has focused on negating or minimizing the psychoactive effects. However, there are indications that higher doses of ketamine could lead to more robust outcomes; numerous subjective accounts of patients' experiences point to the positive effects of insight and perspective into their psychological state. Attention to set and setting, providing a comfortable, quiet environment with relaxing music and ongoing therapeutic presence can minimize dysphoric experiences or facilitate working through them.

In a meta-analysis of 60 studies of the standard ketamine model for the treatment of TRD, the most common acute side effects were headache, dizziness, anxiety, dissociation, elevated blood pressure, and blurred vision, with most side effects resolving shortly after the procedure (Short et al., 2018). Other acute side effects that have been reported are drowsiness, poor coordination, and feeling strange and unreal (Wan et al., 2015).

Longer term-side effects of patients using ketamine under medical supervision remain unknown and mostly unstudied, mainly due to the fact that most controlled studies have not had long-term follow-ups or did not measure long-term adverse effects (Short et al., 2018). However, there is evidence of potential long-term adverse effects gathered from heavy recreational and addicted users of ketamine, as well as patients taking ketamine for pain syndromes. The dose and frequency of ketamine use in addicted patients is much higher than is used to treat psychiatric illness. The adverse effects seen with these heavy users are significant urological pathology, hepatotoxicity, and cognitive deficits. The urological symptoms consist of cystitis with symptoms of pain and frequency, possibly leading to irreversible uropathy and dysfunctional bladder (Chu et al., 2015). There has also been concern about liver toxicity (Wong et al., 2014) in those receiving ketamine.

There is evidence that chronic, daily, high-dose ketamine use impairs short- and long-term memory (Morgan & Curran, 2006; Xiaoyin et al., 2018), especially working and episodic memory (Morgan & Curran, 2012). However, typical doses of ketamine used with patient populations have not shown sustained neurocognitive effects (Koffler et al., 2007; Murrough et al., 2014; Murrough, Burdick, et al., 2015; Shiroma, Albott, et al., 2014).

Ketamine's potential for abuse and addiction has inhibited its acceptance as a standard therapy for TRD. There have been numerous reports of ketamine addiction among recreational users (Jansen, 2004), with some evidence of tolerance and compulsive use in animals (Jansen & Darracot-Cankovic, 2001). Ketamine is not thought to be physically addictive, as there are no physical withdrawal symptoms. However, compulsive ketamine users appear to be addicted to the dissociated state that ketamine can provide, an escape from mundane or painful reality. Nonetheless, in the recent increase in off-label use of ketamine to treat TRD and other psychiatric conditions, there have been few reports of iatrogenic abuse or addiction stemming from ketamine-assisted treatments (Schak et al., 2016). Clinicians are warned to inquire about a history of substance dependence in those who are seeking ketamine therapy.

The FDA (2019) reviewed information about nonmedicinal use of ketamine in the United States. Information is available from the National Survey on Drug Use and Health and Monitoring the Future, the U.S. poison center calls (National Poison Data System), a representative sample of emergency department visits (National Electronic Injury Surveillance System–Cooperative Adverse Drug Event Surveillance), and spontaneous adverse event reports (FDA Adverse Event Reporting System [FAERS]).

Recreational ketamine use is relatively uncommon in the general population, with a reported lifetime prevalence of 1.3% among persons age 12 years and older, which is lower than that for other psychedelics such as ecstasy and LSD. Among 12th graders, the annual prevalence of ketamine use declined from 2.5% in 2000 to 1.2% in 2017. Exposure calls to U.S. poison centers involving ketamine also declined slightly from 2013 to 2017 (from 176 calls in 2013 to 116 calls in 2017), despite the growth in nonveterinary ketamine sales.

Single-substance exposure calls involving ketamine were most commonly associated with minor or moderate health effects, and there were no deaths identified among these calls. In a representative sample of approximately 60 U.S. emergency departments (EDs), there were 44 ketamine-related ED cases in 2016–2017, corresponding to an estimated 669 visits nationally. Of the 44 ketamine-related ED cases, 35 (81.5%) were classified as abuse. Only six (17.1%) of these cases resulted in hospitalization. From 2015 to 2017, the FAERS program received 17 reports of death involving ketamine use. Of note, only one of these reports listed ketamine as the only suspected drug, and the drug–event causal association has not been assessed for any of these cases.

■ Further Questions

Ketamine practices have proliferated and provide frameworks for improving the science and the craft of psychedelic medicine. While ketamine is different from other psychedelics, the pathways toward improving satisfaction and outcomes using ketamine may provide lessons for other psychedelic medications that are less far along in development. Many of the key unanswered questions that arise now in the context of ketamine practices also apply to other psychedelics. What is the optimal role of the therapist? Would doses in the psychedelic range lead to more robust or durable benefits? Are mystical, or ego-dissolving, experiences important in the healing process? How best are ketamine practitioners trained? How best to regulate the field to ensure that these powerful tools are safely and effectively used? How best to prolong the effects of ketamine?

While the importance of set, or client characteristics, is regarded to be important for psychedelic medicine, information to identify people who will benefit most from ketamine is lacking. Clinical responses to ketamine vary within each practice setting and may be associated with personality characteristics, pattern of depression (unipolar vs. bipolar, vegetative vs. agitated, etc.), concomitant medications, substance use, and trauma history. Benzodiazepines and lamotrigine may inhibit some of the benefits of ketamine and warrant further study (Andrade, 2017). Alcohol is a potent inhibitor of ketamine benefits, and active use should be suspended before ketamine treatment.

Setting varies widely across ketamine practices, ranging from IV (or intranasal esketamine) administration without any psychotherapy to close integration of ketamine with psychotherapy during the same session. As mentioned earlier, combining ketamine with cognitive-behavioral therapy (CBT) appears to prolong the beneficial effects of either intervention alone, at least for depression and OCD (Rodriguez et al., 2016; Wilkinson et al., 2017). But in general, models of psychotherapy with ketamine have not been formally researched. CBT, eye movement desensitization and reprocessing (EMDR), internal family systems, acceptance and commitment therapy, and psychodynamic therapy have been utilized in KAP (Wolfson, 2016a). Comparisons of group versus individual therapy will be important, especially since group therapy would be more cost-effective and optimize the use of therapist time. Couple therapy is another setting that is promising for KAP (Van De Veer, Kriya conference, November 13, 2018).

On the other side of the spectrum of psychedelic use, there is evidence that lower doses of ketamine, lower than that used in the NIMH protocol (0.5 mg/kg), are effective in treating depression, and that the oral route can be effective, despite the lower bioavailability (~17%) (Hartberg et al., 2018; Hyde, 2015). In addition, one double-blind, placebo-controlled study in Iran showed that oral (not IV or IM) ketamine, when combined with an antidepressant (sertraline), led to significantly more rapid improvement in moderate to severe depression (measured after 2 weeks), which was sustained after 6 weeks (Arabzadeh et al., 2018).

■ Conclusion

Ketamine, a medication widely used in anesthesia and pain control, and considered a psychedelic in its mind-altering effects, has recently been found to have a proven and unique role in the treatment of depression, and there is promising evidence suggesting benefits for other psychiatric and psychological conditions. There are multiple unanswered questions about the psychiatric use of ketamine, including how best to optimize set, setting, dose, route, frequency, and the role of adjunctive psychotherapy. What patient characteristics and diagnostic entities respond best to ketamine? What are the possible long-term adverse effects of ketamine therapy? The role of KAP, inspired by psychedelic models of healing, shows promise, but much remains to be investigated. Are psychoactive effects important in ketamine's efficacy, or just side effects to be avoided? Insights, facilities, and practices developed for ketamine may help guide the clinical use of other psychedelic medicines.

What is clear is that there are many paradigms in the use of ketamine for psychiatric conditions and treatment needs to be individualized while these best practices are investigated (Bennett, 2019). While other psychedelics may become more widely available through medicalization, legalization, or religious freedom, ketamine is expected to have a durable role based on its unique capacity for transient mind–body dissociation, psychedelic experiences, established safety in medicine, and its rapid efficacy as a short-term antidepressant and antisuicidal agent.

■ References

aan het Rot, M., Collins, K. A., Murrough, J. W., Perez, A. M., Reich, D. L., Charney, D. S., et al. (2010). Safety and efficacy of repeated-dose intravenous ketamine for treatment-resistant depression. *Biological Psychiatry, 67,* 139–145.

Andrade, C. (2017). Ketamine for depression, 5: Potential pharmacokinetic and pharmacodynamic drug interactions. *Journal of Clinical Psychiatry, 78*(7), e858–e861.

Arabzadeh, S., Hakkikazazi, E., Shahmansouri, N., Tafakhori, A., Ghajar, A., Jafarinia, M., et al. (2018). Does oral administration of ketamine accelerate response to treatment in major depressive disorder?: Results of a double-blind controlled trial. *Journal of Affective Disorders, 235,* 236–241.

Bennett, R. (2019). Paradigms of ketamine treatment. *MAPS Bulletin Special Edition, 29*(1), 48–49.

Berman, R. M., Cappiello, A., Anand, A., Oren, D. A., Heninger, G. R., Charney, D. S., et al. (2000). Antidepressant effects of ketamine in depressed patients. *Biological Psychiatry, 47,* 351–354.

Breier, A., Malhotra, A. K., Pinals, D. A., Weisenfeld, N. I., & Pickar, D. (1997). Association of ketamine-induced psychosis with focal activation of the prefrontal cortex in healthy volunteers. *American Journal of Psychiatry, 154,* 805–811.

Chang, L. C., Rajagopalan, S., & Mathew, S. J. (2016). The history of ketamine use and its clinical indications. In S. J. Mathew & C. A. Zarate (Eds.), *Ketamine for treatment-resistant depression: The first decade of progress* (pp. 1–12). Cham, Switzerland: Adis.

Chu, P. S. K., Ng, C. F., & Ma, W. K. (2015). Ketamine uropathy: Hong Kong experience. In D. T. Yew (Ed.), *Ketamine: Use and abuse* (pp. 207–225). Boca Raton, FL: CRC Press.

Clements, J. A., Nimmo, W. S., & Grant, I. S. (1982). Bioavailability, pharmacokinetics, and analgesic activity of ketamine in humans. *Journal of Pharmaceutical Sciences, 71,* 539–542.

Cusin, G., Ionescu, D. F., Pavone, K. J., Akeuju, O., Cassano, P., Taylor, N., et al. (2017). Ketamine augmentation for outpatients with treatment-resistant depression: Preliminary evidence for two-step intravenous dose escalation. *Australian and New Zealand Journal of Psychiatry, 51,* 55–64.

Dakwar, E., Anerella, C., Hart, C. L., Levin, F. R., Mathew, S. J., & Nunes, E. V. (2014). Therapeutic infusions of ketamine: Do the psychoactive effects matter? *Drug and Alcohol Dependence, 136,* 153–157.

Dakwar, E., Hart, C. L., Levin, F. R., Nunes, E. V., & Foltin, R. W. (2017). Cocaine self-administration disrupted by the N-methyl-D-aspartate receptor antagonist ketamine: A randomized, crossover trial. *Molecular Psychiatry, 22,* 76–81.

Dakwar, E., Levin, F., Foltin, R. W., Nunes, E. V., & Hart, C. L. (2014). The effects of subanesthetic ketamine infusions on motivation to quit and cue-induced craving in cocaine-dependent research volunteers. *Biological Psychiatry, 76,* 40–46.

Dakwar, E., Nunes, E. V., Hart, C. L., Foltin, R. W., Mathew, S. J., Carpenter, K. M., et al. (2019). A single ketamine infusion combined with mindfulness-based behavioral modification to treat cocaine dependence: A randomized clinical trial. *American Journal of Psychiatry, 176,* 923–930.

Dakwar, E., Nunes, E. V., Hart, C. L., Hu, M. C., Foltin, R. W., & Levin, F. R. (2018). A subset of psychoactive effects may be critical to the behavioral impact of ketamine on cocaine use disorder: Results from a randomized, controlled laboratory study. *Neuropharmacology, 142,* 270–276.

Daly, E. J., Singh, J. B., Fedgchin, M., Cooper, K., Lim, P., Shelton, R. C., et al. (2018). Efficacy and safety of intranasal esketamine adjunctive to oral antidepressant therapy in treatment-resistant depression: A randomized clinical trial. *JAMA Psychiatry, 75,* 139–148.

Daly, E. J., Trivedi, M. H., Janik, A., Li, H., Zhang, Y., Li, X., et al. (2019). Efficacy of esketamine nasal spray plus oral antidepressant treatment for relapse prevention in patients with treatment-resistant depression: A randomized clinical trial. *JAMA Psychiatry, 76,* 893–903.

Diamond, P. R., Farmery, A. D., Atkinson, S., Haldar, J., Williams, N., Cowen, P. J., et al. (2014). Ketamine infusions for treatment resistant depression: A series of 28 patients treated weekly or twice weekly in an ECT clinic. *Journal of Psychopharmacology, 28,* 536–544.

Domino, E. F. (2010). Taming the ketamine tiger. *Anesthesiology, 113,* 678–684.

Dore, J., Turnipseed, B., Dwyer, S., Turnipseed, A., Andries, J., Ascani, G., et al. (2019). Ketamine assisted psychotherapy (KAP): Patient demographics, clinical data and outcomes in three large practices administering ketamine with psychotherapy. *Journal of Psychoactive Drugs, 51,* 189–198.

Fava, M., Freeman, M. P., Flynn, M., Judge, H., Hoeppner, B. B., Cusin, C., et al. (2020). Double-blind, placebo-controlled, dose-ranging trial of intravenous ketamine as adjunctive therapy in treatment-resistant depression (TRD). *Molecular Psychiatry, 25*(7), 1592–1603.

FDA Briefing Document. (2019). Psychopharmacologic Drugs Advisory Committee (PDAC) and Drug Safety and Risk Management (DSaRM) Advisory Committee Meeting. Retrieved March 13, 2019, from *www.fda.gov/downloads/advisorycommittees/committeesmeetingmaterials/drugs/psychopharmacologicdrugsadvisorycommittee/ucm630970.pdf.*

Feder, A., Parides, M. K., Mourrough, J. W., Perez, A. M., Morgan, J. E., Saxena, S., et al. (2014). Efficacy of intravenous ketamine for treatment of chronic posttraumatic stress disorder: A randomized clinical trial. *JAMA Psychiatry, 71,* 681–688.

Galvez, V., Nikolin, S., Ho, K. A., Alonzo, A., Somogyi, A. A., & Loo, C. K. (2017). Increase in PAS-induced neuroplasticity after a treatment course of intranasal ketamine for depression: Report of three cases from a placebo-controlled trial. *Comprehensive Psychiatry, 73,* 31–34.

George, M. S. (2018). Is there really nothing new under the sun?: Is low-dose ketamine a fast-acting antidepressant simply because it is an opioid? *American Journal of Psychiatry, 175,* 1157–1158.

Ghasemi, M., Kazemi, M. H., Yoosefi, A., Ghasemi, A., Paragomi, P., Amini, H., et al. (2014). Rapid antidepressant effects of repeated doses of ketamine compared with electroconvulsive therapy in hospitalized patients with major depressive disorder. *Psychiatry Research, 215,* 355–361.

Glue, P., Neehoff, S. M., Medlicott, N. J., Gray, A., Kibby, G., & McNaughton, N. (2018). Safety and efficacy of maintenance ketamine treatment in patients with treatment-refractory generalised anxiety and social anxiety disorders. *Journal of Psychopharmacology, 32,* 663–667.

Goldman, N., Frankenthaler, M., & Klepacz, L. (2019). The efficacy of ketamine in the palliative care setting: A comprehensive review of the literature. *Journal of Palliative Medicine, 22,* 1154–1161.

Gouzoulis-Mayfrank, E., Heekeren, K., Neukirch, A., Stoll, M., Stock, C., Obradovic, M., et al. (2005). Psychological effects of (S)-ketamine and N,N,-dimethyltyrptamine (DMT): A double-blind, cross-over study in healthy volunteers. *Pharmacopsychiatry, 38,* 301–311.

Grunebaum, M. F., Galfalvy, H. C., Choo, T. H., Keilp, J. G., Moitra, V. K., Parris, M. S., et al. (2018). Ketamine for rapid reduction of suicidal thoughts in major depression: A midazolam-controlled randomized clinical trial. *American Journal of Psychiatry, 175,* 327–335.

Hartberg, J., Garrett-Walcott, S., & De Gioannis, A. (2018). Impact of oral ketamine augmentation on hospital admissions in treatment-resistant depression and PTSD: A retrospective study. *Psychopharmacology (Berlin), 235,* 393–398.

Hashimoto, K. (2019). Rapid-acting antidepressant ketamine, its metabolites and other candidates: A historical overview and future perspective. *Psychiatry and Clinical Neuroscience, 17,* 613–627.

Hasler, G. (2020). Toward specific ways to combine ketamine and psychotherapy in treating depression. *CNS Spectrums, 25,* 445–447.

Hijazi, Y., & Boulieu, R. (2002). Contribution of CYP3A4, CYP2B6, and CYP2C9 isoforms to N-demethylation of ketamine in human liver microsomes. *Drug Metabolism and Disposition, 30,* 853–858.

Holcomb, H. H., Lahti, A. C., Medoff, D. R., Weller, M., & Tamminga, C. A. (2001). Sequential regional cerebral blood flow brain scans using PET with H2(15)O demonstrate ketamine actions in CNS dynamically. *Neuropsychopharmacology, 25,* 165–172.

Hyde, S. J. (2015). *Ketamine for depression.* Bloomington, IN: Xlibris.

Iglewicz, A., Morrison, K., Nelesen, R. A., Zhan, T., Iglewicz, B., Fairman, N., et al. (2015). Ketamine for the treatment of depression in patients receiving hospice care: A retrospective medical record review of thirty-one cases. *Psychosomatics, 56,* 329–337.

Insel, T. (2014). Post by former NIMH Director Thomas Insel: Ketamine. Retrieved from *www.nimh.nih.gov/about/director/2014/ketamine.shtml.*

Ionescu, D. F., Bentley, K. H., Eikermann, M., Taylor, N., Akeju, O., & Swee, M. B. (2019). Repeat-dose ketamine augmentation for treatment-resistant depression with chronic suicidal ideation: A randomized, double blind, placebo controlled trial. *Journal of Affective Disorders, 243,* 516–524.

Ivan Ezquerra-Romano, I., Lawn, W., Krupitsky, E., & Morgan, C. J. A. (2018). Ketamine for the treatment of addiction: Evidence and potential mechanisms. *Neuropharmacology, 142,* 72–82.

Jansen, K. L. R. (1995). Using ketamine to induce the near-death experience: Mechanism of action and therapeutic potential. *Yearbook for Ethnomedicine and the Study of Consciousness, 4,* 55–79.

Jansen, K. (2004). *Ketamine: Dreams and realities* (2nd ed.). Sarasota, FL: Multidisciplinary Association for Psychedelic Studies (MAPS).

Jansen, K. L. R., & Darracot-Cankovic, R. (2001). The nonmedical use of ketamine: Part 2. A review of problem use and dependence. *Journal of Psychoactive Drugs, 33,* 151–158.

Khorramzadeh, E., & Lofty, A. (1973). The use of ketamine in psychiatry. *Psychosomatics, 14,* 344–346.

Koffler, S. P., Hampstead, B. M., Irani, F., Tinker, J., Kiefer, R-T., Rohr, P., et al. (2007). The neurocognitive effects of 5 day anesthetic ketamine for the treatment of refractory complex regional pain syndrome. *Archives of Clinical Neuropsychology, 22,* 719–729.

Kolp, E., Friedman, H. L., Krupitsky, E., Jansen, K., Sylvester, M., Young, M. S., et al. (2016). Ketamine psychedelic psychotherapy: Focus on its pharmacology, phenomenology, and clinical applications. In P. Wolfson & G. Hartelius (Eds.), *The Ketamine Papers: Science, therapy, and transformation* (pp. 97–197). Santa Cruz, CA: Multidisciplinary Association for Psychedelic Studies (MAPS).

Kolp, E., Friedman, H. L., Young, M. S., & Krupitsky, E. (2006). Ketamine enhanced psychotherapy: Preliminary clinical observations on its effectiveness in treating alcoholism. *Humanistic Psychologist, 34,* 399–422.

Kolp, E., Krupitsky, E., Friedman, H., & Young, M. S. (2009). Entheogen-enhanced transpersonal psychotherapy of addictions: Focus on clinical applications of ketamine for treating alcoholism. In A. Browne-Miller (Ed.), *The Praeger international collection on addictions* (Vol. 3, pp. 403–417). Westport, CT: Praeger.

Kolp, E., Young, M. S., Friedman, H., Krupitzky, E., Jansen, K., & O'Connor, L. (2007). Ketamine enhanced psychotherapy: Preliminary clinical observations on its effects in treating death anxiety. *International Journal of Transpersonal Studies, 26,* 1–17.

Krupitsky, E. (1993/1994). Ketamine psychedelic therapy (KPT) of alcoholism and neurosis. *Yearbook of the European College for the Study of Consciousness, 1993/1994,* 113–122.

Krupitsky, E., Burakov, A., Romanova, T., Dunaevsky, I., Strassman, R., & Grinenko, A. (2002). Ketamine psychotherapy for heroin addiction: Immediate effects and two-year follow-up. *Journal of Substance Abuse Treatment, 23,* 273–283.

Krupitsky, E. M., & Grinenko, A. Y. (1997). Ketamine psychedelic therapy (KPT): A review of the results of ten years of research. *Journal of Psychoactive Drugs, 29,* 165–183.

Krystal, J. H., Sanacora, G., & Duman, R. (2013). Rapid-acting glutamatergic antidepressants: The path to ketamine and beyond. *Biological Psychiatry, 73,* 1133–1141.

Kungurtsev, I. (1991). "Death–rebirth" psychotherapy with ketamine. *Albert Hofmann Foundation Bulletin, 2*(4), 1–6.

Lilly, J. (1978). *The scientist: A novel autobiography.* New York: Lippincott.

Loo, C. (2018). Can we confidently use ketamine as a clinical treatment for depression? *Lancet Psychiatry, 5,* 11–12.

Luckenbaugh, D. A., Niciu, M. J., Ionescu, D. F., Nolan, N. M., Richards, E. M., Brutsche, N. E., et al. (2014). Do the dissociative side effects of ketamine mediate its antidepressant effects? *Journal of Affective Disorders, 159,* 56–61.

Martial, C., Cassol, H., Charland-Verville, V., Pallavicini, C., Sanz, C., Zamberlan, F., et al. (2019). Neurochemical models of near-death experiences: A large-scale study based on the semantic similarity of written reports. *Consciousness and Cognition, 69,* 52–69.

Mathai, D. S., Mathew, S. J., Storch, E. A., & Kosten, T. R. (2018). Revisiting the hallucinogenic potential of ketamine: A case built on current research findings. *Psychiatric Times, 35.* Retrieved from *www.psychiatrictimes.com/view/revisiting-hallucinogenic-potential-ketamine.*

Mattingly, G. W., & Anderson, R. H. (2019). Intranasal esketamine. *Current Psychiatry, 18*(5), 31–38.

McGirr, A., Berlim, M. T., Bond, D. J., Fleck, M. P., Yatham, L. N., & Lam, R. W. (2015). A systematic review and meta-analysis of randomized, double-blind, placebo-controlled trials of ketamine in the rapid treatment of major depressive episodes. *Psychological Medicine, 45,* 693–704.

Metzner, R. (2013). *The toad and the jaguar.* Berkeley, CA: Green Earth Foundation & Regent Press.

Mills, I. H., Park, G. R., Manara, A. R., & Merriman, R. J. (1998). Treatment of compulsive behaviour in eating disorders with intermittent ketamine infusions. *Quarterly Journal of Medicine, 91,* 493–503.

Moore, M., & Alltounian, H. (1978). *Journeys into the bright world.* Rockport, MA: Para Research.

Morgan, C. J., & Curran, H. V. (2006). Acute and chronic effects of ketamine upon human memory: A review. *Psychopharmacology, 188,* 408–424.

Morgan, C. J., & Curran, H. V. (2012). Ketamine use: A review. *Addiction, 107,* 27–38.

Murrough, J. W., Burdick, K. E., Levitch, C. F., Perez, A., Brallier, J. W., Chang, L. C., et al. (2015). Neurocognitive effects of ketamine and association with antidepressant response in individuals with treatment-resistant depression: A randomized controlled trial. *Neuropsychopharmacology, 40,* 1084–1090.

Murrough, J. W., Perez, A. M., Pillemer, S., Stern, J., Parides, M. K., aan het Rot, M., et al. (2013). Rapid and longer-term antidepressant effects of repeated ketamine infusions in treatment-resistant major depression. *Biological Psychiatry, 74,* 250–256.

Murrough, J. W., Soleimani, L., De Wilde, K. E., Collins, K. A., Lapidus, K. A., Iacoviello, B. M., et al. (2015). Ketamine for rapid reduction of suicidal ideation: A randomized controlled trial. *Psychological Medicine, 45,* 3571–3580.

Murrough, J. W., Wan, L.-B., Iacoviello, B., Collins, K. A., Solon, C., Glicksberg, B., et al. (2014). Neurocognitive effects of ketamine in treatment-resistant major depression: Association with antidepressant response. *Psychopharmacology, 231,* 481–488.

Niciu, M. J., Shovestul, B. J., Jaso, B. A., Farmer, C., Luckenbaugh, D. A., Brutsche, N. E., et al. (2018). Features of dissociation differentially predict antidepressant response to ketamine in treatment-resistant depression. *Journal of Affective Disorders, 232,* 310–315.

Papova, V., Daly, E. J., Trivedi, M., Cooper, K., Lane, R., Lim, P., et al. (2019). Efficacy and safety of flexibly dosed esketamine nasal spray combined with a newly initiated oral antidepressant in treatment-resistant depession: A randomized double-blind active-controlled study. *American Journal of Psychiatry, 176,* 428–438.

Pennybaker, S. J., Niciu, M. J., Luckenbaugh, D. A., & Zarate, C. A. (2017). Symptomatology and predictors of antidepressant efficacy in extended responders to a single ketamine infusion. *Journal of Affective Disorders, 208,* 560–566.

Rao, S. S., Wood, D. M., & Dargan, P. I. (2015). Ketamine: Epidemiology of misuse and patterns of acute and chronic toxicity. In D. T. Yew (Ed.), *Ketamine: Use and abuse* (pp. 103–144). Boca Raton, FL: CRC Press.

Rasmussen, K. G., Lineberry, T. W., Galardy, C. W., Kung, S., Lapid, M. I., Palmer, B. A., et al. (2013). Serial infusions of low-dose ketamine for major depression. *Journal of Psychopharmacology, 27,* 444–450.

Rodriguez, C. I., Kegeles, L. S., Flood, P., & Simpson, H. B. (2011). Rapid resolution of obsessions after an infusion of intravenous ketamine in a patient with treatment-resistant obsessive–compulsive disorder: A case report. *Journal of Clinical Psychiatry, 72,* 567–569.

Rodriguez, C. I., Kegeles, L. S., Levinson, A., Feng, T., Marcus, S. M., Vermes, D., et al. (2013). Randomized controlled crossover trial of ketamine in obsessive-compulsive disorder: Proof-of-concept. *Neuropsychopharmacology, 38,* 2475–2483.

Rodriguez, C. I., Wheaton, M., Zwerling, J., Steinman, S. A., Sonnenfeld, D., Galfalvy, H., et al. (2016). Can exposure-based CBT extend IV ketamine's effects in obsessive–compulsive disorder?: An open-label trial. *Journal of Clinical Psychiatry, 77,* 408–409.

Rowland, L. M., Beason-Held, L., Tamminga, C. A., & Holcomb, H. H. (2010). The interactive effects of ketamine and nicotine on human cerebral blood flow. *Psychopharmacology, 208,* 575–584.

Rowland, L. M., Bustillo, J. R., Mullins, P. G., Jung, R. E., Lenroot, R., Landgraf, E., et al. (2005). Effects of ketamine on anterior cingulate glutamate metabolism in healthy humans: A 4-T proton MRS study. *American Journal of Psychiatry, 162,* 394–396.

Ryan, W. C., Marta, C. J., & Koek, R. J. (2016). Ketamine, depression and current research: A review of the literature. In P. Wolfson & G. Hartelius (Eds.), *The Ketamine Papers: Science, therapy, and transformation* (pp. 199–273). Santa Cruz, CA: Multidisciplinary Association of Psychedelic Studies (MAPS).

Sanacora, G., Frye, M. A., McDonald, W., Mathew, S. J., Turner, M. S., Schatzberg, A. F., et al. (2017). A consensus statement of the use of ketamine in the treatment of mood disorders. *JAMA Psychiatry, 74,* 399–405.

Schak, K. M., Vande Voort, J. L., Johnson, E. K., Kung, S., Leung, J. G., Rasmussen, K. G., et al. (2016). Potential risks of poorly monitored ketamine use in depression treatment. *American Journal of Psychiatry, 173*, 215–218.

Schatzberg, A. F. (2019). A word to the wise about esketamine. *American Journal of Psychiatry, 176*, 422–424.

Schenberg, E. E. (2018). Psychedelic-assisted psychotherapy: A paradigm shift in psychiatric research and development. *Frontiers in Pharmacology, 9*, 733.

Shiroma, P. R., Albott, C. S., Johns, B., Thuras, P., Wels, J., & Lim, K. O. (2014). Neurocognitive performance and serial intravenous subanesthetic ketamine in treatment-resistant depression. *International Journal of Neuropsychopharmacology, 17*, 1805–1813.

Shiroma, P. R., Johns, B., Kuskowski, M., Wels, J., Thuras, P., Albott, C. S., & Lim, K. O. (2014). Augmentation of response and remission to serial intravenous subanesthetic ketamine in treatment resistant depression. *Journal of Affective Disorders, 155*, 123–129.

Short, B., Fong, J., Galvez, V., Shelker, W., & Loo, C. K. (2018). Side-effects associated with ketamine use in depression: A systematic review. *Lancet Psychiatry, 5*, 65–78.

Singh, J. B., Fedgchin, M., Daly, E. J., De Boer, P., Cooper, K., Lim, P., et al. (2016). A double-blind, randomized, placebo-controlled, dose-frequency study of intravenous ketamine in patients with treatment-resistant depression. *American Journal of Psychiatry, 173*, 816–826.

Sos, P., Klirova, M., Novak, T., Kohutova, B., Horacek, J., & Palenicek, T. (2013). Relationship of ketamine's antidepressant and psychotomimetic effects in unipolar depression. *NeuroEndocrinology Letters, 34*, 287–293.

Visser, E., & Schug, S. (2006). The role of ketamine in pain management. *Biomedicine and Pharmacotherapy, 60*, 341–348.

Vollenweider, F. X., & Kometer, M. (2010). The neurobiology of psychedelic drugs: Implications for the treatment of mood disorders. *Nature Reviews Neuroscience, 11*, 642–651.

Vollenweider, F. X., Leenders, K. L., Oye, I., Hell, D., & Angst, J. (1997). Differential psychopathology and patterns of cerebral glucose utilisation produced by (S)- and (R)-ketamine in healthy volunteers using positron emission tomography (PET). *European Neuropsychopharmacology, 7*, 25–38.

Vollenweider, F. X., Leenders, K. L., Scharfetter, C., Antonini, A., Maguire, P., Missimer, J., et al. (1997). Metabolic hyperfrontality and psychophathology in the ketamine model of psychosis using positron emission tomography (PET) and [^{18}F]fluorodeoxyglucose (FDG). *European Neuropsychopharmacology, 7*, 9–24.

Wan, L. B., Levitch, C. F., Perez, A. M., Brallier, J. W., Iosifescu, D. V., Chang, L. C., et al. (2015). Ketamine safety and tolerability in clinical trials for treatment-resistant depression. *Journal of Clinical Psychiatry, 76*, 247–252.

Wang, M., & Kaplin, A. (2019). Explaining naltrexone's interference with ketamine's antidepressant effect. *American Journal of Psychiatry, 176*, 410–411.

Williams, N. R., Heifets, B. D., Blasey, C., Sudheimer, K., Pannu, J., Pankow, H., et al. (2018). Attenuation of antidepressant effects of ketamine by opioid receptor antagonism. *American Journal of Psychiatry, 175*, 1205–1215.

Wilkinson, S. T., Ballard, E. D., Bloch, M. H., Mathew, S. J., Murrough, J. W., Feder, A., et al. (2018). The effect of a single dose of intravenous ketamine on suicidal ideation: A systematic review and individual participant data meta-analysis. *American Journal of Psychiatry, 175*, 150–158.

Wilkinson, S. T., Wright, D., Fasula, M. K., Fenton, L., Griepp, M., Ostroff, R. B., et al. (2017). Cognitive behavior therapy may sustain antidepressant effects of intravenous ketamine in treatment-resistant depression. *Psychotherapy and Psychosomatics, 86*, 162–167.

Wink, L. K., O'Melia, A. M., Shaffer, R. C., Pedapati, E., Friedmann, K., Schaefer, T., et al. (2014). Intranasal ketamine treatment in an adult with autism spectrum disorder. *Journal of Clinical Psychiatry, 75*, 835–836.

Wolfson, P. (2016a). Ketamine: Its history, uses, pharmacology, therapeutic practice, and an exploration of its potential as a novel treatment for depression. In P. Wolfson & G. Hartelius (Eds.), *The Ketamine Papers: Science, therapy, and transformation* (pp. 1–23). Santa Cruz, CA: Multidisciplinary Association for Psychedelic Studies (MAPS).

Wolfson, P. (2016b). Psychedelic experiential pharmacology: Pioneering clinical explorations with Salvador Roquet: An interview with Richard Yensen. In P. Wolfson & G. Hartelius (Eds.), *The Ketamine Papers: Science, therapy, and transformation* (pp. 57–68). Santa Cruz, CA: Multidisciplinary Association for Psychedelic Studies (MAPS).

Wolfson, P., & Hartelius, G. (Eds.). (2016). *The Ketamine Papers: Science, therapy, and transformation*. Santa Cruz, CA: Multidisciplinary Association for Psychedelic Studies (MAPS).

Wong, G. L., Tam, Y. H., Ng, C. F., Chan, A. W., Choi, P. C., Chu, W. C., et al. (2014). Liver injury is common among chronic abusers of ketamine. *Clinical Gastroenterology and Hepatology, 12*, 1759–1762.

Xiaoyin, K., Yi, D., Ke, X., Hongbo, H., Dap-
ing, W., Xuefeng, D., et al. (2018). The profile
of cognitive impairments in chronic ketamine
users. *Psychiatry Research, 266,* 124–131.

Yang, C., Shirayama, Y., Zhang, J. C., Ren, Q.,
Yao, W., Ma, M., et al. (2015). R-ketamine:
A rapid-onset and sustained antidepressant
without psychotomimetic side effects. *Translational Psychiatry, 5,* e632.

Yoon, G., Petrakis, I. L., & Krystal, J. H.
(2019). Association of combined naltrexone
and ketamine with depressive symptoms in
a case series of patients with depression and
alcohol use disorder. *JAMA Psychiatry, 76,*
337–338.

Zarate, C. A. Jr., Singh, J. B., Carlson, P. J.,
Brutsche, N. E., Ameli, R., Luckenbaugh, D.
A., et al. (2006). A randomized trial of an *N*-
methyl-D-aspartate antagonist in treatment-
resistant major depression. *Archives of General Psychiatry, 63,* 856–864.

Zhan, Y., Zhang, B., Zhou, Y., Zheng, W., Liu,
W., Wang, C., et al. (2019). A preliminary
study of anti-suicidal efficacy of repeated ketamine infusions in depression with suicidal
ideation. *Journal of Affective Disorders, 251,*
205–212.

Zhang, L.-M., Zhou, W.-W., Ji, Y-J., Li, Y., Zhao,
N., Chen, H-X., et al. (2015). Anxiolytic effects of ketamine in animal models of posttraumatic stress disorder. *Psychopharmacology, 232,* 663–672.

PART IV

Therapeutic Considerations

CHAPTER 18

Set, Setting, and Dose

J. C. CALLAWAY

Introduction

The psychedelic experience is unique. It continues to be researched by modern science, as its role in society continues to mature. This experience results from a chemical interaction between certain alkaloids and specific receptors in the brain. The desired result is often a visionary effect that is typically not well understood. As the term implies (from Greek roots *psyche*, "mind/soul" + *delos*, "to uncover, reveal"), the psychedelic effect is a revealing of the mind/soul. This effect is necessarily from the perspective of the person having the experience, which is often profound and mystical. It invites both theological and scientific philosophies to wonder how an exogenous chemical substance can allow ordinarily hidden parts of the mind to become visible for a few hours. The experience can be equally terrifying under adverse or malicious conditions. Either way, this effect necessarily follows the ingestion or administration of a psychedelic substance, either from plants, fungi, or a purified substance that has been isolated or synthesized in a laboratory. This is the dose. The two other components of a psychedelic experience are the mental set of the individual having the experience and the physical setting of the experience. Together, set, setting and dose provide the context for this effect to occur (see Figure 18.1).

Classic examples of psychedelic substances are mescaline from at least two species of cacti, lysergic acid diethlyamide (LSD) as a semisynthetic product from a laboratory, N,N-dimethyltryptamine (DMT) from many species of plants, and psilocybin from

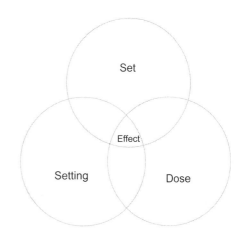

■ FIGURE 18.1. A Venn diagram, not necessarily drawn to scale, representing the relative relationships among set, setting, and dose, to produce a psychedelic effect.

many more species of fungi. Whatever the source, the effect is rightfully referred to as a "trip" to denote this process of unveiling parts of the mind that are not normally available to the waking mind—in essence, a form of mental travel that occurs over time, rather than physical travel. The full effect is typically clear and memorable, as a lifetime's collection of thoughts, memories, and experiences are available for inspection, exploration, and discovery. A fluid sense of self and perception can progress into a transient dissolution of ego. It can be a lot to experience in a short amount of time.

The intensity of the visionary experience and, to some extent, the duration of the effect increase with dose. Eventually, after a few hours, the familiar mentations of life slide back into their well-worn grooves, and the barrier is restored between the waking mind and most of the other stuff. Durable memories tend to linger after the effect, which may have some beneficial influence on subsequent thoughts, actions, and behaviors. A second dosing within a few days will have an attenuated effect, as tolerance rapidly builds after the initial dose of a psychedelic substance. An abstinence of 1 or 2 weeks may be required to reachieve a full effect.

While the mental set of an individual can vary, and naturally does with age and experience, both the dose and the setting can be well defined. In the case of dose, the identity can be characterized to high degree of chemical certainty, weight, and purity. As a technology, a better understanding of the dose increases reliability of the desired outcome by reducing a wide range of additional variables and uncertainties that could distract from the intended effect. A good knowledge of the dose also helps to repeat the desired effect with more confidence and reliability.

For the most part, citizens of modern cultures still lack a coherent vocabulary to describe such a profound experience, and one purpose of this chapter is draw attention to the nuances of dose in the modern development of psychedelic exploration. The academic fields of chemistry and pharmacology have already mapped out many of the basic physical facts for the known psychedelic alkaloids, but these vocabularies are alien to most people, and more accessible concepts are required to further the discussions. As with any new tool or technology, some amount of time is required for awareness to expand into a larger conversation, with useful concepts acquired along the way. For the most part, fear-based politics in modern societies have deterred medical researchers from making more of an effort to investigate this new technology. While their sanctioned value and role in modern cultures remain to be defined, initial applications for psychedelic substances will probably include their use as adjuncts to psychotherapy, especially for treating patients with substance misuse issues and/or severe trauma, and to help people prepare for death (Garcia-Romeu & Richards, 2018; Mithoefer, Grob, & Brewerton, 2016).

■ Set

Essentially, the *set* is the user's current mental state, which may not be easy to understand, much less predict or control. In this discussion, this mainly refers to the mind of the person at the time of the experience. The user's background and cultural context will significantly influence the perception and interpretation of the psychedelic experience. A person's intents and goals are also important components of the mental set. Even the vocabulary of one's own language becomes an issue as the individual attempts to explain the main features of this subjective experience to others. Evaluating the mental set of an individual is a persistent goal of modern psychology, and many features of mental affect can be identified and measured with statistical significance.

The mental set is also influenced by the user's physical state (e.g., age and general health), in addition to an individual's metabolic predisposition, which can also influence the trip. For example, a "fast" metabolizer of harmine may have a different ayahuasca experience than a "slow" metabolizer of this alkaloid (Callaway, 2005a). This means that the user's genetic set can also influence the result of an ayahuasca session in a significant way. With sufficient knowledge of both the dose and the user's somatic state, such a difference can be augmented to some extent by decreasing the dose for the slow metabolizer.

Setting

The *setting* can be broadly described as the physical environment of the experience, which has a significant impact throughout the trip. This is the easiest component to identify, preferably before the trip takes place, and manage for the duration of the experience. Some sort of setting is always present in our lives. In general, a clean, comfortable environment is more conducive to a beneficial experience than an environment with more variation and unpredictability. In general, fewer variables are more conducive to a productive trip than more variables.

Dose

Before the 21st century, with a limited selection of psychedelic substances to discuss, the dose was often assumed. Sometimes the dose and effect are worshiped, typically in a continuation of prehistoric ceremony, where mythological explanations help us understand this mysterious other world. Gradually, as more scientific information arrives, and as more psychedelic molecules are investigated, the nuances of dose become more relevant to a systematic application of a technology that allows us to explore our minds. This consideration is not limited to what the dose is, but to how much of the active substance is present in the dose, how often it is taken, and how the dose is administered. These and other aspects of dose are standard questions for modern pharmacological research.

The dose is a necessary component of the psychedelic experience. Unlike the visions in dream sleep or hallucinatory states of psychoses, a psychedelic trip requires a sufficient amount of an external stimuli to initiate the journey, that is, a dose of psychedelic substance. For this reason, the results of a psychedelic trip do not fulfil the definition of a hallucination, since the effects are caused by an exogenous substance that must be consumed. While there may be a visionary experience as part of the trip, especially at high doses, this is not the same as a hallucination, since the visionary experience is relative to the one having the experience. In extreme cases, a trip may also be judged by others who are not having the experience. In this case, who is to say if the vision is not real or whether one is or is not having the vision?

Knowledge of dose and dosage is a major part of modern pharmacology. Quite a bit is already known about the basic characteristics of psychedelic chemicals that have already been studied in human clinical trials. While dose primarily denotes the identity of a substance, it concerns the actual amount of the substance and how it is administered or consumed. The intensity of the experience, and to some extent the duration, are directly proportional to the dose. While the efficacy of the dose is usually assumed when other information is lacking, the typical situation can be summed up as "This is what we have, let's take it!" However, after adjusting for differences in potency, the psychedelic experience is still not exactly the same between different psychedelic agents because different molecular structures have different receptor binding affinities and binding profiles in the brain, which consequently provide differences in experience for this reason alone.

The effective dose is a function of potency. For example, LSD, as a mind-opening substance, is fully active at 100 µg. By contrast, a solvent, ethanol, can be characterized as a mind-numbing substance, with up to 100 g/day possibly being consumed by an alcoholic. In this comparison, a single daily dose of LSD is about 1 million times more potent than the dosage of alcohol that may be consumed in heavy daily use. Doubling this amount of alcohol could be fatal for most people, while doubling the dose of LSD to 200 µg would mainly result in the death of one's ego for a few precious hours. In pharmacological terms, this means that the safety and therapeutic index of ethanol is low, while the therapeutic index for LSD is extremely high.

Dose: A Physical Substance

In practice, the *dose* is typically assumed to be a sufficient amount of an active substance, sometimes without a certain identity of the active chemical component(s), and only a rough estimation of the amount. Typically, at least one person in the group will know something about the substance, either from direct experience or an analytical report. The physical state of the dose is also important; for example, the consumed substance could be derived from plant(s), fungi, and/or animal(s), or it could be a single molecular species from a laboratory. In general, a known amount of a pure chemical can reproduce the effect with more reliability than a naturally derived product, since there is more potential for unknown variables with the later.

Dose and Route of Administration

The route of administration is another aspect to consider for dose, as the same amount of the same chemical will provide different experiences if the dose is taken orally, smoked, vaporized as a distillate, insufflated as a snuff, administered as an enema, applied topically, or injected as a solution. DMT is a good example of a psychedelic agent that can be consumed in several different ways. Each delivery strategy provides a different type of visionary effect, even if the same amount of DMT is administered to the same individual in each case. For example, the effect from injected or insufflated DMT has a fast onset, which resolves after a few minutes because DMT is rapidly metabolized as it continues to cycle through the liver. As with other drugs, intravenous injection is faster in onset than intramuscular injection. DMT can also be inhaled, as a vapor. This route of administration also has a remarkably fast onset of dramatic visual effects, and baseline consciousness is restored within minutes. While spectacular, this effect may not be long enough to form lasting memories for the extensive narratives that are more typical for orally activated DMT.

DMT can be administered rectally, by enema, or as a suppository (De Smet, 1983). Because rectal absorption allows DMT to pass through the brain before it passes through the liver, enzyme inhibition is not required to experience the visionary effects by this route of administration. In general, rectal absorption is faster than absorption after oral administration, but still slower than injected, inhaled, or insufflated DMT.

The oral activation of DMT in *ayahuasca* provides the slowest onset of effects and the longest duration of action for DMT, with some attenuation in the intensity. I discuss this complex mechanism of action in more detail later in this chapter.

Early Concepts of Chemical Bioactivity

Prior to the 19th century, European scientists generally believed that organic compounds obtained from plants and other living organisms were endowed with a special force that distinguished them from inorganic compounds. This was the natural line between organic substances, which were produced by plants and animals, and inorganic substances. According to this way of thinking, organic matter was endowed with a "vital force" in a concept called "vitalism." In 1828, German chemist Friedrich Wöhler discovered that urea, an organic compound, could be produced in the laboratory from inorganic starting materials. This was the beginning of organic chemistry and the beginning of the end for vitalism and many other superstitions. This is not to say that superstitions are without value, but rather to suggest that superstitions answered important questions until a better answer arrived. This fundamental change in thinking paved the way for a more consistent and reliable philosophy that could be independently verified by others through experimentation and objective observation, and without the additional need of psychopomp or other subjective variables.

Psychoactive Plants and Religion

The deliberate use of psychoactive plants is inseparable from the development of early human cultures in many parts of the New World, especially in Central and South America. Surprisingly few examples of plant-derived psychedelics are found in the literature of the Old World. The ancient Vedic literature from India describes a psychoactive beverage identified as *Soma,* and a similar description of *Haoma* appears in the Avesta literature of ancient Persia, but it is unclear what plants were used to prepare these sacraments. Ancient literature from Greece describes the *Kykeon*, which is also of unknown composition. Perhaps these plants were used to the point of extinction, then replaced with less active ingredients, or even inactive substances, after religious traditions were established. Subsequently, faith, ritual and psychopomp were used to fill in the gaps until these traditions regained new meaning or died out completely.

Finding the Same Methylated Xanthines from Different Plants

It may be difficult to say precisely how or why all of these pharmacological innovations began, yet they did. Before written history, people from around the world sought and found medicinal alkaloids from a wide variety of local plant and fungal species, administered them in every possible way, as both food and/or medicine, with little or no means of communication with other groups of people who discovered and enjoyed the same alkaloids, sometimes from different plants. These discoveries added value to life and could have predated agriculture and the production of ceramics, in most cases.

The prehistoric discovery of caffeine from different plant species is a good example of this botanical serendipity, since caffeine is found in plants that are unique to the Eastern and Western Hemispheres, and it continues to be used by people wherever those plants happen to grow. Also, no new plant sources of caffeine have been discovered. A similar story applies to the alkaloid theophylline, found in tea, as another methylated xanthine that is used as a mild stimulant. Both alkaloids have been engrained into the cultural habits of many modern nations and past civilizations.

Regular use of a dietary stimulant has a direct impact in the individual and society. The mild physical addiction to methylated xanthines reinforces a complex relationship between humans, food, and our daily dose of alkaloids. The habit of drinking tea in England, for example did not exist before tea was imported to England. From the perspective of economic botany, a daily cup of hot tea with added milk and sugar in the afternoon, encouraged people to work long hours at a dull, repetitive task nearly every day. This allowed the Industrial Revolution to begin and to succeed. To drive the point, in addition to other extreme measures, England fought the Opium Wars with China in order to maintain its regular supply of tea. Today, all modern societies are fueled by a wide range of products that contain caffeine, theophylline, and/or other methylated xanthines, just to help us through another day. After all, it is the dose that ultimately attracts and eventually sustains the desire of consumption. For example, those who drink decaffeinated coffee are almost entirely former coffee drinkers, rather than non-coffee drinkers who decided to enjoy decaffeinated coffee.

Finding the Same Psychedelic Alkaloids from Different Plants

Archeological evidence from ancient civilizations in Central and South America clearly demonstrate the religious use of certain plants now known to contain chemicals that can temporarily induce a psychedelic state of mind, such as mescaline, from at least two species of cacti, psilocin and psilocybin from at least 200 species of fungi, and other dimethylated tryptamines from a wide variety of plants and even a few animal species (see Ott, 1993). By eating just a few magic mushrooms, and after the first few adventures into the early human mind, it is easy to imagine how language, philosophies, and theologies may have begun. The discovery and use of psychoactive alkaloids were an inevitable consequence of human curiosity, which naturally drives a systematic exploration of the immediate environment for anything that will provide a benefit, and thus add value to life.

Organized religions and other ceremonial habits probably developed as a effort to harness and utilize this power that is provided by certain plants. Even in modern times, many people still believe that LSD, for example, has miraculous powers of vitalism that go beyond its ability to reveal the mind, as if that were not enough. In fact, chemicals do not contain such power. They can only release that which is already in the mind, and modify information coming into the mind from the setting, during the trip. This is not to say that concepts of spirits, plant teachers, or even molecular teachers are necessarily wrong, but rather to emphasize that an alkaloid, consumed as a dose, is an inanimate configuration of atoms that fits perfectly into a unique profile of receptors in the brain, which affect large swaths of the brain's serotonin system for a few hours.

Psychedelic Plants Were Part of the Columbian Exchange

The knowledge of the psychedelic effect has come to us through certain plants and fungi, and almost entirely through examples from the conquest of the New World. However, the impact of this discovery was mostly ignored or not even noticed by modern civilizations until the later part of the 20th century. The earliest historical information was recorded soon after native contact with Spanish and Portuguese explorers in the late 15th century and 16th century, respectively. By the time of his second voyage to the New World, Christopher Columbus requested his friar, Ramon Pane, to prepare a report on the natives of Hispaniola (today the island comprising Haiti and the Dominican Republic). Pane's report described the shamanic use of *cohoba,* a psychoactive snuff derived from a local plant. As would be established centuries later, *cohoba* is prepared from the DMT-containing seeds of *Anadenanthera peregrina* (L.) Speg., which is remarkably similar to the *yopo* snuff used by the natives of the Orinoco River basin in Colombia and Venezuela, which also contains DMT and other psychoactive alkaloids, and later from archeological sites in the Atacama Desert (see Ott, 1993).

Agents of the Catholic Church recorded most of the early historic information on these practices and always with a dim view of using plants, or anything else, for unsanctioned "divinatory" purposes. Aside from being mentioned in early Church documents, nothing was done with this information. Other new plants were more interesting and easier to exploit by the early Europeans.

The Europeans were not always to blame for the decline of all prehistoric cultures in the Americas, or even the decline of psyche-

delic use in the Americas. For example, archeological evidence from the Atacama Desert in northern Chile provides a clear record of insufflating DMT as snuffs prepared from plants, with elaborate paraphernalia from a culture that flourished and then withered away nearly 700 years before Columbus reached the New World (Torres & Repke, 2006), while much older evidence exists for the use of mescaline-containing cacti in South America.

The Modern Advent of the Classic Psychedelics

Throughout most of the 20th century, only a small collection of molecules was known to elicit the classic psychedelic effect: mescaline (discovered in 1897), LSD (in 1943), DMT (in 1956) and psilocybin (in 1959). With such a short list of molecules, the significance of dose remained a mundane topic. After the effective dose was determined for each of these alkaloids, the topic of dose did not receive much more consideration. In the later part of the 20th century, numerous synthetic variants of mescaline were discovered and rediscovered (Shulgin & Shulgin, 1991), in addition to several novel tryptamine derivatives (Shulgin & Shulgin, 1997), thus increasing the list of psychedelic agents to several hundred distinct molecular species. Receptor binding studies of psychedelic alkaloids began to show significance at certain serotonin receptor subtypes already in the 1950s. Discussions of quantitative structure–activity relationships became possible as the collection of active molecules grew in the 1980s, which allowed a deeper conversation on the very nature of this effect in a few academic laboratories.

Peyote: An Ancient Source of Mescaline

Well before Spanish explorers arrived in Mexico, the Huichol Indians (or Wixáritari) used peyote as a sacred and profound source of knowledge and inspiration (Schaefer & Furst, 1996). No one can provide an exact date to mark the beginning of Huichol culture, but one archeological study examined peyote artifacts from the Shumla

Caves in the Lower Pecos region of southwest Texas and near Cuatro Ciénegas in Coahuila, Mexico, which contained mescaline and were apparently made from peyote and other native plants (Terry et al., 2006). The mean age for the three specimens from Shumla Caves was radiocarbon dated to be 5,195 years before present, while one sample from the Cuatro Ciénegas site was determined to be 835 years before the present. Concerning these samples, authors of that study concluded that "the Shumla Caves' specimens are composed of an aggregate of ground *peyote* mixed with other plant material, i.e., they appear to be manufactured *peyote* effigies, and are definitely not intact *peyote* 'buttons.'" They concluded overall that "this study demonstrates the use of *peyote* by inhabitants of the Lower Pecos region of the Chihuahuan Desert about 6,000 years ago, and confirms its use by inhabitants of the Cuatro Ciénegas region of the Chihuahuan Desert in Late Prehistoric times." This is a lot to consider. Not only had the apparent ceremonial use of peyote existed in this region so long ago, but it continues in this area to this day.

In their fervent quest for gold, silver, and souls, Spanish explorers and Catholic missionaries of the late 16th century were not at all interested in learning about the use of peyote. Despite an aggressive campaign to subjugate the local populations, the Huichol clung to their beliefs and traditions, basing their entire cosmology around the ceremonial use of this small and bitter tasting cactus (Schaefer & Furst, 1996). There are few other surviving examples in the New World that have shown such tenacity. After centuries of direct experience, a good understanding of dose (as a single plant species) was known. Also, since only one plant was involved, the Huichols had no need to conduct further research. Centuries of uninterrupted experience had already refined their way of life.

Mescaline: First from Plants, Then from the Laboratory

By the end of the 19th century, peyote had more secrets to share, especially with a small group of European scientists who were interested in searching for the chemical nature of peyote's psychedelic effect. Peyote is not native to the Old World, yet news of this experience had already reached Germany at a time when the emerging field of organic chemistry had just begun to replace a less objective way of thinking about the world.

Using scientific methods in the late 19th century, a series of alkaloids were isolated from peyote and each alkaloid was systematically ingested at known doses (Heffter, 1898). At that time, the precise chemical identity of these alkaloids was not known, but it was known that each isolated alkaloid was chemically different from the others, and Heffter was able to weigh each dose with a high degree of precision. Only one of these alkaloids provided a psychedelic effect. Eventually enough of one alkaloid was consumed to allow Heffter to experience a full-blown psychedelic effect. This alkaloid named *mescaline* was the first example of a naturally occurring psychedelic substance, ingested as a pure chemical. Despite phenomenal advances in medical science since that time, human experimentation is still the only way to truly know whether a substance is psychedelic.

Mescaline: An Inevitable Discovery

In the 1970s, mescaline was also identified as a major alkaloid in species of *Echinopsis* such as the San Pedro cactus (*Echinopsis pachanoi,* syn. *Trichocereus pachanoi*), which grow in the arid regions of western South America. Both *peyote* and San Pedro cacti have long and distinct histories of ceremonial use in their respective geographic regions of northern Mexico and South America, respectively. However, no known connection existed for the transfer of information between these dispersed cultures. Since people still use these cacti, and since the effect is so unique, it was inevitable that at least one of these species would gain the attention of European explorers, and eventually be passed on to scientists who could isolate and determine the active component(s). It seems inevitable that mescaline would have been discovered by modern scientists.

Evidence for the use of the San Pedro cactus and other other psychedelic plants is featured in prominent stone art work and other artifacts from Chavín de Huantar—the archeological site of a sophisticated pre-Inca culture that developed from 900 B.C.E. to 200 B.C.E., on the central west coast of Peru (Torres, 2008). This is another example of unrelated people finding the same mescaline in different plant species for basically the same purpose, that is, to obtain a dose that reveals the unknown, to make the unknown known because knowing opens up more options than not knowing, and options provide an advantage in the survival game. However, as often happens, the Chavín culture went into decline between 500 and 300 B.C.E., when the larger ceremonial sites were abandoned, with some unfinished, gradually replaced by smaller villages and agricultural land. It was as if too many people had "turned on, tuned in, and dropped out" of a highly structured society that had flourished for centuries, or maybe too few were allowed to handle and dispense the sacrament. Or perhaps too many years of successive droughts occurred, which the elites were unable to explain, predict or control. In any case, Chavín serves as another example of a nascent civilization in the New World that apparently appreciated the psychedelic effect, yet ceased to exist at least 1,700 years before the arrival of Europeans.

LSD: A Semisynthetic Product

Aside from the discovery of mescaline in 1898, and until the accidental discovery of LSD in 1943, there were no other chemicals known to reveal the mind with such profound clarity and reliability. There were also very few scientists who were even interested in this particular topic by the mid-20th century. Access to the required substances, or even access to information on such substances, was not easily had. Since then, LSD has become one of the most remarkable alkaloids in history.

Moreover, a fully effective oral dose for mescaline is near 400 mg, while the fully effective oral dose for LSD is typically near 100 µg. This is a huge difference in potency that begs for a deeper understanding of the varied metabolic pathways that each of these chemicals must travel before arriving to activate receptor sites in the brain. Moreover, the molecular structures of mescaline and LSD are not at all similar. Aside from their chemical identities and their active doses, there was nothing else that was easy to understand about this new area of exploration until the end of the 20th century. Currently, hundreds of psychedelic chemicals have been identified, and a better understanding of both chemical–receptor interactions and brain imaging have begun to provide objective data to complement individuals' observations from the actual experience.

By the 1950s, other psychoactive drugs were already well known to students of the medical sciences (e.g., ethanol in various forms, cocaine, purified opioids, amphetamine, and atropine), but none of these have produced the clarity of mind or lasting memory of an experience that can only be accurately described as psychedelic or mind revealing. Early medical studies with LSD and a few other psychedelic agents led early medical researchers to consider the psychedelic effects to be experimental models of psychosis. As a consequence, the currently disused term *psychotomimetic* (a substance that temporarily mimics some aspects of psychosis) became popular for a time in some research circles. While the chemically induced experience for an ordinary mind is quite different than natural psychosis, this was the first time an ordinary person or medical researcher could experience some aspects of the psychosis for a few hours, and perhaps imagine what it is like to have such a serious mental disorder. Compared to the other available options, this was progress.

Otherwise, the utility and application of this newly discovered technology was not immediately apparent. Some governments sponsored controlled experiments with a wide variety of psychoactive substances in the mid-20th century. Special attention was eventually focused on a few psychedelic chemicals as incapacitating agents and as "truth serums" in sessions known as "brainwashing." LSD was high on that short list (Lee & Shlain, 1985) mostly because the active dose was so low, relative to anything else, and it could be administered in a variety of ways; both overt and covert. It would be naive to think that such efforts do not continue to this day in at least some parts of the world.

Also during the 1950s, other questions were being asked by medical researchers who wanted to learn more about mental illness, in addition to new treatments for alcoholism and other mental disturbances. A relationship of convenience often developed between government and academic projects in order to achieve these varied objectives. After all, governments provided the required context, funding, and permission for most of the psychedelic research that was conducted during the 1950s and 1960s.

Independent from the clandestine government research projects, a small group of individuals from the Harvard University Department of Psychology developed a different perspective in their exploration of this new frontier during the early 1960s and basically made it up as they went along (Leary, Alpert, & Metzner, 1964). An early goal of this research effort was to achieve a reduction in prison recidivism rates by exposing incarcerated individuals to psilocybin. After the project was closed by the university, the group moved to the Millbrook estate, where their focus widened to achieve more elusive goals, such as world peace, love, and cultural change. LSD, the primary chemical used for the postacademic phase of their work, promoted the most salient features of the experience as a consequence of "set and setting." It is not surprising that religious overtones, familiar rituals, and psychopomp were adopted and employed along the way, in order to experience this phenomenal technology in a more familiar context. Gradually, this experience was reconsidered more objectively during the last half of the 20th century, as a specific interaction between exogenous molecules with certain receptors in the brain. This is only the beginning of a long journey that will continue to reveal a better understanding of the mind/soul, as we try to understand how these molecules can reliably expose mental content that is ordinarily hidden.

As a founding concept, set and setting provided a starting point for a much larger conversation, even without much more commentary on the dose. This was appropriate, since these experiences were primarily facilitated by LSD at that time. In general, the active dose was already known with a sufficient degree of certainty, yet the tendency was to explore beyond the minimum effective dose. In other words, a full-blown psychedelic experience was a desirable goal by the 1960s.

■ DMT: Another Inevitable Discovery

Some DMT-containing plants grow in the wet areas of the Amazon Basin, for example, *Psychotria viridis,* while other DMT-containing plants are found in the arid regions of the Atacama Desert, for example, *Anadenanthera colubrina.* Two other DMT-containing mimosa trees, *Anadenanthera peregrina* and *Mimosa tenuiflora* (syn. *Mimosa hostilis*), naturally grow in the arid regions of the Caribbean, South America, and Central America. All of these plants have a long history of human use for visionary purposes (Ott, 1993). These plants are used in several innovative ways in order to overcome the oral inactivity of DMT and to experience the visionary effect. Just as ancient inhabitants of Central and South America discovered and used DMT from a wide variety of plants, given enough time, this molecule was destined to be discovered by modern science. Perhaps like earlier discoveries, the modern discovery of DMT did not occur in a sequence of logical steps.

DMT was a first synthesized in 1931 (Manske, 1931), along with other tryptamine derivatives. This was 15 years before DMT was isolated from the South America beverage known as *vinho de jurema* (Gonçalves de Lima, 1946), yet the isolated DMT was not orally active. It would take more time for scientists to understand the oral activity of DMT in *ayahuasca,* while the oral activity of DMT in *jurema* remains a mystery (Vepsäläinen et al., 2005). The psychedelic activity of DMT was not demonstrated until 1956, after it was isolated from the bark of *Mimosa hostilis* and self-administered by intramuscular injection (Szára, 1956). The mechanism for the oral activity of DMT in ayahuasca was first suggested in 1967, as a passing comment in a publication that mainly focused on DMT-containing snuffs from South America (Holmstedt & Lindgren, 1967).

By 1976, DMT was identified as a naturally occurring transmitter in the mammalian brain (Christian, Harrison, & Pagel, 1976). This gave further support to the transmethylation hypothesis, which proposed a chemical explanation for the hallucinatory symptoms of psychosis in humans (Osmond & Smythies, 1952). One drawback of this explanation is the fact that DMT was also detected in the brains of healthy mammals, and in human cerebrospinal fluid (Christian, Benington, Morin, & Corbett, 1975). To provide an explanation for its presence in healthy humans, DMT was later proposed to be an active neurotransmitter in the visions of natural dream sleep, and that hallucinatory psychosis might be the product of a dysfunctional dream cycle (Callaway, 1988). In any case, there is not yet enough evidence to draw any firm conclusions, and further studies are required to refine or refute these hypotheses. A recently published review on endogenous DMT has extensively covered this topic (Barker, 2018). For a recent general review on DMT, see Mishor, McKenna, and Callaway (2011).

DMT in Ayahuasca

People in the Amazon Basin learned to boil the leaves of *Psychotria viridis* with the *Banisteriopsis cappi* vine to make a powerful psychedelic decoction. This is only one version of a bitter tasting beverage that always contains the harmala alkaloids harmine, harmaline, and tetrahydroharmine (Callaway, 2005b). This innovative technology is used by people throughout northern South America. This topic has been covered extensively in the book entitled *Ayahuasca Analogues* (Ott, 1994).

Among other things, harmala alkaloids from the vine temporarily inhibit the liver enzyme monoamine oxidase A (MAO-A), which would normally destroy DMT when it is consumed orally. With MAO-A inhibited, DMT enters the brain to interact with the serotonin receptors that initiate the visionary effects. Drinking ayahuasca has a different onset profile and effect for DMT. Absorption is a relatively slow process, which takes about 30–40 minutes for the visionary effects to develop. The inhibition of MAO-A typically lasts several hours, which subsequently allows the DMT to remain active for several hours.

However, MAO-A is also responsible for metabolizing the neurotransmitter serotonin. Thus, levels of serotonin continue to increase after MAO-A is inhibited, and DMT must compete with this extra serotonin for the same receptor sites in the brain. For this reason, the effect from ayahuasca is longer in duration and somewhat attenuated, relative to the same amount injected, due to MAO-A inhibition and this extra level of competition between DMT and serotonin in the brain.

There are many other leaves and vines in the forests of the Amazon Basin that have no effect at all, and a systematic process of trial and error that would have resulted in the discovery of this particular plant combination is at least near the edge of being incomprehensible, especially when the goal of that discovery was essentially unknown. There are other technological hurdles to consider. For example, boiling plants to this extent might require ceramics. For now, the mythological explanations are more developed than any scientific speculation. When compared to all the other ways of consuming DMT, ayahuasca presents itself as one of the most complex. By contrast, there are extremely few examples in modern pharmacology in which an enzyme inhibitor is used to allow the oral activity of another chemical that would ordinarily be orally inactive. It is surprising that there is so little interest in the discovery and development of a new drug delivery system that could be useful to modern medicine.

DMT in Snuffs

Various snuffs have been made from the mimosa species *Anadenanthera colubrina* and *Anadenanthera peregrina*. These snuffs contain DMT, 5-methoxy DMT, and 5-hydroxy DMT (bufotenin). The archeological evidence for the preparation and use of these snuffs has been carefully described (Torres & Repke, 2006). Since these alkaloids are insufflated, they do not pass through the liver and are not extensively metabolized before reaching receptors in the brain. Thus, no extra plants are required to make these snuffs active.

DMT in *Vinho de Jurema* (*Mimosa hostilis*)

The beverage *vinho de jurema* contains DMT and is orally active. Only one plant is required to prepare *jurema* (pronounced as "yurema" or "hurema" in English), so a process of trial and error is easier to understand, at least from a practical point of view. Pharmacologically, however, the mechanism of action is still not understood. The presence of DMT in *jurema*, and the subsequent psychedelic activity from drinking this beverage, do not explain the oral activity of DMT in *jurema*. After many years of tedious research, a new class of alkaloids was identified in the bark of *Mimosa hostilis* (syn. *M. tenuiflora*), from which *jurema* is prepared (Vepsäläinen et al., 2005). The first alkaloid to be characterized was named *yuremamine* and represents an entirely new class of alkaloids.

Part of the problem of identifying yuremamine was due to its chemical decomposition to DMT during the isolation process. Eventually, it was realized that the DMT structure is embedded in the larger yuremamine molecule (Vepsäläinen et al., 2005). Perhaps yuremamine acts as a prodrug that can pass unchanged from the digestive tract to the brain, where it is subsequently metabolized to release DMT in the brain. Or perhaps a degrading product can inhibit MAO-A. Whatever the mechanism, the activity suggests the possibility of an entirely new strategy to deliver metabolically sensitive medicines to active sites in the brain.

Unlike the harmala alkaloids in ayahuasca, there are no known MAO-A inhibitors in the bark of *Mimosa hostilis*, or in the beverage *vinho de jurema*, yet DMT and other interesting alkaloids are produced by this plant, and they are found in this beverage, and this beverage is known to provide the visionary effect that is similar to DMT. It will take more time for science to better understand this observation, and provide a rational explanation for the oral activity of DMT in *vinho de jurema*.

▨ Psilocybin in Fungi

For various reasons, women are poorly represented in the modern history of psychedel-ic discovery. The story of María Sabina, a Mazatec shaman from the village of Huatla de Jiménez in Oaxaca, Mexico, is a good example of such a person who could have been overlooked, and one important aspect of her story is worth reporting in this context. Following the discovery of LSD, psilocin and its phosphate ester (psilocybin) were both isolated from the fungus *Psilocybe mexicana*, which was provided by María Sabina for scientific research. To confirm the molecular structure after isolation and identification, psilocybin was subsequently synthesized in the late 1950s (Hofmann, Heim, Brack, & Kobel, 1958). As before, the active component was only identified by human experimentation after preliminary animal tests gave ambiguous results.

To complete this remarkable round of discovery, synthetic tablets of psilocybin were returned to María Sabina, who subsequently confirmed the synthetic dose to be "the same God" she had previously known only through the mushroom. She also remarked on the convenience of having a stable form of her sacrament for times of the year when the mushrooms were difficult to find (Hofmann, 1978). This rare exchange of new and old information rapidly crossed cultural, social, gender, and linguistic barriers at a time when such barriers were typically thick, wide, and opaque at best. This remarkable example speaks volumes to the open mindedness of a few highly educated men from Europe and North America, and how they respected the technology embodied by this frail indigenous woman who lived a humble existence in rural Mexico. This is also a useful commentary on the folly of an artificial argument between the assumed virtues of synthetic versus "natural" psychedelic substances.

While political opinions have been slow to appreciate the value of this discovery, medical science has not lost its fascination with this ancient technology of the mind, and the inherent efficacy of these molecules has not diminished over time. For example, recent clinical trials with psilocybin in patients with end-stage cancer have demonstrated real value for the palliative care of the terminally ill (Grob et al., 2011). It is important for all of us to prepare for the inevitability of death, and the psychedelic experience can help to bring the significance of our mortality into perspective. Promising anecdotal stories and results from preliminary clinical trials offer the hope of efficacious treatments for individuals with substance misuse issues and those who have experienced trauma in their lives.

Psychedelics and Modern Culture

After the discovery of the psychedelic effect by modern science in the 20th century, the next logical step would be the further study and eventual application of this technology. Aside from ethanol, modern cultures had very little capacity to even imagine a use for another mind-altering substance. LSD, for example, was apparently not very useful as truth serum, as everything became truth after a certain point. Eventually, this powerful effect was used to treat alcoholics in the United Kingdom and then in Canada during the 1950s (Lee & Shlain, 1985), apparently with encouraging results. That good work was soon to be terminated after LSD escaped from the lab and dropped directly into popular cultures in the Western Hemisphere during the 1960s. This unsanctioned activity was aggressively persecuted with a fervent authoritative fanaticism that lingers to the present time in most parts of the modern world. This newfound zeal for prosecuting drug crimes was based on a conservative belief that the United States had "lost" the Vietnam War because, for the first time in history, a cadre of potential war conscripts took LSD, smoked *cannabis* and said, "Hell no, we won't go!" It would have been a huge threat to any empire. After all, both governments and modern religions continually inform on, and rely on, conditions of set and setting to propagate their own ideological agendas. For most religions, the soul-revealing properties of a sacrament are primarily a matter of faith. Conversely, and as a matter of fact, a full dose of a psychedelic substance requires no faith at all.

Dose and Tolerance

Additionally, the frequency of dosing will add another layer of pharmacology known as *tolerance*. For most psychedelic agents, tolerance builds rapidly after the first dose, and there is crossover tolerance between other psychedelic substances. For example, the same dose of LSD on a Monday will not produce the same effect on Tuesday. This is not to say that the Tuesday dose is inactive, but that the effect is significantly attenuated. Also, if the equivalent effective dose of psilocybin is consumed on Tuesday, after LSD on Monday, then the effect of psilocybin will also be significantly attenuated. In either case, several days are required after the initial exposure in order to achieve the full effect again. DMT may be an exception to this rule, as repeated doses on the same day do not show significant signs of attenuation in effect (Strassman & Qualls, 1996). The reason for this is not entirely clear, but it may be due to the rapid metabolism of injected DMT and the subsequent lack of time that may be required for a physical tolerance to actually develop.

A special type of tolerance has been reported in long-term users of *ayahuasca* (Callaway et al., 1994). This was observed as an increased density of serotonin uptake receptors on peripheral blood platelets. This type of tolerance is relatively long term and lasts for several weeks, which is different from the crossover tolerance described in the previous paragraph. It also takes about 6 weeks to restore this tolerance. If ayahuasca were an antidepressant, then this rare upregulation of receptor density would be a good indication of a desired therapeutic effect. Unfortunately, antidepressants that act on the serotonin uptake site fail to achieve this sort of effect and are largely ineffective for that and other reasons. If ayahuasca had the research department and marketing reach of a large pharmaceutical company, then we might already have better treatments available for those suffering from depression, anxiety, substance misuse, and other form of mental disorders that are heavily influenced by the serotonin system.

Macro- and Microdosing

Each psychedelic substance has a known effective dose that can be measured to a high degree of accuracy. The effective dose typically endures for a certain amount of time (e.g., LSD at 8–12 hours, psilocybin at 4–6 hours, and DMT at about 30 minutes when injected). While most drugs are administered according to body weight, this parameter has less significance for a psychedelic agent, since the primary effect is on the central nervous system. In other words, body mass index varies to a much larger degree between adults while brain mass is relatively similar, and 100 micrograms of LSD is fully effective in nearly all adults. This also explains the difference in effect for slightly different doses of the same psychedelic substance.

For example, a full dose of LSD will last from 8 to 12 hours. Doubling this will intensify the effect, but the duration of action is much the same as the fully effective dose. Albert Hofmann's first intentional experience with LSD was ignited by 250 µg. He thought this amount would have had no significant effect, as no other chemical was known to be so active at such a low dose. His experience was later described as psychedelic, meaning that his connection to familiar reality was completely detached for a few hours (Hofmann, 1980). Such an overwhelming experience is often life changing, or at least results is some significant changes in thinking about the natural ebb and flow of life.

Psychedelic therapy, as an example of macrodosing, was used to treat intractable conditions such as alcoholism and other forms of substance misuse in the 1950s. The problem was not so much a lack of efficacy for this indication, but the lack of resources to sit with patients for so many hours, the lack of analytical methods that could reliably measure beneficial changes that might occur, and no sort of follow-up program to reinforce beneficial outcomes. It was rather too easy to evaluate abstinence as a primary outcome, but such a blunt observation did not account for the varied shades of mind that make up an individual's mental content. Relapse was a potential problem in the successful cases, as with all treatment modalities, since these "recovered" individuals are often not yet prepared to face the world with their newfound perspective, and typically return to the familiar habits stemming from the original problem. On one level, some progress was made; on other levels, not enough. Aldous Huxley once charac-

terized the psychedelic experience as being neither necessary nor sufficient. In other words, just because a troubled individual had a profound experience, and perhaps gains deep insight into the origins of a personal problem(s), this brief episode of insight is not entirely sufficient to solve a particular problem in the individual's life.

At best, the psychedelic agent acts like a catalyst that can reveal the deepest levels of the mind/soul, and problems in early life can be examined with perspective and clarity for the first time, but a subsequent process of integration is also required to apply this knowledge and make beneficial changes that reinforce the habits of a worthwhile life. But, like a catalyst, it does not do the heavy lifting that is required over longer periods of time (days, weeks, months, etc.) in order to make these lasting changes in thought and behavior.

Macrodosing with a psychedelic agent was also a prominent feature of use, and misuse in the 1960s, particularly by civilian populations in Europe and North America. It is an understatement to say that the widespread, unregulated use of LSD had a significant impact on Western cultures. Again, for example, this was the first time in history that eligible young men publicly proclaimed that they would not go to war. Without the catalytic intervention of LSD, it is unlikely that this change would have happened at all, and certainly not to the degree that it had. Opinions and beliefs on music, dance, visual arts, food, politics, and conventional thoughts on religion were quickly and radically changed during the 1960s, when compared to the cultural changes that mostly did not occur in 1950s. This surprising change in popular attitudes was countered by oppressive laws that attempted to control the uncontrollable, which not only targeted an entire generation but also effectively closed all options for medical research into this remarkable phenomenon. Human medical research with psychedelic substances is still highly restricted and limited in scope.

Microdosing, another aspect of dose, is worthy of some consideration. Broadly speaking, microdosing is the precise dispensing of small amounts of a drug substance. While there are no conclusive definitions of either macro- or microdosing, the former could be at least twice the effective dose, while the later could be less than one-tenth of the effective dose. In the case of LSD, a typical microdose would be near 10 µg, or 10% of an assumed full dose of 100 µg. Microdosing is especially useful for those who have already experienced a full dose, as the effect may be extremely subtle, and could be missed by someone who is not familiar with the full effect. In other words, microdosing can help to focus attention, more as a nootropic agent rather than a psychedelic agent.

The main advantage of low or extremely low doses is the ability to slightly adjust the mental barrier between the conscious and unconscious mind for a few hours, to be more porous, rather than have that barrier erased entirely (i.e., macrodosing). This subtle approach allows the individual to explore unconscious material with more confidence and volition. One could read and write under such conditions, for example, while the idea of reading or writing might seem entirely pointless to an individual who has consumed a full dose of LSD. Ordinary and mundane tasks can be accomplished at lower doses, while insights and new meaning can be realized in microdose sessions. One's focus on conversation, for example, can be enhanced, in order to facilitate a more meaningful exchange of ideas, whether the other person is having same experience or not. This may also be a useful strategy for some individuals with issues that stem from a short attention span.

In a more perfect world, individuals could have access to full-blown psychedelic experiences in comfortable and supervised environment for most of a day, then continue with a series of microdose sessions to resolve specific issues and integrate the information over longer periods of time. This is similar to visiting the dentist for a deep and careful cleaning of the teeth every year or so, followed by a daily routine of brushing and flossing at home. Microdosing, in this analogy, would be equivalent to an occasional mental flossing at home, though not on a daily schedule, while the macrodosing (psychedelic) model would be more analogous to deep dental surgery, which requires a specialized setting and might be experienced only a few times or less during the course of a lifetime.

Conclusion

The efficacy of a psychedelic substance is self-evident, and modern medicine has already begun to consider what value these molecules may have in treating certain patient populations (e.g., in the palliative care of the terminally ill, in patients with substance abuse issues, or people who have experienced severe trauma, to name just a few of the most obvious examples of useful applications).

Following its discovery in 1943, the potent activity of LSD became well known to medical science internationally. This activity, and subsequent interest, inspired a molecule search that led to the identification of serotonin as an endogenous transmitter of chemical information in 1949. This momentous achievement was followed by the discovery of dopamine, which was first synthesized in 1910 in England and subsequently identified in the human brain in 1957. Taken together, these discoveries gave the emerging field of psychiatry a welcomed opportunity to explain behavior as a function of neurochemistry, and proposed deeper questions on the nature of memory, perception, and cognition.

These independently verifiable effects of LSD and other psychedelics in the earliest receptor binding studies led researchers to eventually discover subtypes of neuroreceptors, which furthered a broader understanding of the relationship among neurochemistry, thought, mind, and behavior. This has been an extremely fruitful area for scientific discovery. Yet despite severe administrative restrictions, both the search and research continue as these mysterious molecules continue to lure new generations of researchers to explore the relationships between psychology and neurochemistry. Gradually, as progress continues toward a better understanding of this powerful technology, applications will follow, according to their usefulness to citizens in modern societies.

References

Barker, S. A. (2018). *N,N*-Dimethyltryptamine (DMT), an endogenous hallucinogen: Past, present, and future research to determine its role and function. *Frontiers of Neuroscience,* 6(12), 536.

Callaway, J. C. (1988). A proposed mechanism for the visions of dream sleep. *Medical Hypotheses, 26,* 119–124.

Callaway, J. C. (2005a). Fast and slow metabolizers of hoasca. *Journal of Psychoactive Drugs,* 37(2), 157–161.

Callaway, J. C. (2005b). Various alkaloid profiles in decoctions of *Banisteriopsis caapi. Journal of Psychoactive Drugs,* 37(2), 151–155.

Callaway, J. C., Airaksinen, M. M., McKenna, D. J., Brito, G. S., & Grob, C. S. (1994). Platelet serotonin uptake sites increased in drinkers of ayahuasca. *Psychopharmacology, 116*(3), 385–387.

Christian, S. T., Benington, F., Morin, R. D., & Corbett, L. (1975). Gas–liquid chromatographic separation and identification of biologically important indolealkylamines from human cerebrospinal fluid. *Biochemical Medicine 14,* 191–200.

Christian, S. T., Harrison, R., & Pagel, J. (1976). Evidence for dimethyltryptamine (DMT) as a naturally-occurring transmitter in mammalian brain. *Alabama Journal of Medical Science, 13,* 162–165.

De Smet, P. A. (1983). A multidisciplinary overview of intoxicating enema rituals in the Western hemisphere. *Journal of Ethnopharmacology, 9,* 129–166.

Garcia-Romeu, A., & Richards, W. A. (2018). Current perspectives on psychedelic therapy: Use of serotonergic hallucinogens in clinical interventions. *International Review of Psychiatry, 13,* 1–26.

Gonçalves de Lima, O. (1946). Observacio es sobre o "vinho de Jurema" utilizado pelos indios Pancaru' de Tacaratu' (Pernambuco) [Observations on the "vinho de Jurema" used by the Pancaru' Indians of Tacaratu' (Pernambuco)]. *Ariquivos do Instituto de Pesquisas Agronomicas, 4,* 45–80.

Grob, C. S., Danforth, A. L., Chopra, G. S., Hagerty, M., McKay, C. R., Halberstadt, A. L., et al. (2011). Pilot study of psilocybin treatment for anxiety in patients with advanced-stage cancer. *Archives of General Psychiatry,* 68(1), 71–78.

Heffter, A. (1898). Ueber Pellote: Beiträge zur chemischen und pharmakologischen Kenntniss der Cacteen Zweite Mittheilung. *Naunyn-Schmiedeberg's Archives of Pharmacology,* 40(5–6), 385–429.

Hofmann, A. (1978). History of basic chemical investigation of the sacred mushrooms of Mexico. In J. Ott & J. Bigwood (Eds.), *Teonanacatl: Hallucinogenic mushrooms of North America* (pp. 47–61). Seattle, WA: Madrona.

Hofmann, A. (1980). *LSD: My problem child.* New York: McGraw-Hill.

Hofmann, A., Heim, R., Brack, A., & Kobel, H. (1958). Psilocybin: A psychotropic substance from the Mexican mushroom *Psilocybe mexicana Heim. Experientia,* 14(3), 107–109.

Holmstedt, B., & Lindgren, J.-E. (1967). Chemical constituents and pharmacology of South American snuffs (U.S. Public Health Service Publication No. 1645). In D. McKenna, G. T. Prance, W. Davis, & B. De Leonen (Eds.), *Ethnopharmacologic search for psychoactive drugs* (pp. 339–373). Washington, DC: U.S. Government Printing Office.

Leary, T., Alpert, R., & Metzner, R. (1964). *The psychedelic experience: A manual based on The Tibetan Book of the Dead.* New York: University Books.

Lee, M. A., & Shlain, B. (1985). *Acid dreams: LSD, the CIA and the Sixties Rebellion.* New York: Grove Press.

Manske, R. (1931). A synthesis of the methyltryptamines and some derivatives. *Canadian Journal of Research, 5,* 592–600.

Mishor, Z., McKenna, D., & Callaway, J. (2011). DMT and human consciousness. In M. Winkelman & E. Cardeña (Eds.), *Altering consciousness: Vol. 2. Biological and psychological perspectives* (pp. 85–119). New York: Praeger.

Mithoefer, M. C., Grob, C. S., & Brewerton, T. D. (2016). Novel psychopharmacological therapies for psychiatric disorders: Psilocybin and MDMA [Review]. *Lancet Psychiatry 3*(5), 481–488.

Osmond, H., & Smythies, J. R. (1952). Schizophrenia: A new approach. *Journal of Mental Science, 98,* 309–315.

Ott, J. (1993). *Pharmacotheon: Entheogenic drugs, their plant sources and history.* Kennewick, WA: Natural Products Company.

Ott, J. (1994). *Ayahuasca analogues: Pangaean entheogens.* Kennewick, WA: Natural Products Company.

Schaefer, S. B., & Furst, P. T. (1996). *People of the Peyote: Huichol Indian history, religion, and survival.* Albuquerque: University of New Mexico Press.

Shulgin, A., & Shulgin, A. (1991). *PIHKAL: A chemical love story.* Berkeley, CA: Transform Press.

Shulgin, A., & Shulgin, A. (1997). *TIHKAL: The continuation.* Berkeley, CA: Transform Press.

Strassman, R. J., & Qualls, C. R. (1996). Differential tolerance to biological and subjective effects of four closely spaced doses of N,N-dimethyltryptamine in humans. *Biological Psychiatry,* 39(9), 784–795.

Szára, S. (1956). Dimethyltryptamine: Its metabolism in man: The relation to its psychotic effect to the serotonin metabolism. *Experientia, 12*, 441–442.

Terry, M., Steelman, K. L., Guilderson, T., Dering, P., & Rowe, M. W. (2006). Lower Pecos and Coahuila peyote: New radiocarbon dates. *Journal of Archaeological Science, 33*, 1017–1021.

Torres, C. T. (2008). Chavín's psychoactive pharmacopoeia: The iconographic evidence. In W. J. Conklin & J. Quilter (Eds.), *Chavín art, architecture, and culture* (pp. 239–259). Los Angeles: Cotsen Institute of Archaeology Press, UCLA.

Torres, C. T., & Repke, D. B. (2006). *Anadenanthera: Visionary plant of ancient South America*. New York: Haworth Press.

Vepsäläinen, J. J., Auriola, S., Tukiainen, T., Ropponen, N., & Callaway, J. C. (2005). Isolation and characterization of yuremamine: A new phytoindole. *Planta Medica, 71*, 1053–1057.

CHAPTER 19

The Use of Music in Psychedelic Therapy

MENDEL KAELEN

> Music may be a human invention, but if so, it resembles the ability
> to make and control fire: it is something we invented that transforms
> human life. Indeed, it is more remarkable than fire making in some
> ways because not only is it a product of our brain's mental capacities,
> it also has the power to change the brain. It is thus emblematic of our
> species' unique ability to change the nature of ourselves.
>
> —ANIRUDDH D. PATEL (2003)

▓ Introduction

When we were born into this world, we were
born into a musical world at first. Our very
first relationships were musical relationships
(Stern, 1995). Welcomed by a plethora of
playful high-pitched intonations and soothing lullabies, bathed in a wide spectrum of
melodies and tone colors, we began to give
meaning to this new dance of sensations—
far before we comprehended our first words.
Mothers sing lullabies for their infants universally (Trehub & Trainor, 1998), infant's
music perception abilities precede speech development significantly (Trehub & Trainor,
1998), and some theorists argue that prior
to the evolution of verbal language, humans
communicated through a nonverbal *musical*
language (Mithen, 2007).

Independently of music's exact origins, the
immense significance of music for humans
takes little effort to identify. Sophisticated

musical instruments as old as 20,000 years
(Bibikov, 1978; Lbova, Volkov, Kozhevnikova, & Kulakovskaya, 2013) and 35,000 years
(Conard, Malina, & Münzel, 2009; d'Errico
et al., 2003) have been uncovered. Across
culture and history, music has been assigned
many different functions, including social,
celebratory, medicinal, and with particular
frequency, spiritual (Nettl, 1956). As noted
by ethnomusicologist Bruno Nettl (1956),

> Among many American Indian and some
> Paleo-Siberian tribes, composition is ordinar-
> ily relegated to shamans (medicine-men) or
> other individuals connected with religion in a
> particular way. Indeed, musical and religious
> specialisation are often correlated, and are
> probably the two activities of primitive life in
> which specialisation most commonly occurs.

Like music, the use of psychedelic drugs
(psychedelics) is ancient and universal, too,
and their usage is tightly intertwined with

spirituality (Schultes, Hofmann, & Rätsch, 2001). Furthermore, within the traditional use of psychedelics, music is a prominent component and is considered important in facilitating mental imagery, emotionality, and healing. A good example of this is the singing of songs during ayahuasca-ceremonies by Huni Kuin tribes of Brazil and Shipibo tribes of Peru, of which the anthropologist Marlene Dobkin De Rios (2009) said the following:

> We could only marvel at the pervasive presence of music in a variety of forms, as an integral part of the psychedelic experience. . . . Shamans state that the music they create provokes special types of visions. Healers told me that the particular traditional melodies, *icaros*, that they choose to sing or whistle, would evoke visions they specifically desired their clients to have, to permit them to see the agent responsible for bewitchment, to resolve anxiety created in the wake of psychedelics use, and so on.

This chapter concerns the use of music in psychedelic therapy: An integrative psychotherapeutic approach that combines the administration of a psychedelic medicine (e.g., psilocybin, lysergic acid diethylamide [LSD] or 3,4-methylenedioxymethamphetamine [MDMA]) with introspective music listening and person-centered support. Psychedelic therapy is increasingly demonstrated safe and effective in treating a variety of psychiatric conditions, such as depression, tobacco addiction, alcohol addiction, end-of-life anxiety, and posttraumatic stress disorder (PTSD) (see Lancellotta & Davis, Chapter 10, this volume), and music is a central component in the therapeutic procedures. But why is music considered so important? And how can music best be used during therapy sessions?

In the face of too little research on music and psychedelics, yet a rapidly rising interest in psychedelic therapy, I attempt in this chapter to provide an overview of both historic and contemporary clinical perspectives and research insights on the use of music in psychedelic therapy. I emphasize the significant influence of music on subjective experience and therapy outcomes; the importance of acknowledging its appropriate role within the therapy procedures; and the care, insight, and responsibility needed when using music in psychedelic therapy sessions.

■ The Development of Psychedelic Therapy

In the first half of the 20th century, alongside the discovery of LSD, the ability of psychedelics to quickly and significantly change a person's outlook, personality, mood, and behavior sparked international interest in their psychotherapeutic potentials (Grof, 1980; Hofmann, 1980). Busch and Johnson (1950) were first to report on the therapeutic potential of LSD, describing its effects as increasing the patient's "expressiveness" and as "permitting re-examination of significant experiences of the past, which were sometimes relived with frightening realism." This was the beginning of numerous experiments on the therapeutic use of psychedelics, culminating into an estimated 40,000 patients with mood and addiction disorders who had been treated with LSD and other psychedelics by the late 1960s (Grinspoon & Bakalar, 1981).

Eisner and Cohen (1958) reported that under LSD, "frequently whole sequences unroll before the patient's eyes as though they had been stored on microfilm." Feld, Goodman, and Guido (1958) concluded from their observations that "LSD-25 has the astonishing quality of bringing into focus the patient's repressed emotional attitudes, conflicts, etc., and permits their re-activation." Abramson (1956) remarked that "emotions hitherto camouflaged were brought out, without the intense guilty fears that had kept them submerged." And Pahnke, Kurland, Unger, Savage, and Grof (1970) wrote, "The major dimension of drug-altered reactivity with therapeutic relevance is the affective or emotional sphere: intense, labile, personally meaningful emotionality is uniformly produced, with periodic episodes of overwhelming feeling."

Therapeutic changes were observed to sustain for weeks, months, or longer (Pahnke et al., 1970; Terrill, 1962; Unger, 1963) and were often associated with the "self-transcending" qualities of the experience (Pahnke et al., 1970), later conceptualized as "peak," "transpersonal," or "mystical" experiences (from here on referred to collectively as *peak experiences*). These peak experiences were argued to allow individuals to obtain a significant shift in perspective on themselves, with strong personal meaningfulness, motivating a change in behaviour accordingly (Kurland, Unger, Shaffer, & Savage, 1967). The general consensus arose that it was not the drug that is therapeutic, but specific *experiences* that the drug *can* facilitate (Hoffer, 1965).

However, the experiences psychedelics can facilitate show marked variety across patients and sessions, and naturally have begged the question to researchers and therapists of *how* certain desirable experiences can be more reliably facilitated. In the course of the 1960s, increased awareness emerged of the influence that nondrug variables have on determining the types of experiences patients undergo (i.e., variables other than the drug, such as the mindset of the individual, the social atmosphere, the music and the physical environment) (Fox, 1967; Grof, 1980; Pahnke et al., 1970; Unger, 1963). This is now commonly referred to as the importance of "set and setting," or more generally speaking, "context" (Carhart-Harris et al., 2018), in which *set* refers to the mindset of the individual, including personality, mood, expectations and intentions (i.e., all nondrug variables internal to the individual), whereas *setting* refers to environment in which the drug is taken, including all its interpersonal and sensory qualities (i.e., all nondrug variables external to the individual).

The increased emotional responsiveness under the drug to nondrug variables was increasingly recognized not as an unwanted side effect but as central mechanism of the drug to be utilized for therapeutic objectives. This was attempted by tailoring the design of the setting, such as the environment and the music being played, in such way that these variables became central elements to the therapeutic procedures. By the late 1960s, the foundation of psychedelic therapy was characterized by a strong client-centered approach, including redesigning hospital environments and adapting music and interpersonal support to the highly dynamic individual process of the patient (Fox, 1967; Van Rhijn, 1960).

▤ Motivations for the Use of Music in Psychedelic Therapy

In increased efforts to optimize psychotherapeutic support for patients via the design of setting variables, a striking consistency appeared in the use of music and the emphasis on its "profound significance" (Bonny & Pahnke, 1972; Butterworth, 1962; Hoffer, 1965). Music quickly became a consistent feature during sessions, and first guidelines were developed by Bonny and Pahnke (1972) on the use of music. Sessions were (and remain to the present day) characterized by the patient wearing an eye mask, with music being delivered through headphones. Typically, during psychedelic therapy sessions, music is the most prominent, if not the only, external stimulus present during the peak of the psychedelic therapy sessions.

The prominence of music on the one hand, and the increasing numbers of novel studies and therapists being trained to practice psychedelic therapy on the other, illustrate the growing need for an empirically informed use of music in psychedelic therapy. In what follows, I discuss the key motivations for music use that converge from both historic and contemporary psychedelic therapy research. In summary, these motivations include using music (1) to facilitate peak experiences, (2) to facilitate emotional release, (3) to evoke autobiographical processing and mental imagery, and (4) to provide reassurance (Bonny & Pahnke, 1972; Grof, 1980).

Using Music to Facilitate Peak Experiences

In the 1950s and 1960s, researchers observed that patients who show the strongest improvements often experience feelings of "wonder" and a sense of "transcending" their usual sense of self. Unger (1963) stated, "Nearly invariably, whenever dramatic personality change has been noted following the use of these drugs, it has been associated with this kind of experience, that is one called transcendental or visionary." And Terrill (1962) noted, "When therapeutic changes did occur, they were often of a qualitatively different order than those which occur in traditional psychotherapy. Under the influence of LSD, the individual goes through highly intense and unusual experiences which may very well change the way in which he views life."

A growing body of evidence from modern studies confirms that peak experiences during psychedelic therapy correlate with positive therapy outcomes for a range of psychiatric conditions (Garcia-Romeu, Griffiths, & Johnson, 2014; Griffiths et al., 2008, 2016; Ross et al., 2016). One original motivation to introduce music in psychedelic therapy was to help facilitate peak experiences (Bonny & Pahnke, 1972; Hoffer, 1965; Pahnke et al., 1970; Richards, 2015), and recent research findings provide preliminary support for this. Studies indicate that music-evoked emotions of "wonder" and "transcendence" are enhanced under LSD compared to placebo (Kaelen et al., 2015, 2017). Furthermore, a clinical trial using psilocybin and music to treat depression showed that from the diverse range of subjective experiences patients reported (ranging from increased emotionality and audiovisual effects to anxiety and cognitive struggle), the music experience selectively correlated with peak experiences (feelings of union, bliss, and spirituality) (Kaelen et al. 2018).

Using Music to Facilitate Emotional Release

Initially, researchers viewed music primarily as an "aid in relaxation," but soon they realized that music could support the therapy sessions in different ways, including the promotion of access and the release of therapeutically significant emotionality (Eisner & Cohen, 1958). The uses of music in psychedelic therapy to modulate emotionality are well described by Holzinger (1964), who stated that the patient's ability "to regain fully his emotional expressive abilities" under LSD, "negatively, and especially, positively" is one of the most important therapeutic mechanisms within LSD-assisted psychotherapy. Holzinger continued to describe the main role of music as being "to enhance this ability of the patient to express his feelings."

In psychedelic therapy, patients frequently experience emotional release and typically describe this as an important contribution to their positive therapy outcomes (Belser et al., 2017; Gasser et al., 2014; Watts, Day, Krzanowski, Nutt, & Carhart-Harris, 2017), and population studies relate emotional "breakthrough" experiences under psychedelics, with improvements in well-being (Roseman et al., 2019). Studies indicate that music-evoked emotion is significantly enhanced under psychedelics, and that music plays a significant role in facilitating personally and therapeutically meaningful emotionality within sessions (Kaelen et al., 2018). The following interview excerpts with patients illustrate this point well:

> "Under the influence of psilocybin, [the music] absolutely takes over. Normally when I hear a piece of sad music, or happy music, I respond through choice, but under psilocybin I felt almost that I had no choice but to go with the music."
>
> "And I did feel like [the music] opened up to grief, and I just was very happy for that to happen. It wasn't particularly pleasant in any way, but extraordinarily powerful."

Using Music to Evoke Autobiographical Processing and Mental Imagery

Early researchers reported that LSD has "the astonishing quality" to reactivate patients' "repressed emotional attitudes" (Feld et al., 1958), and that is not uncommon for patients to experience vivid autobiographical reliving (Eisner & Cohen, 1958). One important motivation to introduce music in psychedelic therapy was to promote a "deeper involvement" with these autobiographical processes (Bonny & Pahnke, 1972; Grof, 1980). The combination of psychedelics and music is shown to modulate neural circuitry specialized in mental imagery and personal memory, and is correlated with enhanced vividness of mental imagery and autobiographical memories (Kaelen et al., 2016). Preller and colleagues (2017) demonstrated that meaningfulness perceived in music is enhanced under LSD. In clinical work, the music experience during psychedelic therapy sessions correlates with "insightfulness," a factor that includes loadings from items capturing the experience of vivid personal memories (Kaelen et al., 2018).

Using Music to Provide Reassurance

The experiences that psychedelics facilitate can be extraordinarily profound and may last up to 8 hours (depending on the specific medicine being used), and are dynamic, unpredictable, and, not uncommonly, psychologically challenging at times. Hence, one of the earliest motivations for the use of music was to provide a positive supportive climate in which the individual can feel safe to drop psychological defenses and engage proactively and openly with the unfolding experience. For a significant majority of patients, music has been found helpful in facilitating calm and safety, often including the sensation of music being a source of "support" and "reassurance" (Kaelen et al., 2018). These reassuring effects of music were found to be particularly appreciated in situations in which apprehensions were present, not only prior to the onset of drug effects, but also when reduced arousal and more "mental space" was desired, for example, after emotionally intense periods. The music providing a sense of calm, security, and guidance may form a critical contrasting function to the previously described evocative (i.e., emotionally intensifying) influences of music. The use of music to reduce anxiety and provide comfort has found wide empirical support and utility in a range of other clinical contexts (Finch & Moscovitch, 2016; Mondanaro et al., 2017; Pavlov et al., 2017).

■ Therapeutic Mechanisms of Psychedelics and Music

Important clues as to how psychedelics and music interact therapeutically are emerging gradually from modern clinical research, although significantly more research is needed in this field. My aim in this section is to consolidate these findings into a theoretical framework, integrating neuroscience and psychotherapeutic theory.

The Mind Functions Like a Roadmap

A fundamental objective of the human brain is to maintain homeostasis (i.e., balance), and to acquire learned representations (i.e., predictions) that guide this objective effectively and efficiently (Seth & Friston, 2016). Throughout life, learned representations are assembled into an increasingly complex, hierarchical, inner working model that functions (to introduce a simplifying analogy) like an *inner roadmap*: The acquired representations determine how information is processed, what it means, inform behavior, and produce a sense of self or identity (Apps & Tsakiris, 2014; Carhart-Harris & Friston, 2010). The roadmap functions to provide direction and structure in a highly complex and always-changing world.

Therapy Aims to Update the Roadmap

Yet this experientially derived inner roadmap can also become a source of psychological suffering that individuals attempt to change when seeking help in psychotherapy (Beck, 2020; Young, Klosko, & Weishaar, 2006). Subsequently, it is a goal of all psychotherapies "to influence the client in such a way" (Yapko, 2001), so that new aspects of oneself and new ways of experiencing oneself are discovered and reassembled into an updated self-concept (Beck, 2020; Joyce & Sills, 2014; Rogers, 1966; Young et al., 2006).

Psychedelics (Temporarily) Dissolve the Roadmap

Psychedelics work by temporarily disorganizing the brain's usual functional hierarchy (Carhart-Harris, Erritzoe, et al., 2012; Carhart-Harris, Leech, et al., 2012; Carhart-Harris et al., 2016; Muthukumaraswamy et al., 2013), such that the way information is usually processed and regulated is significantly more flexible (Tagliazucchi, Carhart-Harris, Leech, Nutt, & Chialvo, 2014; Tagliazucchi et al., 2016). In line with many earlier researchers (Busch & Johnson, 1950; Butterworth, 1962; Eisner & Cohen, 1958; Feld et al., 1958; Hoffer, 1965; Pahnke et al., 1970), these modern findings suggest that a central therapeutic function of psychedelic medicine is to provide a relinquishment of emotional control, so that subjective experience can be more freely explored and more fully experienced.

Music Provides Direction in the Absence of the Roadmap

The enhanced mental flexibility and emotional lability that is characteristic of the psychedelic state is considered unspecific (Grof, 1980); that is, psychedelics can facilitate a wide spectrum of subjective experiences, and not all experiences are therapeutic. In the absence of the usually solid meaning-making capacities of the brain, music in this context plays a role in providing direction within the psychedelic experience. Patients often describe the music as a source of "direction and continuity" and as providing "a journey" and a sense of "traveling," as in the following examples (from Kaelen et al., 2018):

> "It felt like the music picked you up and carried you to the next part, and the next piece, and it was the vehicle that moved you."

> "It was like a rollercoaster, you move with the music."

> "I feel the music in large part drove a lot of the experience."

> "The music took you to the places you needed to be."

Music Provides "Experience as Medicine"

Deeply feeling and expressing emotions is argued to be important for psychotherapeutic change (Whelton, 2004), and this aim is central to many (experiential) psychotherapeutic models (Greenberg & Pascual-Leone, 2006). Some research indicates that the patient's level of experiencing emotions (i.e., its "depth") during therapy sessions is predictive for positive therapy outcomes (Greenberg, Korman, & Paivio, 2002; Hendricks, 2002; Orlinsky, Ronnestadm, & Willutzki, 2004). Similarly, in psychedelic therapy, an open attitude toward expressing challenging emotions has frequently been described as important in finding therapeutic resolution, and "openness" to the music-evoked experience, independently of its valence, correlated with reductions in depression after psychedelic therapy (Kaelen et al., 2018).

Compared with other psychotherapy modalities, psychedelic therapy is unique in its capacity to facilitate rapid and sustained therapeutic changes (Bogenschutz et al., 2015; Carhart-Harris et al., 2016; Gasser, Kirchner, & Passie, 2015; Griffiths et al., 2016; Grob et al., 2011; Johnson Garcia-Romeu, Cosimano, & Griffiths, 2014; Johnson, Garcia-Romeu, & Griffiths, 2016; Ross et al., 2016). The promise of psychedelic therapy may be due to its focus on providing a deeply felt and personally meaningful *experience,* in contrast to a focus on changing cognition, behavior, or neurochemistry. This is significant because *learning through experiencing* (i.e., implicit learning) is the foundation for behavior change; it is a core mechanism that brains evolved to adapt themselves in response to the world.

Psychedelics may work therapeutically primarily by engendering implicit learning experiences. Music in this context plays the important role of steering the implicit learning experience into directions that are most psychotherapeutically meaningful: to facilitate reaccessing or newly experiencing internal resources that are therapeutically significant in that moment for the individual, yet difficult to access within the boundaries of the usual self (e.g., directly and deeply experiencing self-worth, existential meaning, absence of drug craving). Subsequently, newly acquired self-representations can be assembled into an updated roadmap, or, as the pioneering humanistic psychologist Carl Rogers (1996) formulated, an *altered self-concept*:

> To perceive a new aspect of oneself is the first step toward changing the concept of oneself. The new element is, in an understanding atmosphere, owned and assimilated into a now altered self-concept. This is the basis, in my estimation, of the behaviour changes that come about as a result of psychotherapy, Once the self-concept changes, the behavior changes to match the freshly perceived self.

▣ Music Is a Form of Nonverbal Communication

There are indeed means other than music to provide direction and implicit learning experiences. The unique value of music in this context, however, is likely due to its nonverbal nature. This significance can be illustrated by the term *affect attunement,* coined by psychologist Daniel N. Stern, which refers to the matching of the caregiver's nonverbal expressions (the changes in intensity and tonality of his or her voice), with the infant's behavior. Affect attunement does not imply the provision of a perfect mirror-image of the infant's experience, but the provision of a reflection in a different modality (i.e., typically sound) of the dynamic contours of the infant's internal feeling states (Stern 1995, 1998).

Stern argued that the very first interpersonal world of human experience, that of the infant interacting with his or her mother, is in essence *a musical relationship.* According to Stern "for the infant, the music comes before the lyrics" and "the entire flow of maternal social behaviors can be likened to a symphony, in which the musical elements are her changing facial expressions, vocalizations, movements, and touches" (Stern, 2010). Affect attunement is believed to guide the awareness of the infant toward the subjective basis underlying his or her own behavior, while maintaining a sense of being securely held and "contained" by the caregiver. Mother–infant affect attunement through musical use of voice is present cross-culturally (Trehub & Trainor, 1998), and is argued to promote emotional learning (Licata, Kristen, & Sodian, 2016; Schore & Schore, 2007; Thompson, 1991).

In psychedelic therapy, the therapeutic actions of music may resemble the process of mother–infant affect attunement. Here, music can be seen as a nonverbal (or even preverbal) language that can provide an attunement to dynamic internal feeling states of the listener, thereby facilitating emotional learning experiences, while simultaneously providing a sense of being securely held and supported. By dramatically enhancing the usual subjective response to music, psychedelics may create a unique therapeutic opportunity for the music to become deeply experiential (i.e., the listener becomes fully *immersed* in the music).

Nonverbal musical language is predominantly process-oriented and abstract, as opposed to being content-oriented and concrete (e.g., movies). This may be particularly significant, as music can thereby reflect and activate intrinsic dynamic feeling states, while allowing the specific autobiographically meaningful content to be spontaneously associated with the music by the mind of the listener. As classical composer Richard Wagner eloquently formulated:

> What music expresses, is eternal, infinite and ideal: it does not express the passion, love, or longing of such-and-such an individual on such-and-such an occasion, but passion, love or longing in *itself,* and this it presents in that unlimited variety of motivations, which is the exclusive and particular characteristic of music, foreign and inexpressible to any other language. (quoted in Storr, 1997)

◼ The Use of Music in Psychedelic Therapy

The main function of music in psychedelic therapy can be conceptualized as providing a source of nonverbal direction, in which the patient can become so deeply *immersed* that the experience unfolds as a "journey" rich with therapeutically meaningful thoughts, emotionality, and imagery, and an important source for implicit learning experiences. For the psychedelic listener, songs become worlds, and this profoundness of the music experience, together with the highly personal and dynamic nature of the psychedelic therapy session, illustrates the importance of therapists, facilitators, and researchers to choose music thoughtfully and on a client-centered basis. Although controlled experiments on the use of music in psychedelic therapy are scarce, observations from clinical work provide insight in key criteria for using music effectively, ethically, and responsibly (Bonny & Pahnke, 1970; Grof, 1980; Kaelen et al., 2018). These criteria include (1) the type of direction provided by the music, (2) adaptation to the session's phase, (3) adaptation to the personal process, (4) understanding the role of silence, (5) preparation of an open mindset, and, finally (6) technical specification for the music delivery.

The Type of Direction

When music is viewed as a source of nonverbal direction, two different and antagonistic categories of therapeutic functions of music can be formulated, according to the degree of direction they provide:

- *Soothing music* ("the sonic blanket"). This function is primarily concerned with providing a soothing, calm, peaceful, safe, and reassuring climate. Soothing music is not emotionally or physiologically activating, it provides a musical ambience that does not strongly demand attention, and it allows the listener to explore various aspects of him- or herself and the experience freely. The degree of direction is low to medium, and is always calming.
- *Deepening music* ("the sonic microscope"). This music intensifies certain subjective experiences. It functions to bring feelings, psychological processes, and memories more strongly into awareness, and for them to be more fully experienced and expressed. Deepening music can be of any emotional valence, and the degree of direction is always medium to high.

Adaptation to the Session's Phase

The music selection for a typical psychedelic therapy session follows the medicine's pharmacodynamics and psychological effects according to a set of five different phases. The duration of each of these phases is dependent on the type of psychedelic medicine and the dosage provided:

1. *Preonset:* Before any effects of the medicine are noticed. Music selection: Soothing.
2. *Onset:* First effects are noticed, building gradually towards peak intensity. Music selection: Combination of soothing and deepening, with positive valence.
3. *Peak:* Effects are felt most strongly. Music selection: Alternate between soothing and deepening functions, matching to the patient's personal process, valence and needs.
4. *Descent:* Effects gradually decline. Music selection: Alternate between soothing and deepening functions, matching to the patient's personal process, valence and needs.
5. *Return:* Effects of the medicine are wearing off, and the patient gradually returns to normal waking consciousness. Music selection: Primarily soothing, or deepening with positive valence, matching to the patient's personal process.

Adaptation to the Personal Process

Hoffer (1965) noted that music can "be very helpful," but that music and other nondrug variables factors "must be looked upon as aids and not as objectives of the experience," and that the music should always be tailored to every patient's unique needs: "Some subjects find music intolerable and visual aids repulsive, and their wishes and feelings must be honoured. They find music extremely distracting and it prevents them from fully experiencing other components of the reaction."

Similarly, strong rejection of or "resistance" to the music is not uncommonly observed during modern clinical trials. In this context, resistance is defined by an attempt to psychologically distance oneself from the music and its influences. Typically, resistance can be recognized by the patient intellectualizing the experience, and/or by feelings of discomfort, irritation and anxiety, and/or a by general sense of the experience being diminished or blocked by the music. This experience can be seen as the opposite of the often-reported music-evoked sense of being on a journey (characterized by dispensing with intellectualization).

Resistance should not be merely understood as an inability of the patient to "be open" but as something much more complex that can occur for a variety of reasons. In fact, it is the therapist's responsibility to understand that resistance occurs for a reason, to uncover this reason, and to respond appropriately. Three different types of *musical resistance* may be defined:

- *Type 1.* The music may be dissonant with the patient's internal experience and therapeutic needs. The music is out of tune with the subjective experience, it is a mismatch, and is experienced as a disruption. Examples (from Kaelen et al., 2018): "I can remember thinking 'this is beautiful music, why am I going to this dark place?' It didn't line up with what had gone on before, you know, that pattern. I just felt as if I was being manipulated, being duped almost"; "I was very aware of the influence of the music, which I found at times intrusive. . . . The music was discordant."
- *Type 2.* The music may be disliked because of a lack of personal connection with

its genre or finding the music aesthetically abrasive. Examples: "I found the first [play-list] a bit of synthetic"; "The piano pieces irritated me; it was like little needles"; "I did struggle with the Brahms and the Bach . . . which I felt were terribly contrived."

• *Type 3.* The music may evoke images, thoughts, or feelings that are challenging and overwhelming, yet the experience may hold therapeutic significance. Examples (from Kaelen et al., 2018): "I didn't like the emotional music in the first experience because I didn't want to cry"; "My response to the music was one of fear, I guess, in part, because I viewed part of the music as this really sombre, serious, negative, cynical way of thinking, like it was my funeral, or like something really profound was about to happen, or death. And it was the music that was informing that feeling."

Each of these three situations requires a different intervention.

• *Intervention for musical resistance type 1 ("therapy as a dialogue").* When resistance arises during a session, a combination of dialogue with the patient and therapeutic intuition can determine the appropriate insight into the situation and response. When the music is dissonant with the patient's subjective state, this is may be the most straightforward scenario, in which the therapist has the responsibility to match the present feeling states and therapeutic needs with music (i.e., optimize affect attunement). Analogous to usual client-centered verbal dialogues in psychotherapy, in which the therapist listens attentively and reflects back to the patient his or her observations in a dynamic and interactive fashion, so do therapists in psychedelic therapy have the responsibility to ensure that music is adequately "attuned" to the patient's dynamically unfolding experience and psychotherapeutic needs.

• *Intervention for musical resistance type 2 ("therapy as a collaboration").* When the music is rejected due to dislike of the music style or qualities, the patient may be encouraged to listen to the music "with new ears," beyond liking or disliking, to redirect the focus on the immediately present imagery, thoughts, and feelings the music is evoking,

which could hold therapeutic significance. The music may also be adapted in order to (1) respect the listener's aesthetics and (2) prevent conflicting patient–therapist power dynamics and promote interpersonal therapeutic alliance.

• *Intervention for musical resistance type 3 ("therapy as an exploration").* When experiences of resistance occur in relation to challenging but therapeutically meaningful psychological material, a constructive relationship with the experience can be increased via client-centered reassurance and encouragement to explore the experience interactively and curiously. In practice, breathing methods, physical contact, and encouragement for emotional release, are often used in these situations.

The Role of Silence

Despite the significance of music in psychedelic therapy, it would be a serious mistake to conclude that all psychedelic therapy sessions should be completely filled with music. Music must be viewed as a therapeutic tool, and like all therapeutic tools, its usage must be informed by insights into when to use and not use the tool. As much as some music can be healing, other music can also be harmful—especially in such a vulnerable state as patients may find themselves in during psychedelic therapy sessions.

Therefore, in addition to deciding between the types of direction given with the music (soothing vs. deepening), therapists must also always ask themselves if it is appropriate to provide (strong) direction in the very first place and whether music is the best means to do so in the given context. The absence of music, at times, may be the strongest therapeutic intervention one can give: Not playing music equals the absence of stimulation and changing of the subjective experience. Although patients may also experience the absence of music as a diminishing of the experience, patients, not uncommonly, describe silence in between songs as important "pit stops" and "breaks on the journey." Silence also provides a heightened opportunity for meaningful therapist-patient interaction and dialogue, and silence may form a critical desensitizing contrast with the periods in which music is played again—making the new music more "freshly" experienced. In previously designed music programs, silence in between songs typically ranges from 1 to 30 seconds, but with longer silent periods of of approximately 1–15 minutes every 20–60 minutes of the session. When working with silence, it is important to brief your patient clearly before the session that there will be periods of silence. If this is not done, the absence of music may be confusing and disruptive to the therapeutic experience.

Preparing for an Open Attitude to the Music

An attitude of openness to the music-evoked experience correlates with positive therapy outcomes (Kaelen et al., 2018) and this mindset must be optimized via adequate preparation prior to the therapy session. This preparation of mindset may in fact determine a significant proportion of the therapeutic experience of music during the session itself. The use of music listening exercises prior to therapy sessions is not explored in current clinical practice, but it may be an effective way to prepare the patient's mindset for the experience. This includes practicing deep listening with eyes closed (fully focused listening) to various styles of music, encouraging full *immersion* into the music (fully experiencing all sensations it evokes), and encouraging curious and proactive engagement with the internal experience, beyond liking or disliking the music. In addition, such exercises can also help therapists gain deeper insight into the musical language and preferences of the individual patient, hence optimizing the music selection, and strengthen the therapeutic alliance.

Music Delivery

The first step in correct music delivery is controlling for the acoustical qualities of the therapy room. Sound-absorbing materials are preferred in the room, on the floors and on the walls, in order to reduce echo and an "acoustical coldness" of the room. Sound pollution of any form, whether it originates from low-quality sound formats, technologies in the room, or human activities inside or outside the room, must be avoided at all costs (e.g., walking, talking, whispering,

doors closing, fiddling with objects, squeaking chairs, paperwork, ventilators). These sounds are "anti-immersive" by definition, as they remind the patient of the room, the session, and, in general, the context of the experience, and move the patient away from the journey inside. Sound pollution can significantly diminish the therapeutic opportunities within the experience, and may at worst induce significant distractions, anxiety, and thought confusion.

In order to enhance the therapeutic influence of music, sound systems, headphones, as well as the music file formats, need to be of sufficiently high quality/fidelity and be positioned specifically in the room. A combination of headphones and speakers may be preferred (both playing the same signal simultaneously), in order to maximize the patient's comfort and agency, to ensure experiential continuity in the event when headphones are taken off, for the music to be felt physically (listening with the body, and not just through the ears), and for the therapist to be able to hear the music simultaneously with the patient (and thereby deepen insight into the patient's process). Speakers need to be positioned such that the "spread" of the sound minimizes localization of the music source within the room (and, hence, awareness of the room). For example, when stereo speakers are used, they need to be positioned equally to the left and the right in front of the listener, and at a sufficient distance (not too close). Volume of the music needs to be loud for deepening music, but never uncomfortably loud; that is, music needs to fill the auditory perception of the listener such that the richness, details, and dynamics of the music can be fully experienced. Soothing music, in particular, when it is ambient music and during pre-onset and return, may at times be played at low volume.

Music needs to be prepared and organized ahead of sessions, and music selection during sessions must never distract the therapists from the relationship with the patient. Ideally, a sufficiently diverse set of playlists of approximately 20 to 60 minutes' duration each, is designed ahead of the session, approximating 15–30 hours of music available in total per session, with easy to interpret labels/tags attached to them to guide selection decisions. Commonly, psychedelic therapists recommend avoidance of familiar music to (1) prevent distractions during the session because of unknown or unwanted associations of the music and to (2) prevent self-selection of familiar music to be used as a potential defense mechanism. There may be an unassessed and unacknowledge significant role for familiar personal music during psychedelic therapy sessions, and a trained music therapist may work with the patient to select the personal music ahead of the session and ensure that boundaries for its selection (when to play the personal music) are clearly communicated. Music programs and digital tools to assist therapists in their music selection, as well as music specifically researched and composed for psychedelic therapy sessions by professional musicians, are available on my websites, *www.mendelkaelen.com* and *www.wavepaths.com*.

Conclusion

Historical and modern research findings suggest that psychedelics and music interact on subjective experience to provide a unique opportunity for experiential learning and psychotherapeutic change. Motivations for music use include (1) support of peak experiences, (2) facilitation of emotional release, (3) promotion of autobiographical processing, and (4) provision of reassurance. A theoretical framework has been outlined in which psychedelics are described as functioning to dissolve the usual psychological control mechanisms, thereby facilitating substantial intensification of the subjective experience of the music. Music here has been suggested to provide an important source of nonverbal direction, including two main types of direction: soothing and deepening.

Effective and ethical use of music has been explained as a mixed function of (1) the type of direction, (2) the phase of the experience, (3) the personal process of the patient, (4) an open attitude toward the music, (5) usage of silence, and (6) technical delivery. The musical experience, in turn, has been argued to act most therapeutically when the patient can fully experientially be immersed in the music, and when openly and interactively engaged with this experience. Music can then facilitate personally meaningful experiences through which new self-concepts can be acquired and integrated as the basis for sustained positive therapeutic changes.

Music is viewed as a powerful therapeutic tool that is part of a wider therapeutic constellation, including the patient–therapist relationship, the room design, and the preparation and integration of the experience. Music influences the therapy's outcomes significantly, and acknowledging the significance of music and the need for further researching the use of music is essential to develop psychedelic therapies empirically, ethically, and effectively. More specifically, significantly more research is needed to assess the influence of different types of musical compositions and acoustic qualities on subjective experience (see, e.g., Barrett et al., 2017), and ways to optimize music selection, as well as ways music can be used to help prepare and integrate psychedelic therapy experiences.

References

Abramson, H. A. (1956). Lysergic acid diethylamide (LSD-25): Xxii. Effect on transference. *Journal of Psychology, 42*(1), 51–98.

Apps, M. A. J., & Tsakiris, M. (2014). The free-energy self: A predictive coding account of self-recognition. *Neuroscience and Biobehavioral Reviews, 41,* 85–97.

Barrett, F. S., Robbins, H., Smooke, D., Brown, J. L., & Griffiths, R. R. (2017). Qualitative and quantitative features of music reported to support peak mystical experiences during psychedelic therapy sessions. *Frontiers in Psychology, 8,* 1238.

Beck, J. S. (2020). *Cognitive behavior therapy: Basics and beyond* (3rd ed.). New York: Guilford Press.

Belser, A. B., Agin-Liebes, G., Swift, T. C., Terrana, S., Devenot, N., Friedman, H. L., et al. (2017). Patient experiences of psilocybin-assisted psychotherapy: An interpretative phenomenological analysis. *Journal of Humanist Psychology, 57,* 354–388.

Bibikov, S. (1978). *A Stone Age orchestra.* New York: Harper & Row.

Bogenschutz, M. P., Forcehimes, A. A. Pommy, J. A., Wilcox, C. E., Barbosa, P. C. R., & Strassman, R. J. (2015). Psilocybin-assisted treatment for alcohol dependence: A proof-of-concept study. *Journal of Psychopharmacology, 29*(3), 289–299.

Bonny, H. L., & Pahnke, W. N. (1972). The use

of music in psychedelic (LSD) psychotherapy. *Journal of Music Therapy, 9*, 64–87.

Busch, A. K., & Johnson, W. C. (1950). L.S.D. 25 as an aid in psychotherapy: Preliminary report of a new drug. *Diseases of the Nervous System, 11*(8), 241–243.

Butterworth, A. T. (1962). Some aspects of an office practice utilizing LSD 25. *Psychiatric Quarterly, 36*, 734–753.

Carhart-Harris, R. L., Bolstridge, M., Day, C. M. J., Rucker, J., Watts, R., Erritzoe, D. E., et al. (2018). Psilocybin with psychological support for treatment-resistant depression: Six-month follow-up. *Psychopharmacology, 235*, 399–408.

Carhart-Harris, R. L., Bolstridge, M., Rucker, J., Day, C. M. J., Erritzoe, D., Kaelen, M., et al. (2016). Psilocybin with psychological support for treatment-resistant depression: An open-label feasibility study. *Lancet Psychiatry, 3*(7), 619–627.

Carhart-Harris, R. L., Erritzoe, D., Williams, T., Stone, J. M., Reed, L. J., Colasanti, A., et al. (2012). Neural correlates of the psychedelic state as determined by fMRI studies with psilocybin. *Proceedings of the National Academy of Sciences of the USA, 109*(6), 2138–2143.

Carhart-Harris, R. L., & Friston, K. J. (2010). The default-mode, ego-functions and free-energy: A neurobiological account of Freudian ideas. *Brain, 133*(4), 1265–1283.

Carhart-Harris, R. L., Leech, R., Williams, T. M. Erritzoe, D., Abbasi, N., Bargiotas, T., et al. (2012). Implications for psychedelic-assisted psychotherapy: Functional magnetic resonance imaging study with psilocybin. *British Journal of Psychiatry, 200*(3), 238–244.

Conard, N. J., Malina, M., & Münzel, S. C. (2009). New flutes document the earliest musical tradition in southwestern Germany. *Nature, 460*, 737–740.

d'Errico, F., Henshilwood, C., Lawson, G., Vanhaeren, M., Tillier, A.-M., Soressi, M., et al., 2003. Archaeological evidence for the emergence of language, symbolism, and music: An alternative multidisciplinary perspective. *Journal of World Prehistory, 17*(1), 1–70.

Dobkin de Rios, M. (2009). *The psychedelic journey of Marlene Dobkin de Rios: 45 years with Shamans, Ayahuasqueros, and Ethnobotanists*. Rochester, VT: Park Street Press.

Eisner, B. G., & Cohen, S. (1958). Psychotherapy with lysergic acid diethylamide. *Journal of Nervous and Mental Disease, 127*(6), 528–539.

Feld, M., Goodman, J., & Guido, J. (1958). Clinical and laboratory observations on LSD-25. *Journal of Nervous and Mental Disease, 126*(2), 176–183.

Finch, K., & Moscovitch, D. A. (2016). Imagery-based interventions for music performance anxiety: An integrative review. *Medical Problems of Performing Artists, 31*(4), 222–231.

Fox, R. P. (1967). A physician's guide to LSD. *GP, 35*(6), 95–100.

Garcia-Romeu, A., Griffiths, R., & Johnson, M. W. (20140. Psilocybin-occasioned mystical experiences in the treatment of tobacco addiction. *Current Drug Abuse Reviews, 7*(3), 157–164.

Gasser, P., Holstein, D., Michel, Y., Doblin, R., Yazar-Klosinski, B., Passie, T., et al. (2014). Safety and efficacy of lysergic acid diethylamide-assisted psychotherapy for anxiety associated with life-threatening diseases. *Journal of Nervous and Mental Disease, 202*(7), 513–520.

Gasser, P., Kirchner, K., & Passie, T. (2015). LSD-assisted psychotherapy for anxiety associated with a life-threatening disease: A qualitative study of acute and sustained subjective effects. *Journal of Psychopharmacology, 29*(1), 57–68.

Greenberg, L. S., Korman, L. M., & Paivio, S. C. 2002. Emotions in humanistic psychotherapy. In D. J. Cain & J. Seeman (Eds.), *Humanistic psychotherapies: Handbook of research and practice* (pp. 499–530). Washington, DC: American Psychological Association.

Greenberg, L. S., & Pascual-Leone, A. (2006). Emotion in psychotherapy: A practice-friendly research review. *Journal of Clinical Psychology, 62*(5), 611–630.

Griffiths, R. R., Johnson, M. W., Carducci, M. A., Umbricht, A., Richards, W. A., Richards, B. D., et al. (2016). Psilocybin produces substantial and sustained decreases in depression and anxiety in patients with life-threatening cancer: A randomized double-blind trial. *Journal of Psychopharmacology, 30*, 1181–1197.

Griffiths, R. R., Richards, W. A., Johnson, M. W., McCann, U. D., & Jesse, R. (2008). Mystical-type experiences occasioned by psilocybin mediate the attribution of personal meaning and spiritual significance 14 months later. *Journal of Psychopharmacology, 22*, 621–632.

Grinspoon, L., & Bakalar, J. B. (1981). *Psychedelic drugs reconsidered* (rev. ed.). New York: Basic Books.

Grob, C. S., Danforth, A. L., Chopra, G. S., Hagerty, M., McKay, C. R., Halberstadt, A. L., et al. (2011). Pilot study of psilocybin treatment for anxiety in patients with advanced-stage cancer. *Archives of General Psychiatry, 68*, 71–78.

Grof, S. (1980). *LSD psychotherapy*. Santa Cruz, CA: MAPS.

Hendricks, M. N. (2002). Focussing-oriented/experiential psychotherapy. In D. J. Cain & J. Seeman (Eds.), *Humanistic psychotherapies: Handbook of research and practice* (pp. 221–251). Washington, DC: American Psychological Association.

Hofmann, A. (1980). *LSD: My problem child.* Santa Cruz, CA: MAPS.

Hoffer, A. (1965). D-lysergic acid diethylamide (LSD): A review of its present status. *Clinical Pharmacology and Therapeutics, 6*(2), 183–255.

Holzinger, R. (1964). LSD-25: A tool in psychotherapy. *Journal of General Psychology, 71,* 9–20.

Johnson, M. W., Garcia-Romeu, A., Cosimano, M. P., & Griffiths, R. (2014). Pilot study of the 5-HT2AR agonist psilocybin in the treatment of tobacco addiction. *Journal of Psychopharmacology, 28*(11), 983–992.

Johnson, M. W., Garcia-Romeu, A., & Griffiths, R. (2016). Long-term follow-up of psilocybin-facilitated smoking cessation. *American Journal of Drug and Alcohol Abuse, 43*(1), 55–60.

Joyce, P., & Sills, C. (2014). *Skills in Gestalt counselling and psychotherapy* (3rd ed.). Thousand Oaks, CA: SAGE.

Kaelen, M., Barrett, F. S., Roseman, L., Lorenz, R., Family, N., Bolstridge, M., et al. (2015). LSD enhances the emotional response to music. *Psychopharmacology, 232*(19), 3607–3614.

Kaelen, M., Roseman, L., Kahan, J., Santos-Ribeiro, A., Orban, C., Lorenz, R., et al. (2016). LSD modulates music-induced imagery via changes in parahippocampal connectivity. *European Neuropsychopharmacology, 26,* 1099–1109.

Kaelen, M., Giribaldi, B., Raine, J., Evans, L., Timmerman, C., Rodriguez, N., et al. (2018). The hidden therapist: Evidence for a central role of music in psychedelic therapy. *Psychopharmacology, 235*(2), 505–519.

Kurland, A. A., Unger, S., Shaffer, J. W., & Savage, C. (1967). Psychedelic therapy utilizing LSD in the treatment of the alcoholic patient: A preliminary report. *American Journal of Psychiatry, 123*(10), 1202–1209.

Lbova, L. V., Volkov, P. V. Kozhevnikova, D. V., & Kulakovskaya, L. V. (2013). Upper Paleolithic "sounding artifacts" from Mesin, Ukraine: Modification marks. *Archaeology, Ethnology and Anthropology of Eurasia, 41*(3), 22–32.

Licata, M., Kristen, S., & Sodian, B. (2016). Mother–child interaction as a cradle of theory of mind: The role of maternal emotional availability. *Social Development, 25*(1), 139–156.

Mithen, S. (2007). *The singing Neanderthals: The origins of music, language, mind, and body.* Cambridge, MA: Harvard University Press.

Mondanaro, J. F., Homel, P., Lonner, B., Shepp, J., Lichtensztein, M., & Loewy, J. V. (2017). Music therapy increases comfort and reduces pain in patients recovering from spine surgery. *American Journal of Orthopedics, 46*(1), E13–E22.

Muthukumaraswamy, S. D., Carhart-Harris, R. L., Moran, R. J., Brookes, M. J., Williams, T. M., Errtizoe, D., et al. (2013). Broadband cortical desynchronization underlies the human psychedelic state. *Journal of Neuroscience, 33*(38), 15171–15183.

Nettl, B. (1956). *Music in primitive culture.* Cambridge, MA: Harvard University Press.

Orlinsky, D. E., Ronnestad, M. H., & Willutzki, U. (2004). Fifty years of psychotherapy process-outcome research: Continuity and change. In M. J. Lambert (Ed.), *Bergin and Garfield's handbook of psychotherapy and behavior change* (5th ed., pp. 307–389). Chicago: Wiley.

Pahnke, W. N., Kurland, A. A., Unger, S., Savage, S., & Grof, S. (1970). The experimental use of psychedelic (LSD) psychotherapy. *Journal of the American Medical Association, 212*(11), 1856–1863.

Patel, A. D. (2003). Language, music, syntax and the brain. *Nature Neuroscience, 6*(7), 674–681.

Pavlov, A., Kameg, K., Cline, T. W., Chiapetta, L., Stark, S., & Mitchell, A. M. (2017). Music therapy as a nonpharmacological intervention for anxiety in patients with a thought disorder. *Issues in Mental Health Nursing, 38*(3), 285–288.

Richards, W. A. (2015). *Sacred knowledge: Psychedelics and religious experiences.* New York: Columbia University Press.

Rogers, C. (1966). *Client-centered therapy.* Washington, DC: American Psychological Association.

Rogers, C. R. (1996). *Way of being.* Boston: Houghton Mifflin.

Roseman, L., Haijen, E., Idialu-Ikato, K., Kaelen, M., Watts, R., & Carhart-Harris, R. (2019). Emotional breakthrough and psychedelics: Validation of the Emotional Breakthrough Inventory. *Journal of Psychopharmacology, 33*(9), 1076–1087.

Ross, S., Bossis, A., Guss, J., Agin-Liebes, G., Malone, T., Cohen, B., et al. (2016). Rapid and sustained symptom reduction following psilocybin treatment for anxiety and depression in patients with life-threatening cancer: A randomized controlled trial. *Journal of Psychopharmacology, 30,* 1165–1180.

Schore, J. R., & Schore, A. N. (2007). Modern attachment theory: The central role of affect regulation in development and treatment. *Clinical Social Work Journal, 36*(1), 9–20.

Schultes, R. E., Hofmann, A., & Ratsch, C. (2001). *Plants of the gods: Their sacred, healing, and hallucinogenic powers* (2nd ed.). Rochester, VT: Healing Arts Press.

Seth, A. K., & Friston, K. J. (2016). Active interoceptive inference and the emotional brain. *Philosophical Transactions of the Royal Society of London. Series B, Biological Sciences, 371.*

Stern, D. N. (1995). *The motherhood constellation: A unified view of parent–infant psychotherapy.* London: Karnac Books.

Stern, D. N. (1998). *The interpersonal world of the infant: A view from psychoanalysis and developmental psychology.* London: Karnac Books.

Stern, D. N. (2010). *Forms of vitality: Exploring dynamic experience in psychology, the arts, psychotherapy, and development.* Oxford, UK: Oxford University Press.

Storr, A. (1997). *Music and the mind.* New York: HarperCollins.

Tagliazucchi, E., Carhart-Harris, R., Leech, R., Nutt, D., & Chialvo, D. R. (2014). Enhanced repertoire of brain dynamical states during the psychedelic experience. *Human Brain Mapping, 35*(11), 5442–5456.

Tagliazucchi, E., Roseman, L., Kaelen, M., Orban, C., Muthukumaraswamy, S. D., Murphy, K., et al. (2016). Increased global functional connectivity correlates with LSD-induced ego dissolution. *Current Biology, 26*(8), 1043–1050.

Terrill, J. (1962). The nature of the LSD experience. *Journal of Nervous and Mental Disease, 135*(5), 425–439.

Thompson, R. A. (1991). Emotional regulation and emotional development. *Educational Psychology Review, 3*(4), 269–307.

Trehub, S. E., & Trainor, L. J. (1998). Singing to infants: Lullabies and play songs. *Advances in Infancy Research, 12,* 43–77.

Unger, S. M. L. (1963). Mescaline, LSD, psilocybin, and personality change: A review. *Psychiatry, 26*(2), 111–125.

Van Rhijn, C. H. (1960). Symbolic presentation. In H. A. Abramson (Ed.), *The use of LSD in psychotherapy* (pp. 151–197). New York: Josiah Macy, Jr. Foundation.

Watts, R., Day, C., Krzanowski, J., Nutt, D., & Carhart-Harris, R. (2017). Patients' accounts of increased "connectedness" and "acceptance" after psilocybin for treatment-resistant depression. *Journal of Humanistic Psychology, 57*(5), 520–564.

Whelton, W. J. (2004). Emotional processes in psychotherapy: Evidence across therapeutic modalities. *Clinical Psychology and Psychotherapy, 11*(1), 58–71.

Yapko, M. D. (2001). *Treating depression with hypnosis: integrating cognitive-behavioral and strategic approaches.* Philadelphia: Routledge.

Young, J. E., Klosko, J. S., & Weishaar, M. E. (2006). *Schema therapy: A practitioner's guide.* New York: Guilford Press.

CHAPTER 20

The Role of the Guide in Psychedelic-Assisted Treatment

MARY COSIMANO

▪ Introduction

The objective in this chapter is to discuss the role of a guide sitting with people during psychedelic-assisted sessions in the Johns Hopkins University Psychedelic Research Program. We address screening and preparation of volunteers, and the nature of the clinical support provided to research study participants before, during, and after psychedelic sessions. This process emphasizes the establishment of trust and rapport with the study team, and familiarity with the research setting and research procedures.

The material that follows is based on my experience as a primary guide in the Johns Hopkins psilocybin studies. It incorporates case material and practical approaches to help guide volunteers safely through what are often challenging, high-dose psilocybin sessions. I have worked as a guide for 20 years, and the approach to facilitating psychedelic experiences presented in this chapter represents my work over that time and the conclusion I have drawn regarding a number of important factors that make this work effective.

Research at Johns Hopkins has primarily involved psilocybin. Nevertheless, the con-
ceptual and technical approach described here applies more generally to other classic hallucinogens, such as lysergic acid diethylamide (LSD), and it draws on research and clinical work from the 1950s through current studies (e.g., Blewett & Chwelos, 1959; Grof, 1980; Leary et al., 1963, 1964). This chapter is a distillation of my understanding of the therapeutic process and doesn't necessarily represent the thinking of my colleagues at the Johns Hopkins University (JHU) Center for Psychedelic and Consciousness Research.

A psychedelic session has the potential to have an important and often profoundly positive effect on an individual's life. Carefully designed and conducted research has shown, for example, that psilocybin not only can significantly diminish depression and anxiety (Carhart-Harris et al., 2018; Griffiths et al., 2016; Grob et al., 2011; Ross et al., 2016), but it may also induce experiences that have a personally meaningful, spiritually significant, and enduring effect on people who have no overt psychological disorder (Griffiths et al., 2006, 2008). Although psychedelics have this potential, it is important that they be used in a carefully structured session conducted by a skilled and experienced guide, often referred to as a *sitter* or *monitor* (Griffiths et al., 2008; Johnson et al., 2008).

This chapter addresses the fundamentals of the process of preparing people for psychedelic sessions, guiding them through the psychedelic experience, and subsequently integrating that experience into their daily lives. The situations that can arise in one of these sessions are as varied and idiosyncratic as the individuals who go through them, and it is impossible to address comprehensively the different contingencies that may arise. The more sessions I have guided, the more I realize that we have no idea what an individual participant's experience will be. This reflects the uniqueness and beauty of these substances. Nevertheless, this chapter deals with a number of important basic considerations that are consistently applicable. The interested reader may want to explore the subject in more depth, and other resources are available in both older (Blewett & Chwelos, 1959; Leary et al., 1964) and more recent manuals (Mithoefer, 2017).

▓ Screening

Determining whether a person is a candidate for psychedelic treatment, and establishing an atmosphere of trust, begins with careful and detailed telephone screening. It is important to identify people who are unlikely to qualify at an early stage in the process, and toward that end, it is necessary to obtain a good deal of information from potential participants, while also answering volunteers' myriad questions regarding the nature, objectives, and procedures of the research protocol. The time taken up by screening varies as a function of the study population, and it can be emotionally challenging. But while obtaining information to ensure the safe and appropriate selection of participants is a major aim of screening, the entire process—beginning with the screening—is conducted in such a way as to maximize trust in the study, and in the research team. The use of psilocybin at this time is limited to approved clinical trials, and therefore this discussion of screening should be understood as reflecting the process of screening appropriate research participants.

Should the use of psilocybin be approved by the U.S. Food and Drug Administration, the protocol may differ in certain details.

The Johns Hopkins studies of people with cancer and depression or anxiety illustrate some of the complexities of screening. In this line of research, for example, study participants have a diagnosis of cancer, and their illness is often considered terminal. Screening of study volunteers involves in-depth discussion of the history of the cancer, including treatments, medications, and side effects, as well as a thorough review of other medical, psychiatric, and family history. There are frequently multiple follow-up calls to give or obtain more details, after preliminary information is reviewed with the study team. A similar thorough approach, although with a different focus, is likewise true of the Johns Hopkins study of psilocybin and depression.

After telephone screening, candidates who appear to meet the inclusion–exclusion criteria and are still interested are invited for an in-house screening. This is an intense, 1- or 2-day process involving medical and psychiatric interviews, physical examination, electrocardiogram (EKG) and blood draws, completion of questionnaires, and interviews with members of the study team.

While there is little risk of physical harm and negligible likelihood of psychological or physical dependence, there may be concerns regarding possible psychological risks involved with these compounds. The use of psychedelics is not appropriate for everyone, and it is essential that volunteers fully understand what is involved. Some potential volunteers, after screening, were uncertain whether the use of psychedelics was something they wanted. In the JHU cancer study, for example, two candidates thought to have a terminal illness were concerned that participation might be too emotionally draining. One decided that she was not up to the experience, as it was more than she wanted to delve into during the last months of her life. The other, although he did not call back for over a month, said that after much thought he was now ready, and that he appreciated having been given the space to make a decision.

After volunteers have been determined to meet the inclusion and exclusion criteria, decide to participate, and give informed consent, they are enrolled in the study and assigned two guides, who will be with them throughout the study. These guides will be present with the participant during all preparatory meetings, psilocybin sessions, and follow-up integration meetings. Although volunteers' most intense relationships are with the guides, the entire study team is a part of their experience. Building trust and rapport is one of the most important contributors to a safe experience, and the more familiar volunteers become with all study personnel, the better they are able to trust the whole process. Once a participant is enrolled in the study, a therapeutic alliance has been established, and the guides begin their journey with the participant.

■ Preparation for a Psychedelic Session

Set and Setting

All participants in the Johns Hopkins psilocybin research studies undergo 6–8 hours of preparation prior to their psilocybin session, with three primary objectives: deveolping trust and rapport with the guides, education regarding session logistics, and psychological preparedness for one or more high-dose psilocybin sessions. Some of these issues are addressed in a paper by Johnson and colleagues (2008). The aim is to begin establishing the set and setting, which are key in laying the groundwork for the best possible outcome (Cohen, 1960; Leary et al., 1963). *Set* refers to a participant's internal mental state, beliefs, and expectations, while the *setting* is the external environment. It is important that psychedelics are used in an environment that feels safe and supportive to the participant.

In the JHU research studies, this preparation is identical for those assigned to the psilocybin condition, and those assigned to a placebo or low dose. This helps preserve the blinded assignment and prepares volunteers for possible placebo sessions, the potential value of which is greater if they are taken seriously. It also reduces the likelihood of a frustrating experience associated with assignment to placebo. This applies to the guide as well. It took a while before I realized that what appeared to be placebo sessions were often difficult. I worried that the

participant would be disappointed, bored, and/or would not have a meaningful experience. Eventually I realized that I wasn't accepting the session for what it was, and therefore began to work consciously to shift that mindset. Now I recognize that however a session presents itself is exactly what it is supposed to be, and it can be an opportunity for growth and meaning.

Especially for individuals who are naive in relation to psychedelics, it is important that they receive an orientation regarding what to expect. Discussion of the possible time and tempo of onset, for example, should make clear that there is no single way that a psilocybin session unfolds, although there are some general guidelines. The onset may be gradual and extended, but on some occasions, it may go very deep, very quickly. Neither is preferable, and both are welcome, interesting, and perfectly safe.

Preparatory meetings always begin with the mention that there has been a wide range of experiences among volunteers over the years, and that these may or may not happen to any given individual, but it is helpful for participants to hear as many scenarios as possible. Just hearing about these scenarios—whether they happen or not—is helpful, and volunteers often later report that they remembered something said by a guide in these preparatory meetings that helped them let go of their fear and go deeper into the experience.

Perceptually, even familiar sights, sounds, and other sensory phenomena may be experienced very differently. Volunteers may experience things in ways that differ considerably from one another, and each individual may experience things quite differently from one session to the next, or across time within a single session. Colors, textures, and music may undergo subtle or striking changes, or they may appear at times entirely unaffected. The perception of time, and of one's body and the environment, may change in striking ways. A sense that time has slowed markedly or disappeared, or become meaningless, may be very strong. It sometimes feels to a volunteer that what is happening will go on forever. In any case, one's attention to the present, to what is happening in the moment, helps one to navigate these alterations in the sense of time. Everything changes in the course of a session, and preoccupation with the passage of time, or with how much time remains in the session, can distract a volunteer from the therapeutic process that is occurring.

Discuss the Logistics of the Psilocybin Session

A discussion of logistics addresses the practical aspects of what participants should expect during the psilocybin session. Much of this material is addressed by Johnson and colleagues (2008). This includes information about what to eat for breakfast (low-fat meal), foods and medications to avoid before and after the session, arrival time, what to wear (comfortable clothes), what to bring (pictures and/or other personally meaningful objects, if desired), note taking, fire alarms, and blood pressure guidelines. We let participants know that we will take their cell phone and shoes—for their safety, and to facilitate the surrendering of control and letting go of the outside world. This also makes it less likely that an individual will attempt to leave the study site prematurely. I sometimes say that this is "so you can't run away," which always brings a laugh and a lightness to the meeting, but there is a truth to it, too, that goes unsaid. Safety medications are located in a locked box in the room, and a physician is always within 5 minutes of the session room in case of emergency.

Participants are told that they will spend the session reclining on a sofa, wearing eyeshades and headphones, and listening to a 6½ hour playlist of music selected specifically for a high-dose psilocybin session. During the preparatory session, they are asked to put on eyeshades and headphones, lie on the sofa, and listen to a track from the playlist. Having done this, it is a familiar experience at the time of the psilocybin session. In one case, this opportunity to practice activated a memory of a truamatic experience from years previously, and a volunteer removed the eyeshades and headphones and sat up immediately after lying on the sofa. I asked her to take the eyeshades home with her, and she bought a set of headphones so she could practice and become comfortable with the therapeutic position. At the subsequent prepatory meeting, she was much more relaxed,

and she was completely comfortable on the day of the psilocybin session.

Preparatory meetings also help familiarize volunteers with the room, and with the location of the private bathroom. After one participant got "lost" in the bathroom, we realized we needed tighter control for their safety, as it is easy for volunteers to get disoriented or lose track of time. We removed the lock from the door, asked them to keep the door open about an inch, and we check on them (calling their name) every minute or so to make sure they are OK. Apart from trips to the bathroom, volunteers are asked to remain reclining throughout the session, although they can move around quite a bit on the sofa, as described below. Some volunteers wanted to dance or do yoga, but our session room is small, and getting up and moving around could present a safety issue. In any case, it is preferable for volunteers to maintain an internal focus. Given this information ahead of time helps to minimize the likelihood of problems during a session.

Volunteers are told that although it is very unlikely, there have been rare occasions on which a participant experiences a loss of bladder control while fully relaxed. They are told that the sofa is covered with flannel sheets, with a waterproof pad underneath. Should incontinence occur, a participant can change into scrubs that are available in the room, and they can bring their own extra clothes to a session should they prefer. On the few occasions when volunteers lost bladder control, they were prepared for the possibility, found it acceptable, and were not embarrassed.

Intention

Intentions are implicit in our studies, with a specific objective or indication (e.g., smoking cessation, cancer-related anxiety or depression, major depressive disorder), and are integral to the experience. Exploration of a volunteer's intention is an essential part of the preparatory meetings. It can facilitate focus and problem solving, and lead to a more therapeutic outcome. However, it may have little influence on the direction taken by the session, and it is important to go wherever the process leads. This often means that the individual should let go of the intention once the session is underway. In our smoking study, for example, we spend the preparatory meetings on the intention to quit smoking, but on the day of the psilocybin session, the guidance is to let go of attempts to direct the session, and go into the experience with an openness to whatever arises.

In a recent study, Haijen and colleagues (2018) found that having an intention is frequently beneficial. The authors noted that "regarding different intentions to have a psychedelic experience . . . 'spiritual connection' measured at baseline was positively associated with Warwick–Edinburgh Mental Well-Being Scale scores at baseline, meaning that individuals who intended to have a psychedelic experience to connect with nature, to have a spiritual experience and/or for therapeutic purposes had overall higher well-being scores at each time-point of measurement."

Whether a participant has a specific (quit smoking, decrease depression) or general (universal love, the will of the universe) intention, it is best to go into the session as just another day, and accept whatever comes up in the moment, as though one has the belief that what is happening is exactly what is supposed to happen. This attitude minimizes the importance of any expectations and makes a positive outcome more likely.

The intention of the guide is equally as important as the intention of the participant. Having a clear intention and being mindful of it determines what one choose to share or not share with the participant. If intentions have not been clairfied, it can be easy to lose focus on the needs of the volunteer. In *Seat of the Soul,* Gary Zukav (1989) states:

> What you share is not as important as why you share it. For example, sharing with the intention to impress people with your generosity, intelligence, or good nature is not the same as sharing with the intention to support another with no strings attached, or sharing because sharing with *love* is healing and natural to us, or consciously sharing with love your presence with others. Your intention for sharing determines the consequences of your sharing and your experiences of sharing.

If the guide's intention is to be present with love, to give one's full attention and listen long enough, the volunteers will open up and have the courage to be vulnerable. When that happens, one will almost always find that at some point one's perception has shifted, and any judgments one had toward them falls away. It has been said that we should listen until we fall in love. This seems to be the case more often than not with our volunteers.

Preparation for Possible Fear and Anxiety

Changes in how one perceives one's own body, or the bodies of others, are common. Sometimes these can be associated with anxiety, or with a fear that something is wrong, medically or otherwise, and informing participants ahead of time of the possibility that this can happen may help them to deal with challenging experiences that come up during the session. These experiences can include, for example, a conviction that one is sick or injured, going crazy, melting, exploding, becoming fragmented, or even dying. Depersonalization, derealization, and paranoia sometimes occur. Paranoia is one of most difficult situations with which a guide might deal, and although there are cerain guidelines, it is important to take special care and be mindful of each case individually. This is always true, but especially with a volunteer with paranoia. Some volunteers may find it helpful to talk a lot, while others prefer to remain quiet. For the guide, knowing when to be somewhat distant and when to be closer is important. This aspect of preparation can feel emotionally heavy at times, and it is helpful for the guides to find ways to lighten it up. Humor can be useful but should not be used in a way that diminishes or avoids the seriousness of the process.

At times, one's perception of self, others, and the world may be painful or frightening, but again, the guide may simply reassure a participant that she or he is OK, and encourage attention to the interesting images and emotions that are present. Many times, these can be beautiful, joyful, and compelling, and one may even feel that one is in the presence of higher beings or ultimate reality. Whether the experience is frightening and painful or pleasant and joyous, volunteers are likely to achieve the most benefit if they are neither attached nor repelled, but rather stay with and accept whatever is happening.

The intellect is rarely helpful in dealing with the emerging material, and cognitive attempts to understand what is happening may be confusing and anxiety-arousing. Participants will need to let go of their expectations, judgments, explanations, and criticisms, and they are advised that it is best to give the intellect a day off, to let go of the thinking mind and its attempts to analyze or direct the experience.

Conversation between Volunteer and Guides during a Session

A psychedelic experience is largely nonverbal and is often described as being *ineffable* (e.g., Richards, 2015). This term was used by William James, who specified four "marks" of mystical experience, the first of which is *ineffability* (James, 1901/1958). By this he meant that "it defies expression, that no adequate report of its contents can be given in words." Hence, psychedelic-assisted therapy is not a verbal process, and as a rule, more than a minimal amount of verbalization can be unproductive, or even counterproductive. Therefore, participants are told in preparatory sessions that conversation is discouraged, and that they should keep their attention focused inward. Talk is likely to be distracting, misleading, and even confusing. The guides may check in with the volunteer on occasion to see how things are going, but this should not be an invitation to engage in a conversation. In fact, if it is experienced by the volunteer as something that would disrupt the inner process, there is no need to speak, and the guides will check back later.

Volunteers are enouraged to talk only if going through a difficult period in the process. On these occasions, as the participant is told beforehand, the only way the guides can know what is happening is if the participant tells them. Psilocybin does not facilitate mind reading, and the guides also need to keep in mind that if they are not sure what a participant is experiencing, it is important to ask rather than to guess. At these times, the aim is not to discuss or try to understand what is happening, but rather to provide emotional support with the process. Frequently, simply acknowledging to the guide and oneself that one is anxious or afraid is sufficient to allow a person to move through the fear and become immersed in the experience. If that is not sufficient, holding the guide's hand and/or repeating a word or mantra often helps.

Nevertheless, there are times when talking seems necessary to move through certain experiences, and the volunteer may need to talk, or be talked to, continuously. The volunteer's need for reassurance that he or she (or the guides) is still "here" is often critical to feeling of safety. This tends to happen in the beginning of a session, and as the volunteer feels safer and relaxes, the anxiety subsides and the volunteer quiets him- or herself, usually rather quickly, although the anxiety sometimes persists for a while.

On one occasion, a participant continued to talk for over an hour despite my and my co-guide's occasional reminders to try to remain quiet and internally focused. Eventually, we realized that talking was important for her, and we let her continue. At the end of the day, she thanked us for letting her talk (she had been aware of our desire that she stop), and she said, "Sometimes you have to tell your story to transcend your story." That was an important lesson for the guides, who need to be mindful of the fact that there are always exceptions to the general "rules."

It is not uncommon for participants to become distracted by trying to decide whether they have let go of their ego. They may say they are not letting go of their ego because they are aware of their surroundings and of themselves. They think ego dissolution means that they are not supposed to be aware of their "self" at all. This frequently happens even when they are experiencing profound states of love and connectedness. From what I have observed over the years, ego dissolution does not mean that one is unaware of the surroundings, of where one is, or of oneself. It may be more accurate to say that at such times, one is a witness to one's experience, but not attached to it.

American writer Ken Wilber said that the objective of spirituality is transcendence of one's ego, not its demolition or repression. Or, as one participant wrote, "Throughout all of this I felt as if my self, my ego, floated: drifted on top of these experiences and I sensed that self and ego are meant to be witness, to bear witness to the glittering, shimmering cathedral of beauty."

Transference and Countertransference

It is helpful to make clear to volunteers that they may at times experience the guides as threatening, malevolent, withholding, angry, demanding, sad, or any other frightening or disturbing attitude. In psychedelic-assisted treatment, it is OK for the volunteer to have any of these transferential reactions, but dwelling on them or acting on them is generally not helpful, and it may be counterproductive. Transference states often arise, but as with other phenomena, the basic approach is to acknowledge them and let them go. Participants might be told in the preparation sessions that if they think a guide harbors strong feelings of some kind toward them, it is useful simply to ask about it. The guides are there for the benefit of the volunteers, and the guides can take care of themselves.

Openness to and Acceptance of the Experience

An essential aspect of preparatory sessions is to prepare a person for the potential effects of psilocybin. This helps to ensure that the individual's mental set will be conducive to a productive session. Gaining volunteers' trust and establishing rapport is accomplished by having them share their life experiences—their joys, sorrows, disappointments—and especially their fears and anxieties. Then, if any of this very personal material comes up during the psilocybin session, they have already talked about it and are more prepared to face and move through whatever surfaces.

A meaningful psychedelic experience often requires that one give up control, fully surrendering to whatever thoughts, emotions, images, and sensations may appear. This is of primary importance, and depends on the volunteers' trust of their guides, of the study staff, and of the study itself. At Johns Hopkins, we introduce our TLO mantra as a means of facilitating this. TLO is a mnemonic intended to help people remember to "Trust, Let go, Be Open"; that is, "Trust us, trust the study design, trust yourself, trust the universe. Let go of what you think should happen, what you want to happen, of your constructs, and Be Open to whatever comes up." Openness to whatever emerges during a psilocybin session is an es-sential part of the psychedelic process. One does not need to like what arises, but it is important to accept it all and allow it to be there, accepting whatever comes up without attaching to it, whether it is difficult or joyful. A number of years after I started guiding, I realized the importance and power in shifting thinking to actually welcome whatever comes up and began incorporating this into these meetings. Everything that comes up is emerging from one's own mind, and it wants to be expressed. It might be frightening, but it cannot cause any harm, and it is most helpful when it is experienced fully in awareness.

The occurrence of a wide range of experiences is a good thing, but only if it is allowed to happen. The emotional material that emerges is frequently intense, and can be expressed in many ways: crying, laughter, groans, screaming, unusual sounds, or body movements. The movements may involve twitching, writhing, thrashing, rocking, and grimacing, among others. One volunteer gyrated as if having orgasms throughout a good deal of the session. Another was on all fours, screaming and moving her body, and afterward she told us she felt she was giving birth and being born.

At times, a psychedelic experience may go in the direction of fear, anxiety, or thoughts of going insane. In their "Handbook for the Therapeutic Use of LSD," Blewett and Chwelos (1959, p. 46) noted, "Nearly all subjects will encounter periods of pronounced anxiety and much of the therapeutic benefit of the experience depends upon learning how to work through the problem areas productive of fear." In any case, the guidelines are the same: Allow the fears, face them, and express them if it seems right, without judging them or fear of being judged. These manifestations of the psychedelic experience may feel painful, disturbing, or unpleasant, but they are not harmful, and they will pass through if they are allowed to do so.

The way one should approach this fear was described by Alan Watts (2019a) as follows:

> The rule for all terrors is head straight into them. When you are sailing in a storm, you do not let a wave hit your boat on the side, you go bow into the wave and ride it. When-

ever you meet a ghost, don't run away because the ghost will capture the substance of your fear and materialize itself out of your own substance. So then whenever confronted with a ghost, walk straight into it and it will disappear. Don't run away. Explore, feel, fear as completely as you can feel it, head straight into it.

Emotional Support and Touching

An important role for the guide is to provide emotional support when it is needed to assist participants in surrendering to difficult emotional experiences. I make it clear that the guides will be there to ensure that the volunteer is safe and provided with the reassurance that is sometimes needed to enable them to relax and go with whatever arises. I instruct them to breathe and to relax if they are afraid of what is emerging, let them know that we will remind them of this during the experience, and ask whether they have any particular words, mantras, or techniques that help them. One volunteer asked me to repeat, "Be still and know" if she found herself anxious or afraid because these words were meaningful to her and helped her relax. "Everything changes" was another thing she found helpful. It is essential that participants feel comfortable and cozy, and understand that the guides' primary goal is their comfort and safety. Here we emphasize that the only way we will know their thoughts and feelings is if they tell us. Do they want more or fewer blankets, louder or softer music? Do they want physical contact or no contact?

Sometimes simple touch can be reassuring and allow participants to go deeper and further. Physical contact may be helpful when one is feeling strong emotions—scared, sad, lonely, joyful. It is important to discuss the option of touch in the preparatory sessions, as there is considerable variation in how people may respond to it. Some people prefer not to be touched, and this should be established beforehand to avoid what might feel intrusive to them. Some people may be accepting of touch but prefer that the guides ask them first, while others would rather have the guides initiate handholding or some other physical contact. They should be told that in no case will there be any sexual touching, or touching while the participant is experiencing sexual feelings or sensations. And volunteers need to know that if at any time they want touching to stop, they can merely say "stop" (Mithoefer, 2017), or pull their hand away.

If they are amenable to touch, I familiarize them with handholding, so that during a session, it is not the first time we have held hands. Some volunteers are uncomfortable the first time in a preparation session, but by the day of the psilocybin session, they are fine with it, and may welcome it. I have found that holding the hand of a participant during the session is an honor and a privilege. The energy that is exchanged in those moments is beyond words. However, this is not something shared in the preparatory meetings because it could influence a participant to think that this is something the guide wants, in which case he or she might ask the guide to hold his or her hand in order to please the guide.

At the conclusion of the preparatory meetings, it is important to determine whether both participants and guides feel they trust each other, and have developed a sufficiently solid rapport to proceed with the session. The guide(s) should explicitly ask the volunteer whether he or she feels ready, and determine whether they themselves feel certain about going ahead. If the volunteer or a guide is not on board, it is important to postpone, or to cancel, the psychedelic session.

The Importance of Preparation

It is impossible to convey to participants who are naive to the effects of psilocybin or LSD, in any meaningful, substantive way, the nature of a psychedelic experience. Moreover, it is a very unusual person who does not experience some anxiety regarding what to expect. Thus, it is essential to ensure the psychological and physical safety of volunteers, and the usefulness of the session, by preparing participants as fully as possible.

More often than not, volunteers' mention the benefits of preparatory meetings in their written and verbal reports. And interestingly, they mentioned not only the guides but also other research team members. The volunteers' experience with the entire team contributes to establishing both the set and setting of a psilocybin session. I observed this in the first four session reports I read, and I hear it over and over again. For example, one volunteer wrote that "the beauty of it all started to feel overwhelming and I felt Roland's words [during her enrollment in the study], 'the mind plays tricks in many ways.' And I remembered our discussion about overwhelm possibly being one of the tricks."

Another volunteer's report addressed a number of the issues we discussed in preparatory meetings. When dealing with "scary" thoughts, I encourage volunteers to "stay with it, to "bring it on," and even to "welcome it," reminding them that they are always safe, and that they will always "come back" no matter how far out they go. I frequently use the boomerang as an example: No matter how far out you go, you will always come back. Boomerang! Thus, this volunteer reported that "when scary thoughts came, I stayed, tried to welcome them, said, 'bring it on' in my mind. Really wanted to go there. Always knew I would come back. Boomerang."

Finally, another volunteer described how the guide's specific suggestions during preparation came back to help her during the psilocybin experience.

> "I felt my fear around the initial intensity. I asked for support and I could hear Mary [the guide] saying the words from above the 'covers of my bed.' The words never brought me out of it, the words helped me feel safe to go deeper into it. The words were the same words she had said to me time and time again over the past three days. 'Trust, let go, release. Dive in. Ask this fear what it wants. Meet this fear.' "

■ During the Session

Once the preparatory meetings have concluded, the volunteer is ready for the psilocybin session. Again, if either the participant or the guides feel they have not developed a good rapport, then the session will not take place. Therefore, it is important to ask participants whether they feel ready, and to check in with yourself, and with the other guide, if there are two guides present. Although this is discussed in the final prepa-

ration, it is important to check again with the participant prior to the session to determine whether he or she is taking any new medications, or if there has been a change in an existing medication regimen. If there are no concerns about current health status or medications, and if the participant and guides are ready, the session can proceed.

Music in Psychedelic Sessions

Music is an important aspect of a psilocybin session. The use of music was first suggested by Al Hubbard (in Blewett & Chwelos, 1959), who maintained that the tempo, timbre, rhythm, and melody provide a sort of structure to the experience, and that emotionally evocative music might lead the process in certain directions. Most playlists consist largely of instrumental music, generally without understandable lyrics, and often largely unfamiliar to the participant. Participants may find some of the music not to their liking, but it is nevertheless there as a kind of safety net, providing emotional support. In the context of a psilocybin experience, people tend to become immersed in the music. Although there are guidelines for selection of music (we have a set playlist at Johns Hopkins), and it is widely considered to be an important part of psychedelic sessions, there is limited research on the contribution of music to outcomes (Barrett et al., 2017; Bonny & Pahnke, 1972; Johnson et al., 2008; Kaelen, Chapter 19, in this volume; Richards, 2015). The majority of our volunteers request the playlist, and once their participation in the study is complete, we can share it with them. It can be a powerful tool to bring them back into their experience at a later date.

The Role of the Guide

My approach is nondirective, much as described by Carl Rogers (1966). This means that I do not offer any direct advice or direction, instead acting with the belief that the person has the answer within, and that answer is most helpful when the participant discovers it on his or her own. The psychedelic experience itself—and not interventions on the part of the guide(s)—appears to be responsible for the healing that takes place. Hence, some prefer the term *sitter* over *guide*, as the basic approach of the sitter is not to guide the volunteer but to facilitate the volunteer's own inner exploration of whatever comes up, in a nondirective manner. This is what brings about the benefits of psilocybin or other hallucinogens, and it requires only the willingness of the participant to follow wherever the experience leads. The guide does not really *guide* the volunteer in any direction other than toward what is inside, and the guide is active primarily in helping the person to surrender when he or she has difficulty doing so. As a guide, one cannot get caught up in what one would like to have happen, or in the idea that as a guide, one can control the direction of the volunteer's experience.

When the volunteer is struggling with what is emerging, supportive encouragement to look at what is happening may be helpful, but interpretations, intellectual analysis, logic, and engaging the participant in conversation typically are not, and may even interfere with the psychedelic process. The "answers" come from within, and often it is the mere presence of the guide that enables volunteers to look within themselves despite the fear. As one participant reported after a psilocybin session, "Had it not been for the two experienced researchers in the room, I probably would have had a full-blown panic attack and lost the larger experience."

Guides must develop the ability to be present with the participant no matter what the nature of the session. I have been at the side of participants literally the entire day, and on other days not at all—and everything in between. It may seem that the days when one is fully engaged with the participant that one's role as guide has been more meaningful or helpful. This is not the case. The guide's presence and attention is just as valuable during the sessions when there is little or no interaction. Our participants have told us that just knowing we were there allowed them to feel safe and go deeper. Sometimes on those days it can be more challenging for the guide to stay focused, but it is important to cultivate the ability to be present at those times as well.

I have found that starting the day with some form of exercise and a good breakfast can greatly assist with the ability to stay fo-

cused and be present as a guide. When I first started guiding, I had a hard time sitting for extended periods of time—I wanted to move around and/or be fed. I began taking a walk and eating a large bowl of oatmeal the morning of session days.

Much of what the guide does is to help out with the participant's basic needs. This includes tasks such as ensuring that the volunteer is comfortable with the room temperature and providing a warm blanket; having drinking water close at hand; providing tissues or an emesis bucket as needed; assisting with getting onto or off of the bed or couch, and escorting the volunteer to the bathroom. Taking care of these things while the participant is otherwise preoccupied is an important part of establishing a safe and supportive setting, and an essential aspect of the guide's role in a psychedelic session. As one volunteer noted after a psilocybin session, "My first experience today seemed to originate out of Brian [guide] covering me with the blanket. This gradually transformed into the vision and sense that Bill and Brian [guides] and I were covered by a blanket-like net that linked us together emotionally and mentally."

Transference and Countertransference in Psilocybin Sessions

If a guide is aware of a developing transferential distortion of her or his relationship with the volunteer, unless it is a serious distortion, it might be left alone, and the patient simply encouraged to stay inside and deal with what is arising. There is a tendency to see the inside world in the external reality, and encouraging the participant to work with it inside is generally best. Sometimes it is enough simply to identify what is happening, nonjudgmentally and nondefensively, and to encourage looking inward.

In turn, guides should be aware of their own emotional state, and be willing to respond simply and directly if volunteers raise questions or concerns about it. Psychedelics can increase an individual's sensitivity to interpersonal cues, and if a volunteer correctly perceives the guide's state (e.g., distance), for the guide to deny it or otherwise distort the emotional reality can be experienced as a breach of trust, significantly disrupting the setting. Simply and directly acknowledging the accuracy of the volunteer's perception may allow the individual to get back into the process in a productive way.

In one case, a research participant sensed that one of the guides seemed distant and preoccupied, which he experienced as frustrating, and as withholding on the part of the sitter. After feeling "stuck" for several minutes, and disappointed in the guide, the volunteer told the guide how he was feeling. On reflection, the guide recognized that, in fact, he was thinking about concerns in his life outside the session. He told the participant and apologized for his preoccupation, and what the volunteer was starting to experience as a "stalemate" was quickly resolved, and the sense of safety and trust was restored. There was no need for extensive discussion or justification of the guide's feelings or attitude, only a validation of the volunteer's perception of interpersonal reality.

Personal Characteristics of the Guide

In thinking about qualities that constitute a "good" guide, I thought of things like knowing all about psilocybin, the history of psychedelic research, different models of treatment, and so on. These are important, but eventually I realized it was the guide's qualities as a person that would benefit the volunteer most. I readily identified a number of essential personal characteristics. Being present and nonjudgmental are among the most important, but so, too, are many others, including awareness, compassion, empathy, respect, honesty, humility, and acceptance. Then I considered the question: Which of those do I possess? The answer is that it varies from day to day depending on my own set, and on the setting. If I just had an argument with my husband, heard of a traumatic event, or hadn't slept well the night before, how might that affect my ability to be present, non-judgmental, and compassionate?

Ethnobotanist and psychedelic researcher Terence McKenna said that he believes all our problems can be boiled down to a single issue: excessive ego. Our work is to shed the ego and come from a place of authenticity, love, connection, presence, and letting go.

I strongly believe a fundamental outcome of the use of psilocybin is for a participant to reconnect to his or her authentic self, to know onself. If that is the major positive outcome of this approach to psilocybin use, it seems that it would also be important for us as guides to be in alignment with that as well. Hence, I am convinced that a desire and willingness to work at knowing one's true, authentic self is one of the most important attributes of an effective guide. The more one knows oneself, the more the other attributes naturally become a part of oneself.

As Gary Zukav (1989) wrote, "You are a micro of a macro. Your soul is a micro of the soul of humankind. . . . You cannot change the macro without first changing the micro. . . . As you change the micro, you simultaneously change the macro of which you are part and to which you are intimately bound. This is the creation of authentic power. The transformation that you create in yourself simultaneously contributes to the transformation of humanity."

I remember sitting in a session with a volunteer who was in a very difficult situation, wondering what I could do or say that would best help the individual to get through it. I really struggled with how I could be "the savior." And then I remember thinking that I'm not the one who knows what's best for the volunteer, and that if I could just step back—get out of myself—that would be best. One needs to be aware that the goal is to minimize, consciously and continuously, the role of the ego.

If we do not know and accept ourselves—all parts of ourselves—we cannot fully accept others, and they will know that, no matter how good we think we are at masking it. As Alan Watts (2019b) said in his talk about how to accept one's dark side:

> "We cannot change anything unless we accept it. . . . If a doctor wishes to help a human being he must be able to accept him as he is and he can do this in reality only when he has already seen and accepted himself as he is. Perhaps this may sound very simple, but simple things are always the most difficult. In actual life it requires the greatest art to be simple, and so acceptance of oneself is the essence of the moral problem and the acid test of one's whole outlook on life."

The Body in Psilocybin Sessions

In contrast to most standard psychodynamic, cognitive, or behavioral approaches to psychotherapy, the body may become very involved in a psilocybin session. This can include sensations (e.g., cold, pain), distortions, or seeming loss of the body schema or body image, along with a wide range of movements. In each case, these are essentially normal expressions of the psychedelic experience, and the participant is generally encouraged to let them occur. As noted previously, many different movements may be experienced, varying in speed, force, duration, and character. They may include movements of isolated body parts (e.g., repetitive movements of a hand) or movement of the entire body. Some appear stereotyped, while others may seem to be a random series of movements of arms, legs, head, and trunk. As noted previously, they may include contractions, trembling, shaking, twitching, writhing, thrashing, rocking, kicking, thrusting, sucking, and grimacing, among others. As with other ways in which the psychedelic experience is expressed, these movements are not harmful, and they pass if they are allowed to occur.

Providing numerous examples in the preparatory meetings can be instrumental in how a participant may interpret these bodily expressions should they occur. In our dose–effect study, a participant's body twitched throughout her entire first session. She was extremely frightened that something was wrong with her physically and unable to relax throughout the entire session. Although we continued to reassure her that she was fine, she said that we had not mentioned that possibility in our preparation meetings, that we had prepared her for going crazy, dying, and meeting monsters, but not the body movements. On the day of her psilocybin session, she was sure there was a problem. She almost dropped out of the study, but after extra integration meetings, she decided to continue. Her next session began with the same body twitches, but this time she was able to relax into them, and had a complete mystical experience. This example stresses the importance of throrough preparatory meetings, as well as the value of ac-

ceptance of whatever occurs, to increase the likelihood of a meaningful experience.

Breath and Breathing and Relaxation

To achieve maximum benefit from the psilocybin sessions, and to access expansive states of consciousness, I believe it is necessary to relax in both body and mind. When stressed, anxious, or afraid, people are often in a state of sympathetic activation and feel unsafe, and they automatically hold themselves in and tense their bodies (Porges, 2007). These states of mind and postures associated with fear and anxiety make it difficult to relax, accept what one is experiencing, and expand one's consciousness. Again, set and setting are important contributors to the psychedelic process; in order to relax, a safe and trusting environment is necessary. Ideally, the preparation meetings have established a milieu of trust, facilitating participants' ability to relax and access deeper and more expansive states of consciousness.

One of the mantras I often use, "Breathe, Relax and Expand," was a result of many participants' observation of the necessity of relaxing. After his first three sessions in our dose–effect study, one participant beautifully captured this:

> "I am again acutely aware of the dramatic effects of relaxing to the drug. Each time I let my shoulders sink into the couch with an exhalation of breath or consciously soften my abdomen and leg muscles, the hallucinated space before me expands to astonishing dimensions, swept across by exquisite lights and shapes. The onset of revelatory experiences, too, seems to correspond to my success in remaining relaxed. In fact, this art of relaxation itself becomes in itself a key part of the revelation. It suddenly seems clear to me that the achievement of a trusting and receptive openness of spirit is bound up with the very essence and purpose of life. Our task in life consists precisely in letting go of fear and expectations in order to give oneself purely to the impact of the present."

Alterations of respiratory rate, depth, and character (e.g., abdominal vs. chest breathing) may serve as indices of the participant's state, and having a volunteer control his or her breath in certain ways may help change an anxious state to one that is more relaxed, in which it is easier to let go and progress through the session, managing difficult moments with greater ease, and eventually getting back a deep and intrinsic connection to what feels like a real self. It may be difficult simply to "try to relax," but the use of diaphragmatic breathing can facilitate a relaxed state. When a volunteer is struggling to let go and experience anxiety or painful emotion, it often helps if he or she focuses on respiration and "breathes into" whatever is happening.

Relaxation has long been known as a way to deal with difficult states during a psychedelic experience. This was first pointed out by Hubbard and subsequently discussed in the first manual for psychedelic psychotherapy (Blewett & Chwelos, 1959). It was also addressed in *The Psychedelic Experience: A Manual Based on* The Tibetan Book of the Dead, by Leary and colleagues (1964), from which were derived John Lennon's lyrics for the Beatles' song "Tomorrow Never Knows" on the album *Revolver*. The lyrics speak to the importance of relaxing and surrendering completely to the experience, of letting go of thoughts and judgments, and letting love flow in.

I believe that the ability to relax allows for this expansiveness and often leads to a sense of the heart opening, allowing deep feelings of love and connection for oneself and others. Both this expansiveness and the sense of love and connection are recurrent themes in psilocybin experiences.

After his psilocybin session, one research participant wrote:

"I was reveling in the undeniable feelings of infinite love. I said [to myself], 'I am love, and all I ever want to be is love.' I repeated this several times and was overwhelmed with the intensity of the love. I was aware of tears flooding my eyes at this point. All the other goals in life seemed completely stupid."

Another participant captured this in his report:

"Once I was past the darkness, I began to feel an increasing feeling of peace and connectedness. . . . I could see the faces of the people that are important to me in my life as if they were on intertwined paths with mine. As their paths intersected mine, I could feel their love and my love for them. I saw the best in each person and couldn't stop smiling. I felt like any conflicts we had were simply misunderstandings. An intense feeling of love and joy emanated from all over my body and I can't imagine feeling any happier. I knew that the worries of everyday life were meaningless and that all that mattered were my connections with the wonderful people who are my family and friends."

The breath may be used for other purposes apart from relaxation. Mithoefer, for example, suggests that some aspects of Holotropic Breathwork (Grof & Grof, 2010) might be used at appropriate times not only to produce a relaxed state but also to allow a volunteer to stay present with emotionally intense experiences.

The Value of Touch

With an understanding of the participant's attitude toward and wishes concerning supportive touching, physical contact may be a much more powerful means of providing reassurance than words. Touch should always be used cautiously and judiciously, and never in a way that might be perceived as sexual or otherwise intrusive. As Mithoefer (2017) notes:

In 3,4-methylenedioxymethamphetamine (MDMA)-assisted psychotherapy, mindful use of touch can be an important catalyst to healing during both the MDMA-assisted sessions and the follow-up therapy. Touch must always be used with a high level of attention and care, with proper preparation and communication, and with great respect for the participant's needs and vulnerabilities. Any touch that has sexual connotations or is driven by the therapist's needs, rather than the participant's, has no place in therapy and can be counter-therapeutic or even abusive. By the same token, withholding nurturing touch when it is indicated can be counter-therapeutic and, especially in therapy involving non-ordinary states of consciousness, may even be perceived by the participant as abuse by neglect. If the participant wants to touch one of the therapists, the therapist allows for and/or provides touch as long as it is appropriate and nonsexual. Nurturing touch that occurs when the participant is deeply re-connecting with times in life when they needed and did not get it can provide an important corrective experience.

Apart from providing comfort and reassurance, simply holding the volunteer's hand may be helpful in other ways, as described by two participants.

> Volunteer A: "I lay down under the covers. The guide put on the headphones and mask and I began to sink deeper and deeper into the bed. Down, down, down I went. Under the covers of my childhood. Mary held my hand and created contact. I thought the contact was there to create support so I would not get overwhelmed. While that was true some of the time, what I felt was true most of the time is that it was more necessary to help me stay in my body, while at the same time my body dissolved. Through the contact I was able to be in both worlds at the same time, hence my whole experience can be integrated and carried through me into the denser planes or reality."

> Volunteer B: "Love and compassion were key elements in the day's journey. The beginning of the movement in this direction, as I best recall, is when Mary took my hand during a particularly evocative and touching musical piece. Up until that time, I had been content to be in my own 'bubble' and had not sought out contact or initiated any communication. The simple touch of the hand was instrumental in helping to open the heart."

The Value of Photographs and Other Personal Items

Volunteers are often encouraged to bring photographs or other personally meaningful items with them to sessions. These can include items such as objects with spiritual or religious significance to the volunteer, stones, a favorite stuffed animal from childhood, artwork, picture books, or other items that may be emotionally engaging. Sometimes these provide reassurance or a sense of familiarity and safety, or they may evoke emotions that are associated with people or situations in their lives. One participant wrote that

> "looking at pictures of family and friends that I had brought with me . . . the guide (MC) showed me my wife. The minute that I started looking at the pictures my heart broke open

and I wept openly and deeply. This was deeply cathartic—while I was crying hard and while some of that was sorrow for pain that had been caused or shared, there was a deep satisfaction and joy that was known because of the love that transcended any difficulty. Said another way, the joy was inseparable from any sadness. The emotional punch that was triggered by looking at the pictures of my family and talking about them with the guides then continued as I looked at the pictures of my two meditation friends and reflected on the deep quality of those relationships."

Sometimes photographs may take an individual in an unanticipated emotional direction:

> "When I looked at photos of my family, instead of feeling pain and loss and sorrow, I felt such joy at their aliveness. In fact, even those who are dead seemed so very alive. I smiled at the photos, and laughed. It seemed that the people in the pictures were imbued with an otherworldly, sweet light. This idea, and the physical and emotional well being that resulted from it, persisted when I lay down again and was long past looking at the photos. People in my mind's eye appeared multi-dimensional, they turned in my inner space and seemed to be very happy in this freedom. They were not flat, static images, but real, dimensional beings with a will of their own. At the end of the session I told Mary and Erin [guides] that I had never smiled at some of these photos but that now I could only smile."

▪ Integration

The therapeutic use of psychedelic substances has as its goal improvement in emotional, behavioral, and/or functional status. Just as the preparatory sessions are an essential precursor to a psilocybin session, the effects of a psychedelic experience may be manifested over a period of weeks, months, or even years following the session.

This is facilitated by what is referred to as *integration*, which begins in the ending stages of a psilocybin session but continues in the days or weeks following that session. The effects of psilocybin or other psychedelics are frequently manifested for some time, and it is important to assist the volunteer to continue processing emotional issues that arose during the session that may continue to emerge. Our first meeting is the day after the psilocybin session, and each participant is asked to write a session report before meeting with us. It is important that they capture their experience without input from their guides.

Moreover, the guide(s) can use one or more integrative sessions to incorporate what has been gained through the experience into the daily life of the volunteer. During this time, the participant may undergo significant changes in his or her sense of self, emotional expression, perspective on other people and the world, and manner of relating to others. The extent to which any individual will require the guide's assistance with this process is as variable as are other aspects of the process. These meetings are the beginning of an ongoing process to make sense of the psilocybin experience. Being able to put words to their often ineffable experience is a powerful way to begin to understand it, but only with those who are familiar with the territory; otherwise, it may be dimisssed as strange or meaningless. So it is important to be mindful of the people with whom you share it.

How can we optimize the outcome of a psychedelic experience? We approach it in a way that is similar to what we recommend before someone goes into a psilocybin session; that is, an individual should live each day with the same attitude as that during a psychedelic experience: that all that happens is welcome, even what is disturbing. He or she is encouraged to ask why certain things have arisen and what can be learned from them. It does not require one to like every situation, but rather to allow and accept it. It is when we try to resist what is happening that we get into trouble. Insanity involves a failure or inability to accept what is.

In integration sessions, the guides should be prepared to help volunteers find answers to questions they may have about their experience, its meaning, and its implications. Guides also provide support and a supportive environment as volunteers work with new insights or perspectives. Interpretations of what happened, or what is happening, or what it is all about, are generally not helpful or indicated, although when it seems

clear that a volunteer is likely to resonate with such comments, they may be useful. As Mithoefer suggests, the use of such interpretations "should be minimized."

A predominantly cognitive or intellectual attitude should be discouraged in favor of a more physical or emotional means of expression. This might include activities such as meditation, physical exercise, breathing exercises, yoga, listening to or playing music, writing about the experience in a journal, and art or other creative activities. Nature is a great healer and integrator. It is often helpful to discuss one's experience with a spouse/partner, friend, family member, or other person with whom one is close, and who is likely to understand. This also may serve to consolidate the experience. Being able to talk about it can also be an effective way to bring one back to the feeling, as if in the session itself.

It is also helpful to encourage an attitude of realistic acceptance of whatever occurred, without exaggerating its significance either positively or negatively. There is a saying: "Don't make an altar at the foot of your experience." It may have felt profoundly positive and liberating, or a session may have been all dark, with no seeming benefit, with this sense continuing into the following day or even longer. After a difficult session, volunteers might be encouraged to realize "if I was able to get through that, I can get through anything." But there may be times when a partially resolved traumatic emotional memory becomes more intense or vivid, or arises more frequently than it did previously. This can nevertheless reflect real progress that might require more active effort toward integration.

Integration of the experience is sometimes enhanced if the participant does something concrete to impress it in his or her mind, to have it as a sort of touchstone to which he or she can return. For example, after his session, one of our participants got a chunk of clay and placed it on an art table in his home. When he felt moved, he would sit with it, contemplate his session, and let it take a life of its own. Although a large majority of participants in the Johns Hopkins psilocybin studies describe their experience as one of the most profound they have ever had (Griffiths et al., 2008), there are some people for whom it may become just another experience as they go back into the routine of their daily lives. The effects of the experience are sometimes subtle and, as is often the case with psychedelics, may take days, weeks, or even years to fully unfold and be incorporated. This may lead some to dismiss the effects of the experience. For example, when her doctor asked how she had been integrating her psilocybin experience a few months previously, one volunteer reported:

> "I'm not sure. . . . I've been trying to stay alert for signs of reorientation, but have only noticed what seem like minor things, for example, unusual fascination with trees and especially their trunks, greater enjoyment of the play of light on the surface of water, uncharacteristic attraction to the intricate patterns of Islamic tile and brick work in photos from a friend's recent vacation."

Her physician responded:

> "Those are all signs that your right brain is much more open. Perhaps your experience may put this into the category of 'minor things' but it does signify a deeper shift inside. If you change the course of a ship's direction by a few degrees it doesn't seem like much at first but in time you end up in a very different place. Sounds like a reorientation of your subconscious."

One of the telephone raters for another volunteer was asked to rate the volunteer's behavior at a 6-month follow-up telephone interview. He remarked that her general demeanor had shifted, and that it appreared that her "life concerns and stress seem to have diminished noticably and significantly." He said that this participant, a young single mother with a terminal diagnosis, had become much more accepting of herself and others, and "much more at ease with who she is and what's going on in her life." He added that the shift was gradual, however, and he likened it to "when you slow-cook something—you let it stew, and then it comes out delicious."

There seems to be no time limit regarding when the integration process is complete, as seen in the case of one of our volunteers,

who wrote the following to us 6 years after his initial psilocybin session, and after returning from a spiritual retreat.

> "Well, one night they lit the candles, shut off the light; this guy came in, settled down . . . and then started to laugh. His eyes were closed, but clearly whatever it was that he was experiencing was influencing him to laugh and laugh. Other meditators (certainly not me, I will say) then started to laugh as well, chuckles at first and then full-blown laughter. And they kind of laughed in unison—it was like all of them were tuning into the same thing at the same time, like a wave of experience.

> "The way they laughed was exactly the way I was laughing out loud during my session with you folks, and it was so obviously similar that I quizzed one of the monks later about what was going on and what they experienced in these sessions. They said that in that extraordinary state of spiritual consciousness everything was so beautiful that any and everything that came into the mind generated such joy that laughing was the result.

> "That was exactly what I experienced under the influence of your drugs! I was in an extraordinary place where yes, the mushroom was producing a wonderful, very colorful abstract movie that danced with the music, but at the same time, I almost certainly was in a heightened consciousness (and spiritual) state that generated the extraordinary "fun" (as I called it) in response to it all.

> "So in my case, at least, in retrospect your experiment was a grand success, something that I have just now learned, six years later."

■ Conclusion

In this chapter I have briefly addressed the most salient features of the process, but there is much that goes beyond its scope. When properly administered, psychedelics have the potential to promote significant and enduring change in individuals' behavior, mood, and other aspects of their psychological state. These substances differ from traditional psychiatric medications in that the safe and effective use of psychedelics requires considerable attention to the set and setting. It is the role of the guide (or sitter) to ensure that the participant is in a situation that will maximize the likelihood of a beneficial outcome. This requires careful preparation and disciplined, compassionate, and empathic attention to the participant and his or her needs that begins before and is sustained throughout the entire session. As the psychedelic experience is winding down, and when it has ended, it becomes important to integrate the experience into the daily life of the individual.

There is much more that I could write about guiding psychedelic sessions and how to approach them, in large part because this is precisely the work I have been involved in and have witnessed for 20 years. I believe that one of the main outcomes of the experimental psilocybin sessions at Johns Hopkins is to enable individuals to know themselves so they can reconnect to their authentic selves, to the selves they once were, or, in some cases, are only now discovering for the first time who they really are. Once they have reconnected to themselves, they can connect to others. I view the connection to ourselves, to others, and to everything as love—our true nature. Psilocybin acts as a key to open our minds and facilitate access to our true nature, to help find meaning to life. The design of the JHU studies, and the implementation of the clinical protocol, appears to help our participants accomplish just that. The role of the guide (or sitter) is instrumental in facilitating these outcomes.

One volunteer's statement sums it up simply and perfectly: "My single strongest memory will be from the first session, when I found myself chasing something that had been eluding me. When I caught it, I discovered that it was me. The subsequent embrace and rejoining seems to me to be the single most powerful event in my life. I feel whole for the first time and able to cope with anything. Apart, 'I' was weak and directionless. Listless, really. But together, I'm strong, capable of anything, and just happier."

■ References

Barrett, F. S., Robbins, H., Smooke, D., Brown, J. L., & Griffiths, R. R. (2017). Qualitative and quantitative features of music reported to support peak mystical experiences during psychedelic therapy sessions. *Frontiers in Psychology, 8*(1238), 1–12 .

Blewett, D. B., & Chwelos, N. (1959). Handbook for the therapeutic use of lysergic acid diethylamide-25: Individual and group procedures. Retrieved from *https://maps.org/research-archive/ritesofpassage/lsdhandbook.pdf*.

Bonny, H. L., & Pahnke, W. N. (1972). The use of music in psychedelic (LSD) psychotherapy. *Journal of Music Therapy, 9*, 64–87.

Carhart-Harris, R. L., Bolstridge, M., Day, C. M. J., Rucker, J., Watts, R., Erritzoe, D. E., et al. (2018). Psilocybin with psychological support for treatment-resistant depression: Six-month follow-up. *Psychopharmacology, 235*, 399–408.

Cohen, S. (1960). Lysergic acid diethylamide: Side effects and complications. *Journal or Nervous and Mental Disease, 130*, 30–40.

Griffiths, R. R., Johnson, M. W., Carducci, M. A., Umbricht, A., Richards, W. A., Richards, B. D., et al. (2016). Psilocybin produces substantial and sustained decreases in depression and anxiety in patients with life-threatening cancer: A randomized double-blind trial. *Journal of Psychopharmacology, 30*, 1181–1197.

Griffiths, R. R., Richards, W. A., Johnson, M. W., McCann, U. D., & Jesse, R. (2008). Mystical-type experiences occasioned by psilocybin mediate the attribution of personal meaning and spiritual significance 14 months later. *Journal of Psychopharmacology, 22*, 621–632.

Griffiths, R. R., Richards, W. A., McCann, U., & Jesse, R. (2006). Psilocybin can occasion mystical-type experiences having substantial and sustained personal meaning and spiritual significance. *Psychopharmacology, 187*, 268–283.

Grob, C. S., Danforth, A. L., Chopra, G. S., Hagerty, M., McKay, C. R., Halberstadt, A. L., et al. (2011). Pilot study of psilocybin treatment for anxiety in patients with advanced-stage cancer. *Archives of General Psychiatry, 68*, 71–78.

Grof, S. (1980). *LSD psychotherapy.* Pomona, CA: Hunter House.

Grof, S., & Grof, C. (2010). *Holotropic Breathwork: A new approach to self-exploration and therapy.* Albany: State University of New York Press.

Haijen, E. C. H. M., Kaelen, M., Roseman, L., Timmermann, C., Kettner, H., Russ, S., et al. (2018). Predicting responses to psychedelics: A prospective study. *Frontiers in Pharmacology, 9*, Article 897.

James, W. (1958). *The varieties of religious experience.* New York: New American Library. (Original work published 1901)

Johnson, M. W., Richards, W. A., & Griffiths, R. R. (2008). Human hallucinogen research:

Guidelines for safety. *Journal of Psychopharmacology, 22,* 603–620.

Leary, T., Litwin, G. H., & Metzner, R. (1963). Reactions to psilocybin administered in a supportive environment. *Journal of Nervous and Mental Disease, 137,* 561–573.

Leary, T., Metzner, R., & Alpert, R. (1964). *The psychedelic experience: A manual based on* The Tibetan Book of the Dead. New York: University Books.

Mithoefer, M. C. (2017). *A manual for MDMA-assisted psychotherapy in the treatment of posttraumatic stress disorder: Version 8.1.* Santa Cruz, CA: Multidisciplinary Association for Psychedelic Studies.

Porges, S. W. (2007). The polyvagal perspective. *Biological Psychiatry, 74,* 116–143.

Richards, W. A. (2015). *Sacred knowledge: Psychedelics and religious experiences.* New York: Columbia University Press.

Rogers, C. (1966). *Client-centered therapy.* Washington, DC: American Psychological Association.

Ross, S., Bossis, A., Guss, J., Agin-Liebes, G., Malone, T., Cohen, B., et al. (2016). Rapid and sustained symptom reduction following psilocybin treatment for anxiety and depression in patients with life-threatening cancer: A randomized controlled trial. *Journal of Psychopharmacology, 30,* 1165–1180.

Watts, A. (2019a, December 19). Turning the head or turning on, part 2. Retrieved September 6, 2020, from *www.alanwatts.org/3-5-9-turning-the-head-or-turning-on-part-2.*

Watts, A. (2019b). Why you must accept your evil side [Video]. YouTube. Retrieved September 6, 2020, from *www.youtube.com/watch?v=_6KKOVjY8rA.*

Zukav, G. (1989). *The seat of the soul.* New York: Fireside.

CHAPTER 21

Comparative Phenomenology and Neurobiology of Meditative and Psychedelic States of Consciousness

Implications for Psychedelic-Assisted Therapy

MILAN SCHEIDEGGER

▨ Comparative Phenomenology of Meditative and Psychedelic States of Consciousness

A variety of Buddhist traditions have independently developed meditation techniques that lead to similar measurable outcomes in terms of predictable and distinctive phenomenological states (Nash & Newberg, 2013). Many types of meditative practices (i.e., breathing, relaxation, concentration, recitations, movement) bring forward altered states of consciousness with psychospiritual significance. Ultimately, mystical-type experiences of self-transcendence may be reached when discursive thinking and subject–object duality are suspended to a degree that the subject is no longer the core organizer of experiential space. This complete dissolution of the self into a sense of unity and interconnectedness with all that exists is a core feature of mystical states commonly referred to as *samadhi, nirvana, kensho,* or *satori* in Eastern spiritual traditions. Notably, students of mysticism have often commented on the similarity of drug-induced psychedelic

experiences to transcendental states attained through advanced levels of deep meditation (Smith, 2000). Psychoactive plant medicines such as ayahuasca, peyote cactus, or psilocybe mushrooms have been traditionally used as "entheogens" by indigenous cultures to support shamanic practices and to induce altered states of consciousness in ritualistic settings (Pahnke, 1966; Schultes, 1969).

Today, drug-induced mystical experiences studied under controlled laboratory conditions provide insights into the phenomenology and neurobiology of these states. Historical references such as William James's experiments with nitrous oxide (James, 1882), Aldous Huxley's experiences with mescaline (Huxley, 1954), Walter Pahnke's (1966) "Good Friday Experiment" with psilocybin, and the work of Robert Masters and Jean Houston (2000) on LSD suggest that drug-induced mystical experiences are experientially indistinguishable from genuine mystical states. Based on previous work by Stace (1960), the phenomenological typology of mystical experiences was further refined by Pahnke into the following experiential categories: (1) sense of unity or oneness; (2) transcendence of time and space; (3) deeply felt positive mood, blessedness, peace; (4) sense of sacredness or awesomeness; (5) objectivity, reality, and intuitive knowledge (noetic quality); (6) paradoxicality; and (7) alleged ineffability, which refer to both the difficulty of grasping the experience by language and logical thinking; (8) transiency; and (9) persisting positive changes in attitude and behavior (Pahnke, 1966). Two classes of mystical states can be further distinguished: In extrovertive experiences, the mind retains habitual sensory content but the objects of perception cease to exist as separate entities from the experiential subject, which typically comes with a profound sense of oneness (i.e., nature mysticism, cosmic consciousness, psychedelic states). In introvertive experiences, consciousness is still preserved but is void of all sensory impressions and the usual sense of individuality, while other differentiated content might still be present (Stace, 1960). Deep introvertive experiences that are devoid of all subject–object dualities, differentiations, and personal psychological characteristics are commonly referred to as "pure consciousness," a transitory state of lucid awareness or pure beingness. Epistemologically, there is no subject of experience in pure consciousness that can take any critical distance toward what is perceived or known, which experientially results in an unmediated implosion of a felt sense of fundamental reality with undoubtable certitude, sometimes also referred to as the "ground of being" (Jones, 2016). This "noetic quality" in terms of an intuitive knowledge with convincing intensity is frequently encountered in mystical states. Both introvertive and extrovertive experiences are receptive and cannot be forced; they may occur spontaneously when experienced meditators surrender and let go of conscious effort. Beyond that, mystical experiences may support the cultivation of selfless awareness and enduring states of transformed consciousness that are less driven by ego-centered cognitions, emotions, desires, and attachments (Jones, 2016).

The natural occurrence of mystical experiences in religious or nonreligious contexts is rare and unpredictable, which makes them difficult to study under controlled empiri-

cal settings. However, several studies show that experiences with a striking similarity to natural occurring mystical states can be reliably induced by psychedelic substances (Barrett & Griffiths, 2017; Griffiths et al., 2018; Pahnke, 1966; Pahnke & Richards, 1966; Smigielski, Kometer, et al., 2019). Comparative phenomenological analysis of psychedelic and meditative states can deepen our understanding of how conscious experience is organized and driven by neuronal processes. However, first-person subjective self-reports are not as quantifiable as neurophysiological data, which necessitates an expanded science of consciousness embracing both first-person subjective experience and third-person neuroscience data (Varela, 1996). Such an integrative research strategy might be aided by the use of neurophenomenological methods of investigation: By examining specifiable meditative or psychedelic states on a microphenomenological level, one may be able to find neural correlates of the most basic types of coherent states of consciousness and subjective experience (Petitmengin & Lachaux, 2013). Due to their refined introspective skills, experienced meditators and trained users of psychoactive substances are expected to generate more stable and reproducible mental states, and give more accurate descriptions compared to naive subjects.

From a phenomenological perspective, altered states of consciousness support the notion that experience is not a rigid, predetermined, and circumscribed entity but rather a flexible and transformable process. Transformative experiences can be achieved by various consciousness-altering techniques such as artistic creativity, ecstasy, psychedelics, trance, meditation, and relaxation (Fischer, 1971). There is converging evidence that both psychedelics and meditation can produce significant alterations of self-experience, ranging from mildly attenuated self-boundaries to states of complete dissolution of the sense of self (Millière et al., 2018). Some drugs have been shown to stimulate parts of the brain that enable depth-mystical experiences to occur, and there may be different neural states for mystical experiences with differentiated content and those without such content. At least some drug-induced altered states (e.g., ketamine, psilocybin, or ayahuasca) share similar neuronal biosignatures as altered states reached by nonpharmacological methods (e.g., meditation): Activity and connectivity in brain regions in cortical midline areas that integrate our coherent sense of self tend to be down-regulated during expanded states of consciousness (Brewer et al., 2011; Carhart-Harris et al., 2012; Palhano-Fontes et al., 2015; Scheidegger et al., 2012). Conversely, sensory information from the periphery is less filtered, which can lead to an extrovertive sense of being united with the entire surrounding, as is the case in nature mysticism or states of cosmic consciousness.

Different phenomenological maps have been proposed to highlight the core experiential organizers of meditative and psychedelic states. In his cartography of ecstatic and meditative states (see Figure 21.1), Roland Fischer (1971) considered the varieties of experience of self-transcendence on the perception–hallucination continuum of increasing *ergotropic arousal* (e.g., creative, psychotropic, and ecstatic experiences) and along the perception–meditation continuum of increasing *trophotropic arousal* (e.g., hypoaroused meditative states). Both directions represent changes in self-referential processing in terms of mutually exclusive psychophysiological alterations of every-

day consciousness. The endpoints of this spectrum are characterized by experiential shifts into a mode of experiencing in which the phenomenal structures of self–other and subject–object are no longer the dominant mode of experience. Such states are also emphasized in non-dual-oriented practices that provide insight into the illusory nature of the subject–object dichotomy that usually structures ordinary dualistic experience.

Lutz and colleagues conceptualized mindfulness as a continuum of practices involving states and processes that can be mapped into a multidimensional phenomenological matrix that serves as a heuristic tool for mapping various styles and stages of mindfulness practice into a multidimensional space (Lutz et al., 2015). During mindfulness meditation, attention to current internal and external experiences is maintained with a nonjudgmental stance, manifesting acceptance, curiosity, and openness (Holzel et al., 2011). Decomposing mindfulness into different dimensions can be used to map multiple practice styles and levels of expertise: Experienced meditators report that they can observe mental processes with increased stability of awareness and less conscious effort, as well as increasing clarity and temporal resolution (Lutz et al., 2015). They develop skills such as meta-awareness that facilitate

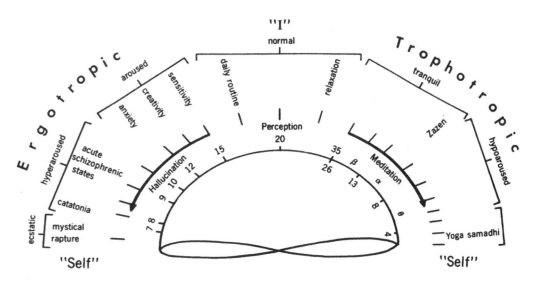

■ **FIGURE 21.1.** Varieties of conscious states mapped on a perception–hallucination continuum of increasing ergotropic arousal (left) and a perception–mediation continuum of increasing trophotropic arousal (right). From Fischer (1971). Reprinted with permission from AAAS.

a detachment from identification with the static sense of self by adopting a nonconceptual and distributed attentional perspective toward the contents of conscious experience (Holzel et al., 2011).

In order to delineate dissociable psychological and neurodynamic effects, different meditation styles such as focused attention or open awareness are most commonly distinguished in empirical studies. The aim of focused attention is to stabilize the mind from distraction by maintaining selective attention on a specific object or physiological process (e.g., breath). Conversely, open awareness promotes a receptive field of nonreactive attitude toward automatic cognitive and emotional interpretations of sensory, perceptual, and endogenous stimuli, developing the scaffolding for a form of meta-awareness (Lutz et al., 2008). Differential influences on perceptual, cognitive, attentional, affective, and self-referential processing in specific brain networks systems are involved in a usual meditation cycle of detecting physiological aspects of present-state feelings, possible distractions, changes in affective reactivity, and in the perspective on the self (Dahl, Lutz, & Davidson, 2015; Fox et al., 2016; Tang, Hölzel, & Posner, 2015; Vago & Silbersweig, 2012). A third category of meditation refers to states of non-dual awareness, which involves the recognition of a background awareness that precedes conceptualization and intention without fragmenting experience into opposing dualities of inside versus outside, self versus other, or good versus bad (Josipovic, 2014). Experientially, non-dual awareness resembles psychedelic states in which the sense of self is expanded or attenuated toward a unified field of experiencing. Accordingly, drug-induced mystical experiences may include both extrovertive and introvertive features (Millière et al., 2018). The extrovertive type usually involves a rich sensory phenomenology, including vivid hallucinations, while the introvertive type may be characterized by states of deep internal absorption and complete loss of self-consciousness into an experience of "emptiness" or "void." When awareness itself becomes the object of attention, the sense of personhood and habitual self-boundaries is attenuated, which is a core phenomenological feature of depth-mystical

experiences (Stace, 1960). In states of pure awareness, consciousness is cleared from habitual activity and sources of noise, or even completely devoid of any sensory and conceptual content, and may be presenting consciousness in its simplest form. According to anecdotal reports, some psychedelic drugs such as nitrous oxide, ketamine, or 5-methoxy-N,N-dimethyltryptamine (5-MeO-DMT), especially at high doses, have been reported to induce virtually contentless states similar to the descriptions of pure consciousness from mystical traditions or near-death/out-of-body experiences of pure light (Barsuglia et al., 2018; James, 1882; Krupitsky & Grinenko, 1997). A recently proposed multidimensional model of self-loss in global states of consciousness suggests that states of drug-induced ego dissolution may vary according to not only the extent to which narrative and multisensory aspects of self-consciousness are inhibited, but also the richness or sparsity of their phenomenology: While some forms of self-loss induced by psychedelics may involve a rich sensory phenomenology, others are more similar to descriptions of pure consciousness and may be almost devoid of sensory content (Millière et al., 2018).

Psychedelic-Induced Transformative Experiences and Mindfulness-Related Capabilities

Several studies revealed that under supportive conditions, psychedelics can induce personally meaningful and profound psychospiritual experiences, with a striking resemblance to genuine mystical states. An important historical reference to the empirical investigation of drug-induced mysticism is the so-called "Good Friday" Experiment (Pahnke, 1966). During the broadcast of a church service in the Marsh Chapel at the University of Boston, students of theology received either 30 mg of psilocybin or 200 mg of nicotinic acid (active placebo) in a double-blind study design. Psychometric assessments revealed that psilocybin subjects experienced significantly stronger mystical phenomena than controls that ranked among the most significant experiences of their lives even in the long-term follow-up (Doblin,

1991). A high degree of persisting positive changes were reported by the experimental group compared to the control group. In a replication and extension of the "Good Friday" experiment, Griffiths and colleagues found that psilocybin, when administered to healthy subjects under supportive conditions, can occasion personally meaningful and spiritually significant mystical-type experiences with sustained positive changes in attitudes, mood, and behavior (Griffiths et al., 2006, 2008, 2011). Most notably, the occurrence of mystical experiences during the psilocybin session was predictive of high ratings of spiritual significance and personal meaning in the long-term follow-up (Griffiths et al., 2008). Consistent with participant claims of hallucinogen-occasioned increases in aesthetic appreciation, imagination, and creativity, lasting increases in the personality trait of openness were found in participants who had mystical experiences during their psilocybin session (MacLean, Johnson, & Griffiths, 2011). In summary, the studies by Griffiths and colleagues show that under double-blind conditions that provided significant controls for expectancy bias, psilocybin can occasion complete mystical experiences in the majority of people studied. These effects are dose-dependent (Griffiths et al., 2011), specific to psilocybin compared to a psychoactive control substance (methylphenidate) (Griffiths et al., 2008), and have enduring impact on the moods, attitudes, and behaviors of participants (Barrett & Griffiths, 2017; Griffiths et al., 2008).

It is widely agreed that the psychological disposition and the beliefs of the subject (set) and the physical environment (setting) are important to shape the content and quality of drug-induced experiences. In a standard hospital setting, fewer mystical experiences were reported after acute administration of 200 μg LSD in healthy subjects compared to psilocybin in a supportive setting (Liechti et al., 2016). The occurrence of mystical experiences may be higher in spiritually inclined participants who are already predisposed to have these experiences (Smigielski, Kometer, et al., 2019) or may be facilitated by environmental factors such as the music played during the session (Kaelen et al., 2018). Indeed, recent studies indicate enduring positive changes in psychological functioning in participants of psilocybin-assisted mindfulness practices (Griffiths et al., 2018; Smigielski, Kometer, et al., 2019). At 6 months, participants who received high doses of psilocybin in combination with meditation and spiritual practices showed large, significant positive changes on longitudinal measures of interpersonal closeness, gratitude, life meaning/purpose, forgiveness, death transcendence, daily spiritual experiences, religious faith and coping (Griffiths et al., 2018). Compared to the studies by Griffiths and colleagues designed as individual sessions, psilocybin was recently administered to experienced meditators in a group setting (Smigielski, Kometer, et al., 2019). The study successfully tested the feasibility of a mindfulness retreat combining the use of psychedelics with contemplative practice and showed that psilocybin may facilitate profound altered states of self-consciousness compared to meditation only. The 5-day retreats were held in a meditation center located in an aesthetically pleasing Swiss mountain setting, where the participants followed a structured meditative discipline known in the Zen tradition as *sesshin*. After 3 days of preparatory silent meditation, a single dose of psilocybin (315 μg/kg orally [p.o.] vs. placebo) was administered in a double-blind way on day 4, followed by meditative integration on day 5. Psilocybin-induced responses, valued equivalent to the strongest lifetime mystical experience, increased acute meditation depth and postretreat level of mindfulness, with positive changes in attitudes and behaviors reported in the 4-month follow-up evaluation (Smigielski, Kometer, et al., 2019).

The reviewed findings support the conclusions from previous studies that under supportive conditions, psilocybin may induce profound, valuable experiences that in their content seem to be phenomenologically contingent with naturally occurring mystical-type states as conceptualized by Stace and Hood (Hood, 1975). In deep mediation such experiences mostly occur unpredictably and at low rates (4–8%) (Austin, 2013; Paloutzian & Park, 2013), while at moderate to high doses, psilocybin seems to induce such positive states of self-transcendence at comparably high rates (up to ~60–70%)

(Griffiths et al., 2011; Pahnke, 1966; Studerus et al., 2012). However, the same dose may also occasion a dissolution of the ego that is associated with negative emotions, thought disturbances, or panic (~10–30%) (Griffiths et al., 2011; Studerus et al., 2012). Around one-third of participants from the study by Griffiths and colleagues (2011) experienced strong anxiety at higher dose during a psilocybin session, while anxiety scores in experienced meditators were not significantly elevated in a group retreat setting (Smigielski, Kometer, et al., 2019). As a valuable therapeutic skill, mindfulness allows for a more detached and less judgmental stance toward difficult thoughts and emotions, and might help to manage some distressing aspects of psychedelic experiences, and thereby potentially increase the safety and tolerability of psychedelic-assisted therapy. Results from meditation retreats without psychedelic drug administration suggested beneficial effects on measures of anxiety, depression, and stress, as well as measures of emotional regulation and quality of life. Changes in mindfulness, compassion, nonattachment, and acceptance are discussed as potential mechanisms of action (Khoury et al., 2017; Montero-Marin et al., 2016). Taken together, these converging observations suggest that the group retreat format may become a suitable setting for psychedelic-assisted therapy or mindfulness practice. The group setting may positively contribute to transformative experiences through the reassuring presence of others, social bonding and group cohesion. Furthermore, this is in line with the traditional ritualistic contexts in which hallucinogenic substances were used among indigenous people.

Currently, the Amazonian plant tea ayahuasca is spreading all over the world as an alternative medicine, with increasing numbers of Westerners seeking treatment in established retreat centers in South America (Tupper, 2008). Traditionally, ayahuasca is used in ritualistic settings as herbal medicine for curative and religious purposes by indigenous and mestizo people (Labate, Cavnar, & Gearin, 2016; Schultes, 1969). In Brazil, syncretic religious traditions such as Santo Daime, União do Vegetal, and Barquinha evolved around the sacramental ingestion of ayahuasca, incorporating Christian, animistic, and shamanistic practices and belief systems (Labate, 2016). Interestingly, a recent study with the main psychoactive ingredient of ayahuasca, *N,N*-dimethyltryptamine (DMT), revealed striking phenomenological similarities between the DMT state and near-death-experiences, including the subjective feeling of transcending one's body and entering an alternative realm, perceiving and communicating with sentient "entities" and themes related to death and dying (Timmermann et al., 2018). This potentially explains why ayahuasca plays a central role as "entheogen" to support shamanic trance states in indigenous rituals, or why it is popularized for psychospiritual development in neoshamanic contexts. It has also been shown that the therapeutic effects of ayahuasca relate to its ability to enhance mindfulness capacities such as the ability for "decentering" and reduced inner reactivity or judgmental processing of experiences. These changes are comparable to outcomes of conventional mindfulness trainings without drug administration (Soler et al., 2016). Compared to a standard 8-week mindfulness-based stress reduction (MBSR) course, four weekly ayahuasca sessions were found to increase acceptance capacities, even without the specific goal of improving these skills (Soler et al., 2018). Another observational study assessed subacute and long-term effects of ayahuasca in a ceremonial setting and found changes in affect, satisfaction with life, and mindfulness abilities to be related to the level of ego dissolution experienced during the ceremony (Uthaug et al., 2018). In summary, these findings indicate that the acute transformative effects and intermediate outcomes of psychedelics such as psilocybin or ayahuasca are highly context-sensitive and might benefit from a mindfulness-based supportive framework.

■ Comparative Neurobiology of Psychedelic and Meditative States of Self-Transcendence

By altering brain chemistry and habitual information processing, drugs may disrupt ordinary consciousness and produce some of the necessary conditions for meditative or mystical states to occur. While the addictive potential of commonly abused drugs mostly relies on dopaminergic stimulation, which is associated with pleasurable states, ego inflation, and addictive craving, classical psychedelics preferentially activate the serotonin system, which mediates prosocial emotions, ego dissolution, and self-transcendence (Nour et al., 2016; Previc, 2009). The effects produced by classical psychedelics such as psilocybin, mescaline, LSD, and DMT are principally mediated through the serotonergic 5-HT$_{1A/2A}$ receptors (Nichols, 2016). Interestingly, the variability in 5-HT$_{1A}$ receptor density in the brain was found to be inversely correlated with scores for self-transcendence, which underscores the role of the serotonin system in mediating spiritual experiences (Borg et al., 2003).

It was recently discovered, that resting-state brain activity is organized into multiple, large-scale functional connectivity networks that enable efficient neuronal communication between different brain hubs that subserve complex mental functions (Fox et al., 2005). Serotonergic psychedelics share the common biomechanism of increased excitability of the prefrontal cortex via 5HT$_{2A}$ receptor agonism (Vollenweider & Kometer, 2010). Due to these widespread changes in neuronal excitability, both short-lived and persisting connectivity networks emerge between brain regions during the psychedelic state that normally do not show significant functional association (Petri et al., 2014; Tagliazucchi et al., 2014). The breakdown between conventional pathways of neuronal communication and the formation of novel functional associations is in line with a recent hypothesis that psychedelics lead to entropic activity within the brain (Carhart-Harris et al., 2014). During the drug-induced high-entropy state, brain activity is less constrained and allows for a larger repertoire of states that succeed in a more random fashion. The observed increase in entropy may be related to the temporary removal of some of the restrictions that are necessary for sustaining ordinary consciousness, resulting in a more flexible mental state. Phenomenologically, this slightly higher entropy state is perceived as experientially richer but not as informative as normal waking consciousness: The way meaning is attributed to things is broadened, expanding the sense of reality, including experiential novelty or even bizarreness. This higher entropy state is associated with increased cognitive flexibility, creativity, and imagination (Gallimore, 2015).

Accumulated evidence highlights common neurobiological signatures for meditative states of self-transcendence and psychedelic states of ego dissolution, in particular through modulations of activity and connectivity in the default mode network (DMN; Brewer et al., 2011; Carhart-Harris et al., 2012; Kometer et al., 2015; Palhano-Fontes et al., 2015). The DMN is a large-scale network that functionally integrates distant brain nodes and mediates a variety of self-related cognitions such as mind wandering, autobiographical memory, self-reflective thought, envisioning the future, and considering the perspective of others (Raichle, 2015). A recent review and meta-analysis of meditation neuroimaging studies found attenuation of either activity or functional connectivity in key nodes of the DMN, particularly in the medial prefrontal cortex (Brewer et al., 2011; Farb, Segal, & Anderson, 2013; Farb et al., 2007; Scheibner et al., 2017) and in the posterior cingulate cortex (Brewer et al., 2011; Brewer & Garrison, 2014; Ives-Deliperi, Solms, & Meintjes, 2011; Pagnoni, 2012; Scheibner et al., 2017) across different types of meditation, which has been interpreted as indicating diminished self-referential processing (Tang et al., 2015). Abnormalities in the DMN are linked to symptom severity in various psychiatric disorders, with adaptive changes in DMN function following effective treatments (Fox & Greicius, 2010). Accordingly, the DMN was proposed as a biomarker for monitoring the therapeutic effects of meditation (Simon & Engström, 2015).

Network modulations of cortical midline structures involved in self-referential processing may facilitate states of self-transcendence, a proposed key treatment mediator in psychedelic-assisted therapies. In support of this notion, changes in DMN activity and functional integrity were found under ayahuasca, psilocybin, and LSD (Carhart-Harris et al., 2012, 2016; Kometer et al., 2015; Palhano-Fontes et al., 2015; Speth et al., 2016). Using positron emission tomography (PET) imaging, neurometabolic changes in fronto-limbic-parieto-striatal networks, including prefrontal and DMN regions, were associated with psilocybin-induced experiences of oceanic self-boundlessness (Vollenweider & Geyer, 2001; Vollenweider et al., 1997). Recent reviews exploring the neural correlates of drug-induced ego dissolution (Millière, 2017; Millière et al., 2018) particularly highlight increased functional connectivity between the DMN and a task-positive network (Carhart-Harris et al., 2013), decreased integrity of the DMN (Carhart-Harris et al., 2016) and salience network (Lebedev et al., 2015), decreased connectivity between the parahippocampal and retrosplenial cortices (Carhart-Harris et al., 2016), increased entropic brain activity, and signaling complexity and diversity (Atasoy et al., 2017; Lebedev et al., 2016; Schartner et al., 2017). Converging evidence from functional magnetic resonance imaging (fMRI) and electrocortical studies (electroencephalographic/magnetoencephalographic [EEG/MEG]) reveals decreased activity and low-frequency oscillatory power localized to DMN areas, which may be related to a decrease in long-range neural communication between these and other brain areas, while local and basic perceptual processing is relatively preserved (Muthukumaraswamy et al., 2013). After psilocybin, oscillatory power decreases in the posterior cingulate cortex (PCC) correlated with ratings of disintegration of the self (Muthukumaraswamy et al., 2013), and reduced synchronization of low-frequency δ oscillations in the retrosplenial cortex, the parahippocampus, and the lateral orbitofrontal area, correlated with the intensity levels of spiritual experience and insightfulness (Kometer et al., 2015). Enhanced mindfulness capacities after ayahuasca intake were associated with modulations in glutamatergic neurotransmission in the posterior DMN (Sampedro et al., 2017). It was further suggested that general effects of psychedelics involve the temporary disruption of the habitual neural hierarchy, replacing the predominant top-down control of the frontal cortex with bottom-up dynamics of lower brain areas (Alonso et al., 2015; Riba et al., 2004). In conclusion, transient changes in oscillatory activity, network integrity, brain entropy, and signaling complexity seemingly drive the phenomenological characteristics of drug-induced altered states of consciousness.

Psychedelic states are characterized by blurring between self- and other-related and external versus internal information processing and hence share a phenomenological similarity with states of non-dual awareness. A study of non-dual awareness in meditators showed increased functional connectivity patterns between habitually anticorrelated intrinsic and extrinsic information processing systems such as the central precuneus and the dorsolateral prefrontal cortex that might correspond to a state of unity of awareness in which extrinsic and intrinsic experiences are increasingly synergistic rather than competing (Josipovic, 2014). Decreases in connectivity of the central precuneus to the angular gyrus were identified that may be contributing to experiences of spatial extendedness, as the two areas are together involved in integrating spatial reference frames (Josipovic, 2014). A similar pattern of increased correlation between the DMN and habitually anticorrelated networks has been observed during various other forms of meditation (Berkovich-Ohana et al., 2015; Brewer et al., 2011). Notably, increased DMN to task-positive functional connectivity networks was also found in psychosis and after psilocybin administration, which share some phenomenological similarities in terms of decreased separateness of internally and externally focused states (Carhart-Harris et al., 2013). Increasing evidence from neurobehavioral studies suggests that the effects of psychedelic drugs arise, at least in part, from their common capacity to disrupt thalamo-cortical gating of external and internal information to the cortex (Vollenweider & Geyer, 2001). According to the cortico-striato-thalamo-cortical (CSTC) model of information processing, deficient gating of sensory and cognitive information is thought to result in loss of coherent ego experience due to overloading with excessive exteroceptive and interoceptive stimuli and difficulty in distinguishing self from nonself (Vollenweider & Geyer, 2001). The CSTC model posits that the thalamus plays a key role in controlling or gating information to the cortex and is thereby fundamentally involved in the regulation of the level of awareness and attention (Vollenweider & Geyer, 2001). This notion is particularly well in line with the information integration theory of consciousness, which highlights the role of the thalamo-cortical system in the integration of information (Tononi, 2004). It was recently suggested that one possible construal of nondual awareness is in terms of the breakdown between endogenous and exogenous stimuli leading to a temporary loss of experiential boundary between self and world. On the other hand, purely conscious states could be defined as states of extreme absorption involving high sensory gating, whose sparse phenomenal content has little overlap with the rich phenomenology of ordinary wakeful experience (Millière et al., 2018).

The effects of psilocybin-assisted mindfulness training on self-consciousness and brain default mode network connectivity were recently assessed in a randomized, double-blind, placebo-controlled neuroimaging study of 38 experienced meditators following a single administration of psilocybin (315 µg/kg p.o.) during a 5-day mindfulness retreat (Smigielski, Scheidegger, et al., 2019). Brain dynamics were quantified pre- and postretreat by fMRI during the resting state and two meditation forms, focused attention and open awareness. The analysis of functional connectivity identified psilocybin-related alterations in self-referential processing regions such as the DMN, with increased anteroventral DMN integrity at rest and decouplings of anteroposterior and frontoparietal DMN connectivity during open awareness. Notably, the postintervention reduction in connectivity between medial prefrontal and PCC was associated with positively experienced ego dissolution during the psilocybin-assisted mindfulness session. Moreover, both experiential and brain connectivity markers were predictive of positive changes in psychosocial functioning of participants 4 months later (Smigielski, Scheidegger, et al., 2019). This is well in line with a neural model of recently proposed mystical experiences based on modulation of brain networks that are involved in self-referential processing and maintenance of a sense of the self in space and time (Barrett & Griffiths, 2017). The separation of the self from the body is a well-known mystical experience,

and converging patterns of altered brain activity in the temporoparietal junction, which integrates bodily and sensory modalities, have been associated with psychedelic and meditation-induced out-of-body-experiences. In deep meditative states, activity in the part of the parietal lobe that determines our spatiotemporal orientation and bodily sense of distinction between oneself and the rest of the world was found to be decreased. At the same time, parts of the limbic system in the temporal lobes that are tagging events as biologically significant were activated (Newberg & Iversen, 2003). The involvement of temporoparietal brain areas in self-transcendence is further evidenced by out-of-body experiences (Blanke & Mohr, 2005; Blanke et al., 2002) and brain lesion mapping with pre- and postneurosurgery personality assessments (Urgesi et al., 2010). The functional elimination of neural input to the brain-orienting system in the parietal lobes can cause a transient blurring of demarcation between self and world, resulting in a state of self-transcendence that is experienced as highly significant and ineffable.

In conclusion, both meditation- and psychedelic-induced states of transcendence of usual body, space, and time perception may rely on altered communication between self-referential processing networks in the brain. Consistent with the idea that psychedelics induce disintegration and desegregation of functional brain networks, decreased DMN integrity and functional coupling between the frontal cortex and the PCC, medial temporal, and parietal networks may be a marker of altered brain state that is consistent with mystical experiences during meditation or psychedelics (Barrett & Griffiths, 2017; Winkelman, 2017). The striking phenomenological similarity of mystical-type experiences across cultures and areas may be partially explained by common underlying brain mechanisms that give rise to this innate human mental capacity. However, it must be critically noted that the few examples of drug- and non-drug-induced mystical experiences that have been empirically investigated so far allow only very limited conclusions about the biological basis of the broad and complex spectrum of psychospiritual experiences.

▨ Shared Psychological Mechanisms Related to Mindfulness Practice and Psychedelic Experiences

Both meditative practices and psychedelic experiences share common psychological mechanisms that may be mediating increased levels of well-being. Although previous sections focused more on attenuation of self-referential processing, both meditation and psychedelics may also increase various other aspects of self-experience. For instance, mindfulness training was found to be associated with a more positive self-representation, higher self-esteem, and self-acceptance (Crescentini & Capurso, 2015). A recent review about the use of psychedelics and entactogens in clinical trials, and recreational and ceremonial settings, highlights positive effects on mood, well-being, prosocial behaviors, empathy, cognitive flexibility, creativity, openness, value orientations, nature-relatedness, spirituality, self-transcendence, and mindfulness-related capabilities (Jungaberle et al., 2018). Enhanced skills in navigating altered states of consciousness such as clarity of awareness, self-inquiry, change in perspective, disidentification, meta-awareness, cognitive reappraisal, emotion regulation, and self-compassion may represent other converging mechanisms underlying the transformative effects of mindfulness practice (Guendelman, Medeiros, & Rampes, 2017; Vago & Silbersweig, 2012) and psychedelic-assisted therapies (Millière et al., 2018; Scheidegger, 2020; Walsh & Thiessen, 2018).

Experientially, psychedelics typically evoke a heightened state of introspection characterized by increased awareness, dreamlike visions and geometric patterns, intense emotions, and recollection of autobiographical memories. Occasionally, psychedelic experiences also include visionary experiences with symbolic, archetypal, and psychospiritual contents (Shanon, 2002). Insight into maladaptive behavioral, emotional, and cognitive patterns reflect the general action of psychedelics as psychointegrative medicines. Contrary to other psychotropic drugs such as opioids, benzodiazepines, or antipsychotics that tend to emotionally numb and narrow the field of consciousness, psychedelics usually increase the level of mental clarity and emotional awareness compared to everyday consciousness. This parallels the mindfulness practice of *self-inquiry*, which is defined as the process of investigating the dynamics and nature of conscious experience (Dahl et al., 2015). A central mechanism of self-inquiry is to undo maladaptive cognitive patterns by exploring the dynamics of perception, emotion, and cognition, and generating insights into one's internal models of the self, others, and the world. Thus, dysfunctional thoughts and emotions can be better recognized, restructured, and integrated, which accelerates and deepens transformative processes. In mindfulness practice, cognitive reappraisal and perspective taking are hypothesized to be important mechanisms used to target maladaptive psychological processes and replace them with more adaptive patterns. *Cognitive reappraisal* is an important strategy in the regulation of emotion and refers to the process of changing how we think about situations and events in such a way that our response to them is altered (Dahl et al., 2015). Conversely, mindfulness-based *emotion regulation* emphasizes accepting, allowing, or being nonjudgmental or nonevaluative about an experience in the present moment. Mindfulness skills practice improves patients' ability to effectively tolerate and cope with negative emotional states by extinguishing fear responses and avoidance behaviors previously elicited by these stimuli (Murakami et al., 2015). Complemented with mindfulness-based emotion regulation, lowered intensity and frequency of negative affect, and improved positive mood states through attentional deployment, cognitive–emotional reappraisal and response modulation might be achieved as an outcome of psychedelic-assisted therapy.

Another way of understanding psychedelic-assisted therapy is to compare it with the technique of behavioral exposure: Anxiety is usually best resolved through repeated exposure to the feared object or context. Comparably, psychedelic experiences share the same sequence of exposing the patient to the entire possible spectrum of intense feelings and mental states. If the subject is able to surrender to the often described psychedelic state of confronting innermost fears, this challenging initial phase is usually followed by a sudden transformation of the experience into emotional relief, insightful reflections, states of self-transcendence, and changed worldview and outlook on life (Frecska, Bokor, & Winkelman, 2016). In analogy to behavioral exposure therapy that aims at decreasing fear responses, a state of nonspecific stress resistance could be achieved. Through repeated exposures to the psychedelic state, the mind trains its intrinsic capability to deal with difficult emotions that may finally lead to a more relaxed and accepting attitude toward general human suffering. Mindfulness meditation resembles this exposure situation because practitioners turn toward their emotional experience, bring acceptance to bodily and affective responses, and refrain from engaging in internal reactivity toward it, which leads to states of greater equanimity. Hence, mindfulness training was suggested to enhance the ability to extinguish conditioned fear by structurally and functionally affecting the brain network that supports safety signaling (Tang et al., 2015).

Clinical studies have shown that a diminished ability to step back and observe one's internal processes of thinking and feeling has an important role in a variety of psychiatric conditions, including depression and anxiety (Dahl et al., 2015). Reversing states of experiential fusion through cognitive distancing, decentering, and the cultivation of meta-awareness were identified to mediate treatment effects of mindfulness-based interventions (Bernstein et al., 2015). This aligns with the Buddhist notion that identification with a static concept of self causes psychological distress, and that disidentification from a narrow self-concept through enhanced meta-awareness results in the freedom to experience a more genuine way of being (Olendzki, 2010). Interestingly, ayahuasca was found to elevate levels of mindfulness, self-compassion, and decentering that refer to the capacity to observe thoughts and emotions as transitory mental events without being trapped by them (Sampedro et al., 2017; Soler et al., 2016). However, psychedelic-induced states of enhanced mindfulness and cognitive flexibility are short-lived and strongly support the notion for concomitant psychotherapy to train patients to stabilize and maintain more balanced states of mind that allow for better adaptation to their environment.

■ Converging Roles of Mindfulness and Psychedelics for Mental Health Care: Implications for Psychedelic-Assisted Psychotherapy

Based on the scientific literature reviewed here, the use of psychedelic substances as tools that can intensify, deepen, and accelerate psychotherapeutic processes may be of significant value in the treatment of numerous mental health conditions. However, elicitation of a drug-induced peak experience probably lacks sustained transformative effects if it is not embedded in a real-world learning environment, where novel insights, attitudes, and behaviors can be consolidated. The cultivation of mindfulness ameliorates psychiatric and stress-related symptoms and is therefore increasingly being incorporated into psychotherapeutic interventions (Holzel et al., 2011). Mindfulness-based treatment frameworks may therefore provide essential skills to integrate, maintain, and further stabilize more adaptive states of consciousness following drug-induced transformative experiences. Although beneficial effects of mindfulness practice and psychedelics on mental health and well-being have previously been reported, there is little systematic research on the psychological and neurobehavioral mechanisms that underlie their potentially transformative effects (Gu et al., 2015; Jungaberle et al., 2018; Vago & Silbersweig, 2012).

States of attenuated self-referential processing are of particular clinical relevance for psychedelic-assisted therapy: Although the field of consciousness is usually narrowed in depressive, anxious, obsessive–compulsive, or addictive states, it can be broadened toward more flexible and less biased modes of conscious awareness following transformative experiences. Negative emotional biases related to critical self-referential processing are particularly well resolved through mindfulness training that develops skills such as meta-awareness, self-regulation, and a positive relationship between self and other that transcends self-focused needs and increases prosocial characteristics (Vago & Silbersweig, 2012). Likewise, improvements in mindfulness-related capabilities may be enhanced not only by meditation practices but also through distinctive features of transformative experiences induced by ayahuasca or psilocybin (Griffiths et al., 2018; Soler et al., 2016). While the meditation expert has learned to navigate purposefully through different states of consciousness, mental illness is characterized as the loss of freedom to navigate skillfully toward more adaptive mental states. With progression toward peak or breakthrough states of ego dissolution and self-transcendence, therapeutic transformation or unlearning of previously conditioned self-referential behaviors and attitudes is facilitated. Through expanded states of consciousness, patients may become increasingly aware of how to navigate their own consciousness and break out from maladaptive states through increased meta-awareness and cognitive flexibility. The induction of transformative experiences and mindfulness-related capabilities is therefore expected to contribute to the noted increases in well-being and mood following exposure to psychedelics. From a conceptual perspective, it makes sense to assume that through attenuation of ego boundaries and expansion of consciousness toward states of self-transcendence, a transient state of release from clinical symptoms is induced. This follows logically from the notion that symptoms arise at the interface between the individual and his or her environment, signaling a homeostatic imbalance with a need for behavioral adjustment or removal of noxious influences. When ego boundaries are dissolved to a degree that the conceptual distinction between external and internal world is suspended, there is no interface for the generation of symptoms anymore. With progressive reorientation in body, space, and time, the process-related dynamics of symptom formation and possible avenues for their resolution become more evident to the patient. From this clinical epistemological perspective, it can be argued that drug-induced states of self-transcendence provide unique chances to gain metacognitive awareness into the intrinsic dynamic of root causes and processes underlying the formation of symptoms and open a psychotherapeutic window for adaptation, transformation, and personal growth.

In order to further investigate enduring positive, trait-level changes in psychological functioning following transformative experiences, the model of so-called "quantum change" has been proposed (Miller, 2004). Broadly, two general kinds differentiated by the qualitative nature of the acute experience have been distinguished: the sudden, dramatic, mystical type, similar to common reports of near-death experiences, and the enduring insightful type, centering on insight, something lying more within the conceptual world of psychotherapy (Miller, 2004). To reach meaningful breakthrough experiences with transformative potential may require a capacity to surrender or let go of psychological resistance (Richards, 2015). The willingness to surrender and the dispositional trait of absorption were both associated with stronger mystical-type experiences in meditators or in response to psychedelics (Carhart-Harris et al., 2018; Russ & Elliott, 2017; Studerus et al., 2012). In the early treatment paradigm of psychedelic therapy, high doses of psychedelic drugs have been used to induce breakthrough experiences with an overwhelming impact on the patient's worldview and self-concept, with beneficial long-term outcomes (Majić, Schmidt, & Gallinat, 2015; Pahnke et al., 1970). Clinical researchers have found favorable outcomes in treatment of anxiety and depression resulting from a life-threatening diagnosis (Griffiths et al., 2016; Ross et al., 2016), and addictive behaviors such as nicotine or alcohol dependence (Bogenschutz et al., 2015; Garcia-Romeu, Griffiths, & Johnson, 2014) are associated with subjects undergoing a psychedelic-induced mystical experience. Outside of clinical settings, mystical-type experiences among psychedelic users were found to predict changes in well-being (Carhart-Harris et al., 2018). Hence, the mystical experience was proposed as a behavioral marker for the underlying therapeutic mechanism of psychedelics (Nichols, Johnson, & Nichols, 2017).

Notably, significant numbers of Buddhist retreatants were drawn to spiritual practice following psychedelics (Tart, 1991). Likewise, participants of the "Good Friday" Experiment, when interviewed more than 20 years later, reported that their psilocybin experience had contributed to their spiritual lives (Doblin, 1991). However, the stabilization of transient insights from altered states into enduring altered traits is one of the great challenges facing all transformative disciplines (Smith, 2000). Due to their mutually exclusive psychophysiology, ordinary and altered states of consciousness cannot occur at the same time, which raises questions of transfer and stabilization: How can brief transformative moments of altered perception be integrated within the boundaries of everyday consciousness? To further develop and maintain mindfulness-related capabilities, sustainable therapeutic transformation strongly relies on concomitant mental training; otherwise, short-term beneficial effects are likely to fade away. Although an older literature suggests that administration of psychedelics in a psychotherapeutic context may produce enduring decreases in psychopathology and increases in positive worldview and dispositional characteristics (Passie, 2007), it has to be critically noted that there is little evidence for enduring changes on well-validated trait measures of disposition or personality in healthy subjects (Doblin, 1991; Griffiths et al., 2008, 2011; Leary, Litwin, & Metzner, 1963; Studerus et al., 2011). By contrast, long-term effects of contemplative practices on well-being do not appear to be necessarily mediated by intense experiences but rather by improving self-regulation through attention control, emotion regulation, and self-awareness, thereby supporting more healthy functioning by transforming habitual patterns of responding (Tang et al., 2015).

Since both psychedelics and meditation attenuate the habitual perceptual, affective, and conceptual distinctions among self, others, and the environment, resulting states of self-transcendence are closely related to characteristics such as altruism, kindness, respect, trust, empathy, compassion, and prosocial behaviors (Belser et al., 2017; Kreplin, Farias, & Brazil, 2018; Luberto et al., 2018; Watts et al., 2017). These empathogenic effects can serve basically to develop increased levels of relational embeddedness, self-acceptance, and self-compassion through direct experience of corrective emotions. In settings that are supportive for cultivating mindfulness, psilocybin-induced, mystical-type experiences were found to fa-

cilitate enduring trait-level increases in prosocial attitudes and behaviors such as interpersonal closeness, gratefulness, forgiveness, and purposefulness (Griffiths et al., 2018). Peak meditative states of awakening that create deep transformations of consciousness and behavior involve a shift from egocentric toward more allocentric frames of reference that need to be further stabilized for the attainment of stable well-being and prosocial orientations (Austin, 2013). Most notably, patients undergoing psilocybin treatment for depression reported that medications and some short-term talk therapies tended to reinforce their sense of disconnection and avoidance, whereas treatment with psilocybin encouraged connection and acceptance (Watts et al., 2017). With increased levels of connectedness to the self, others, and the environment (Carhart-Harris et al., 2017; Forstmann & Sagioglou, 2017), self-destructive behavioral patterns can be attenuated, and general improvement in relationship homeostasis may be reached. This facilitates the individual's resolution of dysfunctional habits that underlie the dynamics of self-destructive and addictive behaviors by experiencing greater self-acceptance and increased capacity to regulate painful emotions (Lafrance et al., 2017). Indeed, Kuyken and colleagues (2010) found that positive effects of mindfulness-based cognitive therapy interventions on depressive symptoms were mediated by the enhancement of self-compassion across treatment. Cultivating self-compassion and self-kindness brings understanding toward oneself in instances of perceived inadequacy or suffering. The notion of common humanity puts one's experiences into the perspective of larger human experience rather than as separating and isolating (Neff, 2003).

Based on converging evidence from contemplative science and psychedelic research, a novel treatment paradigm is proposed here, that follows the distinct model of transformation-based therapy (Scheidegger, 2020). In conventional substitution-oriented approaches, the root cause of psychological illness is primarily treated as a result of deficient brain metabolism that needs to be substituted with drugs on a daily basis. In contrast, the goal of transformation-based therapy is to move the patient from a suboptimal state into a more adaptive state of consciousness that needs to be further stabilized by concurrent psychotherapy. The therapeutic focus is less on the resolution of specific symptoms, and their substitution by means of psychotropic drugs, than on empowering the innate dynamic capacity of the patient to regain sustained access to more adaptive states of consciousness that are naturally followed by symptom resolution on many levels. The concept of transformation-based therapy, as introduced here, is well in line with process-oriented adaptations of third-wave cognitive-behavioral therapies (CBT). While standard CBT is more outcome-oriented, modifying psychiatric symptoms as directly as possible, the third wave of CBT emphasizes a set of new behavioral and cognitive approaches such as emotions, relationships, values, mindfulness, acceptance, and metacognition (Hayes & Hofmann, 2017). As reviewed earlier, the therapeutic effects of psychedelics on psychological functioning are particularly aligned with mindfulness-based approaches that aim to increase acceptance, self-compassion, present-moment and metacognitive awareness, and psychological flexibility in the service of achieving core life values. Adaptive changes in value orientation are likely to follow from recognition of maladaptive orientations (e.g., self-centeredness, addictive cravings, experiential avoidance). Accordingly, a process-oriented view on therapeutic transformation is encouraged, starting with the assessment of the current state of stagnation and identifying the direction for adaptive change by encouraging an awareness of the patient's potential for self-direction. Psychedelics may become particularly useful to support this process of self-discovery, creation of meaning, and enrichment of the patient's self-awareness toward the attainment of insight, sense of agency, identity, self-esteem, emotional awareness, and increased psychological well-being.

References

Alonso, J. F., Romero, S., Mañanas, M. À., & Riba, J. (2015). Serotonergic psychedelics temporarily modify information transfer in humans. *International Journal of Neuropsychopharmacology, 18*(8), pyv039.

Atasoy, S., Roseman, L., Kaelen, M., Kringelbach, M. L., Deco, G., & Carhart-Harris, R. L. (2017). Connectome-harmonic decomposition of human brain activity reveals dynamical repertoire re-organization under LSD. *Scientific Reports, 7*(1), Article No. 17661.

Austin, J. H. (2013). Zen and the brain: Mutually illuminating topics. *Frontiers in Psychology, 4*, Article No. 784.

Barrett, F. S., & Griffiths, R. R. (2017). Classic hallucinogens and mystical experiences: Phenomenology and neural correlates. *Current Topics in Behavioral Neurosciences, 22*(8), 3–38.

Barsuglia, J., Davis, A. K., Palmer, R., Lancelotta, R., Windham-Herman, A.-M., Peterson, K., et al. (2018). Intensity of mystical experiences occasioned by 5-MeO-DMT and comparison with a prior psilocybin study. *Frontiers in Psychology, 9*, Article No. 2459.

Belser, A. B., Agin-Liebes, G., Swift, T. C., Terrana, S., Devenot, N., Friedman, H. L., et al. (2017). Patient experiences of psilocybin-assisted psychotherapy: An interpretative phenomenological analysis. *Journal of Humanistic Psychology, 57*(4), 354–388.

Berkovich-Ohana, A., Wilf, M., Kahana, R., Arieli, A., & Malach, R. (2015). Repetitive speech elicits widespread deactivation in the human cortex: The "Mantra" effect? *Brain and Behavior, 5*(7), 1–13.

Bernstein, A., Hadash, Y., Lichtash, Y., Tanay, G., Shepherd, K., & Fresco, D. M. (2015). Decentering and related constructs: A critical review and metacognitive processes model. *Perspectives on Psychological Science, 10*(5), 599–617.

Blanke, O., & Mohr, C. (2005). Out-of-body experience, heautoscopy, and autoscopic hallucination of neurological origin Implications for neurocognitive mechanisms of corporeal awareness and self-consciousness. *Brain Research Reviews, 50*(1), 184–199.

Blanke, O., Ortigue, S., Landis, T., & Seeck, M. (2002). Stimulating illusory own-body perceptions. *Nature, 419*, 269–270.

Bogenschutz, M. P., Forcehimes, A. A., Pommy, J. A., Wilcox, C. E., Barbosa, P. C. R., & Strassman, R. J. (2015). Psilocybin-assisted treatment for alcohol dependence: A proof-of-concept study. *Journal of Psychopharmacology, 29*(3), 289–299.

Borg, J., Andrée, B., Soderstrom, H., & Farde, L. (2003). The serotonin system and spiritual experiences. *American Journal of Psychiatry, 160*(11), 1965–1969.

Brewer, J. A., & Garrison, K. A. (2014). The posterior cingulate cortex as a plausible mechanistic target of meditation: Findings from neuroimaging. *Annals of the New York Academy of Sciences, 1307*(1), 19–27.

Brewer, J. A., Worhunsky, P. D., Gray, J. R., Tang, Y.-Y., Weber, J., & Kober, H. (2011). Meditation experience is associated with differences in default mode network activity and connectivity. *Proceedings of the National Academy of Sciences of the USA, 108*(50), 20254–20259.

Carhart-Harris, R. L., Erritzoe, D., Haijen, E., Kaelen, M., & Watts, R. (2017). Psychedelics and connectedness. *Psychopharmacology, 29*(4), 1–4.

Carhart-Harris, R. L., Erritzoe, D., Williams, T., Stone, J. M., Reed, L. J., Colasanti, A., et al. (2012). Neural correlates of the psychedelic state as determined by fMRI studies with psilocybin. *Proceedings of the National Academy of Sciences of the USA, 109*(6), 2138–2143.

Carhart-Harris, R. L., Leech, R., Erritzoe, D., Williams, T. M., Stone, J. M., Evans, J., et al. (2013). Functional connectivity measures after psilocybin inform a novel hypothesis of early psychosis. *Schizophrenia Bulletin, 39*(6), 1343–1351.

Carhart-Harris, R. L., Leech, R., Hellyer, P. J., Shanahan, M., Feilding, A., Tagliazucchi, E., et al. (2014). The entropic brain: A theory of conscious states informed by neuroimaging research with psychedelic drugs. *Frontiers in Human Neuroscience, 8,* Article No. 20.

Carhart-Harris, R. L., Muthukumaraswamy, S., Roseman, L., Kaelen, M., Droog, W., Murphy, K., et al. (2016). Neural correlates of the LSD experience revealed by multimodal neuroimaging. *Proceedings of the National Academy of Sciences of the USA, 113*(17), 4853–4858.

Carhart-Harris, R. L., Roseman, L., Haijen, E., Erritzoe, D., Watts, R., Branchi, I., et al. (2018). Psychedelics and the essential importance of context. *Journal of Psychopharmacology, 32*(7), 725–731.

Crescentini, C., & Capurso, V. (2015). Mindfulness meditation and explicit and implicit indicators of personality and self-concept changes. *Frontiers in Psychology, 6*(1083), Article No. 44.

Dahl, C. J., Lutz, A., & Davidson, R. J. (2015). Reconstructing and deconstructing the self: Cognitive mechanisms in meditation practice. *Trends in Cognitive Sciences, 19*(9), 515–523.

Doblin, R. (1991). Pahnke's "Good Friday" experiment: A long-term follow-up and methodological critique. *Journal of Transpersonal Psychology, 23*(1), 1–28.

Farb, N. A. S., Segal, Z. V., & Anderson, A. K. (2013). Mindfulness meditation training alters cortical representations of interoceptive attention. *Social Cognitive and Affective Neuroscience, 8*(1), 15–26.

Farb, N. A. S., Segal, Z. V., Mayberg, H., Bean, J., McKeon, D., Fatima, Z., et al. (2007). Attending to the present: Mindfulness meditation reveals distinct neural modes of self-reference. *Social Cognitive and Affective Neuroscience, 2*(4), 313–322.

Fischer, R. (1971). A cartography of the ecstatic and meditative states. *Science, 174,* 897–904.

Forstmann, M., & Sagioglou, C. (2017). Lifetime experience with (classic) psychedelics predicts pro-environmental behavior through an increase in nature relatedness. *Journal of Psychopharmacology, 31*(8), 975–988.

Fox, K. C. R., Dixon, M. L., Nijeboer, S., Girn, M., Floman, J. L., Lifshitz, M., et al. (2016). Functional neuroanatomy of meditation: A review and meta-analysis of 78 functional neuroimaging investigations. *Neuroscience and Biobehavioral Reviews, 65,* 208–228.

Fox, M. D., & Greicius, M. (2010). Clinical applications of resting state functional connectivity. *Frontiers in Systems Neuroscience, 4,* Article No. 19.

Fox, M. D., Snyder, A. Z., Corbetta, M., Van Essen, D. C., & Raichle, M. E. (2005). The human brain is intrinsically organized into dynamic, anticorrelated functional networks. *Proceedings of the National Academy of Sciences of the USA, 102*(27), 9673–9678.

Frecska, E., Bokor, P., & Winkelman, M. (2016). The therapeutic potentials of ayahuasca: Possible effects against various diseases of civilization. *Frontiers in Pharmacology, 7,* Article No. 35.

Gallimore, A. R. (2015). Restructuring consciousness—the psychedelic state in light of integrated information theory. *Frontiers in Human Neuroscience, 9*(20), Article No. 346.

Garcia-Romeu, A., Griffiths, R. R., & Johnson, M. W. (2014). Psilocybin-occasioned mystical experiences in the treatment of tobacco addiction. *Current Drug Abuse Reviews, 7*(3), 157–164.

Griffiths, R. R., Johnson, M. W., Carducci, M. A., Umbricht, A., Richards, W. A., Richards, B. D., et al. (2016). Psilocybin produces substantial and sustained decreases in depression and anxiety in patients with life-threatening cancer: A randomized double-blind trial. *Journal of Psychopharmacology, 30*(12), 1181–1197.

Griffiths, R. R., Johnson, M. W., Richards, W. A., Richards, B. D., Jesse, R., Maclean, K. A., et al. (2018). Psilocybin-occasioned mystical-type experience in combination with meditation and other spiritual practices produces enduring positive changes in psychological functioning and in trait measures of prosocial attitudes and behaviors. *Journal of Psychopharmacology, 32,* 49–69.

Griffiths, R. R., Johnson, M. W., Richards, W. A., Richards, B. D., McCann, U., & Jesse, R. (2011). Psilocybin occasioned mystical-type experiences: Immediate and persisting dose-related effects. *Psychopharmacology, 218*(4), 649–665.

Griffiths, R., Richards, W., Johnson, M., McCann, U., & Jesse, R. (2008). Mystical-type experiences occasioned by psilocybin mediate the attribution of personal meaning and spiritual significance 14 months later. *Journal of Psychopharmacology, 22*(6), 621–632.

Griffiths, R. R., Richards, W. A., McCann, U., & Jesse, R. (2006). Psilocybin can occasion mystical-type experiences having substantial and sustained personal meaning and spiritual significance. *Psychopharmacology, 187*(3), 268–283.

Gu, J., Strauss, C., Bond, R., & Cavanagh, K. (2015). How do mindfulness-based cognitive therapy and mindfulness-based stress reduction improve mental health and wellbeing?: A systematic review and meta-analysis of mediation studies. *Clinical Psychology Review, 37,* 1–12.

Guendelman, S., Medeiros, S., & Rampes, H. (2017). Mindfulness and emotion regulation: Insights from neurobiological, psychological, and clinical studies. *Frontiers in Psychology, 8,* 220.

Hayes, S. C., & Hofmann, S. G. (2017). The third wave of cognitive behavioral therapy and the rise of process-based care. *World Psychiatry, 16*(3), 245–246.

Holzel, B. K., Lazar, S. W., Gard, T., Schuman-Olivier, Z., Vago, D. R., & Ott, U. (2011). How does mindfulness meditation work?: Proposing mechanisms of action from a conceptual and neural perspective. *Perspectives in Psychological Science, 6*(6), 537–559.

Hood, R. W. (1975). The construction and preliminary validation of a measure of reported mystical experience. *Journal for the Scientific Study of Religion, 14*(1), 29–41.

Huxley, A. (1954). *The doors of perception.* New York: Harper & Brothers.

Ives-Deliperi, V. L., Solms, M., & Meintjes, E. M. (2011). The neural substrates of mindfulness: An fMRI investigation. *Social Neuroscience, 6*(3), 231–242.

James, W. (1882). Subjective effects of nitrous oxide. *Mind, 7,* 186–208.

Jones, R. H. (2016). *Philosophy of mysticism: Raids on the ineffable.* Albany: State University of New York Press.

Josipovic, Z. (2014). Neural correlates of nondual awareness in meditation. *Annals of the New York Academy of Sciences of the USA, 1307*(1), 9–18.

Jungaberle, H., Thal, S., Zeuch, A., Rougemont-Bücking, A., Heyden, von, M., Aicher, H., et al. (2018). Positive psychology in the investigation of psychedelics and entactogens: A critical review. *Neuropharmacology, 142,* 179–199.

Kaelen, M., Giribaldi, B., Raine, J., Evans, L., Timmerman, C., Rodriguez, N., et al. (2018). The hidden therapist: Evidence for a central role of music in psychedelic therapy. *Psychopharmacology, 235*(2), 505–519.

Khoury, B., Knäuper, B., Schlosser, M., Carrière, K., & Chiesa, A. (2017). Effectiveness of traditional meditation retreats: A systematic review and meta-analysis. *Journal of Psychosomatic Research, 92,* 16–25.

Kometer, M., Pokorny, T., Seifritz, E., & Vollenweider, F. X. (2015). Psilocybin-induced spiritual experiences and insightfulness are associated with synchronization of neuronal oscillations. *Psychopharmacology (Berlin), 232,* 3663–3676.

Kreplin, U., Farias, M., & Brazil, I. A. (2018). The limited prosocial effects of meditation: A systematic review and meta-analysis. *Scientific Reports, 8*(1), 2403.

Krupitsky, E. M., & Grinenko, A. Y. (1997). Ketamine psychedelic therapy (KPT): A review of the results of ten years of research. *Journal of Psychoactive Drugs, 29*(2), 165–183.

Kuyken, W., Watkins, E., Holden, E., White, K., Taylor, R. S., Byford, S., et al. (2010). How does mindfulness-based cognitive therapy work? *Behaviour Research and Therapy, 48*(11), 1105–1112.

Labate, B. C. (2016). *Ayahuasca, ritual and religion in Brazil.* New York: Routledge.

Labate, B. C., Cavnar, C., & Gearin, A. K. (2016). *The world ayahuasca diaspora.* New York: Routledge.

Lafrance, A., Loizaga-Velder, A., Fletcher, J., Renelli, M., Files, N., & Tupper, K. W. (2017). Nourishing the spirit: Exploratory research on ayahuasca experiences along the continuum of recovery from eating disorders. *Journal of Psychoactive Drugs, 49*(5), 427–435.

Leary, T., Litwin, G. H., & Metzner, R. (1963). Reactions to psilocybin administered in a supportive environment. *Journal of Nervous and Mental Disease, 137*(6), 561–573.

Lebedev, A. V., Kaelen, M., Lövdén, M., Nilsson, J., Feilding, A., Nutt, D. J., et al. (2016). LSD-induced entropic brain activity predicts subsequent personality change. *Human Brain Mapping, 37*(9), 3203–3213.

Lebedev, A. V., Lövdén, M., Rosenthal, G., Feilding, A., Nutt, D. J., & Carhart-Harris, R. L. (2015). Finding the self by losing the self: Neural correlates of ego-dissolution under psilocybin. *Human Brain Mapping, 36*(8), 3137–3153.

Liechti, M. E., Dolder, P. C., & Schmid, Y. (2016). Alterations of consciousness and mystical-type experiences after acute LSD in humans. *Psychopharmacology, 29*(Suppl. 2), 1–12.

Luberto, C. M., Shinday, N., Song, R., Philpotts, L. L., Park, E. R., Fricchione, G. L., et al. (2018). A systematic review and meta-analysis of the effects of meditation on empathy, compassion, and prosocial behaviors. *Mindfulness, 9*(3), 708–724.

Lutz, A., Jha, A. P., Dunne, J. D., & Saron, C. D. (2015). Investigating the phenomenological matrix of mindfulness-related practices from a neurocognitive perspective. *American Psychologist, 70*(7), 632–658.

Lutz, A., Slagter, H. A., Dunne, J. D., & Davidson, R. J. (2008). Attention regulation and monitoring in meditation. *Trends in Cognitive Sciences, 12*(4), 163–169.

MacLean, K. A., Johnson, M. W., & Griffiths, R. R. (2011). Mystical experiences occasioned by the hallucinogen psilocybin lead to increases in the personality domain of openness. *Journal of Psychopharmacology, 25*(11), 1453–1461.

Majić, T., Schmidt, T. T., & Gallinat, J. (2015). Peak experiences and the afterglow phenomenon: When and how do therapeutic effects of hallucinogens depend on psychedelic experiences? *Journal of Psychopharmacology, 29*(3), 241–253.

Masters, R., & Houston, J. (2000). *The varieties of psychedelic experience*. New York: Simon & Schuster.

Miller, W. R. (2004). The phenomenon of quantum change. *Journal of Clinical Psychology, 60*(5), 453–460.

Millière, R. (2017). Looking for the self: Phenomenology, neurophysiology and philosophical significance of drug-induced ego dissolution. *Frontiers in Human Neuroscience, 11*, 245.

Millière, R., Carhart-Harris, R. L., Roseman, L., Trautwein, F.-M., & Berkovich-Ohana, A. (2018). Psychedelics, meditation, and self-consciousness. *Frontiers in Psychology, 9*, Article No. 1475.

Montero-Marin, J., Puebla-Guedea, M., Herrera-Mercadal, P., Cebolla, A., Soler, J., Demarzo, M., et al. (2016). Psychological effects of a 1-month meditation retreat on experienced meditators: The role of non-attachment. *Frontiers in Psychology, 7*, Article No. 1935.

Murakami, H., Katsunuma, R., Oba, K., Terasawa, Y., Motomura, Y., Mishima, K., et al. (2015). Neural networks for mindfulness and emotion suppression. *PLOS ONE, 10*(6), e0128005.

Muthukumaraswamy, S. D., Carhart-Harris, R. L., Moran, R. J., Brookes, M. J., Williams, T. M., Erritzoe, D., et al. (2013). Broadband cortical desynchronization underlies the human psychedelic state. *Journal of Neuroscience, 33*(38), 15171–15183.

Nash, J. D., & Newberg, A. (2013). Toward a unifying taxonomy and definition for meditation. *Frontiers in Psychology, 4*, 806.

Neff, K. (2003). Self-compassion: An alternative conceptualization of a healthy attitude toward oneself. *Self and Identity, 2*, 101–185.

Newberg, A. B., & Iversen, J. (2003). The neural basis of the complex mental task of meditation: neurotransmitter and neurochemical considerations. *Medical Hypotheses, 61*(2), 282–291.

Nichols, D. E. (2016). Psychedelics. *Pharmacological Reviews, 68*(2), 264–355.

Nichols, D. E., Johnson, M. W., & Nichols, C. D. (2017). Psychedelics as medicines: An emerging new paradigm. *Clinical Pharmacology and Therapeutics, 101*(2), 209–219.

Nour, M. M., Evans, L., Nutt, D., & Carhart-Harris, R. L. (2016). Ego-dissolution and psychedelics: Validation of the Ego-Dissolution Inventory (EDI). *Frontiers in Human Neuroscience, 10*, 269.

Olendzki, A. (2010). *Unlimiting mind: The radically experiential psychology of Buddhism*. New York: Simon & Schuster.

Pagnoni, G. (2012). Dynamical properties of BOLD activity from the ventral posteromedial cortex associated with meditation and attentional skills. *Journal of Neuroscience, 32*(15), 5242–5249.

Pahnke, W. N. (1966). Drugs and mysticism. *International Journal of Parapsychology, 8*(2), 295–314.

Pahnke, W. N., Kurland, A. A., Unger, S., Savage, C., & Grof, S. (1970). The experimental use of psychedelic (LSD) psychotherapy. *Journal of the American Medical Association, 212*(11), 1856–1863.

Pahnke, W. N., & Richards, W. A. (1966). Implications of LSD and experimental mysticism. *Journal of Religion and Health, 5*(3), 175–208.

Palhano-Fontes, F., Andrade, K. C., Tofoli, L. F., Santos, A. C., Crippa, J. A. S., Hallak, J. E. C., et al. (2015). The psychedelic state induced by ayahuasca modulates the activity and connectivity of the default mode network. *PLOS ONE, 10*(2), e0118143.

Paloutzian, R. F., & Park, C. L. (Eds.). (2013). *Handbook of the psychology of religion and spirituality*. New York: Guilford Press.

Passie, T. (2007). Contemporary psychedelic therapy: An overview. In M. J. Winkelman & T. B. Roberts (Eds.), *Psychedelic medicine* (Vol. 1, pp. 45–68). Westport CT: Praeger.

Petitmengin, C., & Lachaux, J.-P. (2013). Micro-cognitive science: Bridging experiential and neuronal microdynamics. *Frontiers in Human Neuroscience, 7*, Article No. 617.

Petri, G., Expert, P., Turkheimer, F., Carhart-Harris, R., Nutt, D., Hellyer, P. J., & Vaccarino, F. (2014). Homological scaffolds of brain functional networks. *Journal of the Royal Society, Interface, 11*(101), Article No. 20140873.

Previc, F. H. (2009). *The dopaminergic mind in human evolution and history*. New York: Cambridge University Press.

Raichle, M. E. (2015). The brain's default mode network. *Annual Review of Neuroscience, 38*(1), 433–447.

Riba, J., Anderer, P., Jané, F., Saletu, B., & Barbanoj, M. J. (2004). Effects of the South American psychoactive beverage ayahuasca on regional brain electrical activity in humans: A functional neuroimaging study using low-resolution electromagnetic tomography. *Neuropsychobiology, 50*(1), 89–101.

Richards, W. A. (2015). *Sacred knowledge: Psychedelics and religious experiences*. New York: Columbia University Press.

Ross, S., Bossis, A., Guss, J., Agin-Liebes, G., Malone, T., Cohen, B., et al. (2016). Rapid and sustained symptom reduction following psilocybin treatment for anxiety and depression in patients with life-threatening cancer: A randomized controlled trial. *Journal of Psychopharmacology, 30*(12), 1165–1180.

Russ, S. L., & Elliott, M. S. (2017). Antecedents of mystical experience and dread in intensive meditation. *Psychology of Consciousness: Theory, Research, and Practice, 4*(1), 38–53.

Sampedro, F., de la Fuente Revenga, M., Valle, M., Roberto, N., Domínguez-Clavé, E., Elices, M., et al. (2017). Assessing the psychedelic "after-glow" in ayahuasca users: Post-acute neurometabolic and functional connectivity changes are associated with enhanced mindfulness capacities. *International Journal of Neuropsychopharmacology, 20*(9), 698–711.

Schartner, M. M., Carhart-Harris, R. L., Barrett, A. B., Seth, A. K., & Muthukumaraswamy, S. D. (2017). Increased spontaneous MEG signal diversity for psychoactive doses of ketamine, LSD and psilocybin. *Scientific Reports, 7*, 1–12.

Scheibner, H. J., Bogler, C., Gleich, T., Haynes, J.-D., & Bermpohl, F. (2017). Internal and external attention and the default mode network. *NeuroImage, 148*, 381–389.

Scheidegger, M. (2020). Psychedelic medicines and their role in shifting the paradigm from pharmacological substitution towards transformation-based psychiatry. In B. C. Labate & C. Cavnar (Eds.), *Ayahuasca healing and science* (2nd ed.). Cham, Switzerland: Springer.

Scheidegger, M., Walter, M., Lehmann, M., Metzger, C., Grimm, S., Boeker, H., et al. (2012). Ketamine decreases resting state functional network connectivity in healthy subjects: Implications for antidepressant drug action. *PLOS ONE, 7*(9), e44799.

Schultes, R. E. (1969). Hallucinogens of plant origin. *Science, 163*, 245–254.

Shanon, B. (2002). *The antipodes of the mind*. New York: Oxford University Press.

Simon, R., & Engström, M. (2015). The default mode network as a biomarker for monitoring the therapeutic effects of meditation. *Frontiers in Psychology, 6*(70), Article No. 776.

Smigielski, L., Kometer, M., Scheidegger, M., Krähenmann, R., Huber, T., & Vollenweider, F. X. (2019). Characterization and prediction of acute and sustained response to psychedelic psilocybin in a mindfulness group retreat. *Scientific Reports, 9*(1), Article No. 14914.

Smigielski, L., Scheidegger, M., Kometer, M., & Vollenweider, F. X. (2019). Psilocybin-assisted mindfulness training modulates self-consciousness and brain default mode network connectivity with lasting effects. *NeuroImage, 196*, 1–38.

Smith, H. (2000). *Cleansing the doors of perception*. New York: Tarcher.

Soler, J., Elices, M., Dominguez-Clavé, E., Pascual, J. C., Feilding, A., Navarro-Gil, M., et al. (2018). Four weekly ayahuasca sessions lead to increases in "acceptance" capacities: A comparison study with a standard 8-week mindfulness training program. *Frontiers in Pharmacology, 9*, Article No. 224.

Soler, J., Elices, M., Franquesa, A., Barker, S., Friedlander, P., Feilding, A., et al. (2016). Exploring the therapeutic potential of ayahuasca: Acute intake increases mindfulness-related capacities. *Psychopharmacology, 233*(5), 823–829.

Speth, J., Speth, C., Kaelen, M., Schloerscheidt, A. M., Feilding, A., Nutt, D. J., et al. (2016). Decreased mental time travel to the past correlates with default-mode network disintegration under lysergic acid diethylamide. *Journal of Psychopharmacology, 30*(4), 344–353.

Stace, W. T. (1960). *Mysticism and philosophy*. New York: Macmillan.

Studerus, E., Gamma, A., Kometer, M., & Vollenweider, F. X. (2012). Prediction of psilocybin response in healthy volunteers. *PLOS ONE, 7*(2), e30800.

Studerus, E., Kometer, M., Hasler, F., & Vollenweider, F. X. (2011). Acute, subacute and long-term subjective effects of psilocybin in healthy humans: A pooled analysis of experimental studies. *Journal of Psychopharmacology, 25*(11), 1434–1452.

Tagliazucchi, E., Carhart-Harris, R., Leech, R., Nutt, D., & Chialvo, D. R. (2014). Enhanced repertoire of brain dynamical states during the psychedelic experience. *Human Brain Mapping, 35*(11), 5442–5456.

Tang, Y.-Y., Hölzel, B. K., & Posner, M. I. (2015). The neuroscience of mindfulness meditation. *Nature Reviews Neuroscience, 16*(4), 213–225.

Tart, C. (1991). Influences of previous psychedelic drug experiences on students of Tibetan Buddhism: A preliminary exploration. *Journal of Transpersonal Psychology, 23*(2), 139–173.

Timmermann, C., Roseman, L., Williams, L., Erritzoe, D., Martial, C., Cassol, H., et al. (2018). DMT models the near-death experience. *Frontiers in Psychology, 9*, 1–12.

Tononi, G. (2004). An information integration theory of consciousness. *BMC Neuroscience, 5*, 42.

Tupper, K. W. (2008). The globalization of ayahuasca: Harm reduction or benefit maximization? *International Journal on Drug Policy, 19*(4), 297–303.

Urgesi, C., Aglioti, S. M., Skrap, M., & Fabbro, F. (2010). The spiritual brain: Selective cortical lesions modulate human self-transcendence. *Neuron, 65*(3), 309–319.

Uthaug, M. V., van Oorsouw, K., Kuypers, K. P. C., van Boxtel, M., Broers, N. J., Mason, N. L., et al. (2018). Sub-acute and long-term effects of ayahuasca on affect and cognitive

thinking style and their association with ego dissolution. *Psychopharmacology, 235*(10), 2979–2989.

Vago, D. R., & Silbersweig, D. A. (2012). Self-awareness, self-regulation, and self-transcendence (S-ART): A framework for understanding the neurobiological mechanisms of mindfulness. *Frontiers in Human Neuroscience, 6*, Article No. 296.

Varela, F. J. (1996). Neurophenomenology: A methodological remedy for the hard problem. *Journal of Consciousness Studies, 3*(4), 330–349.

Vollenweider, F. X., & Geyer, M. A. (2001). A systems model of altered consciousness: Integrating natural and drug-induced psychoses. *Brain Research Bulletin, 56*(5), 495–507.

Vollenweider, F. X., & Kometer, M. (2010). The neurobiology of psychedelic drugs: Implications for the treatment of mood disorders. *Nature Reviews Neuroscience, 11*(9), 642–651.

Vollenweider, F. X., Leenders, K. L., Scharfetter, C., Maguire, P., Stadelmann, O., & Angst, J. (1997). Positron emission tomography and fluorodeoxyglucose studies of metabolic hyperfrontality and psychopathology in the psilocybin model of psychosis. *Neuropsychopharmacology, 16*(5), 357–372.

Walsh, Z., & Thiessen, M. S. (2018). Psychedelics and the new behaviourism: Considering the integration of third-wave behaviour therapies with psychedelic-assisted therapy. *International Review of Psychiatry, 10*(4), 1–7.

Watts, R., Day, C., Krzanowski, J., Nutt, D., & Carhart-Harris, R. (2017). Patients' accounts of increased "connectedness" and "acceptance" after psilocybin for treatment-resistant depression. *Journal of Humanistic Psychology, 57*(5), 520–564.

Winkelman, M. J. (2017). The mechanisms of psychedelic visionary experiences: Hypotheses from evolutionary psychology. *Frontiers in Neuroscience, 11*, Article No. 539.

CHAPTER 22

Adverse Effects

KELAN THOMAS and BENJAMIN MALCOLM

▓ Introduction

The "classic hallucinogen" psychedelics can be divided into two chemical categories, tryptamines (e.g., psilocybin, lysergic acid diethylamide [LSD], N,N-dimethyltryptamine [DMT]) and phenethylamines (e.g., mescaline), which have profound psychotropic effects due to 5-hydroxytryptamine 2A (5-HT_{2A}) receptor agonist activity. The "other hallucinogenic" compounds include phenethylamine amphetamine derivatives such as 3,4-methylenedioxymethamphetamine (MDMA) that affect monoamine transporters and receptors or have entirely separate pharmacological activity at glutamate and opioid receptors, such as ketamine and ibogaine. There are also hundreds of synthetic phenethylamine and tryptamine compounds invented by chemists such as Alexander Shulgin and David Nichols, who have inspired the next generation of medicinal chemists to continue developing novel designer psychedelic analogues. In this chapter the "classic hallucinogens" are considered together, while "other hallucinogens" are discussed separately due to their unique pharmacology and risk profiles.

Psychedelics have been consumed in traditional religious contexts from natural sources (psilocybin mushrooms, morning glory seeds, ayahuasca, and peyote) for millennia, but anthropological literature provides minimal insight on adverse effects. The recreational use of synthetic psychedelics in the United States, such as LSD in the 1960s and MDMA in the 1980s, resulted in more reports of harm, including case reports of death. It was recognized that deaths in nonmedical recreational contexts were likely linked to confounding variables, which led to the development of a conceptual harm reduction framework for psychedelic use accounting for "set and setting." Mental preparation and carefully controlled environments were vital for reliably reducing the risks of psychological harm and behavioral consequences secondary to unsafe consumption environments (Johnson, Richards, & Griffiths, 2008).

Strategies that can minimize the risk of harm from challenging psychedelic experiences include careful preparation of mind*set* prior to a session, along with providing a safe *setting* for the experience to unfold and supportive integration afterwards. During a session, providing reassurance and a calming presence with acceptance, compassion, and caring should help to assuage any abreactions as they emerge. Encouraging someone to trust, to let go and be open for a connection with what they are feeling, without any resistance, may help the person navigate the more difficult aspects of the experience with nonjudgmental curiosity. In the case of more severe distressed reactions, when someone may be a danger to him- or herself or others, then anxiolytics and antipsychotics may also be an appropriate intervention.

In the recent clinical trials with hallucinogens, conducted in more intentional controlled settings since the 1990s, the participants have been thoroughly screened for mental illness risk, and there have not been any life-threatening adverse drug events reported in these studies. However, guidelines for safety with hallucinogen research suggest that the most commonly expected adverse effects are psychological, including anxiety, distress, delusions, fear, panic, and paranoia, which are anticipated acute, transient effects even in controlled settings. These guidelines also suggest the risk of physiological toxicity is relatively low but may include nausea, dizziness, hypertension, tachycardia, hyperreflexia, tremors, weakness, paresthesia, mydriasis, and blurred vision (Johnson et al., 2008). In an attempt to comprehensively review the adverse effects of psychedelics, toxicology literature associated with unsafe recreational environments was also selectively reviewed for reports of adverse effects that may be generalizable to a therapeutic setting, but more robust evidence from clinical trial research is emphasized in this chapter.

Classic Hallucinogens (Psilocybin, LSD, DMT, Mescaline)

Acute Adverse Effects

Psychiatric

Anxiety. Transient anxiety (17–100%) and psychological discomfort (32%) reported in seven recent psilocybin-assisted therapy clinical trials (*n* = 135) resolved 6–8 hours after psilocybin administration. During the days and months following these psilocybin sessions, significant reductions on various psychiatric ratings scales measuring anxiety, such as the State–Trait Anxiety Inventory (STAI), Hospital Anxiety and Depression Scale (HADS), and Hamilton Anxiety Rating Scale (HAM-A), demonstrated that these adverse effects were transient and isolated to the acute psilocybin effects (Thomas, Malcolm, & Lastra, 2017).

Transient anxiety (23%), emotional distress (36%), and affect lability (14%) were also reported in a recent LSD-assisted therapy clinical trial for anxiety associated with life-threatening diseases (*n* = 12) during 22 experimental dosing sessions. The day after these sessions, some participants still reported mild emotional distress (9%), which resolved within a couple of days after LSD administration. During the months following the two LSD sessions in the trial, there were actually significant reductions in anxiety, with STAI rating scale scores decreased by ~10 points (Gasser et al., 2014; Gasser, Kirchner, & Passie, 2015).

In a study of LSD's subjective effects in 16 healthy volunteers, only ~13% of participants reported transient anxiety that resolved within hours. Researchers attributed this reaction to overall elevated Five-Dimensional Altered States of Consciousness Scale (5D-ASC) scores, with higher subscale scores for anxious ego dissolution (+25%), disembodiment (+45%), and impaired control and cognition (+40%) compared with placebo (Schmid et al., 2015a).

In an older study of mescaline (5 mg/kg) and LSD (1.5 µg/kg) investigating cross-tolerance and subjective effects with 10 healthy volunteers, mescaline demonstrated peak subjective effects about an hour later that abated more gradually than LSD effects, and the mescaline-related alterations in mood, anxiety, difficulty thinking and perceptual distortions were rated less intense than LSD peak effects (Wolbach, Isbell, & Miner, 1962).

Bolus doses of 0.2–0.4 mg/kg of intravenous (IV) DMT have been administered to experienced hallucinogen users, with nearly all participants reporting intense dissociation and transient anxiety "rush" symptoms that for many were quickly replaced by euphoric effects (Strassman, 1996; Strassman, Qualls, Uhlenhuth, & Kellner, 1994). Another study of an IV DMT 0.2–0.3 mg/kg bolus followed by flexible continuous infusions up to 0.02 mg/kg/minute for 84 minutes had 20% of participants drop out due to the infusion's "intense unpleasant psychological effects" (Gouzoulis-Mayfrank et al., 2005). No adverse psychological sequelae were reported after 24 hours, and one explanation for these acute infusion adverse effects is that DMT displays a lack of acute tolerance, differentiating it from other classical psychedelics such as psilocybin, mescaline, or LSD (Strassman, Qualls, & Berg, 1996).

Psychotic Thinking. Psychotic-like symptoms, such as confusion or thought disorder (7–75%) and paranoia (2–8%) were also reported in the recent psilocybin-assisted therapy clinical trials, which resolved 6–8 hours after psilocybin administration (Thomas et al., 2017). In an epidemiological survey study soliciting details about 1,993 psilocybin mushroom users' worst "bad trip," 2.7% received medical care in a hospital setting during acute effects and 7.6% sought professional help for enduring psychological symptoms, including three cases with onset of enduring psychotic symptoms and three cases with a suicide attempt (Carbonaro et al., 2016).

Psychotic-like symptoms were also reported for LSD-assisted therapy, such as feeling abnormal (41%), illusions (73%) and hallucinations (5%). The day after these LSD sessions, some participants still reported mild related adverse events such as feeling abnormal (5%) and illusions (5%), but no flashback phenomena or prolonged effects were noted, and these symptoms resolved a couple days after LSD administration (Gasser et al., 2015). In another study with healthy volunteers, LSD also increased prepulse inhibition (PPI) of the acoustic startle response by ~15%, which was similar to the sensorimotor gating deficits observed in schizophrenia (Schmid et al., 2015a).

Researchers studying IV DMT studied subjective phenomena via the Hallucinogen Rating Scale (HRS) found that reality testing was often impaired with high-dose (0.4 mg/

kg) DMT. The DMT experience was acutely hyperreal, superseding dreams or waking reality, but subjects returned to their baseline mental state approximately 15 minutes after administration (Strassman et al., 1994).

Neurological

General. Headaches were the most common neurological adverse effect reported by 28–50% of the participants in the psilocybin clinical trials (Thomas et al., 2017). There also appeared to be dose-dependent relationship with headaches in other subjective psilocybin effect studies, since 24 hours after taking psilocybin, the healthy volunteers reported escalating rates of headache by dosage: placebo = 2.5%, 115 µg/kg = 12.5%, 215 µg/kg = 22.5%, and 315 µg/kg = 37.5% (Studerus, Kometer, Hasler, & Vollenweider, 2011).

Only one case of a treatment-emergent moderate headache (8%) was reported in the LSD-assisted therapy clinical trial (*n* = 12), along with gait disturbance (32%), feeling cold (45%), and hyperhidrosis (14%) during the LSD sessions (Gasser et al., 2014). A pharmacokinetic study with 16 healthy volunteers also revealed adverse effects of headache (50%) and imbalance (31%). This study also described LSD's temporal effect on body temperature, in which mean temperature decreased by ~0.1°C during the first 30 minutes, then increased by ~0.6°C to a nadir (37.8°C) 3 hours after LSD administration, which subsequently decreased over the next 24 hours (Dolder, Schmid, Haschke, Rentsch, & Liechti, 2015). A pharmacological functional magnetic resonance imaging (fMRI) study of subjective effects in healthy volunteers (*n* = 24) revealed that 17% experienced transient mild headaches after drug effects wore off, and one participant experienced transient sleep disturbances for 2 nights after LSD administration (Preller et al., 2018).

One participant in a study of IV DMT abstained from completing the crossover phase of the study due to headache and mild orthostasis until the next day following a DMT infusion, although both resolved completely without intervention (Gouzoulis-Mayfrank et al., 2005).

In a study comparing LSD and mescaline, both drugs increased pupillary dilation and body temperature, but slowed the kneejerk reaction; mescaline demonstrated a larger effect size than LSD for these three physiological measures (Wolbach et al., 1962).

Fatigue. A psilocybin dose–effects study demonstrated 50–70% higher general inactivation (inactivation, tiredness, and drowsiness) mean subscale scores on the Adjective Mood Rating Scale (AMRS) for these moderate- and high-dose conditions during acute psilocybin effects (Hasler, Grimberg, Benz, Huber, & Vollenweider, 2004). There was also a dose-dependent effect on fatigue in other subjective effect studies, since 24 hours after psilocybin administration, the healthy volunteers reported higher rates of fatigue by dosage: placebo = 12.5%, 115 µg/kg = 40%, 215 µg/kg = 35%, and 315 µg/kg = 60% (Studerus et al., 2011).

Difficulty concentrating (63%) and exhaustion (44%) reported during the first 10 hours after LSD administration in a study of LSD subjective effects with 16 healthy volunteers completely resolved after 72 hours (Schmid, Enzler, et al., 2015).

Cognitive Impairment. Cognitive testing in healthy volunteers, assessed by the Frankfurt Attention Inventory (FAIR), demonstrated a dose-dependent psilocybin-induced impairment on sustained attention in which Quality and Continuity subscale mean scores were 50% lower for both moderate (215 µg/kg) and high (315 µg/kg) psilocybin doses during peak effects (Hasler et al., 2004).

Seizures. There have been no seizures reported in recent psilocybin or LSD clinical trials, but one study analyzed 2000–2016 data from the American Association of Poison Control Centers database and found hyperthermia for 2% and seizures for 0.8% of recreational psilocybin mushroom exposure calls (*n* = 5,883) to poison centers. For recreational LSD exposure calls (*n* = 3,554) to poison control centers in the study, hyperthermia was identified in 3.8% and seizures in 4% of these calls (Leonard, Anderson, & Klein-Schwartz, 2018).

Cardiovascular

Acutely elevated cardiac vital signs during peak effects ~2 hours after psilocybin administration was one of the most commonly reported adverse effects (11–76%) from psilocybin clinical trials, with mean peak systolic blood pressure (SBP) in the range of ~140–155 mmHg, mean peak diastolic blood pressure (DBP) in the range of ~80–90 mmHg, and mean peak heart rate (HR) in the range of ~70–90 bpm (Thomas et al., 2017).

There were no significant main effects for low, moderate, and high doses of psilocybin on electrocardiogram (EKG) interval changes or mean arterial pressure (MAP) in healthy volunteers over placebo, but in post hoc testing the peak SBP and MAP were ~20–25 mmHg higher for high-dose psilocybin than for placebo (Hasler et al., 2004). These transient and moderate elevations in SBP and HR have not been associated with any serious adverse cardiac events in these supervised experimental studies. Despite the cardiac safety in controlled clinical trials, there have been a couple of rare recreational psilocybin mushroom case reports of myocardial infarction, with one resulting in the death of 24-year-old heart transplant recipient (Lim, Wasywich, & Ruygrok, 2012).

Cardiac vital signs during plateau effects 4 hours after LSD administration were unchanged from baseline in the LSD-assisted therapy clinical trial (Gasser et al., 2014). However, the study of 16 healthy volunteers demonstrated that mean peak SBP (+20 mmHg), DBP (+12 mmHg) and HR (+15 bpm) were all higher than placebo 1–2 hours after LSD administration and remained elevated until the 6-hour time point (Schmid, Enzler, et al., 2015). These transient and moderate elevations in BP and HR have not been associated with any serious adverse cardiac events in these studies. Despite the cardiac safety in recent clinical trials, a recent review of LSD toxicity case reports concluded there have been two LSD overdose sudden cardiac death cases (Nichols & Grob, 2018). In one case it was determined that the decedent had taken LSD 320 mg based on plasma concentration, which is >1000-fold higher than the therapeutic dosage range, while the other case was also presumed to have had excessively high dosing, with insufficient data to extrapolate exact dosage (Nichols & Grob, 2018).

In an older study of mescaline (5 mg/kg) and LSD (1.5 mcg/kg) investigating cross-tolerance and subjective effects with 10 healthy volunteers, LSD and mescaline both demonstrated increased HR and SBP, with LSD having a greater mean difference in effect on these measures (Wolbach et al., 1962).

DMT rapidly and transiently increased BP and HR in a dose-dependent manner that closely mimicked blood concentrations when given IV. The average HR increased by ~25 bpm (beats per minute) and MAP increased by ~18 mmHg in response to the 0.4 mg/kg dose, which resolved to baseline 15 minutes after the infusion ended (Strassman & Qualls, 1994).

Gastrointestinal

Nausea, one of the most common gastrointestinal adverse effects, was reported by 14–33% of participants in the psilocybin clinical trials (Thomas et al., 2017). Emesis was reported by one participant each in two of the trials (Bogenschutz et al., 2015; Griffiths et al., 2016).

Nausea (25%) and lack of appetite (31%) were reported by participants in a healthy volunteer LSD subjective effects study, but these were not reported in the LSD-assisted therapy clinical trial (Gasser et al., 2015; Schmid, Enzler, et al., 2015).

Acute mescaline intoxication may present with symptoms of nausea, vomiting, diarrhea, abdominal pain, and cramps that usually resolve 8–10 hours after ingestion, but there have been rare reports of abdominal pain persisting for 3–4 days (Teitelbaum & Wingeleth, 1977).

Renal

There have been no renal adverse effects reported in recent psilocybin or LSD clinical trials, but one study analyzed 2000–2016 data from the American Association of Poison Control Centers database and found that creatinine increased for 0.4%, rhabdomyolysis for 0.3%, and creatinine

phosphokinase (CPK) was elevated for 1% of recreational psilocybin mushroom exposure calls ($n = 5,883$) to poison centers. For recreational LSD exposure calls ($n = 3,554$) to poison control centers in the study, creatinine was increased for 1.4%, rhabdomyolysis for 1.1%, and CPK was elevated for 5%, but there was only one reported case of acute renal failure (Leonard et al., 2018).

Chronic Adverse Effects

Psychiatric

Mood Symptoms. Among 110 healthy volunteers who participated in eight psilocybin subjective drug effect studies, 8% reported symptoms of occasional mood swings and concentration problems that resolved after a few weeks. However, one volunteer required referral to a psychotherapist due to his irritability, anxiety, and depressive feelings that were subsequently stabilized after a few sessions of psychotherapy (Studerus et al., 2011).

A U.S. population sample (2008–2011) study evaluated associations between lifetime use of psilocybin ($n = 14,438$) and mental health outcomes, which demonstrated a lower likelihood (adjusted odds ratio [aOR] 0.7–0.8) of past-year serious psychological distress, inpatient mental health treatment, depression diagnosis, or prescription for psychiatric medication (Johansen & Krebs, 2015). There was no association between lifetime LSD use ($n = 12,806$) and adverse mental health outcomes, but LSD past-year use actually demonstrated a lower likelihood of serious psychological distress (aOR = 0.8), and inpatient (aOR = 0.5), or outpatient (aOR = 0.7) mental health treatment (Johansen & Krebs, 2015). In their earlier study of a 2001–2004 U.S. population sample there was an association between lifetime LSD use ($n = 17,486$) and lower likelihood of past-year outpatient mental health treatment and medication prescribed (both aORs = 0.9). Past-year LSD use was also associated with a lower likelihood of serious psychological distress in the worst month of the past year (aOR = 0.7) (Krebs & Johansen, 2013).

This same U.S. population sample (2008–2011) study also revealed associations between lifetime mescaline/peyote use (n = 5,595) and greater likelihood of past-year symptoms of major depressive episode (aOR = 1.2), but not an actual diagnosis of depression during the past year. Interestingly, when lifetime peyote use (n = 2,512) was analyzed independently, there was no association with past-year symptoms of major depressive episode or diagnosis of depression (Johansen & Krebs, 2015). In their earlier study of the 2001–2004 U.S. population sample, they found an association between lifetime mescaline/peyote use (n = 6,254) and lower likelihoods (aORs 0.6 and 0.9) of past-year medication prescribed, medication needed though not received, agoraphobia, and serious psychological distress in the worst month of the past year (Krebs & Johansen, 2013).

Hallucinogen Persisting Perceptual Disorder. The diagnostic criteria for hallucinogen persisting perceptual disorder (HPPD) include reexperiencing perceptual changes from previous hallucinogen intoxication that caused functional impairment (Halpern, Lerner, & Passie, 2018). The authors suggest there may be two distinct forms of HPPD; Type 1 with very brief "flashbacks" estimated to occur in 1 in 20 regular users, and Type 2 with more chronic, waxing and waning visual disturbances over months to years that cause distress or impairment for 1 in 50,000 hallucinogen users. In a survey-based investigation of 2,455 respondents with extensive drug histories (median of five different drugs used), about 24% reported at least one drug-free abnormal visual experience (e.g., trail, patterns, movement) on a constant or near-constant basis, while 4% found these experiences distressing enough consider treatment, and only 1% actually sought treatment (Baggott, Coyle, Erowid, Erowid, & Robertson, 2011).

Psychotic Thinking. The Krebs and Johansen (2013) U.S. population sample (2001–2004) study of psychedelics and mental health did not identify any association between lifetime use of psilocybin (n = 14,413), LSD (n = 17,486), or mescaline/peyote (n = 6,254), and nonaffective psychosis or visual phenomena consistent with "flashbacks" or HPPD. However, lifetime use of psilocybin (aOR = 0.6) and mescaline/peyote (aOR = 0.7) both demonstrated a lower likelihood of one specific psychotic symptom, which was "felt force taking over mind." Bogenschutz and Ross (2018) suggested that older reports of LSD-induced psychosis prompted them and other modern psychedelic researchers during the past 20 years to exclude participants with a personal or family history of psychotic spectrum illness and, to date, no cases of persisting psychosis have been reported in these more recent psilocybin or LSD clinical trials (Bogenschutz & Ross, 2018).

An older survey review of 44 U.S. physicians by Cohen (1960), who provided data for roughly 5,000 people with 50,000 LSD or mescaline sessions, described three mescaline cases of severe anxiety, one case of prolonged psychosis reaction for several days that resolved, and four physicians reported fleeting recurrences of the mescaline state after a period of complete recovery. For LSD, rates of attempted suicide were estimated to be 1.2, completed suicide 0.4, and prolonged psychotic reactions (>48 hours) at 1.8 per 1,000 psychiatric patients treated with LSD, while LSD experimental research subjects were estimated to have prolonged psychosis in only 0.8 per 1,000 subjects and no suicide attempts. About a decade later, Malleson (1971) attempted to replicate this survey study with 73 U.K. physicians, who provided data for roughly 4,300 patients with 49,000 LSD sessions, and he estimated the attendant suicide rate to be 0.7 and prolonged psychosis (>48 hours) at 9 per 1,000 LSD-treated psychiatric patients, with about two-thirds of the psychosis cases fully resolved during the subsequent weeks to months (Malleson, 1971).

Cardiovascular

There have been no reports of valvular heart disease with classic psychedelics in the medical literature to date, but a recent trend of "microdosing" LSD or psilocybin every few days for extended intervals may theoretically increase the risk of valvular heart disease due to consistent 5-HT$_{2B}$ receptor agonism (Nichols, 2016). Over the years, there have been several 5-HT$_{2B}$ agonists (e.g., fenfluramine and pergolide) withdrawn from the

U.S. market due to mitogenesis of interstitial cells from cardiac valve tissue that may potentially lead to valvular heart disease and sudden cardiac death (Roth, 2007). Research of psychedelic microdosing should closely monitor for cardiac valvulopathy, which can lead to subsequent valvular regurgitation.

Teratogenicity

A thorough review of the teratogenicity case reports, including reports of 161 children of parents who took LSD before or during pregnancy, concluded there was no clear evidence of LSD-related teratogenicity in humans or animals (Long, 1972). Another genetic toxicology review of LSD by M. M. Cohen, the same researcher who first published a study of *in vitro* LSD chromosomal damage that led to a popular media panic, also concluded that LSD was neither teratogenic nor oncogenic (Cohen & Shiloh, 1977).

A cytogenetic study comparing 57 peyote-consuming Huichol Indians to 50 Huichol controls who did not use peyote revealed no detectable abnormalities in the chromosomes of lymphocytes sampled. The treating physician for the population also observed no increase in congenital abnormalities at birth despite consistent consumption of peyote by mothers during pregnancy (Dorrance, Janiger, & Teplitz, 1975).

Drug Interactions

Coadministration of certain psychiatric medications that also bind to 5-HT$_{2A}$ receptors, such as buspirone and antipsychotics (chlorpromazine, haloperidol, risperidone), have reduced the subjective effects of psilocybin by ~40–99%, which could theoretically decrease the efficacy of psychedelic-assisted therapy with classic psychedelics (Keeler, 1967; Pokorny, Preller, Kraehenmann, & Vollenweider, 2016; Vollenweider, Vollenweider-Scherpenhuyzen, Babler, Vogel, & Hell, 1998).

Psilocin is metabolized by UGT1A9 and UGT1A10 glucuronidation, so coadministration of medications inhibiting these enzymes may theoretically increase dose-related adverse effects of psilocybin (Manevski et al., 2010). Based on *in vitro* data, it has been proposed that LSD is metabolized by cytochrome P450 enzymes; therefore, various enzyme inhibitors may theoretically increase dose-related adverse effects of LSD (Klette, Anderson, Poch, Nimrod, & ElSohly, 2000).

The harmala alkaloid monoamine oxidase inhibitors (MAOIs) (harmine, harmaline, tetrahydroharmine) are routinely combined with DMT in the Amazonian sacrament ayahuasca (see discussion of ayahuasca below) without precipitation of serotonin syndrome or other severe harm. Harmala alkaloids have also been combined with other psychedelics and have the general effect of prolonging or intensifying the subjective experience (Ott, 1999). However, the safety of combining psychedelics other than DMT with harmala alkaloids is not well documented, and cases of death have occurred when combining DMT analogues such as 5-methoxy-N,N-dimethyltryptamine (5-MeO-DMT) with harmala alkaloids (International Center for Ethnobotanical Education, Research, and Service [ICEERS], 2017).

Harm Reduction and Risk Management

• Hallucinogen research guidelines for safety recommend reassurance and deescalation by the therapists guiding the session as the best strategy for managing psychological adverse effects, but in the rare cases of severe acute distress, the medication of choice would be a benzodiazepine such as diazepam 10 mg (Johnson et al., 2008). The benzodiazepine should reduce severe psychological distress and corresponding cardiovascular symptoms of tachycardia and hypertension related to a panic attack.

• In the case of severe psychotic symptoms, antipsychotics such as risperidone and olanzapine may be considered, but these should be a last resort due to their own neurological adverse effect profiles with extrapyramidal symptoms. Haloperidol should be avoided entirely, based on a study demonstrating that IV haloperidol 0.21 mg/kg pretreatment in healthy volunteers actually exacerbated psilocybin's subjective effects of anxious ego dissolution, loss of thought control, and ideas of reference (Vollenweider, Vollenweider-Scherpenhuyzen, et al., 1998).

• Monitor for development of valvular heart disease with chronic use.

Novel Designer Psychedelics

The number of psychedelic substances in the illicit marketplace continues to grow at a rapid rate with novel designer psychedelics that include phenethylamines (2C- and -NBOMe derivatives), synthetic cathinones (mephedrone, methylone), tryptamines and DMT analogues (DiPT, 5-MeO-DMT), ketamine analogues (methoxetamine), as well as other research chemicals. Most lack basic scientific data regarding dose–response relationships or adverse effects in controlled environments.

Several of these novel psychedelics have been implicated in fatal adverse events. Compounds such as NBOMe are potent and active at even microgram dosage ranges, with several reported fatalities (Morini et al., 2017). There have been cases in which 2,5-dimethoxy-4-(n)-propylphenethylamine (2C-P) was mistaken for 2,5-dimethoxy-4-bromophenethylamine (2C-B), resulting in severe serotonergic toxicity (Stoller et al., 2017). Cathinones, also known as "bath salts," and the dissociative methoxetamine have also led to fatalities (Botanas, Bryan de la Pena, Kim, Lee, & Cheong, 2019; Busardo, Kyriakou, Napoletano, Marinelli, & Zaami, 2015). Ultimately, there may be therapeutic potential in novel designer psychedelics, although extreme caution should be exercised until they are studied further in controlled settings.

MDMA

MDMA is a ring-substituted phenylethylamine classified as both a psychedelic and as a psychostimulant. Similar to psychostimulant *d*-amphetamine, MDMA is able to release both dopamine and norepinephrine from presynaptic nerve terminals. However, unlike *d*-amphetamine, MDMA primarily releases serotonin from presynaptic nerve terminals. It also binds to postsynaptic 5-HT$_{2A}$ receptors, 5-HT, norepinephrine (NE), and dopamine (DA) reuptake pumps, and has neurohormonal effects resulting in vasopressin and oxytocin release.

Acute Adverse Effects

Psychiatric

Several Phase II trials (*n* = 103) have investigated MDMA use in posttraumatic stress disorder (PTSD) populations, including some participants who had comorbid depressive or anxiety disorders. In a pooled analysis, MDMA active doses (75–125 mg) were associated with 72% reporting anxiety, which was ~24% higher frequency than controls (0–40 mg) during experimental sessions (Mithoefer et al., 2019). During the weeks between the first MDMA administration and before open-label experimental Session 3, 24% of the active dose group reported anxiety, which was ~14% higher than controls; depressed mood, irritability, and panic attacks were reported ~6–8% higher for the active dose group than for controls (only one with depressed mood). Suicidal ideation was transiently increased during the treatment period and occurred 28% more frequently in the active dose group than in controls (25% vs. 7%), but this may not be related to MDMA effects since suicidal ideation was already ~30% more frequent in the active dose group at baseline even before MDMA dosing (46% vs. 17%). There was no suicidal behavior during the MDMA treatment period. After two MDMA psychotherapy sessions, the active dose group also experienced a 22-point greater reduction from baseline on Clinician-Administered PTSD Scale, DSM-IV version (CAPS-IV) total PTSD scores than controls, with 54.2% of the active dose group in remission compared to only 22.6% of controls, which suggests substantial resolution of anxiety symptoms (Mithoefer et al., 2019). Lorazepam or zolpidem, respectively, have been used to manage residual anxiety or insomnia symptoms in the week after MDMA use (Oehen, Traber, Widmer, & Schnyder, 2013; Ot'alora et al., 2018).

Neurological

General. MDMA active doses (75–125 mg) were associated with 64% frequency of jaw tightness and 40% with dizziness during experimental sessions, which were ~24 and ~21% higher than controls, respectively (Mithoefer et al., 2019).

Hyperthermia. Temperature responses have been measured in response to MDMA use in a number of laboratory studies and collectively support a dose-dependent effect on body temperature. Doses <1 mg/kg produced negligible and statistically insignificant changes in body temperature, doses of 1–1.9 mg/kg produced significant changes of around 0.4°C, while doses >2 mg/kg produced temperature increases of 0.4–1°C. Most cases of MDMA-induced hyperthermia are responsive to cooler environments and aggressive cooling (ice packs or ice baths) and occur in thermally stressful environments (hot tubs or dance clubs) (Parrott, 2012b).

Neuroendocrine. MDMA promotes the release of antidiuretic hormone (ADH), which can cause the syndrome of inappropriate ADH (SIADH), characterized by excessive water reabsorption and hyponatremia. Excessive water intake can also exacerbate this risk, which may lead to hyponatremic encephalopathy and sudden death. Severe hyponatremia also increases the risk for seizures; thus, persons predisposed to hyponatremia or low sodium may be at increased risk for complications of MDMA (Campbell & Rosner, 2008).

Seizures. MDMA has never precipitated a seizure in clinical trials, although it has led to seizures in individuals with a history of epilepsy and new onset seizures in uncontrolled nonclinical settings. MDMA may cause seizures by a number of mechanisms, including lowering sodium levels via vasopressin release, increasing core body temperature, and excessive release of monoamines (Giorgi et al., 2006).

Cardiovascular

A handful of studies demonstrated that MDMA increases BP and HR in a dose-dependent manner, and peak effects are not significantly different than oral doses of amphetamine 40 mg or methamphetamine 40 mg (Hysek et al., 2014; Kirkpatrick et al., 2012; Kolbrich et al., 2008; Mas et al., 1999). Maximum differences in cardiovascular parameters were observed 60–120 min-

utes after MDMA ingestion and were ~40 mmHg for SBP, ~25 mmHg for DBP, and ~30 bpm for HR higher than placebo (Hysek et al., 2014; Kirkpatrick et al., 2012; Kolbrich et al., 2008; Mas et al., 1999). The pooled data from Phase II PTSD clinical trials demonstrated that MDMA active doses 75–125 mg had a higher mean increase in peak SBP ~18 mmHg, DBP ~7 mmHg, and HR ~20 bpm than control doses 0–40 mg; there was one serious adverse event of exacerbated ventricular asystole reported with the 125-mg dose (Mithoefer et al., 2019). In some cases, hypertensive effects can also be pronounced to the point of hypertensive crisis (Vollenweider, Gamma, Liechti, & Huber, 1998).

Gastrointestinal

MDMA active doses (75–125 mg) have been reported to cause acute nausea (~40%) and lack of appetite (49%) that were ~21–26% higher than those in controls (0–40 mg) (Mithoefer et al., 2019).

Chronic Adverse Effects

Psychiatric

MDMA neurotoxicity is complex, and the neurotoxic potential of MDMA has been a controversial subject in the scientific community for decades. Along with the multiple problematic aspects in generalizing data from ecstasy users to clinical MDMA use, data misrepresentation, questionable methodologies, a political agenda, and biased government funding has plagued MDMA neurotoxicity research (Grob, 2000). Human neuroimaging studies have consistently demonstrated that heavy recreational ecstasy use is associated with reduced serotonin reuptake transporter (SERT) densities, while other studies have found that deficits are correlated with total lifetime use, intensity of use, and concurrent drug use (Parrott, 2012a). Recent PTSD clinical trials have not reported any psychotic or mood symptoms as adverse effects, but MDMA and other psychostimulants are known to potentially exacerbate underlying neuropsychiatric conditions such as bipolar disorder and schizophrenia (Vaiva et al., 2001).

There are many possible mechanisms of short and long-term MDMA-induced neurotoxicity, including the production of toxic metabolites or monoamine depletion; therefore, excessive use with concurrent drugs may increase the neurotoxic potential (e.g., MDMA + methamphetamine or alcohol) (Green, King, Shortall, & Fone, 2012).

Neurological

Cognitive Impairment. In clinical laboratory studies of humans there has been a lack of evidence for persistent short- or long-term deficits (Mithoefer, Jerome, & Doblin, 2003). Doses of 1.7 mg/kg were used safely in the clinical laboratory setting without evidence of neurotoxicity such as changes in SERT density or memory problems (Grob, 2000; Mithoefer et al., 2003; Vollenweider, Jones, & Baggott, 2001). Animal models of MDMA-induced 5-HT toxicity have demonstrated long-term damage to 5-HT neurons, but problems with interspecies scaling have led some to call into question the validity of extrapolating deficits observed in animals to humans (Green et al., 2012).

Parkinson's Disease. In 2002, prominent neurological researcher George Ricaurte published an article in *Science* stating that common recreational doses of MDMA were able to produce severe dopaminergic toxicity in primates (Ricaurte, Yuan, Hatzidimitriou, Cord, & McCann, 2002). He went on to conclude that "[MDMA] may put these individuals at increased risk for developing Parkinsonism." It was later discovered that the adverse effects described were due to methamphetamine administration rather than MDMA, and his paper was subsequently retracted from the scientific literature (LeVay, 2008; Mithoefer et al., 2003; Ricaurte, Yuan, Hatzidimitriou, Cord, & McCann, 2003).

Teratogenicity

MDMA is known to be able to traverse the placenta and is presumed to be teratogenic (Mohamed, Ben Hamida, Cassel, de Vasconcelos, & Jones, 2011). There are no high-quality data available to inform safety risks during pregnancy, although heavy ecstasy use is likely deleterious to the fetus. A prospective case–control study followed polydrug users during pregnancy and found that mothers who used ecstasy had children with psychomotor retardation that persisted up to the 2-year study endpoint (Singer et al., 2012, 2016). The average mother enrolled in the study had used MDMA 171 times in her lifetime prior to pregnancy, many mothers used weekly, and MDMA-using mothers also ingested significantly more tobacco, marijuana, cocaine, amphetamines, LSD, and mushrooms during their pregnancy than mother's who did not use ecstasy.

Drug Interactions

Antidepressants that inhibit the serotonin reuptake pump (selective serotonin reuptake inhibitor [SSRI], serotonin–norepinephrine reuptake inhibitor [SNRI], tricyclic antidepressant [TCA]) have been demonstrated to greatly diminish or even abolish the psychedelic effects of MDMA in healthy volunteers (Farre et al., 2007; Hysek, Simmler, et al., 2012; Liechti & Vollenweider, 2000; Segura et al., 2005; Tancer & Johanson, 2007).

The combined use of psychostimulants such as amphetamines or cathinones with MDMA is known to lead to pharmacodynamic interactions, including increased cardiovascular and neuropsychiatric toxicity (Mohamed et al., 2011; Rietjens, Hondebrink, Westerink, & Meulenbelt, 2012). Alcohol (0.8 g/kg ethanol) has been demonstrated to increase plasma concentrations of MDMA ~10% and impair psychomotor coordination (Hernandez-Lopez et al., 2002). Cannabis is frequently combined with ecstasy in a recreational setting and may help reduce negative effects associated with the comedown of MDMA, such as irritability or aggression, although it may also increase anxiety, impulsivity, or psychotic symptoms (Mohamed et al., 2011).

Monoamines are metabolized by monoamine oxidase (MAO) and inhibition of this enzyme using MAOIs is contraindicated with MDMA. Concurrent use of MAOIs and ecstasy has led to cases of death and is considered the most dangerous drug interaction (Pilgrim, Gerostamoulos, & Drummer, 2011; Pilgrim, Gerostamoulos, Woodford,

& Drummer, 2012; Smilkstein, Smolinske, & Rumack, 1987).

MDMA is metabolized by cytochrome P450 2D6 (*CYP2D6*) to the active metabolite 3,4-methylenedioxyamphetamine (MDA). Inhibition of *CYP2D6* via concurrent drug administration or a poor metabolizer genotype for the *CYP2D6* enzyme is associated with increased plasma concentrations and prolonged effects of MDMA (de la Torre et al., 2005; Hysek, Simmler, et al., 2012; Schmid, Rickli, et al., 2015). However, the contribution to toxicity of *CYP2D6* status may be minimal due to MDMA inhibiting *CYP2D6* itself and rendering all users temporarily to have reduced *CYP2D6* function (Schmid et al., 2016). It has been hypothesized that inhibition of other hepatic enzymes such as *CYP1A2, 2C19,* or *2B6* may play a larger role in toxic reactions than *CYP2D6* (Schmid et al., 2016). Nevertheless, cases of prolonged effects, harm, and death have been reported with the use of the strong *CYP2D6, 3A4,* and *2B6* inhibitor ritonavir (Henry & Hill, 1998; Papaseit et al., 2012; Rietjens et al., 2012). Therefore, serious caution is warranted with drugs that strongly inhibit CYP enzymes or inhibit multiple CYP enzymes simultaneously.

Harm Reduction and Risk Management

• Caution or avoidance is recommended in persons with a history of epilepsy or seizure disorder and with medications known to lower the seizure threshold.

• MDMA may not be appropriate for persons with uncontrolled hypertension, history of stroke, myocardial infarction, heart failure, arrhythmias, or other advanced cardiovascular conditions.

• Clonidine or carvedilol were able to attenuate the hemodynamic and thermodynamic effects of MDMA without reducing the psychotropic effects. Either drug could be useful in the management of MDMA-induced hypertensive crisis (Hysek, Brugger, et al., 2012; Hysek, Schmid, et al., 2012).

• Avoid drugs with interaction potential such as MAOIs or *CYP2D6* inhibitors.

• Taper and discontinuation of antidepressants at least 2 weeks prior to MDMA use is recommended to avoid loss of efficacy.

▣ Ayahuasca

Ayahuasca is a traditional plant brew sacrament containing DMT and MAOIs that has been used historically in Amazonian shamanic rituals.

Acute Adverse Effects

Psychiatric

Clinical studies of healthy volunteers demonstrate a dose-dependent increase in all domains of the HRS (except Volition), while the Addiction Research Center Inventory (ARCI) has demonstrated increases in Morphine–Benzedrine, LSD, and Amphetamine scales demonstrating ayahuasca's increased euphoria, somatic–dysphoric, and stimulating effects, respectively (Dos Santos, Osorio, Crippa, & Hallak, 2016b). Other studies of healthy volunteers have described transient dissociation, dysphoria, and anxiety of 20-minutes duration or suspiciousness and menace that resolved as ayahuasca's acute effects resolved (Dos Santos, 2013b; Riba et al., 2001). High doses of ayahuasca have been reported to carry a risk of adverse psychological reactions such as panic or traumatization (Gable, 2007).

One neuroimaging study of experienced ayahuasca users (*n* = 10) observed increases in the Young Mania Rating Scale (YMRS) by ~8 points and in the Brief Psychiatric Rating Scale (BPRS) by ~8 points that returned to baseline 200 minutes after ayahuasca administration (de Araujo et al., 2012). In a preliminary report of six persons with major depression, ayahuasca produced nonsignificant increases in the BPRS that correlated with reports of disorientation/confusion, conceptual disorganization, emotional withdrawal, and psychomotor retardation (Osorio Fde et al., 2015). Another open-label study of persons with recurrent depression (*n* = 17) treated with ayahuasca observed acute and transient increases in Clinician-Administered Dissociative States Scale (CADSS) scores by ~20 points 80 minutes after administration. These participants were reported to be calm and relaxed during the acute drug effects, as demonstrated by a decrease in the Anxious Depression BPRS subscale mean score by ~4 points, in the

HAM-D by ~11 points, and the MADRS by ~6 points from baseline to 180 minutes after ayahuasca administration (Sanches et al., 2016). A recent randomized, placebo-controlled trial for treatment-resistant depression (*n* = 29) demonstrated nonsignificant score increases on the CADSS and BPRS during the ayahuasca session (Palhano-Fontes et al., 2019).

Cardiovascular

The cardiovascular effects of ayahuasca were examined in 18 healthy volunteers. HR and SBP were not significantly increased, but DBP increased by ~9 mmHg (Riba et al., 2003). Other studies have reported HR >100 bpm and SBP >140 mmHg, although no antihypertensive rescue interventions were required, and episodes of tachycardia or hypertension lasted 15–30 minutes on average when potential tolerance to cardiovascular effects was observed (Dos Santos, 2013a, 2013b).

Gastrointestinal

The traditional sacrament ayahuasca is notorious for causing gastrointestinal distress, involving intense eructation, nausea, vomiting, or diarrhea in a large percentage of users. An open-label depression study reported emesis in 47% of volunteers, and a randomized trial also reported nausea (71%) and vomiting (57%) at even higher rates (Palhano-Fontes et al., 2019; Sanches et al., 2016). In the ayahuasca tradition, these effects are thought to be cleansing/healing (*limpia*) and are collectively known as purging (*la purga*) (dos Santos, 2013a).

Drug Interactions

Ayahuasca is unique among psychedelic sacraments, as its effect is produced from the combination of MAOIs found in the *Banisteriopsis caapi* vine and DMT from *Psychotria viridis* or *Diplopterys cabrerana*. Due to its MAOI properties, serious drug and dietary interactions are of concern among persons who participate in ayahuasca ceremonies.

Monoamine oxidase A (MAO-A) is an enzyme that breaks down the neurotransmitters 5-HT, DA, and NE. Drug and dietary interaction potential with MAOIs was originally described with pharmaceutical MAOIs in combination with many drugs, but particularly other antidepressants (Gillman, 2016; Youdim, Edmondson, & Tipton, 2006). This is why the recent ayahuasca depression trials all had participants taper and discontinue antidepressants at least 2 weeks prior to the ayahuasca session.

The resulting toxidrome known as serotonin syndrome is life threatening and can cause death. Potential for severe drug interactions has been confirmed with at least one case report detailing severe physiological responses from the combination of ayahuasca with SSRIs (Callaway & Grob, 1998). An analysis of calls to U.S. Poison Control Centers from 2005 to 2015 revealed 538 exposure calls related to ayahuasca, with clinical manifestations including hallucination (35%), tachycardia and agitation (both 34%), hypertension (16%), and mydriasis (13%). Twenty-eight (5%) cases required emergent intubation, and three persons died. There were 12 reports of seizure, four of cardiac arrest, and seven of respiratory arrest. While poison control calls did not allow analysis of concomitant drug use, the symptoms and outcomes reported are consistent with serotonin syndrome in severe cases (Heise & Brooks, 2017). Therefore, it is reasonable to determine contraindicated medications with harmala alkaloids or ayahuasca by extrapolating from MAOI contraindications (see Table 22.1).

Prior to ayahuasca use, it is the interacting drugs' pharmacokinetics (opposed to ayahuasca's) that should inform the recommendation of how long to avoid use. A general rule of thumb is to wait at least five elimination half-lives from the time of last drug ingestion to the time of ayahuasca use. While this is the minimum time period that is predicted to be safe, consideration of longer periods of abstinence should be given due to individual variability in elimination of various drugs or the presence of long-acting active metabolites.

The pharmacokinetics and reversibility of MAO inhibition induced by harmala alkaloids in ayahuasca carries important practical implications for understanding and avoiding drug and dietary interactions. For example, the half-life of harmine and

TABLE 22.1. Potential Adverse Drug–Drug Interactions Due to MAOIs in Ayahuasca

Psychiatric medications	Allergy, cough, and cold	Appetite suppressants
• Antidepressants: SSRIs, SNRIs, clomipramine, imipramine, St. John's wort • Lithium • Attention-deficit/hyperactivity disorder stimulants: amphetamine salts, methylphenidate • Ziprasidone	• Chlorpheniramine • Dextromethorphan • Pseudoephedrine	• Caffeine (high doses) • Coca or cocaine • *Ma huang* (ephedra) • Phentermine

Opioid analgesics	Phenethylamines	Shamanic sacraments
• Meperidine • Methadone • Propoxyphene • Tramadol	• Cathinones: mephedrone, methylone, methylenedioxypyrovalerone • 2Cx, Dox, and NBOMe analogues • Mescaline • MDMA	• 5-MeO-DMT • *Kambo* • Tobacco purges/cleanses

harmaline ranges from 2 to 3 hours, while the half-life of tetrahydroharmine is approximately 8 hours (Callaway et al., 1999). Therefore, it is predicted that after 48 hours, there would be very little MAO inhibition provided by harmala alkaloids and interacting foods or drugs could be resumed shortly thereafter. Harmine is both a substrate and an inhibitor of the *CYP2D6* enzyme, with differences in peak harmine concentrations for poor and extensive *CYP2D6* metabolizers (Callaway, 2005).

Reports of death in connection with ayahuasca ceremonies or retreat centers tend to feature the concurrent or successive use of different natural or pharmaceutical medicines, often with intense purgative effects or strong drug interaction potential. Deaths are likely due to arrhythmias or seizures induced by electrolyte abnormalities, or from serotonin syndrome. Factors that appear to increase the risk of ayahuasca use involve the use of alternative MAOIs such as those from *Peganum harmala* (Syrian rue), alternative psychedelics or additional plants in the brew (e.g., 5-MeO-DMT instead of *N,N*-DMT), concomitant use of contraindicated drugs with MAOIs, concurrent tobacco cleanses, or other shamanic sacraments, such as the frog venom *kambo* (Crittenden, 2015; dos Santos, 2013a; Heise & Brooks, 2017; ICEERS, 2017; Ott, 1999; Plucinska, 2015).

Dietary Interaction

MAO in the small intestine and liver is responsible for degrading other biogenic amines (besides DMT) as one of the body's natural defense mechanisms. Although tyramine, an amino acid that is normally metabolized by MAO, has a vasopressor effect when ingested in the setting of MAO inhibition, it can result in dangerously high blood pressure. Effects of tyramine intake in persons taking ayahuasca have not been described. Table 22.2 lists common food and beverage items that contain tyramine and should be avoided with MAOIs, or at least limited to <5 g/day intake.

Chronic Adverse Effects

Psychiatric

There is little evidence of psychological risk with intermittent long-term use of ayahuasca (Dos Santos, Balthazar, Bouso, & Hallak, 2016). Longitudinal studies in healthy volunteers do not demonstrate adverse effects and do demonstrate decreased psychopathology scores. To date, ayahuasca has been tested in a few small studies of addiction and treatment-resistant depression without serious psychiatric adverse effects (Dos Santos, Osorio, et al., 2016). Ayahuasca or DMT use is not appropriate for persons with a history

TABLE 22.2. Potential Adverse Reactions of Tyramine-Containing Foods and Drinks to MAOIs in Ayahuasca

Food	Drink
• Aged cheeses	• Tap beers
• Air-dried, aged, or fermented meats, sausages, or salami	• Nonpasteurized beer
	• Chianti
• Pickled herring	• Vermouth
• Soy sauce	• Kombucha
• Sauerkraut	• Acidophilus milk
• Fava beans and other broad bean pods	• Caffeinated beverages
• Tofu	
• Concentrated yeast extract	
• Food that is spoiled	
• Overripe fruits	
• Miso soup	
• Chocolate	

of bipolar or psychotic disorders, and there have been several reports of psychological crises precipitated by ayahuasca in these persons (Dos Santos, Bouso, & Hallak, 2017). However, ayahuasca is not thought to cause schizophrenia, as rates of psychotic episodes in the União do Vegetal (UDV) do not differ from population averages (Gable, 2007).

Teratogenicity

Ayahuasca use in pregnancy is controversial, although pregnant women who worship with South American ayahuasca churches such as the Santo Daime and UDV have a historical precedent of using ayahuasca without apparent ill effects to their children (Dos Santos, 2013b; Labate & Feeney, 2012).

Harm Reduction and Risk Management

• Avoid drugs and food with interaction potential for appropriate lengths of time prior to ayahuasca use.

• Persons using ayahuasca may be instructed to sit up or to lie on their sides during the experience to reduce aspiration risk should vomiting occur.

• Caution use in persons who are older, medically frail, or particularly susceptible to electrolyte abnormalities,

• Avoid other intense purgatives or shamanic sacraments that may pose risk of electrolyte abnormalities or drug interactions.

■ Ibogaine

Ibogaine is an indolylalkylamine psychedelic with a distinct mechanism of action and safety profile. It binds to opioid (μ, κ, δ), N-methyl-D-aspartate (NMDA) glutamate, σ and nicotinic receptors, as well as monoamine transporters (Litjens & Brunt, 2016). Ibogaine is metabolized to the long-acting active metabolite noribogaine. While it is touted for its potent addiction interrupting properties, especially with opioids, several cardiac-related deaths have been reported with ibogaine use. It appears that the presence or absence of withdrawal symptoms secondary to substance use disorders, individual pharmacokinetics (*CYP2D6* phenotype), dose of ibogaine administered, concurrent drug use, and preexisting medical conditions may all substantially influence the safety of ibogaine (Alper, Stajic, & Gill, 2012). Therefore, while psychological risk precautions are similar to other psychedelic-assisted psychotherapy modalities, additional medical precautions are warranted to reduce physiological risks associated with ibogaine use.

Acute Adverse Effects

Psychiatric

Few studies have systematically reported on neuropsychiatric side effects of ibogaine, as the majority of the literature has focused on reporting outcomes related to withdrawal and detoxification from drugs of abuse, particularly opioids. Ibogaine carries an anecdotal reputation of eliciting a challenging or unpleasant psychological experience relative to other psychedelics. In one phenomenological analysis of subjective ibogaine experiences in drug-dependent persons, strongly unpleasant physical effects, heightened memory retrieval associated with drug abuse, and dream-like visions were reported (Schenberg et al., 2017). Rarely, mania or psychosis have occurred after ibogaine use (Houenou, Homri, Leboyer, & Drancourt, 2011; Marta, Ryan, Kopelowicz, & Koek, 2015).

Neurological

Acute neurological adverse effects reported with ibogaine occur commonly when using ibogaine to treat drug dependence. A couple of studies have indicated adverse effects consistent with transient cerebellar dysfunction, including mild tremors, ataxia, dizziness, nystagmus, and dysmetria. Cerebellar dysfunction occurred within the first 2 hours after administration, with resolution by 24 hours (Mash et al., 2001). Another study utilized a dose–response design with noribogaine (60, 120, or 180 mg) and reported three severe adverse events (nausea, vomiting, and headache), in which headache and visual impairment (increased intensity of light) were also the most common neuropsychiatric side effects (Glue et al., 2016b).

Several case reports have documented severe neurological adverse effects such as muscle spasms, tonic–clonic seizures, decorticate posturing, and coma with permanent cognitive deficits after ibogaine use (Alper et al., 2012; Litjens & Brunt, 2016).

Cardiovascular

Cardiotoxicity is a well-documented and severe adverse effect associated with the use of ibogaine or iboga. Ibogaine binds to the hERG potassium channel on cardiac myocytes, which can prolong the QTc interval and increases the risk of monomorphic ventricular tachyarrhythmias such as *torsades de pointes* (TdP) (Alper et al., 2012, 2016). In a dose–response study of noribogaine in opioid-dependent persons ($n = 27$), there was a dose-dependent effect on the QTc interval with average increases of ~16, 28, and 42 milliseconds (msec) in the 60, 120, and 180 mg dose groups, respectively. Two participants had a QTc interval >480 msec, and two had QTc interval increases >60 msec (Glue et al., 2016b). A similarly designed study using lower doses in healthy volunteers had one participant with a QTc interval increase >60 msec approximately 24 hours postadministration of noribogaine 10 mg (Glue et al., 2015b). Additional effects such as bradycardia, cardiopulmonary arrest, and pulmonary embolism have been reported to occur with close temporal association to ibogaine use (Alper et al., 2012).

Due to the wide ranges in reports of ibogaine doses administered, variability in dosing effects, and dose-dependent cardiotoxic effects, it is unclear what the optimal dose is in the management of detoxification when considering risks versus benefits. One study of 50 ECG-monitored persons being detoxified from opioids with ibogaine reported using 18–20 mg/kg as a flood dose without any fatalities, but lower doses of 8–12 mg/kg may also be effective with less risk (Malcolm, Polanco, & Barsuglia, 2018; Mash et al., 2001).

In a case series, one subject died after receiving a dose of 29 mg/kg ibogaine, highlighting the risk of overdosing (Alper, Lotsof, Frenken, Luciano, & Bastiaans, 1999). Similarly, another study of 14 persons that used a mean dose of 31.4 mg/kg had one participant die during treatment (Noller, Frampton, & Yazar-Klosinski, 2018). Forensically, there have been 12 fatalities due to ibogaine that reported a mean dose of 14.3 ± 6.1 mg/kg (range 4.5–29 mg/kg), which is within the recommended therapeutic range, but concurrent use of drugs of abuse and other confounding medical risk factors (e.g., advanced cardiac disease) were common in these deaths (Alper et al., 2012).

Gastrointestinal

Several studies in both drug-dependent and healthy volunteers have reported nausea in response to ibogaine administration (Glue et al., 2015; Mash et al., 2001). Vomiting commonly occurs during ibogaine use as a single episode in response to motion (Alper et al., 1999). Prolonged vomiting may indicate the presence of significant withdrawal if treating an opioid-dependent subject and further increase the risk of medical complications due to electrolyte imbalance.

Teratogenicity

Clinical guidelines for use of ibogaine list pregnancy as a medical exclusionary criterion due to lack of evidence (Dickinson et al., 2016). In an experiment investigating uterine contractility in response to ibogaine administration, it was found that lower doses stimulated contraction of uterine smooth muscle, while larger doses inhibited it, although it is unclear whether this is clinically significant (Orescanin-Dusic et al., 2018).

Drug Interactions

Concurrent use of other medications that also have the ability to prolong the QTc interval would increase the risk of arrhythmias from ibogaine. Methadone is commonly used for opioid use disorder and is also associated with severe QTc prolongation; therefore, it is recommended to switch to a different opioid agent at least 1 week prior to using ibogaine in opioid-dependent persons (Glue et al., 2016a).

Ibogaine is able to potentiate opioid signaling, despite lacking characteristic opioid effects such as pupil constriction, which may raise lethality if opioids are used simultaneously or subsequently (Alper et al., 2012). Also, ibogaine appears to have the ability to sensitize persons to other drugs of abuse such as cocaine or methamphetamine, which would increase risks if used concurrently and have been reported to cause death in combination (Addy, 2012; Szumlinski, Maisonneuve, & Glick, 2000).

Drugs that inhibit the metabolic enzyme *CYP2D6* may increase ibogaine associated toxicity and one study demonstrated that pretreatment with the *CYP2D6* inhibitor paroxetine 20 mg was able to increase exposure to ibogaine/noribogaine by ~2 fold (Glue et al., 2015b); therefore, *CYP2D6*-poor metabolizers may also have increased risks with ibogaine.

Harm Reduction and Risk Management

• Ibogaine is not appropriate for persons with cardiac diseases such as congenital long QTc syndrome, history of myocardial infarction, angina, coronary artery disease, or other advanced cardiac conditions.

• Clinical guidelines for ibogaine use recommend evaluation of medical history, ECG, electrolyte and liver function no greater than 2.5 times the upper limit of normal prior to ibogaine use, as well as telemetry (continuous ECG monitoring), pulse oximetry, and vital sign monitoring during the experience (Dickinson et al., 2016).

• Protocols, personnel, and equipment required for emergent cardiac resuscitation should be in place prior to ibogaine use (Brown & Alper, 2018).

• Ibogaine should not be used for detoxification from alcohol or benzodiazepines.

• Ibogaine should not be used concurrently with drugs of abuse such as alcohol, cocaine, or methamphetamine, or with medications that can prolong the QTc interval or inhibit *CYP2D6*.

▪ Ketamine

Ketamine is an arylcyclohexylamine derivative metabolized to active metabolite norketamine by *N*-demethylation (Zhao et al., 2012). Ketamine is an NMDA receptor antagonist that provides a "trapping block" of excitatory glutamatergic transmission (Ghasemi et al., 2014). Earlier studies of ketamine for mood disorders utilized a racemic mixture of R- and S-ketamine, while the recently approved esketamine nasal spray for treatment-resistant depression is purely the S- enantiomer. There have been few head-to-head data to determine any safety differences between the racemic mixture and esketamine; therefore, adverse effects are collectively discussed in this section (Andrade, 2017a).

Acute Adverse Effects

Psychiatric

A review of 61 clinical studies with nearly 450 patients using IV ketamine infusion for treating depression demonstrated increased dissociation, psychotomimetic effects, and manic symptoms based on CADSS, BPRS, and YMRS, respectively (Ryan, Marta,

& Koek, 2014). The peak scores on these scales were higher than placebo by ~7 points for CADSS, ~3 points for BPRS, and ~3 points for YMRS during the infusion, but all resolved by 4 hours after administration (Murrough et al., 2013; Zarate et al., 2006). In this comprehensive review of ketamine in depression, only three participants discontinued for worsening mood and one for increased anxiety from randomized controlled trials, but from open-label trials there was also a panic attack, a suicide attempt during the washout period before an infusion, and a "mild" hypomanic episode after the third infusion (Ryan et al., 2014). The most common adverse reaction from the intranasal esketamine U.S. Food and Drug Administration (FDA)–approval trials for depression was dissociation for 41% versus 9% with placebo, while anxiety was 13% versus 6%, and euphoric mood was 4% versus 1%, respectively (Janssen Pharmaceuticals Inc., 2019). Due to black box warnings of dissociation and sedation, the Spravato Risk Evaluation and Mitigation Strategy (REMS) requires at least 2 hours of monitoring after intranasal administration in a clinic. There are also additional black box warnings for potential abuse or misuse, and suicidality for pediatric and young adult patients taking antidepressants (Janssen Pharmaceuticals Inc., 2019).

Neurological

Adverse effects reported in ketamine clinical trials for depression included headache, dizziness, nausea, metallic taste, blurred vision, diplopia, imbalance, paresthesia, weakness, fatigue, drowsiness, and poor memory that resolved a short time after the infusion ended (Katalinic et al., 2013; Ryan et al., 2014). In the recent esketamine FDA approval trials, the most common neurological adverse reactions were dizziness (29%), vertigo (23%), sedation (23%), headache (20%), dysgeusia (19%), hypoesthesia (18%), and lethargy (11%) (Janssen Pharmaceuticals Inc., 2019).

Cardiovascular

Transient elevations in cardiac vital signs were commonly reported after ketamine administration for patients with depression (Ryan et al., 2014). In an analysis of three IV ketamine depression trials ($n = 97$), there were mean increases from baseline in SBP (19.6 mmHg) and DBP (13.4 mmHg), where 14.3% of participants received antihypertensive rescue medication for these ketamine-induced hemodynamic changes (Wan et al., 2015). In two intranasal esketamine trials, the maximum mean increase from baseline in SBP (16–19 mmHg), DBP (8–10 mmHg) and HR (9 bpm) peaked 40 minutes after administration and resolved within 2 hours (Canuso et al., 2018; Daly et al., 2018). In these intranasal esketamine FDA approval trials, ~10% experienced substantially increased SBP ≥40 mmHg and ~13% had increased DBP ≥25 mmHg (Janssen Pharmaceuticals Inc., 2019). Ventricular extrasystole and syncope episodes were the two adverse events that led to early discontinuation during intranasal esketamine trials (Canuso et al., 2018; Daly et al., 2018). In the ketamine review, hypertensive episodes unresponsive to β-blockers, and bradycardia with hypotension were the cardiac-related adverse events that led to treatment discontinuation in three participants from the trials (Ryan et al., 2014)

Gastrointestinal

Nausea is another common dose-related adverse effect of ketamine and esketamine reported by 15–35% of participants in major depressive disorder clinical trials, while vomiting was reported for 9% in the esketamine FDA approval trials (Canuso et al., 2018; Daly et al., 2018; Janssen Pharmaceuticals Inc., 2019; Ryan et al., 2014).

Chronic Adverse Effects

Psychiatric

Mood Symptoms. In the review of ketamine for depression there was one report of a manic episode for a patient with treatment-resistant depression who received 34 doses of ketamine at variable intervals over a year, but there were no reports of mania in the National Institute of Mental Health (NIMH) bipolar depression ketamine clinical trials (Ryan et al., 2014).

Psychotic Thinking. A study of 150 individuals stratified by frequent, infrequent, and ex-ketamine recreational users, along with polydrug users and non-drug-user controls, demonstrated that frequent recreational ketamine users (mean 20.1 days/month) exhibited higher scores on psychosis-like self-report measures, including unusual experiences, cognitive disorganization, conviction in delusions, and preoccupation with delusions and dissociative symptoms (Morgan, Muetzelfeldt, & Curran, 2009).

Neurological

A field-based snowball sampling study investigated the effects of recreational ketamine use on cognitive performance and determined that both regular users (mean 13.5 days/month) and infrequent users (< 2 days/month) demonstrated poor performance on immediate and delayed recall of prose during the acute ketamine effects, but the regular users also had impaired episodic and semantic memory 3 days after using ketamine (Curran & Monaghan, 2001). In a 3-year follow-up, the same ketamine users had semantic memory improvements that correlated with a reduction in ketamine use frequency, but there was persisting impairment in episodic memory (Morgan, Monaghan, & Curran, 2004). In the largest study with 150 individuals evenly distributed for frequent, infrequent, and ex-ketamine users, along with polydrug users and non-drug-user controls, they determined that frequent ketamine users (mean 20.1 days/month) also exhibited greater cognitive impairments in recognition memory, working memory, and planning (Morgan et al., 2009).

Genitourinary

In a review of 61 clinical trials there was only one report of cystitis, and it was deemed unrelated to the ketamine infusion (Ryan et al., 2014). The esketamine FDA approval trials reported that esketamine-treated patients had increased daytime urinary frequency (3%) and an overall higher rate of lower urinary tract symptoms (LUTS) than placebo-treated patients (Janssen Pharmaceuticals Inc., 2019). A Hong Kong (2000–2007) retrospective analysis of 59 recreational ketamine users referred to urology for LUTS showed that 71% had cystoscopy demonstrating various degrees of epithelial inflammation similar to chronic interstitial cystitis, 51% had hydronephrosis on ultrasonography, and 7% had features suggestive of papillary necrosis on radiological imaging (Chu et al., 2008). A 2009–2010 survey-based study of 1,285 past-year ketamine users in the United Kingdom determined that 27% experienced LUTS, with frequent urination (17%), lower abdominal pain (11%), burning/stinging during urination (8.1%), incontinence (3.3%), and blood in urine (1.5%), which were significantly related to dose and frequency of ketamine use. Among these users with LUTS, 51% reported improvement in symptoms upon cessation of use, with 4% reporting deterioration despite ketamine cessation (Winstock, Mitcheson, Gillatt, & Cottrell, 2012). The precise pathological mechanism for this adverse effect remains unclear, but evidence from ketamine recreational users and intranasal esketamine clinical trials highlights the importance of continued monitoring for LUTS during long-term administration of ketamine.

Teratogenicity

Esketamine intranasal spray is not recommended in pregnancy due to a lack of human data, along with animal data suggesting potential skeletal malformations and neuroapoptosis with ketamine (Janssen Pharmaceuticals Inc., 2019).

Drug Interactions

Ketamine efficacy may be diminished by medications that act on glutamate systems, such as memantine, lamotrigine and clozapine (Andrade, 2017b). Drugs that induce or inhibit *CYP2B6* and *CYP3A4* may reduce or increase, respectively, the clinical effects of oral ketamine (Andrade, 2017b). Concurrent use with drugs such as ethanol, opioids, barbiturates, and benzodiazepines may intensify central nervous system (CNS) or respiratory depression, which has led to fatalities. Drugs such as cocaine or amphetamines may also increase ketamine's risk of acute cardiotoxicity (European Monitoring Center for Drugs and Drug Addiction, 2002).

Harm Reduction and Risk Management

• Avoid drugs that have pharmacodynamic interactions by interfering with glutamate or enhancing γ-aminobutyric acid (GABA) neurotransmission.

• Avoid drugs with pharmacokinetic interactions that inhibit or induce *CYP3A4*, *CYP2C9* or *CYP2B6* enzyme metabolism of oral ketamine.

• Monitor for development of LUTS with chronic use.

▨ Conclusion

Hallucinogenic adverse effects are primarily related to psychological reactions during the acute phase of administration and seem to be minimized by the carefully prepared therapeutic environments provided in more recent clinical trials. Routine medical monitoring in psychedelic-assisted therapy treatment should also help to mitigate any risks from acute cardiovascular changes. Two rare, but serious conditions with routine chronic use that warrant careful monitoring include cardiac valvulopathy with the classic hallucinogens and LUTS with ketamine. This comprehensive summary of potential adverse effects should provide the clinician with the necessary knowledge to recognize and mitigate these risks.

▨ References

Addy, P. H. (2012). Acute and post-acute behavioral and psychological effects of salvinorin A in humans. *Psychopharmacology (Berl)*, 220(1), 195–204.

Alper, K., Bai, R., Liu, N., Fowler, S. J., Huang, X. P., Priori, S. G., et al. (2016). hERG blockade by iboga alkaloids. *Cardiovasc Toxicol*, 16(1), 14–22.

Alper, K. R., Lotsof, H. S., Frenken, G. M., Luciano, D. J., & Bastiaans, J. (1999). Treatment of acute opioid withdrawal with ibogaine. *Am J Addict*, 8(3), 234–242.

Alper, K. R., Stajic, M., & Gill, J. R. (2012). Fatalities temporally associated with the ingestion of ibogaine. *J Forensic Sci*, 57(2), 398–412.

Andrade, C. (2017a). Ketamine for depression, 3: Does chirality matter? *J Clin Psychiatry*, 78(6), e674–e677.

Andrade, C. (2017b). Ketamine for depression, 5: Potential pharmacokinetic and pharmacodynamic drug interactions. *J Clin Psychiatry*, 78(7), e858–e861.

Baggott, M. J., Coyle, J. R., Erowid, E., Erowid, F., & Robertson, L. C. (2011). Abnormal visual experiences in individuals with histories of hallucinogen use: A Web-based questionnaire. *Drug Alcohol Depend*, 114(1), 61–67.

Bogenschutz, M. P., Forcehimes, A. A., Pommy, J. A., Wilcox, C. E., Barbosa, P. C., & Strassman, R. J. (2015). Psilocybin-assisted treatment for alcohol dependence: A proof-of-concept study. *J Psychopharmacol*, 29(3), 289–299.

Bogenschutz, M. P., & Ross, S. (2018). Therapeutic applications of classic hallucinogens. *Curr Top Behav Neurosci, 36*, 361–391.

Botanas, C. J., Bryan de la Pena, J., Kim, H. J., Lee, Y. S., & Cheong, J. H. (2019). Methoxetamine: A foe or friend? *Neurochem Int, 122*, 1–7.

Brown, T. K., & Alper, K. (2018). Treatment of opioid use disorder with ibogaine: Detoxification and drug use outcomes. *Am J Drug Alcohol Abuse, 44*(1), 24–36.

Busardo, F. P., Kyriakou, C., Napoletano, S., Marinelli, E., & Zaami, S. (2015). Mephedrone related fatalities: A review. *Eur Rev Med Pharmacol Sci, 19*(19), 3777–3790.

Callaway, J. C. (2005). Fast and slow metabolizers of hoasca. *J Psychoactive Drugs, 37*(2), 157–161.

Callaway, J. C., & Grob, C. S. (1998). Ayahuasca preparations and serotonin reuptake inhibitors: A potential combination for severe adverse interactions. *J Psychoactive Drugs, 30*(4), 367–369.

Callaway, J. C., McKenna, D. J., Grob, C. S., Brito, G. S., Raymon, L. P., Poland, R. E., et al. (1999). Pharmacokinetics of hoasca alkaloids in healthy humans. *J Ethnopharmacol, 65*(3), 243–256.

Campbell, G. A., & Rosner, M. H. (2008). The agony of ecstasy: MDMA (3,4-methylenedioxymethamphetamine) and the kidney. *Clin J Am Soc Nephrol, 3*(6), 1852–1860.

Canuso, C. M., Singh, J. B., Fedgchin, M., Alphs, L., Lane, R., Lim, P., et al. (2018). Efficacy and safety of intranasal esketamine for the rapid reduction of symptoms of depression and suicidality in patients at imminent risk for suicide: Results of a double-blind, randomized, placebo-controlled study. *Am J Psychiatry, 175*(7), 620–630.

Carbonaro, T. M., Bradstreet, M. P., Barrett, F. S., MacLean, K. A., Jesse, R., Johnson, M. W., et al. (2016). Survey study of challenging experiences after ingesting psilocybin mushrooms:

Acute and enduring positive and negative consequences. *J Psychopharmacol, 30*(12), 1268–1278.

Chu, P. S., Ma, W. K., Wong, S. C., Chu, R. W., Cheng, C. H., Wong, S., et al. (2008). The destruction of the lower urinary tract by ketamine abuse: A new syndrome? *BJU Int, 102*(11), 1616–1622.

Cohen, M. M., & Shiloh, Y. (1977). Genetic toxicology of lysergic acid diethylamide (LSD-25). *Mutat Res, 47*(3–4), 183–209.

Cohen, S. (1960). Lysergic acid diethylamide: side effects and complications. *J Nerv Ment Dis, 130*, 30–40.

Crittenden, G. (2015). What really happened when a 32-year-old Canadian died after a tobacco purge in the Amazon? Retrieved from *http://reset.me/story/what-really-happened-when-a-32-year-old-canadian-died-after-a-tobacco-purge-in-the-amazon.*

Curran, H. V., & Monaghan, L. (2001). In and out of the K-hole: A comparison of the acute and residual effects of ketamine in frequent and infrequent ketamine users. *Addiction, 96*(5), 749–760.

Daly, E. J., Singh, J. B., Fedgchin, M., Cooper, K., Lim, P., Shelton, R. C., et al. (2018). Efficacy and safety of intranasal esketamine adjunctive to oral antidepressant therapy in treatment-resistant depression: A randomized clinical trial. *JAMA Psychiatry, 75*(2), 139–148.

de Araujo, D. B., Ribeiro, S., Cecchi, G. A., Carvalho, F. M., Sanchez, T. A., Pinto, J. P., et al. (2012). Seeing with the eyes shut: Neural basis of enhanced imagery following ayahuasca ingestion. *Hum Brain Mapp, 33*(11), 2550–2560.

de la Torre, R., Farre, M., Mathuna, B. O., Roset, P. N., Pizarro, N., Segura, M., et al. (2005). MDMA (ecstasy) pharmacokinetics in a CYP2D6 poor metaboliser and in nine CYP2D6 extensive metabolisers. *Eur J Clin Pharmacol, 61*(7), 551–554.

Dickinson, J., McAlpin, J., Wilkins, C., Fitzsimmons, C., Guion, P., Paterson, T., et al. (2016). Clinical guidelines for ibogaine-assisted detoxification (Version 1.1). Retrieved from *https://s3.ca-central-1.amazonaws.com/ibosafe-pdf-resources/ibogaine/clinical+guidelines+for+ibogaine-assisted+detoxification.pdf.*

Dolder, P. C., Schmid, Y., Haschke, M., Rentsch, K. M., & Liechti, M. E. (2015). Pharmacokinetics and concentration–effect relationship of oral LSD in humans. *Int J Neuropsychopharmacol, 19*(1), pyv072.

Dorrance, D. L., Janiger, O., & Teplitz, R. L. (1975). Effect of peyote on human chromosomes: Cytogenetic study of the Huichol Indians of Northern Mexico. *JAMA, 234*(3), 299–302.

Dos Santos, R. G. (2013a). A critical evaluation of reports associating ayahuasca with life-threatening adverse reactions. *J Psychoactive Drugs, 45*(2), 179–188.

Dos Santos, R. G. (2013b). Safety and side effects of ayahuasca in humans—an overview focusing on developmental toxicology. *J Psychoactive Drugs, 45*(1), 68–78.

Dos Santos, R. G., Balthazar, F. M., Bouso, J. C., & Hallak, J. E. (2016). The current state of research on ayahuasca: A systematic review of human studies assessing psychiatric symptoms, neuropsychological functioning, and neuroimaging. *J Psychopharmacol, 30*(12), 1230–1247.

Dos Santos, R. G., Bouso, J. C., & Hallak, J. E. C. (2017). Ayahuasca, dimethyltryptamine, and psychosis: A systematic review of human studies. *Ther Adv Psychopharmacol, 7*(4), 141–157.

Dos Santos, R. G., Osorio, F. L., Crippa, J. A., & Hallak, J. E. (2016). Antidepressive and anxiolytic effects of ayahuasca: A systematic literature review of animal and human studies. *Rev Bras Psiquiatr, 38*(1), 65–72.

European Monitoring Center for Drugs and Drug Addiction. (2002). Report on the risk assessment of ketamine in the framework of the joint action on new synthetic drugs (92-9168-123-7). Retrieved from *www.emcdda.europa.eu/publications/risk-assessments/ketamine_en.*

Farre, M., Abanades, S., Roset, P. N., Peiro, A. M., Torrens, M., O'Mathuna, B., et al. (2007). Pharmacological interaction between 3,4-methylenedioxymethamphetamine (ecstasy) and paroxetine: Pharmacological effects and pharmacokinetics. *J Pharmacol Exp Ther, 323*(3), 954–962.

Gable, R. S. (2007). Risk assessment of ritual use of oral dimethyltryptamine (DMT) and harmala alkaloids. *Addiction, 102*(1), 24–34.

Gasser, P., Holstein, D., Michel, Y., Doblin, R., Yazar-Klosinski, B., Passie, T., et al. (2014). Safety and efficacy of lysergic acid diethylamide-assisted psychotherapy for anxiety associated with life-threatening diseases. *J Nerv Ment Dis, 202*(7), 513–520.

Gasser, P., Kirchner, K., & Passie, T. (2015). LSD-assisted psychotherapy for anxiety associated with a life-threatening disease: A qualitative study of acute and sustained subjective effects. *J Psychopharmacol, 29*(1), 57–68.

Ghasemi, M., Kazemi, M. H., Yoosefi, A., Ghasemi, A., Paragomi, P., Amini, H., et al. (2014). Rapid antidepressant effects of repeated doses of ketamine compared with electroconvulsive therapy in hospitalized patients with major depressive disorder. *Psychiatry Res, 215*(2), 355–361.

Gillman, P. K. (2016). Monoamine oxidase inhibitors: A review concerning dietary tyramine and drug interactions. *PsychoTropical Comment, 16*(6), 1–97.

Giorgi, F. S., Lazzeri, G., Natale, G., Iudice, A., Ruggieri, S., Paparelli, A., et al. (2006). MDMA and seizures: A dangerous liaison? *Ann NY Acad Sci, 1074*, 357–364.

Glue, P., Cape, G., Tunnicliff, D., Lockhart, M., Lam, F., Gray, A., et al. (2016a). Switching opioid-dependent patients from methadone to morphine: Safety, tolerability, and methadone pharmacokinetics. *J Clin Pharmacol, 56*(8), 960–965.

Glue, P., Cape, G., Tunnicliff, D., Lockhart, M., Lam, F., Hung, N., et al. (2016b). Ascending single-dose, double-blind, placebo-controlled safety study of noribogaine in opioid-dependent patients. *Clin Pharmacol Drug Dev, 5*(6), 460–468.

Glue, P., Lockhart, M., Lam, F., Hung, N., Hung, C. T., & Friedhoff, L. (2015a). Ascending-dose study of noribogaine in healthy volunteers: Pharmacokinetics, pharmacodynamics, safety, and tolerability. *J Clin Pharmacol, 55*(2), 189–194.

Glue, P., Winter, H., Garbe, K., Jakobi, H., Lyudin, A., Lenagh-Glue, Z., et al. (2015b). Influence of CYP2D6 activity on the pharmacokinetics and pharmacodynamics of a single 20 mg dose of ibogaine in healthy volunteers. *J Clin Pharmacol, 55*(6), 680–687.

Gouzoulis-Mayfrank, E., Heekeren, K., Neukirch, A., Stoll, M., Stock, C., Obradovic, M., et al. (2005). Psychological effects of (S)-ketamine and N,N-dimethyltryptamine (DMT): A double-blind, cross-over study in healthy volunteers. *Pharmacopsychiatry, 38*(6), 301–311.

Green, A. R., King, M. V., Shortall, S. E., & Fone, K. C. (2012). Lost in translation: Preclinical studies on 3,4-methylenedioxymethamphetamine provide information on mechanisms of action, but do not allow accurate prediction of adverse events in humans. *Br J Pharmacol, 166*(5), 1523–1536.

Griffiths, R. R., Johnson, M. W., Carducci, M. A., Umbricht, A., Richards, W. A., Richards, B. D., et al. (2016). Psilocybin produces substantial and sustained decreases in depression and anxiety in patients with life-threatening cancer: A randomized double-blind trial. *J Psychopharmacol, 30*(12), 1181–1197.

Grob, C. S. (2000). Deconstructing ecstasy: The politics of MDMA research. *Addiction Research, 8*(6), 549–588.

Halpern, J. H., Lerner, A. G., & Passie, T. (2018). A review of hallucinogen persisting perception disorder (HPPD) and an exploratory study of subjects claiming symptoms of HPPD. *Curr Top Behav Neurosci, 36*, 333–360.

Hasler, F., Grimberg, U., Benz, M. A., Huber, T., & Vollenweider, F. X. (2004). Acute psychological and physiological effects of psilocybin in healthy humans: A double-blind, placebo-controlled dose–effect study. *Psychopharmacology (Berl), 172*(2), 145–156.

Heise, C. W., & Brooks, D. E. (2017). Ayahuasca exposure: Descriptive analysis of calls to US Poison Control Centers from 2005 to 2015. *J Med Toxicol, 13*(3), 245–248.

Henry, J. A., & Hill, I. R. (1998). Fatal interaction between ritonavir and MDMA. *Lancet, 352*(9142), 1751–1752.

Hernandez-Lopez, C., Farre, M., Roset, P. N., Menoyo, E., Pizarro, N., Ortuno, J., et al. (2002). 3,4-Methylenedioxymethamphetamine (ecstasy) and alcohol interactions in humans: Psychomotor performance, subjective effects, and pharmacokinetics. *J Pharmacol Exp Ther, 300*(1), 236–244.

Houenou, J., Homri, W., Leboyer, M., & Drancourt, N. (2011). Ibogaine-associated psychosis in schizophrenia: A case report. *J Clin Psychopharmacol, 31*(5), 659.

Hysek, C. M., Brugger, R., Simmler, L. D., Bruggisser, M., Donzelli, M., Grouzmann, E., et al. (2012). Effects of the alpha(2)-adrenergic agonist clonidine on the pharmacodynamics and pharmacokinetics of 3,4-methylenedioxymethamphetamine in healthy volunteers. *J Pharmacol Exp Ther, 340*(2), 286–294.

Hysek, C. M., Schmid, Y., Rickli, A., Simmler, L. D., Donzelli, M., Grouzmann, E., et al. (2012). Carvedilol inhibits the cardiostimulant and thermogenic effects of MDMA in humans. *Br J Pharmacol, 166*(8), 2277–2288.

Hysek, C. M., Simmler, L. D., Nicola, V. G., Vischer, N., Donzelli, M., Krahenbuhl, S., et al. (2012). Duloxetine inhibits effects of MDMA ("ecstasy") *in vitro* and in humans in a randomized placebo-controlled laboratory study. *PLOS ONE, 7*(5), e36476.

Hysek, C. M., Simmler, L. D., Schillinger, N., Meyer, N., Schmid, Y., Donzelli, M., et al. (2014). Pharmacokinetic and pharmacodynamic effects of methylphenidate and MDMA administered alone or in combination. *Int J Neuropsychopharmacol, 17*(3), 371–381.

International Center for Ethnobotanical Education, Research, and Service. (2017). Risks associated with combining *Bufo Alvarius* with ayahuasca. Retrieved from *http://news.iceers.org/2017/05/alert-bufo-alvarius-and-ayahuasca*.

Janssen Pharmaceuticals Inc. (2019, May). *Spravato (esketamine)* [prescribing information]. Titusville, NJ: Author.

Johansen, P. O., & Krebs, T. S. (2015). Psychedelics not linked to mental health problems or suicidal behavior: A population study. *J Psychopharmacol, 29*(3), 270–279.

Johnson, M., Richards, W., & Griffiths, R. (2008). Human hallucinogen research: Guidelines for safety. *J Psychopharmacol, 22*(6), 603–620.

Katalinic, N., Lai, R., Somogyi, A., Mitchell, P. B., Glue, P., & Loo, C. K. (2013). Ketamine as a new treatment for depression: A review of its efficacy and adverse effects. *Aust NZ J Psychiatry, 47*(8), 710–727.

Keeler, M. H. (1967). Chlorpromazine antagonism of psilocybin effect. *Int J Neuropsychiatry, 3*(1), 66–71.

Kirkpatrick, M. G., Gunderson, E. W., Perez, A. Y., Haney, M., Foltin, R. W., & Hart, C. L. (2012). A direct comparison of the behavioral and physiological effects of methamphetamine and 3,4-methylenedioxymethamphetamine (MDMA) in humans. *Psychopharmacology (Berl), 219*(1), 109–122.

Klette, K. L., Anderson, C. J., Poch, G. K., Nimrod, A. C., & ElSohly, M. A. (2000). Metabolism of lysergic acid diethylamide (LSD) to 2-oxo-3-hydroxy LSD (O-H-LSD) in human liver microsomes and cryopreserved human hepatocytes. *J Anal Toxicol, 24*(7), 550–556.

Kolbrich, E. A., Goodwin, R. S., Gorelick, D. A., Hayes, R. J., Stein, E. A., & Huestis, M. A. (2008). Physiological and subjective responses to controlled oral 3,4-methylenedioxymethamphetamine administration. *J Clin Psychopharmacol, 28*(4), 432–440.

Krebs, T. S., & Johansen, P. O. (2013). Psychedelics and mental health: A population study. *PLOS ONE, 8*(8), e63972.

Labate, B. C., & Feeney, K. (2012). Ayahuasca and the process of regulation in Brazil and internationally: Implications and challenges. *Int J Drug Policy, 23*(2), 154–161.

Leonard, J. B., Anderson, B., & Klein-Schwartz, W. (2018). Does getting high hurt?: Characterization of cases of LSD and psilocybin-containing mushroom exposures to national poison centers between 2000 and 2016. *J Psychopharmacol, 32*, 1286–1294.

LeVay, S. (2008). *When science goes wrong: Twelve tales from the dark side of discovery.* New York: Penguin Group.

Liechti, M. E., & Vollenweider, F. X. (2000). The serotonin uptake inhibitor citalopram reduces acute cardiovascular and vegetative effects of 3,4-methylenedioxymethamphetamine ("Ecstasy") in healthy volunteers. *J Psychopharmacol, 14*(3), 269–274.

Lim, T. H., Wasywich, C. A., & Ruygrok, P. N. (2012). A fatal case of "magic mushroom" ingestion in a heart transplant recipient. *Intern Med J, 42*(11), 1268–1269.

Litjens, R. P., & Brunt, T. M. (2016). How toxic is ibogaine? *Clin Toxicol (Phila), 54*(4), 297–302.

Long, S. Y. (1972). Does LSD induce chromosomal damage and malformations?: A review of the literature. *Teratology, 6*(1), 75–90.

Malcolm, B. J., Polanco, M., & Barsuglia, J. P. (2018). Changes in withdrawal and craving scores in participants undergoing opioid detoxification utilizing ibogaine. *J Psychoactive Drugs, 50*, 256–265.

Malleson, N. (1971). Acute adverse reactions to LSD in clinical and experimental use in the United Kingdom. *Br J Psychiatry, 118*(543), 229–230.

Manevski, N., Kurkela, M., Hoglund, C., Mauriala, T., Court, M. H., Yli-Kauhaluoma, J., et al. (2010). Glucuronidation of psilocin and 4-hydroxyindole by the human UDP-glucuronosyltransferases. *Drug Metab Dispos, 38*(3), 386–395.

Marta, C. J., Ryan, W. C., Kopelowicz, A., & Koek, R. J. (2015). Mania following use of ibogaine: A case series. *Am J Addict, 24*(3), 203–205.

Mas, M., Farre, M., de la Torre, R., Roset, P. N., Ortuno, J., Segura, J., et al. (1999). Cardiovascular and neuroendocrine effects and pharmacokinetics of 3, 4-methylenedioxymethamphetamine in humans. *J Pharmacol Exp Ther, 290*(1), 136–145.

Mash, D. C., Kovera, C. A., Pablo, J., Tyndale, R., Ervin, F. R., Kamlet, J. D., et al. (2001). Ibogaine in the treatment of heroin withdrawal. *Alkaloids Chem Biol, 56*, 155–171.

Mithoefer, M. C., Feduccia, A. A., Jerome, L., Mithoefer, A., Wagner, M., Walsh, Z., et al. (2019). MDMA-assisted psychotherapy for treatment of PTSD: Study design and rationale for phase 3 trials based on pooled analysis of six phase 2 randomized controlled trials. *Psychopharmacology (Berl), 236*, 2735–2745.

Mithoefer, M., Jerome, L., & Doblin, R. (2003). MDMA ("ecstasy") and neurotoxicity. *Science, 300*, 1504–1505.

Mohamed, W. M., Ben Hamida, S., Cassel, J. C., de Vasconcelos, A. P., & Jones, B. C. (2011). MDMA: Interactions with other psychoactive drugs. *Pharmacol Biochem Behav, 99*(4), 759–774.

Morgan, C. J., Monaghan, L., & Curran, H. V. (2004). Beyond the K-hole: A 3-year longitudinal investigation of the cognitive and subjective effects of ketamine in recreational users who have substantially reduced their use of the drug. *Addiction, 99*(11), 1450–1461.

Morgan, C. J., Muetzelfeldt, L., & Curran, H. V. (2009). Ketamine use, cognition and psychological wellbeing: A comparison of frequent, infrequent and ex-users with polydrug and non-using controls. *Addiction, 104*(1), 77–87.

Morini, L., Bernini, M., Vezzoli, S., Restori, M., Moretti, M., Crenna, S., et al. (2017). Death after 25C-NBOMe and 25H-NBOMe consumption. *Forensic Sci Int, 279*, e1–e6.

Murrough, J. W., Perez, A. M., Pillemer, S., Stern, J., Parides, M. K., aan het Rot, M., et al. (2013). Rapid and longer-term antidepressant effects of repeated ketamine infusions in treatment-resistant major depression. *Biol Psychiatry, 74*(4), 250–256.

Nichols, D. E. (2016). Psychedelics. *Pharmacol Rev, 68*(2), 264–355.

Nichols, D. E., & Grob, C. S. (2018). Is LSD toxic? *Forensic Sci Int, 284*, 141–145.

Noller, G. E., Frampton, C. M., & Yazar-Klosinski, B. (2018). Ibogaine treatment outcomes for opioid dependence from a twelve-month follow-up observational study. *Am J Drug Alcohol Abuse, 44*(1), 37–46.

Oehen, P., Traber, R., Widmer, V., & Schnyder, U. (2013). A randomized, controlled pilot study of MDMA (+/-3,4-methylenedioxymethamphetamine)-assisted psychotherapy for treatment of resistant, chronic post-traumatic stress disorder (PTSD). *J Psychopharmacol, 27*(1), 40–52.

Orescanin-Dusic, Z., Tatalovic, N., Vidonja-Uzelac, T., Nestorov, J., Nikolic-Kokic, A., Mijuskovic, A., et al. (2018). The effects of ibogaine on uterine smooth muscle contractions: Relation to the activity of antioxidant enzymes. *Oxid Med Cell Longev, 2018*, Article 5969486.

Osorio Fde, L., Sanches, R. F., Macedo, L. R., dos Santos, R. G., Maia-de-Oliveira, J. P., Wichert-Ana, L., et al. (2015). Antidepressant effects of a single dose of ayahuasca in patients with recurrent depression: A preliminary report. *Rev Bras Psiquiatr, 37*(1), 13–20.

Ot'alora, G. M., Grigsby, J., Poulter, B., Van Derveer, J. W., III, Giron, S. G., Jerome, L., et al. (2018). 3,4-methylenedioxymethamphetamine-assisted psychotherapy for treatment of chronic posttraumatic stress disorder: A randomized phase 2 controlled trial. *J Psychopharmacol, 32*, 1295–1307.

Ott, J. (1999). Pharmahuasca: Human pharmacology of oral DMT plus harmine. *J Psychoactive Drugs, 31*(2), 171–177.

Palhano-Fontes, F., Barreto, D., Onias, H., Andrade, K. C., Novaes, M. M., Pessoa, J. A., et al. (2019). Rapid antidepressant effects of the psychedelic ayahuasca in treatment-resistant depression: A randomized placebo-controlled trial. *Psychol Med, 49*, 655–663.

Papaseit, E., Vazquez, A., Perez-Mana, C., Pujadas, M., de la Torre, R., Farre, M., et al. (2012). Surviving life-threatening MDMA (3,4-methylenedioxymethamphetamine, ecstasy) toxicity caused by ritonavir (RTV). *Intensive Care Med, 38*(7), 1239–1240.

Parrott, A. C. (2012a). MDMA and 5-HT neurotoxicity: The empirical evidence for its adverse effects in humans—no need for translation. *Br J Pharmacol, 166*(5), 1518–1520; discussion 1521–1512.

Parrott, A. C. (2012b). MDMA and temperature: A review of the thermal effects of "Ecstasy" in humans. *Drug Alcohol Depend, 121*(1–2), 1–9.

Pilgrim, J. L., Gerostamoulos, D., & Drummer, O. H. (2011). Deaths involving MDMA and the concomitant use of pharmaceutical drugs. *J Anal Toxicol, 35*(4), 219–226.

Pilgrim, J. L., Gerostamoulos, D., Woodford, N., & Drummer, O. H. (2012). Serotonin toxicity involving MDMA (ecstasy) and moclobemide. *Forensic Sci Int, 215*(1–3), 184–188.

Plucinska, J. (2015). A British tourist has been killed at a Peruvian ayahuasca ceremony. Retrieved from *http://time.com/4154455/peru-ayahuasca-murder-amazon-hallucinogen*.

Pokorny, T., Preller, K. H., Kraehenmann, R., & Vollenweider, F. X. (2016). Modulatory effect of the 5-HT1A agonist buspirone and the mixed non-hallucinogenic 5-HT1A/2A agonist ergotamine on psilocybin-induced psychedelic experience. *Eur Neuropsychopharmacol, 26*(4), 756–766.

Preller, K. H., Schilbach, L., Pokorny, T., Flemming, J., Seifritz, E., & Vollenweider, F. X. (2018). Role of the 5-HT2A receptor in self- and other-initiated social interaction in lysergic acid diethylamide-induced states: A pharmacological fMRI study. *J Neurosci, 38*(14), 3603–3611.

Riba, J., Rodriguez-Fornells, A., Urbano, G., Morte, A., Antonijoan, R., Montero, M., et al. (2001). Subjective effects and tolerability of the South American psychoactive beverage ayahuasca in healthy volunteers. *Psychopharmacology (Berl), 154*(1), 85–95.

Riba, J., Valle, M., Urbano, G., Yritia, M., Morte, A., & Barbanoj, M. J. (2003). Human pharmacology of ayahuasca: Subjective and cardiovascular effects, monoamine metabolite excretion, and pharmacokinetics. *J Pharmacol Exp Ther, 306*(1), 73–83.

Ricaurte, G. A., Yuan, J., Hatzidimitriou, G., Cord, B. J., & McCann, U. D. (2002). Severe dopaminergic neurotoxicity in primates after a common recreational dose regimen of MDMA ("ecstasy"). *Science, 297*(5590), 2260–2263.

Ricaurte, G. A., Yuan, J., Hatzidimitriou, G., Cord, B. J., & McCann, U. D. (2003). Retraction. *Science, 301*(5639), 1479.

Rietjens, S. J., Hondebrink, L., Westerink, R. H., & Meulenbelt, J. (2012). Pharmacokinetics and pharmacodynamics of 3,4-methylenedioxymethamphetamine (MDMA): Interindividual differences due to polymorphisms and drug-drug interactions. *Crit Rev Toxicol, 42*(10), 854–876.

Roth, B. L. (2007). Drugs and valvular heart disease. *N Engl J Med, 356*(1), 6–9.

Ryan, W. C., Marta, C. J., & Koek, R. J. (2014). Ketamine and depression. *International Journal of Transpersonal Studies, 33*(2), 40–74.

Sanches, R. F., de Lima Osorio, F., Dos Santos, R. G., Macedo, L. R., Maia-de-Oliveira, J. P., Wichert-Ana, L., et al. (2016). Antidepressant effects of a single dose of ayahuasca in patients with recurrent depression: A SPECT study. *J Clin Psychopharmacol, 36*(1), 77–81.

Schenberg, E. E., de Castro Comis, M. A., Alexandre, J. F. M., Tófoli, L. F., Chaves, B. D. R., & da Silveira, D. X. (2017). A phenomenological analysis of the subjective experience elicited by ibogaine in the context of a drug dependence treatment. *Journal of Psychedelic Studies, 1*, 74–83.

Schmid, Y., Enzler, F., Gasser, P., Grouzmann, E., Preller, K. H., Vollenweider, F. X., et al. (2015). Acute effects of lysergic acid diethylamide in healthy subjects. *Biol Psychiatry, 78*(8), 544–553.

Schmid, Y., Rickli, A., Schaffner, A., Duthaler, U., Grouzmann, E., Hysek, C. M., et al. (2015). Interactions between bupropion and 3,4-methylenedioxymethamphetamine in healthy subjects. *J Pharmacol Exp Ther, 353*(1), 102–111.

Schmid, Y., Vizeli, P., Hysek, C. M., Prestin, K., Meyer Zu Schwabedissen, H. E., & Liechti, M. E. (2016). CYP2D6 function moderates the pharmacokinetics and pharmacodynamics of 3,4-methylene-dioxymethamphetamine in a controlled study in healthy individuals. *Pharmacogenet Genomics, 26*(8), 397–401.

Segura, M., Farre, M., Pichini, S., Peiro, A. M., Roset, P. N., Ramirez, A., et al. (2005). Contribution of cytochrome P450 2D6 to 3,4-methylenedioxymethamphetamine disposition in humans: Use of paroxetine as a metabolic inhibitor probe. *Clin Pharmacokinet, 44*(6), 649–660.

Singer, L. T., Moore, D. G., Fulton, S., Goodwin, J., Turner, J. J., Min, M. O., et al. (2012). Neurobehavioral outcomes of infants exposed to MDMA (Ecstasy) and other recreational drugs during pregnancy. *Neurotoxicol Teratol, 34*(3), 303–310.

Singer, L. T., Moore, D. G., Min, M. O., Goodwin, J., Turner, J. J., Fulton, S., et al. (2016). Motor delays in MDMA (ecstasy) exposed infants persist to 2 years. *Neurotoxicol Teratol, 54*, 22–28.

Smilkstein, M. J., Smolinske, S. C., & Rumack, B. H. (1987). A case of MAO inhibitor/MDMA interaction: Agony after ecstasy. *J Toxicol Clin Toxicol, 25*(1–2), 149–159.

Stoller, A., Dolder, P. C., Bodmer, M., Hammann, F., Rentsch, K. M., Exadaktylos, A. K., et al. (2017). Mistaking 2C-P for 2C-B: What a difference a letter makes. *J Anal Toxicol, 41*(1), 77–79.

Strassman, R. J. (1996). Human psychopharmacology of N,N-dimethyltryptamine. *Behav Brain Res, 73*(1–2), 121–124.

Strassman, R. J., & Qualls, C. R. (1994). Dose-response study of N,N-dimethyltryptamine in humans: I. Neuroendocrine, autonomic, and cardiovascular effects. *Arch Gen Psychiatry, 51*(2), 85–97.

Strassman, R. J., Qualls, C. R., & Berg, L. M. (1996). Differential tolerance to biological and subjective effects of four closely spaced doses of N,N-dimethyltryptamine in humans. *Biol Psychiatry, 39*(9), 784–795.

Strassman, R. J., Qualls, C. R., Uhlenhuth, E. H., & Kellner, R. (1994). Dose–response study of N,N-dimethyltryptamine in humans: II. Subjective effects and preliminary results of a new rating scale. *Arch Gen Psychiatry, 51*(2), 98–108.

Studerus, E., Kometer, M., Hasler, F., & Vollenweider, F. X. (2011). Acute, subacute and long-term subjective effects of psilocybin in healthy humans: A pooled analysis of experimental studies. *J Psychopharmacol, 25*(11), 1434–1452.

Szumlinski, K. K., Maisonneuve, I. M., & Glick, S. D. (2000). Differential effects of ibogaine on behavioural and dopamine sensitization to cocaine. *Eur J Pharmacol, 398*(2), 259–262.

Tancer, M., & Johanson, C. E. (2007). The effects of fluoxetine on the subjective and physiological effects of 3,4-methylenedioxymethamphetamine (MDMA) in humans. *Psychopharmacology (Berl), 189*(4), 565–573.

Teitelbaum, D. T., & Wingeleth, D. C. (1977). Diagnosis and management of recreational mescaline self poisoning. *Journal of Analytical Toxicology, 1*(1), 36–37.

Thomas, K., Malcolm, B., & Lastra, D. (2017). Psilocybin-assisted therapy: A review of a novel treatment for psychiatric disorders. *J Psychoactive Drugs, 49*(5), 446–455.

Vaiva, G., Boss, V., Bailly, D., Thomas, P., Lestavel, P., & Goudemand, M. (2001). An "accidental" acute psychosis with ecstasy use. *J Psychoactive Drugs, 33*(1), 95–98.

Vollenweider, F. X., Gamma, A., Liechti, M., & Huber, T. (1998). Psychological and cardiovascular effects and short-term sequelae of MDMA ("ecstasy") in MDMA-naive healthy volunteers. *Neuropsychopharmacology, 19*(4), 241–251.

Vollenweider, F. X., Jones, R. T., & Baggott, M. J. (2001). Caveat emptor: Editors beware. *Neuropsychopharmacology, 24*(4), 461–463.

Vollenweider, F. X., Vollenweider-Scherpenhuyzen, M. F., Babler, A., Vogel, H., & Hell, D. (1998). Psilocybin induces schizophrenia-like psychosis in humans via a serotonin-2 agonist action. *NeuroReport, 9*(17), 3897–3902.

Wan, L. B., Levitch, C. F., Perez, A. M., Brallier, J. W., Iosifescu, D. V., Chang, L. C., et al. (2015). Ketamine safety and tolerability in clinical trials for treatment-resistant depression. *J Clin Psychiatry, 76*(3), 247–252.

Winstock, A. R., Mitcheson, L., Gillatt, D. A., & Cottrell, A. M. (2012). The prevalence and natural history of urinary symptoms among recreational ketamine users. *BJU Int, 110*(11), 1762–1766.

Wolbach, A. B., Jr., Isbell, H., & Miner, E. J. (1962). Cross tolerance between mescaline and LSD-25, with a comparison of the mescaline and LSD reactions. *Psychopharmacologia, 3*, 1–14.

Youdim, M. B., Edmondson, D., & Tipton, K. F. (2006). The therapeutic potential of monoamine oxidase inhibitors. *Nat Rev Neurosci, 7*(4), 295–309.

Zarate, C. A., Jr., Singh, J. B., Carlson, P. J., Brutsche, N. E., Ameli, R., Luckenbaugh, D. A., et al. (2006). A randomized trial of an *N*-methyl-D-aspartate antagonist in treatment-resistant major depression. *Arch Gen Psychiatry, 63*(8), 856–864.

Zhao, X., Venkata, S. L., Moaddel, R., Luckenbaugh, D. A., Brutsche, N. E., Ibrahim, L., et al. (2012). Simultaneous population pharmacokinetic modelling of ketamine and three major metabolites in patients with treatment-resistant bipolar depression. *Br J Clin Pharmacol, 74*(2), 304–314.

PART V

Indications and Purpose

CHAPTER 23

Utility of Psychedelics in the Treatment of Psychospiritual and Existential Distress in Palliative Care
A Promising Therapeutic Paradigm

ANTHONY P. BOSSIS

▨ Introduction

Throughout the course of human clinical research with psychedelics (hallucinogens), from the first wave of studies in the mid-20th century to the reemergence in the early 21st century, a primary focus has been on their therapeutic utility in treating persons suffering the emotional distress associated with a terminal illness. The end of life is often marked by feelings of demoralization, meaninglessness, despair, and hopelessness. The effects of psychedelic-generated states of consciousness have been demonstrated to markedly reduce depression, anxiety, and existential distress associated with cancer and advanced terminal disease. From the early 1960s through the mid-1970s, the therapeutic application of the compounds LSD (lysergic acid diethylamide) and DPT (N,N-dipropyltryptamine) to alleviate the emotional end-of-life anguish of patients with cancer provided the first glimpse into the therapeutic and promising transformative features of this unique treatment model. Following a hiatus of over three decades,

researchers conducting clinical research trials with the psychedelic compound psilocybin (4-phosphoryloxy-N,N-dimethyltryptamine) and LSD have again begun exploring the safety and efficacy of psychedelics to effectively treat the often-debilitating psychological symptoms associated with a life-threatening illness. This chapter reviews the history and treatment model of serotonergic psychedelic research in individuals with life-threatening illness, presents the rationale for this novel approach by documenting the psychological and existential distress that often accompanies end-of-life experiences, and offers therapeutic implications for palliative care.

▨ Psychological Distress in Palliative and End-of-Life Care

Death is not the opposite of life, but a part of it.
—HARUKI MURAKAMI

For individuals coping with cancer or other potentially life-threatening diseases, the course of illness may be accompanied by anxiety, depression, hopelessness, severe personal anguish, and a marked degree of spiritual and existential suffering (Jones, Huggins, Rydall, & Rodin, 2003; Mitchell et al., 2011; Rodin et al., 2009). For some, this may lead to demoralization syndrome, characterized as "hopelessness, helplessness, meaninglessness, and existential distress" (Kissane, Clarke, & Street, 2001, p. 13). Murata (2003) describes this "spiritual pain" at the end-of-life as "a pain caused by the extinction of the being and meaning of the self" (p. 15). Spiritual and existential variables are significant determinants of quality of life in advanced or end-of-life illness (Boston, Bruce, & Schreiber, 2011; Edwards, Pang, Shiu, & Chan, 2010). Psychological and existential distress associated with advanced disease has been associated with a desire for a hastened death (Chochinov, Wilson, & Lander, 1998; Kelly et al., 2002; Rodin et al., 2009); moreover, suicide in individuals with advanced-stage cancer has been found to be is twice as high than that in the general population (Chochinov et al., 1998).

The biopsychosocial model of medicine (Engel, 1977) broadened the earlier biomedical model to include psychological and social dimensions of human experience. In recent years, the emerging appreciation of the effect of spirituality on health and notably on end-of-life experience has resulted in the expanded *biopsychosocial–spiritual* model (Sulmasy, 2002). When terminal illness is considered within this framework, an individual's spiritual personal history is regarded as an important variable, with implications for impacting health care outcomes along with biological, psychological, and social dimensions (Puchalski et al., 2009). The biopsychosocial–spiritual model posits that effective clinical health care include meaning-making and transcendent aspects as fundamental dimensions of human experience.

The World Health Organization (WHO, 2011) defines *palliative care* as an approach that (1) affirms life and regards dying as a normal process; (2) neither hastens nor postpones death; (3) integrates the psychological and spiritual aspects of patient care; and (4) encourages life review to help patients recog-

nize purpose, value, and meaning. Reports by the Institute of Medicine (IOM; 2014), the WHO (2011), the National Cancer Network (Holland & Bultz, 2007), and the National Consensus Project for Quality Palliative Care (Puchalski et al., 2009) collectively acknowledge the clinical significance of the spiritual and existential domain of well-being and call for the evaluation and effective treatment of this sphere of suffering patients in palliative care. Despite a decades-long call by the IOM for improvement in end-of-life care, reports of myriad symptoms have increased during the last year of life, including a 26% increase in depression (Singer et al., 2015). The call for effective and novel therapies to alleviate end-of-life emotional suffering provides the rationale and impetus for the reemergence of clinical trials in psychedelic research in palliative care.

■ Search for Meaning and Transcendence

Man is not destroyed by suffering; he is destroyed by suffering without meaning.
—VIKTOR FRANKL

The urge to transcend self-conscious selfhood is a principle appetite of the soul.
—ALDOUS HUXLEY

Central to emotional well-being at the end of life is the capacity to find connection to something more enduring or greater than oneself through meaning making and transcendent experience. *Meaning* and *transcendence* are among the most cited variables influencing emotional well-being in palliative care (Puchalski et al., 2009; Vachon, Fillion, & Achille, 2009). Although coping with a life-threatening illness may be beset with emotional suffering, the end-of-life experience has the potential to trigger a search for meaning (Folkman, 2010; Greenstein & Breitbart, 2000; McClain, Rosenfeld, & Breitbart, 2003). The search for meaning is understood as a basic foundation of human consciousness (Frankl, 1984; Yalom, 1980). Terror management theory, a theoretical model derived from the writings of Ernest Becker, notably *The Denial of Death* (1973), suggests that although awareness of death may generate terror or anxiety, this anxiety may be effectively managed by a search for meaning (Greenberg, Pyszczynski, & Solomon, 1986). Meaning making in advanced cancer has demonstrated improved spiritual well-being and overall quality of life, while reducing levels of psychological distress (Lin & Bauer-Wu, 2003; McMillan & Weitzner, 2000; Morita, Tsunoda, Inoue, & Chihara, 2000). Meaning-enhancing interventions have also been shown to decrease wishes for a desire for a hastened death (Breitbart et al., 2010; Wilson et al., 2007) whereas a loss of meaning has been associated with an enhanced desire for a hastened death (Meier et al., 1998). The cultivation of meaning presents an opportunity for personal growth, improved interpersonal and family relationships, and greater spiritual well-being, with a heightened appreciation for living fully in the final years, months, or days of one's life (Lee, 2008; Lee, Cohen, Edgar, Laizner, & Gagnon, 2004). Viktor Frankl, Holocaust survivor and founder of logotherapy, a psychotherapeutic model focused on meaning making, wrote, "Meaning can be found in life literally up to the last moment, up to the last breath, in the face of death" (1988, p. 76).

Self-transcendence, the ability to extend self-experience beyond the immediate framework of illness to achieve new and novel perspectives, offers an opportunity for psychological and spiritual well-being at the end of life (Coward, 1991; Coward & Reed, 1995; Puchalski, Kilpatrick, McCullough, & Larson, 2003; Vachon et al., 2009). Abraham Maslow (1971, p. 269) defined *transcendence* as "the very highest and most inclusive or holistic levels of human consciousness, behaving and relating, as ends rather than means, to oneself, to significant others, to human beings in general, to other species, to nature, and to the cosmos." Through self-transcendence, self-boundaries can be expanded *inwardly,* through self-acceptance and meaning; *outwardly,* through reaching out to others and to nature; *temporally,* through integrating past and future into the present; and *transpersonally,* through connecting with dimensions in consciousness beyond the discernible world (Reed, 2003, 2009). Eric Cassell (1982, pp. 643–644), in his seminal article on the nature of suffering wrote:

Transcendence is probably the most powerful way in which one is restored to wholeness after an injury to personhood. When experienced, transcendence locates the person in a far larger landscape. The suffering is not isolated by pain but is brought closer to a transpersonal source of meaning and to the human community that shares those meanings. Such an experience need not involve religion in any formal sense; however, in its transpersonal dimension, it is deeply spiritual. . . . Everyone has a transcendent dimension, a life of the spirit. The quality of being greater and more lasting than an individual life gives this aspect of the person its timeless dimension. The profession of medicine appears to ignore the human spirit. When I see patients in nursing homes who have become only bodies, I wonder whether it is not their transcendent dimension that they have lost.

Broadhurst and Harrington (2016) found that dying patients' naturally occurring transcendent experiences led to a sense of spiritual well-being and comfort, helped with unresolved interpersonal conflicts, and contributed to a peaceful death. Transcendence is underscored in this consensus operational definition of healing by a leading group of scholars, including Elisabeth Kübler-Ross, Cicely Saunders, Eric Cassell, and Bernard Siegel: "*Healing is the personal experience of the transcendence of suffering*" (Egnew, 2005 p. 258; original emphasis).

◼ A Brief History of Psychedelics

It is true that my discovery of LSD was a chance discovery, but it was the outcome of planned experiments and these experiments took place in the framework of systematic pharmaceutical, chemical research. It could better be described as serendipity.

—ALBERT HOFMANN

The category of drugs known as classic hallucinogens are primarily mediated through agonist action at serotonin (5-HT_{2A}) receptor sites, although there is not a complete understanding of mechanisms associated with shifts in subjective states of consciousness (Passie, Seifert, Schneider, & Emrich, 2002; Presti & Nichols, 2004). Neuroimaging findings suggest alterations in connectivity within the default mode network, a group of regions in the brain characterized by functions of a self-referential nature (Carhart-Harris et al., 2012, 2016). The serotonergic classic hallucinogens are divided into two classes of alkaloids: the tryptamines and the phenethylamines. Psilocybin, LSD, DMT (N,N-dimethyltryptamine), and DPT belong to the class of tryptamines. The compound mescaline falls within the class of phenethylamines. The serotonergic compounds that have been used in clinical research to treat the emotional distress associated with a life-threatening or terminal illness are LSD, psilocybin, and DPT. For a comprehensive appraisal of the neuropsychopharmacological mechanisms of action of psychedelic compounds, the reader is referred to Nichols (2004).

The subjective effects of classic serotonergic psychedelics generally include alterations— often significant in scope—in consciousness, mood, cognition, and sensory perception. These nonordinary states of consciousness may produce feelings of euphoria, insight, and states of awareness often described as unitive or transcendent in nature. The effects are dependent, in part, on variables related to the individual and environment—the "set and setting" — in which the compounds are taken (Leary, Metzner, & Alpert, 1964). *Set* refers to the mindset of the individual, his or her psychosocial history, personality organization, and intention, attitude, and expectations regarding the drug-administered session. *Setting* defines the social and physical context of the environment in which the psychedelic is taken.

Hallucinogen, the commonly used term for this class of compounds in the medical nomenclature, is misrepresentative in part given that the primary effects are not the production of hallucinations. The term *psychedelic* (mind-manifesting or mind-revealing) coined by British psychiatrist Humphry Osmond in a letter to Aldous Huxley in 1956 (Horowitz & Palmer, 1977) derives from the Greek ψυχή δηλείν (*psyche* meaning soul or mind and *delos* meaning "make visible, manifest, or reveal"). *Entheogen*, from the Greek ἔνθεος and γενέσθαι ("becoming divine within" or "becoming god within") is used in the context of these drugs having the capacity to induce transcendent, spiritual, or mystical experiences (Wasson, Hofmann, & Ruck, 2008).

Historical Use of Psychedelics

Psychedelic compounds are believed to have been used in plant form for millennia and throughout the world within specific indigenous cultures primarily for healing and visionary purposes (Schultes, Hofmann, & Rätsch, 2001). Over 3,500 years ago in ancient India, *Soma*, a Vedic drink believed to be extracted from the mushroom *Amanita muscaria*, was used ritually for its entheogenic properties. Of the more than 1,000 holy hymns found in the *Rig Veda*, the ancient sacred text of Hinduism, 120 are devoted exclusively to this entheogenic sacrament (Schultes et al., 2001; Wasson & Ingalls, 1971). In ancient Greece, at the site of Eleusis and the Eleusinian Mysteries, *Kykeon*, a drink thought to include an ergot-like alkaloid entheogenic substance, was believed to have been used for the facilitation of transformative experience (Wasson, Kramrisch, Ott, & Ruck, 1986; Wasson et al., 2008). It is thought that *Paspalum distichum*, an ergot collected from wild grass from the Mediterranean region in Greece and similar to the *ololiuhqui* potion prepared from specific species of morning glories (*Turbina corymbosa*), was the psychedelic ingredient of *Kykeon*. For nearly 2000 years, beginning in approximately 1600 B.C.E., the secret rites at Eleusis were celebrated in honor of the myth of Demeter and Persephone (see Figure 23.1). Cicero, a participant in the rites at Eleusis wrote, "Not only have we found there the reason to live more joyously, but also that we may die with greater hope" (in Hofmann, 2000, p. 33). On the influence of the Mysteries on Plato, Wasson and colleagues (2008) wrote:

> Plato tells us that beyond this ephemeral and imperfect existence here below, there is another ideal world of Archetypes, where the original, the true, the beautiful pattern of things exists for evermore. Poets and philosophers for millennia have pondered and discussed his conception. It is clear to me where Plato found his "Ideas"; it was clear to those who were initiated into the Mysteries among his contem-

poraries too. Plato had drunk of the potion in the Temple of Eleusis and had spent the night seeing the great Vision. (pp. 29–30)

Over 2,000 years ago in Central America and in Mexico, the use of psilocybin mushrooms, known by the ancient Aztecs as *teonanactl* ("flesh of the gods") were utilized in religious ritual (Schultes et al., 2001; see Figure 23.2). The mescaline-containing peyote cactus was used by indigenous cultures of Mexico for what is believed to be thousands of years (El-Seedi, DeSmet, Beck, Possnert, & Bruhn, 2005; Schultes et al., 2001). Finally, among these few examples, *ayahuasca,* a drink containing the alkaloid DMT and called "vine of the soul" by the Quechuan indigenous peoples, has been used in the Andes and highlands of South America since pre-Columbian years (Dobkin de Rios, 1984; Schultes et al. 2001).

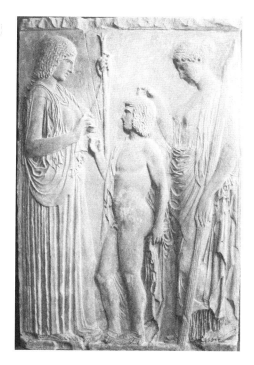

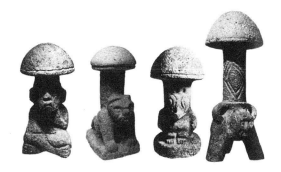

■ FIGURE 23.2. Various Pre-Columbian *Psilocybe* mushroom stones, approximately 1 foot tall—1000 B.C.E. to 500 C.E. (Public domain).

Early Psychiatric Research with Psychedelics

In 1897, Arthur Heffter, the first Western researcher to identify a psychedelic compound, isolated the naturally occurring alkaloid mescaline from the peyote cactus (Bruhn, De Smet, El-Seedi, & Beck, 2002). In 1938, Albert Hofmann serendipitously discovered LSD and in 1943 he accidently ingested the synthesized compound, having a firsthand subjective experience of the drug's dramatic consciousness-altering effects (Hofmann, 1979). Psilocybin mushrooms were introduced to America in 1957 by amateur mycologist Gordon Wasson in a *Life* magazine article about his experience that drew widespread attention (see Figure 23.3). For years, Wasson, a vice president at J. P. Morgan and Company, and his wife Valentina, a New York pediatrician, had studied the ceremonial use of mushrooms used in Mexico and Central America and had been in search of the hallucinogenic mushroom. On the evenings of June 29 and 30, 1955, Gordon Wasson, with friend and photographer Allan Richardson, participated in a mushroom ceremony (*velada*) in the village of Oaxaca, Mexico. The ceremony was led by a shaman (*curandera*) named Marina Sabina (Wasson, in an effort to protect her identity, used the pseudonym Eva Mendez in his article). The mushrooms, identified as *Psilocybe* mushrooms by mycologist Roger Heim, a friend of Wasson, were sent to Sandoz Pharmaceutical laboratories in Switzerland, where Albert Hofmann subsequently isolated and

■ FIGURE 23.1. The Eleusinian Relief. At left, Demeter, presents Triptolemus with sheaves of wheat to bestow on humanity. At right, Persephone, blesses Triptolemus with her left hand. Circa 440 B.C.E. Archaeological Museum of Eleusis, Eleusis, Greece. *Photo:* Anthony P. Bossis.

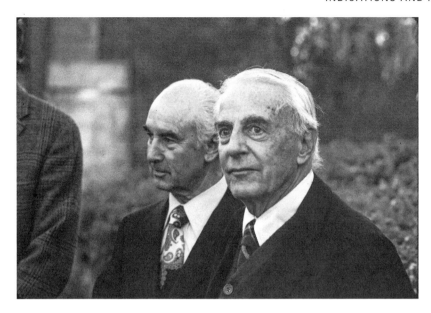

■ FIGURE 23.3. Albert Hofmann (left) and Gordon Wasson (right), Second International Conference on Hallucinogenic Mushrooms, Port Townsend, Washington, October 28, 1977. *Photo:* Jeremy Bigwood.

synthesized the alkaloid psilocybin (Grof & Halifax, 1977; Metzner, 2004).

As clinical research with hallucinogens began in the mid-20th century, two therapeutic models emerged: the *psychedelic* model, using a moderate to high dose of psychedelic medicine, with the objective of inducing a transcendent, peak, or mystical experience, and the *psycholytic* model, utilizing lower doses, with the aim of facilitating the therapeutic process within a psychoanalytically oriented setting. Research initially focused on the *psychotomimetic* model, with the belief that psychedelics could aid in inducing psychotic-like symptoms. Following the research came the development of the *mysticomimetic* model, with the theory that these medicines have the capacity to generate transcendent or mystical-type experiences. Clinical studies followed with depressive, anxiety, neurotic, and obsessive–compulsive disorders. During the first wave of psychedelic research spanning the 1950s through the mid-1970s, over 1,000 scientific or scholarly articles were published with over 40,000 subjects (Grinspoon & Balakar, 1979). The two most promising therapeutic applications to emerge, setting the stage for

the recent reemergence of psychedelic research in the 2000s, were for the treatment of alcoholism and for the existential and psychological distress associated with terminal cancer.

■ Psychedelics and Mystical Experience

To the extent that all mystical or peak-experiences are the same in their essence and have always been the same, all religions are the same in their essence and have always been the same. This something common we may call the "core-religious experience" or the "transcendent experience."
—ABRAHAM MASLOW

The most beautiful and profound emotion we can experience is the sensation of the mystical. It is the sower of all true science. He to whom this emotion is a stranger, who can no longer wonder and stand rapt in awe, is as good as dead.
—ALBERT EINSTEIN

Apart from the therapeutic applications of psychedelics, arguably the most fascinating finding is the capacity of these substances to generate mystical, peak, or numinous states of consciousness.

Historical Perspective of Mystical Experience

Mystical experiences have occurred naturally and cross-culturally throughout human history and are described by mystics, saints, and a growing proportion of the general population, with a Pew Research survey showing nearly half of the American population reporting personal mystical experiences (Heimlich, 2009). Mystical experience is marked by not only by belief but also direct experience. The *philosophia perennis* ("perennial philosophy") proposes that at the core of the world religions exists a universal, fundamental, mystical truth regarding the nature of self, consciousness, and ultimate reality. Rudolph Otto (1923) described the numinous experience in *The Idea of the Holy* as a *mysterium tremendum et fascinans,* or "an awe-inspiring mystery." From the mystical schools of Neo-Platonism and Gnosticism through the Abrahamic (Judaism, Christianity, and Islam) and Eastern (Buddhism, Hinduism, Taoism) religions, this philosophical model proposes that there is a truth or knowledge achievable via direct mystical insight. Naturally occurring mystical experiences are associated with historical figures, including Plotinus, Shankara, Rumi, St. Teresa of Avilla, Pseudo-Dionysius the Areopagite, Gregory of Nyssa, Gershom Scholem, and Meister Eckhart. Spiritually, the mystical experience is considered the supreme state of consciousness, characterized by union, or *unio mystica,* with transcendent or ultimate reality and represented by myriad names in the religious lexicon, including the *Ground of Being, God, Brahman, Christ Consciousness,* or the *Tao.* States of consciousness described as reflecting this transcendent reality include *samadhi* in Hinduism, *theosis* in Eastern Orthodox Christian theology, and *satori* or *kensho* (Japanese for seeing into one's "essence or true nature" (Aitken, 1982) in Zen Buddhism. Contemplative practices that highlight direct experience include *Zazen* in Zen Buddhism, *Vipassana* in Buddhism, and Centering Prayer and *Hesychasm* derived from early Christian practices.

The Varieties of Religious Experience, William James's (1902/1919) groundbreaking treatise on the psychology of religious experience, brought the topic into the purview of psychology, creating a theoretical foundation for further inquiry and research. James described the characteristics of religious experience:

> (1) *ineffability:* difficulty or impossibility to describe the experience, that it must be directly experienced; (2) *noetic quality:* an experience of receiving "knowledge," "illuminations, revelations, full of significance and importance"; (3) *transiency:* "Mystical states cannot be sustained for long"; the experiences by their nature are transient and brief; and (4) *passivity:* the individual feels "as if he were grasped and held by a superior power" (pp. 380–381).

A second and integral book on religious experience in the first years of the 20th century, and one that influenced William James, is Richard Maurice Bucke's *Cosmic Consciousness: A Study in the Evolution of the Human Mind* (1901). Following a personal and naturally occurring mystical experience, Bucke, a prominent Canadian psychiatrist, began studying the history and phenomenology of religious experience. Using the term *cosmic consciousness,* he characterized this state as a "consciousness of the cosmos, that is, of the life and order of the universe" with the subjectivity of a "sense of immortality, a consciousness of eternal life, . . . [a] moral exaltation, an indescribable feeling of elevation, elation, and joyousness, and a quickening of the moral sense" (p. 8). Bucke described his personal experience as "a sense of immense joyousness accompanied or immediately followed by an intellectual illumination quite impossible to describe" with the insight that the cosmos as "not dead matter but a living Presence, that the soul of man is immortal" and "that the foundation principle of the world is what we call love and that the happiness of every one is in the long run absolutely certain" (p. 8). Bucke described a loss of fear of death among his many lasting personal changes. In addition to his own experience and descriptions from contemporary vignettes, Bucke provided writings from historical figures including Buddha, Jesus, Paul, Dante, Blake, Walt Whitman, and de Balzac. The works by James and Bucke established a foundation for essential writings on mystical or religious experience by Evelyn Underhill (1911/2001), Rudolf Otto (1923), Carl Jung (1938/1949), and W. T. Stace (1960).

In *The Perennial Philosophy* (1945), Aldous Huxley, the English writer famous for his novel *Brave New World*, highlighted the universality of mystical experience in the world religions. For Huxley, the mystical or religious experience establishes the philosophical core and arguably the *sine qua non* of religion. Abraham Maslow (1971, p. 164), the American psychologist, characterizing these transcendent or religious states of consciousness as *peak experiences,* described them as "the feeling of ecstasy and wonder and awe, the loss of placement in time and space with, finally, the conviction that something extremely important and valuable had happened, so that the subject was to some extent transformed and strengthened even in his daily life by such experiences."

Psychedelic-Generated Mystical Experience Research

The first research protocol to explore the utility of psychedelics as a method to evaluate the nature of mystical experience was Walter Pahnke's (1963) "Good Friday" Experiment conducted on Christian Good Friday at Boston University's Marsh Chapel in 1962. In a double-blind study of 20 theology students, Pahnke, seeking to investigate whether psychedelic-generated mystical experiences were as "genuine" as those that are naturally occurring, administered psilocybin (30 mg) to 10 theology students and nicotinic acid to 10 others. A private chapel within Marsh Chapel adorned with religious symbols and stained-glass windows served as the setting, with instructions to the subjects to surrender to "unexplored realms of experience" and to avoid resisting the experience even if anxiety-provoking images or content were to arise (p. 96). Derived from accounts of naturally occurring mystical experiences, including those described in the works on mysticism by William James (1919) and Walter T. Stace (1960), Pahnke developed the Mystical Experience Questionnaire (MEQ; Pahnke, 1963; Pahnke & Richards, 1966) with the following primary subjective features: sense of unity, transcendence of time and space, sense of sacredness,

noetic quality, deeply felt positive mood, ineffability, paradoxicality, transiency, and persisting positive changes in attitude and/or behavior (see Table 23.1 for a complete definition).

Pahnke (1963) reported that between 30 and 40% of the students receiving psilocybin had a complete mystical experience versus none for the students who had the nicotinic acid. However, in all categories of mystical experience, average scores of the psilocybin group were higher than the control group, with the positive effects sustained at 6 months (Pahnke, 1963, 1966). Pahnke concluded that psilocybin subjects had a statistically significant and different experience than the controls and had "experienced phenomena which were indistinguishable from, if not identical with" (1963, p. 234) naturally occurring mystical experience. Despite limitations associated with research design standards of the era, the findings established that psilocybin had safely facilitated a mystical experience similar to naturally occurring mystical experiences (Doblin, 1991). Pahnke's study has been described as "perhaps the most famous study in the study of religion" (Hood, Hill, & Spilka, 2009, p. 356).

Decades later, Doblin (1991) conducted a retrospective follow-up study, interviewing seven of the original psilocybin subjects and nine of the controls who had participated at Marsh Chapel. Remarkably, Doblin reported that "all psilocybin subjects participating in the long-term follow-up, but none of the controls, still considered their original experience to have had genuinely mystical elements and to have made a uniquely valuable contribution to their spiritual lives" (p. 23). Doblin's study, however, revealed that one agitated participant who had taken psilocybin had left the supervised location and was administrated chlorpromazine, an antipsychotic drug to sedate him, a fact not documented in the original paper.

Over four decades later, building on the work by Pahnke, researchers at Johns Hopkins University began a series of studies investigating the capacity of psilocybin to safely generate mystical experiences. The first trial compared psilocybin (30 mg/70 kg) with methylphenidate (40 mg/70 kg) in a group of 36 psychedelic-naïve, healthy individuals reporting regular participation in

TABLE 23.1. Subjective Features of Mystical Experience (Pahnke, 1963; Pahnke & Richards, 1966)

- *Unity:* Sense of oneness achieved through ego/self-transcendence. Although the usual sense of identity, or ego, fades away, consciousness and memory are not lost; instead, one becomes aware of being part of a dimension much greater than oneself.

- *Transcendence of time and space:* The subject feels beyond past, present, and future, and beyond ordinary three-dimensional space in a realm of eternity or infinity. A sense of timelessness, when past and future collapse into the present moment—an infinite realm, with no space boundaries.

- *Deeply felt positive mood:* Joy, blessedness, peace, and love to an overwhelming degree of intensity, often accompanied by tears.

- *Sense of sacredness:* Nonrational intuitive response of awe and wonder in the presence of inspiring reality. Core elements are awe, humility, and reverence, but the terms of traditional theology or religion need not necessarily be used in the description.

- *Noetic quality (objectivity and reality):* As named by William James, this is a feeling of insight or illumination that, on an intuitive, nonrational level and with a tremendous force of certainty, subjectively has the status of Ultimate Reality. This knowledge is not an increase of facts but is a gain in psychological, philosophical, or theological insight.

- *Ineffability:* Experience is felt to be beyond words, nonverbal, and impossible to describe, yet most persons who insist on ineffability do in fact make elaborate attempts to communicate the experience.

- *Paradoxicality:* A sense of reconciliation of opposites.

- *Transiency:* The psychedelic peak does not last in its full intensity but instead passes into an afterglow and remains only as a memory.

- *Persisting positive changes in attitudes and behavior:* Toward self, others, life, and the experience itself.

spiritual activities in a double-blind crossover study (Griffiths, Richards, Johnson, McCann, & Jesse, 2008; Griffiths, Richards, McCann, & Jesse, 2006). Drawing on the concepts of set and setting, guidelines were utilized for the preparation, medication, and follow-up integration sessions to enhance safety and optimize the probability of mystical or peak experience (Johnson, Richards, & Griffiths, 2008). Utilizing a revised version of the Pahnke–Richards MEQ (Unity, Transcendence of Time and Space, Sacredness, Noetic Quality, Ineffability and Paradoxicality, and Deeply Felt Positive Mood), the study demonstrated that 61% of the participants in the psilocybin group endorsed criteria for a "complete mystical experience" versus 11% of the methylphenidate group. A complete mystical experience was defined as a score of 60% or higher on each dimension of the MEQ. The study found the experiences to have substantial and sustained personal meaning and spiritual significance in the volunteers (Griffiths et al., 2006). Two months following the medication session, 71% and 33% of the participants rated the psilocybin session as among the top five most spiritually significant experience of their lives and the single most spiritually significant experience of their life, respectively, compared with 8% of the methylphenidate group, who rated it as among the top five spiritually significant but with none rating it the single most significant experience. Adverse effects included 31% of the psilocybin group reporting significant fear during some portions of the medication session. In a 14-month follow-up, 67% of the volunteers rated their experience in the psilocybin session as among the top five most spiritually significant experience of their lives and 58% as among the five most meaningful experiences (Griffiths et al., 2008).

A follow-up trial (Griffiths et al., 2011) evaluated the effects of psilocybin with 18 healthy individuals in a double-blind, dose-dependent study evaluating effects at 5, 10, 20, and 30 mg/70kg. The authors found that 72% of the participants endorsed criteria for a complete mystical experience at either or both of the two highest psilocybin dose sessions. Aside from transient "episodes of psychological struggle" during parts of the high-dose session, no adverse effects were reported (Griffiths et al., 2011, p. 664). Collectively, these studies (Griffiths et al., 2006, 2008, 2011; Pahnke, 1963) demonstrated that psilocybin, when administered in interpersonally supportive sessions with carefully screened participants, and following guidelines tailored to preparation, medication, and integration sessions, can reliably and safely facilitate mystical experiences.

Psychedelic Research for Terminal Cancer: 1962–1977

The soul is neither born, nor does it ever die; nor having once existed, does it ever cease to be. The soul is without birth, eternal, immortal, and ageless. It is not destroyed when the body is destroyed.

—BHAGAVAD GITA

If the use of psychedelic psychotherapy for the dying patient ever should become widespread in our society, there would probably be a change in our whole approach toward death. There might be less fear and more acceptance of this part of the life process.

—WALTER PAHNKE

Prior to the start of the first wave of studies with terminal cancer patients, two individuals, while not directly involved with the research, are noteworthy figures in the history of psychedelic medicine for the dying: Valentina Pavlovna Wasson and Aldous Huxley. As noted, Valentina Wasson and her husband Gordon Wasson had visited Mexico numerous times in search of, and eventually participating in, ritual mushroom ceremonies. In 1957, Valentina, in an interview in *This Week* magazine, suggested that hallucinogenic mushrooms could be helpful in treating the suffering associated with terminal illness. In 1974, Stanislav Grof and colleagues at Maryland Psychiatric Research Center discovered the article in the Wasson home library, years after beginning their psychedelic research with the dying and unaware of Valentina's prescient ideas (Grof & Halifax, 1977).

Following his arrival in Hollywood, California, in 1937 and the publication of *The Perennial Philosophy,* Aldous Huxley (1945) had his first psychedelic experience

in 1953, receiving mescaline from Humphry Osmond, a psychiatrist conducting psychedelic research in Saskatchewan, Canada (see Figure 23.4). Huxley documented his impactful experience in the *Doors of Perception* (1954), a book whose influence on the emerging cultural and recreational use of psychedelics later troubled Huxley, who had preferred that psychedelics remain within the circle of artists, writers, researchers, and poets. Huxley's interest in psychedelics for spiritual inquiry is reflected in this letter to Christian monk and mystic Thomas Merton in January 1959 (in Horowitz & Palmer, 1977):

> [Psychedelic experience] helped me to understand many of the obscure utterances to be found in the writings of the mystics, Christian and Oriental. An unspeakable sense of gratitude for the privilege of being born into this universe. ("Gratitude is heaven itself," says Blake—and I know now exactly what he was talking about.) A transcendence of the ordinary subject–object relationship. A transcendence of the fear of death. A sense of solidarity with the world and its spiritual principle and the conviction that, in spite of the pain, evil, and all the rest, everything is somehow all right. Finally, an understanding, not intellectual, but in some sort total, an understanding with the entire organism, of the affirmation that God is Love. (pp. 158–159)

His interest in death and dying deepened by the loss of his first wife, Maria, in 1955, Huxley developed a fascination in the use of

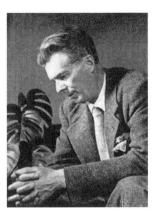

FIGURE 23.4. Aldous Huxley, 1954. (Public domain).

psychedelic-generated mystical experience for the dying. In a correspondence to Osmond, Huxley expressed interest in research that would involve the "administration of LSD to terminal cancer cases, in the hope that it would make dying a more spiritual, less strictly physiological process" (Bisbee et al., 2018, p. 373). In his final novel, *Island,* Huxley (1972) writes of a utopian society where a psilocybin compound called moksha medicine (*moksha* from the Sanskrit meaning "liberation") is used as a sacrament for spiritual insight and is suggestive of helping the dying.

As Huxley was dying at home on November 22, 1963, he asked that his second wife, Laura, inject him with LSD, which she later wrote was consistent with taking the *moksha* medicine he had written about in *Island.* Following the LSD administration, Laura read to him from a manuscript of the yet unpublished *The Psychedelic Experience: A Manual Based on The Tibetan Book of the Dead* (Leary et al., 1964), based on the *Bardo Thodol,* commonly known as *The Tibetan Book of the Dead:*

> You are going forward and up, you are going towards the light. Willing and consciously you are going, you are doing this beautifully. You are going towards the light, you are going towards a greater love. Light and free. Forward and up. You are going towards the best, the greatest love, and it is so easy and you are doing it beautifully. Going forward and up towards the light, into the light, into complete love. (in Horowitz & Palmer, 1977, pp. 264–265)

Noting that November 22, 1963, was also the day of the assassination of President John F. Kennedy, Laura writes in her book *This Timeless Moment* (1968/1991) that "both John F. Kennedy and Aldous Huxley had waged a common fight against ignorance and bad will; both dedicated their lives to helping humanity to understand and love itself" (in Horowitz & Palmer, 1977. p. 259).

Eric Kast/Chicago Medical School

The first studies to take place in the early 1960s investigating the therapeutic use of classic hallucinogens in patients with terminal cancer were led by Eric Kast at the Chicago Medical School. Kast investigated the efficacy of LSD in patients with pain and terminal cancer, not on emotional distress, but on its potential analgesic and pain control properties (Kast & Collins, 1964). Kast hypothesized that LSD could possibly reduce the subjective experience of pain through the "attenuation of anticipation" of pain arising from the sensory distortion of somatic experience. The study compared the analgesic effects of 100 µg of LSD to the pain medications dihydromorphinone (Dilaudid) and meperidine (Demerol) in 50 patients suffering from "intolerable pain"—39 with advanced or terminal cancer and 11 with nonmalignant severe pain syndromes. In their findings, Kast and Collins reported that while the therapeutic action of LSD was slower, LSD demonstrated superior pain control compared with narcotic analgesia and "showed a protracted and more effective action than either of the other drugs" (Kast & Collins, 1964, p. 291). While Kast's study predates the gate control theory of pain (Melzack & Wall, 1965), a theory highlighting the significance of psychological factors *along with* neural mechanisms in the subjective perception of pain experience, Kast's results underscore its eventual clinical and theoretical relevance. Notably, the study demonstrated that along with pain reduction, there were improvements in attitudes toward death and dying. The authors note that patients often disregarded the seriousness of their terminal situation, instead focusing on the beauty of a variety of images and impressions, noting that it "is conceivable that relevance of meaningful sensory input can for protracted periods of time outweigh the fear of dying" (Kast & Collins, 1964, p. 291).

Due to the positive changes in patients' emotional and coping responses to death and dying, Kast turned his attention in follow-up studies to include evaluation of the emotional domain of distress (Kast, 1966, 1967). Observing the changes in attitudes regarding death in a study with 128 patients, all within 2 months of death at time of their participation, Kast noted that "patients were so strikingly unconcerned about death or any other anticipatory concern" that even though a "patient was able to state that death was near, that the situation was hopeless," the patient "felt that this did not matter" (Kast 1967, p. 654). Kast again found a reduction in subjective reports of pain within 3 hours of LSD administration, lasting an average of 12 hours. In some patients, pain intensity was reduced up to 3 weeks following LSD administration, long after drug action, pointing to the alteration in the perception of pain as mediated through psychological and cognitive factors rather than through direct pain analgesia. Elaborating on the possible therapeutic physical pain-reducing factors, Kast (1967) wrote that LSD "seems to deprive the patient of his ability to concentrate on one specific sensory input, even if the input is of urgent survival value" and that "the meaning of pain . . . and its frightful psychic resonance (such as possible doom and destruction) is greatly alleviated" (p. 648). Kast theorized that "LSD obliterates the individual's ego boundaries. In consequence, a geographic separation can more easily be made between the self and the ailing part" (p. 648).

In a follow-up study evaluating 80 patients with terminal malignant disease and all having a life expectancy of weeks or months, patients received 100 µg LSD (Kast, 1966). As in the prior study, Kast (1966) noted the effects consisted of a "lessening of patients' physical distress and a lifting of their mood and outlook" (p. 87). Unlike in the prior studies, he felt the necessity to terminate some of the patient's drug effects with intramuscularly administered chlorpromazine, reporting "only ten patients were able to tolerate the experience for more than ten hours without having some frightening image that necessitated termination" (p. 82). Likely contributing to the necessity of terminating the LSD sessions prematurely was that these early studies did not fully acknowledge the therapeutic context—*set and setting*—or utilize therapeutic guidelines specific to preparation, medication session monitoring, and follow-up integration that would be a vital component of all subsequent research with the dying.

In all, Kast evaluated the effects of LSD on 258 patients, 247 of whom had terminal cancer. No medical complications were noted in any of the studies, and the collective findings showed a reduction in pain severity and depressive feelings, improved sleep, and,

most notably, a lessening of fear related to the progression of disease, dying, and pending death. Kast poignantly noted that "patients who had been listless and depressed were touched to tears by the discovery of a depth of feeling they had not thought themselves capable" (1966, p. 86), and that the experience generated by LSD "creates a new will to live and a zest for experience which against a background of dismal darkness and preoccupying fear produces an exciting and promising outlook. In human terms the short but profound impact upon the dying patient is impressive" (p. 86). While lacking the preparatory and integration sessions associated with set and setting that would be an integral aspect of all subsequent psychedelic research, Kast's research established a foundation and cultivated medical interest in the application of psychedelics with the dying.

Sidney Cohen

Following the studies at Chicago Medical School, Sidney Cohen, a psychiatrist at University of California at the Los Angeles School of Medicine, began investigating the effects of LSD in terminal cancer on only a few individuals. Cohen, previously acquiring LSD from Sandoz Laboratories, had already, since the mid-1950s, been working with Betty Eisner, evaluating the use of LSD as an adjunct for psychotherapy. Cohen was a member of a group of scientists and writers in southern California in the 1950s investigating the use of LSD as a method for facilitating psychotherapy and exploring and enhancing the understanding of mystical or religious experience. This small community of intellectuals, spiritual seekers, and artists included Aldous Huxley; Anaïs Nin, the essayist and novelist; Humphry Osmond, the Canadian psychiatrist who conducted LSD research with alcoholics; Gerald Heard, the British philosopher, writer, and friend of Huxley; Oscar Janiger, a Los Angeles psychiatrist who had been administering LSD in his private practice; and Alan Watts, the Anglican priest turned Zen and psychedelic writer and prominent figure of the emerging Zen Buddhist and psychedelic culture. Huxley and Heard, in particular, were fascinated by the parallels between psychedelic-generated experience and accounts of religious experiences found in the mystic traditions. Both men were closely associated with the Vedanta Society of Southern California founded by Swami Prabhavananda. It is noteworthy to acknowledge the influence of this growing intellectual and spiritual community on the early development of interest with psychedelics, both in the emerging literary and research worlds.

Cohen never published his findings in the scientific literature, but he did speak and write about what he felt was confirmation of Kast's findings regarding the promise that psychedelics held for the dying. Referring to the amelioration of physical pain, Cohen (1965, p. 78) wrote in *Harper's* magazine that "it would seem that LSD does not act directly on the part of the brain that receives pain impulses. Instead, it appears to alter the meaning of the pain, and in doing so, diminishes it." The ability to alter the meaning and hence the perception of the physical pain through the altered and transpersonal state of consciousness brought on by the LSD is captured in this comment by a terminal cancer patient with whom Cohen had worked: "The pain is changed. I know that when I pressed here yesterday, I had an unendurable pain. I couldn't even stand the weight of a blanket. Now I press hard—it hurts, it hurts all right—but it doesn't register as terrifying" (p. 77). Cohen wrote, "Death must become a more human experience. To preserve the dignity of death and prevent the living from abandoning or distancing themselves from the dying is one of the great dilemmas of modern medicine" (p. 77).

Spring Grove State Hospital/Maryland Psychiatric Research Center

Beginning in 1967, investigators of a psychedelic research program at the Spring Grove State Hospital in Baltimore, Maryland (which later became the Maryland Psychiatric Research Center), began exploring the clinical efficacy of LSD and DPT upon the psychological and existential distress of patients with terminal cancer. Since 1963, the group had been conducting research investigating the efficacy of LSD and DPT with alcoholics under the direction of Sanford Unger and Albert Kurland. The decision to turn their attention to the therapeutic use of psychedelics with the dying came about after a hospital staff member was diagnosed with metastatic breast cancer and her emotional distress was successfully treated with LSD (Richards, 1980). Utilizing the guidelines already employed with the alcoholism study, Sidney Wolf, a psychologist with the alcohol treatment team, worked closely with their colleague and served as her guide during her high-dose (200 µg) LSD session. The successful treatment of her emotional distress was reflected by improvements in mood, perspective on life and pending death, and relationships with her family. Following is an excerpt from her journal (in Grof & Halifax, 1977, p. 23):

> Mainly I remember two experiences. I was alone in a timeless world with no boundaries. There was no atmosphere; there was no color, no imagery, but there may have been light. Suddenly I recognized that I was a moment in time, created by those before me and in turn the creator of others. This was my moment, and my major function had been completed. By being born, I had given meaning to my parents' existence. Again, in the void, alone without the time–space boundaries. Life reduced itself over and over again to the least common denominator. I cannot remember the logic of the experience, but I became poignantly aware that the core of life is love. At this moment, I felt that I was reaching out to the world—to all people—but especially to those closest to me. I wept long for the wasted years, the search for identity in false places, the neglected opportunities, the emotional energy lost in basically meaningless pursuits. [And in reflecting on the totality of the experience, she wrote,] What has changed for me? I am living now, and being. I can take it as it comes. I am still me, but more at peace. My family senses this and we are closer. All who know me well say this has been a good experience.

Observing the therapeutic changes of their colleague's experience with LSD, the team at Spring Grove, led by Walter Pahnke until his early and untimely death in 1971, and then by Stanislav Grof and William Richards, began the development of research protocols with LSD and DPT with terminal cancer patients. Unlike Kast's research, the clear objective of the Spring Grove research was to facilitate a "psychological peak experience" (consistent with the mystical experience criteria in Table 23.1) that was theorized to be associated with a positive clinical outcome (Grof, Goodman, Richards, & Kurland, 1973; Kurland, Pahnke, Unger, Savage, & Grof, 1971; Pahnke, Kurland, Goodman, & Richards, 1969; Richards, Rhead, DiLeo, Yensen, & Kurland, 1977). Utilizing the protocol from the treatment of alcoholism studies at Spring Grove, the treatment team addressed guidelines of "set and setting," careful medication session monitoring, and preparatory and postmedication integration therapeutic sessions. The development and implementation of these guidelines organized around the objective of facilitating a psychological peak or mystical experience is a watershed development in psychedelic clinical research and continues to serve as the foundation for present-day clinical trials with psilocybin and other psychedelic compounds (Griffiths et al., 2016; Grob et al., 2011; Johnson et al., 2008; Ross et al., 2016).

A primary objective of preparatory sessions was to foster a sense of trust and rapport between patient and session guides, which was found to minimize adverse effects, particularly fear and anxiety during the medication session (Grof et al., 1973; Johnson et al., 2008; Pahnke et al., 1969). Therapists reviewed the patient's history (developmental, interpersonal, psychosocial, and family), unresolved relational conflicts, religious orientation, coping response to the terminal cancer diagnosis, and expectation for the sessions. The experimental drug sessions took place in a comfortable living-room-like setting with soft lighting, rugs, art and flowers—all to establish a relaxed nonmedical atmosphere. The patient was encouraged to bring family photographs or personal items. Vital to the setting was the inclusion of carefully selected music played through headphones—primarily classical— to help facilitate the release of emotional expression and the surrender to the internal unfolding experience (Bonny & Pahnke, 1972; Kurland et al., 1971; Richards, 1980). The patient would lay down on a couch or bed with headphones and eyeshades to encourage inward attention during the totality of the experience. The nondirective but emotionally present and focused position of the

therapist team (usually a male–female dyad) during the experimental drug session included offers of interpersonal support, guidance, and assurance when needed. Ideally, there was minimal verbal exchange during the nonordinary states of consciousness experienced by the patient. If panic or anxiety was experienced in response to any images or rising emotions, therapists provided assurance, encouraging the patient to accept or "move into" the experience or image, ideally resulting in an insightful experience (Richards, 1980). A period of follow-up therapeutic integration sessions exploring psychological material arising from the medication session typically began the evening of the session or the following day.

From 1967 through the mid-1970s, the investigators at Spring Grove published a series of research, clinical, and theoretical papers (Grof, 1980; Grof et al., 1973; Kurland, Pahnke, Unger, Savage, & Goodman, 1969; Pahnke, 1969; Pahnke et al., 1969, 1970; Richards, Grof, Goodman, & Kurland, 1972; Richards et al., 1979). The first data to be published (Pahnke et al., 1969) were from an open-label study of 22 patients with terminal cancer, utilizing 200–300 µg LSD. The primary inclusion criterion was a depressive reaction secondary to a cancer diagnosis. Additional inclusion factors were anxiety, emotional withdrawal, and physical pain. The categories of the MEQ were slightly revised and characterized as "psychological-peak experience" (Unity, Transcendence, Deeply Felt Positive Mood, Sacredness, Meaningfulness of Psychological and/or Philosophical Insight, and Ineffability), with Pahnke and colleagues noting that "the most therapeutically useful kind of LSD experience, and therefore the immediate aim of the LSD session itself, is the psychedelic peak experience" (1969, p. 146). Pre- and post-LSD sessions measured for depression, anxiety, emotional tension, psychological isolation, fear of death, and necessity for pain medication. The findings demonstrated that of the 22 patients, "14 showed improvement in varying degrees while eight remained essentially unchanged" (p. 148). In approximately two-thirds of the patients, the authors note a "meaningful positive change and in 6 of these 14 patients a dramatic improvement" (p. 148). Of significance, the data suggested a correlation between psychedelic peak or mystical experience and clinical improvement, reflected in the finding that five of the six who improved most dramatically met criteria for an intense psychedelic peak experience (a score of five out of six on the "Positive Psychedelic Content" measure). Pahnke (1969, p. 12) reflected on the experiences of this first group of patients:

> The most dramatic effects came in the wake of a psychedelic mystical experience. There was a decrease in fear, anxiety, worry, and depression. Sometimes the need for pain medications was lessened, but mainly because the patient was able to tolerate what pain he had more easily. There was an increase in serenity, peace, and calmness. Most striking was a decrease in the fear of death. It seems as if the mystical experience, by opening the patient to usually untapped ranges of human consciousness, can provide a sense of security that transcends even death. Once the patient is able to release all the psychic energy which he has tied to the fear of death and worry about the future, he seems able to live more meaningfully in the present. He can turn his attention to the things which have the most significance in the here and now.

Additional findings were published (Grof et al., 1973) in an open-label study of 31 patients with terminal cancer utilizing LSD with a dose range of 200–500 μg. Inclusion criteria were depression, anxiety, isolation, and pain secondary to the terminal cancer diagnosis. A survival expectancy of 3 months was a requirement for inclusion. A 13-point rating scale developed by Pahnke and Richards (Emotional Condition Rating Scale [ECRS]; 1966) was administered pre- and postmedication sessions, and the prior psychological peak experience scale was utilized. Preparatory sessions occurred over a 2- to 3-week period for an average total of about 10 hours. Of the 31 patients, 29% (nine patients) showed *dramatic improvement*; 41.9% (13 patients) showed *moderate improvement*; 22.6% (seven patients) were *unchanged*; and 6.4% (2 patients) showed *negative effects* on the measures, although the authors describe this minor negative rating as negligible. As in the prior study by Pahnke and colleagues (1969), most signifi-

cant improvements were associated with a higher or intense psychological peak experience, described as an "experience of unity, usually preceded by agony and death and followed by spiritual rebirth" (Grof et al., 1973, p. 141) and that "increased acceptance of death usually followed sessions in which the patients' reported deep religious and mystical experiences" (p. 143). The authors concluded that "the most dramatic therapeutic results have been, however, observed in association with the psychedelic peak experience that appears to be a new and rather powerful mechanism responsible for profound personality changes" (p. 142). As in the Kast studies, there were reduced ratings in subjective physical pain typically lasting longer than the drug action.

In an effort to minimize the length of the experimental session (LSD sessions typically lasted 6–12 hours) and the subsequent physical impact upon debilitated cancer patients, research led by William Richards utilizing DPT, a shorter acting serotonergic hallucinogen, was tried with terminal cancer patients (Richards, 1978, 1980; Richards et al., 1977, 1979). In addition to shorter acting properties, there was hope it would prove less controversial in the midst of the sensationalist media coverage of LSD in the late 1960s and early 1970s (Richards et al., 1979). A few publications present data on a slightly different number of patients from the same cohort: Data on 34 patients were provided in Richards and colleagues (1977); 30 patients in Richards and colleagues (1979); and 28 patients in Richards (1978). The criteria for psychological peak or mystical experience were the six domains of Unity, Transcendence of Time and Space, Objectivity and Reality (Noetic Quality), Sense of Sacredness, and the final domain of Ineffability and Paradoxicality (Richards, 1978; Richards et al., 1977). Measures administered in these studies were the previously used ECRS, the Mini-Mult (an abbreviated version of the Minnesota Multiphasic Personality Inventory [MMPI]), and the Personal Orientation Inventory (POI). DPT was administered intramuscularly, and dosage was determined by body weight and assessments of psychological resistance (Richards et al., 1979). As in the LSD protocols, eye shades and headphones were used, and therapists were present throughout the experience of nonordinary states of consciousness providing interpersonal verbal and physical support (hand holding) when indicated. On the ECRS, only the scales for Depression and Anxiety reached significance greater than .05 at $p = .03$ and $p = .01$, respectfully. On the Mini-Mult, six of the 11 scales met statistical significance for clinical improvement including that of Depression. On the POI, the scales of Time Competence and Inner Directness reached statistical positive change, defined as the patients living more in the present moment with less rumination or worry over past or future events and being more self-assertive and confident. The scales for Self-Regard, Self-Acceptance, and Capacity for Intimate Contact were found to indicate a positive significance at .02, .005, and .02, respectively. These findings were evaluated at 1-week post-DPT session. Consistent with prior findings, the results demonstrated that clinical improvements were correlated with those patients classified as "peakers" (those who had scored higher on the psychedelic peak or MEQ) versus "nonpeakers" (who did not have the full peak or mystical experience). Similar content and range of nonordinary altered states of consciousness were reported in the DPT studies, as in the LSD studies. The difference between DPT and LSD was most acutely seen in the rapidity of onset, total drug duration, and abruptness of termination. Whereas LSD peak content and intensity occurred at about the third to fifth hour, the DPT peak intensity was reached in approximately 10–15 minutes, which the group felt could be a disadvantage given the shorter time to acclimate to the dramatic changes in consciousness. The drug was well tolerated, with no serious adverse reactions (Richards et al., 1979). Consistent with LSD studies, observations from the DPT sessions echoed insights that the psychedelic drug did not provide a specific drug effect per se, but rather the combination of set and setting, and the unique phenomenology associated with a transpersonal experience allowed an opportunity for personal psychological or spiritual growth within the context of a terminal illness.

With growing sensationalist media coverage on the emerging recreational and non-medical use of psychedelics, the cultural climate grew increasingly challenging for funding and governmental support of psychedelic research in the United States. The studies finally ended in the mid-1970s following the passage of the Controlled Substance Act of 1970, which had placed hallucinogens into Schedule 1 of the U.S. Drug Enforcement Administration's classification system of regulated substances. Near the end of the trials, the investigators turned to psilocybin in a comparison model to DPT in a few patients. The final cancer patient from this consequential era of psychedelic research received psilocybin in a session guided by William Richards in the Spring of 1977 (W. Richards, personal communication, August 25, 2018).

The preliminary research findings from Chicago Medical School through the studies at Spring Grove State Hospital/Maryland Psychiatric Research Center offered a cautiously promising and novel clinical approach for the treatment of the psychological, spiritual, and existential distress in a population of dying patients. While limited by the absence of currently held standard research practices such as double-blind, randomized, and placebo-controlled conditions, these early findings established a foundation for psychedelic therapy, notably, the psychedelic peak or mystical experience model arising from the studies at Spring Grove and Maryland Psychiatric Research Center. These studies also posited the association between the mystical/psychological peak experience and positive outcomes in cancer distress, a significant finding that continues to hold clinical and research implications decades later (Griffiths et al., 2016; Grof et al., 1973; Pahnke et al., 1969; Richards et al., 1977, 1979; Ross et al., 2016). William Richards estimates the final number of patients from the Spring Grove/Maryland Research Center studies receiving LSD to be at 50, with 40 receiving DPT, and less than 4 receiving psilocybin (Richards, 1980; personal communication, August 25, 2018). (Due to the publication of myriad reports from this group, with some reports reanalyzing or covering previously described patient data, the precise total number of patients enrolled in the cancer studies varies slightly across reports.)

On the significance of the mystical experience in the transformation of the dying patient, Pahnke (1969, p. 15) wrote:

Our experiments have indicated that deep within every human being there are vast untapped resources of love, joy, and peace. One aspect of the psychedelic mystical experience is a release of these positive feelings with subsequent decrease in negative feelings of depression, despair, and anxiety. But this shift in mood is not enough to account for our most dramatic finding—loss of the fear of death. In fact, the experience of deeply felt positive mood may be more the result than the cause of this change in attitude toward death. Our data show that these feelings are released most fully when there is complete surrender to the ego-loss experience of positive ego transcendence, which is often experienced as a moment of death and rebirth. At this point, unless the patient previously had experienced mystical consciousness spontaneously, he becomes intensely aware of completely new dimensions of experience which he might never before have imagined possible. From his own personal experience, he now knows that there is more to the potential range of human consciousness than we ordinarily realize. This profound and awe-inspiring insight sometimes is experienced as if a veil had been lifted and can transform attitudes and behavior. Once a person has had this vision, life and death can be looked at from a new perspective.

In 1976, in the waning days of the research studies, the CBS television news magazine *60 Minutes* aired a segment featuring an interview with terminal cancer patient Kenneth Pugh, a patient from the Spring Grove studies. Pugh described the LSD-generated experience as helping him accept his pending death without terror, cope with his physical pain, and improve his ability to speak about his dying and death with his family (in Phifer, 1977, pp. 287–288):

It's all blackness at first, and all of a sudden, it's just like-like Panavision. It just opens up. I had no bad experiences whatsoever. None. I had nothing to fear. I didn't see horrible animals or gargoyles or anything of this nature. I heard beautiful music. I saw beautiful scenery. My first encounter, when I went into this world, I was only seven years old. I was a child. It took me that far back at first. We played as we did when we were children. At

one point, I found myself standing on the top of a mountain. There were three people there; and I was one, and Christ was the other, and the Holy spirit was the other; and we were standing with our arms around each other. This, to me, was a very moving experience. It gave me a feeling of everything's okay, it's all going to end well.

Following the prohibition of psychedelics, Kurland and colleagues (1971) prophetically glimpsing the future, wrote in a summary titled "The Year 2000" that "one can visualize, thirty years hence, that these techniques may be more generally applied" and "for those whom death may approach prematurely through some disease process for which no remedy is available, the preparation for dying may be made an experience of meaning and resolution, adding dignity and stature to both the patient and those close to him" (p. 105). Not until 2011, 40 years following these written words, would the next clinical research publication on psychedelics in dying persons be published.

■ Contemporary Research

When the psyche is not under that obligation
to live in time and space alone, and obviously,
it doesn't, then to that extent the psyche is
not submitted to those laws, and that means a
practical continuation of life, of a sort of psychical
existence, beyond time and space.
                                        —CARL G. JUNG

Following a hiatus of over 30 years, research with classic serotonergic hallucinogens in individuals with cancer or other life-threatening illness resumed in the 2000s with four double-blind, randomized, placebo-controlled clinical trials, three in the United States utilizing psilocybin (Griffiths et al., 2016; Grob et al., 2011; Ross et al., 2016) and one study in Switzerland investigating LSD (Gasser, Holstein, et al., 2014; Gasser, Kirchner, & Passie, 2014). Collectively, the four studies comprised 104 patients, including cancer patients (Griffiths et al., 2016; Grob et al., 2011; Ross et al., 2016) and patients with a variety of life-threatening illnesses (Gasser, Holstein, et al., 2014a; Gasser, Kirchner, & Passie, 2014b). All patients had coexisting anxiety disorders.

University of California, Los Angeles; Johns Hopkins University; New York University School of Medicine

While the studies with cancer distress in the United States in the 1960s and 1970s utilized LSD or DPT, the three American trials in the 2010's used psilocybin for distress associated with cancer. Psilocybin, the psychoactive compound in many species of mushrooms, metabolizes to psilocin, an agonist at 5-HT_{2A} and 5-HT_{2C} receptors, and was used for its unique properties and safety in the new trials with cancer patients (Grob, Bossis, & Griffiths, 2013). The psilocybin trials in the United States took place at the University of California, Los Angeles (UCLA), the Johns Hopkins University School of Medicine, and the New York University (NYU) School of Medicine and were all supported by the Heffter Research Institute (*www.heffter.org*). All three sites utilized established guidelines of set and setting, notably interpersonally supportive preparatory sessions, medication session monitoring, and postmedication therapeutic integration sessions first developed at Spring Grove/Maryland Psychiatric Center (Grof & Halifax, 1977; Johnson et al., 2008; Richards et al., 1979).

The first of these psilocybin studies on the safety and efficacy of psychedelics with terminal illness in the 21st century was conducted by Grob and colleagues (2011) at Harbor–UCLA Medical Center. In this pilot study, 12 patients diagnosed with advanced-stage cancer and a coexisting DSM-IV-diagnosed anxiety disorder (acute stress disorder, generalized anxiety disorder due to cancer, or adjustment disorder) were administered either 0.2 mg/kg of psilocybin or the placebo niacin (250 mg) in two separate experimental medication sessions, several weeks apart, with each subject acting as his or her own control in a crossover design. Subjects' ages ranged from 36 to 58 years and 11 participants were women. Primary cancers included breast cancer, colon cancer, and ovarian cancer. By the time of publication of the study, 10 of the 12 had died. All participants are now deceased.

Primary measure data from the Beck Depression Inventory (BDI), Profile of Mood States (POMS), and State–Trait Anxiety Inventory (STAI) were collected at the following time points: (1) the day prior to the experimental sessions (psilocybin and niacin); (2) at the end of the day of the experimental sessions; (3) the day following the experimental sessions; (4) 2 weeks after each experimental session; (5) and monthly for 6 months. Changes in consciousness were measured by the Five-Dimensional Altered States of Consciousness Profile (5D-ASC).

Although the psilocybin dose was less than the comparatively higher doses of psychedelics in the earlier research and in the subsequent trials at Johns Hopkins University and NYU, potentially limiting the intensity or scope in altered states of consciousness, the results showed acute trends in reductions in anxiety and depression. Statistically significant changes in depression were noted at the 6-month follow-up point, and significant anxiety reductions were observed at the 1- and 3-month follow-up time points. Scores on the BDI decreased by almost 30% from the first medicine session to 1 month following the second session and were sustained at the 6-month time point. On the STAI Anxiety measure, statistically significant reductions were reached at the 1- and 3-month time points. While not statistically significant, there were trends in improved mood on the POMS measure. On the 5D-ASC, psilocybin showed differences in subjects' experience, the greatest being Oceanic Boundlessness. The authors note that participants reported a greater quality-of-life experience and improvements in coping with the psychological stressors of terminal cancer, notably closer relational and empathic bonds to family, including an increased openness to address their end-of-life status. In addition to demonstrating trends in reducing anxiety and depression, the UCLA study was pivotal in establishing safety and feasibility, receiving U.S. Food and Drug Administration (FDA) regulatory approval and setting a foundation for future studies.

Following the findings from UCLA, in December 2016, teams at Johns Hopkins University School of Medicine (Griffiths et al., 2016) and NYU School of Medicine (Ross et al., 2016) each published a paper demonstrating robust and positive findings utilizing psilocybin with cancer patients with coexisting anxiety, depression, and psychosocial distress. The research papers, published together in a special issue of the *Journal of Psychopharmacology*, were accompanied by 11 editorials by American and European leaders in palliative care, addiction, psychiatry, and drug policy. Together, the two studies included 80 cancer patients, with approximately 80% of the patients demonstrating decreases in anxiety, depression, and measures of existential distress with these improvements sustained at a minimum of 6 months. Medical exclusionary criteria included epilepsy, renal disease, diabetes, abnormal liver function, and severe cardiovascular disease. Psychiatric exclusionary criteria included a personal or immediate family history of schizophrenia, bipolar disorder, delusional disorder, paranoid disorder, and schizoaffective disorder. In both randomized, double-blind, crossover trials, the 30-item MEQ (Barrett, Johnson, & Griffiths, 2015; MacLean, Leoutsakos, Johnson, & Griffiths, 2012) was administered to assess for mystical experience. Significantly, both *studies demonstrated the mystical experience to be a mediating factor and predictor in enduring changes in outcome measures, including anxiety and depressive outcomes.*

In the Johns Hopkins study, Griffiths and colleagues (2016) included 51 participants, all diagnosed with a potentially life-threatening cancer diagnosis and 65% having recurrent or metastatic disease. Types of cancer included breast, gastrointestinal, genitourinary, aerodigestive, and hematological malignancies. All volunteers had a DSM-IV diagnosis of either anxiety or mood disorder (adjustment disorder with anxiety or mixed anxiety and depression, dysthymic disorder, generalized anxiety disorder, major depressive disorder, and dual diagnosis of an anxiety disorder and major depression). Using a crossover design, the study compared a low dose of psilocybin (1 or 3 mg/70 kg), categorized as "placebo-like" versus a high dose of psilocybin (22 or 30 mg/70 kg) on the primary outcome measures of anxiety and depressed mood, and myriad secondary measures reflecting quality of life, spiritual well-being, death acceptance, death transcendence, purpose in life, optimism, and meaningfulness. Each participant served as his or her own control and was randomized to receive either the low or high dose of psilocybin in two separate medication sessions 5 weeks apart, with half receiving the low dose first and half receiving the high dose first. The first medication session occurred approximately 1 month after enrollment and after approximately 8 hours of preparatory sessions. Therapeutically relevant outcome data were collected from the participants at the following time points: (1) baseline: immediately following enrollment into the study; (2) 5 weeks after Session 1; (3) 5 weeks after Session 2; and (4) 6 months after Session 2. No serious adverse effects (SAEs) attributed to the administration of psilocybin were reported. There were transient and moderate elevations in systolic and/or diastolic blood pressure following psilocybin administration. The authors report that 32 and 26% of the participants in the high-dose session experienced some type of transient psychological discomfort and an episode of anxiety, respectively.

Measures evaluating the subjective experiences generated by psilocybin were the Hallucinogen Rating Scale; the 5-D-ASC; the States of Consciousness Questionnaire; the Mysticism Scale, and the MEQ. The primary outcome variables of depression and anxiety were measured by the clinician-rated Hamilton Rating Scale for Depression (GRID-HAM-D) and the Hamilton Anxiety Rating Scale (HAM-A), respectfully.

The results demonstrated that the high dose of psilocybin generated large and sustained positive effects on both primary variables of depression and anxiety, and increases in measures of quality of life, life meaning, death acceptance, and optimism. The reductions in depression and anxiety were sustained at the 6-month follow-up, with clinical response at 78% and 83%, respectively. The overall rate of symptom remission at 6 months was 65% for depression and 57% for anxiety. On the depression measure, 5 weeks after the high dose of psilocybin and before crossover, 92% of participants showed a clinically significant response (i.e., ≥50% decrease relative to baseline) compared with 32% response rate of the participants who took a low dose in the first medication session. At 6 months, 79% of the high-dose first group had a sustained clinical response on the depression outcome. For the anxiety outcome measure at 5 weeks, 76% of the high-dose first group showed a clinically significant response versus 24% of the low-dose first group, with 83% of the high-dose first group continuing to show a clinically significant response at 6 months.

In addition to the two primary measures, 9 of the 15 secondary measures met the most conservative criteria for demonstrating positive psilocybin effects at the 6-month follow-up (defined as showing a significant between-group difference 5 weeks after the first session, as well as a difference between assessments after the first and second session in the group that had low-dose first). These nine secondary psychiatric measures are the BDI; the Hospital Anxiety and Depression Scale (HADS; Depression scale); the STAI (State–Trait Anxiety Inventory); the Profile of Mood States (POMS; Mood Disturbance); the Brief Symptom Inventory; the McGill Quality of Life Questionnaire (MQOL; Overall Quality of Life), MQOL (Meaningful Existence); the Life Attitude Profile—Revised (LAP-R; Death Acceptance); and the Life Orientation Test Revised (LOT-R; Optimism). Figure 23.5 graphically shows six of these plus the two primary measures.

On the Persisting Effects Questionnaire (PEQ), high-dose psilocybin generated significant improvement versus low-dose on attitudes about life and self, mood, social effects, behavior, and spirituality, with these effects sustained at the 6-month follow-up. At 6 months, 67% rated the high-dose psilocybin experience among the five most meaningful experiences of their lives, including the single most meaningful experience; 70% rated the high-dose psilocybin as one of the top five most spiritually significant life events, including the single most spiritually significant event, and 83% rated the high-dose psilocybin experience as increasing their well-being or life satisfaction.

Of theoretical and clinical significance was the association of a mystical experience (MEQ) with a majority of the enduring changes in therapeutic outcome measures. This significant association between mystical experience and therapeutic outcome was sustained following an analysis to control for overall intensity of drug effect, further positing mystical experience as playing a mediating role in positive therapeutic outcomes in emotional distress associated with a life-threatening illness.

The NYU clinical trial (Ross et al., 2016) included 29 patients with a cancer diagnosis in a double-blind, placebo-controlled, randomized, crossover design comparing psilocybin (0.3 mg/kg) to niacin (250 mg) on primary outcome measures of anxiety and depression, imbedded in psychological support and brief therapy. Nearly two-thirds of the patients (62%) had advanced cancers (Stages 3 or 4). Types of cancer included breast, reproductive, and hematological. The participants' psychiatric diagnoses (Structured Clinical Interview for DSM-IV [SCID-IV]) included adjustment disorder with anxiety and depressed mood, chronic (14%), adjustment disorder with anxiety, chronic (71%), and generalized anxiety disorder (14%). The protocol provided two experimental sessions, one with psilocybin and the other with niacin, with each patient serving as his or her own control with 7 weeks between experimental sessions. Patients were randomized to either the psilocybin-first or the niacin-first group, and the two groups were compared before and following the 7-week crossover. The first medication session (either psilocybin or niacin) took place following 6 hours of preparation over a roughly 3- to 4-week period. Clinical data for the primary measures were collected at the following time points: (1) baseline (2–4 weeks prior to Dose 1); (2) 1 day prior to Dose 1; (3) 1 day after Dose 1; (4) 2 weeks after Dose 1; (5) 6 weeks after Dose 1; (6) 7 weeks following Dose 1 (which was 1 day prior to Dose 2 and crossover); (7) 1 day after Dose 2; 6 weeks after Dose 2; and (8) 26 weeks after Dose 2.

Primary outcome measures were the anxiety and depression measures for the HADS: HADS Anxiety (HAD-A); HADS Depression (HAD-D); and HADS Total/Combined (HAD-T); the BDI; and the STAI for State (STAI-S) and Trait (STAI-T) Anxiety. Secondary measures included assessing cancer-related distress, quality of life, and spiritual well-being: Demoralization (DEM); Hopelessness Assessment and Illness (HAI); Death Anxiety Scale (DAS): and Death Transcendence Scale (DTS); World Health Organization Quality of Life Scale (WHO-Brief); and the Functional Assessment of Chronic Illness Therapy—Spiritual Well-Being (FACIT-SWB). Subjective drug effects were assessed with the MEQ30 and PEQ. There were no serious medical or psychiatric SAEs reported.

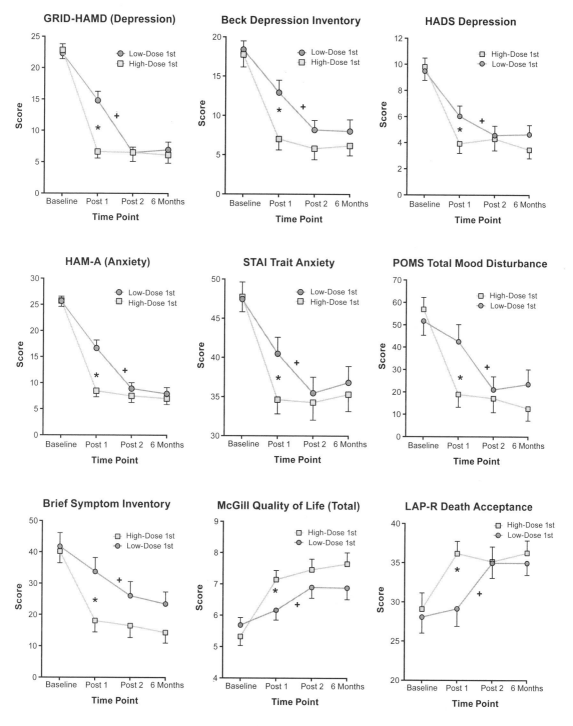

FIGURE 23.5. Effects of psilocybin on selected outcome measures assessed at baseline, 5 weeks after Session 1 (Post 1), 5 weeks after Session 2 (Post 2), and at 6-month follow-up. Data points show means. Circles represent the group that received a low dose on the first session and a high dose on the second session; squares represent the group that received a high dose on the first session and a low dose on the second session. Star symbols indicate a significant difference between the two groups at the post-Session 1 time point ($p < .05$, planned comparison). Cross symbols indicate a significant difference between the post-Session 1 and post-Session 2 time points in the low-dose first (high-dose second) group ($p < .05$, planned comparison).

The results indicated that on the primary outcome variables of depression and anxiety, the psilocybin-first group demonstrated immediate, substantial, and sustained clinical benefits versus the niacin-first group at the 7-week time point before the crossover (Figure 23.6). The magnitude of differences between the psilocybin and control groups measured by Cohen's *d* effect sizes was large across all primary measures assessed at all five time points before the crossover. For primary outcome measures, the psilocybin-first group showed significant within-group decreases in anxiety and depression immediately after (day after) receiving psilocybin, with reductions sustaining significance at all subsequent time points, including the final time point at approximately 8 months. The niacin-first group showed significant reductions in five of the six primary measures *only after* receiving psilocybin in the second medication session, and these reductions persisted until the end of study.

Psilocybin demonstrated antidepressive and antianxiety response rates, with 83% of volunteers in the psilocybin-first group (vs. 14% in the niacin-first group) meeting criteria for an antidepressant response (≥ 50% decrease relative to baseline with BDI) and 58% of volunteers in the psilocybin-first group (vs. 14% in niacin-first group) meeting criteria for an anxiolytic response (≥ 50 % decrease relative to baseline with HADS-A) at the 7-week crossover. On the secondary outcome measures, psilocybin compared to niacin demonstrated improvements in spiritual well-being and quality of life, while yielding reductions in demoralization and hopelessness. These changes were observed 2 weeks post-dose 1 and sustained at 6.5 months. At the 26-week time point, 70 and 52% of the study volunteers rated what they believed to be the psilocybin session as the singular or top five most personally meaningful, or the singular or top most spiritually significant experience of their lives, respectively. At the final time point, 87% of the study volunteers reported increased life satisfaction or general well-being that they attributed to the psilocybin-generated experience. Common adverse effects included nonclinically significant elevations in blood pressure and heart rate (76%); headache (28%); nausea (14%); and transient or epi-sodic anxiety (17%). As of this writing, 12 of the participants have died.

As with prior research with heathy volunteers (Griffiths et al., 2006, 2008, 2011), the NYU trial, along with the Johns Hopkins cancer-anxiety trial, demonstrated the capacity of psilocybin to safely generate mystical experiences. Moreover, the NYU and Johns Hopkins trials, consistent with prior psychedelic research with cancer-associated psychological distress (Richards et al., 1977), found that the mystical experience as measured by the MEQ30 was shown to be a mediating factor in the positive therapeutic primary outcomes of anxiety and depression in cancer distress.

To enhance the generalizability of the conclusions, future multisite studies would ideally employ a larger sample size with a more diverse sample relative to race, ethnicity, sexual orientation, economic class, and educational level that is representative of the general population. Additionally, further research should include not just patients with cancer, but patients with a broad spectrum of diagnoses that is more representative of the palliative care population. While physical pain secondary to cancer was evaluated, there were no significant findings, although it is important to note that patients with pain continued their pain medications during the sessions. Additional challenges or limitations include the difficulty of effective blinding due to the unique and often profound shifts in consciousness that psychedelics can generate. Another is the crossover design, limiting effective analyses of measures after the crossover.

LSD Clinical Trial in Solothurn, Switzerland

The first study to investigate the therapeutic efficacy and safety of LSD in patients with a life-threatening disease and experiencing psychological distress since the research at Spring Grove in the mid-1960s was a Phase II double-blind, randomized, active placebo-controlled pilot study conducted by Gasser, Holstein, and colleagues (2014) in Switzerland. Consistent with contemporary research, the trial implemented guidelines specific to the model of set and setting. The study included 12 patients with anxiety associated with a life-threatening disease,

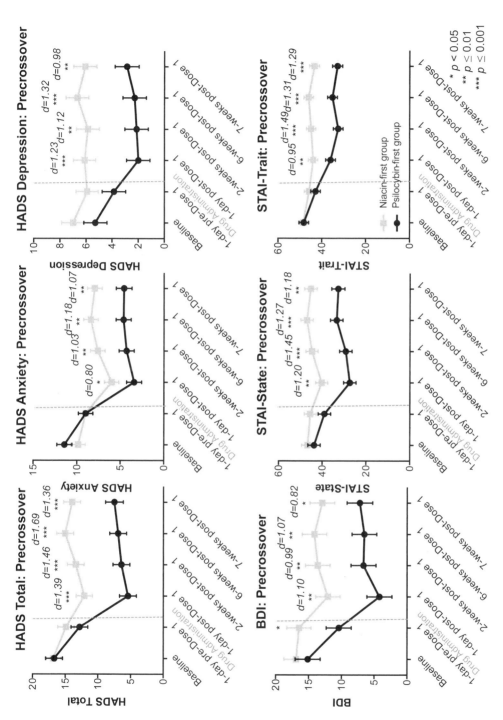

FIGURE 23.6. Primary outcome variables: cancer-related anxiety and depression (precrossover). Means (±SE) for primary outcome measures are shown in the two treatment groups at the following time points: baseline, 1 day predose 1, 1 day postdose 1, 2 weeks postdose 1, 6 weeks postdose 1, and 7 weeks postdose 1. Asterisks indicate significance level of between-group *t*-tests. Effect sizes, represented as Cohen's *d*, are shown above time points at which the treatment groups differ. Closed points represent significant within-group differences relative to scores at baseline.

including breast and gastric cancers, non-Hodgkin's lymphoma, celiac disease, and Parkinson's disease. One participant had prior experience with LSD. At study admission, all volunteers scored greater than 40 on either the State or Trait scale of the STAI. Half of the patients were diagnosed (SCID) with generalized anxiety disorder (GAD). Other comorbid psychiatric diagnoses among the patients were major depression (63%), dysthymia (18%), posttraumatic stress disorder (PTSD; 8%), and panic disorder (27%). Patients were randomized to either a group receiving a moderate oral dose of 200 µg of LSD (N = 8) or an active placebo of 20 µg of LSD (N = 4). The authors note one active placebo patient was excluded from analysis following the completion of all study procedures after "a correction in the diagnosis of the qualifying disease state" no longer met inclusion criteria (Gasser, Holstein, et al 2014, p. 517). The authors note the 20-µg dose was likely chosen to produce short-lived and mild effects, but not the therapeutic effects typically seen at higher doses of LSD. Both groups (high-dose LSD and low-dose LSD) received two LSD sessions 2 to 3 weeks apart embedded within two preparatory and six integrative psychotherapy sessions. Following the unblinding that occurred 2 months after the second medication session, the active placebo group could, if desired, cross over and receive an open-label treatment with 200 µg of LSD.

The primary outcome measure for anxiety was the STAI Anxiety measure Form X, a self-report for state and trait anxiety symptoms. Secondary outcome measures were the European Cancer Quality of Life Questionnaire (EORTC-QLQ-30), the Symptom Checklist-90—Revised (SCL-90-R), and the HADS. Outcome measure data was collected at (1) baseline; (2) 1 week after each drug administration session; (3) 2-month follow-up; and (4) 12-month follow-up.

On the primary outcome measure for anxiety at the 2-month follow-up, the findings demonstrated positive trends in the STAI in reductions in trait and state anxiety, with effect sizes of 1.1 and 1.2, respectively. These reduction in the STAI for both state and trait anxiety were also sustained at 12 months. In contrast, all of the active placebo participants experienced increases in trait anxiety. The authors note that secondary measures were not analyzed for significance because of "concerns of multiplicity" (Gasser, Holstein, et al., 2014, p. 6) and sample size and challenges with blinding, given the robust effects of LSD, were study limitations.

There were no serious adverse effects attributed to LSD (anxiety, psychotic, or perceptual disorders). There were mild fluctuations in heart rate and blood pressure but of no clinical significance. Patients reporting mild-to-moderate emotional distress were 36% for the high-dose sessions and 33% for the low-dose active placebo sessions. There were six reports of adverse effects, such as emotional distress, that persisted until the next day.

In addition to the four quantitative studies (Gasser, Holstein, et al., 2014; Griffiths et al., 2016; Grob et al., 2011; Ross et al., 2016), three qualitative studies were completed from cancer patient narratives, two from the NYU psilocybin trial (Belser et al., 2017; Swift et al., 2017) and one from the LSD trial (Gasser et al., 2014b). An additional review evaluated thematic content of four patients from the NYU study (Malone et al., 2018). By identifying themes with psilocybin session experiences, these studies offer cogent insights into the potential mechanisms of therapeutic change. Utilizing a phenomenological analysis of verbatim transcripts recorded in semistructured interviews with 13 cancer patients in the 2016 NYU trial, Belser and colleagues (2017) identified myriad themes from the volunteers' subjective experiences, including forgiveness, improved interpersonal functioning, enhanced appreciation of relationships, cultivation of insight regarding death, and revised life priorities. Accompanying these experiences were feelings of joy, bliss, ineffability, unity and interconnectedness, and strong feelings of love. Swift and colleagues (2017), in a separate qualitative analysis from the same cohort, identified additional themes, one in particular categorized as an "uncoupling from cancer," which was described as experiencing a distinct emotional "separation" or nonattachment from cancer, resulting in an enhanced capacity to identify with other qualities of self-experience and values of personhood. In the qualitative study of the LSD trial, Gasser and colleagues (2015) cite increased access to emotions, reduced fear of death, increased quality of life, and increased equanimity among the lasting benefits articulated by study volunteers. The reader is referred to these qualitative studies for more details.

Collectively, the four clinical trials between 2011 and 2016, totaling 104 patients, demonstrated the safe utility of psilocybin (Griffiths et al., 2016; Grob et al., 2011; Ross et al., 2016) and LSD (Gasser, Holstein, et al., 2014) in carefully screened and interpersonally supported settings for patients diagnosed with cancer or life-threatening illness. Aside from mild-to-moderate elevations in blood pressure, headache, and nausea, there were no serious medical or psychiatric adverse effects or events requiring medical intervention in any of these trials. None of the patients in these four studies reported hallucinogen persisting perception disorder (HPPD). On the occasion of difficult or challenging experience, the recent trials (Gasser, Holstein, et al., 2014; Griffiths et al., 2016; Grob et al., 2011; Ross et al., 2016) affirm prior findings that while fear, panic, paranoia, and states of heightened anxiety may occur during a drug session, these reactions can be well managed with empathic, calm, reassurance from the therapists (Johnson et al., 2008), These encounters within the drug-administered experience often lead to therapeutic insight when subjects are carefully and empathically supported and encouraged to accept the unfolding changes in consciousness with concomitant reassurance that they are safe and the effects of the drug are temporary.

▨ Phenomenology and Implications for Palliative Care

If you die before you die, then you won't die when you die.

—INSCRIPTION, ST. PAUL'S MONASTERY, MOUNT ATHOS, GREECE

Our true nature is the nature of no birth and no death. Only when we touch our true nature can we transcend the fear of non-being, the fear of annihilation.

—THICH NHAT HANH

The development of the psychedelic treatment model for the treatment of emotional suffering associated with a life-threatening diagnosis or the end of life offers a promising approach to the discipline of palliative care. Conventional psychopharmacotherapies may take weeks to prove efficacy, if at all, and then only with daily compliance with the pharmacological compound in providing symptom relief. The psychedelic treatment model by comparison has demonstrated the ability for a single dose and experiential session, embedded within a brief course of preparation and psychotherapeutic integration, to generate shifts in consciousness, providing the opportunities for *experiences* found to provide personally transformative and *enduring* effects. Rather than the sole reduction of symptoms, this model offers the potential for therapeutic change through the occasion to explore existential and spiritual dimensions of human experience. Psychedelic treatment does not therefor solely rely on a drug effect per se, but rather on insights and memories from the unique phenomenology of transpersonal experience that allows the possibility to discover new perspectives regarding the nature of self, death, and consciousness.

Thematic analyses on spirituality within palliative care include meaning making and transcendence among the most cited variables (Vachon et al., 2009). The psychedelic treatment model, by demonstrating the capacity to enhance personal meaning (Griffiths et al., 2006, 2008, 2011) and with self-transcendence comprising a primary feature of mystical experience (Griffiths et al., 2006, 2008; Pahnke, 1969), potentially establishes an ideally effective theoretical and clinical response to the existential plight of the palliative care patient. Of the cancer patients from the Johns Hopkins and NYU clinical trials, 67 and 70%, respectively, rated the psilocybin experience as among the five most meaningful experience of their lives, including the single most meaningful experience (Griffiths et al., 2016; Ross et al., 2016). Meaning making in advanced cancer has been determined to lead to enhanced spiritual well-being and overall quality of life, while reducing levels of psychological distress and a desire to hasten death (Lin & Bauer-Wu, 2003; Morita et al., 2000).

The opportunity for the end-of-life patient, through self-transcendence, to identify not solely with the failing body, but instead, to identify with something more enduring provides novel opportunities for therapeutic or ontological insight on the nature of self, body, or death. For the dying patient whose body is failing, the insight that "I am not only this body" or "I am not this cancer" offers transformative and therapeutic potential. Through the unique phenomenological typographies of transpersonal states comes the possibility for locating awareness of self from alternative vantage points in consciousness, potentially cultivating newfound possibilities. Themes emergent from these transpersonal states, such as psychospiritual death–rebirth experiences, become highly salient to those with life-threatening diseases and may challenge prior assumptions: What is death? What is consciousness? Where is consciousness? What happens to consciousness upon physical death? What, if anything, is enduring?

Descriptions of transcendent experiences suggestive of states of consciousness associated with dying or postdeath phenomena have been reported by persons in psychedelic cancer distress studies (Belser et al., 2017; Grof, 2006; Malone et al., 2018; Swift et al., 2017). Research on near-death experiences (NDEs) includes accounts of NDEs in language similar to experiences of mystical and psychedelic-generated consciousness (Grof, 2006; Moody, 1975; Ring, 1984). NDEs are defined as intense psychological and often transcendent experiences associated with life-threatening conditions, trauma, or with closeness to death (Greyson & Stevenson, 1980; Moody, 1975). In a study investigating similarities of the subjective experience of psychedelics and the descriptive measures of NDEs, Timmermann and colleagues (2018) administered the serotonergic psychedelic compound DMT versus a placebo to 13 healthy volunteers, who then completed a validated measure of NDEs. The findings revealed significant increases in the phenomenological features of NDEs of those having received DMT versus placebo, suggesting a commonality in the phenomenology and possible neurobiology between psychedelic and actual NDEs.

Grof (2006, p. 294) writes that for the end-of-life patient after psychedelic therapy, "death, instead of being the ultimate end of everything, suddenly appeared as a transition to a different type of existence. These patients perceived the alternative of consciousness continuing beyond physical death as much more plausible than of its ceasing at the time of biological death," and that

> individuals who experienced psycho-spiritual death and rebirth saw the experience as a foretaste of what would happen at the time of biological death. They reported [that] they no longer feared death. Deep experiences of cosmic unity, convincing past life memories, and certain other transpersonal forms of consciousness seemed to render physical death less important and threatening. These experiences could also profoundly transform the attitudes of patients who were facing death in a matter of months, weeks, or days. (p. 292)

Therapeutic implications are associated with not only mystical or peak experience but also other domains of experience within the psychedelic model, including the archetypal and psychodynamic dimensions (Pahnke & Richards, 1966; Richards, 1979). The archetypal dimension comprises visionary experiences or phenomena of religious or philosophical meaning that may include religious symbols, features from mythology, and historic figures such as Christ or Buddha. The psychodynamic experience offers the opportunity for substantial therapeutic benefit for a person with a life-threatening illness or at the end of life. Through psychodynamically oriented themes contained in an autobiographical review of one's life during psychedelic-generated experiences, individuals may experience emotionally charged memories of current and past relationships, unresolved conflicts or traumas, or the prospect of processing themes of guilt, anger, or regret. The opportunity for "letting go," forgiveness (for self and others), or resolution of family or early attachment dynamics has highly significant therapeutic value (Richards, 1979). Qualitative reports and clinical vignettes of psychedelic research narratives contain descriptions of increased closeness to family members, equanimity, greater acceptance of death, greater appreciation of time living, and gratitude (Belser et al., 2017; Grof, 2006; Swift et al., 2017).

A common theme reported from subjective states of psychedelic experiences is that of encountering multidimensional experiences of love: loving-kindness to self, to other persons throughout one's life history, and a sense of universal, divine, or cosmic love, what I find akin to the Greek work *agape*. In a letter to Humphry Osmond regarding a personal psychedelic experience, Huxley wrote, "What came through the closed door was the realization—not the knowledge, for this wasn't verbal or abstract—but the direct, total awareness, from the inside, so to say, of Love as the primary and fundamental cosmic fact" (in Bisbee et al., 2018, pp. 216–217). On the phenomenology of NDEs, Ring (2006, p. 187; original emphasis) notes, "And of all lessons of the near-death experience, none is greater than the importance, indeed the primacy, of love. And what the near-death experience teaches about love is that everything *is* love, and is made of love, and comes from love."

Patrick Mettes, a participant with whom I had the privilege to work in the NYU cancer study, who died 16 months after his psilocybin session, had spoken and written in detail about the powerful subjective experience of love he had experienced during his psilocybin session. Patrick was diagnosed with cholangiocarcinoma, cancer of the bile ducts, which had metastasized to his lungs. He reported his experience of love during his psilocybin session as vital in contributing to equanimity and acceptance in the months before his death. He spoke of experiencing consciousness as "filled with love, it *was* love" and "like nothing I've experienced before." The following is an excerpt from what Patrick wrote the evening of and the morning after his psilocybin session (in Grob et al., 2013, p. 304):

> From here on, love was the only consideration. Everything that happened, anything and everything that was seen or heard centered on love. It was and is the only purpose. Love seemed to emanate from a single point of light. . . . It was so pure. The sheer joy . . . the bliss was indescribable. And in fact, there are no words to accurately capture my experience . . . my state . . . this place. I know I've had no earthly pleasure that's ever come close to this feeling . . . no sensation, no image of beauty, nothing during my time on earth has felt as pure and joyful and glorious as the height of this journey.
> I was beginning to wonder if man spent too much time and effort at things unimport-

ant . . . trying to accomplish so much . . . when really, it was all so simple. No matter the subject, it all came down to the same thing: Love. Earthly matters such as food, music, architecture, anything, everything . . . aside from love, seemed silly and trivial.
> I thought about my cancer but only briefly. I took a tour of my lungs. I could see some things but it was more a matter of feeling the inside of my lungs. I remember breathing deeply to help facilitate the "seeing." There were nodules but they seemed rather unimportant. . . . I was being told (without words) to not worry about the cancer. . . . It's minor in the scheme of things . . . simply an imperfection of your humanity and that the more important matter . . . the real work to be done is before you. Again love. Undoubtedly, my life has changed in ways I may never fully comprehend. But I now have an understanding . . . an awareness that goes beyond intellect . . . that my life, that every life, and all that is the universe, equals one thing . . . love.

For over half of a century, and working with over 450 research participants, clinical researchers have investigated the utility of serotonergic psychedelics in treating the psychosocial and existential suffering associated with cancer and other life-threatening illnesses. When administered in carefully screened, interpersonally supportive and monitored clinical research conditions, therapy with the compounds LSD, DPT, and psilocybin has demonstrated the ability to produce enhanced emotional well-being and marked reductions in interpersonal, psychospiritual, and existential distress. The mechanisms of action are multidetermined, complex, and likely attributed to a synergistic combination of variables including the actions of the medicine and the set and setting.

Of significance is the emergence of the psychological peak or mystical experience treatment model, with findings that have empirically demonstrated positive therapeutic outcomes associated with the occurrence of a mystical or peak experience. Psilocybin has been found to safely generate mystical experience in healthy volunteers (Griffiths et al., 2006, 2008, 2011; Pahnke, 1963), and therapeutic outcomes have been correlated with mystical experience in smoking cessation (Garcia-Romeu, Griffiths, & Johnson, 2014; Johnson, Garcia-Romeu, Cosimano,

& Griffiths, 2014) and treatment of alcoholism (Bogenschutz et al., 2015).

Relevant to palliative care is a growing body of empirical evidence that psychedelic-generated mystical or psychological peak experience may be a safe and effective treatment model for the treatment of psychological and existential distress in patients with cancer (Griffiths et al., 2016; Grof et al., 1973; Pahnke, 1969; Richards, 1978; Richards et al., 1977; Ross et al., 2016). Specifically, Griffiths and colleagues (2016) and Ross and colleagues (2016) have demonstrated that mystical experiences have a mediating role in the reduction of anxiety and depression in patients with a diagnosis of life-threatening cancer. Further research will ideally continue to investigate the association between mystical/peak experience and positive therapeutic outcomes in life-threatening and end-of-life distress.

Furthermore, the scientific study of mystical experience poses intriguing opportunities to advance knowledge on the phenomenology and neurobiology of mystical states, possibly providing a tool for exploring questions arising in consciousness research: Is consciousness a direct result of complex function and processes as suggested by the materialistic view? Or is consciousness nonlocal, emerging and existing in part outside biology? Does it elegantly and in synergistic fashion work in concert with the brain, but not be confined by it? Does it continue to exist when the brain dies as some NDE research explores? How can both ancient wisdom and modern science work collaboratively advancing the science of consciousness?

Implications for the psychedelic treatment model in palliative care provide a broad range of potential positive effects: (1) improved psychological, spiritual, and existential well-being; (2) enhanced ability to cognitively or emotionally reframe the impact of cancer, dying, and death; (3) increased capacity for appreciation of time living; (4) increased feelings of connectedness to nature; (5) enhanced capacity to attend to unfinished business and unresolved interpersonal conflicts; (6) improved relational functioning; (7) the possibility through transpersonal states of consciousness to form new understandings regarding death (i.e., understanding death as "not the end" but a transition of some manner in continuing consciousness); (8) increased sense of meaning and purpose; and (9) increased acceptance and peace with death (Grob et al., 2013).

▓ Conclusion

φύσις κρύπτεσθαι φιλεῖ.
[Nature loves to be hidden.]
                                    —HERACLITUS

If you bring forth what is within you, what you bring forth will save you. If you do not bring forth what is within you, what you do not bring forth will destroy you.

                              —JESUS, *Gospel of Thomas*

Despite advances in chemotherapies and the treatment of pain and other end-of-life symptoms, there remains a paucity of identified therapeutic approaches aimed at treating the psychospiritual and existential distress of the dying patient or those diagnosed with a life-threatening illness. The need for successful psychotherapies is underscored by surveys showing that one-third to nearly one-half of cancer patients report significant levels of psychosocial distress (National Comprehensive Cancer Network, 2013; Zabora, BrintzenhofeSzoc, Curbow, Hooker, & Piantadosi, 2001). Research findings demonstrate that enhanced spiritual or existential well-being is associated with decreased levels of emotional distress in patients with advanced cancer (McClain et al., 2003; Park, Edmondson, Fenster, & Blank, 2008) and has been found to buffer against depression, hopelessness, and desire for a hastened death (Fernsler, Klemm, & Miller, 1999; Kandasamy, Chaturvedi, & Desai, 2011; Nelson, Rosenfeld, Breitbart, & Galietta, 2002).

The psychedelic therapy model represents a potential paradigm shift for the fields of hospice and palliative care. This is a promising development, particularly given the call for effective and novel treatments amid the paucity of psychotherapies aimed at the relief of this domain of distress of the sick or dying patient. With continued prudent research methodologies focused on efficacy and safety, careful medical and psychiatric screening of research participants, and specialized and comprehensive training of clinicians, future multisite trials ideally will eventually lead to the rescheduling of these compounds for palliative and hospice care.

Moving into the 21st century, we are witnessing an evolution in the cultural conversation on the end of life, reflected by a marked increase in academic conferences and publications, popular interest reflected by books and media, and the emergence of events such as Death Cafes, where attendees engage over dinner to discuss myriad aspects of death and dying. The openness draws from multidisciplinary and cross-cultural sources including religious and spiritual traditions, indigenous cultures, palliative and hospice care, thanatology, and scientific investigations into the nature of consciousness. The aging baby-boomer generation, gradually reaching into older age, is undoubtedly driving much of this new and focused awareness. Despite death and dying still seeming to be a cultural taboo, these recent developments do suggest a positive change. The development of psychedelic psychotherapies may ideally contribute to this shift in our national conversation on the art of dying and, consequently, on the art of living.

The therapeutic effects of the psychedelic mystical experience treatment model offer limitless possibilities for insight and healing for the person negotiating advanced illness or the end of life. These may include profound transpersonal or spiritual experiences with allusions of consciousness existing beyond death of the physical body, or simply, but remarkably, a profound sense of gratitude for having lived this single human life, albeit with its joy and sorrow. Insights from the therapeutic use of psychedelics may not only diminish anguish for the dying but also allow for the end of life to be imbued with greater acceptance, meaning, equanimity, and even a sense of wonder.

▪ References

Aitken, R. (1982). *Taking the path of Zen.* San Francisco: North Point Press.

Barrett, F. S., Johnson, M. W., & Griffiths, R. R. (2015). Validation of the revised mystical experience questionnaire in experimental sessions with psilocybin. *Journal of Psychopharmacology, 29*(11), 1182–1190.

Becker, E. (1973). *The denial of death.* New York: Free Press.

Belser, A. B., Agin-Liebes, G., Swift, T. C., Terrana, S., Devenot, N., Friedman, H. L., et al. (2017). Patient experiences of psilocybin-assisted psychotherapy: An interpretative phenomenological analysis. *Journal of Humanistic Psychology, 57*(4), 354–388.

Bisbee, C., Bisbee, P., Dyck, E., Farrell, P., Sexton, J., & Spisak, J. (2018). *Psychedelic prophets.* Montreal, Canada: McGill–Queens University Press.

Bogenschutz, M. P., Forcehimes, A. A., Pommy, J. A., Wilcox, J. E., Barbosa, P. C. R., & Strassman, R. J. (2015). Psilocybin-assisted treatment for alcohol dependence: A proof-of-concept study. *Journal of Psychopharmacology, 29*(3), 289–299.

Bonny, H., & Pahnke, W. N. (1972). The use of music in psychedelic (LSD) therapy. *Journal of Music Therapy, 9,* 64–87.

Boston, P., Bruce, A., & Schreiber, R. (2011). Existential suffering in the palliative care setting: An integrated literature review. *Journal of Pain and Symptom Management, 41,* 604–618.

Breitbart, W., Rosenfeld, B., Gibson, C., Pessin, H., Poppito, S., Nelson, C., et al. (2010). Meaning-centered group psychotherapy for patients with advanced cancer: A pilot randomized controlled trial. *Psycho-Oncology, 19,* 21–28.

Broadhurst, K., & Harrington, A. (2016). A thematic literature review: The importance of providing spiritual care for end-of-life patients who have experienced transcendence phenomena. *American Journal of Hospice and Palliative Medicine, 33*(9), 881–893.

Bruhn, J. G., De Smet, P. A., El-Seedi, H. R., & Beck, O. (2002). Mescaline use for 5700 years. *Lancet, 359,* 1866.

Bucke, R. M. (1901). *Cosmic consciousness: A study in the evolution of the human mind.* Philadelphia: Innes & Sons.

Carhart-Harris, R. L., Bolstridge, M., Rucker, J., Day, C. J., Erritzoe, D., Kaelen, M., et al. (2016). Psilocybin with psychological support for treatment-resistant depression: An open-label feasibility study. *Lancet Psychiatry, 3,* P619–P627.

Carhart-Harris, R. L., Erritzoe, D., Williams, T., Stone, J. M., Reed, L. J., Colasanti, A., et al. (2012). Neural correlates of the psychedelic state as determined by fMRI studies with psilocybin. *Proceedings of the National Academy of Sciences of the USA, 109*(6), 2138–2143.

Cassell, E. J. (1982). The nature of suffering and

the goals of medicine. *New England Journal of Medicine, 306*(11), 639–645.

Chochinov, H. M., Wilson, K. G., & Lander, S. (1998). Depression, hopelessness, and suicidal ideation in the terminally ill. *Psychosomatics, 39,* 336–370.

Cohen, S. (1965, September). LSD and the anguish of dying. *Harper's,* pp. 69–78.

Coward, D. (1991). Self-transcendence and emotional well-being in women with advanced breast cancer. *Nursing Forum, 18,* 857–863.

Coward, D., & Reed, P. G. (1995). Self-transcendence: A resource for healing at the end of life. *Issues in Mental Health Nursing, 17,* 275–288.

Dobkin de Rios, M. (1984). *Visionary vine: Hallucinogenic healing in the Peruvian Amazon.* Prospect Heights, IL: Waveland Press.

Doblin, R. (1991). Pahnke's "Good Friday experiment"; A long-term follow-up and methodological critique. *Journal of Transpersonal Psychology, 23*(1), 1–28.

Edwards, A., Pang, N., Shiu, V., & Chan, C. (2010). The understanding of spirituality and the potential role of spiritual care in end-of-life and palliative care: A meta-study of qualitative research. *Palliative Medicine, 24*(8), 753–770.

Egnew, T. R. (2005). The meaning of suffering: Transcending suffering. *Annals of Family Medicine, 3*(3), 255–262.

El-Seedi, H. R., De Smet, P., Beck, O., Possnert, G., & Bruhn, J. G. (2005). Prehistoric peyote use: Alkaloid analysis and radiocarbon dating of archaeological specimens of *Lophophora* from Texas. *Journal of Ethnopharmacology, 101,* 238–242.

Engel, G. (1977). The need for a new medical model: A challenge for biomedicine. *Science, 8,* 129–136.

Fernsler, J., Klemm, P., & Miller, M. (1999). Spiritual well-being and demands of illness in people with colorectal cancer. *Cancer Nursing, 22,* 134–140.

Folkman, S. (2010). Stress, coping, and hope. *Psycho-Oncology, 19*(9), 901–908.

Frankl, V. E. (1984). *Man's search for meaning.* Boston: Beacon Press.

Frankl, V. E. (1988). *The will to meaning: Foundations and applications of logotherapy.* New York: Penguin.

Garcia-Romeu, A., Griffiths, R. R., & Johnson, M. W. (2014). Psilocybin-occasioned mystical experiences in the treatment of tobacco addiction. *Current Drug Abuse Reviews, 7*(3), 157–164.

Gasser, P., Holstein, D., Michel, Y., Doblin, R., Yazar-Klosinski, B., Passie, T., et al. (2014). Safety and efficacy of lysergic acid diethylam-

ide-assisted psychotherapy for anxiety associated with life-threatening diseases. *Journal of Nervous and Mental Disease, 202,* 513–520.

Gasser, P., Kirchner, K., & Passie, T. (2015). LSD-assisted psychotherapy for anxiety associated with a life-threatening disease: A qualitative study of acute and sustained subjective effects. *Journal of Psychopharmacology, 29*(1), 57–68.

Greenberg, J., Pyszczynski, T., & Solomon, S. (1986). The causes and consequences of a need for self-esteem: A terror management theory. In R. F. Baumeister (Ed.), *Public self and private self* (pp. 189–212). New York: Springer-Verlag.

Greenstein, M., & Breitbart, W. (2000). Cancer and the experience of meaning: A group psychotherapy program for people with cancer. *American Journal of Psychotherapy, 54,* 486–500.

Greyson, B., & Stevenson, I. (1980). The phenomenology of near-death experiences. *American Journal of Psychiatry, 137,* 1193–1196.

Griffiths, R. R., Johnson, M. W., Carducci, M. A., Umbricht, A., Richards, W. A., Richards, B. D., et al. (2016). Psilocybin produces substantial and sustained decreases in depression and anxiety in patients with life-threatening cancer: A randomized double-blind trial. *Journal of Psychopharmacology 30,* 1181–1197.

Griffiths, R. R., Johnson, M. W., Richards, W. A., Richards, B. D., McCann, U., & Jesse, R. (2011). Psilocybin occasioned mystical-type experiences: Immediate and persisting dose-related effects. *Psychopharmacology, 218*(4), 649–665.

Griffiths, R. R., Richards, W. A., Johnson, M. W., McCann, U., & Jesse, R. (2008). Mystical-type experiences occasioned by psilocybin mediate the attribution of personal meaning and spiritual significance 14 months later. *Journal of Psychopharmacology, 22*(6), 621–632.

Griffiths, R. R., Richards, W. A., McCann, U., & Jesse, R. (2006). Psilocybin can occasion mystical experiences having substantial and sustained personal meaning and spiritual significance. *Psychopharmacology, 187,* 268–283.

Grinspoon, L., & Bakalar, J. B. (1979). *Psychedelic drugs reconsidered.* New York: Basic Books.

Grob, C. S., Bossis, A. P., & Griffiths, R. R. (2013). Use of the classical hallucinogen psilocybin for treatment of existential distress associated with cancer. In B. I. Carr & J. Steel (Eds.), *Psychological aspects of cancer* (pp. 291–308). New York: Springer.

Grob, C. S., Danforth, A. L., Chopra, G. S., Hagerty, M., McKay, C. R., Halberstadt, A.

L., et al. (2011). Pilot study of psilocybin treatment for anxiety in patients with advanced-stage cancer. *Archive of General Psychiatry, 68,* 71–78.

Grof, S. (1980). *LSD psychotherapy.* Pomona, CA: Hunter House.

Grof, S. (2006). *The ultimate journey: Consciousness and the mystery of death.* Ben Lomond, CA: Multidisciplinary Association for Psychedelic Studies.

Grof, S., Goodman, L. E., Richards, W. A., & Kurland, A. A. (1973). LSD-assisted psychotherapy in patients with terminal cancer. *International Pharmacopsychiatry, 8,* 129–144.

Grof, S., & Halifax, J. (1977). *The human encounter with death.* New York: Dutton.

Heimlich, R. (2009). Mystical experiences. Retrieved from *www.pewresearch.org/fact-tank/2009/12/29/mystical-experiences.*

Hofmann, A. (1979). *LSD: My problem child.* Los Angeles: Tarcher.

Hofmann, A. (2000). The message of the Eleusinian Mysteries for today's world. In R. Forte (Ed.), *Entheogens and the future of religion.* San Francisco: Council on Spiritual Practices.

Holland, J. C., & Bultz, B. D. (2007). The NCCN guidelines for distress management: A case for making distress the sixth vital sign. *Journal of National Comprehensive Cancer Network, 5,* 3–7.

Hood, R. W., Hill, P. C., & Spilka, B. (2009). *The psychology of religion: An empirical approach.* New York: Guilford Press.

Horowitz, M., & Palmer, C. (1977). *Moksha.* Los Angeles: Tarcher.

Huxley, A. (1945). *The perennial philosophy.* New York: Harper & Brothers.

Huxley, A. (1954). *The doors of perception.* London: Clarke, Irwin, & Co.

Huxley, A. (1972). *Island.* New York: Harper & Row.

Huxley, L. (1991). *This timeless moment: A personal view of Aldous Huxley.* San Francisco: Mercury House. (Original work published 1968)

Institute of Medicine. (2014). *Dying in America: Improving quality and honoring individual preferences near the end of life.* Washington, DC: National Academies Press.

James, W. (1919). *The varieties of religious experience.* New York: Longmans, Green. (Original work published 1902)

Johnson, M. W., Garcia-Romeu, A., Cosimano, M. P., & Griffiths, R. R. (2014). Pilot study of the 5-HT2AR agonist psilocybin in the treatment of tobacco addiction. *Journal of Psychopharmacology, 28*(11), 983–992.

Johnson, M. W., Richards, W. A., & Griffiths, R. R. (2008). Human hallucinogen research: Guidelines for safety. *Journal of Psychopharmacology, 22,* 603–620.

Jones, J. M., Huggins, M. A., Rydall, A. C., & Rodin, G. M. (2003). Symptomatic distress, hopelessness, and the desire for hastened death in hospitalized cancer patients. *Journal of Psychosomatic Research, 55,* 411–418.

Jung, C. (1949). *Psychology and religion.* New Haven, CT: Yale University Press. (Original work published 1938)

Kandasamy, A., Chaturvedi, S., & Desai, G. (2011). Spirituality, distress, depression, anxiety, and quality of life in patients with advanced cancer. *Indian Journal of Cancer, 48,* 55–58.

Kast, E. C. (1966). LSD and the dying patient. *Chicago Medical School Quarterly, 26,* 80–87.

Kast, E. C. (1967). Attenuation of anticipation: A therapeutic use of lysergic acid diethylamide. *Psychiatric Quarterly, 41*(4), 646–657.

Kast, E. C., & Collins, V. (1964). A study of lysergic acid diethylamide as an analgesic agent. *Anesthesia and Analgesia, 43,* 285–291.

Kelly, B., Burnett, P., Pelusi, D., Badger, S., Varghese, F., & Robertson, M. (2002). Terminally ill cancer patients' wish to hasten death. *Palliative Medicine, 16,* 339–345.

Kissane, D., Clarke, D. M., & Street, A. F. (2001). Demoralization syndrome: A relevant psychiatric diagnosis for palliative care. *Journal of Palliative Care, 17,* 12–21.

Kurland, A. A., Pahnke, W. N., Unger, S., Savage, C., & Goodman, E. (1969). Psychedelic psychotherapy (LSD) in the treatment of the patient with a malignancy. In A. Cerletti & F. J. Bove (Eds.), *The present status of psychotropic drugs: Pharmacological and clinical aspects* (pp. 432–434). Amsterdam, the Netherlands: Excerpta Medica.

Kurland, A., Pahnke, W., Unger, S., Savage, C., & Grof, S. (1971). Psychedelic LSD research. In W. Evans & N. Kline (Eds.), *Psychotropic drugs in the year 2000* (pp. 86–108). Springfield, IL: Charles C Thomas.

Leary, T., Metzner, R., & Alpert, R. (1964). *The psychedelic experience: A manual based on The Tibetan Book of the Dead.* New York: Citadel Press.

Lee, V. (2008). The existential plight of cancer: Meaning making as a concrete approach to the intangible search for meaning. *Supportive Care in Cancer, 16,* 779–785.

Lee, V., Cohen, R., Edgar, L., Laizner, A. M., & Gagnon, A. J. (2004). Clarifying "meaning" in the context of cancer research: A systematic literature review. *Palliative and Supportive Care, 2*(3), 291–304.

Lin, H. R., & Bauer-Wu, S. M. (2003). Psychospiritual well-being in patients with advanced cancer: An integrative review of the literature. *Journal of Advanced Nursing, 44,* 69–80.

MacLean, K. A., Leoutsakos, J. K., Johnson, M. W., & Griffiths, R. R. (2012). Factor analysis of the Mystical Experience Questionnaire: A study of experiences occasioned by the hallucinogen psilocybin. *Journal for the Scientific Study of Religion, 51,* 721–737.

Malone, T. V., Mennenga, S. E., Guss, J., Podrebarac, S. K., Owens, L. T., Bossis, A. P., et al. (2018). Individual experiences in four cancer patients following psilocybin-assisted psychotherapy. *Frontiers in Pharmacology, 9,* 1–6.

Maslow, A. H. (1971). *The farther reaches of human nature.* New York: Arkana/Penguin Books.

McClain, C. S., Rosenfeld, B., & Breitbart, W. (2003). Effect of spiritual well-being on end-of-life despair in terminally-ill cancer patients. *Lancet, 361,* 1603–1607.

McMillan, S. C., & Weitzner, M. (2000). How problematic are various aspects of quality of life in patients with cancer at the end of life? *Oncology Nursing Forum, 27,* 817–823.

Meier, D. E., Emmons, C. A., Wallenstein, S., Quill, T., Morrison, R. S., & Cassel, C. K. (1998). A national survey of physician-assisted suicide and euthanasia in the United States. *New England Journal of Medicine, 338,* 1193–1201.

Melzack, R., & Wall, P. D. (1965). Pain mechanisms: A new theory. *Science, 150,* 971–979.

Metzner, R. (2004). *Teonanacatl: Sacred mushroom of visions.* Verona, CA: Four Trees Press.

Mitchell, A. J., Chan, M., Bhatt, H., Halton, M., Grassi, L., Johansen, C., et al. (2011). Prevalence of depression, anxiety, and adjustment disorder in oncological, hematological, and palliative-care settings: A meta-analysis of 94 interview-based studies. *Lancet Oncology, 12,* 160–174.

Moody, R. (1975). *Life after life: The investigation of a phenomenon survival of bodily death.* New York: HarperCollins.

Morita, T., Tsunoda, J., Inoue, S., & Chihara, S. (2000). An exploratory factor analysis of existential suffering in Japanese terminally ill cancer patients. *Psycho-Oncology, 9,* 164–168.

Murata, H. (2003). Spiritual pain and its care in patients with terminal cancer: Construction of a conceptual framework by philosophical approach. *Palliative and Supportive Care, 1,* 15–21.

National Comprehensive Cancer Network. (2013). Distress during cancer care. Retrieved from *www.nccn.org/patients/guidelines/content/PDF/distress-patient.pdf.*

Nelson, C. J., Rosenfeld, B., Breitbart, W., & Galietta, M. (2002). Spirituality, religion, and depression in the terminally ill. *Psychosomatics, 43,* 213–220.

Nichols, D. E. (2004). Hallucinogens. *Pharmacology and Therapeutics, 101,* 131–181.

Otto, R. (1923). *The idea of the holy.* London: Oxford University Press.

Pahnke, W. (1963). *Drugs and mysticism: an analysis of the relationship between psychedelic drugs and the mystical consciousness.* Thesis presented to the President and Fellows of Harvard University for the PhD in Religion and Society, Cambridge, MA.

Pahnke, W. (1966). The contribution of the psychology of religion to the therapeutic use of psychedelic substances. In H. Abramson (Ed.), *The use of LSD in psychotherapy and alcoholism* (pp. 629–649). New York: Bobbs-Merrill.

Pahnke, W. N. (1969). The psychedelic mystical experience in the human encounter with death. *Harvard Theology Review, 62,* 1–21.

Pahnke, W. N., Kurland, A. A., Goodman, L. E., & Richards, W. A. (1969). LSD-assisted psychotherapy with terminal cancer patients. *Current Psychiatric Therapy, 9,* 144–152.

Pahnke, W. N., Kurland, A. A., Unger, S., Savage, C., Wolf, S., & Goodman, L. E. (1970). Psychedelic therapy (utilizing LSD) with cancer patients. *Journal of Psychedelic Drugs, 3,* 63–75.

Pahnke, W., & Richards, W. (1966). Implications of LSD and experimental mysticism. *Journal of Religion and Health, 5*(3), 175–208.

Park, C. L., Edmondson, D., Fenster, J. R., & Blank, T. O. (2008). Meaning making and psychological adjustment following cancer: The mediating roles of growth, life meaning, and restored just-world beliefs. *Journal of Consulting Psychology, 76,* 863–875.

Passie, T., Seifert, J., Schneider, U., & Emrich, H. M. (2002). The pharmacology of psilocybin. *Addiction Biology, 7,* 357–364.

Phifer, B. (1977). A review of the research and theological implications of the use of psychedelic drugs with terminal cancer patients. *Journal of Drug Issues, 7*(3), 287–292.

Presti, D. E., & Nichols, D. E. (2004). Biochemistry and neuropharmacology of psilocybin mushrooms. In R. Metzner (Ed.), *Teonanacatl: Sacred mushroom of vision.* El Verano, CA: Four Trees Press.

Puchalski, C., Ferrell, B., Virani, R., Otis-Green, S., Baird, P., Bull, J., et al. (2009). Improving the quality of spiritual care as a dimension of palliative care: The report of the consensus conference. *Journal of Palliative Medicine, 12,* 885–904.

Puchalski, C. M., Kilpatrick, S. D., McCullough,

M. E., & Larson, D. B. (2003). A systematic review of spiritual and religious variables in *Palliative Medicine, American Journal of Hospice and Palliative Care, Hospice Journal, Journal of Palliative Care,* and *Journal of Pain and Symptom Management. Palliative and Supportive Care, 1,* 7–13.

Reed, P. (2003). A nursing theory of self-transcendence. In M. J. Smith & P. Liehr (Eds.), *Middle range theory for advanced practice nursing* (pp. 145–166). New York: Springer.

Reed, P. (2009). Demystifying self-transcendence for mental health nursing practice and research. *Archives of Psychiatric Nursing, 23*(5), 397–400.

Richards, W. A. (1978). Mystical and archetypal experiences of terminal patients in DPT-assisted psychotherapy. *Journal of Religion and Health, 17*(2), 117–126.

Richards, W. A. (1980). Psychedelic drug-assisted psychotherapy with persons suffering from terminal cancer. *Altered States of Consciousness, 5*(4), 309–319.

Richards, W., Grof, S., Goodman, L., & Kurland, A. (1972). LSD-assisted psychotherapy and the human encounter with death. *Journal of Transpersonal Psychology, 4,* (121), 121–150.

Richards, W. A., Rhead, J. C., DiLeo, F. B., Yensen, R., & Kurland, A. A. (1977). The peak experience variable in DPT-assisted psychotherapy with cancer patients. *Journal of Psychedelic Drugs, 9,* 1–10.

Richards, W., Rhead, J., Grof, S., Goodman, L., DiLeo, F., & Rush, L. (1979). DPT as an adjunct in brief psychotherapy with cancer patients. *Omega—Journal of Death and Dying, 10,* 9–26.

Ring, K. (1984). *Heading toward omega: In search of the meaning of the near-death experience.* New York: Morrow.

Ring, K. (2006). *Lessons from the light: What we can learn from the near-death experience.* Needham, MA: Moment Point Press.

Rodin, G., Lo, C., Mikulincer, M., Donner, A., Gagliese, L., & Zimmermann, C. (2009). Pathways to distress: The multiple determinants of depression, hopelessness, and the desire for hastened death in metastatic cancer patients. *Social Science and Medicine, 68,* 562–569.

Ross, S., Bossis, A., Guss, J., Agin-Liebes, G., Malone, T., Cohen, B., et al. (2016). Rapid and sustained symptom reduction following psilocybin treatment for anxiety and depression in patients with life-threatening cancer:

A randomized controlled trial. *Journal of Psychopharmacology, 30,* 1165–1180.

Schultes, R. E., Hoffman, A., & Rätsch, C. (2001). *Plants of the gods: Their sacred, healing, and hallucinogenic powers* (rev. ed.). Rochester, VT: Healing Arts Press.

Singer, A., Meeker, D., Teno, J., Lynn, J., Lunney, J., & Lorenz, K. (2015). Symptom trends in the last year of life from 1998–2010. *Annals of Internal Medicine, 162*(2), 175–183.

Stace, W. T. (1960). *Teaching of the mystics.* New York: New American Library.

Sulmasy, D. P. (2002). A biopsychosocial–spiritual model for the care of patients at the end of life. *The Gerontologist, 42,* 24–33.

Swift, T., Belser, A. B., Agin-Liebes, G., Terrana, S., Devenot, N., Friedman, H. L., et al. (2017). Cancer at the dinner table: Experiences of psilocybin-assisted psychotherapy for the treatment of cancer-related distress. *Journal of Humanistic Psychology, 57*(5), 488–519.

Timmermann, C., Roseman, L., Williams, L., Erritzoe, D., Martial, C., Cassol, H., et al. (2018). DMT models the near-death experience. *Frontiers in Psychology, 9,* 1424.

Underhill, E. (1911). *Mysticism: A study of the nature and development of man's spiritual consciousness.* Oxford, UK: Oneworld.

Vachon, M., Fillion, L., & Achille, M. (2009). A conceptual analysis of spirituality at the end of life. *Journal of Palliative Medicine, 12,* 53–57.

Wasson, G., Hofmann, A., & Ruck, C. (2008). *The road to Eleusis: Unveiling the secret of the mysteries.* Berekely, CA: North Atantic Books.

Wasson, G., Kramrisch, S., Ott, J., & Ruck, C. (1986). *Persephone's quest: Entheogens and the origins of religion.* New Haven, CT: Yale University Press.

Wasson, R. G., & Ingalls, D. H. (1971). The soma of the Rig Veda: What was it? *Journal of the American Oriental Society, 91,* 169–187.

Wilson, K. G., Chochinov, H. M., Skirko, M. G., Allard, P., Chary, S., Gagnon, P. R., et al. (2007). Depression and anxiety disorders in palliative cancer care. *Journal of Pain and Symptom Management, 33,* 118–129.

World Health Organization. (2011). WHO definition of palliative care. Retrieved from *www.who.int/cancer/palliative/definition/en.*

Yalom, I. (1980). *Existential psychotherapy.* New York: Basic Books.

Zabora, J., BrintzenhofeSzoc, K., Curbow, B., Hooker, C., & Piantadosi, S. (2001). The prevalence of psychological distress by cancer site. *Psycho-Oncology, 10,* 19–28.

CHAPTER 24

Classic Psychedelics for Treatment of Alcohol Use Disorder

MICHAEL P. BOGENSCHUTZ and SARAH E. MENNENGA

▓ Introduction

The Public Health Impact of Alcohol Use Disorder

Of all misused substances, alcohol is perhaps the most damaging in the United States and globally (Hasin et al., 2007; Nutt, King, & Phillips, 2010; Rehm et al., 2009). Alcohol use disorders (AUDs) affect approximately 12% of the U.S. population at some point in their lifetimes (Hasin et al., 2007). Alcohol use was responsible for approximately 4.6% of global disability-adjusted life years and 36.4% of neuropsychiatric disability-adjusted life years in 2004 (Rehm et al., 2009). In the U.S. population, alcohol accounted for 12.1% of disability-adjusted life years among men and 4.6% among women (Rehm et al., 2009). The economic cost of alcohol use as been estimated at $185 billion annually in the United States alone (Volkow & Li, 2005).

Limitations of Current Treatments for AUD

A number of pharmacological and behavioral treatments have been developed that have some efficacy for AUD. Roughly one-third of participants in AUD studies achieve abstinence or remission during the first year following treatment, and the majority of those will eventually relapse (Willenbring, 2014). Recent meta-analyses have shown small to moderate effect sizes of pharmacological and brief interventions for AUD (Berglund, 2005; Ferri, Amato, & Davoli, 2006; Kaner et al., 2018; McQueen et al., 2011; Pani et al., 2014; Rösner et al., 2010a, 2010b), and the combination of multiple treatment modalities appears to provide limited additional benefit (Anton et al., 2006; Fiellin et al., 2006; Willenbring, 2014).

▓ Historical Background of Classic Psychedelics for Treatment of AUD

Following the accidental discovery of the psychoactive effects of lysergic acid diethylamide (LSD) in 1943 (Hofmann, 1979), the 1950s through the early 1970s saw an explosion of research on classic psychedelics. Clinical scientists explored the use of classic psychedelics to facilitate treatment of alcohol and drug addiction, anxiety and depression associated with the end of life, obsessive–compulsive disorder, and other conditions. In the field of addiction, the primary focus was the use of LSD in the treatment of AUD. Psychedelic treatment of AUD was subject of numerous studies, as summarized below, until clinical research on psychedelics came to halt in the early 1970s.

After a hiatus of some 30 years, the past decade has witnessed renewed interest in the use of psychedelics to treat addiction. Early-stage clinical trials of psilocybin for addiction to nicotine (Johnson et al., 2014) and alcohol dependence (Bogenschutz et al., 2015) have recently been completed, and controlled trials are currently underway examining the efficacy of psilocybin in treatment of addiction to alcohol, nicotine, and cocaine. Observational studies of sacramental use of plant materials containing classic psychedelics (peyote containing mescaline, or ayahuasca containing N,N-dimethyltryptamine [DMT]) suggest that these practices are associated with decreased disordered use of substances and few if any detrimental effects (Albaugh & Anderson, 1974; Barbosa et al., 2012; Doering-Silveira et al., 2005; Fabregas et al., 2010; Garrity, 2000; Halpern et al., 2005, 2008; Kunitz & Levy, 1994; Lu et al., 2009; Roy, 1973). Ayahuasca is being used to treat addictions in treatment programs in Latin America and the Caribbean, but efficacy studies have not been published. The relative safety of classic psychedelics (particularly psilocybin and LSD) in clinical research settings has been well documented (Johnson, Richards, & Griffiths, 2008), and promising early-stage trials have spurred interest in the use of psilocybin to treat anxiety and depression associated with life-threatening cancer (Griffiths et al., 2016; Ross et al., 2016), as well as major depression (Carhart-Harris, Bolstridge, et al., 2016).

Psychopharmacology of Classic Psychedelics

Definition of Classic Psychedelics

Classic psychedelics have been characterized in a number of different ways, and finding clear definition that distinguishes them from other classes of drugs has proved difficult. Generally, classic psychedelics include drugs that meet the following three fundamental criteria: (1) produce alterations in perception, cognition, affect, sense of meaning, and/or sense of self; (2) yield similar discriminative stimulus effects; and (3) exert their primary actions through agonist activity at the serotonin-2A (5-HT_{2A}) receptor (Glennon, Rosecrans, & Young, 1983; Halberstadt, 2015; Nichols, 2016). The information presented here focuses primarily on the classic psychedelics that have demonstrated promise for treatment of AUD or related indications. This includes the synthetic chemical LSD, which has been the most widely studied of the classic psychedelics for treatment of AUD (Mangini, 1998). Also included is psilocybin, a naturally occurring prodrug to the psychedelic compound psilocin, which has become the primary focus of ongoing clinical trials for the treatment of AUD (Bogenschutz et al., 2015, 2018). Other psychedelics such as dipropyltryptamine (DPT) (Grof et al., 1973), the mescaline-containing peyote cactus (Albaugh & Anderson, 1974; Blum, Futterman, & Pascarosa, 1977), and DMT-containing ayahuasca brews (Barbosa et al., 2018; Brierley & Davidson, 2012; Grob et al., 1996; McKenna, 2004) have been researched as potential adjuncts to AUD treatment, and are discussed in this chapter as well.

Basic Biological Mechanisms of Classic Psychedelics

Not long after Albert Hofmann accidentally discovered LSD's consciousness-altering effects, the serotonin molecule was identified in several different tissues, including the brain of rats and rabbits (Twarog & Page, 1953). By this time, it was widely accepted that LSD produced effects thought to be similar to those experienced by patients with schizophrenia, and these effects were postulated to be the result of LSD's actions in the brain. It was quickly recognized that LSD was structurally related to serotonin, resulting in development of the earliest hypotheses regarding serotonin's role in psychiatric illnesses, and also the mechanism by which LSD produced its mind-altering effects (Woolley & Shaw, 1954).

Over the next several decades, as understanding of brain function and neuroscience methods improved, the basic biological mechanisms of LSD and other classic psychedelics were widely studied. From these studies was formed a rich literature on the acute impact of LSD and other classic psychedelics on the brain and cognition, and several comprehensive reviews on the psychopharmacology of classic psychedelics have been published (Halberstadt, 2015; Nichols, 2004). Here we provide a brief overview of the existing research, with a focus on the mechanisms of action that may be relevant to treatment of AUD. How the acute effects of psychedelics relate to long-term change in complex behaviors such as AUD is still largely unknown, although several hypotheses have been proposed and are discussed below.

The 5-HT_{2A} receptor has been shown to mediate the acute subjective effects of classic psychedelics, which all act as full or partial 5-HT_{2A} agonists (Glennon, Titeler, & McKenney, 1984; Halberstadt, 2015; Halberstadt & Geyer, 2011; Nichols, 2016; Vollenweider et al., 1998). In humans, administration of a 5-HT_{2A} antagonist blocks the acute subjective effects of psilocybin (Vollenweider et al., 1998), and the intensity of psilocybin's psychedelic effects is positively associated with anterior cingulate and medial prefrontal cortical 5-HT_{2A} receptor occupation by psilocin, the active metabolite of psilocybin (Quednow, Geyer, & Halberstadt, 2010). Canonical signaling through the 5-HT_{2A} receptor leads to activation of phospholipase C (PLC), formation of inositol trisphosphate (IP3) and diacylglycerol (DAG), and eventually mobilization of calcium from intracellular stores through the G-protein $G\alpha q$ (Nichols & Nichols, 2008). However, the 5-HT_{2A} receptor exhibits ligand-dependent functional selectivity for alternative signal transduction pathways, as well as for receptor endocytosis, recycling, and phosphorylation (Raote, Bhattacharyya, & Panicker, 2013). Several other signaling pathways can be initiated by 5-HT_{2A} receptor activation, including β-arrestin-2, Src, extracellular signal-regulated kinase (ERK), p38 mitogen-activated protein (MAP) kinase, phospholipase A_2, Akt, and phospholipase D (Kurrasch-Orbaugh et al., 2003a; Gonzalez-Maeso et al., 2007; Schmid & Bohn, 2010;

Barclay et al., 2011; Halberstadt, 2015). Activation of more than one signaling pathway may underlie the 5-HT_{2A}-dependent effects of psychedelics, since canonical PLC–DAG–IP3 signaling is not sufficient to produce behavioral responses in rodents (Rabin et al., 2002; Kurrasch-Orbaugh et al., 2003b; Gonzalez-Maeso et al., 2007).

Modern neuroimaging techniques have been utilized to examine how classic psychedelics alter network connectivity and oscillatory synchronization. Ample evidence (reviewed in (Bogenschutz & Nichols, 2019) indicates that psychedelics temporarily impact cortical sensory and sensorimotor gating via cortico-striato-thalamo-cortical (CTSC) feedback loops (Geyer & Vollenweider, 2008; Vollenweider & Geyer, 2001; Vollenweider et al., 2007), producing "hyperfrontality" (Gouzoulis-Mayfrank et al., 1999; Hermle et al., 1992; Hermle, Gouzoulis-Mayfrank, & Spitzer, 1998; Riba et al., 2006). CTSC feedback loops are credited with integration of incoming information in the form of neural activity across the cortex (Geyer & Vollenweider, 2008), giving rise to conscious awareness and guiding attention (Edelman, 2003; Geyer & Vollenweider, 2008; Vollenweider et al., 2007; Tononi, 2004).

Increased functional connectivity between the default mode network and the task-positive network has also been shown following psilocybin administration (Carhart-Harris et al., 2013), suggesting a breakdown of separation between internal and external stimuli as central to psychedelic states. Psilocybin-induced reduction in cortical oscillatory synchronization across a broad range of frequencies, predominantly in the default mode network, and a general breakdown of network organization has been reported (Muthukumaraswamy et al., 2013). These findings are consistent with the hypothesis that psychedelics disrupt the organization of spontaneous cortical activity at rest (Carhart-Harris et al., 2012).

The claustrum has been put forth as a region ideally situated to coordinate activation of the default mode network with related cortical networks (Reser et al., 2014; Seeley et al., 2007; Torgerson et al., 2015), indicating that it is a likely mediator of psychedelic impact on default mode network–task positive network connectivity. Carhart-Harris and colleagues (2016b) expanded on this by showing that LSD-induced desynchronization coupled with enhanced connectivity in the primary visual cortex is associated with visual effects of psychedelics, whereas reduced functional connectivity in the parrahippocampal region is associated with reports of ego dissolution and altered meaning. Together, these results suggest that classic psychedelics temporarily produce widespread temporary disruption of interactions between brain networks responsible for perception of self, environment, and meaning, consistent with the reported subjective effects of these drugs.

To date, studies of psychedelic impact on network connectivity have focused on acute effects rather than persisting changes. It is difficult to speculate how these short-term changes might lead to persistent changes relevant to AUD; however, such widespread temporary disruption of function is likely to produce a lasting impact, especially within the context of a psychotherapeutic intervention. An ongoing Phase II clinical trial of psilocybin-assisted psychotherapy for AUD will be the first study to examine changes in resting state and functional connectivity from pre–AUD treatment to 1-day posttreatment with a classic psychedelic (ClinicalTrials.gov Identifier: NCT02061293).

Acute Subjective Effects of Classic Psychedelics

The acute subjective effects of classic psychedelics have proven difficult to measure and describe. These compounds rarely occasion true hallucinations, but rather tend to temporarily distort perception and cognition in ways that are unique to this class of drugs and markedly different from normal waking consciousness. Grinspoon and Balakar (1997) described the subjective effect of psychedelics in the following way: "Without causing physical addiction, craving, major physiological disturbances, delirium, disorientation, or amnesia, [it] more or less reliably produces thought, mood, and perceptual changes otherwise rarely experienced except in dreams, contemplative and reli-

gious exaltation, flashes of vivid involuntary memory, and acute psychosis."

Numerous operational definitions of the subjective effects of psychedelics have been developed in the form of self-report questionnaires and validated following treatment with several different psychedelic compounds. These scales are reliably impacted by administration of classic psychedelics and have exhibited predictive value in studies of AUD and other psychiatric indications. The Five-Dimensional Altered States of Consciousness Scale (5D-ASC; Dittrich, 1998) has 94 items and yields five primary dimensions: Oceanic Boundlessness, Dread of Ego Dissolution, Visionary Restructuralization, Acoustic Alterations, and Altered Vigilance. The Hallucinogen Rating Scale (HRS) was developed and validated at the University of New Mexico by Rick Strassman and colleagues (1994) in studies of intravenous DMT, and later validated in ayahuasca users (Riba et al., 2001). The HRS comprises 99 items divided into six subscales: Intensity, Somaesthesia, Affect, Perception, Cognition, and Volition. The Mystical Experience Questionnaire (MEQ) has been used extensively to measure mystical-type states of consciousness in psychedelic administration experiments (Griffiths et al., 2006; Pahnke, 1969; Richards et al., 1977; Turek, Soskin, & Kurland, 1974). This scale includes 43 items from the Pahnke–Richards MEQ, designed to capture features of the classic mystical experience: internal and external unity, transcendence of space and time, ineffability and paradoxicality, sense of sacredness, sense of ultimate truth or reality (noetic quality), and positive mood (Griffiths et al., 2006). A briefer, 30-item version of the MEQ was developed from factor analysis in a large survey sample (MacLean, Leoutsakos, Johnson, & Griffiths, 2012) and subjected to confirmatory factor analysis supporting a four-factor structure (Barrett, Johnson, & Griffiths, 2015). The Mysticism Scale assesses "mystical" dimensions of the psychedelic experience with 32 items that produce three factors titled Interpretation, Introvertive, and Extrovertive (Hood et al., 2001). This questionnaire has been used in studies of non-drug-induced mystical experiences and has also been used in the psilocybin work of Griffiths and colleagues (2006). Finally, in recent years questionnaires have been developed to tap additional aspects of the psychedelic experience, such as the Emotional Breakthrough Inventory (Roseman et al., 2019) and the Challenging Effects Questionnaire (Barrett et al., 2016).

◼ Use of Classic Psychedelics for AUD

LSD

Several authors have reviewed the research literature on LSD-assisted treatment of AUD (Abuzzahab & Anderson, 1971; Halpern, 1996; Mangini, 1998; Dyck, 2006; Grinspoon & Balakar, 1997). From the 1950s through the early 1970s, dozens of publications reported on the effects of LSD in the treatment of AUD. Clinical outcome studies and uncontrolled trials had encouraging results, particularly when the psychedelic model was used (Abuzzahab & Anderson, 1971). At least a dozen trials included a control group of some kind (Krebs & Johansen, 2012; Miller & Wilbourne, 2002), but these studies were of variable quality and generally underpowered, and most did not demonstrate a significant treatment effect. However, when a meta-analysis was done (Krebs & Johansen, 2012) of the six randomized controlled trials of LSD for AUD that reported drinking outcomes (Smart et al., 1966; Hollister, Shelton, & Krieger, 1969; Ludwig et al., 1969; Bowen, Soskin, & Chotlos, 1970; Pahnke et al., 1970; Tomsovic & Edwards, 1970), a consistent treatment effect was seen favoring LSD. These studies included 325 participants who received LSD in a single high-dose session (210 to 800 μg), and 211 who received control treatment (placebo, low-dose LSD, ephedrine, or amphetamine). In the meta-analysis, 59% of the LSD-treated participants were significantly improved at the first posttreatment follow-up compared to 38% of the control participants (odds ratio 1.96, $p = .0003$). The effect was homogeneous across the six studies, and it remained significant at 6-month follow-up. Although these findings are not conclusive evidence of efficacy, they provide strong support for renewed clinical investigation of LSD and other classic psychedelics for the treatment of AUD.

DPT

More limited research was conducted on the use of DPT in the treatment of AUD (Grof et al., 1973; Rhead et al., 1977). DPT is a classic psychedelic (Fantegrossi,, Murnane, & Reissig, 2008), structurally very similar to DMT. Its psychoactive effects last from 1 to 6 hours, depending on the dose, when given by intramuscular injection (Rhead et al., 1977). In a single-group pilot study involving 51 participants, Grof and colleagues (1973) reported highly significant improvement in clinical outcomes among the 47 participants (92%) who received between 1 and 6 DPT (mean 1.9) sessions and completed followup at 6 months. Subsequently, a randomized trial conducted by the same group evaluated the effects of DPT treatment relative to those of "conventional treatment" (psychotherapy similar to that received by the DPT group, but without the DPT sessions) and "routine hospital treatment" (Rhead et al., 1977). Although posttreatment psychological outcomes suggested more favorable response in the DPT-treated group, the DPT-treated participants and the other groups did not differ in clinical outcomes assessed at 6-month follow-up, and at 12 months, the conventional treatment group had better drinking outcomes and social functioning than the other two groups. This study suffered from methodological limitations including differential dropout among the groups and very high overall dropout rates both during treatment and in the follow-up period (only 37% of participants assessed at 12 months).

Psilocybin

The physiological and psychoactive effects of psilocybin were characterized within a few years of its isolation (Isbell, 1959; Leary, Litwin, & Metzner, 1963), and it was used to some extent in both psychedelic and psycholytic models of treatment (Metzner, 2005). With the exception of a cohort of alcoholic patients treated with both psilocybin and LSD (Rydzyński et al., 1968; Rydzyński & Gruszczyński, 1978), we are not aware of any published studies of psilocybin used to treat AUD prior to one published by the first author (M. P. B.) and colleagues in 2015. In this single-group, proof-of-concept study,

10 volunteers with DSM-IV alcohol dependence received 12 weeks of manualized therapy that included motivational enhancement therapy and sessions devoted to preparation for and debriefing from the psilocybin sessions. Psilocybin was administered (21 mg/70 kg or 28 mg/70 kg orally) in supervised sessions scheduled at weeks 4 and 8 of the treatment. Participants' responses to psilocybin were qualitatively similar to those described in normal volunteers (Griffiths et al., 2006, 2008, 2011), but some of the participants had a relatively mild response to the doses used. Drinking decreased nonsignificantly in the first 4 weeks of treatment (when participants had not yet received psilocybin), but decreased significantly following psilocybin administration at week 4. Improvement was maintained during 36 weeks of follow-up. The intensity of self-reported effects during the first psilocybin session at week 4 strongly predicted decrease in drinking during weeks 5–8 (r = .76 to r = .89). Based on these promising results, a larger double-blind trial (NCT02061293) to investigate efficacy and mechanisms is now underway. The ongoing study includes 93 participants randomly assigned to psilocybin versus diphenhydramine control, using a 12-week treatment model similar to that of the proof-of-concept study. The study uses a somewhat higher dose range for psilocybin (25–40 mg/70 kg). Following a 36-week, double-blind follow-up period, participants are eligible for a third medication session in which all participants receive psilocybin, with an additional 3 months of follow-up. Based on patient reports, intensely meaningful experiences leading to dramatic improvement in drinking and other areas of life have included not only mystical-type content, but in some cases also feature predominantly autobiographical content, cathartic experiences, intensely dysphoric struggles, and experiences of forgiveness and love (Bogenschutz et al., 2018).

Ayahuasca

Ayahuasca is a psychedelic tea containing the classic psychedelic DMT and β-carbolines (principally harmine, harmaline, and tetrahydroharmine). The harmine and harmaline are monoamine oxidase inhibitors that render DMT orally active (Callaway et al., 1996; McKenna, Towers, & Abbott, 1984). Ayahuasca has been used by indigenous peoples of the Amazon Basin for centuries, and is used sacramentally by organized religions including the União do Vegetal (UDV) and Santo Daime (McKenna, 2007). Ayahuasca is currently being used in treatment centers and in shamanic or "neoshamanic" contexts for the treatment of addiction, posttraumatic stress disorder, and other conditions (Labate & Cavnar, 2011; Liester & Prickett, 2012). Although many individuals have reported that ayahuasca has facilitated their recovery from addiction, to our knowledge, only observational studies have been published (Berlowitz et al., 2019; Giovannetti et al., 2020; Thomas et al., 2013), and controlled trials have not been published. A preclinical study showed that ayahuasca specifically blocked acquisition and reinstatement of behavioral sensitization to alcohol in mice (Oliveira-Lima et al., 2015). A second study demonstrated that ayahuasca blocked both acquisition and reinstatement of conditioned place preference for ethanol (Cata-Preta et al., 2018).

Cross-sectional studies have consistently shown low rates of alcohol misuse among members of religious groups using ayahuasca (Barbosa et al., 2016, 2018; Doering-Silveira et al., 2005; Fabregas et al., 2010; Halpern et al., 2008). Halpern and colleagues (2008) conducted structured interviews of 34 American Santo Daime members regarding the effects of church participation. Twenty-four of the 36 members had a history of substance use disorder, of which 22 were in full remission. The five individuals who had a history of alcohol dependence all reported that church involvement played a pivotal role in their recovery. In two case–control studies, Fabregas and colleagues (2010) found that ritual users of ayahuasca had lower scores on the Addiction Severity Index (ASI) Alcohol Use and Psychiatric subscales compared to a control group. In a recent survey of 1,947 adult Brazilian UDV members, Barbosa and colleagues (2018) found that the rates of current AUD were much lower than Brazilian norms, and that both years of UDV membership and number of ayahuasca sessions in the past 12 months were negative predictors of AUD. However, in a recent large, non-representative, online survey, ayahuasca users were found to a significantly higher average score on the Alcohol Use Identification Test (mean = 9.41, SD = 5.91, n = 458) than nonusers of psychedelics (mean = 8.45, SD = 5.50, n = 68,775), although the ayahuasca users scored lower than users of other psychedelics (mean = 10.33, SD = 5.94, n = 16,615). This finding suggests that antiaddictive effects of ayahuasca and other psychedelics likely depend on the intentions of the users and the context of their use.

Peyote

The peyote cactus (*Lophophora williamsii*), the San Pedro cactus (*Trichocereus pachanoi*), and a number of other cacti contain psychoactive quantities of the classic psychedelic mescaline (Gabermann, 1978; Ogunbodede et al., 2010). Peyote buttons have been harvested by Native peoples in North America for over 5,000 years (El-Seedi et al., 2005). Peyote is used sacramentally by groups including the Huichol of northern Mexico (Meyerhoff, 1974) and the Native American Church (NAC) (Stewart, 1987). It is widely believed that taking peyote in the context of NAC ceremonies helps alcoholics achieve and maintain sobriety (Albaugh & Anderson, 1971; Garrity, 2000; Kunitz & Levy, 1994; Lu et al., 2009). Proposed psychological mechanisms include cathartic experiences (Albaugh & Anderson, 1971) and improved self-understanding and motivation for sobriety (Garrity, 2000). However, we are not aware of any published quantitative studies of alcohol use among NAC members.

▦ Possible Mechanisms of Action

The basic pharmacology thought to underlie the acute consciousness-altering effects of classic psychedelics has been well studied and is briefly described on pages 477–478. The temporary changes in perception and cognition resulting from psychedelic administration have been shown to be predictive of long-term cognitive and behavioral changes; however, very little is known about the mechanism(s) underlying these persisting effects. Several theories about how psyche-

delics may be creating long-term positive behavioral change have been proposed and are described below. These include modulation of 5-HT$_{2A}$ receptors, signaling at 5-HT$_{2A}$ in conjunction with modulatory effects at other receptors, the induction of neuroplasticity via release of neurotrophic factors. These theories are not mutually exclusive and may all play a role in the widespread and complex effects seen following administration of classic psychedelics.

The Possible Role of 5-HT$_{2A}$ Receptor Modulation

Administration of classic psychedelics (including LSD, 2,5-dimethoxy-4-iodoamphetamine [DOI], 2,5-dimethoxy-4-methylamphetamine [DOM], and psilocin) to rodents results in behavioral tolerance corresponding with down-regulation of cortical 5-HT$_{2A}$ receptors (Buckholtz et al., 1990; Buckholtz, Zhou, & Freedman, 1988; Gresch et al., 2005; Leysen, Janssen, & Niemegeers, 1989). Tolerance to the subjective effects of psychedelics is seen in humans as well (Nichols, 2004), suggesting that administration of classic psychedelics leads to 5-HT$_{2A}$ receptor down-regulation in human cortex. The prototypical classic psychedelic DOI has been shown to produce receptor endocytosis followed by delayed receptor recycling after 7.5 hours, compared to only 2.5 hours following 5-HT-induced 5-HT$_{2A}$ endocytosis (Raote, Bhattacharya, & Panicker, 2007, Raote et al., 2013). These findings indicate that the classic psychedelics may have a unique ability to modulate 5-HT$_{2A}$ receptor expression at the cell membrane not seen following signaling through endogenous ligands.

Increased fronto-limbic 5-HT$_{2A}$ receptor binding is associated with increased anxiety and difficulty coping with stress (Frokjaer et al., 2008), both of which are linked to higher risk for relapse in substance use disorders (Lu & Richardson, 2014; Schellekens et al., 2015; Seo & Sinha, 2014; Sinha, 2012; Sinha & Li, 2007). It has thus been proposed that down-regulation of 5-HT$_{2A}$ receptors may be therapeutic in patients with AUD, potentially via changes in anxiety and stress responsivity (Bogenschutz & Johnson, 2016). Questions remain, however, regarding whether cortical 5-HT$_{2A}$ down-regulation alone is sufficient to reduce drinking in human AUD populations. For example, while the 5-HT$_{2A}$ antagonist ritanserin and amperozide were shown to suppress alcohol consumption in rodents (Johnson, 2008), treatment with ritanserin was not effective at reducing drinking clinical trials (Johnson et al., 1996; Wiesbeck et al., 1999). Moreover, mixed results have been reported regarding associations between 5-HT$_{2A}$ expression and AUD (Thompson et al., 2012; Underwood et al., 2008).

Possible Modulatory Roles of Other Receptors

In addition to their actions at 5-HT$_{2A}$ receptors, the classic psychedelics also all act as agonists at the 5-HT$_{2C}$ receptor, and some (e.g., LSD, DMT, and 5-methoxy-*N*,*N*-dimethyltryptamine [5MeO-DMT]) have agonist activity at the 5-HT$_{1A}$ receptor, potentially contributing to their acute consciousness-altering and/or long-term therapeutic effects (Halberstadt & Geyer, 2011). There is also evidence that glutamatergic neurotransmission plays a role in the subjective effects of classic psychedelics, particularly the metabotropic glutamate receptor mGluR2. Antagonism at this receptor has been shown to potentiate the DOI-induced rodent head twitch response, used as a proxy for psychedelic effects in humans, whereas mGluR2 agonists tend to attenuate the response (Gewirtz & Marek, 2000). 5-HT$_{2A}$ and mGluR2 receptors have been shown to form functional heterodimers, although it is unknown whether these receptor complexes exist in the brain (Fribourg et al., 2011; Gonzalez-Maeso et al., 2008).

LSD is also a partial dopamine D$_2$ receptor agonist and is known to synergistically enhance D$_2$ signaling (Giacomelli et al., 1998). LSD's actions at D$_2$ receptors are thought to underlie the second temporal phase of LSD's acute effects, beginning about 1 hour after LSD administration (Marona-Lewicka, Thisted, & Nichols, 2005). Moreover, functional interactions between 5-HT$_{2A}$ and D$_2$ receptors have been demonstrated in transfected HEK293 cells and in ventral and dorsal striatum (Albizu et al., 2011; Borroto-Escuela et al., 2010). Interestingly, while LSD and DOI enhance dopamine D$_2$ promotor recognition and signaling through D$_2$–5-HT$_{2A}$ heteroreceptors, serotonin antagonizes D$_2$ signaling through this complex (Borroto-Escuela et al., 2010, 2014), suggesting additional ligand-dependent functional selectivity at this receptor complex.

Neurotrophic Factors and Induction of Neuroplasticity

Neuroplasticity refers to changes in neural pathways and synapses in response to environment, behavior, thoughts, emotions, and other incoming stimuli (Pascual-Leone et al., 2011). The barrage of stimuli encountered across the lifespan, coupled with the brain's ability to respond and adapt to changing demands, is thought to give rise to human individuality. Neuroplasticity encompasses the ability of individual synapses to change in function, as well as the malleability of entire networks of connections, and it is largely regarded as the neurocorrelate of learning and memory. The idea of *metaplasticity*, the plasticity of neuroplasticity, was introduced in the mid-1990s (Abraham & Bear, 1996; Deisseroth et al., 1995), and is described as a sliding threshold for synaptic modification, which itself can be modified. Abraham and Bear state that metaplasticity is a change in the ability to induce subsequent synaptic plasticity. The metaplastic mechanisms described so far, while necessary for adaptive learning and memory, also present an opportunity for runaway, or maladaptive, learning to occur. Mechanisms by which an individual may encounter problems with maintaining metaplastic homeostasis (Roth-Alpermann et al., 2006), and how those problems might translate to behavioral abnormalities are only just beginning to be explored.

Much of the existing research on anxiety, depression, and addiction has centered on changes and imbalances in individual systems and neurotransmitters. Several brain regions known to be involved in memory, reward, and emotion (hippocampus, amygdala, prefrontal cortex, and others) exhibit multiple forms of neuroplasticity, and there are large bodies of evidence implicating aberrant neuroplasticity in animal models of stress, depression, and addiction. This collection of work has led to the development of the neuroplasticity hypotheses of addiction (Kalivas & O'Brien, 2008; Kalivas & Volkow, 2011; Thomas, Kalivas, & Shaham, 2008), depression (Massart, Mongeau, & Lanfumey, 2012; Serafini et al., 2012; Wainwright & Galea, 2013), and anxiety (Boyle, 2013). These hypotheses state that the disparities seen in each of these disorders are secondary to a disruption of homeostatic metaplasticity.

Most of the known pharmacological effects of psilocybin and other classic psychedelics involve activation of signal transduction pathways classically associated with increased neuroplastic potential. IP3/DAG production associated with 5-HT_{2A} receptor activation leads to an increase in intracellular calcium, capable of triggering synaptic remodeling. Growth and differentiation of new neurons and remodeling of existing neurons associated with release of brain-derived neurotropic factor (BDNF), is seen in rodents following psilocybin administration (Ly et al., 2018). Activation of p38/MAPK and the Ras-Raf-MEK-ERK pathway are also both possible via activation of the 5-HT_{2A} receptor and other receptors activated by psychedelic drugs (Barclay et al., 2011; Gonzalez-Maeso et al., 2007; Halberstadt, 2015; Kurrasch-Orbaugh et al., 2003a, 2003b; Schmid & Bohn, 2010). This, along with evidence that activation of the α subunit and canonical IP3/DAG signaling pathway of 5-HT_{2A}, may not be sufficient for the psychedelic effects of psilocybin (Kurrasch-Orbaugh, Parrish, et al., 2003; Kurrasch-Orbaugh, Watts, et al., 2003), implicate 5-HT_{2A} Gβγ-mediated ERK1 and 2 activation as a potential mechanism for the psychedelic and long-term therapeutic effects of these drugs.

In line with this evidence, it is possible that psychedelic compounds are providing therapeutic benefit by inducing a temporary state in which the neuroplastic potential of several brain regions is increased. This widespread increase in neuroplastic potential, a nonspecific metaplastic effect, may serve to reset a system in which learning has gone awry. This equal-opportunity boost to neuroplastic potential could serve to allow self-correction of individual systems-level imbalances, perhaps explaining why these compounds seem to be exerting such long-lasting and widely applicable mental health benefits. This could possibly also explain why existing pharmaceuticals, which are aimed at correcting secondary imbalances at the synaptic level, are falling short of a widespread, long-lasting cure. Another implication of this theory is that set and setting of the psychedelic experience are crucial in determining clinical outcome. Under this framework, the initial thoughts and experiences that happen shortly after drug administration should have a high potential to shape an individual's thought patterns going forward.

The Role of Subjective Experience

Clinical trials for various psychiatric indications have examined the role of acute subjective experiences induced by psychedelics in long-term beneficial change (Bogenschutz et al., 2015; Garcia-Romeu, Griffiths, & Johnson, 2015; Griffiths, 2016; Ross et al., 2016). Following treatment with psilocybin, decreased alcohol consumption has been shown to be associated with higher scores on the Mystical factor of the MEQ, the HRS Intensity subscale, and the G-ASC dimension of the 5D-ASC (a composite comprising scores on the Oceanic Boundlessness, Visual Restructuralization, and the Dread of Ego Dissolution factors) (Bogenschutz et al., 2015). Higher HRS Intensity scores and total scores on the MEQ have also been associated with greater improvement in drinking-related outcomes such as craving and self-efficacy (Bogenschutz et al., 2015). Better smoking cessation outcomes have been seen in participants who exhibited scores on the MEQ that qualified their experience as a "complete" mystical experience (Garcia-Romeu et al., 2015), and a greater reduction in anxiety- and depression-related outcomes have been seen in cancer patients who reported higher total scores on the MEQ (Griffiths, 2016; Ross et al., 2016). A recent animal study showed a single-dose LSD-induced reduction of alcohol consumption in mice, indicating that subjective experience may not fully explain the impact of psychedelics in AUD treatment (Alper et al., 2018). Whether subjective effects are part of the causal chain of psilocybin-induced improvements or simply a proximal indicator of another mechanism is unknown. However, these results implicate the strength of the acute subjective effects of psilocybin in human participants as a strong and useful indicator of clinical improvement in several addiction-related outcomes.

Persisting Psychological Changes

There is evidence that classic psychedelics produce enduring changes in personality and other psychological domains that may be relevant to addiction. Although personality traits are generally thought to be established by adulthood, a single administration of high-dose psilocybin was shown to enhance the personality trait of openness (MacLean, Johnson, & Griffiths, 2011), a finding that is consistent with subjective reports of study participants. Psychological assessments performed on members of UDV, a Brazilian religion that regularly uses the DMT-containing brew ayahuasca/hoasca, have shown enhanced mood and cognition, lower rates of recent alcohol use, and increased agreeableness and openness in UDV members relative to a comparison group (Barbosa et al., 2016). Interestingly, while UDV members showed lower rates of recent alcohol use, they also showed higher rates of past alcohol use to intoxication. Another report indicated that while lifetime rates of tobacco and alcohol use were higher than population norms in UDV members between 25 and 34 years old, current tobacco use disorder and AUD were less prevalent in the UDV sample (Barbosa et al., 2018). Additionally, naturalistic use of psychedelics by criminal offenders with a history of substance use has been shown to be associated with lower rates of corrections supervision failure, suggesting that use of psychedelics may be protective against criminal recidivism (Hendricks et al., 2014) in substance-using populations. While these findings do not provide direct evidence for mechanisms underlying psychedelic treatment of AUD, they warrant further investigation.

Likelihood of a Complex Mechanism

For nearly a century, neuroscience and pharmacology have operated under a dogma surrounding the nature of drug effects. Drug effects have long been described as a generally linear process beginning with receptor interactions and continuing through downstream signaling pathways that ultimately impact the structure and function of cells and neural networks. The concept that receptors for drugs exist at the surface of cells dates back to the late 1800s and early 1900s, followed in the mid-1900s by the concepts of receptor affinity, agonists, and antagonists. The last 50+ years have seen numerous findings that challenge and add complexity to this picture, including (but not limited to) the concept of inverse and protean agonists, the possibility of receptor oligomerization, and the roles of allosteric modulation, posttranslational modifications, functional selectivity, and novel signaling molecules (reviewed in Hill, 2006). Nonetheless, modern drug discovery still favors a model by which a drug's interaction with a particular receptor/signaling pathway is responsible for its clinical utility. More than a decade ago it was suggested that fully embracing the complexity of potential drug–target interactions would greatly benefit drug discovery, particularly for psychiatric indications (Agid et al., 2007).

Psychedelics are a prime example of how the dominant conceptual framework can impact the study of existing compounds and even hinder the discovery of novel mechanisms relevant to their effects. The 5-HT$_{2A}$ receptor has long been considered to be the primary "mechanism" by which classic psychedelics exert their temporary consciousness-altering effects; thus, it has also been the focus of research into the mechanism underlying their long-term clinical benefits. It is becoming increasingly clear, however, that the mechanism(s) responsible for the acute and persisting effects of psychedelics are complex and likely to involve actions at multiple receptors and signaling proteins, as well as interactions with the external and internal environment. The concept that "set and setting" influence the outcome of psychedelic treatment is widely accepted by clinicians working in this field. However, there has been very little research on how psychological states (e.g., intentions, expectations) and environmental factors (including behavioral interventions) may interact with a psychedelic drug such as psilocybin to produce a treatment effect.

Psychedelics have attracted attention as potential treatments for depression, end-of-life existential distress, and several other psychiatric and medical indications, in addition to substance use disorders. It is therefore unlikely that the therapeutic mechanism(s) of psychedelics are specific to AUD or even addiction in general. Case reports of individuals who have undergone psilocybin-assisted treatment for AUD credit the varied and personalized nature of psilocybin experiences as the basis of their therapeutic value (Bogenschutz et al., 2018). As we stated earlier, it is possible that each of the potential mechanisms described here plays a role in psychedelic treatment of AUD. The evidence to date suggests that classic psychedelics exert numerous effects that may collectively be capable of producing a long-term therapeutic benefit in patients with AUD.

▮ Conclusions and Future Directions

Taken as a whole, the evidence suggests that classic psychedelics hold great interest as potential treatments for addiction, particularly given the limited efficacy of existing treatments. The existing efficacy data are promising, although very preliminary except in the case of LSD treatment of AUD. The extensive literature on safety of psychedelics in clinical research contexts also supports continued exploration of their efficacy. Psychedelics have molecular targets consistent with antiaddictive effects, and some preclinical studies have demonstrated clinically relevant effects. The model of one or several doses of a drug leading to long-term change and benefit is of enormous potential and, within psychiatry, unique to psychedelics.

Although plausible biological mechanisms have been proposed and are being investigated, at this point, the strongest evidence is for the role of highly significant and meaningful experiences (and their objective correlates) as mediators of therapeutic effects. Such experiences have been shown to be associated with positive outcome following psilocybin administration in normal volunteers, cancer patients with anxiety and depression around the end of life, and major depression, as well as AUD and cigarette addiction (Bogenschutz et al., 2015; Carhart-Harris, Bolstridge, et al., 2016; Griffiths et al., 2016; Johnson et al., 2014; Ross et al., 2016). It is consistent with the extensive literature arguing for the role of transformative experiences, variously described as "conversion experiences" (James, 1902), "spiritual awakenings," (Alcoholic Anonymous, 2001; Forcehimes, 2004) or "quantum change" (Miller & C'de Baca, 2001) experiences in facilitation of sudden and dramatic changes in human lives, including but not limited to addictive behavior. However, it has never before been possible to occasion such experiences reliably with a medicine. This is a unique mechanism among pharmacotherapies, and one that is fascinating from both biological and psychological perspectives. Given the limitations of our current understanding of the effects of classic psychedelics in AUD, there are many lines of investigation that could contribute important and clinically relevant knowledge. Although the effects of psilocybin in addition have been impressive in the limited work that has been done, it cannot be assumed that all classic psychedelics have the same clinical effects. Further efficacy trials with psilocybin, and other classic psychedelics (especially LSD and ayahuasca/pharmahuasca) for AUD, as well as nicotine, cocaine, and opioid use disorder, should be developed. Depending on the status of drug development for other indications and the prospects for off-label use, a program of trials leading to the submission of an New Drug Application (NDA) for psychedelic-assisted treatment of AUD may be necessary to allow empirically supported treatment with psilocybin or another psychedelic if there is clear evidence for efficacy. Little work has been done on mechanisms of action (e.g., psychological mediators of persisting psychological and behavioral change, neuroimaging studies of persisting effects on brain structure and function, and the possible role of genetic, epigenetic, and other biomarkers in moderating response to psychedelics). Further thought should be given to optimizing the integration of the classic psychedelic treatment with psychosocial treatments, and possibly with other medications. If psychedelic-assisted treatment proves effective for AUD, is important to investigate whether efficacy depends on the nature of concurrent psychosocial treatment accompanying classic psychedelic. This is critical in terms of understanding both efficacy and the psychological mechanisms of action. Previous and current methods have minimized the number of doses (sessions) provided. If one or two sessions are effective, additional "booster" sessions might or might not further improve outcomes. Finally, since all drugs have risks, continued attention to safety is critical, including optimizing screening, preparation, use of ancillary medications, and debriefing and follow-up following sessions. In view of the almost complete neglect of clinical research on classic psychedelics during a period of enormous progress in the neuroscience of addiction, it is both daunting and inspiring to observe how many basic questions remain unanswered regarding psychedelic-assisted treatment of AUD.

■ References

Abraham, W. C., & Bear, M. F. (1996). Metaplasticity: The plasticity of synaptic plasticity. *Trends in Neurosciences, 19*, 126–130.

Abuzzahab, F. S., Sr., & Anderson, B. J. (1971). A review of LSD treatment in alcoholism. *International Pharmacopsychiatry, 6*, 223–235.

Agid, Y., Buzsáki, G., Diamond, D. M., Frackowiak, R., Giedd, J., Girault, J.-A., et al. (2007). How can drug discovery for psychiatric disorders be improved? *Nature Reviews Drug Discovery, 6*, 189–201.

Albaugh, B., & Anderson, P. (1974). Peyote in the treatment of alcoholism among American Indians. *American Journal of Psychiatry, 131*, 1247–1250.

Albizu, L., Holloway, T., Gonzalez-Maeso, J., & Sealfon, S. C. (2011). Functional crosstalk and heteromerization of serotonin 5-HT2A and dopamine D2 receptors. *Neuropharmacology, 61*, 770–777.

Alcoholics Anonymous. (2001). *Alcoholics anonymous* (4th ed.). New York: Alcoholics Anonymous World Services.

Alper, K., Dong, B., Shah, R., Sershen, H., & Vinod, K. Y. (2018). LSD administered as a single dose reduces alcohol consumption in C57BL/6J mice. *Frontiers in Pharmacology, 9*, 994.

Anton, R. F., O'Malley, S. S., Ciraulo, D. A., Cisler, R. A., Couper, D., Donovan, D. M., et al. (2006). Combined pharmacotherapies and behavioral interventions for alcohol dependence: The COMBINE study: A randomized controlled trial. *Journal of the American Medical Association, 295*, 2003–2017.

Barbosa, P. C., Mizumoto, S., Bogenschutz, M. P., & Strassman, R. J. (2012). Health status of ayahuasca users. *Drug Testing and Analysis, 4*, 601–609.

Barbosa, P. C., Strassman, R. J., Da Silveira, D. X., Areco, K., Hoy, R., Pommy, J., et al. (2016). Psychological and neuropsychological assessment of regular hoasca users. *Comprehensive Psychiatry, 71*, 95–105.

Barbosa, P. C. R., Tofoli, L. F., Bogenschutz, M. P., Hoy, R., Berro, L. F., Marinho, E. A. V., et al. (2018). Assessment of alcohol and tobacco use disorders among religious users of ayahuasca. *Frontiers in Psychiatry, 9*, 136.

Barclay, Z., Dickson, L., Robertson, D. N., Johnson, M. S., Holland, P. J., Rosie, R., et al. (2011). 5-HT2A receptor signalling through phospholipase D1 associated with its C-terminal tail. *Biochemical Journal, 436*, 651–660.

Barrett, F. S., Bradstreet, M. P., Leoutsakos, J. S., Johnson, M. W., & Griffiths, R. R. (2016). The Challenging Experience Questionnaire: Characterization of challenging experiences with psilocybin mushrooms. *Journal of Psychopharmacology, 30*, 1279–1295.

Barrett, F. S., Johnson, M. W., & Griffiths, R. R. (2015). Validation of the revised Mystical Experience Questionnaire in experimental sessions with psilocybin. *Journal of Psychopharmacology, 29*, 1182–1190.

Berglund, M. (2005). A better widget?: Three lessons for improving addiction treatment from a meta-analytical study. *Addiction, 100*, 742–750.

Berlowitz, I., Walt, H., Ghasarian, C., Mendive, F., & Martin-Soelch, C. (2019). Short-term treatment effects of a substance use disorder therapy involving traditional Amazonian medicine. *Journal of Psychoactive Drugs, 51*, 323–334.

Blum, K., Futterman, S. L., & Pascarosa, P. (1977). Peyote, a potential ethnopharmacologic agent for alcoholism and other drug dependencies: Possible biochemical rationale. *Clinical Toxicology, 11*, 459–472.

Bogenschutz, M. P., Forcehimes, A. A., Pommy, J. A., Wilcox, C. E., Barbosa, P. C., & Strassman, R. J. (2015). Psilocybin-assisted treatment for alcohol dependence: A proof-of-concept study. *Journal of Psychopharmacology, 29*, 289–299.

Bogenschutz, M. P., & Johnson, M. W. (2016). Classic hallucinogens in the treatment of addictions. *Progress in Neuro-Psychopharmacology and Biological Psychiatry, 64*, 250–258.

Bogenschutz, M. P., & Nichols, D. E. (2019).

The pharmacology of hallucinogens. In S. C. Miller, D. Fiellin, R. N. Rosenthal, & R. Saitz (Eds.), *The ASAM principles of addiction medicine* (6th ed., pp. 230–251). Philadelphia: Wolters Kluwer.

Bogenschutz, M. P., Podrebarac, S. K., Duane, J. H., Amegadzie, S. S., Malone, T. C., Owens, L. T., et al. (2018). Clinical interpretations of patient experience in a trial of psilocybin-assisted psychotherapy for alcohol use disorder. *Frontiers in Pharmacology, 9,* 100.

Borroto-Escuela, D. O., Romero-Fernandez, W., Narvaez, M., Oflijan, J., Agnati, L. F., & Fuxe, K. (2014). Hallucinogenic 5-HT2AR agonists LSD and DOI enhance dopamine D2R protomer recognition and signaling of D2-5-HT2A heteroreceptor complexes. *Biochemical and Biophysical Research Communications, 443,* 278–284.

Borroto-Escuela, D. O., Romero-Fernandez, W., Tarakanov, A. O., Marcellino, D., Ciruela, F., Agnati, L. F., et al. (2010). Dopamine D2 and 5-hydroxytryptamine 5-HT($_2$A) receptors assemble into functionally interacting heteromers. *Biochemical and Biophysical Research Communications, 401,* 605–610.

Bowen, W. T., Soskin, R. A., & Chotlos, J. W. (1970). Lysergic acid diethylamide as a variable in the hospital treatment of alcoholism: A follow-up study. *Journal of Nervous and Mental Disease, 150,* 111–118.

Boyle, L. M. (2013). A neuroplasticity hypothesis of chronic stress in the basolateral amygdala. *Yale Journal of Biology and Medicine, 86,* 117–125.

Brierley, D. I., & Davidson, C. (2012). Developments in harmine pharmacology—implications for ayahuasca use and drug-dependence treatment. *Progress in Neuro-Psychopharmacology and Biological Psychiatry, 39,* 263–272.

Buckholtz, N. S., Zhou, D., & Freedman, D. X. (1988). Serotonin2 agonist administration down-regulates rat brain serotonin2 receptors. *Life Sciences, 42,* 2439–2445.

Buckholtz, N. S., Zhou, D. F., Freedman, D. X., & Potter, W. Z. (1990). Lysergic acid diethylamide (LSD) administration selectively down-regulates serotonin2 receptors in rat brain. *Neuropsychopharmacology, 3,* 137–148.

Callaway, J. C., Raymon, L. P., Hearn, W. L., McKenna, D. J., Grob, C. S., Brito, G. S., et al. (1996). Quantitation of *N,N*-dimethyltryptamine and harmala alkaloids in human plasma after oral dosing with ayahuasca. *Journal of Analytical Toxicology, 20,* 492–497.

Carhart-Harris, R. L., Bolstridge, M., Rucker, J., Day, C. M., Erritzoe, D., Kaelen, M., et al. (2016). Psilocybin with psychological support for treatment-resistant depression: An open-label feasibility study. *Lancet Psychiatry, 3,* 619–627.

Carhart-Harris, R. L., Erritzoe, D., Williams, T., Stone, J. M., Reed, L. J., Colasanti, A., et al. (2012). Neural correlates of the psychedelic state as determined by fMRI studies with psilocybin. *Proceedings of the National Academy of Sciences of the USA, 109,* 2138–2143.

Carhart-Harris, R. L., Leech, R., Erritzoe, D., Williams, T. M., Stone, J. M., Evans, J., et al. (2013). Functional connectivity measures after psilocybin inform a novel hypothesis of early psychosis. *Schizophrenia Bulletin, 39,* 1343–1351.

Carhart-Harris, R. L., Muthukumaraswamy, S., Roseman, L., Kaelen, M., Droog, W., Murphy, K., et al. (2016). Neural correlates of the LSD experience revealed by multimodal neuroimaging. *Proceedings of the National Academy of Sciences of the USA, 113,* 4853–4858.

Cata-Preta, E. G., Serra, Y. A., Moreira-Junior, E. D. C., Reis, H. S., Kisaki, N. D., Libarino-Santos, M., et al. (2018). Ayahuasca and its DMT- and beta-carbolines-containing ingredients block the expression of ethanol-induced conditioned place preference in mice: Role of the treatment environment. *Frontiers in Pharmacology, 9,* 561.

Deisseroth, K., Bito, H., Schulman, H., & Tsien, R. W. (1995). A molecular mechanism for metaplasticity. *Current Biology, 5,* 1334–1338.

Dittrich, A. (1998). The standardized psychometric assessment of altered states of consciousness (ASCs) in humans. *Pharmacopsychiatry, 31,* 80–84.

Doering-Silveira, E., Grob, C. S., De Rios, M. D., Lopez, E., Alonso, L. K., Tacla, C., et al. (2005). Report on psychoactive drug use among adolescents using ayahuasca within a religious context. *Journal of Psychoactive Drugs, 37,* 141–144.

Dyck, E. (2006). "Hitting highs at rock bottom": LSD treatment for alcoholism, 1950–1970. *Social History of Medicine, 19,* 313–329.

Edelman, G. M. (2003). Naturalizing consciousness: A theoretical framework. *Proceedings of the National Academy of Sciences of the USA, 100,* 5520–5524.

El-Seedi, H. R., De Smet, P. A., Beck, O., Possnert, G., & Bruhn, J. G. (2005). Prehistoric peyote use: Alkaloid analysis and radiocarbon dating of archaeological specimens of *Lophophora* from Texas. *Journal of Ethnopharmacology, 101,* 238–242.

Fabregas, J. M., Gonzalez, D., Fondevila, S.,

Cutchet, M., Fernandez, X., Barbosa, P. C., et al. (2010). Assessment of addiction severity among ritual users of ayahuasca. *Drug and Alcohol Dependence, 111,* 257–261.

Fantegrossi, W. E., Murnane, K. S., & Reissig, C. J. (2008). The behavioral pharmacology of hallucinogens. *Biochemical Pharmacology, 75,* 17–33.

Ferri, M., Amato, L., & Davoli, M. (2006). Alcoholics Anonymous and other 12-step programmes for alcohol dependence. *Cochrane Database of Systatic Reviews, 3,* CD005032.

Fiellin, D. A., Pantalon, M. V., Chawarski, M. C., Moore, B. A., Sullivan, L. E., O'Connor, P. G., et al. (2006). Counseling plus buprenorphine-naloxone maintenance therapy for opioid dependence. *New England Journal of Medicine, 355,* 365–374.

Forcehimes, A. A. (2004). De profundis: Spiritual transformations in Alcoholics Anonymous. *Journal of Clinical Psychology, 60,* 503–517.

Fribourg, M., Moreno, J. L., Holloway, T., Provasi, D., Baki, L., Mahajan, R., et al. (2011). Decoding the signaling of a GPCR heteromeric complex reveals a unifying mechanism of action of antipsychotic drugs. *Cell, 147,* 1011–1023.

Frokjaer, V. G., Mortensen, E. L., Nielsen, F. A., Haugbol, S., Pinborg, L. H., Adams, K. H., et al. (2008). Frontolimbic serotonin 2A receptor binding in healthy subjects is associated with personality risk factors for affective disorder. *Biological Psychiatry, 63,* 569–576.

Gabermann, V. (1978). [Estimation of mescaline and pellotine in *Lophophora coulter* plants (Cactaceae) by means of the oscillographic polarography]. *Biokhimiia, 43,* 246–251.

Garcia-Romeu, A., Griffiths, R., & Johnson, M. W. (2015). Psilocybin-occasioned mystical experiences in the treatment of tobacco addiction. *Current Drug Abuse Reviews, 7,* 157–164.

Garrity, J. F. (2000). Jesus, peyote, and the holy people: Alcohol abuse and the ethos of power in Navajo healing. *Medical Anthropology Quarterly, 14,* 521–542.

Gewirtz, J. C., & Marek, G. J. (2000). Behavioral evidence for interactions between a hallucinogenic drug and Group II metabotropic glutamate receptors. *Neuropsychopharmacology, 23,* 569–576.

Geyer, M. A., & Vollenweider, F. X. (2008). Serotonin research: Contributions to understanding psychoses. *Trends in Pharmacological Sciences, 29,* 445–453.

Giacomelli, S., Palmery, M., Romanelli, L., Cheng, C. Y., & Silvestrini, B. (1998). Lysergic acid diethylamide (LSD) is a partial agonist of

D2 dopaminergic receptors and it potentiates dopamine-mediated prolactin secretion in lactotrophs *in vitro*. *Life Sciences, 63,* 215–222.

Giovannetti, C., Garcia Arce, S., Rush, B., & Mendive, F. (2020). Pilot evaluation of a residential drug addiction treatment combining traditional Amazonian medicine, ayahuasca and psychotherapy on depression and anxiety. *Journal of Psychoactive Drugs*. [Epub ahead of print]

Glennon, R. A., Rosecrans, J. A., & Young, R. (1983). Drug-induced discrimination: A description of the paradigm and a review of its specific application to the study of hallucinogenic agents. *Medical Research Reviews, 3,* 289–340.

Glennon, R. A., Titeler, M., & McKenney, J. D. (1984). Evidence for 5-HT$_2$ involvement in the mechanism of action of hallucinogenic agents. *Life Sciences, 35,* 2505–2511.

Gonzalez-Maeso, J., Ang, R. L., Yuen, T., Chan, P., Weisstaub, N. V., Lopez-Gimenez, J. F., et al. (2008). Identification of a serotonin/glutamate receptor complex implicated in psychosis. *Nature, 452,* 93–97.

Gonzalez-Maeso, J., Weisstaub, N. V., Zhou, M., Chan, P., Ivic, L., Ang, R., et al. (2007). Hallucinogens recruit specific cortical 5-HT(2A) receptor-mediated signaling pathways to affect behavior. *Neuron, 53,* 439–452.

Gouzoulis-Mayfrank, E., Schreckenberger, M., Sabri, O., Arning, C., Thelen, B., Spitzer, M., et al. (1999). Neurometabolic effects of psilocybin, 3,4-methylenedioxyethylamphetamine (MDE) and d-methamphetamine in healthy volunteers: A double-blind, placebo-controlled PET study with [^{18}F]FDG. *Neuropsychopharmacology, 20,* 565–581.

Gresch, P. J., Smith, R. L., Barrett, R. J., & Sanders-Bush, E. (2005). Behavioral tolerance to lysergic acid diethylamide is associated with reduced serotonin-2A receptor signaling in rat cortex. *Neuropsychopharmacology, 30,* 1693–1702.

Griffiths, R. (2016). A single dose of psilocybin produces substantial and enduring decreases in anxiety and depression in patients with a life-threatening cancer diagnosis: A randomized double-blind trial. *Neuropharmacology, 40,* S90–S91.

Griffiths, R. R., Johnson, M. W., Carducci, M. A., Umbricht, A., Richards, W. A., Richards, B. D., et al. (2016). Psilocybin produces substantial and sustained decreases in depression and anxiety in patients with life-threatening cancer: A randomized double-blind trial. *Journal of Psychopharmacology, 30,* 1181–1197.

Griffiths, R. R., Johnson, M. W., Richards, W.

A., Richards, B. D., McCann, U., & Jesse, R. (2011). Psilocybin occasioned mystical-type experiences: Immediate and persisting dose-related effects. *Psychopharmacology (Berlin)*, *218*, 649–665.

Griffiths, R., Richards, W., Johnson, M., McCann, U., & Jesse, R. (2008). Mystical-type experiences occasioned by psilocybin mediate the attribution of personal meaning and spiritual significance 14 months later. *Journal of Psychopharmacology*, *22*, 621–632.

Griffiths, R. R., Richards, W. A., McCann, U., & Jesse, R. (2006). Psilocybin can occasion mystical-type experiences having substantial and sustained personal meaning and spiritual significance. *Psychopharmacology (Berlin)*, *187*, 268–283; discussion 284–292.

Grinspoon, L., & Balakar, J. B. (1997). *Psychedelic drugs reconsidered*. New York: Lindesmith Center.

Grob, C. S., McKenna, D. J., Callaway, J. C., Brito, G. S., Neves, E. S., Oberlander, G., et al. (1996). Human psychopharmacology of hoasca, a plant hallucinogen used in ritual context in Brazil. *Journal of Nervous and Mental Disease*, *184*, 86–94.

Grof, S., Soskin, R. A., Richards, W. A., & Kurland, A. A. (1973). DPT as an adjunct in psychotherapy of alcoholics. *International Pharmacopsychiatry*, *8*, 104–115.

Halberstadt, A. L. (2015). Recent advances in the neuropsychopharmacology of serotonergic hallucinogens. *Behavioural Brain Research*, *277*, 99–120.

Halberstadt, A. L., & Geyer, M. A. (2011). Multiple receptors contribute to the behavioral effects of indoleamine hallucinogens. *Neuropharmacology*, *61*, 364–381.

Halpern, J. H. (1996). The use of hallucinogens in the treatment of addiction. *Addiction Research*, *4*, 177–189.

Halpern, J. H., Sherwood, A. R., Hudson, J. I., Yurgelun-Todd, D., & Pope, H. G. (2005). Psychological and cognitive effects of long-term peyote use among Native Americans. *Biological Psychiatry*, *58*, 624–631.

Halpern, J. H., Sherwood, A. R., Passie, T., Blackwell, K. C., & Ruttenber, A. J. (2008). Evidence of health and safety in American members of a religion who use a hallucinogenic sacrament. *Medical Science Monitor*, *14*, SR15–SR22.

Hasin, D. S., Stinson, F. S., Ogburn, E., & Grant, B. F. (2007). Prevalence, correlates, disability, and comorbidity of DSM-IV alcohol abuse and dependence in the United States: Results from the National Epidemiologic Survey on Alcohol and Related Conditions. *Archives of General Psychiatry*, *64*, 830–842.

Hendricks, P. S., Clark, C. B., Johnson, M. W., Fontaine, K. R., & Cropsey, K. L. (2014). Hallucinogen use predicts reduced recidivism among substance-involved offenders under community corrections supervision. *Journal of Psychopharmacology*, *28*, 62–66.

Hermle, L., Couzoulis-Moyfronk, E., & Spitze, M. (1998). Blood flow and cerebral laterality in the mescaline model of psychosis. *Pharmacopsychiatry*, *31*, 85–91.

Hermle, L., Ftinfgeld, M., Oepen, G., Botsch, H., Borchardt, D., Gouzoulis, E., et al. (1992). Mescaline-induced psychopathological, neuropsychological, and neurometabolic effects in normal subjects: Experimental psychosis as a tool for psychiatric research. *Society of Biological Psychiatry*, *32*, 976–991.

Hill, S. J. (2006). G-protein-coupled receptors: Past, present and future. *British Journal of Pharmacology*, *147*(Suppl. 1), S27–S37.

Hofmann, A. (1979). How LSD originated. *Journal of Psychedelic Drugs*, *11*, 53–60.

Hollister, L. E., Shelton, J., & Krieger, G. (1969). A controlled comparison of lysergic acid diethylamide (LSD) and dextroamphetmine in alcoholics. *American Journal of Psychiatry*, *125*, 1352–1357.

Hood, R. W., Ghorbani, N., Watson, P. J., Ghramaleki, A. F., Bing, M. N., Davison, H. K., et al. (2001). Dimensions of the Mysticism Scale: Confirming the three-factor structure in the United States and Iran. *Journal for the Scientific Study of Religion*, *40*, 691–705.

Isbell, H. (1959). Comparison of the reactions induced by psilocybin and LSD-25 in man. *Psychopharmacologia*, *1*, 29–38.

James, W. (1902). *The varieties of religious experience*., Cambridge, MA: Harvard University Press.

Johnson, B. A. (2008). Update on neuropharmacological treatments for alcoholism: Scientific basis and clinical findings. *Biochemical Pharmacology*, *75*, 34–56.

Johnson, B. A., Jasinski, D. R., Galloway, G. P., Kranzler, H., Weinreib, R., Anton, R. F., et al. (1996). Ritanserin in the treatment of alcohol dependence—a multi-center clinical trial. *Psychopharmacology (Berlin)*, *128*, 206–215.

Johnson, M. W., Garcia-Romeu, A., Cosimano, M. P., & Griffiths, R. R. (2014). Pilot study of the 5-HT2AR agonist psilocybin in the treatment of tobacco addiction. *J Psychopharmacology*, *28*, 983–992.

Johnson, M., Richards, W., & Griffiths, R. (2008). Human hallucinogen research: Guidelines for safety. *Journal of Psychopharmacology*, *22*, 603–620.

Kalivas, P. W., & O'Brien, C. (2008). Drug addiction as a pathology of staged neuroplasticity. *Neuropsychopharmacology, 33*, 166–180.

Kalivas, P. W., & Volkow, N. D. (2011). New medications for drug addiction hiding in glutamatergic neuroplasticity. *Molecular Psychiatry, 16*, 974–986.

Kaner, E. F., Beyer, F. R., Muirhead, C., Campbell, F., Pienaar, E. D., Bertholet, N., et al. (2018). Effectiveness of brief alcohol interventions in primary care populations. *Cochrane Database System Reviews, 2*, CD004148.

Krebs, T. S., & Johansen, P. O. (2012). Lysergic acid diethylamide (LSD) for alcoholism: Meta-analysis of randomized controlled trials. *Journal of Psychopharmacology, 26*, 994–1002.

Kunitz, S. J., & Levy, J. E. (1994). *Drinking careers: A twenty-five year study of three Navajo populations.* New Haven, CT: Yale University Press.

Kurrasch-Orbaugh, D. M., Parrish, J. C., Watts, V. J., & Nichols, D. E. (2003). A complex signaling cascade links the serotonin2A receptor to phospholipase A2 activation: The involvement of MAP kinases. *Journal of Neurochemistry, 86*, 980–991.

Kurrasch-Orbaugh, D. M., Watts, V. J., Barker, E. L., & Nichols, D. E. (2003). Serotonin 5-hydroxytryptamine 2A receptor-coupled phospholipase C and phospholipase A2 signaling pathways have different receptor reserves. *Journal of Pharmacology and Experimental Therapeutics, 304*, 229–237.

Labate, B. C., & Cavnar, C. (2011). The expansion of the field of research on ayahuasca: Some reflections about the ayahuasca track at the 2010 MAPS "Psychedelic Science in the 21st Century" conference. *International Journal of Drug Policy, 22*, 174–178.

Leary, T., Litwin, G. H., & Metzner, R. (1963). Reactions to psilocybin administered in a supportive environment. *Journal of Nervous and Mental Disease, 137*, 561–573.

Leysen, J. E., Janssen, P. F. M., & Niemegeers, C. J. E. (1989). Rapid desensitization and down-regulation of 5-HT$_2$ receptors by DOM treatment. *European Journal of Pharmacology, 163*, 145–149.

Liester, M. B., & Prickett, J. I. (2012). Hypotheses regarding the mechanisms of ayahuasca in the treatment of addictions. *Journal of Psychoactive Drugs, 44*, 200–208.

Lu, L., Liu, Y., Zhu, W., Shi, J., Liu, Y., Ling, W., et al. (2009). Traditional medicine in the treatment of drug addiction. *American Journal of Drug and Alcohol Abuse, 35*, 1–11.

Lu, Y. L., & Richardson, H. N. (2014). Alcohol, stress hormones, and the prefrontal cortex: A proposed pathway to the dark side of addiction. *Neuroscience, 277*, 139–151.

Ludwig, A., Levine, J., Stark, L., & Lazar, R. (1969). A clinical study of LSD treatment in alcoholism. *American Journal of Psychiatry, 126*, 59–69.

Ly, C., Greb, A. C., Cameron, L. P., Wong, J. M., Barragan, E. V., Wilson, P. C., et al. (2018). Psychedelics promote structural and functional neural plasticity. *Cell Reports, 23*, 3170–3182.

MacLean, K. A., Johnson, M. W., & Griffiths, R. R. (2011). Mystical experiences occasioned by the hallucinogen psilocybin lead to increases in the personality domain of openness. *Journal of Psychopharmacology, 25*, 1453–1461.

Maclean, K. A., Leoutsakos, J. M., Johnson, M. W., & Griffiths, R. R. (2012). Factor analysis of the Mystical Experience Questionnaire: A study of experiences occasioned by the hallucinogen psilocybin. *Journal for the Scientific Study of Religion, 51*, 721–737.

Mangini, M. (1998). Treatment of alcoholism using psychedelic drugs: A review of the program of research. *Journal of Psychoactive Drugs, 30*, 381–418.

Marona-Lewicka, D., Thisted, R. A., & Nichols, D. E. (2005). Distinct temporal phases in the behavioral pharmacology of LSD: Dopamine D2 receptor-mediated effects in the rat and implications for psychosis. *Psychopharmacology (Berlin), 180*, 427–435.

Massart, R., Mongeau, R., & Lanfumey, L. (2012). Beyond the monoaminergic hypothesis: Neuroplasticity and epigenetic changes in a transgenic mouse model of depression. *Philosophical Transactions of the Royal Society, 367*, 2485–2494.

McKenna, D. J. (2004). Clinical investigations of the therapeutic potential of ayahuasca: Rationale and regulatory challenges. *Pharmacology and Therapeutics, 102*, 111–129.

McKenna, D. J. (2007). The healing vine: Ayahuasca as medicine in the 21st century. In M. J. Winkelman & T. B. Roberts (Eds.), *Psychedelic medicine: New evidence for hallucinogenic substances as treatments* (Vol. 1, pp. 21–44). Westport, CT: Praeger.

McKenna, D. J., Towers, G. H., & Abbott, F. (1984). Monoamine oxidase inhibitors in South American hallucinogenic plants: Tryptamine and beta-carboline constituents of ayahuasca. *Journal of Ethnopharmacology, 10*, 195–223.

McQueen, J., Howe, T. E., Allan, L., Mains, D., & Hardy, V. (2011). Brief interventions for heavy alcohol users admitted to general hospital wards. *Cochrane Database Systems Review, 8*, CD005191.

Metzner, R. (2005). *Sacred mushroom of visions:*

Teonanácatl: A sourcebook on the psilocybin mushroom. Rochester, VT: Park Street Press

Meyerhoff, B. (1974). *Peyote hunt*. Ithaca, NY: Cornell University Press.

Miller, W. R., & C'de Baca, J. (2001). *Quantum change: When epiphanies and sudden insights transform ordinary lives*. New York: Guilford Press.

Miller, W. R., & Wilbourne, P. L. (2002). Mesa Grande: A methodological analysis of clinical trials of treatments for alcohol use disorders. *Addiction, 97*, 265–277.

Muthukumaraswamy, S. D., Carhart-Harris, R. L., Moran, R. J., Brookes, M. J., Williams, T. M., Errtizoe, D., et al. (2013). Broadband cortical desynchronization underlies the human psychedelic state. *Journal of Neuroscience, 33*, 15171–15183.

Nichols, D. E. (2004). Hallucinogens. *Pharmacology and Therapeutics, 101*, 131–181.

Nichols, D. E. (2016). Psychedelics. *Pharmacological Reviews, 68*, 264–355.

Nichols, D. E., & Nichols, C. D. (2008). Serotonin receptors. *Chemical Reviews, 108*, 1614–1641.

Nutt, D. J., King, L. A., & Phillips, L. D. (2010). Drug harms in the UK: A multicriteria decision analysis. *Lancet, 376*, 1558–1565.

Ogunbodede, O., McCombs, D., Trout, K., Daley, P., & Terry, M. (2010). New mescaline concentrations from 14 taxa/cultivars of *Echinopsis* spp. (Cactaceae) ("San Pedro") and their relevance to shamanic practice. *Journal of Ethnopharmacology, 131*, 356–362.

Oliveira-Lima, A. J., Santos, R., Hollais, A. W., Gerardi-Junior, C. A., Baldaia, M. A., Wuo-Silva, R., et al. (2015). Effects of ayahuasca on the development of ethanol-induced behavioral sensitization and on a post-sensitization treatment in mice. *Physiology and Behavior, 142*, 28–36.

Pahnke, W. N. (1969). Psychedelic drugs and mystical experience. *International Journal of Psychiatry in Clinical Practice, 5*, 149–162.

Pahnke, W. N., Kurland, A. A., Unger, S., Savage, C., & Grof, S. (1970). The experimental use of psychedelic (LSD) psychotherapy. *Journal of the American Medical Association, 212*, 1856–1863.

Pani, P. P., Trogu, E., Pacini, M., & Maremmani, I. (2014). Anticonvulsants for alcohol dependence. *Cochrane Database of Systematic Reviews, 2*, CD008544.

Pascual-Leone, A., Freitas, C., Oberman, L., Horvath, J. C., Halko, M., Eldaief, M., et al. (2011). Characterizing brain cortical plasticity and network dynamics across the age-span in health and disease with TMS-EEG and TMS-fMRI. *Brain Topography, 24*, 302–315.

Quednow, B. B., Geyer, M. A., & Halberstadt, A. L. (2010). Serotonin and schizophrenia. In C. P. Muller & B. Jacobs (Eds.), *Handbook of the behavioral neurobiology of serotonin* (pp. 585–620). London: Academic Press.

Rabin, R. A., Regina, M., Doat, M., & Winter, J. C. (2002). 5-HT$_{2A}$ receptor-stimulated phosphoinositide hydrolysis in the stimulus effects of hallucinogens. *Pharmacology, Biochemistry and Behavior, 72*, 29–37.

Raote, I., Bhattacharyya, A., & Panicker, M. M. (2007). Serotonin 2A (5-HT$_{2A}$) receptor function: Ligand-dependent mechanisms and pathways. In A. Chattopadhyay (Ed.), *Serotonin receptors in neurobiology* (pp. 105–132). Boca Raton, FL: CRC Press/Taylor & Francis.

Raote, I., Bhattacharyya, S., & Panicker, M. M. (2013). Functional selectivity in serotonin receptor 2A (5-HT2A) endocytosis, recycling, and phosphorylation. *Molecular Pharmacology, 83*, 42–50.

Rehm, J., Mathers, C., Popova, S., Thavorncharoensap, M., Teerawattananon, Y., & Patra, J. (2009). Global burden of disease and injury and economic cost attributable to alcohol use and alcohol-use disorders. *Lancet, 373*, 2223–2233.

Reser, D. H., Richardson, K. E., Montibeller, M. O., Zhao, S., Chan, J. M., Soares, J. G., et al. (2014). Claustrum projections to prefrontal cortex in the capuchin monkey (*Cebus apella*). *Frontiers in Systems Neuroscience, 8*, 123.

Rhead, J. C., Soskin, R. A., Turek, I., Richards, W. A., Yensen, R., Kurland, A. A., et al. (1977). Psychedelic drug (DPT)-assisted psychotherapy with alcoholics: A controlled study. *Journal of Psychedelic Drugs, 9*, 287–300.

Riba, J., Rodriguez-Fornells, A., Strassman, R. J., & Barbanoj, M. J. (2001). Psychometric assessment of the Hallucinogen Rating Scale. *Drug and Alcohol Dependence, 62*, 215–223.

Riba, J., Romero, S., Grasa, E., Mena, E., Carrio, I., & Barbanoj, M. J. (2006). Increased frontal and paralimbic activation following ayahuasca, the pan-Amazonian inebriant. *Psychopharmacology (Berlin), 186*, 93–98.

Richards, W. A., Rhead, J. C., Dileo, F. B., Yensen, R., & Kurland, A. A. (1977). The peak experience variable in DPT-assisted psychotherapy with cancer patients. *Journal of Psychedelic Drugs, 9*, 1–10.

Roseman, L., Haijen, E., Idialu-Ikato, K., Kaelen, M., Watts, R., & Carhart-Harris, R. (2019). Emotional breakthrough and psychedelics: Validation of the Emotional Breakthrough Inventory. *Journal of Psychopharmacology, 33*, 1076–1087.

Rösner, S., Hackl-Herrwerth, A., Leucht, S., Lehert, P., Vecchi, S., & Soyka, M. (2010a).

Acamprosate for alcohol dependence. *Cochrane Database of Systematic Reviews, 9,* CD004332.

Rösner, S., Hackl-Herrwerth, A., Leucht, S., Vecchi, S., Srisurapanont, M., & Soyka, M. (2010b). Opioid antagonists for alcohol dependence. *Cochrane Database of Systematic Reviews, 12,* CD001867.

Ross, S., Bossis, A., Guss, J., Agin-Liebes, G., Malone, T., Cohen, B., et al. (2016). Rapid and sustained symptom reduction following psilocybin treatment for anxiety and depression in patients with life-threatening cancer: A randomized controlled trial. *Journal of Psychopharmacology, 30,* 1165–1180.

Roth-Alpermann, C., Morris, R. G. M., Korte, M., & Bonhoeffer, T. (2006). Homeostatic shutdown of long-term potentiation in the adult hippocampus. *Proceedings of the National Academy of Sciences of the USA, 103,* 11039–11044.

Roy, C. (1973). Indian peyotists and alcohol. *American Journal of Psychiatry, 130,* 329–330.

Rydzyński, Z., Cwyna, R. S., Grzelak, L., & Jagiello, W. (1968). Preliminary report on the experience with psychosomimetic drugs in the treatment of alcoholism. *Activas Nervosa Superior (Praha), 10,* 273.

Rydzyński, Z., & Gruszczyński, W. (1978). Treatment of alcoholism with psychotomimetic drugs: A follow-up study. *Activas Nervosa Superior (Praha), 20,* 81–82.

Schellekens, A. F., De Jong, C. A., Buitelaar, J. K., & Verkes, R. J. (2015). Co-morbid anxiety disorders predict early relapse after inpatient alcohol treatment. *European Psychiatry, 30,* 128–136.

Schmid, C. L., & Bohn, L. M. (2010). Serotonin, but not *N*-methyltryptamines, activates the serotonin 2A receptor via a ss-arrestin2/Src/Akt signaling complex *in vivo. Journal of Neuroscience, 30,* 13513–13524.

Seeley, W. W., Menon, V., Schatzberg, A. F., Keller, J., Glover, G. H., Kenna, H., et al. (2007). Dissociable intrinsic connectivity networks for salience processing and executive control. *Journal of Neuroscience, 27,* 2349–2356.

Seo, D., & Sinha, R. (2014). The neurobiology of alcohol craving and relapse. *Handbook of Clinical Neurology, 125,* 355–368.

Serafini, G., Pompili, M., Innamorati, M., Giordano, G., Montebovi, F., Sher, L., et al. (2012). The role of microRNAs in synaptic plasticity, major affective disorders and suicidal behavior. *Neuroscience Research, 73,* 179–190.

Sinha, R. (2012). How does stress lead to risk of alcohol relapse? *Alcohol Research: Current Reviews, 34*(4), 432–440.

Sinha, R., & Li, C. S. (2007). Imaging stress- and cue-induced drug and alcohol craving: Association with relapse and clinical implications. *Drug and Alcohol Review, 26,* 25–31.

Smart, R. G., Storm, T., Baker, E. F., & Solursh, L. (1966). A controlled study of lysergide in the treatment of alcoholism: 1. The effects on drinking behavior. *Quarterly Journal of Studies on Alcohol, 27,* 469–482.

Stewart, O. (1987). *The peyote religion: A history.* Norman: University of Oklahoma Press.

Strassman, R. J., Qualls, C. R., Uhlenhuth, E. H., & Kellner, R. (1994). Dose–response study of *N,N*-dimethyltryptamine in humans: II. Subjective effects and preliminary results of a new rating scale. *Archives of General Psychiatry, 51,* 98–108.

Thomas, G., Lucas, P., Capler, N. R., Tupper, K. W., & Martin, G. (2013). Ayahuasca-assisted therapy for addiction: Results from a preliminary observational study in Canada. *Current Drug Abuse Reviews, 6,* 30–42.

Thomas, M. J., Kalivas, P. W., & Shaham, Y. (2008). Neuroplasticity in the mesolimbic dopamine system and cocaine addiction. *British Journal of Pharmacology, 154,* 327–342.

Thompson, P. M., Cruz, D. A., Olukotun, D. Y., & Delgado, P. L. (2012). Serotonin receptor, SERT mRNA and correlations with symptoms in males with alcohol dependence and suicide. *Acta Psychiatrica Scandinavica, 126,* 165–174.

Tomsovic, M., & Edwards, R. V. (1970). Lysergide treatment of schizophrenic and nonschizophrenic alcoholics: A controlled evaluation. *Quarterly Journal of Studies on Alcohol, 31,* 932–949.

Tononi, G. (2004). An information integration theory of consciousness. *BMC Neuroscience, 5,* 42.

Torgerson, C. M., Irimia, A., Goh, S. Y., & Van Horn, J. D. (2015). The DTI connectivity of the human claustrum. *Human Brain Mapping, 36,* 827–838.

Turek, I. S., Soskin, R. A., & Kurland, A. A. (1974). Methylenedioxyamphetamine (MDA) subjective effects. *Journal of Psychiatric Drugs, 6,* 7–14.

Twarog, B. M., & Page, I. H. (1953). Serotonin content of some mammalian tissues and urine and a method for its determination. *American Journal of Physiology, 175,* 157–161.

Underwood, M. D., Mann, J. J., Huang, Y. Y., & Arango, V. (2008). Family history of alcoholism is associated with lower 5-HT2A receptor binding in the prefrontal cortex. *Alcoholism: Clinical and Experimental Research, 32,* 593–599.

Volkow, N. D., & Li, T. K. (2005). Drugs and

alcohol: Treating and preventing abuse, addiction and their medical consequences. *Pharmacology and Therapeutics, 108*, 3–17.

Vollenweider, F. X., Csomor, P. A., Knappe, B., Geyer, M. A., & Quednow, B. B. (2007). The effects of the preferential 5-HT2A agonist psilocybin on prepulse inhibition of startle in healthy human volunteers depend on interstimulus interval. *Neuropsychopharmacology, 32*, 1876–1887.

Vollenweider, F. X., & Geyer, M. A. (2001). A systems model of altered consciousness: Integrating natural and drug-induced psychoses. *Brain Research Bulletin, 56*, 495–507.

Vollenweider, F. X., Vollenweider-Scherpenhuyzen, M. F., Babler, A., Vogel, H., & Hell, D. (1998). Psilocybin induces schizophrenia-like psychosis in humans via a serotonin-2 agonist action. *NeuroReport, 9*, 3897–3902.

Wainwright, S. R., & Galea, L. A. (2013). The neural plasticity theory of depression: Assessing the roles of adult neurogenesis and PSA-NCAM within the hippocampus. *Neural Plasticity, 2013*, Article 805497.

Wiesbeck, G. A., Weijers, H. G., Chick, J., Naranjo, C. A., & Boening, J. (1999). Ritanserin in relapse prevention in abstinent alcoholics: Results from a placebo-controlled double-blind international multicenter trial. *Alcoholism: Clinical and Experimental Research, 23*, 230–235.

Willenbring, M. L. (2014). Treatment of heavy drinking and alcohol use disorder. In R. K. Ries, D. A. Fiellin, S. C. Miller, & R. Saitz (Eds.), *The ASAM principles of addiction medicine* (pp. 375–388). New York: Wolters Kluwer.

Woolley, D. W., & Shaw, E. (1954). A biochemical and pharmacological suggestion about certain mental disorders. *Proceedings of the National Academy of Sciences of the USA, 40*, 228–231.

CHAPTER 25

Psychedelics in the Treatment of Addiction

MATTHEW W. JOHNSON

Introduction

In the original heyday of psychedelic research from the 1950s through the 1970s, when over 1,000 papers were published describing the treatment of over 40,000 patients with psychedelics (Grinspoon, 1981), one of the main therapeutic targets of interest was the treatment of addiction. Specifically, most of this research focused on using lysergic acid diethylamide (LSD) in the treatment of alcoholism, although in some cases the classic psychedelics mescaline (e.g., Smith, 1958, 1959) and dipropyltrypamine (Rhead et al., 1977) were also used to treat alcoholism. The initial hypothesis for using psychedelics for alcoholism was that they might serve to mimic delirium tremens, which sometimes prompted sobriety (Chwelos, Blewett, Smith, & Hoffer, 1959; Dyck, 2006; Smith, 1958). The logic was that classic psychedelics are relatively safe in the physiological domain, in contrast to delirium tremens, which could be fatal. However, rather than dysphoric reactions, these researchers often observed positive, mystical-type effects (i.e., involving distinct qualities including a strong

sense of unity; closely related to, or perhaps synonymous with the concepts "peak experience" and "transcendental experience") and insightful effects that seemed to prompt sobriety in response to psychedelic drug administration. A number of studies investigated LSD in the treatment of alcoholism. These varied both in their methods and in their initially reported conclusions regarding efficacy, with some studies showing positive trends for LSD that did not reach statistical significance at relatively small sample sizes. These factors led reviewers to conclude that efficacy was undetermined (e.g., Abuzzahab & Anderson, 1971; Mangini, 1998). However, within the last decade, a meta-analysis of the only studies from the older era that randomly assigned patients to either an LSD or control condition (six original studies; a total of 536 patients) showed significant and substantial decreases in alcohol misuse at the first follow-up (at least 1 month after treatment) in the participants receiving LSD compared to the control participants (Krebs & Johansen, 2012). Renewed work along these lines, using the classic psychedelic psilocybin to treat alcohol use disorder,

493

has shown promising preliminary results in an open-label pilot study (Bogenschutz et al., 2015). For a far more detailed review of past and current research using psychedelics specifically to treat alcohol use disorder, see Chapter 24, this volume, coauthored by Michael P. Bogenschutz and Sarah E. Mennenga.

In early research examining psychedelics in the treatment of alcoholism, the observation that treatment outcomes depend on the nature of the subjective experience following psychedelic administration (Chwelos et al., 1959; Dyck, 2006; Smith, 1958) suggests something profound and possibly paradigm-shifting about this treatment model (Johnson, 2018b). It suggests that, unlike typical addiction medications, the efficacy of psychedelics in treating alcoholism might not rely on the ability of the medication to directly modify alcohol reinforcement, craving, or withdrawal at the neurobiological level governing alcohol effects. Rather, the psychedelic may occasion powerfully plastic biological, mental, and behavioral states during or after the period of drug action, in which heightened learning may occur, prompting persistent behavior change long after the biological effects of the medication have been resolved. This paradigm might afford some remarkable distinctions in comparison to traditional psychiatric medications. First, a single or a few administrations can be associated with persisting behavioral change, as shown in studies by colleagues and myself, which found that a single high dose of psilocybin led to lasting reductions in depression and anxiety among cancer patients, still persistent when examined at 6 months posttreatment in some studies (Griffiths et al., 2016; Grob et al., 2011; Ross et al., 2016). This differs strongly for the typical model necessitating regular (e.g., daily) administration of psychiatric medication as with typical antidepressants and anxiolytics. A second fundamental way in which the psychedelic therapy paradigm is distinguished may be in its generality. A powerful plastic state with enhanced potential for learning is one that may not only be applicable for the treatment of alcohol use disorders, but also applicable to behavioral change generally, including other substance use disorders, the focus of this chapter.

Heroin

The idea that psychedelics held clinical potential for substances of abuse beyond alcohol goes back to the earlier era of research. One early study tested whether LSD might have therapeutic potential in the treatment of opioid dependence (Savage & McCabe, 1973). This study was with 78 heroin-using individuals who were inmates under parole/probation supervision by the State of Maryland. Participants were randomized to either a psychedelic therapy condition involving a single administration of LSD (300–450 µg) during a 6-week residential stay at a "halfway house" or a comparison condition involving attendance at an outpatient clinic, daily urine testing for opiates, and weekly group therapy sessions. The LSD group showed significantly lower urinalysis-confirmed heroin use at every time point examined, including the 12-month posttreatment assessment, at which continuous abstinence rates were 25% in the LSD group versus 5% in the comparison group. A fascinating component of the report consisted of participant comparisons of LSD effects with heroin effects. One participant stated, "Heroin has a numbing-like effect on you. It tends to relax you and somewhat takes you out and away from your surroundings and yourself. LSD makes you more aware of yourself and puts you right into whatever has been troubling you." Echoing a similar theme, another participant stated, "Comparing LSD to heroin is like comparing a speck of dust with a mountain. The difference is that heroin helps you to turn from yourself and LSD show you how to face yourself." A third stated, "The two experiences of heroin and LSD are like night and day. Heroin is night, a time to sleep and with sleep, nothing comes but a dream. But with LSD, it is like dawn, a new awakening, it expands your mind, it gives you a brand-new outlook on life."

A major caveat in interpreting the results of this study, as acknowledged by the study's authors, is that the groups differed on other aspects of treatment aside from LSD treatment, including a 6-week residential stay for the LSD group. However, these preliminary data were promising, and it is a shame that 45 years have passed since their publication, with no follow-up studies. With the United States now facing an epidemic of opioid dependence and associated fatalities (Kolodny et al., 2015), the present is an ideal time for revisiting the use of psychedelics in the treatment of opioid use disorders.

■ Tobacco

Based on these early data suggesting antiaddiction efficacy of classic psychedelics across multiple target drugs of abuse, my colleagues and I embarked on a study using the classic psychedelic psilocybin as a smoking cessation medication. Tobacco addiction seemed an intriguing target for a number of reasons. Although there was preliminary evidence of antiaddiction efficacy of classic psychedelics for alcoholism and opioid dependence, those are addictions to drugs that are extremely intoxicating. Tobacco addiction is similar in that it is unquestionably a drug addiction, with all of the hallmark features present to one degree or another in other forms of drug addiction, including drug-mediated reinforcement, craving, withdrawal, preference for immediate drug reward over delayed but arguably more highly valued consequences such as improved health, and high rates of relapse among those attempting to quit (Bickel, Johnson, Koffarnus, MacKillop, & Murphy, 2014; Hughes, 2006; Johnson, Bickel, & Baker, 2007). However, tobacco addiction differs from alcohol, opioids, and many other drugs of abuse, in that it is not associated with substantial behavioral intoxication and associated current quality-of-life destruction, at least as typically consumed in the form of modern cigarettes (Hughes, 2006). This begs an interesting question: Are psychedelics potentially effective in addiction treatment because they somehow allow the person to reevaluate the life disintegration that often comes with highly impairing drugs? Put another way, do they prompt something like a "rock bottom" experience, with accompanying realization about the harms one has done to him- or herself and loved ones? If so, perhaps tobacco addiction would not be sensitive to psychedelic treatment. Rarely does one lose a job, ruin a career, or lose a spouse due to his or her tobacco addiction, as is

known to happen with highly intoxicating drugs such as alcohol and opioids. In some sense, one might consider tobacco addiction a "purer" form of addiction, in that it constitutes more of a straightforward competition between short- versus long-term interests. Life is relatively unimpaired for the vast majority of years of a smoking career, but then an increased probability of serious illness and premature death typically come after decades of smoking. Could psychedelic sessions be efficacious in helping individuals resolve such competing motivations at play in addiction, in the absence of severe current life destruction? Cigarette smoking seemed a fascinating test case.

Aside from serving an intriguing model system of addiction, cigarette smoking is, of course, of interest because it is responsible for far more deaths than any other drug. In the United States, smoking is responsible for approximately five to seven times more deaths than alcohol, and approximately 26 times more deaths than all illicit drugs combined (Danaei et al., 2009; Mokdad, Marks, Stroup, & Gerberding, 2004). Although smoking cessation medications are approved by the U.S. Food and Drug Administration (FDA) and show greater efficacy than placebo, the large majority of individuals fail to maintain abstinence in the long term for any given quit attempt with these medications (e.g., Hughes, Shiffman, Callas, & Zhang, 2003; Jorenby et al., 2006). Therefore, there is a dire unmet need for more effective medications, particularly given the overwhelming mortality associated with smoking.

In order to evaluate safety and test the waters for feasibility and potential efficacy of the approach, we conducted an open-label pilot study in 15 nicotine-dependent, treatment-resistant tobacco cigarette smokers (Johnson, Garcia-Romeu, Cosimano, & Griffiths, 2014). Participants (10 men and five women) with a mean age of 51 years, had been smoking for a mean of 31 years. They reported a mean of six previous serious quit attempts using a variety of methods, and currently smoked an average of 19 cigarettes per day. They provided breath and urine samples that showed carbon monoxide and cotinine levels, respectively, that confirmed their status as smokers. Participants underwent a 15-week program including manualized cognitive-behavioral therapy (CBT) for smoking cessation and up to three psilocybin sessions. After four preparatory sessions in which CBT content and specific preparation for receiving psilocybin were provided, the first psilocybin session occurred on the participant's predesignated target quit date. This session involved the administration of a moderately high dose (20 mg/70 kg) of psilocybin. Additional psilocybin sessions were provided at 2 and 8 weeks after the target quit date. For these last two sessions, the default plan was to administer a high dose (30 mg/70 kg) unless the moderately high dose seemed of sufficient strength in the judgment of the participant (only one participant deviated from the default plan). Between and after these psilocybin session days, volunteers visited the laboratory on a weekly basis. During these visits, CBT content was provided.

No serious adverse events attributable to psilocybin occurred during the study. At the 6-month posttarget quit date, 12 out of 15 participants (80%) were biologically verified (via breath carbon monoxide and urine cotinine analysis) as smoking abstinent. Nine of the 15 participants (60%) met the threshold criteria to qualify as having had a "complete" mystical-type experience (a subjective experience sensitive to psychedelic effects, as described in the Introduction) on the States of Consciousness Questionnaire in at least one of their multiple sessions (Garcia-Romeu, Griffiths, & Johnson, 2014). Those who were smoking abstinent at 6 months had significantly higher mystical-type experience scores as measured by the States of Consciousness Questionnaire on their session days. Moreover, a significant negative relationship was shown between mystical-type experience score on the States of Consciousness Questionnaire on their session days, and the degree of cigarette craving reduction at study intake to the 6-month follow-up. At a very long-term follow-up 2.5 years after the target quit date, 12 of the original 15 participants were qualitatively interviewed regarding their experience in the study (Noorani, Garcia-Romeu, Swift, Griffiths, & Johnson, 2018). Participants described the psilocybin sessions as leading to insights into self-identity and reasons for smoking, and a lasting sense of interconnectedness, awe, and curiosity. These psilocybin effects were reported to have overshadowed tobacco withdrawal symptoms. Moreover, aside from smoking, participants reported increases in prosocial behavior and aesthetic appreciation.

Volunteers were reassessed with breath and urine samples at their 12-month follow-up and at the very long-term follow-up, which was on average 2.5 years after the target quit date. Biologically confirmed abstinence rates were 67 and 60% at these two time points, respectively. Although the open-label and nonrandomized nature of the design precludes any definitive conclusions regarding the efficacy of psilocybin per se, these results were very promising. Consider that at approximately 6 months posttarget quit date, over-the-counter nicotine replacement therapy is associated with an approximately 7% abstinence rate (Hughes et al., 2003), sustained-release bupropion is associated with an approximately 20% abstinence rate (Jorenby et al., 2006), and varenicline is associated with an approximately 30% abstinence rate (Jorenby et al., 2006). So, if the question was whether the approach was promising enough to warrant the time and resources for conducting a more rigorous follow-up, the answer was a resounding "yes."

We are now conducting a comparative efficacy trial that randomizes treatment-resistant smokers to a single psilocybin session (concurrent with the target quit date) or the transdermal nicotine patch (per FDA guidelines, beginning 24 hours after their target quit date). Both treatment arms are run in combination with a 13-week program of the same manualized CBT used in our pilot study. Before their target quit date, and after 24 hours of nicotine abstinence, participants undergo functional magnetic resonance imaging (fMRI), during which they complete a variety of tasks including the Multi-Source Interference Task (MSIT), a measure of cognitive control. Participants complete the task again, 24 hours after their target quit date. Interim results were presented at the 80th Annual Scientific Meeting of the College on Problems of Drug Dependence (Johnson, 2018a) and the 2018 meeting of the Society of Biological Psychiatry (McKenna et al., 2018). Interim results show substantially higher cotinine-verified 12-month abstinence rates in the psilocybin group (50%, *n* = 10) compared to the nicotine patch group (*n* = 9, 20%), continuing to suggest promising results for psilocybin in smoking cessation. MSIT results showed significant pre- versus post-target quit date reductions in the reaction time congruency effect in psilocybin participants (*n* = 9), but there was no change in the nicotine patch group (*n* = 7). For psilocybin participants, MSIT congruency effect reaction time was significantly and positively correlated with superior parietal cortex activation during the task for the prepsilocybin scan, but not for the postpsilocybin scan. These preliminary neurocognitive analyses suggest significantly improved cognitive control and a reduction of fMRI response in the superior parietal cortex the day after quitting for the psilocybin group, suggesting psilocybin may improve smoking cessation outcomes by enhancing cognitive control. This study is ongoing. If results continue to suggest promise in using psilocybin in smoking cessation, the approach should be tested in additional, rigorous studies.

▥ Cocaine

Cocaine use disorder is a clinical target of psychedelic therapy under investigation by Peter Hendricks (2018) at the University of Alabama at Birmingham. Although dozens of compounds have been tested over the last few decades, no medication has been approved by the FDA for the treatment of cocaine use disorder. This ongoing double-blind study plans to randomize 40 individuals with cocaine use disorder to receive either 25 mg/70 kg psilocybin or a psychoactive comparison compound (100 mg diphenhydramine) on a single session day. Like the aforementioned cigarette smoking cessation research, in the weeks preceding the drug administration session, preparatory meetings take place involving both CBT content for the treatment of cocaine use disorder and specific preparation for a high-dose psilocybin session. Also, like the current smoking cessation trial, fMRI is conducted both be-

fore the psilocybin session day and the day after psilocybin in order to determine potential neurobiological correlates of treatment success that might underlie potential psilocybin efficacy for cocaine abstinence. Weekly CBT-based sessions continue for 4 weeks following the psilocybin. A final follow-up session is conducted about 6 months after the end of active treatment (i.e., the last CBT-based session).

Interim results from the cocaine use disorder trial were recently presented at the 80th annual scientific meeting of the College on Problems of Drug Dependence (Hendricks, 2018). Although very preliminary, with 10 participants thus far (six randomized to psilocybin, and four randomized to diphenhydramine; relatively well matched on demographics at this preliminary stage), results were promising regarding both safety and potential efficacy for cocaine abstinence. No serious adverse events were attributable to study medication. Although the groups were statistically indistinguishable in their urinalysis-confirmed cocaine abstinence at baseline assessment, the psilocybin group had a mean of 100% cocaine-abstinent days during the final 90- to 180-day assessment period, while the control group had a mean of approximately 86% cocaine-abstinent days during the same time period, which was a statistically significant difference. Urinalysis was performed at the 180-day follow-up, providing confirmation regarding abstinence during the several days preceding the follow-up visit. To be clear, results for both groups thus far are better than one would expect for cocaine use disorder treatment. Perhaps the careful preparation, rapport building, and willingness to take a bold step such as psychedelic therapy might be part of the mix for both groups that may account for promising preliminary results.

Regarding long-term changes other than cocaine abstinence, the psilocybin group, compared to the control group, showed substantial increases in ratings of life satisfaction at each of the follow-up visits and reported substantially reduced stress at the majority of follow-up visits. It is possible that such changes are related to addiction recovery, either as a cause or a consequence. Regarding the nature of their session day experiences, the psilocybin group showed substantially higher ratings on all factors of mystical-type experience, a construct of subjective experience known to be sensitive to psilocybin effects, as discussed earlier in regard to smoking cessation. In this study, mystical-type experience was assessed on session days (after psilocybin effects had largely resolved) using the validated 30-item Mystical Experience Questionnaire (MEQ-30; Barrett, Johnson, & Griffiths, 2015). These psychometrically distinct factors include (1) unity, noetic quality, and sacredness; (2) positive mood; (3) transcendence of time and space; and (4) ineffability. The psilocybin group also showed substantially higher ratings on all factors of the Challenging Experience Questionnaire, a measure validated to assess subjectively difficult reactions to psilocybin, sometimes colloquially referred to as "bad trips" but often valued as learning experiences within supervised psychedelic therapy sessions (Barrett, Bradstreet, Leoutsakos, Johnson, & Griffiths, 2016). These psychometrically distinct factors include grief, fear, death, insanity, isolation, physical distress, and paranoia. Therefore, session content very much appeared to be in line with expectations regarding the administration of a high dose of psilocybin within a psychedelic therapy context. Moreover, every patient in the psilocybin group indicated that the session was among either the single most meaningful experience of his or her lifetime (two volunteers) or among the five most meaningful experience of his or her lifetime (four volunteers). One of the four volunteers in the control group indicated that the session was among the meaningful experience of his or her lifetime (none in the other category). This response from a control group participant clearly suggests that placebo effects and/or the nonpharmacological aspects of the intervention can play a powerful role in shaping the experience. Although very preliminary, study results thus far suggest that examining psychedelic therapy for cocaine use disorder is a credible and promising line of research. Given the incredible amount of resources over the last few decades devoted to finding an effective medication for the treatment of cocaine use disorder, and the fact that no medication has been approved by the FDA, continued prom-

ising results would be exciting and might address a critical unmet need.

Conclusions

While we await more definitive results for the lines of research using psilocybin to treat tobacco and cocaine use disorders, the emerging possibility of an approach with cross-addiction generality is looking more realistic. On the short list of research that needs to be conducted is to revisit the use of psychedelics in the treatment of opioid use disorder, particularly given the modern opioid epidemic (Kolodny et al., 2015). One could also test the treatment on a whole host of target drugs of abuse, including methamphetamine. Moreover, it is plausible that antiaddiction effects are not limited to drugs of abuse. Credibility for this argument is lent by the finding discussed in the Introduction regarding persisting reductions in depression and anxiety in cancer patients (Griffith et al., 2016; Grob et al., 2011; Ross et al., 2016). As I have postulated previously (Johnson, 2018b; Pollan, 2018), it may be that depression, anxiety, and other psychiatric disorders that are not nominally considered addictions may in fact constitute addictions as broadly defined; that is, they involve a narrowed mental and behavioral repertoire in which one is stuck in a certain pattern, focused on a certain activity to the suboptimal exclusion of other aspects of the environment and life. Whether that pattern of behavior is in the self-administration of tobacco, alcohol, cocaine, opioids, or other drugs, or whether it is the cyclical, self-perpetuating thoughts of self-hatred, inevitable failure, or worry that can come with mood and anxiety disorders, it may be that psychedelics have the ability to at least temporarily allow one to see outside of those narrow patterns, to recognize the suboptimality of these patterns, and therefore become motivated and learn to adopt more optimal patterns of living. This broad view of psychedelics as behavior-change agents may constitute a paradigm shift in psychiatry (Johnson, 2018b; Kuhn, 1962). Although each disorder needs to be empirically tested, and more research is needed at the psychological and biological levels to understand the mechanisms of this broad behavior-change potential, it already seems justified to test the ability of psychedelic therapy to treat disorders including anorexia, obesity, gambling disorder, and sexual impulse control disorders. I hope that the field of psychedelic research will sufficiently expand, both in terms of attracting qualified scientists and acquiring federal funding, in order to fully test the potential of psychedelics as behavior-change agents.

◪ Acknowledgments

I thank Peter S. Hendricks, PhD, for helpful clarifications regarding his presentation at the College on Problems of Drug Dependence, and Nora Belblidia for assistance with manuscript preparation. I have advisory relationships with the following organizations: AWAKN Life Sciences Inc., Beckley Psychedelic Ltd., Entheogen Biomedical Corp., Field Trip Psychedelics Inc., Mind Medicine Inc., Otsuka Pharmaceutical Development & Commercialization Inc., and Silo Pharma, Inc.

◪ References

Abuzzahab, F. S., Sr., & Anderson, B. J. (1971). A review of LSD treatment in alcoholism. *International Pharmacopsychiatry, 6*(4), 223–235.

Barrett, F. S., Bradstreet, M. P., Leoutsakos, J. S., Johnson, M. W., & Griffiths, R. R. (2016). The Challenging Experience Questionnaire: Characterization of challenging experiences with psilocybin mushrooms. *Journal of Psychopharmacology, 30*(12), 1279–1295.

Barrett, F. S., Johnson, M. W., & Griffiths, R. R. (2015). Validation of the revised Mystical Experience Questionnaire in experimental sessions with psilocybin. *Journal of Psychopharmacology, 29*(11), 1182–1190.

Bickel, W. K., Johnson, M. W., Koffarnus, M. N., MacKillop, J., & Murphy, J. G. (2014). The behavioral economics of substance use disorders: Reinforcement pathologies and their repair. *Annual Review of Clinical Psychology, 10*, 641–677.

Bogenschutz, M. P., Forcehimes, A. A., Pommy, J. A., Wilcox, C. E., Barbosa, P. C., & Strassman, R. J. (2015). Psilocybin-assisted treatment for alcohol dependence: A proof-of-concept study. *Journal of Psychopharmacology, 29*(3), 289–299.

Chwelos, N., Blewett, D. B., Smith, C. M., & Hoffer, A. (1959). Use of d-lysergic acid diethylamide in the treatment of alcoholism. *Quarterly Journal on Studies of Alcohol, 20,* 577–590.

Danaei, G., Ding, E. L., Mozaffarian, D., Taylor, B., Rehm, J., Murray, C. J., et al. (2009). The preventable causes of death in the United States: Comparative risk assessment of dietary, lifestyle, and metabolic risk factors. *PLOS Medicine, 6*(4), e1000058.

Dyck, E. (2006). "Hitting highs at rock bottom": LSD treatment for alcoholism, 1950–1970. *Social History of Medicine, 19,* 313–329.

Garcia-Romeu, A., Griffiths, R. R., & Johnson, M. W. (2014). Psilocybin-occasioned mystical experiences in the treatment of tobacco addiction. *Current Drug Abuse Reviews, 7*(3), 157–164.

Griffiths, R. R., Johnson, M. W., Carducci, M. A., Umbricht, A., Richards, W. A., Richards, B. D., et al. (2016). Psilocybin produces substantial and sustained decreases in depression and anxiety in patients with life-threatening cancer: A randomized double-blind trial. *Journal of Psychopharmacology, 30*(12), 1181–1197.

Grinspoon, L. (1981). LSD reconsidered. *The Sciences, 21,* 20–23.

Grob, C. S., Danforth, A. L., Chopra, G. S., Hagerty, M., McKay, C. R., Halberstadt, A. L., et al. (2011). Pilot study of psilocybin treatment for anxiety in patients with advanced-stage cancer. *Archives of General Psychiatry, 68*(1), 71–78.

Hendricks, P. S. (2018, June). *Psilocybin treatment of cocaine use disorder.* Presentation at the Drug Addiction Treatment with Classic Psychedelics, College on Problems of Drug Dependence 80th Annual Scientific Meeting, San Diego, CA.

Hughes, J. R. (2006). Should criteria for drug dependence differ across drugs? *Addiction, 101,* 134–141.

Hughes, J. R., Shiffman, S., Callas, P., & Zhang, J. (2003). A meta-analysis of the efficacy of over-the-counter nicotine replacement. *Tobacco Control, 12*(1), 21–27.

Johnson, M. W. (2018a, June). *Psilocybin treatment of tobacco use disorder.* Presentation at the Drug Addiction Treatment with Classic Psychedelics, College on Problems of Drug Dependence 80th Annual Scientific Meeting, San Diego, CA.

Johnson, M. W. (2018b). Psychiatry might need some psychedelic therapy (Introduction to issue: The renaissance in psychedelic research). *International Review of Psychiatry, 30,* 285–290.

Johnson, M. W., Bickel, W. K., & Baker, F. (2007). Moderate drug use and delay discounting: A comparison of heavy, light, and never smokers. *Experimental and Clinical Psychopharmacology, 15*(2), 187–194.

Johnson, M. W., Garcia-Romeu, A., Cosimano, M. P., & Griffiths, R. R. (2014). Pilot study of the 5-HT2AR agonist psilocybin in the treatment of tobacco addiction. *Journal of Psychopharmacology, 28*(11), 983–992.

Jorenby, D. E., Hays, J. T., Rigotti, N. A., Azoulay, S., Watsky, E. J., Williams, K. E., et al. (2006). Efficacy of varenicline, an α4β2 nicotinic acetylcholine receptor partial agonist, vs placebo or sustained-release bupropion for smoking cessation: A randomized controlled trial. *Journal of the American Medical Association, 296*(1), 56–63.

Kolodny, A., Courtwright, D. T., Hwang, C. S., Kreiner, P., Eadie, J. L., Clark, T. W., et al. (2015). The prescription opioid and heroin crisis: A public health approach to an epidemic of addiction. *Annual Review of Public Health, 36*, 559–574.

Krebs, T. S., & Johansen, P.-Ø. (2012). Lysergic acid diethylamide (LSD) for alcoholism: Meta-analysis of randomized controlled trials. *Journal of Psychopharmacology, 26*(7), 994–1002.

Kuhn, T. S. (1962). *The structure of scientific revolutions* (3rd ed.). Chicago: University of Chicago Press.

Mangini, M. (1998). Treatment of alcoholism using psychedelic drugs: A review of the program of research. *Journal of Psychoactive Drugs, 30*(4), 381–418.

McKenna, M., Fedota, J., Garcia-Romeu, A., Johnson, M., Griffiths, R., & Stein, E. (2018). T263: Psilocybin improves cognitive control and downregulates parietal cortex in treatment-seeking smokers. *Biological Psychiatry, 83*(9), S231–S232.

Mokdad, A. H., Marks, J. S., Stroup, D. F., & Gerberding, J. L. (2004). Actual causes of death in the United States, 2000. *Journal of the American Medical Association, 291*(10), 1238–1245.

Noorani, T., Garcia-Romeu, A., Swift, T. C., Griffiths, R. R., & Johnson, M. W. (2018). Psychedelic therapy for smoking cessation: Qualitative analysis of participant accounts. *Journal of Psychopharmacology, 32*(7), 756–769.

Pollan, M. (2018). *How to change your mind: What the new science of psychedelics teaches us about consciousness, dying, addiction, depression, and transcendence.* New York: Penguin Press.

Rhead, J. C., Soskin, R. A., Turek, I., Richards, W. A., Yensen, R., Kurland, A. A., et al. (1977). Psychedelic drug (DPT)-assisted psychotherapy with alcoholics: A controlled study. *Journal of Psychedelic Drugs, 9*, 287–300.

Ross, S., Bossis, A., Guss, J., Agin-Liebes, G., Malone, T., Cohen, B., et al. (2016). Rapid and sustained symptom reduction following psilocybin treatment for anxiety and depression in patients with life-threatening cancer: A randomized controlled trial. *Journal of Psychopharmacology, 30*(12), 1165–1180.

Savage, C., & McCabe, O. L. (1973). Residential psychedelic (LSD) therapy for the narcotic addict: A controlled study. *Archives of General Psychiatry, 28*(6), 808–814.

Smith, C. M. (1958). A new adjunct to the treatment of alcoholism: The hallucinogenic drugs. *Quarterly Journal of Studies on Alcohol, 19*, 406–417.

Smith, C. M. (1959). Some reflections on the possible therapeutic effects of the hallucinogens with special reference to alcoholism. *Quarterly Journal of Studies on Alcohol, 20*, 292–301.

CHAPTER 26

The Treatment of Depressive Disorders with Psychedelics

DAVE KING and JONNY MARTELL

Depression: Epidemiology and Impact

Depression ranks among the most burdensome social and medical challenges of the modern world. It is extremely common, affecting approximately 10–15% of the general population at least once during the lifetime (Bromet et al., 2011; Lim et al., 2018). The total number of people in the world with depression was estimated at 322 million in 2015, an increase of almost 20% from estimates made in 2005, and prevalence rates are projected to continue increasing over the next 30 years (Heo et al., 2008; World Health Organization, 2017). The impact on society is massive. In 2016, depressive disorders were the third largest cause of years lost to disability globally (World Health Organization, 2018). Global illness burden in depression has grown by 37% over the past two decades and, by 2030, depression is expected to be the leading cause of illness burden (Heo et al., 2008; Murray et al., 2012). Already, it is the largest contributor to suicide, which is the second leading cause of death among 15–29 year olds (World Health Organization, 2017; 2018).

Depression is not a simple illness. Three-fourths of all depressed patients experience insomnia, while nearly half of young depressed adults report the opposite (i.e. hypersomnia; Nutt, Wilson, & Paterson, 2008). Some suffer from depression for decades, while others experience only a single episode. Since depressed patients present with such a wide variety of symptoms, it is challenging to describe precisely what depression is. Some authors have proposed that depression is best understood as the tendency to enter into, and inability to recover from, negative mood states, rather than as a specific constellation of negative mood symptoms (Holtzheimer & Mayberg, 2011).

In some cases, depressive episodes may be a presenting feature of underlying endocrinological, inflammatory, gastrointestinal, metabolic, neurodegenerative, substance misuse, or neoplastic disorders (Schulz & Arora, 2015). Depression is also closely associated with several other psychiatric conditions. Nearly two-thirds of patients with schizophrenia may also exhibit signs of depression (e.g., Gozdzik-Zelazny, Borecki, & Pokorski, 2011). In bipolar disorder, patients alternate between episodes of depression and of mania, characterized by elevated mood, pressure of speech, decreased need for sleep and, in some instances, psychosis.

Due to this clinical distinction with major depressive disorder (MDD), patients with bipolar disorder are typically excluded from current trials on depressed patients.

■ Early Studies of Psychedelic-Assisted Therapies for Depression

Two years after the first publication on the discovery and effects of lysergic acid diethylamide (LSD) in humans, Condrau (1949) reported that LSD is capable of inducing feelings of euphoria and might have potential as an antidepressant medication. In a sample of five "depressives" receiving "daily increasing" doses of LSD, Condrau reported that two patients showed clinical benefit. The following year saw publication of the first paper on the use of LSD in combination with psychotherapy (Busch & Johnson, 1950), which reported results comparable to those of Condrau. A third paper (Savage, 1952), also reported a limited response to LSD as a treatment for depressive illness. These early case series are anecdotal, but they do reveal that LSD was recognized as a potential treatment for depression soon after the first publication reporting its discovery.

Bossis (Chapter 23, this volume) addresses in detail the literature on psychedelic-assisted therapies for end-of-life anxiety and depression, a topic systematically reviewed by Reiche and colleagues (2018). Two historical studies on end-of-life depression are nonetheless germane. In the earlier study, patients with terminal cancer were administered substantial doses of LSD, up to 500 µg; 71% of these patients showed pronounced or moderate improvements after treatment (Grof, Goodman, Richards, & Kurland, 1973). In a later study, Richards and colleagues (1980) used the psychedelic drug dipropyltryptamine (DPT) as an adjunct to psychotherapy in cancer patients suffering from psychological distress. They also reported significant decreases in depression after treatment. Like many studies at the time, neither was placebo-controlled. Ten hours of psychotherapeutic preparation for the experimental session and postintegrative psychotherapeutic aftercare were provided to subjects in both studies.

In a systematic review of 21 studies published between 1949 and 1973, Rucker, Jelen, Flynn, Frowde, and Young (2016) reported that clinician-judged improvement was observed in more than three-fourths of patients with unipolar mood disorders after treatment with psychedelic drugs in a variety of therapeutic contexts. The studies reviewed were suboptimal; most lacked adequate controls and standardized assessment tools (i.e., improvements were qualitatively judged by clinicians using vague criteria). They covered a broad range of mood and anxiety disorders and, in the majority of cases, used out-of-date terminology such as "neurotic" and "psychoneurotic" disorders. These cases are not entirely compatible with contemporary diagnoses, but of the 11 studies concerning cohorts classified as "depressives," "depressive reactions," and "depressive neuroses," improvement was reported for just under three-fourths of the 137 participants.

The most comprehensive early studies reported were those conducted at the Spring Grove State Hospital and the Maryland Psychiatric Research Center (Rucker et al., 2016). The therapeutic methodology reported in these papers included weekly interviews with patients 4–8 weeks prior to dosing, the presence of a male and a female therapist, the use of music and visual stimuli as a therapeutic aids, and prolonged follow-up sessions to help integrate and work through the material experienced during the dosing session (Savage, Fadiman, Mogar, & Allen, 1966; Savage, Hughes, & Mogar, 1967). In both studies, symptom improvement was reported to be around 80% of patients. Unlike much of the research that preceded these studies, they included a control group and used randomized group selection.

Almost all the early studies of psychedelic-assisted therapies for depression are considered methodologically or statistically unfit by contemporary standards, and most of the disorders they investigated are now understood and classified differently. Compounding this, many contemporary studies exclude certain patient populations included in some older trials, such as those with a history of psychosis. One upcoming randomized controlled trial (RCT) of psilocybin in London will select patients with treatment-resistant depression, but older studies recruited patients without complete access to the wide range of antidepressant treatments available today. For these reasons, contemporary psychedelic research involves somewhat different clinical populations than those selected by earlier studies. Although there is insufficient historical evidence to say with confidence that psychedelic therapies are effective treatments for depression as it is known today, there is at least enough to indicate the possibility, and to justify ongoing investigation.

Today, significant methodological challenges remain. Placebo control groups are used to measure the collateral therapeutic value of the intervention minus the drug, but these have the greatest rigor when the placebo is difficult to distinguish from the active drug. If the identity of the treatment is evident, the conditions of participant and investigator blinding fail, and the experiment becomes vulnerable to *ascertainment bias*. Participants who recognize that they have received the inactive placebo may be less willing to report improvement (*patient ascertainment bias*), and investigators who recognize the group to which a patient has been allocated may unconsciously report more favorable outcomes for patients receiving the active drug (*observer bias*). It is difficult to achieve blinding in studies of psychoactive drugs by using placebos, since the nature of psychoactive drugs is to affect acute and observable changes in mood, perception, and behavior.

Far more so than for other drugs, whether psychoactive or not, the content and quality of the psychedelic experience is inextricably related to the environment in which it takes place, and the state of mind of subjects as they enter it. These are known, respectively, as *setting* and *set*. The RCT seeks to isolate the therapeutic contribution of specific variables, but when the efficacy of the drug is dependent on a range of environmental and individual variables, it becomes problematic to extrapolate study data to other settings.

These methodological problems illuminate the reasons why older psychedelic research had such a difficult time integrating the study design of the RCT. This is explored by the historian Matthew Oram (2014, 2016).

Underground Psychedelic Psychotherapy

The 1971 United Nations Convention on Psychotropic Substances was the first international treaty to address the regulation of LSD and other classical psychedelics. It stated that the scientific and medical use of psychedelic drugs should be exempt from prohibition, so long as the researchers and research projects were duly authorized by government approval. However, an interlaced barrier to research was woven rapidly from domestic drug control policies, political moves to delegitimize the social groups that predominantly used psychedelic drugs, and difficulties in merging psychedelic research protocols with the requirements of the RCT trial. Psychedelic science was unfunded, unpopular, and unpublishable for several decades. During this time, many therapists accustomed to psychedelic-assisted therapies continued treatment unlawfully, believing that it was in their patients' best interests (Fischer, 2015; Metzner, 2013; Stolaroff, 2004). There is little in the way of data to scientifically evaluate the risks and benefits of this underground work, but it is notable that so many therapists were moved to risk imprisonment in their pursuit of the practice.

Some research and training programs did receive government approval to explore the therapeutic benefits of psychedelic therapies after prohibition. From 1988 to 1994, the Swiss Medical Association for Psycholytic Therapy was granted permission to train psychiatrists in LSD- and 3,4-methylenedioxymethamphetamine (MDMA)-assisted psychotherapy, under the direction of Dr. Samuel Widmer. When this program was aborted and psycholytic therapy was prohibited once again, many of its trainees took their therapy underground, just as others had when the drugs were first restricted (Fischer, 2015).

In 2015, a former director of the White House Office of Drug Abuse Policy, Dr. Peter Bourne, expressed regret for not making sufficient efforts to reduce the regulatory burdens placed on psychedelic science during his time in office under Jimmy Carter's presidency. In his letter to *The New Yorker*, he wrote that "had we been able to lift the ban on scientific research into medical applications, doctors would probably now have a far better understanding of brain function, and the unnecessary suffering of many terminally ill patients could have been alleviated."

Contemporary Studies of Psychedelic-Assisted Therapies for Depression

As of June 2018, several large-scale RCTs investigating psychedelic-assisted therapies for treatment-resistant depression were underway, but no results have yet been published (Rucker, Iliff, & Nutt, 2018). Contemporary clinical evidence is limited to a handful of open-label studies and a small number of RCTs with psychologically distressed end-of-life cohorts, which are unlikely to be representative of other depressed patient populations.

Recent clinical data on psychedelic treatments in depressed patients have been limited to psilocybin and ayahuasca. Ayahuasca is a psychedelic concoction used in traditional ritual and medical contexts by various indigenous communities native to the Amazon basin. Of the numerous chemical constituents of ayahuasca, the primary psychedelic component is dimethyltryptamine (DMT). In a Brazilian inpatient psychiatric unit, ayahuasca was administered open-label to six subjects with diagnoses of recurrent MDD as an investigative treatment for an acute depressive episode (Osório et al., 2015). This study was designed to test feasibility and safety of ayahuasca in this patient group rather than to assess efficacy. However, the intervention was found to induce potent and rapid-onset anxiolytic and antidepressant effects, with reductions in mean depression scores of up to 82% after 1 day. Unlike the majority of contemporary clinical studies with psychedelics, the ayahuasca was not administered in conjunction with psychotherapy, nor were any posttreatment psychotherapeutic sessions reported.

An open-label pilot study evaluated the feasibility and safety of psilocybin in 12 patients with moderate-to-severe treatment-resistant depression (Carhart-Harris, Bolstridge, et al., 2016). Three-fourths of

subjects met criteria for severe or very severe depression, and almost all (92%) had received psychotherapy at some point prior to enrollment. According to patient estimates, the average duration of depressive illness was 17.8 years. An initial low dose (10 mg) of psilocybin was administered to test tolerability. In a subsequent session, high-dose (25 mg) psilocybin was provided, with therapists present and with curated music playing. All subjects received psychological support before, during, and after the drug treatment.

The study suggested that psilocybin could be safely administered to depressed patients, with no reported serious adverse outcomes. However, mild adverse effects were common and included transient initial anxiety; transient confusion or thought disorder; mild, transient nausea; transient headache; and mild, transient paranoia. Although it was not designed to investigate efficacy, the study reported rapid and enduring reductions in symptoms, with large effect sizes. Every patient showed reductions in depression severity at 1 week after treatment, two-thirds met criteria for treatment response, and more than half met criteria for remission. Three months after treatment, 58% showed enduring treatment response, and 42% remained in clinical remission. Controlled research is required to assess whether these findings are reliable.

Data from RCTs on psychedelic interventions for psychological distress in patients with terminal illness are limited but support the case for further investigation. Griffiths and colleagues (2016) assessed the therapeutic value of high-dose psilocybin to treat existential distress in 51 patients with life-threatening cancer, using a randomized crossover design with low-dose psilocybin as an active placebo. All subjects received a number of drug-free preparatory and follow-up sessions, one high-dose drug session, and one low-dose drug session. More than two-thirds of participants had a diagnosis involving depressed mood, but it should be stressed that depressive symptoms in this cohort are likely not representative of treatment-resistant depression in otherwise healthy subjects, and we should be cautious to not extrapolate these data. What may be an effective treatment in patients who are terminally ill may well not confer the same benefits to other patient populations.

Clinician-rated measures of depression were used to assess clinical response and symptom remission. After the first dosing session, 92% of subjects receiving high-dose psilocybin showed clinical response to treatment compared to 32% of those receiving the low-dose active placebo, and symptom remission was observed in 60 and 16%, respectively. Six months after treatment, three-fourths of subjects showed enduring response to treatment, regardless of whether they had received psilocybin on the first or the second dosing session. Approximately two-thirds of patients were in symptom remission overall.

A similar RCT involving 29 patients with life-threatening cancer, using niacin as a placebo, reported "rapid and sustained" reductions of depressive symptoms following psilocybin-assisted psychotherapy (Ross et al., 2016). Seven weeks after the first dosing session, 83% of the psilocybin group showed treatment response, compared to 14% of those who had been administered niacin. At the 6-month follow-up, approximately 80% of the study group members were in clinical remission.

These data should, however, be interpreted with caution. For instance, there is a strong placebo response in depression, reported consistently between 30 and 40% (Brown, 1994), and placebo response is a predictor of treatment response. One study reported that placebo-mediated opioid release in brain regions related to emotion, stress regulation, and the pathophysiology of MDD predicted 43% of the variance in response to antidepressants (Peciña et al., 2015). Considering the close relationship between placebo response theory and the set and setting theory of psychedelic action (Hartogsohn, 2016), it may prove challenging to unpick the true efficacy of psychedelic drugs as antidepressants, particularly when this class of compounds has been shown to enhance suggestibility (Carhart-Harris et al., 2015). This is compounded by what has been dubbed the *decline effect*—the tendency of experimental effect sizes to decrease in significance over years of replication (Schooler, 2011). The *winner's curse* contributes to this uncertainty, reflecting a bias of scientific publications to report the most significant data. Furthermore, the *Hawthorne effect* refers to the tendency of study groups to respond differently to treatment relative to patient groups that are not involved as research participants (McCambridge, Witton, & Elbourne, 2014). Improvement of patients in clinical trials may be affected by the increased attention and observation they receive.

Suggested Mechanisms: Context and Connection

Understanding the mechanisms by which psychedelic therapy might work in depressive disorders is important in order to optimize and refine treatment models. Several observations are worth holding in mind. First, a tension exists between the hope of finding a unifying theory of psychedelic drug effects (Swanson, 2018) and the need to remain open to various insufficiently scrutinized phenomenological aspects of the therapy (Roseman, Nutt, & Carhart-Harris, 2018). Second, these mechanisms might not be specific to depression. The apparent therapeutic versatility of psychedelics suggests they might address a more fundamental problem (Alexander, 2010; Kessler, 2016) common to numerous neurotic mental health conditions (Carhart-Harris, Muthukumaraswamy, et al., 2016; Griffiths & Grob, 2010). A candidate construct in achieving this is a renewed sense of connectedness (Watts, Day, Krzanowski, Nutt, & Carhart-Harris, 2017). Finally, the context of a psychedelic experience is of importance to therapeutic outcomes (Carhart-Harris, Erritzoe, Haijen, Kaelen, & Watts, 2018). Disambiguating and testing facets of context are challenging tasks in controlled trials. Attention to variables such as ritual, expectation, and suggestion evoke principles of shamanic healing or a kind of "applied mysticism" (Grob, 1994), and these do not sit easily with clinical trial methodology. Psychedelic therapy seems to operate "on a frontier between spirituality and science that is as provocative as it is uncomfortable" (Pollan, 2018).

That *context* is so crucial may be understood in light of recent neurobiological hypotheses relating to the proplasticity effects of serotonin 2A agonism (Branchi, 2011;

Carhart-Harris & Nutt, 2017). Carhart-Harris and Nutt (2017) present findings to support the notion that a key function of 5-HT$_{2A}$ receptor signaling is to mediate plasticity and associated adaptation to the environment in early life and extreme adversity (i.e. when change is most functionally advantageous). Via serotonin 2a receptor agonism, the psychedelic experience is exquisitely sensitive to environmental context. Where the importance of this synergistic effect of context and pharmacological action was neglected historically, results of psychedelic therapy was found wanting (Oram, 2014). The emphasis on environmental context and quality of experience within contemporary psychedelic research reflects a much-needed paradigm shift in a medical culture historically resistant to the nonmaterial aspects of pharmacotherapy (Hartogsohn, 2016).

What follows focuses primarily on research derived from the Imperial College pilot study of psilocybin, with psychological support for treatment-resistant depression. These have supported the centrality of the "peak" experience to therapeutic outcomes (Roseman, Demetriou, et al., 2018; Roseman, Nutt, et al., 2018) and the synergistic effect of the music (Kaelen et al., 2018), and identified themes related to connectedness and acceptance as central to the process of change (Watts et al., 2017). Finally, we explore the construct of ego dissolution for its relationship to the mystical experience and the greater sense of connectedness. These proposed mechanisms are speculative given the relative infancy of the current research renaissance.

The Peak Experience

The earlier wave of psychedelic research held the so-called "mystical" experience as a sine qua non for therapeutic success (Grinspoon & Bakalar, 1979). It is a notoriously difficult area to study for various epistemological and practical reasons (Majić, Schmidt, & Gallinat, 2015), but it remains a significant preoccupation of the current research renaissance. In the Imperial College pilot study, Roseman and colleagues (Roseman, Demetriou, et al., 2018; Roseman, Nutt, et al., 2018) showed that the occurrence and scale of Oceanic Boundlessness, linked to Stace's

"mystical experience" (Studerus, Gamma, & Vollenweider, 2010), predicted long-term reductions in depressive symptoms This finding echoed those of other studies in which mystical experiences predicted long-term outcomes, including, of note, the New York University and Johns Hopkins trials of psilocybin for end-of-life depression and anxiety (Bogenschutz et al., 2015; Griffiths et al., 2016; Johnson, Garcia-Romeu, & Griffiths, 2017; MacLean, Johnson, & Griffiths, 2011; Ross et al., 2016).

This measure of mystical experience was significantly more predictive of improvement in depressive symptoms compared with perceptual changes, a point the authors invoke in endorsing the term *psychedelic* over *hallucinogen*. The finding justifies the emphasis placed on inducing peak-type experiences in psychedelic therapy and challenges the notion that such subjective experiences might be unwanted and extraneous side effects of serotonin 2A receptor agonism (Goodwin, 2016).

The Afterglow

Everything glistened and sparkled in a new light.
The world was as if newly created.
                                        —HOFMANN (2005)

Examining the acute psychedelic state prompts consideration of the subsequent time course of subjective experiences and its role in therapeutic change. The "afterglow" phenomenon, described by Pahnke (1969) as a state of "elevated and energetic mood with a relative freedom from concerns of the past and from guilt and anxiety," lasts for days to several weeks after a psychedelic experience. It is thought to represent a particularly fertile window for psychotherapeutic intervention and integration of material arising in the dosing session. This was supported in a study of healthy volunteers drinking ayahuasca: Postacute (24 hours postdosing) functional brain connectivity changes correlated with an increase in certain traits associated with mindfulness (Sampedro et al., 2017), itself a potential marker of cognitive flexibility (Moore & Malinowski, 2009)

Postacute functional magnetic resonance imaging (fMRI) scans of patients in the Imperial College pilot study revealed decreased amygdala cerebral blood flow correlated with reduced depressive symptoms (Carhart-Harris et al., 2017). Increased ventromedial prefrontal cortex–bilateral inferior lateral parietal cortex resting-state functional connectivity (RSFC) predicted treatment response at 5 weeks, as did a reduction in parahippocampal–prefrontal cortex RSFC. This in turn was predicted by the acute mystical or "peak" experience. More generally, these imaging results point toward the acute disintegration in default mode network functional connectivity of the psychedelic experience being remediated in the post-acute period, a process likened to a "reset" mechanism. Other studies point to more enduring psychological effects of the peak experience in terms of personal meaningfulness and spiritual significance 14 months later (Griffiths et al., 2008) and in bringing about changes in the personality domain of openness over a year later (MacLean et al., 2011). However, people volunteering to take part in such studies likely display significant trait openness at baseline in contrast to depressed populations. In the depressed population of the Imperial College pilot study, pronounced increases in extraversion and openness were found at 3-month follow-up (Erritzoe et al., 2018). It is unclear whether such longer-term changes in either population are underpinned by conspicuous anatomical (Carlos Bouso et al., 2015) or functional brain changes, or whether they result from an "epistemic transformation" that has ambiguous neural correlates.

Recent *in vitro* and *in vivo* studies of psychedelics reveal their ability to increase neuritogenesis (production of new projections from existing neuronal cell bodies), spinogenesis, and synaptogenesis, promoting plasticity via an evolutionarily conserved mechanism (Ly et al., 2018). Given the evidence for the atrophy of prefrontal cortex neurons in the pathophysiology of depression (Pittenger & Duman, 2008), the ability of psychedelics (and ketamine) to reverse such a process via structural and functional neural plasticity is of great interest.

Although it is not yet fully understood how single doses of psychedelics maintain their therapeutic value in some people for long periods after the drug has been cleared from the body, several further areas of investigation have provided clues. For instance, psychedelics may modulate changes in serotonin receptor binding. The literature indicates a selective reduction of serotonergic activity at 5-HT_{2A} receptors in depressed patients and the importance of 5-HT_{2A} receptor activity in the regulation of mood and facial recognition, supporting the hypothesis of antidepressant activity by 5-HT_{2A} receptor agonists such as psychedelic drugs (Nichols, 2016). However, it is important to remember that some 5-HT_{2A} receptor antagonists, such as mirtazapine, also show antidepressant action in some patients, perhaps reflecting the biological heterogeneity of depressive disorders. Psychedelics have also been associated with robust anti-inflammatory outcomes in a variety of models (Szabo, 2015), suggesting that they may help treat underlying inflammatory causes and contributions present in some subsets of depressed patients (Pariante, 2017). Furthermore, these drugs also modulate neuroendocrine pathway activity, potentially acting to regulate glucocorticoid-driven responses to stress and inflammation (Schindler, Wallace, Sloshower, & D'Souza, 2018). The extent to which these biological effects account for the clinical effects of psychedelic therapy remains to be seen.

Meaning-Amplifying Properties of Psychedelics

On mescaline, Huxley (1963) wrote that "objects were all but quivering under the pressure of significance by which they were charged." He was alluding to an important and possibly overlooked mediating mechanism in the action of psychedelics: their ability to enhance meaning (Hartogsohn, 2018). This property is supported by research (Carhart-Harris et al., 2015; Kaelen et al., 2015; Preller et al., 2017) and shines a fresh light on the breadth of psychedelics' applicability if one considers that the placebo response can be deconstructed as a "meaning response" (Moerman & Jonas, 2002). Although contested by some, it follows that the personal significance of mystical experiences and insights induced by the psychedelic experience will be amplified over and beyond what would be acquired by nonpsychedelic means. This disparity is further magnified when contrasting the meaning-enhancing aspect of psychedelics' mode of action with selective serotonin reuptake inhibitor (SSRI) antidepressants—medication that, for many, blunts their experience of emotions (Price, Cole, & Goodwin, 2009).

The meaning or suggestibility-enhancing property of psychedelics can pose awkward philosophical and ethical questions about the "veracity" of patients' experiences. Hartogsohn (2018) challenges such stances, putting forth the case that it is perhaps unethical *not* to exploit this property of psychedelics if they effectively alleviate patients' suffering. It is also important to consider the role that broader culture can play in the efficacy of psychedelics, giving rise to a cultural feedback loop: people's acute and longer-term responses to psychedelics feed back into the cultural context via media portrayals and public opinion that in turn affect the set or expectations of patients/ users, and so the cycle continues (Carhart-Harris et al., 2018).

The Role of Music

Music has come to be considered an integral aspect of the psychedelic therapy treatment model. Bonny and Pahnke (1972) discussed how music complements therapeutic objectives "1) by helping the patient relinquish usual controls and enter more fully into his inner world of experience; 2) by facilitating the release of intense emotionality; 3) by contributing toward a peak experience; 4) by providing continuity in an experience of timelessness; 5) by directing and structuring the experience." Music-evoked emotion (Kaelen et al., 2015), mental imagery (Kaelen et al., 2016), and the personal meaningfulness of music (Preller et al., 2017) are significantly modified by psychedelics, and recent qualitative studies of psychedelic therapy point to the important influence of music in patients' experiences (Belser et al., 2017; Watts et al., 2017). Kaelen and colleagues' (2018) study of participants' experience in the Imperial College pilot study was the first to quantify and qualify the influence of music on the acute experience and therapeutic outcomes. Crucially, it points to an optimal music experience as being an essential prerequisite for therapeutic success.

Three key variables related to the subjective experience of the music positively predicted the extent to which patients reported having mystical experiences: (1) liking—the degree to which the music was liked, (2) resonance—the degree to which it resonated with their emotional state, and (3) openness—the degree to which they could be open to the music-evoked experience. In addition, resonance and openness were predictors of the degree to which people reported insightfulness. All three variables were positively related to reductions in depressive symptom scores at 1 week, whereas intensity of drug effects was not, pointing toward a synergistic effect of music and the drug on therapeutic outcomes.

The ability of psychedelics to disrupt brain mechanisms regulating emotions (Carhart-Harris, Muthukumaraswamy, et al., 2016; Muthukumaraswamy et al., 2013; Tagliazucchi et al., 2016) might form a basis for the amplified emotional response to evocative musical stimuli seen in the study. In conjunction with psychedelics' capacity to facilitate a loosening of psychological control via ego dissolution and enhanced suggestibility (Carhart-Harris et al., 2015), music might act synergistically to (re-)activate personally meaningful memories, thoughts, and associated emotions. Confrontation with and exploration of salient emotions is important for therapeutic change across a range of psychotherapeutic models (Whelton, 2004) and is being borne out by qualitative research in psychedelic research trials (Belser et al., 2017; Watts et al., 2017). Psychedelic therapy arguably stands out for the speed and intensity with which this is brought about by the work of the drug and music.

"Connectedness"—and Acceptance

Watts and colleagues' (2017) 6-month follow-up phenomenological analysis of patients' experiences in the Imperial College pilot study is one of several recent qualitative studies of recent psychedelic therapy trials (Belser et al., 2017; Gasser, Kirchner, & Passie, 2015). Given their greater accessibility and proximity to lived experiences of patients, a focus on psychological mechanisms is a welcome counterpart to cognitive neuroscientific approaches. The two major themes the study revealed as explaining therapeutic change were a movement from a sense of disconnection to connection and from emotional avoidance to acceptance, conceived of as expansions, outward and inward, respectively. For many, a renewed sense of connectedness to self, others, and the world at large was felt acutely during the treatment itself but was also experienced for weeks to months later. Similar themes emerged from the New York University study: feelings of connection to loved ones or "relational embeddedness" and a shift "from feelings of separateness to interconnectedness" (Belser et al., 2017). The construct of connectedness is particularly appealing for its mechanistic resonance with neuroimaging research revealing the enhanced global connectivity and unconstrained cognition of the "entropic" brain in which rigid, inflexible, and excessively self-referential thinking of an overactive default mode network might be temporarily loosened (Carhart-Harris et al., 2014).

Feeling connected to others and the natural world are viewed as important mediators of psychological well-being (Cervinka, Röderer, & Hefler, 2012; Lee, Dean, & Jung, 2008) and instrumental to recovery in mental health (Leamy, Bird, Le Boutillier, Williams, & Slade, 2011), whereas a sense of disconnection is thought to contribute to numerous mental health disorders, especially depression (Karp, 1997). An increased connection to nature was found post psilocybin use (Forstmann & Sagioglou, 2017; Lyons & Carhart-Harris, 2018) and correlated with the amount of past psychedelic use and the intensity of "ego dissolution" (Nour, Evans, Nutt, & Carhart-Harris, 2016). It is hypothesised that these must follow on from a primary (re-)connection to self, as personally salient features of the acute experience must be integrated first (Carhart-Harris et al., 2018); if not, spiritual bypassing may be the result.

In keeping with motifs central to depth psychology and therapeutic models asserting the importance of assimilating problematic experiences (Stiles, 2001), the second change process was described as moving from a position of avoidance to a position of greater acceptance of painful emotions. Depression was characterized by rumination narrowing patients' emotional repertoires; avoidance or repression of painful emotions, and avoidance of traumatic memories. In their move toward acceptance, many patients experienced greater affective intensity during the session and a diminution of intensely painful emotions once they surrendered to them; in some cases, patients revisited childhood trauma and/or, in contrast, past experiences of love. Many patients' experiences of these emotions were more embodied, often through sobbing, experienced cathartically for the first time in many years. After the session, patients reported broader repertoires of emotions.

Patients contrasted these processes of change with traditional treatments- both psychological and pharmacological- that were experienced as reinforcing the sense of disconnection and emotional avoidance underlying their depression. In keeping with this phenomenological distinction with antidepressants, Roseman and colleagues' (2018) analysis of postacute fMRI data on these patients' responsiveness to emotional stimuli supports a model of psychedelics' therapeutic action that is very different than SSRIs (Carhart-Harris & Nutt, 2017). Their results revealed increased amygdala responsiveness to emotional stimuli; more specifically, right amygdala increases in response to fearful versus neutral faces predicted clinical improvements at 1 week. (Opposing trends in amygdala reactivity to emotional stimuli in the *acute* psychedelic phase with *healthy* patients deserve cautious interpretation given likely impaired task performance acutely, but point to the complex temporal nature of this neurobiological mechanism [Kraehenmann et al., 2015]). Roseman and colleagues' (finding is in contrast to SSRIs' purported action in altering negative emotional biases (Harmer, Duman, & Cowen, 2017) via a *dampening* of amygdala reactivity (Ma, 2015). Doubts exist as to whether chronically administered SSRIs might induce a dampening of amygdala reactivity to *all* emotionally salient stimuli, as suggested by the high rates of emotional blunting experienced in treated patients (Price et al., 2009) and the poor impact of these medications on anhedonia (McCabe, Mishor, Cowen, & Harmer, 2010). If SSRIs are to be conceived as more palliative in their approach to depression, psychedelic therapy offers an alternative paradigm for those patients who fail to respond to SSRIs.

Ego Dissolution

William James (1902/1985) saw the loss of a sense of self as integral to the mystical experience, itself a key facet of psychedelic therapy. Alterations to one's sense of self or ego are a defining feature of higher- dose psychedelic experience (Carhart-Harris et al., 2014) and similar to James, in LSD therapy, Grof (1980) asserts the importance for therapeutic outcomes of a strong effect: of "ego death and . . . loss of boundaries between the subject and the objective world, with ensuing feelings of unity." Various studies have started to elucidate the neurobiological mechanisms underpinning this ego disturbance or "dissolution." A study using LSD revealed decreased connectivity between the parahippocampus and retrosplenial cortex that correlated strongly with ratings of ego dissolution and "altered meaning," suggesting this circuit's importance for the maintenance of "self" or "ego" and its processing of meaning (Carhart-Harris, Muthukumaraswamy, et al., 2016). With psilocybin, positive correlations were found between the magnitude of the decreases in posterior cingulate cortex (PCC) α power and ratings of ego disintegration (Muthukumaraswamy et al., 2013). More generally, the increased global functional connectivity of the "psychedelic brain" is correlated with ego dissolution (Tagliazucchi et al., 2016), making it "a candidate neural correlate of the unitive experience— i.e. connectedness in its acute form" (Carhart-Harris et al., 2018).

Although ego dissolution as a construct needs further validation work among more heterogeneous populations (Millière, 2017; Nour et al., 2016), it is an important phenomenological aspect of the psychedelic experience with historical pedigree and a growing understanding of its neurobiological substrates. Important foci for future research might be how the ego- dissolving properties of the psychedelic state play out over time in relation to a sense of connectedness, and whether these correlate with particular anatomical and functional brain changes.

Conclusion

We do not yet know whether psychedelic drugs will have a prominent place in the psychiatric medicine cabinets of the future. The data so far show only that they can be used with relative safety by depressed patients under clinical supervision. Multiple Phase II and Phase III trials are still required to assess their efficacy as antidepressant treatments. There is a Phase II dose-ranging study underway of psilocybin for treatment-resistant depression (vs. placebo) across seven European sites. Also underway is a Phase II trial in moderately severe depression (vs. the SSRI escitalopram) that will look more specifically at differential mechanisms with regard amygdala activation.

The data presently available strongly support further research. Although many of the contemporary trials on psychedelics with psychological support for depressive disorders have not been designed to test efficacy, they have nonetheless tended to show significant and sustained therapeutic responses. From a theoretical perspective, there are good reasons to expect psychedelic therapies to have antidepressant potential. Psychedelic drugs modulate many systems known to be dysregulated in depressive disorders, from neuroendocrine axes (Schindler et al., 2018) to inflammation (Szabo, 2015). They may promote the growth and plasticity of brain cells (Ly et al., 2018), improve feelings of connectedness (Watts et al., 2017), and enhance meaning (Hartogsohn, 2018). Time will tell whether these substances can offer effective and affordable solutions to depression. For now, we may be cautiously optimistic.

References

Alexander, B. K. (2010). *The globalisation of addiction: A study in poverty of the spirit.* Oxford, UK: Oxford University Press.

Belser, A. B., Agin-Liebes, G., Swift, T. C., Terrana, S., Devenot, N., Friedman, H. L., et al. (2017). Patient experiences of psilocybin-assisted psychotherapy: An interpretative phenomenological analysis. *Journal of Humanistic Psychology, 57,* 354–388.

Bogenschutz, M. P., Forcehimes, A. A., Pommy, J. A., Wilcox, C. E., Barbosa, P., & Strassman,

R. J. (2015). Psilocybin-assisted treatment for alcohol dependence: A proof-of-concept study. *Journal of Psychopharmacology, 29*(3), 289–299.

Bonny, H. L., & Pahnke, W. N. (1972). The use of music in psychedelic (LSD) psychotherapy. *Journal of Music Therapy, 9*, 64–87.

Bourne, P. (2015, March 9). Letters. Retrieved from *www.newyorker.com/magazine/2015/03/09/letters-from-the-march-9-2015-issue.*

Branchi, I. (2011). The double edged sword of neural plasticity: Increasing serotonin levels leads to both greater vulnerability to depression and improved capacity to recover. *Psychoneuroendocrinology, 36*, 339–351.

Bromet, E., Andrade, L. H., Hwang, I., Sampson, N. A., Alonso, J., de Girolamo, G. et al. (2011). Cross-national epidemiology of DSM-IV major depressive episode. *BMC Medicine, 9*(1).

Brown, W. A. (1994). Placebo as a treatment for depression. *Neuropsychopharmacology, 10*, 265–269.

Busch, A. K., & Johnson, W. C. (1950). L.S.D. 25 as an aid in psychotherapy: Preliminary report of a new drug. *Diseases of the Nervous System, 11*(8), 241–243.

Carhart-Harris, R. L., Bolstridge, M., Rucker, J., Day, C. M. J., Erritzoe, D., Kaelen, M., et al. (2016). Psilocybin with psychological support for treatment-resistant depression: An open-label feasibility study. *Lancet Psychiatry, 3*(7), 619–627.

Carhart-Harris, R. L., Erritzoe, D., Haijen, E., Kaelen, M., & Watts, R. (2018). Psychedelics and connectedness. *Psychopharmacology, 235*, 547–550.

Carhart-Harris, R. L., Kaelen, M., Whalley, M. G., Bolstridge, M., Feilding, A., & Nutt, D. J. (2015). LSD enhances suggestibility in healthy volunteers. *Psychopharmacology (Berlin), 252*, 785–794.

Carhart-Harris, R. L., Leech, R., Hellyer, P. J., Shanahan, M., Feilding, A., Tagliazucchi, E., et al. (2014). The entropic brain: A theory of conscious states informed by neuroimaging research with psychedelic drugs. *Frontiers in Human Neuroscience, 8*, 20.

Carhart-Harris, R. L., Muthukumaraswamy, S., Roseman, L., Kaelen, M., Droog, W., Murphy, K., et al. (2016). Neural correlates of the LSD experience revealed by multimodal neuroimaging. *Proceedings of the National Academy of Sciences of the USA, 113*, 4853–4888.

Carhart-Harris, R. L., & Nutt, D. J. (2017). Serotonin and brain function: A tale of two receptors. *Journal of Psychopharmacology, 31*(9), 1091–1120.

Carhart-Harris, R. L., Roseman, L., Bolstridge, M., Demetriou, L., Pannekoek, J. N., Wall, M. B., et al. (2017). Psilocybin for treatment-resistant depression: fMRI-measured brain mechanisms. *Scientific Reports, 7*, Article 13187.

Caroseman, L., Haijen, E., Erritzoe, D., Watts, R., Branchi, I., et al. (2018). Psychedelics and the essential importance of context. *Journal of Psychopharmacology, 32*, 725–731.

Carlos Bouso, J., Palhano-Fontes, F., Rodriguez-Fornells, A., Ribeiro, S., Sanches, R., Crippa, J., et al. (2015). Long-term use of psychedelic drugs is associated with differences in brain structure and personality in humans. *European Neuropsychopharmacology, 25*, 483–492.

Cervinka, R., Röderer, K., & Hefler, E. (2012). Are nature lovers happy?: On various indicators of well-being and connectedness with nature. *Journal of Health Psychology, 17*, 379–388.

Condrau, G. (1949). Clinical experiences in mental illness with lysergic acid-diethylamide. *Acta Psychiatrica et Neurologica, 24*(1), 9–32.

Erritzoe, D., Roseman, L., Nour, M. M., MacLean, K., Kaelen, M., Nutt, D. J., et al. (2018). Effects of psilocybin therapy on personality structure. *Acta Psychiatrica Scandinavica, 138*, 368–378.

Fischer, F. M. (2015). *Therapy with substance?: Psycholytic psychotherapy in the twenty first century.* London: Muswell Hill Press.

Forstmann, M., & Sagioglou, C. (2017). Lifetime experience with (classic) psychedelics predicts pro-environmental behavior through an increase in nature relatedness. *Journal of Psychopharmacology, 31*(8), 975–988.

Gasser, P., Kirchner, K., & Passie, T. (2015). LSD-assisted psychotherapy for anxiety associated with a life-threatening disease: A qualitative study of acute and sustained subjective effects. *Journal of Psychopharmacology, 29*(1), 57–68.

Goodwin, G. M. (2016). Psilocybin: Psychotherapy or drug? *Journal of Psychopharmacology, 30*(12), 1201–1202.

Gozdzik-Zelazny, A., Borecki, L., & Pokorski, M. (2011). Depressive symptoms in schizophrenic patients. *European Journal of Medical Research, 16*(12), 549–552.

Griffiths, R. R., & Grob, C. S. (2010). Hallucinogens as medicine. *Scientific American, 303*, 76–79.

Griffiths, R. R., Johnson, M. W., Carducci, M. A., Umbricht, A., Richards, W. A., Richards, B. D., et al. (2016). Psilocybin produces substantial and sustained decreases in depression and anxiety in patients with life-threatening cancer: A randomized double-blind trial. *Jour-*

nal of Psychopharmacology, 30(12), 1181–1197.

Griffiths, R. R., Richards, W. A., Johnson, M. W., McCann, U. D., & Jesse, R. (2008). Mystical-type experiences occasioned by psilocybin mediate the attribution of personal meaning and spiritual significance 14 months later. Journal of Psychopharmacology, 22, 621–632.

Grinspoon, L., & Bakalar, J. B. (1979). Psychedelic drugs reconsidered. New York: Basic Books.

Grob, C. S. (1994). Psychiatric research with hallucinogens: What have we learned? Yearbook for Ethnomedicine and the Study of Consciousness, 3, 91–112.

Grof, S. (1980). LSD psychotherapy. Alameda, CA: Hunter House.

Grof, S., Goodman, L. E., Richards, W. A., & Kurland, A. A. (1973). LSD-assisted psychotherapy in patients with terminal cancer. International Pharmacopsychiatry, 8, 129–144.

Harmer, C. J., Duman, R. S., & Cowen, P. J. (2017). How do antidepressants work?: New perspectives for refining future treatment approaches. Lancet Psychiatry, 4, 409–418.

Hartogsohn, I. (2016). Set and setting, psychedelics and the placebo response: An extrapharmacological perspective on psychopharmacology. Journal of Psychopharmacology, 30, 1259–1267.

Hartogsohn, I. (2018). The meaning-enhancing properties of psychedelics and their mediator role in psychedelic therapy, spirituality, and creativity. Frontiers in Neuroscience, 12, 129.

Heo, M., Murphy, C. F., Fontaine, K. R., Bruce, M. L., & Alexopoulos, G. S. (2008). Population projection of US adults with lifetime experience of depressive disorder by age and sex from year 2005 to 2050. International Journal of Geriatric Psychiatry, 23(12), 1266–1270.

Hofmann, A. (2005). LSD: My problem child. Sarasota, FL: Multidisciplinary Association for Psychedelic Studies.

Holtzheimer, P. E., & Mayberg, H. S. (2011). Stuck in a rut: Rethinking depression and its treatment. Trends in Neurosciences, 34, 1–9.

Huxley, A. (1963). The doors of perception: Heaven and hell. New York: Harper & Row.

James, W. (1985). The varieties of religious experience: A study in human nature. London: Penguin Classics. (Original work published 1902)

Johnson, M. W., Garcia-Romeu, A., & Griffiths, R. R. (2017). Long-term follow-up of psilocybin-facilitated smoking cessation. American Journal of Drug and Alcohol Abuse, 45, 55–60.

Kaelen, M., Barrett, F. S., Roseman, L., Lorenz, R., Family, N., Bolstridge, M., et al. (2015). LSD enhances the emotional response to music. Psychopharmacology (Berlin), 232, 3607–3614.

Kaelen, M., Giribaldi, B., Raine, J., Evans, L., Timmerman, C., Rodriguez, N., et al. (2018). The hidden therapist: Evidence for a central role of music in psychedelic therapy. Psychopharmacology (Berlin), 235, 505–519.

Kaelen, M., Roseman, L., Kahan, J., Santos-Ribeiro, A., Orban, C., Lorenz, R., et al. (2016). LSD modulates music-induced imagery via changes in parahippocampal connectivity. European Neuropsychopharmacology, 26, 1099–1109.

Karp, D. A. (1997). Speaking of sadness: Depression, disconnection, and the meanings of illness. New York: Oxford University Press.

Kessler, D. A. (2016). Capture: Unravelling the mystery of mental suffering. New York: Harper Wave.

Kraehenmann, R., Preller, K. H., Scheidegger, M., Pokorny, T., Bosch, O. G., Seifritz, E., et al. (2015). Psilocybin-induced decrease in amygdala reactivity correlates with enhanced positive mood in healthy volunteers. Biological Psychiatry, 78(8), 572–581.

Leamy, M., Bird, V., Le Boutillier, C., Williams, J., & Slade, M. (2011). Conceptual framework for personal recovery in mental health: Systematic review and narrative synthesis. British Journal of Psychiatry, 199(6), 445–452.

Lee, R. M., Dean, B. L., & Jung, K. R. (2008). Social connectedness, extraversion, and subjective well-being: Testing a mediation model. Personality and Individual Differences, 45, 414–419.

Lim, G. Y., Tam, W. W., Lu, Y., Ho, C. S., Zhang, M. W., & Ho, R. C. (2018). Prevalence of depression in the community from 30 countries between 1994 and 2014. Science Reports, 8, 2861.

Ly, C., Greb, A. C., Cameron, L. P., Wong, J. M., Barragan, E. V., Wilson, P. C., et al. (2018). Psychedelics promote structural and functional neural plasticity. Cell Reports, 23, 3170–3182.

Lyons, T., & Carhart-Harris, R. L. (2018). Increased nature relatedness and decreased authoritarian political views after psilocybin for treatment-resistant depression. Journal of Psychopharmacology, 32, 811–819.

Ma, Y. (2015). Neuropsychological mechanism underlying antidepressant effect: A systematic meta-analysis. Molecular Psychiatry, 20, 311–319.

MacLean, K. A., Johnson, M. W., & Griffiths, R. R. (2011). Mystical experiences occasioned by the hallucinogen psilocybin lead to increases in the personality domain of openness. *Journal of Psychopharmacology, 25*, 1453–1461.

Majić, T., Schmidt, T. T., & Gallinat, J. (2015). Peak experiences and the afterglow phenomenon: When and how do therapeutic effects of hallucinogens depend on psychedelic experiences? *Journal of Psychopharmacology, 29*, 241–253.

McCabe, C., Mishor, Z., Cowen, P. J., & Harmer, C. J. (2010). Diminished neural processing of aversive and rewarding stimuli during selective serotonin reuptake inhibitor treatment. *Biological Psychiatry, 67*, 439–445.

McCambridge, J., Witton, J., & Elbourne, D. R. (2014). Systematic review of the Hawthorne effect: New concepts are needed to study research participation effects. *Journal of Clinical Epidemiology, 67*, 267–277.

Metzner, R. (2013). *The toad and the jaguar: A field report of underground research on a visionary medicine:* Bufo alvarius *and 5-methoxy-dimethyltryptamine.* Berkeley, CA: Regent Press.

Millière, R. (2017). Looking for the self: Phenomenology, neurophysiology and philosophical significance of drug-induced ego dissolution. *Frontiers in Human Neuroscience, 11*, 245.

Moerman, D. E., & Jonas, W. B. (2002). Deconstructing the placebo effect and finding the meaning response. *Annals of Internal Medicine, 136*(6), 471–476.

Moore, A., & Malinowski, P. (2009). Meditation, mindfulness and cognitive flexibility. *Consciousness and Cognition, 18*(1), 176–186.

Murray, C. J. L., Vos, T., Lozano, R., Naghavi, M., Flaxman, A. D., Michaud, C., et al. (2012). Disability-adjusted life years (DALYs) for 291 diseases and injuries in 21 regions, 1990–2010: A systematic analysis for the Global Burden of Disease Study 2010. *The Lancet, 380*, 2197–2223.

Muthukumaraswamy, S. D., Carhart-Harris, R. L., Moran, R. J., Brookes, M. J., Williams, T. M., Errtizoe, D., et al. (2013). Broadband cortical desynchronization underlies the human psychedelic state. *Journal of Neuroscience, 33*(38), 15171–15183.

Nichols D. E. (2016). Psychedelics. *Pharmacology Review, 68*, 264–355.

Nour, M. M., Evans, L., Nutt, D., & Carhart-Harris, R. L. (2016). Ego-dissolution and psychedelics: Validation of the Ego-Dissolution Inventory (EDI). *Frontiers in Human Neuroscience, 10*, 269.

Nutt, D. J., Wilson, S., & Paterson, L. (2008). Sleep disorders as core symptoms of depression. *Dialogues in Clinical Neuroscience, 10*(3), 329–336.

Oram, M. (2014). Efficacy and enlightenment: LSD psychotherapy and the drug amendments of 1962. *Journal of the History of Medicine and Allied Sciences, 69*(2), 221–250.

Oram, M. (2016). Prohibited or regulated?: LSD psychotherapy and the United States Food and Drug Administration. *History of Psychiatry, 27*(3), 290–306.

Osório, F. de L., Sanches, R. F., Macedo, L. R., Dos Santos, R. G., Maia-de-Oliveira, J. P., Wichert-Ana, L., et al. (2015). Antidepressant effects of a single dose of ayahuasca in patients with recurrent depression: A preliminary report. *Revista Brasileira de Psiquiatria, 37*(1), 13–20.

Pahnke, W. N. (1969). Psychedelic drugs and mystical experience. *International Journal of Psychiatry in Clinical Practice, 5*(4), 149–162

Pariante, C. M. (2017). Why are depressed patients inflamed?: A reflection on 20 years of research on depression, glucocorticoid resistance and inflammation. *European Neuropsychopharmacology, 27*(6), 554–559.

Peciña, M., Bohnert, A. S. B., Sikora, M., Avery, E. T., Langenecker, S. A., Mickey, B. J., et al. (2015). Association between placebo-activated neural systems and antidepressant responses. *JAMA Psychiatry, 72*(11), 1087–1094.

Pittenger, C., & Duman, R. S. (2008). Stress, depression, and neuroplasticity: A convergence of mechanisms. *Neuropsychopharmacology, 33*, 88–109.

Pollan, M. (2018). *How to change your mind: What the new science of psychedelics teaches us about dying, addiction, depression, and transcendence.* London: Allen Lane.

Preller, K. H., Herdener, M., Pokorny, T., Planzer, A., Kraehenmann, R., Stämpfli, P., et al. (2017). The fabric of meaning and subjective effects in LSD-induced states depend on serotonin 2A receptor activation. *Current Biology, 27*, 451–457.

Price, J., Cole, V., & Goodwin, G. M. (2009). Emotional side-effects of selective serotonin reuptake inhibitors: Qualitative study. *British Journal of Psychiatry, 195*, 211–217.

Reiche, S., Hermle, L., Gutwinski, S., Jungaberle, H., Gasser, P., & Majić, T. (2018). Serotonergic hallucinogens in the treatment of anxiety and depression in patients suffering from a life-threatening disease: A systematic review. *Progress in Neuro-Psychopharmacology and Biological Psychiatry, 81*, 1–10.

Richards, W. A., Rhead, J. C., Grof, S., Goodman, L. E., Di Leo, F., & Rush, L. (1980). DPT as an adjunct in brief psychotherapy with cancer patients. *OMEGA—Journal of Death and Dying, 10*(1), 9–26.

Roseman, L., Demetriou, L., Wall, M. B., Nutt, D. J., & Carhart-Harris, R. L. (2018). Increased amygdala responses to emotional faces after psilocybin for treatment-resistant depression. *Neuropharmacology, 81*, 1–10.

Roseman, L., Nutt, D. J., & Carhart-Harris, R. L. (2018). Quality of acute psychedelic experience predicts therapeutic efficacy of psilocybin for treatment-resistant depression. *Frontiers in Pharmacology, 8*, 974.

Ross, S., Bossis, A., Guss, J., Agin-Liebes, G., Malone, T., Cohen, B., et al. (2016). Rapid and sustained symptom reduction following psilocybin treatment for anxiety and depression in patients with life-threatening cancer: A randomized controlled trial. *Journal of Psychopharmacology, 30*(12), 1165–1180.

Rucker, J. J. H., Iliff, J., & Nutt, D. J. (2018). Psychiatry and the psychedelic drugs: Past, present and future. *Neuropharmacology, 142*, 200–218.

Rucker, J. J. H., Jelen, L. A., Flynn, S., Frowde, K. D., & Young, A. H. (2016). Psychedelics in the treatment of unipolar mood disorders: A systematic review. *Journal of Psychopharmacology, 30*, 1220–1229.

Sampedro, F., Revenga, M. D. L. F., Valle, M., Roberto, N., Domínguez-Clavé, E., Elices, M., et al. (2017). Assessing the psychedelic "after-glow" in ayahuasca users: Post-acute neurometabolic and functional connectivity changes are associated with enhanced mindfulness capacities. *International Journal of Neuropsychopharmacology, 20*, 698–711.

Savage, C. (1952). Lysergic acid diethylamide (LSD-25): A clinical–psychological study. *American Journal of Psychiatry, 108*, 896–900.

Savage, C., Fadiman, J., Mogar, R., & Allen, M. H. (1966). The effects of psychedelic (LSD) therapy on values, personality, and behavior. *International Journal of Neuropsychiatry, 2*, 241–254.

Savage, C., Hughes, M. A., & Mogar, R. (1967). Effectiveness of psychedelic (LSD) therapy: A preliminary report. *British Journal of Social Psychology, 2*, 59–66.

Schindler, E. A. D., Wallace, R. M., Sloshower, J. A., & D'Souza, D. C. (2018). Neuroendocrine associations underlying the persistent therapeutic effects of classic serotonergic psychedelics. *Frontiers in Pharmacology, 9*, 177.

Schooler, J. (2011). Unpublished results hide the decline effect. *Nature, 470*, 437.

Schulz, P. E., & Arora, G. (2015). Depression. *Continuum (Minneapolis, Minn.), 21*, 756–771.

Stiles, W. B. (2001). Assimilation of problematic experiences. *Psychotherapy: Theory, Research, Practice, Training, 38*, 462–465.

Stolaroff, M. J. (2004). *The secret chief revealed.* Sarasota, FL: Multidisciplinary Association for Psychedelic Studies.

Stotland, N. L. (1998). *Speaking of sadness: Depression, disconnection, and the meanings of illness* [Book review]. *Women's Health Issues, 8.*

Studerus, E., Gamma, A., & Vollenweider, F. X. (2010). Psychometric evaluation of the altered states of consciousness rating scale (OAV). *PLOS ONE, 5*(8), e12412.

Swanson, L. R. (2018). Unifying theories of psychedelic drug effects. *Frontiers in Pharmacology, 9*, 172.

Szabo, A. (2015). Psychedelics and immunomodulation: Novel approaches and therapeutic opportunities. *Frontiers in Immunology, 6*, 358.

Tagliazucchi, E., Roseman, L., Kaelen, M., Orban, C., Muthukumaraswamy, S. D., Murphy, K., et al. (2016). Increased global functional connectivity correlates with lsd-induced ego dissolution. *Current Biology, 26*, 1043–1050.

Watts, R., Day, C., Krzanowski, J., Nutt, D., & Carhart-Harris, R. (2017). Patients' accounts of increased "connectedness" and "acceptance" after psilocybin for treatment-resistant depression. *Journal of Humanistic Psychology, 57*(5), 520–564.

Whelton, W. J. (2004). Emotional processes in psychotherapy: Evidence across therapeutic modalities. *Clinical Psychology and Psychotherapy, 11*(1), 58–71.

World Health Organization. (2001). The World Health Report 2001: Mental health, new understanding, new hope. Retrieved from *www.who.int/whr/2001/en/whr01_en.pdf.*

World Health Organization. (2017). *Depression and other common mental disorders: Global health estimates.* Geneva: Author.

World Health Organization. (2018). *Global health estimates 2016: Disease burden by cause, age, sex, by country and by region, 2000–2016.* Geneva: Author.

CHAPTER 27

Hallucinogens in Headache

EMMANUELLE A. D. SCHINDLER

◼ Introduction to Migraine and Cluster Headache

Headache is one of the most common medical complaints, makes proper diagnosis and timely treatment of headache disorders a public health priority. The headache attack is the primary identifying feature of any specific headache disorder and almost (but not) always involves pain. Headache pain stems from meningeal, vascular, cervical, facial, and dental structures, which are innervated by the trigeminal and high cervical nerves (Charles, 2018). Autonomic nuclei and ganglia are also activated during certain headache attacks to produce features such as ptosis, lacrimation, and rhinorrhea (Goadsby, 2012). Dilation of carotid artery branches is also a result of autonomic activation and the release of inflammatory peptides (Goadsby & Edvinsson, 1994; Sarchielli et al., 2006); it is not the cause of headache pain, as previously believed. Other neurological features of headache attacks, such as aura, involve cortical signaling and may occur independent of pain (Close, Eftekhari, Wang, Charles, & Russo, 2018).

One of the more common primary headache disorders is migraine headache, the prevalence of which approximates 15% (Burch, Rizzoli, & Loder, 2018; Lipton, Stewart, Diamond, Diamond, & Reed, 2001). Migraine is also the number one cause of disability worldwide in persons under age 50 (GBD Disease and Injury Incidence, 2017). Migraine has strong familial ties and clinical associations with cerebrovascular and gastrointestinal disease, as well as epilepsy and mental health (Barbas & Schuyler, 2006; Cecchi et al., 2018; McLean & Mercer, 2017). One of the most painful headache disorders is cluster headache, which has a prevalence between 0.1 and 0.5% (Russell, 2004). Cluster attacks involve periorbital pain so severe that the disorder has been nicknamed "suicide headache" (Horton, 1952). Cluster headache has remarkable associations with circadian biology, occurring (or worsening) at certain times of year and individual attacks occurring at specific times of day (Rozen & Fishman, 2012). Table 27.1 summarizes characteristics of migraine and cluster headaches, which, though distinct, have several areas of overlap. The prevalence of concomitant migraine in patients with cluster headache has a widely reported range (Andersson, 1985; D'Amico et al., 1997; Taga, Russo, Manzoni, & Torelli,

TABLE 27.1. Distinctions and Overlap between Migraine and Cluster Headaches

Feature	Migraine headache and attacks	Cluster headache and attacks
Prevalence	12–15% (Burch et al., 2018; Lipton et al., 2001)	Estimates range from 0.1 to 0.5% (Russell, 2004)
Age of onset	Childhood and young adulthood (D'Amico et al., 1997)	May begin in childhood (uncommon), though more commonly begins in young adulthood (May et al., 2018)
Gender ratio	More women than men (3:1) (Barbas & Schuyler, 2006)	More men than women (4:1) (Goadsby, 2012)
Heritability	• Up to four times risk with affected first-degree relative (migraine with aura[a]) (Barbas & Schuyler, 2006) • Rare migraine variants, such as autosomal-dominant familial hemiplegic migraine, have known genetic mutations (i.e., *CACNA1A, ATP1A2*) (Barbas & Schuyler, 2006)	Familial association exists though genetic studies are variable (Barbas & Schuyler, 2006; May et al., 2018)
Central pathology	• Trigeminal nerve and brainstem (Maniyar, Sprenger, Monteith, Schankin, & Goadsby, 2014; May et al., 2018; Weiller et al., 1995) • Hypothalamus (Schulte, Allers, & May, 2017), thalamus (Lendvai & Kinfe, 2017), and pituitary (Shabas, Sheikh, & Gilad, 2017) • Cortex (Brennan & Pietrobon, 2018; Close et al., 2018) (particularly relevant to migraine with aura[a])	• Posterior hypothalamus (Bartsch, Paemeleire, & Goadsby, 2009; Cohen & Goadsby, 2006; May & Goadsby, 2001) • Pituitary lesions may present with cluster phenotype (Favier et al., 2007)
Duration and Frequency	• Between 4 and 72 hours (Headache Classification Committee, 2013) • Typically no more than one daily attack	• Between 15 minutes and 3 hours (Headache Classification Committee, 2013) • Up to eight daily attacks
Pain	• Moderate to severe in intensity • Dull, throbbing, pulsing • Often unilateral, but can encompass large portions of the head	• Severe in intensity • Ripping, boring, drilling • Primarily focused around one eye
Associated symptoms	• Photophobia, phonophobia, nausea, and/or vomiting are diagnostic of attacks (Headache Classification Committee, 2013) • Autonomic features may be seen, particularly in older patients (Kelman, 2006) and those with seasonal variation (Shin, Park, Shim, Oh, & Kim, 2015)	• Ipsilateral autonomic features are characteristic of attacks: ptosis, lacrimation, conjunctival injection, nasal congestion, rhinorrhea (Headache Classification Committee, 2013) • Nausea, vomiting, and photophobia present in up to half of patients (Taga et al., 2017; Vikelis & Rapoport, 2016)
Effect of movement	• Aggravation of attacks with movement • Patients prefer to lie down and remain still	• Restlessness is classic during attacks (Headache Classification Committee, 2013) • Patients may pace, rock, or rub/hit their head to soothe pain during attacks (Goadsby, 2012) • Self-injury, including attempted suicide, may occur (Rothrock, 2006)

(continued)

TABLE 27.1. *(continued)*

Feature	Migraine headache and attacks	Cluster headache and attacks
Circadian relationship	May show seasonal and/or diurnal variation (Shin et al., 2015)	• Attacks usually occur at predictable times of day (Rozen & Fishman, 2012) • Cycles[b] often occur during the same time each year (Rozen & Fishman, 2012)
Triggers	Stress, lack of sleep, menstruation, alcohol, chocolate, etc. (numerous triggers reported) (Pellegrino, Davis-Martin, Houle, Turner, & Smitherman, 2018)	Alcohol, strong smells, bright or flashing lights, weather changes, jetlag, high altitude (May et al., 2018; Rozen & Fishman, 2012)
Acute treatment	Nonsteroidial anti-inflammatory, acetaminophen, triptan (oral, intranasal, injectable) (Marmura, Silberstein, & Schwedt, 2015)	High-flow oxygen, triptan (intranasal, injectable), sphenopalatine ganglion stimulation (Robbins, Starling, Pringsheim, Becker, & Schwedt, 2016)
Preventive treatment	Topiramate, valproic acid, beta-blockers, tricyclic antidepressants, onabotulinum toxin (Loder, Burch, & Rizzoli, 2012)	Verapamil, lithium, suboccipital steroid injection (Robbins et al., 2016)

[a]*Aura* is a stereotyped neurological symptom that occurs before or during the pain component of migraine. The most common auras are visual scotoma, sensory disturbance, and aphasia.
[b]*Cycles* or *periods* in cluster headache are intervals of times lasting weeks to months, during which attacks occur. This is applicable to the episodic form of cluster headache.

2017), though the coexistence of these two disorders may not be uncommon when considering migraine that is remission.

▣ Conventional Headache Treatment

Patients with infrequent headache attacks may only require an abortive medication to manage their disease, but those whose attacks occur more often should take preventive measures (Diener, Charles, Goadsby, & Holle, 2015). The attack frequency at which a preventive medication is started varies among headache disorders and individual patients. For migraine headache, the threshold for starting a preventive is approximately once weekly. Patients with cluster headache usually take a preventive medication during their cycle or if they have chronic (year-round) cluster headache (Goadsby, 2012). The response to any single existing preventive headache medication is only about 50% (Diener et al., 2015; Klapper, Klapper, & Voss, 2000; Schindler et al., 2015; Schurks et al., 2006). Side effects and exclusion due to cardiovascular, cerebrovascular, or other significant medical history may further limit the ability to try a medication or reach clini-

cally effective doses (Gonzalez-Hernandez, Marichal-Cancino, MaassenVanDenBrink, & Villalon, 2018; May et al., 2018). Approximately 5% of patients seen in headache clinics have refractory migraine headache despite adequate trials of conventional medications (Irimia, Palma, Fernandez-Torron, & Martinez-Vila, 2011). In cluster headache, approximately 10–20% of patients are refractory to medical therapy (May, 2005). Patients with cluster headache are further limited in their use of abortive therapy, as the frequency of cluster attacks often exceeds the recommended daily use (e.g., maximum two daily injections of sumatriptan). Oxygen inhalation at high rates (12–15 L/minute) is an effective abortive therapy for cluster headache that may be used multiple times daily, though acquiring this treatment may be hindered by lack of physician training or insurance coverage (O'Brien et al., 2017).

The new line of monoclonal antibodies targeting calcitonin gene-related peptide (CGRP) signaling is promising for those headache patients for whom other treatment options have failed (Schuster & Rapoport, 2017). Postmarketing analysis will determine the long-term safety of this novel therapy, as, in addition to its role in headache, CGRP has protective roles in the cardiovascular and gastrointestinal systems (Gonzalez-Hernandez et al., 2018; Kamada et al., 2006). When pharmacotherapeutic options fail, external devices (e.g., vagal nerve stimulator), implanted extracranial devices (e.g., sphenopalatine stimulator), and implanted intracranial devices (e.g., deep brain stimulation [DBS]) may be tried for headache treatment (Bartsch, Paemelire, & Goadsby, 2009). For instance, posterior hypothalamic DBS has a preventive efficacy of up to two-thirds in refractory cluster headache, though the procedure is highly invasive and has been reported to result in death (Starr et al., 2007). Patients with migraine and cluster headache who remain significantly debilitated by their disease have sought novel means to control their pain, including nonapproved medications, alternative therapies, and illicit substances (Andersson, Persson, & Kjellgren, 2017; Schindler et al., 2015). This practice has led to anecdotal evidence for the therapeutic utility of hallucinogens in headache, not only speaking to the existence of a unique therapeutic drug class but also highlighting the unmet needs of a significant number of headache sufferers.

▪ Effects of Hallucinogens in Headache

Much of the literature regarding use of hallucinogens in headache is in regard to cluster headache. Cases and survey analyses report on the unique ability of the classic indoleamine hallucinogens to terminate cluster periods, induce remission, and prolong the duration of remission (Schindler et al., 2015; Sewell, Halpern, & Pope, 2006; Matharu, van Vliet, Ferrari, & Goadsby, 2005; Sempere, Berenguer-Ruiz, & Almazan, 2006). Moreover, in contrast to standard therapies, hallucinogens produce these lasting effects after a single dose or a few doses (Schindler et al., 2015; Sewell et al., 2006; Matharu et al., 2005; Sempere et al., 2006). Psilocybin (most commonly in the form of *Psilocybe* mushroom) was reported to be completely effective as a preventive in cluster headache in approximately half of those who tried it; psilocybin was at least moderately effective in approximately 70% (Schindler et al., 2015;

Sewell et al., 2006). Another tryptamine hallucinogen, *N*,*N*-dimethyltryptamine (DMT), was reported to have at least moderate efficacy in preventing attacks in approximately half of those who tried it (Schindler et al., 2015). The synthetic ergot hallucinogen, lysergic acid diethylamide (LSD), and a similar naturally occurring hallucinogenic compound found in certain flowering plant seeds, lysergic acid amide (LSA), were also reported to have preventive efficacies approximating 80 and 60%, respectively in cluster headache (Schindler et al., 2015; Sewell et al., 2006). LSD and psilocybin were also identified by patients as agents that extend the remission period in cluster headache (Schindler et al., 2015; Sewell et al., 2006).

Given the relative short duration of attacks (typically under 1 hour), oral ingestion of a drug is not ideal for acute treatment of cluster headache. Nevertheless, psilocybin was reported to offer at least partial abortive efficacy in approximately 90% of those who tried it (Schindler et al., 2015; Sewell et al., 2006); complete efficacy was reported in about 35% (Schindler et al., 2015). LSD was an effective abortive in one of two patients who reported taking it for such purposes (Sewell et al., 2006). Unless patients have particularly long attacks (e.g., 2–3 hours), an oral hallucinogen (or congener) would not be expected to provide significant relief. Furthermore, the need for abortive therapy several times daily, as is often required in cluster headache, would not make such compounds ideal abortive agents. It is noted through these patient experiences, however, that hallucinogens do have acute effects.

When patients with cluster headache have used hallucinogens to manage their condition, a range of doses is used. Subthreshold doses, such as 0.1 g dried *P. cubensis* up to full psychedelic doses, such as 300 µg LSD, are reported to have therapeutic effects (Schindler et al., 2015). A congener of LSD that lacks significant psychedelic effects, 2-bromo-lysergic acid diethylamide (BOL-148 or BOL), was reported in a survey (Schindler et al., 2015) and shown in an open-label case series (Karst, Halpern, Bernateck, & Passie, 2010) to have lasting therapeutic effects in cluster headache. Another nonhallucinogenic ergot derivative similar to LSD, lisuride, has been reported in cases to have lasting effects in cluster headache after limited exposure (Raffaelli, Martins, & Dos Santos, 1983). A synthetic tryptamine compound with reduced psychotropic effects, 5-methoxy-N,N-diallyl-tryptamine (5-MeO-DALT), has also been used by cluster headache patients, with single doses terminating attacks for up to 2 weeks (Post, 2014).

A popular regimen for terminating an active cluster period or inducing remission from chronic cluster headache is three doses, each separated by 5 days (Schindler et al., 2015; Sewell et al., 2006). Occasionally, patients have reported full remission from cluster headache after such a treatment, though some may require intermittent dosing separated by weeks to months as prophylaxis (Matharu et al., 2005; Schindler et al., 2015). Additional formal investigation of these sustained effects after limited dosing is required to understand this very unique ability of the drug class.

Though not as extensive as the evidence in cluster headache, there are also reports of headache-suppressing effects in migraine headache with LSD (Sewell & Gottschalk, 2011) and BOL (Richards, Chapman, Goodell, & Wolff, 1958; Sicuteri, 1963). A reexamination of these findings is warranted given the prevalence of migraine and the burden it produces on a worldwide scale. The overlap that exists between migraine and cluster headache (see Table 27.1) certainly makes a therapeutic effect conceivable. The existing anecdotal evidence in headache disorders is strongly supportive of a therapeutic effect, though further formal investigation is needed to fully characterize and understand the outcomes of hallucinogens in headache. Currently, there are preliminary clinical trials investigating the effects of psilocybin (NCT02981173, NCT04280055) and LSD (NCT03781128) in cluster headache and psilocybin in migraine (NCT03341689). These studies will serve as validation for the anecdotally reported effects and inform the goals and design of future research.

Safety of Hallucinogens in Headache

Hallucinogens and their congeners are generally well tolerated when used for headache management, though a range of adverse effects has been reported. Survey analysis identified "sickness," "wooziness," and abdominal discomfort in patients with cluster headache who take hallucinogens for treatment (Schindler et al., 2015). Psilocybin is also reported to produce headache or worsen existing headache (Johnson, Sewell, & Griffiths, 2012), though this transient effect does not preclude an eventual therapeutic result (Sewell et al., 2006). Patients administrated BOL for cluster headache treatment reported a "flabby" or "light drunk" feeling (Karst et al., 2010). In an isolated case, BOL produced LSD-like psychotropic effects in a "moderately anxious" man, though, interestingly, when given chlorpromazine to reverse this, he had a resumption of peak "visual illusions, 'cloudy' mentation and color misinterpretation" (Richards et al., 1958). These responses suggest paradoxical reactions to BOL and the antipsychotic in a susceptible individual. Lisuride may cause nausea hypotension, myalgia, and cold extremities (Raffaelli et al., 1983). 5-MeO-DALT was reported to induce drowsiness, lightheadedness, and "very mild closed-eye visuals" (Post, 2014).

In contrast to other preventive headache medications, which are taken daily or multiple times daily, transient psychotropic effects or discomfort from intermittent hallucinogen (or congener) use may be considered relatively benign. Despite a generally safe profile, the use of hallucinogens in headache or any other condition must be considered carefully. In the ongoing cluster and migraine headache studies, a strict set of criteria for study participation is followed, and comprehensive physical and psychiatric evaluations are performed prior to patient acceptance. For instance, psychotic and manic disorders are exclusionary to the studies, as are cardiac conduction defects, hormonal imbalances, and other conditions that may place subjects at risk. The range of potential adverse effects from nausea and anxiety to psychosis and hallucinogen persisting perception disorder (Martinotti et al., 2018) is reviewed with candidates prior to study participation. Subjects are monitored during experimental sessions and receive repeated follow-up contacts to ensure safety and tolerability of the intervention. Given the range of possible effects and the relevance of set and setting, such safety measures must continue as hallucinogens are investigated, whether it be in headache disorders or other conditions (Johnson, Richards, & Griffiths, 2008).

Source of Headache-Suppressing Effects

The source of hallucinogens' lasting effects in headache is unknown. The drugs are quickly metabolized and do not remain present through the period of efficacy, making the effects of this drug class unique. This contrasts the lasting effects attained after single exposure to, say, the novel anti-CGRP drugs, which remain present in the body between monthly or quarterly injections. The serotonergic system is central to headache disorders (Bahra, Matharu, Buchel, Frackowiak, & Goadsby, 2001; Sommer, 2006) and thus, the serotonergic actions of hallucinogens might be implicated in their therapeutic effects. What distinguishes these compounds from existing serotonergic headache medicines (e.g., sumatriptan, dihydroergotamine, methysergide, amitriptyline) has yet to be uncovered. That hallucinogens induce sensory and perceptual alterations is certainly distinctive, though reports of headache relief with subthreshold doses (Schindler et al., 2015; Sewell et al., 2006), as well as compounds such as BOL (Karst et al., 2010; Richards et al., 1958; Schindler et al., 2015; Sicuteri, 1963), lisuride (Raffaelli et al., 1983) and 5-MeO-DALT (Post, 2014), suggest that psychedelic effects are not required for the headache-suppressing effects.

An area that is relevant to both headache and hallucinogens is the neuroendocrine system. First, there is a clear role for hypothalamic involvement in headache disorders. Compared to healthy controls, posterior hypothalamic gray-matter volume of patients with cluster headache is increased (May et al., 1999). The inferior posterior hypothalamus is activated during cluster attacks (Cohen & Goadsby, 2006; May & Goadsby, 2001) and serves as a target of DBS therapy in refractory cases (Bartsch et al., 2009). In migraine headache, the posterior hypothalamus is implicated in acute headache pain,

while the anterior region subtends chronification (Schulte, Allers, & May, 2017). Psilocybin decreases hypothalamic activity in humans as measured by blood oxygen level-dependent (BOLD) functional MRI (Carhart-Harris et al., 2012). Relative changes in subcortical activation have also been identified with psilocybin exposure (Gouzoulis-Mayfrank et al., 1999; Kraehenmann et al., 2015; Vollenweider et al., 1997), which is further relevant to headache, as regions such as the thalamus, pituitary, and brainstem are key to headache pathology (Favier et al., 2007; Lendvai & Kinfe, 2017; Maniyar, Sprenger, Monteith, Schankin, & Goadsby, 2014; Shabas, Sheikh, & Gilad, 2017). Whether limited dosing of a psychedelic (or congener) may alter hypothalamic or other functions in the long term could be investigated with sequential imaging, coupled with a trigger challenge, such as alcohol or nitroglycerin (May, Bahra, Buchel, Frackowiak, & Goadsby, 1998).

One of the many functions of the hypothalamus is the setting of the biological clock. There are seasonal and circadian rhythms to many headache disorders, with cluster headache exemplifying this cyclical nature quite clearly (Rozen & Fishman, 2012). Fall and spring are times of the year during which cluster periods tend to begin or when symptoms worsen in those with chronic cluster headache (Rozen & Fishman, 2012). Individual cluster attacks also have the propensity to occur at predictable times of day (Rozen & Fishman, 2012), particularly overnight during rapid eye movement (REM) sleep (Dodick, Eross, Parish, & Silber, 2003; Kudrow, McGinty, Phillips, & Stevenson, 1984; Sahota & Dexter, 1990). Animal studies have shown that LSD postpones REM sleep onset and reduces REM duration in a dose-dependent manner (Brooks, 1975; Depoortere & Loew, 1971; Hobson, 1964; Kay & Martin, 1978). BOL had the same effects (Depoortere & Loew, 1972), though to a lesser degree than LSD (Depoortere & Loew, 1971) at the dose tested. There are mixed findings on the effects of LSD on REM sleep in humans (Muzio, Roffwarg, & Kaufman, 1966; Toyoda, 1964), though in at least one patient, LSD delayed the first REM period the night of drug administration and increased REM duration the night after drug administration (Green, 1965). That LSD and BOL may affect REM sleep (Brooks, 1975; Depoortere & Loew, 1971; Hobson, 1964; Kay & Martin, 1978) might suggest that one of their therapeutic benefits in cluster headache stems from manipulation of the sleep period during which attacks often occur. Extending polysomnogram measures after exposure to a hallucinogen (or congener) would further characterize potential lasting effects on sleep architecture.

One of the circadian hormones, melatonin, may also serve as a means to measure the effects of hallucinogens in headache disorders. In cluster headache, melatonin is reduced in peripheral blood (Chazot et al., 1984; Leone et al., 1995) and released on a phase-advanced schedule (Chazot et al., 1984). Nightly supplementation has been identified as a potential therapy for cluster headache (Leone, D'Amico, Moschiano, Fraschini, & Bussone, 1996), as well as migraine (Leite Pacheco et al., 2018) and posttraumatic (Kuczynski, Crawford, Bodell, Dewey, & Barlow, 2013) headache. In animals, urinary excretion of melatonin was delayed after a single exposure to a substituted amphetamine hallucinogen (±-1-(2,5-dimethoxy-4-iodophenyl)-2-aminopropane) [DOI]), an effect that persisted for 8 days (Kennaway, Moyer, Voultsios, & Varcoe, 2001). This effect may serve as a corrective measure in the timing of melatonin release in patients with cluster headache, though additional human studies are required to fully understand this relationship.

Headache disorders are complex and perhaps best understood as network disorders (Brennan & Pietrobon, 2018). Neuroplastic changes have also been recognized in headache, including migraine (Brennan & Pietrobon, 2018), cluster (Naegel et al., 2014), tension-type (Chen, He, Xia, Guo, & Zheng, 2016), and posttraumatic (Mustafa et al., 2016) headaches. This said, the recent revelation of neuroplasticity induced by hallucinogens (Ly et al., 2018) is highly relevant to their therapeutic effects in headache. The specific involvement of serotonin 2A, mTOR, and TrkB signaling in hallucinogens' neuroplastic effects (Ly et al., 2018) is directly applicable to headache as well, as each has associations with headache and/or pain (Guo, Deng, Bo, & Yang, 2017; Kwon

et al., 2017; Sommer, 2006). These recent findings have added to the range of processes that may be targeted in uncovering the mechanism(s) of action of hallucinogens and their congeners in headache. Indeed, given the heterogeneity that exists within individual headache disorders, an available array of treatment options is most desirable.

▪ Conclusion

Anecdotal evidence for the therapeutic benefits of hallucinogens, such as LSD and psilocybin, and their congeners, such as BOL and 5-MeO-DALT, in cluster and migraine headache has provided a wealth of information and additional support for the growing recognition of the therapeutic value of this group of compounds. Much investigation is required to understand more fully the effects and safety of hallucinogens in treating headache. Ongoing formal studies of the effects of psilocybin in headache disorders will provide the first controlled scientific data with regard to headache-suppressing effects and serve as the basis for additional investigations. The source for the long-lasting therapeutic effects of hallucinogens in headache remains unknown, though the activity of these compounds in the same neuroanatomical locations and functional processes that are aberrant in headache provides a number of foci for consideration and future study. Importantly, while the search to understand the various and unique effects of hallucinogens continues, the powerful nature of these compounds, which has brought them both fame and infamy, must be respected and factored into every aspect of their use.

▪ References

Andersson, M., Persson, M., & Kjellgren, A. (2017). Psychoactive substances as a last resort—a qualitative study of self-treatment of migraine and cluster headaches. *Harm Reduction Journal, 14*, 60.

Andersson, P. G. (1985). Migraine in patients with cluster headache. *Cephalalgia, 5*, 11–16.

Bahra, A., Matharu, M. S., Buchel, C., Frackowiak, R. S., & Goadsby, P. J. (2001). Brainstem activation specific to migraine headache. *Lancet, 357*, 1016–1017.

Barbas, N. R., & Schuyler, E. A. (2006). Heredity, genes, and headache. *Seminars in Neurology, 26,* 507–514.

Bartsch, T., Paemeleire, K., & Goadsby, P. J. (2009). Neurostimulation approaches to primary headache disorders. *Current Opinion in Neurology, 22,* 262–268.

Brennan, K. C., & Pietrobon, D. (2018). A systems neuroscience approach to migraine. *Neuron, 97,* 1004–1021.

Brooks, D. C. (1975). The effect of LSD upon spontaneous PGO wave activity and REM sleep in the cat. *Neuropharmacology, 14,* 847–857.

Burch, R., Rizzoli, P., & Loder, E. (2018). The prevalence and impact of migraine and severe headache in the United States: Figures and trends from government health studies. *Headache, 58,* 496–505.

Carhart-Harris, R. L., Erritzoe, D., Williams, T., Stone, J. M., Reed, L. J., Colasanti, A., et al. (2012). Neural correlates of the psychedelic state as determined by fMRI studies with psilocybin. *Proceedings of the National Academy of Sciences of the USA, 109,* 2138–2143.

Cecchi, G., Paolucci, M., Ulivi, M., Assenza, F., Brunelli, N., Rizzo, A. C., et al. (2018). Frequency and clinical implications of hypercoagulability states in a cohort of patients with migraine with aura. *Neurological Sciences, 39,* 99–100.

Charles, A. (2018). The pathophysiology of migraine: Implications for clinical management. *Lancet Neurology, 17,* 174–182.

Chazot, G., Claustrat, B., Brun, J., Jordan, D., Sassolas, G., & Schott, B. (1984). A chronobiological study of melatonin, cortisol growth hormone and prolactin secretion in cluster headache. *Cephalalgia, 4,* 213–220.

Chen, B., He, Y., Xia, L., Guo, L. L., & Zheng, J. L. (2016). Cortical plasticity between the pain and pain-free phases in patients with episodic tension-type headache. *Journal of Headache Pain, 17,* 105.

Close, L. N., Eftekhari, S., Wang, M., Charles, A. C., & Russo, A. F. (2018). Cortical spreading depression as a site of origin for migraine: Role of CGRP. *Cephalalgia, 39,* 428–434.

Cohen, A. S., & Goadsby, P. J. (2006). Functional neuroimaging of primary headache disorders. *Expert Review of Neurotherapeutics, 6,* 1159–1171.

D'Amico, D., Centonze, V., Grazzi, L., Leone, M., Ricchetti, G., & Bussone, G. (1997). Coexistence of migraine and cluster headache: Report of 10 cases and possible pathogenetic implications. *Headache, 37,* 21–25.

Depoortere, H., & Loew, D. M. (1971). Alterations in sleep–wakefulness cycle in rats following treatment with (+)-lysergic acid diethylamide (LSD-25). *British Journal of Pharmacology, 41,* 402P–403P.

Depoortere, H., & Loew, D. M. (1972). Proceedings: Alterations in the sleep–wakefulness cycle in rats after administration of (-)-LSD or BOL-148: A comparison with (+)-LSD. *British Journal of Pharmacology, 44,* 354P–355P.

Diener, H. C., Charles, A., Goadsby, P. J., & Holle, D. (2015). New therapeutic approaches for the prevention and treatment of migraine. *Lancet Neurology, 14,* 1010–1022.

Dodick, D. W., Eross, E. J., Parish, J. M., & Silber, M. (2003). Clinical, anatomical, and physiologic relationship between sleep and headache. *Headache, 43,* 282–292.

Favier, I., van Vliet, J. A., Roon, K. I., Witeveen, R. J. W., Verschuuren, J. J. C. H., Ferrari, M. D., et al. (2007). Trigeminal autonomic cephalgias due to structural lesions: A review of 31 cases. *Archives of Neurology, 64,* 25–31.

GBD Disease and Injury Incidence and Prevalence Collaborators. (2017). Global, regional, and national incidence, prevalence, and years lived with disability for 328 diseases and injuries for 195 countries, 1990–2016: A systematic analysis for the Global Burden of Disease Study 2016. *Lancet, 390,* 1211–1259.

Goadsby, P. J. (2012). Trigeminal autonomic cephalalgias. *Continuum, 18,* 883–895.

Goadsby, P. J., & Edvinsson, L. (1994). Human *in vivo* evidence for trigeminovascular activation in cluster headache: Neuropeptide changes and effects of acute attacks therapies. *Brain: A Journal of Neurology, 117*(Pt. 3), 427–434.

Gonzalez-Hernandez, A., Marichal-Cancino, B. A., MaassenVanDenBrink, A., & Villalon, C. M. (2018). Side effects associated with current and prospective antimigraine pharmacotherapies. *Expert Opinion on Drug Metabolism and Toxicology, 14,* 25–41.

Gouzoulis-Mayfrank, E., Schreckenberger, M., Sabri, O., Arning, C., Thelen, B., Spitzer, M., et al. (1999). Neurometabolic effects of psilocybin, 3,4-methylenedioxyethylamphetamine (MDE) and d-methamphetamine in healthy volunteers: A double-blind, placebo-controlled PET study with [^{18}F]FDG. *Neuropsychopharmacology, 20,* 565–581.

Green, W. J. (1965). The effect of LSD on the sleep-dream cycle: An exploratory study. *Journal of Nervous and Mental Disease, 140,* 417–426.

Guo, J. Q., Deng, H. H., Bo, X., & Yang, X. S. (2017). Involvement of BDNF/TrkB and ERK/CREB axes in nitroglycerin-induced rat migraine and effects of estrogen on these signals in the migraine. *Biology Open, 6,* 8–16.

Headache Classification Committee of the International Headache Society. (2013). The International Classification of Headache Disorders, 3rd edition (beta version). *Cephalalgia, 33,* 629–808.

Hobson, J. A. (1964). The effect of LSD on the sleep cycle of the cat. *Electroencephalography and Clinical Neurophysiology, 17,* 52–56.

Horton, B. T. (1952). Histaminic cephalgia. *Lancet, 72,* 92–98.

Irimia, P., Palma, J. A., Fernandez-Torron, R., & Martinez-Vila, E. (2011). Refractory migraine in a headache clinic population. *BMC Neurology, 11,* 94.

Johnson, M., Richards, W., & Griffiths, R. (2008). Human hallucinogen research: Guidelines for safety. *Journal of Psychopharmacology, 22,* 603–620.

Johnson, M. W., Sewell, R. A., & Griffiths, R. R. (2012). Psilocybin dose-dependently causes delayed, transient headaches in healthy volunteers. *Drug and Alcohol Dependence, 123,* 132–140.

Kamada, K., Gaskin, F. S., Yamaguchi, T., Carter, P., Yoshikawa, T., Yusof, M., et al. (2006). Role of calcitonin gene-related peptide in the postischemic anti-inflammatory effects of antecedent ethanol ingestion. *American Journal of Physiology: Heart and Circulatory Physiology, 290,* H531–H537.

Karst, M., Halpern, J. H., Bernateck, M., & Passie, T. (2010). The non-hallucinogen 2-bromo-lysergic acid diethylamide as preventative treatment for cluster headache: An open, non-randomized case series. *Cephalalgia, 30,* 1140–1144.

Kay, D. C., & Martin, W. R. (1978). LSD and tryptamine effects on sleep/wakefulness and electrocorticogram patterns in intact cats. *Psychopharmacology, 58,* 223–228.

Kelman, L. (2006). Migraine changes with age: IMPACT on migraine classification. *Headache, 46,* 1161–1171.

Kennaway, D. J., Moyer, R. W., Voultsios, A., & Varcoe, T. J. (2001). Serotonin, excitatory amino acids and the photic control of melatonin rhythms and SCN c-FOS in the rat. *Brain Research, 897,* 36–43.

Klapper, J. A., Klapper, A., & Voss, T. (2000). The misdiagnosis of cluster headache: A non-clinic, population-based, Internet survey. *Headache, 40,* 730–735.

Kraehenmann, R., Preller, K. H., Scheidegger, M., Pokorny, T., Bosch, O. G., Seifritz, E., et al. (2015). Psilocybin-induced decrease in amygdala reactivity correlates with enhanced positive mood in healthy volunteers. *Biological Psychiatry, 78,* 572–581.

Kuczynski, A., Crawford, S., Bodell, L., Dewey, D., & Barlow, K. M. (2013). Characteristics of post-traumatic headaches in children following mild traumatic brain injury and their response to treatment: A prospective cohort. *Developmental Medicine and Child Neurology, 55,* 636–641.

Kudrow, L., McGinty, D. J., Phillips, E. R., & Stevenson, M. (1984). Sleep apnea in cluster headache. *Cephalalgia, 4,* 33–38.

Kwon, M., Han, J., Kim, U. J., Cha, M., Um, S. W., Bai, S. J., et al. (2017). Inhibition of mammalian target of rapamycin (mTOR) signaling in the insular cortex alleviates neuropathic pain after peripheral nerve injury. *Frontiers in Molecular Neuroscience, 10,* 79.

Leite Pacheco, R., de Oliveira Cruz Latorraca, C., Adriano Leal Freitas da Costa, A., Luiza Cabrera Martimbianco, A., Vianna Pachito, D., & Riera, R. (2018). Melatonin for preventing primary headache: A systematic review. *International Journal of Clinical Practice, 72,* e13203.

Lendvai, I. S., & Kinfe, T. M. (2017). Migraine improvement after anterior thalamic deep brain stimulation for drug-resistant idiopathic generalized seizure: A case report. *Headache, 57,* 964–966.

Leone, M., D'Amico, D., Moschiano, F., Fraschini, F., & Bussone, G. (1996). Melatonin versus placebo in the prophylaxis of cluster headache: A double-blind pilot study with parallel groups. *Cephalalgia, 16,* 494–496.

Leone, M., Lucini, V., D'Amico, D., Moschiano, F., Maltempo, C., Fraschini, F., et al. (1995). Twenty-four-hour melatonin and cortisol plasma levels in relation to timing of cluster headache. *Cephalalgia, 15,* 224–229.

Lipton, R. B., Stewart, W. F., Diamond, S., Diamond, M. L., & Reed, M. (2001). Prevalence and burden of migraine in the United States: Data from the American Migraine Study II. *Headache, 41,* 646–657.

Loder, E., Burch, R., & Rizzoli, P. (2012). The 2012 AHS/AAN guidelines for prevention of episodic migraine: A summary and comparison with other recent clinical practice guidelines. *Headache, 52,* 930–945.

Ly, C., Greb, A. C., Cameron, L. P., Wong, J. M., Barragan, E. V., Wilson, P. C., et al. (2018). Psychedelics promote structural and functional neural plasticity. *Cell Reports, 23,* 3170–3182.

Maniyar, F. H., Sprenger, T., Monteith, T., Schankin, C., & Goadsby, P. J. (2014). Brain activations in the premonitory phase of nitroglycerin-triggered migraine attacks. *Brain: A Journal of Neurology, 137,* 232–241.

Marmura, M. J., Silberstein, S. D., & Schwedt, T. J. (2015). The acute treatment of migraine in adults: The American Headache Society evidence assessment of migraine pharmacotherapies. *Headache, 55,* 3–20.

Martinotti, G., Santacroce, R., Pettorruso, M., Montemitro, C., Spano, M. C., Lorusso, M., et al. (2018). Hallucinogen persisting perception disorder: Etiology, clinical features, and therapeutic perspectives. *Brain Science, 8,* 47.

Matharu, M. S., van Vliet, J. A., Ferrari, M. D., & Goadsby, P. J. (2005). Verapamil induced gingival enlargement in cluster headache. *Journal of Neurology, Neurosurgery and Psychiatry, 76,* 124–127.

May, A. (2005). Cluster headache: Pathogenesis, diagnosis, and management. *Lancet, 366,* 843–855.

May, A., Ashburner, J., Buchel, C., McGonigle, D. J., Friston, K. J., Frackowiak, R. S., et al. (1999). Correlation between structural and functional changes in brain in an idiopathic headache syndrome. *Nature Medicine, 5,* 836–838.

May, A., Bahra, A., Buchel, C., Frackowiak, R. S., & Goadsby, P. J. (1998). Hypothalamic activation in cluster headache attacks. *Lancet. 352,* 275–278.

May, A., & Goadsby, P. J. (2001). Hypothalamic involvement and activation in cluster headache. *Current Pain and Headache Reports, 5,* 60–66.

May, A., Schwedt, T. J., Magis, D., Pozo-Rosich, P., Evers, S., & Wang, S. J. (2018). Cluster headache. *Nature Reviews Disease Primers, 4,* Article 18006.

McLean, G., & Mercer, S. W. (2017). Chronic migraine, comorbidity, and socioeconomic deprivation: Cross-sectional analysis of a large nationally representative primary care database. *Journal of Comorbidity, 7,* 89–95.

Mustafa, G., Hou, J., Tsuda, S., Nelson, R., Sinharov, A., Wilkie, Z., et al. (2016). Trigeminal neuroplasticity underlies allodynia in a preclinical model of mild closed head traumatic brain injury (cTBI). *Neuropharmacology, 107,* 27–39.

Muzio, J. N., Roffwarg, H. P., & Kaufman, E. (1966). Alterations in the nocturnal sleep cycle resulting from LSD. *Electroencephalography and Clinical Neurophysiology, 21,* 313–324.

Naegel, S., Holle, D., Desmarattes, N., Theysohn, N., Diener, H.-C., Katsarava, Z., et al. (2014). Cortical plasticity in episodic and chronic cluster headache. *Neuroimage: Clinical, 6,* 415–423.

O'Brien, M., Ford, J. H., Aurora, S. K., Govindan, S., Tepper, D. E., & Tepper, S. J. (2017). Economics of inhaled oxygen use as an acute therapy for cluster headache in the United States of America. *Headache, 57,* 1416–1427.

Pellegrino, A. B. W., Davis-Martin, R. E., Houle, T. T., Turner, D. P., & Smitherman, T. A. (2018). Perceived triggers of primary headache disorders: A meta-analysis. *Cephalalgia, 38,* 1188–1198.

Post, M. D. (2014). Treatment of cluster headache symptoms using synthetic tryptamine, N,N-diallyl-5 methoxytryptamine. Retrieved from *https://figshare.com/articles.*

Psilocybin for the treatment of cluster headache. (2016). Retrieved from *https://figshare.com/articles.*

Psilocybin for the treatment of migraine headache. (2017). Retrieved from *https://figshare.com/articles.*

Raffaelli, E., Jr., Martins, O. J., & Dos Santos, P. D. F. A. (1983). Lisuride in cluster headache. *Headache, 23,* 117–121.

Richards, N., Chapman, L. F., Goodell, H., & Wolff, H. G. (1958). LSD-like delirium following ingestion of a small amount of its brom analog (BOL-148). *Annals of Internal Medicine, 48,* 1078–1082.

Robbins, M. S., Starling, A. J., Pringsheim, T. M., Becker, W. J., & Schwedt, T. J. (2016). Treatment of cluster headache: The American Headache Society evidence-based guidelines. *Headache, 56,* 1093–1106.

Rothrock, J. (2006). Cluster: A potentially lethal headache disorder. *Headache, 46,* 327.

Rozen, T. D., & Fishman, R. S. (2012). Cluster headache in the United States of America: Demographics, clinical characteristics, triggers, suicidality, and personal burden. *Headache, 52,* 99–113.

Russell, M. B. (2004). Epidemiology and genetics of cluster headache. *Lancet Neurology, 3,* 279–283.

Sahota, P. K., & Dexter, J. D. (1990). Sleep and headache syndromes: A clinical review. *Headache, 30,* 80–84.

Sarchielli, P., Alberti, A., Baldi, A., Coppola, F., Rossi, C., Pierguidi, L., et al. (2006). Proinflammatory cytokines, adhesion molecules, and lymphocyte integrin expression in the internal jugular blood of migraine patients without aura assessed ictally. *Headache, 46,* 200–207.

Schindler, E. A., Gottschalk, C. H., Weil, M. J., Shapiro, R. E., Wright, D. A., & Sewell, R. A. (2015). Indoleamine hallucinogens in cluster headache: Results of the Clusterbusters Medication Use Survey. *Journal of Psychoactive Drugs, 47,* 372–381.

Schulte, L. H., Allers, A., & May, A. (2017). Hypothalamus as a mediator of chronic migraine: Evidence from high-resolution fMRI. *Neurology, 88,* 2011–2016.

Schurks, M., Kurth, T., de Jesus, J., Jonjic, M., Rosskopf, D., & Diener, H. C. (2006). Cluster headache: Clinical presentation, lifestyle features, and medical treatment. *Headache, 46,* 1246–1254.

Schuster, N. M., & Rapoport, A. M. (2017). Calcitonin gene-related peptide-targeted therapies for migraine and cluster headache: A review. *Clinical Neuropharmacology, 40,* 169–174.

Sempere, A. P., Berenguer-Ruiz, L., & Almazan, F. (2006). [Chronic cluster headache responding to psilocybin]. *Revista de Neurologia, 43,* 571–572.

Sewell, R. A., & Gottschalk, C. H. (2011). Problem child is no headache. *Headache, 51,* 306–307.

Sewell, R. A., Halpern, J. H., & Pope, H. G., Jr. (2006). Response of cluster headache to psilocybin and LSD. *Neurology, 66,* 1920–1922.

Shabas, D., Sheikh, H. U., & Gilad, R. (2017). Pituitary apoplexy presenting as status migrainosus. *Headache, 57,* 641–642.

Shin, Y. W., Park, H. J., Shim, J. Y., Oh, M. J., & Kim, M. (2015). Seasonal variation, cranial autonomic symptoms, and functional disability in migraine: A questionnaire-based study in tertiary care. *Headache, 55,* 1112–1123.

Sicuteri, F. (1963). Prophylactic treatment of migraine by means of lysergic acid derivatives. *Triangle, 6,* 116–125.

Sommer, C. (2006). Is serotonin hyperalgesic or analgesic? *Current Pain and Headache Reports, 10,* 101–106.

Starr, P. A., Barbaro, N. M., Raskin, N. H., & Ostrem, J. L. (2007). Chronic stimulation of the posterior hypothalamic region for cluster headache: Technique and 1-year results in four patients. *Journal of Neurosurgery, 106,* 999–1005.

Taga, A., Russo, M., Manzoni, G. C., & Torelli, P. (2017). Cluster headache with accompanying migraine-like features: A possible clinical phenotype. *Headache, 57,* 290–297.

Toyoda, J. (1964). The effects of chlorpromazine and imipramine on the human nocturnal sleep electroencephalogram. *Folia Psychiatrica et Neurologica Japonica, 18,* 198–221.

Vikelis, M., & Rapoport, A. M. (2016). Cluster headache in Greece: An observational clinical and demographic study of 302 patients. *Journal of Headache and Pain, 17,* 88.

Vollenweider, F. X., Leenders, K. L., Scharfetter, C., Maguire, P., Stadelmann, O., & Angst, J. (1997). Positron emission tomography and fluorodeoxyglucose studies of metabolic hyperfrontality and psychopathology in the psilocybin model of psychosis. *Neuropsychopharmacology, 16,* 357–372.

Weiller, C., May, A., Limmroth, V., Jüptner, M., Kaube, H., Schayck, R. V., et al. (1995). Brain stem activation in spontaneous human migraine attacks. *Nature Medicine, 1,* 658–660.

PART VI

Mystical/Religious Experiences and Philosophical Considerations

CHAPTER 28

Mystical/Religious Experiences with Psychedelics

WILLIAM A. RICHARDS

◼ Introduction

Experiential discoveries of realms within human consciousness often described as "sacred," "awesome," or "holy," with and without the facilitation of psychedelic substances, have been and continue to be reported within the histories of the major world religions. Often, they are reported by quite ordinary people, some of whom may not even view themselves as "religious" or be associated with religious institutions. Perhaps there are common neurological, biochemical, and/or energetic substrates that correlate with these awe-filled states of awareness. Researchers in the future may be able to describe these factors more clearly than we can at our current stage of trying to decipher the enigmas of consciousness and the relationships between the brain and the human mind. Tantalizing clues include the knowledge that our bodies naturally manufacture dimethyltryptamine (DMT), usually in minute quantities, a molecule very similar in structure to psilocybin, that may play a role in the occurrence of some so-called "non-drug-facilitated" experiences often labeled *religious* or *mystical* (Barker et al., 2013; Strassman, 2001).

As will subsequently be surveyed, these inspiring and sometimes frightening experiences range from (1) states of perceptual or aesthetic enhancement to (2) cathartic experiences of personal insight and rebirth/forgiveness, to (3) states in which the everyday self (often called the "ego") beholds, approaches, encounters and often interacts with transpersonal content, often called *visionary* or *archetypal,* to (4) unitive states that most psychedelic researchers and other scholars in the psychology of religion today call *complete mystical consciousness.*

The content of the experiential domains themselves appears very similar, if not identical, regardless of whether the alternative state of consciousness seemed to occur spontaneously, was encountered during the implementation of meditative procedures, occurred during the action of a psychedelic substance, or was facilitated by some other technology (e.g., sensory deprivation or overload, natural childbirth, fasting, sleep deprivation, athletic feats. artistic performance). This range of experiences was encompassed in Abraham Maslow's term *peak experiences* (1964). They have also been discussed in books by many other authors, notably including William James (1902), James Bissett

Pratt (1920), Walter T. Stace (1960), Robert Masters & Jean Houston (1966), Marghanita Laski (1968), Stanislav Grof (1975), and the present writer (Richards, 2015).

The usual religious word for these many different states of consciousness is *revelation*. In medicine, some prefer to refer to such experiences simply as "nonordinary" or "alternative" states of mind, aware that similar, though often more disorganized, experiences sometimes also are reported by persons we diagnose as psychotic. When such experiences occur, the person in whose consciousness the content is unfolding typically feels that "truth" is being manifested and "deeper" or "higher" insights into the nature of the mind (or "reality") are being encountered or manifested. Some would refer to these diverse human experiences as stages on a continuum of "enlightenment," as if some internal rheostat is revealing more and more light or truth, both about the growing edges and opportunities of one's personal or spiritual development and frontiers regarding the ultimate nature of what may be called "mind," "consciousness," or "reality."

On the basis of an expanding professional literature, including carefully designed protocols with double-blind, controlled features (e.g., Griffiths et al., 2004, 2006, 2016, 2017; Grob et al., 2011; Ross et al., 2016), it appears that the potential significance of these sacred epiphanies extends beyond the inspiring wonder and memories of beauty, meaning, and sometimes transient terror that they leave in their wake. Recent psychedelic research has documented, and continues to demonstrate, potent positive changes in attitudes and behavior in the days, months, and years following many of these experiences. Some changes are dramatic, as illustrated by St. Paul's vision on the Road to Damascus and his subsequent leadership in the formative stages of Christianity; others are more subtle, reflected in shifts toward more humanistic values, increased genuineness in interpersonal relationships, and gradual increases in compassion, tolerance, of diversity and care for the planet on which we discover ourselves. Some experiences, often called *sacred* or *religious*, may indeed effect "quantum change" (Miller & C'de Baca, 2001), rapidly accelerating the processes of psychotherapy and/or psychological and spiritual development. This is why an increasing number of mental health professionals find themselves investigating the promise of psychedelic substances as powerful tools in facilitating substantial changes in human distress, notably in the treatment of addictions, depression, and states of anxiety, and perhaps in changing the ways in which we approach the process of dying and death itself.

■ An Overview of States of Consciousness with Potential Religious Import

Shifts in Sensory Perception

Though some would consider sensory changes in an artistic rather than a religious context, they are worthy of note. The dead grass, as reflected in Van Gogh's paintings, is seen as golden grain, scintillating in the sunlight; a wrinkled human face suddenly reflects wisdom and the richness of a life fully lived; a tree is transformed from a mere object in the environment to a living being, reflecting intelligence in nature. Such changes in perception are known to occur with open eyes following the ingestion of low or threshold doses of psychedelic substances, as well as in more intense alternative states of awareness. They are also reported in sensory modalities other than vision, for example, when one claims to "enter into the structure of music" or feels an intuitive sense of a nonverbal message within a composer's musical composition.

Personal Psychodynamic Experiences

As is well known in many forms of psychotherapy and in religious circles with an emphasis on "conversion" (typically in the evangelical Protestant tradition in Christianity), emotions of formerly repressed grief, guilt, and anger can be experienced in remarkable intensity, often culminating in feelings of relief, forgiveness, and fresh and/or new beginnings. Psychedelic substances in relatively low dosage (called *psycholytic therapy* in Europe) are known to facilitate the occurrence of these experiences, and are therefore believed to have promise in "accelerating psychotherapy."

Visionary/Archetypal Experiences

In this fascinating experiential realm, the ego (or everyday personality) encounters vibrant mental imagery, often including gods, goddesses, angels, demons, dragons, precious gemstones, elaborate architectural forms, other civilizations, and similar content. Such imagery is often reported as having a strong sense of substance, portentousness, and reality, evoking responses of awe and humility.

Not infrequently the images encountered appear to arise from traditions unfamiliar to the person experiencing them and his or her enculturation, supporting Carl Jung's concept of a "collective unconscious" within us all, perhaps encoded in our DNA.

Archetypes (i.e., "foundation stones" of psychic structure) thus are "beheld" and approached (sometimes with "fear and trembling"). As in a dream sequence, this may lead to a dialogue, an epiphany, a message received, or a lesson learned. Such experiences tend to vividly remain in memory and may be facilitative of changes in attitudes or behavior. This is the realm of the vision of the Christ or the Buddha, of the Virgin Mary, Quan Yin or Fatima Zahra, of Jung's "Wise old man," "Great Mother," and "Child"; it is also the terrain in which various mythological figures, including angels, demons, elves, witches, guardian deities, extraterrestrials, and so forth, may be visualized and encountered. Sometimes these visual encounters may progress further, as reflected in reports of "entering into the essence of the image" and "becoming it" or "going through the image" as a portal into unitive mystical states of awareness.

Mystical Consciousness

By general consensus among psychedelic researchers and many psychologists of religion, complete *mystical consciousness* tends to be defined as a state of awareness preceded by the "death" of the ego, followed by a unitive immersion in an experiential realm beyond time and space (often called "eternal" or "infinite"), then followed by the "rebirth" of the ego back into the everyday world. Like experiences labeled "visionary/archetypal." they include deep positive emotion, feelings of sacredness/awe/reverence, and claims of ineffability. But they also tend to be characterized by reports of union/unity and of convincing intuitive knowledge. In the literature of world religions there are many terms that point to this revelatory state: *moksha* and *samadhi* in Hinduism, *nirvana* and *satori* in Buddhism, *sekhel mufla* in Judaism, *the beatific vision* in Christianity, *baqá wa faná* in Islam, or *wu wei* in Taoism. Though fine distinctions can be found in many of the individual attempts to describe such experiences, many scholars consider those descriptions as evidence in support of a "perennial philosophy," a state of being intrinsic to the core of each human mind that has been discovered and rediscovered throughout the ages (Hood, 2006; Huxley, 1945; Kelly et al., 2007; Richards, 2015; Stace, 1960).

Before psychedelic substances became implemented as research tools in the psychology of religion, the academic literature on mysticism tended to distinguish between "Western Mysticism," with an emphasis on the personal relationship with the Divine (as in Visionary/Archetypal experiences) and "Eastern Mysticism," with its emphasis on unitive consciousness—in Hinduism, the "drop of water of the atman merging with the ocean of Brahman" or perhaps in the concept of Protestant theologian Paul Tillich (1951) of God as "the ground of Being." Now, through psychedelic research, it appears that most human beings, whether born in the East or the West, may be capable of experiencing both of these incredibly profound states of human consciousness given carefully determined dosage, personal openness, supportive preparation, and skillful guidance.

Similarly, the findings of psychedelic research support two ways in which the unity in mystical states may be approached. During the transition in consciousness to "internal unity," typically occurring when relaxed with closed eyes, awareness of the everyday self fades, while consciousness itself continues and expands through various so-called "dimensions of being" until a nontemporal unitive state prevails. "External unity" is reported to occur with open eyes through focused sensory perception, moving through various transformations until the perceiver and the perceived seem to merge and the insight "All is one" becomes convincingly dominant. Some have described this in the language of physicist/philosopher Alfred North Whitehead (1978), as if the energy or subatomic particles that make up reality themselves become conscious and somehow resonate with one another.

These mystical states of consciousness are typically claimed to be very convincing and self-validating. They are claimed to be "more real" than everyday awareness and somehow to be beyond our usual concepts of time, space, and substance.

Psychedelics in the History of Religions

Not only have various seers, prophets, and mystics in the histories of most world religions reported visionary insights, but some scholars have also posited that revelatory states of consciousness may be found at the very origins of religious systems of belief and practice. They point to the references to *soma* in the Hindu Rigveda and *homa* in ancient Zoroastrian literature, the drink called *kykeon* in the Greek mystery religions, drunk by Plato and others, and even the *manna* that the early Israelites consumed in the early mornings enroute to Canaan (Hofmann, 1983/2009; Merkur, 2001; Ruck, 2006; Smith, 2000; Wasson et al., 1986, 1978/1998). Native Americans are thought to have used mescaline from the peyote cactus for spiritual purposes for at least 5,500 years (El-Seedi et al., 2005). Cave paintings of human-like figures with mushrooms, found on the Tassili Plateau in Northern Algeria, believed to indicate early psychedelic use, have been dated to 5000 B.C.E. (Samorini, 1992). One theologian, on the basis of his research in ancient languages, has posited that some references to Jesus in early Christianity were actually references to a sacred psychoactive mushroom (Allegro, 1970). A scholar of the classics has presented evidence that the eucharist in early Christianity may have contained an active psychedelic substance (Muraresku, 2020).

An Indian Sanskrit scholar notes a practice called *aushadi* as "the most powerful and rapid method of awakening" (Saraswati, 1984). It entails the use of "specific herbs" that "can bring about either partial or full awakening." Although he distances himself from "drugs like marijuana, LSD [lysergic acid diethylamide] and so on," he notes the critical importance of pursuing this path only with "a guru or qualified guide," akin to the guidelines employed today in implementing psychedelic interventions in ways that ensure safety and promote efficacy. Religions in the 21st century that employ psychedelic substances in their practices include the Native American Church, indigenous groups in Central America and beyond that use psilocybin-containing mushrooms as a sacrament, and religions based in Brazil and neighboring countries in South America that honor the use of DMT in the form of the brew called ayahuasca.

The Discovery of Religious/Mystical Experiences in Modern Psychedelic Research and the Importance of Interpersonal Support

In the earliest days of modern psychedelic research, when LSD and similar substances were administered to volunteer subjects by investigators who lacked knowledge of the critical importance of psychological set, and the physical and interpersonal setting (environment), experiences dominated by panic, paranoia, and confusion often occurred. Thus, it was believed that these substances were "psychotomimetic" and caused "model psychoses." This led to hypotheses that they might be employed to facilitate an experience similar to *delirium tremens*, a "hitting bottom experience" that might motivate an alcoholic to work toward sobriety and/or somehow facilitate helpful changes in brain chemistry for some persons (Dyck, 2008), or that they might provide new perspectives to help us better understand schizophrenia and bipolar disorders (Leuner, 1962).

As the importance of set and setting was gradually recognized and implemented, so-called "psychotomimetic" experiences decreased and positive, highly valued "mysticomimetic" experiences increased in research centers on both sides of the Atlantic (Chwelos et al., 1959). With this change came many proposed uses of psychedelics in accelerating psychotherapy with diverse forms of psychopathology and a gradual confidence that these substances were not capriciously unpredictable in their effects, and could be administered safely to medically screened volunteers (Aaronson & Osmond, 1970; Abramson, 1967; Crocket et al., 1963; Johnson et al., 2008).

In contemporary psychedelic research and treatment, regardless of dosage, it has become accepted that ethical use of these psychoactive substances requires the prior establishment of significant rapport with volunteer subjects, skillful though not intrusive support during the period of drug action, should it be needed, and initial assistance in integrating and applying whatever new experiential insights may occur during the period of drug action to the routines of everyday living. For most people to be able to relinquish ego controls sufficiently to explore and permit the full experiencing of intense alternative states of consciousness, especially those deemed to have a religious or mystical nature, a safe and secure set and setting is now a basic research requirement.

■ The Potential "Fruits for Life" of Religious/Mystical Experiences

The intensification and acceleration of processes well known in psychodynamic forms of psychotherapy, such as the resolution of various conflicts, of guilt and grief, tends to take place when psychedelics are administered in relatively low or moderate dosage. Personal memories emerge, sometimes from early childhood, frequently accompanied by intense emotional catharsis, often culminating in new insights and feelings of relief, freedom, and relaxation. Treatment with psychedelics in this *psycholytic* (mind-releasing) format typically has been implemented with a series of sessions, sometimes several times in a week for several months. The content of most sessions is "in the realm of the ego," that is, the history of the individual person from birth to the present (e.g., Frederking, 1955; Leuner 1981; Sandison, 1954).

As the critical importance of a supportive set and setting became recognized, it was discovered that higher dosage often facilitated the occurrence of states of consciousness beyond the ego (or personal life history) that were often called "peak," "religious," or "mystical." Though psychological insights and catharsis focused on life-history events

or syndromes still sometimes occurred either prior to or following the transcendental states of mind, the memories of the transcendental states themselves began to become recognized as a uniquely powerful factor in the healing process. Claims of changes in self-concept were reported, including intuitive convictions of intrinsic worth, loss of estrangement and a sense of belonging to the human family, being able to receive and give love and forgiveness, and a vision of reality that offered meaning and ensured safety in the midst of life challenges. The "higher power" of Alcoholics Anonymous was often claimed to have been encountered, along with a convincing awareness of inner strengths and resources that hitherto had been fictitious or speculative at best. This has become recognized as a potent factor in the psychedelic treatment of addictions to alcohol, narcotics, cocaine and nicotine (Bogenschutz et al., 2018; Johnson et al., 2014).

In evaluating the potential significance of mystical experiences, the pragmatic philosopher and psychologist William James (1902) first called attention to the "fruits for life" that often are claimed to follow and, in one degree or another, influence attitudes and behavior in the months and years following their occurrence. This theme was continued by Walter Pahnke in his definition of *mystical consciousness*, which included "persisting positive change in attitudes and behavior" (Pahnke & Richards, 1966).

The therapeutic potency of mystical experiences has been especially noteworthy in projects of research with psychedelic substances and persons with terminal illnesses. Patients with cancer have not only reported decreases in depression and anxiety following glimpses of transcendence during the action of psychedelics, but they have also claimed loss of a fear of death, decreased preoccupation with pain, and increased capacity to nurture and appreciate genuine interpersonal relationships (Griffiths et al., 2016; Richards, 1978; Richards et al., 1972, 1977; Ross et al., 2016). What is especially unique about this high-dose approach to treatment, which is designed to facilitate transcendental forms of consciousness, is that often a single administration of the psychedelic substance, or at most three administrations, constitutes a significant intervention.

Future Investigations and Applications

In terms of applied treatment in the future, it may well be that both low-dose "psycholytic" and high-dose "psychedelic" sessions will be employed by clinicians. Though appreciative of the psychotherapeutic impact of transcendental experiences in high-dose psychedelic interventions, some investigators historically preferred to continue administering the substances in serial sessions in low or moderate doses, focusing on psychological dynamics in the mainstream of psychoanalytic thought (Leuner, 1981). A Dutch psychiatrist, G. W. Arendsen-Hein (1963), valuing and integrating both psychedelic and psycholytic approaches, coined the term *psychodelytic* therapy to refer to applied clinical usage in mental health treatment outside of a research context.

The study of transcendental states of human consciousness, often labeled "religious" or "mystical," may well be of importance beyond their applications in medical treatment. These inspiring revelatory states may also have their place in education and in religious study and practice (Richards, 2015). Initial studies are in process, exploring their potential value in enhancing meditative practices and in the training of clergy and other professional religious leaders. Ultimately, such research may provide clues—scientific, philosophical and spiritual—that may assist us in deciphering the mysteries of consciousness itself.

References

Aaronson, B., & Osmond, H. (Eds.). (1970). *Psychedelics: The uses and implications of hallucinogenic drugs.* New York: Doubleday Anchor.

Abramson, H. A. (Ed.). (1967). *The use of LSD in psychotherapy and alcoholism.* Indianapolis, IN: Bobbs-Merrill.

Allegro, J. M. (1970). *The sacred mushroom and the cross: A study of the nature and origins of Christianity within the fertility cults of the Ancient Near East.* Garden City, NY: Doubleday.

Arendsen-Hein, G. W. (1963). Treatment of the neurotic patient, resistant to the usual techniques of psychotherapy, with special reference to LSD. *Topical Problems of Psychotherapy, 4,* 50–57.

Barker, S. A., Borjigin, J., Lomnicka, I., & Strassman, R. (2013). Dimethyltryptamine hallucinogens, their precursors and major metabolites in rat pineal gland microdialysate. *Biomedical Chromatography, 27*(12), 1690–1700.

Bogenschutz, M. P., Podrebarac, S. K., Duane, J. H., Amegadzie, S. S., Malone, T. C., Owens, L. T., et al. (2018). Clinical interpretations of patient experience in a trial of psilocybin-assisted psychotherapy for alcohol use disorder. *Frontiers in Pharmacology, 9,* 100.

Chwelos, N., Blewett, D. B., Smith, C., & Hoffer, A. (1959). Use of LSD-25 in the treatment of chronic alcoholism. *Quarterly Journal of Studies on Alcoholism, 20,* 415–672.

Crocket, R., Sandison, R. A., & Walk, W. (Eds.). (1963). *Hallucinogenic drugs and their psychotherapeutic use.* London: Lewis.

Dyck, E. (2008). *Psychedelic psychiatry: LSD from clinic to campus.* Baltimore: Johns Hopkins University Press.

El-Seedi, H. R., De Smet, P. A., Beck, O., Possnert, G., & Bruhn, J. G. (2005). Prehistoric peyote use: Alkaloid analysis and radiocarbon dating of archaeological specimens of *Lophophora* from Texas. *Journal of Ethnopharmacology, 101*(1–3), 238–242.

Frederking, W. (1955). Intoxicant drugs (mescaline and lysergic acid diethylamide) in psychotherapy. *Journal of Nervous and Mental Disease, 121*(3), 262–266.

Griffiths, R. R., Johnson, M. W., Carducci, M. A., Umbricht, A., Richards, W. A., Richards, B. D., et al. (2016). Psilocybin produces substantial and sustained decreases in depression and anxiety in patients with life-threatening cancer: A randomized double-blind trial. *Journal of Psychopharmacology, 30,* 1181–1197.

Griffiths, R. R., Johnson, M. W., Richards, W. A., Richards, B. D., Jesse, R., MacLean, K. A., et al. (2017). Psilocybin-occasioned mystical-type experiences in combination with meditation and other spiritual produces enduring positive changes in psychological functioning and trait measures of prosocial attitudes and behavior. *Journal of Psychopharmacology, 32*(1), 49–69.

Griffiths, R. R., Richards, W. A., McCann, U., & Jesse, R. (2006). Psilocybin can occasion mystical-type experiences having substantial and sustained personal meaning and spiritual significance. *Psychopharmacology, 187*(3), 268–283.

Grob, C. S., Danforth, A. L., Chopra, G. S., Hagerty, M., McKay, C. R., Halberstadt, A., et al. (2011). Pilot study of psilocybin treatment for anxiety in patients with advanced-stage cancer. *Archives of General Psychiatry, 68*(1), 71–78.

Grof, S. (1975). *Realms of the human uncon- scious: Observations from LSD research.* New York: Viking.

Hofmann, A. (2009). *LSD, my problem child: Reflections on sacred drugs, mysticism and science.* Sarasota, FL: Multidisciplinary Asso- ciation of Psychedelic Studies. (Original work published 1983)

Hood, R. W. (2006). The common core thesis in the study of mysticism. In P. McNamara (Ed.), *Where God and science meet* (pp. 119–138). Westport, CT: Praeger.

Huxley, A. (1945). *The perennial philosophy.* New York: Harper.

James, W. (1902). *The varieties of religious expe- rience.* New York: Modern Library.

Johnson, M. W., Garcia-Romeu, A., Cosimano, M., & Griffiths, R. R. (2014). Pilot study of the 5-HT2A R agonist psilocybin in the treat- ment of tobacco addiction. *Journal of Psycho- pharmacology, 28*(11), 983–992.

Johnson, M. W., Richards, W. A., & Griffiths, R. R. (2008). Human hallucinogen research: Guidelines for safety. *Journal of Psychopa- thology, 22*(6), 603–619.

Kelly, E. F., Kelly, E. W., Crabtree, A., Gauld, A., Grosso, M., & Greyson, B. (2007). *Irreducible mind: Toward a psychology for the 21st cen- tury.* Lanham, MD: Rowman & Littlefield.

Laski, M. (1968). *Ecstasy: A study of some secu- lar and religious experiences.* Westport, CT: Greenwood Publishing Group.

Leuner, H. (1962). *Die Experimentelle Psychose: Ihre Psychopharmakologie, Phänomenolo- gie und Dynamik in Beziehung zur Person: Einer Konditional-Genetischen und Funktio- nalen Psychopathologie der Psychose.* Berlin: Springer.

Leuner, H. (1981). *Halluzinogene: Psychische Grenzzustände in Forschung und Psychother- apie.* Bern, Switzerland: Hans Huber.

Maslow, A. H. (1964). *Religions, values and peak experiences.* Columbus: Ohio State Uni- versity Press.

Masters, R. E. L., & Houston, J. (1966). *The va- rieties of psychedelic experience.* New York: Dell.

Merkur, D. (2001). *The psychedelic sacrament: Mana, meditation and mystical experience.* Rochester, VT: Park Street Press.

Miller, W. R., & C'de Baca, J. (2001). *Quantum change: When epiphanies and sudden insights transform ordinary lives.* New York: Guilford Press.

Muraresku, B. G. (2020). *The immortality key: The secret history of the religion with no name.* New York: St. Martin's Press.

Pahnke, W. N., & Richards, W. A. (1966). Im- plications of LSD and experimental mysticism. *Journal of Religion and Health, 5,* 175–208.

Pratt, J. B. (1920). *The religious consciousness: A psychological study.* New York: Macmillan.

Richards, W. A. (1978). Mystical and archetypal experiences of terminal patients in DPT-as- sisted psychotherapy. *Journal of Religion and Health, 17*(2), 117–126.

Richards, W. A. (2015). *Sacred knowledge: Psychedelics and religious experiences.* New York: Columbia University Press.

Richards, W. A., Grof, S., Goodman, L. E., & Kurland, A. A. (1972). LSD-assisted psycho- therapy and the human encounter with death. *Journal of Transpersonal Psychology, 4,* 121– 150.

Richards, W. A., Rhead, J. C., DiLeo, F. B., Yensen, R., & Kurland, A. A. (1977). The peak experience variable in DPT-assisted psy- chotherapy with cancer patients. *Journal of Psychedelic Drugs, 9,* 1–10.

Ross, S., Bossis, A., Guss, J., Agin-Liebes, G., Malone, T., Cohen, B., et al. (2016). Rapid and sustained symptom reduction following psilocybin treatment for anxiety and depres- sion in patients with life-threatening cancer: A randomized controlled trial. *Journal of Psy- chopharmacology, 30,* 1165–1180.

Ruck, C. A. P. (2006). *Sacred mushrooms of the goddess: Secrets of Eleusis.* Berkeley, CA: Ronin.

Samorini, G. (1992). The oldest representations of hallucinogenic mushrooms in the world. *In- tegration, 2*(3), 69–78.

Sandison, R. A. (1954). Psychological aspects of the LSD treatment of neuroses. *Journal of Mental Science, 100,* 508–515.

Saraswati, S. (1984). *Kundalini Tantra.* Munger, India: Bihar School of Yoga.

Smith, H. (2000). *Cleansing the doors of percep- tion: The religious significance of entheogenic plants and chemicals.* New York: Tarcher/ Putnam.

Stace, W. T. (1960). *Mysticism and philosophy.* Philadelphia: Lippincott.

Strassman, R. (2001). *DMT: The spirit molecule.* Rochester, VT: Park Street Press.

Tillich, P. (1951). *Systematic theology: Volume 1.* Chicago: University of Chicago Press.

Wasson, R. G., Hofmann, A., & Ruck, C. A. P. (1998). *The road to Eleusis: Unveiling the secret of the mysteries.* Los Angeles: William Dailey Rare Books. (Original work published 1978)

Wasson, R. G., Kramrich, S., Ott, J., & Ruck, C. A. (1986). *Persephone's quest: Entheogens and the origins of religion.* New Haven, CT: Yale University Press.

CHAPTER 29

Philosophical Considerations Concerning the Use of Hallucinogens in Psychiatric Treatment

CANDICE L. SHELBY

▪ Introduction

One result of what Max Weber first called the "disenchantment of the world,"[1] the replacement of the belief in spiritual beings, absolute moral truth, and a just God, with a naturalistic understanding of our existence and meaning making, has been a kind of existential insecurity. William James (1917) says that a kind of essential sadness

> lies at the heart of every merely positivistic, agnostic, or naturalistic scheme of philosophy. . . . For naturalism, fed on recent cosmological speculations, mankind is in a position similar to that of a set of people living on a frozen lake, surrounded by cliffs over which there is no escape, yet knowing that little by little the ice is melting, and the inevitable day drawing near when the last film of it will disappear, and to be drowned ignominiously will be the human creature's portion. The merrier the skating, the warmer and more sparkling the sun by day, and the ruddier the bonfires at night, the more poignant the sadness with which one must take in the meaning of the total situation. (pp. 142–143)

If this is so, it is no wonder that patients are seeking treatments for anxiety and depression at record rates (Campbell, 2017); nor it is a surprise that clinical success has in these areas been persistently elusive (Turner & Rosenthal, 2008). As James (1917) also says, this kind of "soul sickness," is not easy to unseat. Neither drugs, nor talking about it, nor a change of place or activities, nor, as is often recommended, a conscious effort to "buck up and get going" go very far toward healing this kind of sickness. The healing of this mind of malaise, as with any change in our fundamental beliefs or attitudes, James says, "must come to the individual with the force of a revelation" (p. 114).

What James means is that for something to really change someone's mind, it must not merely be conveyed intellectually; it must hit at the very foundations of a person's emotional life, and one's entire perspective. For many, this kind of change has been sought through prayer, religious ceremonies, and/or meditative practices. For most sufferers in the Western World in recent decades, though, the most prevalent (and profitable) approach offered has been pharmaceuticals and/or talk therapy. Sadly, neither of these approaches has proven very successful at alleviating symptoms.

One approach that has been consistently successful, both throughout history in various parts of the world and recently in the West in scientifically studied contexts, involves the use of plant-based or synthesized hallucinogens. Lysergic acid diethylamide (LSD), 3,4-methylenedioxymethamphetamine (MDMA), psilocybin, ayahuasca, ibogaine, and other compounds have been effectively employed in the treatment of depression, anxiety, posttraumatic stress disorder (PTSD), and addictions of various kinds. Before being prohibited, beginning in the 1960s, these substances had been fairly widely employed in several countries in psychotherapy; and since permissions have once again begun to be granted to use these compounds in research studies, sufferers from an array of disorders have been treated with noteworthy success (Grob et al., 2011). [2] So, the questions arise, what do these substances do that other, more standard treatments do not do, and why is their therapeutic use regarded with such skepticism? In what follows, I argue that misgivings about psychedelic and psycholytic approaches are unwarranted, and that, in fact, these approaches should be embraced. Making that case, though, will require, in addition to consideration of how they might work to bring about psychological healing, reflection on fundamental concepts such as mind, self, identity, and mystical experience.

Consciousness, Mind, and Self

Philosophers have argued for at least 375 years about the natures of the mind and the self. According to Descartes and his long train of followers, the mind is a certain kind of entity, immaterial, freestanding and separate from the body. Although this kind of conception stems from a religious worldview and may in principle not be supported by empirical evidence, it is intuitively plausible and continues to remains popular even among some philosophers. On this sort of dualistic account, in principle, it would seemingly be impossible to change the mind's processing by making changes in the body, since the mind is essentially a different kind of stuff from the physical. A range of sometimes very creative explanations of how

physical changes could correspond to mental changes, given this radical difference, have been offered through the centuries. Perhaps most famous, or infamous, among these is Descartes' suggestion that mind and body interact in the pineal gland. On this picture, although the cognitive structures of the mind do receive input from the senses, those structures themselves are not alterable by physical or bodily changes. Immediately upon disseminating these ideas to his peers, however, Descartes was met with skepticism about the logical coherence of such interaction. Thomas Hobbes (and a long train of followers), for instance, rejected outright the notion that there exist two fundamentally different kinds of stuff constituting mind and body, insisting instead that mind is material. The brain is moved by transmitted impulses, Hobbes thought, then various bits move around various others, producing changes that we vainly think of as independent thinking. The dichotomy of either reifying the mind or eliminating it as a "real" entity was thus firmly established.

This dramatic division between conceptions of minds and bodies continued into the 20th century as scientists and philosophers began to consider the nature of consciousness. Some philosophers think of consciousness as a brute element of the universe, much like energy/matter, so that our brains do something, but whatever that something is, it is not producing consciousness. Perhaps brain activities and consciousness align, and they certainly seem to correlate in at least certain ways, but they are not the same kinds of things. Consciousness is, as David Chalmers says, unlike visual processing or auditory processing, a "hard problem," because even if we were to know in the most minute detail how the processing of sensory inputs occur, this would say nothing about why those inputs are *experienced*. Consciousness is categorically different from physical processes, and therefore cannot be explained in terms of them. Most philosophers, however, have thought of consciousness as either reducing to physical phenomena, or in terms of black-box functions of physical phenomena, or as illusory; more recently, some have characterized consciousness as emergent from physical phenomena. I will not bother outlining the myriad details distinguishing the plethora of versions of these various theories here. Let us instead simply consider what neuroscience currently tells us about how brains function in the broadest sense, and use those insights to determine whether the kinds of change in consciousness that hallucinogens can bring about in a therapeutic setting would threaten the integrity of mind, self, or identity.

To begin with, then, one popular understanding of how the conscious mind works is, as Neal Levy (2018) puts it, akin to how a CEO operates in a business organization, with one central organizer delegating tasks to other mechanisms in the brain, but without ever giving up ultimate decision-making authority. On this kind of view, it would seem that the CEO is some sort of stable entity that, through its ultimate power over all the moving parts, constitutes the essence of the mind of an individual. Significant changes to an entity so conceived would mean a change in identity, which, as we shall see, many thinkers fear greatly (usually in connection with life after death issues; we consider those below). As it turns out, however, nothing like the CEO metaphor is supported by recent research. Rather, the view that the evidence suggests has come to be that the brain is modular, composed of many anatomically or functionally defined regions that constitute separate mechanical systems, each inflexibly performing a single task, sometimes with competing goals and often with no direct communication between them. This would imply that the mind is not an entity at all but something more like interacting levels of mostly unconscious processes. On this sort of view, one might worry that anarchy would seem to follow, and so it might appear a wonder that we (or any organisms with complex structures, for that matter) could even manage to stay alive, much less to think about things and experience the world as a particular self.

But we do. So the question then becomes how that might happen. Following neuroscientists such as Michael Gazzaniga (2018), some philosophers have argued that consciousness—and indeed for Gazzaniga, a morally responsible self—emerges from various "layers" of independent systems, each of which follows its own autonomous laws, operates on its own temporal and spa-

tial scales, and interacts preferentially with the layers just above or below it (Bassett & Gazzaniga, 2011).[3] That is, the mental, in one way or another, emerges from physical body/brain system dynamics. Although the term *emerge* has, since the mid-20th century, been rejected by many philosophers because of unclarities and old baggage associated with it, the term is widely used by physicists and neuroscientists, and I use it here, explaining and dismissing what I take to be the most significant objections offered against the notion that the mental emerges from the physical.

First of all, it is essential to understand that conscious experience relies on the development of neural systems initially directed by genetic encoding, but which is affected at every stage by interactions with the system's local and global environments, and is deeply dependent on activity-based learning. The brain, in other words, is essentially a dynamically evolving system with basic default structures and functions dictated by genetic coding, but it is refined at every turn by interaction with the environment in which it unfolds. Multipotential neural structures develop into functional units but are constrained in their development by many factors, including environmental stimuli and activity, and these structures in turn subserve other systems at higher levels of organization.

So far, so good. Now we can see how a complex brain comprising a multitude of modules processing a huge mass of information might develop. But we have done nothing to account for the seeming unity of the consciousness that arises out of that multitude of independently operating functional entities; indeed, if anything, we ought to expect from what has been said at best a well-organized automaton, and at worst the anarchic mess of competing subsystems mentioned earlier. But an anarchic mess would seemingly self-destruct and certainly would not appear to be able to account for the kind of consciousness whose integrity might be threatened by treatment with hallucinogenic compounds. The unity that appears fundamental among the characteristics of consciousness seems to be explained by a mostly left-hemisphere lateralized module that is commonly referred to as the default mode network (DMN), although Michael Gazanniga seems to refer to the same module with his term the "interpreter." This module, although it is well connected to other parts of the brain, is not the CEO of earlier philosophical speculation. It is a module. It does not sit as some kind of brain matter homunculus, some place which at which all processing "finishes," controlling what all other parts of the brain do. Rather this network operates to make the activities of various other modules, which may or may not be coordinated or even coherent with one another, make sense in conscious experience with the "usual flow" of how things go. In other words, this module provides phenomenological unity. It creates the autobiography that constitutes a particular take on the world, develops a narrative about why we do what we do, functions in the creation of theory of mind, which we use with one another, and evokes a sense of self, or ego. The DMN, of course, comprises neurons, as do all other modules, each of which is composed of molecules, each of which has its own composition, and so forth, and it comprises part of a larger system, and systems of systems, which constitute what we experience as a conscious mind. This module, with its own systems-level operations, can evidently influence or control other modules—for example, it might stop me from eating the greasy French fries that I am considering—but it can also be influenced by other modules and end up providing me with a story of why it is OK today to eat those fries if I do in fact end up doing so.

Now we have a problem, though, and one that accounts for many of the various philosophical views of consciousness and mind that have been offered. How is it that a "higher" layer of organization can control a "lower" level if it is dependent on that lower level for its existence? This kind of question caused barrels of ink to be spilled at the end of the 20th century, with attempts to explain the mind/brain relation coming from all directions. Reductionists led the charge but were quickly challenged by eliminativist, supervenience, and epiphenomenalist approaches. Some philosophers, dissatisfied with the contortions of common sense that some of these views required, and recognizing that we clearly do control our behaviors with something more complex than individual neurons or individual neural circuits, have avoided the causal question altogether, and focused on different kinds of issues. Functionalists, for instance, recognize that what a thing is depends on its role relative to other entities and systems with which it interacts. In their view, in accordance with the view of the emergentist, a neuron is not a neuron unless it plays the role of one in a system in which there are roles for neurons. Likewise, an "interpreter" cannot exist unless it has a role to play in a system in which it has a place. But within the complex systems that are human brain circuits (and brains, conscious minds, and selves), each element has a role to play, and in fact exists only because of its relations with all the others.

Philosophical and scientific objections to this picture arise largely, as was suggested earlier, because of the issue of causation. What causes what? Can causation be "top-down," as well as "bottom-up"? Can it be cyclical? Reductionists and supervenience theorists consider these questions to be nonstarters (although they admit that causation can *seem* to be other than bottom-up; in their view, however, that is just a matter of misinterpretation of the phenomena). Epiphenomenalists maintain that the mind has no causal efficacy whatsoever. Emergentism is rejected by all of these groups either on the grounds that it is "spooky," that something seems to come from nothing, or on the grounds of overdetermination. If the neurons at the "bottom" are really the cause of an act or an experience, then something constituted of those neurons cannot also be the cause of that act or experience. That is just an incoherence, these philosophers say. The problem, though, seems to be not with the emergentist account of what happens, but rather with the notion of causation in use. The intuitive understanding of "cause" (and the one that underlies that ever-hawked distinction between correlation and causation) is a linear one derived from a Newtonian conception of the universe. On that understanding there can, by definition, be no such thing as top-down or cyclical causation, with emergent processes influencing (constraining or altering) the processes that brought the emergent ones about to begin with. But that understanding is simply a mistake. Many kinds of causal questions may be asked, but people tend to conflate them. When we ask, "What caused X?," we might be asking about the structures that made it possible for X to happen, or we might be asking about the mechanics of how X happened, among other things. As philosopher J. L. Mackie (1974) points out, when the fireman looks to see what caused the kitchen to burn down, he might seek an answer in terms of an overheated frying pan, the lack of a sprinkler system, curtains flapping from an open window, sufficient oxygen in the room, no one being at home to stop it, or all of these together in a particular sort of relationship. What counts as a cause depends largely on what question one asks. And in complex dynamic systems, with multiple scales of organization, massive parallel processing, and preponderant feedback loops, we should not be surprised to find that this is the case.

But if dynamic, mutually causal systems are the way to explain how consciousness and the sense of a persisting self are generated, how should we understand hallucinogen-induced experiences? Are they even real? Should we consider them as psychiatric treatments at all, or rather, as some say, as something more akin to a spiritual revelation? What would that latter even mean? Do the changes brought about by such experiences, particularly by psychedelic ones, because of the way that they are brought about, in a revolutionary manner rather than bit by bit over time, threaten the identity of a patient, making the treatments too radical to condone? None of us think that the changes we all undergo over a decade or two threaten our identity, but if those same changes happened over a day, would our view be different? These kinds of considerations, despite their supporters' enthusiasm for them, fail to undermine the value or medicinal nature of treatment involving psychedelic substances; in fact, quite the contrary is true. The very questions that arise in the philosophical assessment of the healing that is brought about by psychedelic-assisted therapies show that these therapies are some of the best on offer as approaches to true healing. In order to make that case, let us consider some of the arguments on offer by opponents to this view.

Changing the Brain

"Those drugs change the brain" is one objection that people often make to the use of hallucinogens. Yes, they do. But so do the billions of dollars' worth of antidepressants and anxiolytic medications dispensed every year. And so does meditation, exercise, water, and being awake. The difference generally alluded to here, though, is that while pharmaceutical drugs make a controllable difference with regard to certain, contained aspects of the self (Aristotle would call them "accidental properties"), and talk therapies bring about basically the same kinds of changes, only very gradually, hallucinogens make profound global changes to the brain and one's "take" on the world, and thereby in some way make some sort of objectionable changes to one's identity.

A few things could be said in response to this kind of charge. First, not all treatment involving hallucinogens is psychedelic therapy, in which significant doses are given in order to trigger intense, transformational experiences all at once. Although it is this model that has been most researched, it is not the only type of hallucinogen-assisted therapy extant. Psycholytic therapy, or the use of lower doses of hallucinogens for the purpose of increasing the impact of ordinary-length therapeutic sessions, has also been used both in the United States and in Europe, both prior to their prohibition in the last 1960s and since research has begun again. Ketamine-assisted therapy is, in fact, increasingly used in therapeutic sessions in the United States. Second, it is simply not true that pharmaceutical psychoactive drugs are controllable and therefore safe, while hallucinogens are not. It is not just that no one is certain of how these widely prescribed pharmaceuticals work, leaving their prescription to trial and error; what is more, people often have adverse reactions to them. It is now firmly established, for example, that antidepressants are associated with suicidal ideation in many teenagers. Third, it is not the case that pharmaceutical compounds make only (positive) localized differences in the brain. As is well known, many people have experienced severe problems with addiction to anxiolytic medications, especially those in the benzodiazepine class of drugs (e.g., consider the

1982 movie *I'm Dancing as Fast as I Can,* focused on one woman's attempts to recover from tolerance to and dependence on Valium). Furthermore, a recent *New York Times* article included interviews with numerous individuals who experienced debilitating effects from trying to withdraw from antidepressants (Carey & Geveloff, 2018). And, as science writer Robert Whitaker has pointed out, this is just what should be expected. Given our brains' (and our general) adaptability, long-term use of antidepressants can result in patients' experiencing worsening of depression; extra serotonin will eventually affect the expression of genes that determine the number of serotonin receptors, and fewer receptors for serotonin will make the patient worse off than before he or she began the treatment (Whitaker, 2010). Finally, if the permanence or semipermanence of changes in the brain is the argument against the therapeutic use of hallucinogens, then it misses the mark altogether, for not only do other types of drug treatments create changes just as long-lasting but so also do talk therapy and cognitive-behavioral therapy, when successful, and that is a good thing. Surely our conception of healing when we naively visit a surgeon, medical doctor, or psychiatrist, is not simply to control our symptoms for as long as we stay in treatment. That may be the best option available in some cases, but it is not the definition of "healing." We seek "to get better."

With the assistance of hallucinogens in therapeutic settings, many people by their own accounts do get better, for at least three potential sets of reasons, some or all of which may be related to the specific mechanism of action of a particular compound. One reason that profound shifts in emotional memory may come about in patients with PTSD through the use of MDMA, for example, concerns the biochemistry of the extinction of fear memory. Patients with PTSD have certain of their memories deeply entangled with fear responses. One way to think about how the changes that treatment with MDMA are brought about is through the phenomenon of fear extinction. Numerous research groups have focused on the effects that the serotonin 5-HT_{2A} receptors on individual neurons have on enhancing fear extinction memory. By creating a greater availability of serotonin, some researchers have found, the fearful emotional component of such memories is loosened, and the fear can be extinguished when an organism is exposed to the source of the fear, without the expected attendant negative event (Young, Andero, Ressler, & Howell, 2015; Young et al., 2017). When 5-HT_{2A} receptors were blocked in experiments, the fear memory extinction enhancement associated with administration of MDMA was found to disappear, so the conclusion was drawn that these receptors were the key to understanding MDMA's effectiveness. But its effect on these receptors cannot be the whole of the story, for MDMA also enhances release and reception of dopamine, norepinephrine, the hormones oxytocin and cortisol, and other signaling molecules, all of which are involved in modulating emotional memory circuits. For this reason, although the receptor level is one way of understanding how MDMA may be operating, and it is certainly interesting and worthy of further study, it does not seem up to the task of explaining how these memories continue to be emotionally undisruptive for the long term after treatment, as they have recently been shown to be in humans.

Perhaps a better level of analysis for providing an answer to the question that we seek to answer—"Why do patients with PTSD seem to be truly healed through MDMA-assisted therapy?"—is the neural systems level. At this level we can ask whether all those molecules MDMA affects operate by extinguishing the fear memory that causes PTSD symptoms, or whether they interfere with the reconsolidation of memories that have been disrupted during administration of the compound. Although some researchers, as just mentioned, drew the conclusion that extinction was the phase in which MDMA did its work, a research group at the University of Colorado recently put that hypothesis to the test, and found that MDMA may instead operate by modifying fear memory during reconsolidation (Hake et al., 2019). This set of experiments showed that MDMA, when administered during the reconsolidation phase, but not when administered prior to the extinction phase or at any other time outside the reconsolidation phase, resulted in a delayed and persistent diminution in conditioned fear. This result fits with earlier research that indicated propranolol affects the reconsolidation of emotional memories (Lonergan et al., 2013). Presumably, the way these substances work is that memories (tightened synaptic strengths between the neurons involved) originally created with the involvement of powerful negative inputs from emotion-producing modules are loosened during the treatment, then reconsolidated without those inputs. This would provide a mechanism for explaining how MDMA could change patients' experiences of their formerly fear-laden memories in a long-term way, without relapse.

A second reason why psychedelics may have such powerful effects on changing patients' overall outlook and mood long after treatment could be that learning occurs when patients experience new insights due to higher connectivity among different parts of the brain during the time that the medication is active in the system (Carhart-Harris et al., 2016). That is to say, rather than associations between ideas, and ideas and feelings running along the usual, well-worn lines, particularly with respect to the "DMN," during exposure to certain compounds, processing in the brain becomes much more integrated, allowing decidedly different perspectives to arise. Learning that happens from experiencing things in profoundly different ways from the usual may be maintained long after the treatment event due to the profundity of the insight (which would imply a large-scale change in one's overall conceptual framework) and/or powerful emotional experiences that may accompany those insights, as indicated in the James quotes in the opening paragraphs.

Finally, depression of the default mode network is correlated with the experience of "ego dissolution," or a feeling of the diminution or disappearance of the normal sense of self, in favor of a more encompassing sense of the unity of all things (Carhart-Harris et al., 2016). This is discussed more in the sections below. In each of these cases, brain systems are indeed changed, as are the systems that emerge from those systems, such as those responsible for conscious awareness during the time of treatment, and at a higher level of complexity and on a longer time scale, one's personal identity.

But, surely, not just these, but all powerful experiences, and indeed one might argue, all nontrivial learning changes conceptual frameworks and the self. That is a good thing. After all, many of us pay large sums to have our children changed through both profound experiences (travel to foreign places) and university training, and people for many centuries have practiced various forms of prayer and meditation in order to achieve the sense(s) of unity that use of hallucinogens can create under the right circumstances. Only in the case of conceiving of the self as a static entity that in some way forever defines an individual would changes in the self in any of these ways be understandable as some kind of threat to identity. For dynamic systems such as the organisms that we are, change is central to what it means to grow, to mature, and to develop wisdom.

■ Mysticism and Mystical Experience

"This isn't medical treatment at all!" some (medical doctors) might say with respect to hallucinogen-assisted psychotherapies. "What is happening here is a personal change, or a spiritual or mystical experience—brought about with the use of substances perhaps—but since its success depends on setting, guidance, and all kinds of things other than the ingestion of the drugs themselves, whatever it is, it is not medical treatment." Through this sort of reasoning, some have come to the conclusion that hallucinogen-assisted therapies ought to be left out of medical discourse. I do not see why such treatments cannot be both physiological medical treatments and mystical or spiritual experiences (or some other kind of experience that has positive outcomes), if the emergent view of mind outlined above is correct. In that view (the one, after all, suggested by the Greek etymology of *psyche*), it is medicine that has the incorrect understanding of mind, and therefore the incorrect (or at least incomplete) understanding of how mental health can be achieved. Surely spiritual or mystical (if there is a difference) experience must be *experienced* in order to exist, and unless one is an unrepentant dualist, that means it must be in some sense physiologically based, but including emergent levels beyond just the neurons, ions, and whatnot that compose the brain. That is not to say that the spiritual, or mystical, is not a special category of experience; in fact, it seems to be. But this in no way implies that such experiences cannot form an important part of psychiatric treatment.

Mystical experience, since before recorded history, has been sought as a way of providing guidance in developing meaning and purpose in life, as well as for curing illness of all kinds, both physical and psychic, so before moving on, let us take a moment to consider its character. Accounts of mystical experience can be found throughout the literatures of diverse cultures around the world. Several characteristics of mystical experience are cited nearly universally. Perhaps the fullest list of such characteristics was identified by William T. Stace (1961). First of all, mystical experiences involve some type of undifferentiated unity. Stace distinguishes two types of unity: (1) internal unity (i.e., undifferentiated awareness, unitary consciousness) and (2) external unity (i.e., a sense of unity with the surrounding environment). The first, which Stace refers to as "introvertive unity," we can characterize as nondiscursive consciousness, in which experience itself is undifferentiated. The second, which he calls "extrovertive unity," involves the perception, as Stace puts it, that "all is one," that everything in existence is connected. The experience of unity can happen with eyes closed and other sensory information blocked, or by experiencing the sensed world only as though transfigured—as though through an opening of the "doors of perception," in Aldous Huxley's term. Extrovertive mystical unity also involves a sense of the inner subjectivity of all (i.e., a sense of a living presence in all things; a sense of objectivity and reality (that the experience is not merely one's own, but is an encounter with objective truth); a sense of "blessedness, joy, happiness, satisfaction, etc.," as well as a feeling that what one is apprehending is somehow sacred (i.e., worthy of reverence, divine, or holy). This sort of mystical experience is also, according to Stace, marked by paradoxicality (i.e., needing to use illogical or contradictory statements to describe the experience), which for many involve an attendant feeling of the ineffability of the experience (Stace, 1961).

Although this last characteristic is the most tentatively included by many writers (which may be because the impossibility of expressing something and the difficulty of talking about paradoxes are related, but do not amount to the same thing), it is described by William James (1917) as the "handiest of the marks" by which to identify mystical experience. He agrees with Stace that mystical experience does not have the quality of a mere subjective feeling, but instead is marked by the noetic, as though it is revealing something objectively true and right about of the nature of things themselves. James also notes that these experiences are transient, and that they are passively undergone, that is, without a sense of the experiencer's being in control once it begins, although it can be deliberately instigated.

More specific to our own aim here, Walter Pahnke (1971), well-known researcher in the clinical uses of LSD, specified a list of nine elements characteristic of mystical experiences, whether spontaneously or chemically generated. His list overlaps with those of the philosophers, but he adds to theirs a feeling of transcendence of time and space, and persisting positive changes in attitudes and behavior. With respect to the last, I cannot see how that could be a characteristic of the mystical experience itself, since such experiences by Pahnke's own lights are transient, but in his much more specifically psychological account, we can consider the persisting positive changes a side effect of mystical experience, and for our purposes, one of the most important ones listed.

Note that nothing about the mystical experience as analyzed by either of our philosophers, as Pahnke shows with his clinic-based research, depends on free-floating souls or spirits, or the Divine (unless one counts all of existence together as something divine, a position taken by some philosophers and scientists alike). If the concept were referential in that way, there would be no way to know whether anyone had ever had a mystical experience, as there is, as far as we know, no way to know whether there are spirits or the Divine (again, monism aside). It is, first and essentially, an *experience*. Pahnke refers to it specifically as a psychological experience, and Einstein spoke of it as an emotion. These characterizations suggest that mystical experience, whether the result of interoception alone or of interoception together with sensory perceptions, is the result of the operation of some level of the complex system that involves our atoms, molecules, cells, and systems of cells; our bodies, our selves, and our environments. In short, it need not require any more or fewer ontological assumptions than does any other psychological experience. As Robin Carhart-Harris's group showed, depressing the activity of the DMN allows all kinds of normally anticorrelated modules to communicate with one another, opening the doors to all kinds of connections not normally available to experience to become conscious, including quite plausibly a feeling of unity both in consciousness itself (becoming more oneself, as it is sometimes put), and in a sense of the unity of all things.[5]

■ The Self

Even if I have answered the objection that the mystical can also be psychological, and that psychiatric treatment with hallucinogens should not be rejected on the grounds that it is not properly a treatment at all, there still remains the question of whether psychedelic (in particular) experiences are objectionable on the ground that they alter or perhaps even dissolve the self, undermining the whole idea of psychiatric healing. As I mentioned earlier, this cannot be a viable objection unless we think of the self as a static entity that forever defines a person.

But for the purposes of answering the self-dissolving (and hence psychiatric healing-undermining) objection, there are at least two different senses in which we can think of the self. We can think of the self as simply whatever is consciously aware, a sense that babies seem to have from birth, a particular point of view, perhaps brought about in usual cases by proprioception, interoception, and perspective in sensory perception. It is what Descartes referred to when he said about himself, "I am a thinking thing," although whether he ever actually did or could achieve consciousness in just this sense is extremely doubtful. Kant, too, thought of our morality as arising from an "I" completely

separate from psychology, preferences, inclinations, or motivations of any kind. That is one sense of "self."

There is also, though, the "who" one is, the set of attitudes, character traits, dispositions, and, at an ever higher level of organization, the identity by which one recognizes oneself as one among others in the world, the "kind of person" one is, the persona, or ego. In this sense, the young child, whose personality, as we say, "is developing," hardly has any sense of self in this way. The child is very open to new ways of doing things, can learn any language (and thus any way of being in the world) as well as any other, and does not have any highly habituated responses, ways of solving problems, or strong sense of autobiography. As time goes on, however, and the default neural network becomes better established, and pruning events reduce the number of interconnections among modules in the brain, so do we become more "expert" at all kinds of things, develop dispositions to see things in certain ways, to solve problems in certain ways, and to think about "who we are" in the autobiographical sense, developing a temporal sense of self. Our memories say much about who we are in this sense, and so do our projects. The successful predictions that we have made in the past create attractor wells for similar situations in the future, so much so that we just automatically perceive situations in the familiar ways, and sometimes see things (e.g., explanations of our actions, or malicious intent) where there is nothing. But all this happens within a context of a world, including a social world, that gives us constant feedback. That feedback constrains our predictions in the future, as well as our understanding of who we are as social beings. Like every other level of organization, this system operates on its own spatial and temporal scales, according to an autonomous set of rules. Self in this sense emerges over a years-long time frame, and involves social relations, as well as awareness of our own conscious as the locus of all experience.

Although the loss of the self in the second sense is tragic when it disappears permanently, as we recognize in extreme cases of retrograde amnesia, for example, self in this sense is not threatened by use of hallucinogens. These substances, as discussed earlier, can certainly contribute to *changes* in the self in the second sense, but they do not have as a side effect permanent amnesia. Hallucinogen-assisted therapies instead have their effect by suppressing one module in particular, the DMN, which results in the softening or dissolution of the sense of self (ego), not in forgetting the past that in part creates that ego. Consciousness, with the suppression of the activity of the default neural network is, in the term of the 1960s, *expanded*. For some, this is a mystical experience; for others, it is more of a shift in perspective, but in the vast majority of cases of those included in research studies completed so far, it is something positive, and lastingly positive for that very self that seems to be dissolved during the experience. Roland Griffiths reports, for instance, that subjects in his well-known psilocybin study expressed increased satisfaction with their social relations over a year after the treatment was completed. Many claimed that they were "more prosocial, more generous, and more loving," and Griffiths comments that "caretaking of self and others emerges from this experience" (in Miller, 2017, p. 145). So, while the use of hallucinogens in psychotherapy may indeed be vulnerable to the charge that it "changes the self" or causes one to "lose oneself," this is only a threat if one fails to be clear about what these terms mean. Loss of self in the sense that it happens during hallucinogen-assisted therapies is a positive thing that is in fact often actively sought and characterized as a good thing in many religious and meditative traditions, as well as in a variety of other activities, such as extreme sports, playing music, and sex.

Conclusion

William James cites the case of a man he treated with a sort of "spiritual cure." The man reported satisfaction and overall improvement in his quality of life and his view of himself, despite the fact that he did not receive traditional talk therapy or anything like the pharmaceuticals that are widely used today. He reported that his experience was of personal growth. And, in his own words, "I may say that the growth has all been toward the elimination of selfishness.

I do not mean simply the grosser, more sensual forms, but those subtler and generally unrecognized kinds, such as express themselves in sorrow, grief, regret, envy, etc." (James, 1917, p. 126). If that is a sense in which one can say that self was lost, it is not a bad thing. Indeed, it may be the cure for the very "essential sadness" that James recognized over 100 years ago as the unintended consequence of our culture's rationalism.

Notes

1. Weber used the German word *Entzauberung*, which is translated into English as "disenchantment," but which literally means rather "de-magic-ation."

2. Also see Bogenschutz et al. (2015), Grob, Bossis, and Griffiths (2013), Johnson and Griffiths (2017), and Sessa (2017).

3. There is an abundance of research connecting the default mode network (DMN) to social aspects of cognition and behavior. For just one meta-review, see Mars et al. (2012).

4. I also argue for this position from a philosophical view in Shelby (2016).

5. For a lengthier discussion of mystical experience in the medical, psychiatric, and psychological treatment of illness, see journalist Michael Pollan's (2018) *How to Change Your Mind: What the New Science of Psychedelics Teaches Us About Consciousness, Dying, Addiction, Depression, and Transcendence.*

References

Bassett, D. S., & Gazzaniga, M. S. (2011). Understanding complexity in the human brain. *Trends in Cognitive Sciences, 15*(5), 200–209.

Bogenschutz, M. P., et al. (2015). Psilocybin-assisted treatment for alcohol dependence: A proof-of-concept study. *Journal of Psychopharmacology, 29*(3), 289–299.

Campbell, D. (2017). NHS prescribed record number of antidepressants last year. Retrieved from *www.theguardian.com/society/2017/jun/29/nhs-prescribed-record-number-of-antidepressants-last-year.*

Carey, B., & Geveloff, R. (2018, April 7). Many people taking antidepressants discover that they cannot quit. Retrieved from *www.nytimes.com/2018/04/07/health/antidepressants-withdrawal-prozac-cymbalta.html.*

Carhart-Harris, R. L., et al. (2016). Neural correlates of the LSD experience revealed by multimodal neuroimaging. *Proceedings of the National Academy of Sciences of the USA, 113*(17), 4853–4858.

Gazzaniga, M. (2018). On determinism and human responsibility. In G. D. Caruso & O. Flanagan (Eds.), *Neuroexistentialism: Meaning, morals, and purpose in the age of neuroscience* (pp. 223–234). New York: Oxford University Press.

Grob, C. S., Bossis, A. P., & Griffiths, R. R. (2013). Use of the classic hallucinogen psilocybin for treatment of existential distress associated with cancer. In B. I. Carr & J. Steel (Eds.), *Psychological aspects of cancer: A guide to emotional and psychological consequences of cancer, their causes, and their management* (pp. 291–308). New York: Springer.

Grob, C. S., et al. (2011). Pilot study of psilocybin treatment for anxiety in patients with advanced-stage cancer. *Archives of General Psychiatry, 68*(1), 71–78.

Hake, H. S., et al. (2019). 3,4-Methylenedioxymethamphetamine (MDMA) impairs the extinction and reconsolidation of fear memory in rats. *Physiology and Behavior, 199,* 343–350.

James, W. (1917). *The varieties of religious experience: A study in human nature: Being the Gifford Lectures on Natural Religion delivered at Edinburgh in 1901–1902.* New York: Longmans, Green, and Co.

Johnson, M. W., & Griffiths, R. R. (2017). Potential therapeutic effects of psilocybin. *Neurotherapeutics, 14*(3), 734–740.

Levy, N. (2018). Choices without choosers. In G. D. Caruso & O. Flanagan (Eds.), *Neuroexistentialism: Meaning, morals, and purpose in the age of neuroscience* (pp. 111–125). New York: Oxford University Press.

Lonergan, M. H., Olivera-Figueroa, L. A., Pitman, R. K., & Brunet, A. (2013). Propranolol's effects on the consolidation and reconsolidation of long-term emotional memory in healthy participants: A meta-analysis. *Journal of Psychiatry and Neuroscience, 38,* 221–231.

Mackie, J. L. (1974). *The cement of the universe: A study of causation.* Oxford, UK: Clarendon Press

Mars, R. B., et al. (2012). On the relationship between the "default mode network" and the social brain. *Human Neuroscience, 6,* 1–9.

Miller, R. L. (2017). *Psychedelic medicine: The healing powers of LSD, MDMA, psilocybin, and ayahuasca.* Rochester, VT: Park Street Press

Pahnke, W. (1971). The psychedelic mystical experience in the human encounter with death. *Harvard Theological Review, 62,* 1–21.

Pollan, M. (2018). *How to change your mind: What the new science of psychedelics teaches us about consciousness, dying, addiction, depression, and transcendence.* New York: Penguin Press.

Sessa, B. (2017). MDMA and PTSD treatment: PTSD: From novel pathosociology to innovative therapeutics. *Neuroscience Letters, 649,* 176–180.

Shelby, C. L. (2016). *Addiction: A philosophical perspective.* New York: Palgrave Macmillan.

Stace, W. T. (1961). *Mysticism and philosophy.* London: Macmillan.

Turner, E., & Rosenthal, R. (2008). Efficacy of antidepressants. *British Medical Journal, 336,* 516–517.

Whitaker, R. (2010). *Anatomy of an epidemic.* New York: Crown Publishing Group.

Young, M. B., Andero, R., Ressler, K. J., & Howell, L. L. (2015). 3,4-Methylenedioxymethamphetamine facilitates fear extinction learning. *Translational Psychiatry, 5*(9), e634.

Young, M. B., et al. (2017). Inhibition of serotonin transporters disrupts the enhancement of fear memory extinction by 3,4-methylenedioxymethamphetamine (MDMA). *Psychopharmacology, 234*(19), 2883–2895.

Author Index

Subject Index

Note. *f*, *n*, or *t* following a page number indicate a figure, a note, or a table.